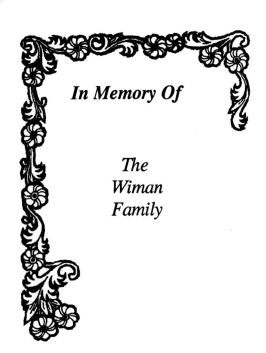

NURSING DIAGNOSES AND INTERVENTIONS FOR THE ELDERLY

NURSING DIAGNOSES AND INTERVENTIONS FOR THE ELDERLY

MERIDEAN MAAS, PhD, RN, FAAN

KATHLEEN BUCKWALTER, PhD, RN, FAAN

MARY A. HARDY, PhD, RN, C

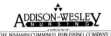

ADDISON-WESLEY NURSING

A Division of The Benjamin/Cummings Publishing Company, Inc.

Redwood City, California • Fort Collins, Colorado • Menlo Park, California
Reading, Massachusetts • New York • Don Mills, Ontario • Wokingham, U.K.
Amsterdam • Bonn • Sydney • Singapore • Tokyo • Madrid • San Juan

Executive Editor: Debra Hunter
Sponsoring Editor: Mark McCormick
Production Supervisor: Janet Vail
Production Coordination: The Book Company
Text and Cover Design: The Book Company
Copy Editor: Melissa Andrews

Cover photo: Earth Scenes © Sean Morris

Copyright © 1991 by Addison-Wesley Nursing
A division of The Benjamin/Cummings Publishing Company, Inc.

Library of Congress Cataloging-in-Publication Data

Nursing diagnoses and interventions for the elderly / [editors]
    Meridean Maas, Kathleen C. Buckwalter, Mary A. Hardy.
        p.   cm.
    Includes index and bibliographical references.
    ISBN 0-201-12679-6
    1. Geriatric nursing.   2. Nursing assessment.   I. Maas, Meridean.
II. Buckwalter, Kathleen Coen.   III. Hardy, Mary Anderson.
    [DNLM: 1. Geriatric Nursing.   2. Nursing Process.]
RC954.N885   1991
610.73'65—dc20
DNLM/DLC
for Library of Congress   90-14406
                                                           CIP

ISBN 0-201-12679-6

ABCDEFGHIJ-KE-9543210

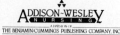

THE BENJAMIN/CUMMINGS PUBLISHING COMPANY, INC.

Addison-Wesley Nursing
A Division of The Benjamin/Cummings Publishing Company, Inc.
390 Bridge Parkway
Redwood City, California 94065

To Ada K. Jacox, PhD, RN, FAAN;
Myrtle Kitchell Aydelotte, PhD, RN, FAAN;
Joan King, PhD, RN;
and Geraldene Felton, EdD, RN, FAAN;
our valued friends, mentors, and colleagues.
Their inspiration, guidance, and support will
always be valued.

M.M., K.B., and M.H.

Foreword

PHYLLIS B. KRITEK, RN, PhD, FAAN

FOR PEOPLE IN SEARCH OF SYMBOLS OF NURSING'S coming of age in the United States, this book is such a symbol. Few expressions of the national crisis in health care delivery reflect our collective uncertainty as poignantly as the health needs of the dependent elderly. We are awash in demographics and descriptors. We swing between vectors of denial and despair in addressing this health care challenge. The authors of this book transcend this pattern. They also reframe the challenge. In doing so, they demonstrate the potential inherent in nursing to substantively improve the quality of life for elderly persons.

The nursing diagnosis movement is first a movement toward a common language system, a concept delineation process. We know something as real only when we have focused upon it long enough to name, explore, and understand it to some degree. The tragic inadequacies in the care of the dependent elderly are in part a function of conceptual neglect or lack of information. We simply have not focused long enough to understand the complexities of health in the elderly. This book sets a steady focus and uses nursing's emerging language system to assure a continuing exploration. It is a model of creative scholarly dialogue.

This book will be warmly welcomed to many libraries. For nurse educators, it is the text they wish someone would write. For nursing students, it is not only a pragmatic guide for nursing practice, it is also a model of competent scholarship, offering a clear statement of premises, delineation of supporting and differing viewpoints, acknowledgment of the limits of current knowledge, intellectual respect for inherent complexity, and descriptions of knowledge needed for the future.

Nurses who daily face the challenge of planning and delivering care to dependent elderly persons will soon find this book a new companion in their lives. Indeed, gerontological nurses and their copies of this book could quickly become inseparable. The book is indispensable. It is what we need in every nursing home, every hospital unit admitting elderly patients during an acute crisis, every home care agency. We need it where those nurses who plan and deliver care can reach out and grab a book both germane and scholarly, intelligent and practical. We need it where good nurses are trying to deliver to dependent elderly persons the best quality care nursing can provide.

As the authors and editors note, this book is a beginning. It initiates a dialogue. We will collectively be enhanced by it. Both what it is and how it is done are sources of professional enrichment. It is also, therefore, an invitation to every nurse who learns from it to join the dialogue, to increase and enhance the discourse. I thank the authors and editors for their efforts on our collective behalf. And I look forward, with you, the readers, to the continuing dialogue.

Preface

SINCE THE FIRST NATIONAL CONFERENCE ON THE Classification of Nursing Diagnoses was held in St. Louis in 1973, interest in nursing diagnosis among nurses in all practice settings and roles has grown steadily. The impact of the nursing diagnosis movement has reached every aspect of the profession, especially clinical practice and research. The increasing use of nursing diagnoses in clinical practice has stimulated research to identify, develop and describe the prevalence of diagnoses among specific populations of clients, to validate and refine the taxonomy of diagnoses, to evaluate and sharpen diagnostic skills, and to test the outcomes of intervention strategies.

Purpose of the Book

This book is devoted to a discussion of nursing diagnoses and interventions for the dependent elderly. As such, the diagnoses selected for the volume are not exhaustive but represent a severely underdeveloped knowledge base. Rather, we have chosen diagnoses based on existing research of prevalence in the population and on our judgments as to the diagnoses that most need to be developed and shared with nurses.

Although most of the diagnoses have been accepted for clinical testing by the North American Nursing Diagnosis Association (NANDA) (Carroll-Johnson, 1989), some are specific types of more general diagnoses; e.g., Potential for Poisoning: Drug Toxicity is viewed as a specific type of Potential for Injury. Other diagnoses that have not been approved by NANDA (e.g., Impaired Swallowing and Translocation Syndrome) are included because they are frequent and difficult to manage problems that nurses encounter among the dependent elderly. Our intent is to expand the conceptual and operational development of the diagnoses and interventions to increase their clinical usefulness and to promote further development by nurse clinicians and researchers. The explicated diagnoses, etiologies, and signs and symptoms are compared with those accepted by NANDA wherever possible.

Organization

In the Foreword, Kritek addresses the questions that have been raised about the approach used to develop this book as well as implications for the emerging nursing diagnosis taxonomy. Within each of the eleven units in the book, each representing one of Gordon's Functional Health Patterns, there is an overview and a chapter on normal aging. Each of the chapters within a unit is organized as follows:

Jacox provides, in the Epilogue, a discussion of salient issues regarding nursing diagnosis and management of the institutionalized elderly and the emergence of a standard nomenclature for nursing diagnoses. The implications she outlines for theory building, research, and clinical practice raise more questions for debate and resolution.

Pedagogy

The aspects of normal aging that begin every Functional Health Pattern unit may be used to evaluate pathological parameters for each diagnosis. It is important that readers realize, however, that the elderly are not a homogeneous population, especially those over the age of 80 years. What were once thought of as changes "normal" to aging are now thought of as "usual" (Rowe and Kohn, 1987). Based on a synthesis of the literature, each of the forty-three diagnosis chapters presents a conceptual definition and a theoretical discussion of a diagnosis, including etiology and signs and symptoms. Diagnoses are presented using the problem label (P), the etiology (E), and the defining characteristics or signs and symptoms (S) structural criteria developed by Gordon (1987).

Significance of the diagnosis for the elderly population is discussed in terms of prevalence, consequences if not treated, predispositions or risk factors, and the importance for nurses to diagnose and treat the elderly. The research base for the diagnosis and a critique of assessment tools are also presented, if available. Case studies are used to illustrate the assessment data, the process of assessment and diagnosis, including differential diagnosis wherever appropriate.

The majority of chapters highlight one intervention for each diagnosis or subdiagnosis and illustrate its use by referring to the case study. Other relevant interventions are discussed briefly and many are cross-referenced to a more detailed discussion in another chapter. The criteria for selection of interventions were drawn from those developed by Bulechek and McCloskey (1985). Wherever possible, the research base for the intervention is described. Desired outcomes for the intervention strategy are presented along with the evaluation process to be used. Readers should be cautioned, however, against interpreting interventions as "treatments of choice" because an adequate research base to predict a "cause and effect" relationship is often lacking.

Instead, nurses must use their judgment in choosing intervention strategies for the highly complex, rapidly changing, and often multi-causal problems presented by the elderly. Each chapter includes a summary and recommendations for future development and testing of the diagnosis and interventions.

Theoretical Base

Although Gordon's (1982) Functional Health Patterns, a middle range typology, are used to order and group the diagnoses and the editors subscribe to the view that nursing diagnoses are concepts representing a factor isolating level of theory building; we did not otherwise explicitly adopt or attempt to force any particular nursing theory or model on the authors. This factor may account for the varying approaches used by authors. We believe that the development of nursing diagnoses is more likely to be enriched and expanded by this eclectic theoretical approach. This is in spite of our awareness that the conceptual framework developed by the Nurse Theorists' Group has been adopted by NANDA as the organizing framework for the nursing diagnosis taxonomy. We opted to avoid the premature closure that a more explicit use of one particular model might produce.

Contributors

The authors were identified by the editors as doing research and/or having published in the area of the diagnosis. The editors are grateful to each of these contributing authors who raised important questions and provided their scholarship to make this book a reality. Perhaps we have benefited more than anyone from the challenge to ourselves and the authors to extend knowledge about diagnosis and intervention for the elderly.

Acknowledgments

To our husbands, Dick and Jody, and our children, Robin, Richard, Regan, Jody, Andrea, Abigail, Christina, and Anderson. Their patience, support, and tolerance of this endeavor in the face of sometimes chaotic family situations enabled us to proceed with this project in a less guilt-ridden manner.

To the staff of the Blue and Gold Cafe, Belle Plaine, Iowa, a spot halfway between our respective homes, who provided us with the space to work on this book and a hot cup of coffee while we did so.

To each of the authors who contributed their expertise and actually made this book a reality.

To Nancy Evans and Debra Hunter, publishing editors, who were so helpful and supportive throughout the project, from the initial idea to its completion.

To all our colleagues and staff at the College of Nursing, The University of Iowa, especially Nancy Goldsmith, who so ably assisted in the preparation and processing of the manuscript.

To Gail Ardery, Jackie Stolley, and Beth Weitzel, who helped us unselfishly with editing and proofing.

To Laura Lenz, who was indispensable. She typed, processed, retyped, and reprocessed the manuscript in the most professional manner. In our view, her technical and organizational competence is unequalled.

Finally to Dolores Rose, who collaborated with us and diligently assisted with the preparation of each page of the manuscript.

Reviewers

The authors express their thanks to the following reviewers:

Joan Arnold
Karen Beaver
Barbara Bowers
Valarie Bradbury
Helen Clark
Gail Day
Bobbye Gorenberg
Patricia Holly
Barbara Hoshiko
Laurel Breen Jaussen
Marianne Johnson
Kathy Kelly
Ilene Lubkin
Neville Nkongho
Ruth Ouimette
Mary Alice Pratt
Jennifer Schaller-Ayers
Rachel Scott
Neville Strumph
Beryl Thomas
Robyn Tyler
Mary Opal Wolanin

References

Bulechek G, McCloskey JC (editors): *Nursing Interventions: Treatments for Nursing Diagnoses.* Saunders, 1985.

Gordon M: *Nursing Diagnosis: Process and Application.* McGraw-Hill, 1982.

McLane A (editor): *Classification of Nursing Diagnoses: Proceedings of the 7th National Conference.* Mosby, 1987.

Rowe J, Kahn R: Human aging: Usual and successful. *Science* 1987; 237:143–149.

Contributors

Jackie Akins
Iowa Veterans Home

Mary Blegen
College of Nursing
The University of Iowa

Gloria Bulechek
College of Nursing
The University of Iowa

Donna Bunten
Veterans Administration Medical Center, Knoxville, Iowa

Diane Cesarone
Joint Commission on Accreditation of Health Care Organizations

Patricia Clinton
College of Nursing
The University of Iowa

Donelle Cusack
Veterans Administration Medical Center, Knoxville, Iowa

Marguerite Dixon
College of Nursing
University of Illinois at Chicago

Cynthia M. Dougherty
University of Washington

Janice Drury
Department of Nursing
Iowa Veterans Home

Linda Eastman
College of Nursing
The University of Iowa

Jo Ann Eland
College of Nursing
The University of Iowa

Janis B. Eldridge
Private Practice, Springfield, MA

Jan Elsen
The University of Iowa Hospitals and Clinics

Richard J. Fehring
College of Nursing
Marquette University

Rita A. Frantz
College of Nursing
The University of Iowa

Orpha J. Glick
College of Nursing
The University of Iowa

Teresa A. Gyldenvand
College of Nursing
The University of Iowa

Geri Richards Hall
The University of Iowa Hospitals and Clinics

Margo A. Halm
The University of Iowa Hospitals and Clinics

Barbara Hammer
Pardoc Memorial Hospital, Hendersonville, NC

Mary A. Hardy
College of Nursing
The University of Iowa

Ada Jacox
Center for Nursing and Health Services Research
University of Maryland

Karlene M. Kerfoot
St. Lukes Episcopal Hospital, Houston, Texas

Janie Knipper
The University of Iowa Hospitals and Clinics

Phyllis B. Kritek
School of Nursing
University of Wisconsin-Milwaukee

John Lantz
School of Nursing
San Diego State University

Colleen C. Love
Atascadero State Hospital
Atascadero, California

Susan MacLean
College of Nursing
Rush University, Chicago

Audrey McLane
Marquette University, Milwaukee

Ruth McShane
University of Wisconsin, Milwaukee

Diane Munns
Veterans Affairs Outpatient Clinic
Santa Barbara, California

Pedro Natividad
Army Nurse Corps, Fort Knox, Kentucky

Lucyanne Nolan
Veterans Administration Medical Center, Augusta, Georgia

Karen O'Heath
The University of Chicago Hospital

Carla J. Parent
Lafayette Clinic, Detroit

Cathy Penn
St. Lukes Hospital, Cedar Rapids, Iowa

Kathy Rajcevich
Audie L. Murphy Memorial Veterans Hospital, San Antonio, Texas

Barbara Rakel
The University of Iowa Hospitals and Clinics

Marilyn Rantz
Lakeland Nursing Home, Elkhorn, WI

JoAnn L. Reinboth
Grand View College, Des Moines

Jean Reese
College of Nursing
The University of Iowa

Deanne Remer
School of Nursing
Mercy Hospital Medical Center, Des Moines

Dolores Rose
Health Services Research Center
The University of Iowa

Jo Ellen R. Ross
College of Nursing
The University of Iowa

Janet Specht
Iowa Veterans Home

Jerry Stamper
San Jose State University

Julie Tackenburg
University of Arizona Medical Center

Luann Tandy
Veterans Administration Medical Center, Knoxville, Iowa

Marilyn Ter Maat
Rehab Hospital of the Pacific, Honolulu

Marita Titler
The University of Iowa Hospitals and Clinics

Trish Tunink
Alzheimer's Association, Des Moines

Connie Higgins Vogel
Prairie Rose Mental Health Center, Harlan, Iowa

Karen Wadle
Veterans Administration Medical Center, Knoxville, Iowa

Bonnie McDonald Wakefield
Veterans Administration Medical Center, Iowa City

Carol A. Watson
Mercy Medical Center, Cedar Rapids, Iowa

Kay Weiler
College of Nursing
The University of Iowa

Elizabeth A. Weitzel
MEDICAP, Marshalltown, Iowa

Ann L. Whall
University of Michigan, Ann Arbor

Gwen Whiting
Research Network, Evanston, Illinois

James Z. Wilberding
Veterans Administration Medical Center, Seattle

Brief Contents

Contents

Introduction

Nursing Diagnoses and Interventions for the Dependent Elderly: Epidemiologic Rationale

MERIDEAN MAAS, PhD, RN, FAAN

KATHLEEN BUCKWALTER, PhD, RN, FAAN

DOLORES ROSE, MA, RN

MARY HARDY, PhD, RN, C

THROUGHOUT THE 20TH CENTURY THE ELDERLY (OVER age 65) population of the United States has steadily increased. At present, about 70% of the population can expect to live beyond age 65. Another 17% will survive to age 85, a percentage that will increase to over 50% according to projections for the year 2050 (Brody, 1982). The female population age 85 and older will triple between 1980 and 2030. This segment of the population is more often single or widowed and thus at increased risk of needing long-term care assistance (Davis, 1986). These elderly may live within the community in a variety of settings ranging from high rises for the elderly to their own homes, or they may be institutionalized. Many, if not most, will be in a dependent role at least sometime during their remaining years, whether they are hospitalized, placed in a nursing home, or cared for at home by professionals and/or family caregivers.

Along with the rapid growth in the percentage of population age 65 and older there has been an even more dramatic increase in the number of long-term care facilities. Currently, in the United States approximately 5% of the over-65 population and 20% of the over-85 population reside in long-term care facilities (American Association of Retired Persons, 1986). The number of elderly residents in nursing homes increased 17% from 1977 to 1985 (Hing, 1987), and the number and percentage of the dependent elderly population is also expected to increase during the next several decades. If current trends continue, the older population in nursing homes will double in the next 35 years, from 1.3 million in 1985 to 2.8 million in 2020 (American Association of Retired Persons, 1986).

These demographic trends have and will continue to affect both the future of long-term care services and the nurses who diagnose and treat responses to illness in the elderly. In particular, the demand for quality nursing home care will be enormous. Nurses must be aware of and be able to meet a complex and interdependent array of psychosocial, spiritual, environmental, and physical needs of long-term care residents.

Because of the deinstitutionalization movement, many elderly individuals were discharged from mental institutions and relocated in community long-term care facilities over the last two decades (Liptzin, 1986). In fact, today's nursing homes have been labeled modern day "geropsychiatric ghettos," and many of the most challenging problems faced by nurses in these facilities are related to the emotional and behavioral disturbances and cognitive impairments of residents (Liptzin, 1986). It is estimated that 70% to 80% of nursing home residents have psychiatric problems (Roybal, 1984; Rovner and Rabins, 1985). Mental problems may influence whether an elderly person is able to manage at home or needs to enter a nursing home. Moreover, mental problems can develop after institutionalization. Therefore, this book has included a number of relevant psychosocial nursing diagnoses, such as Altered Thought Processes: Dementia; Reactive Depression; Body Image Disturbance; Powerlessness; Fear; Anxiety; Self-Esteem Disturbance; Dysfunctional Grieving; Social Isolation; Ineffective Individual Coping; and Potential for Violence. The elaboration of assessment and intervention strategies is intended to prepare nurses to correct some of the inattention to psychosocial problems in the elderly. Careful attention to the signs and symptoms that distinguish mental illness diagnoses should help prevent misdiagnosis and inappropriate treatment.

Most dependent elderly also experience a number of chronic physical conditions that affect their functional health status and ability to perform activities of daily living. Elderly persons usually have one or more chronic illnesses. Responses to these illnesses combined with the functional losses associated with aging require nursing diagnosis and treatment if the elderly are to achieve optimal adaptation and control over aspects of daily living.

The nursing diagnoses that are the most common functional responses to chronic physical illness are also reflected in the content of the book and include Self-Care Deficit; Diversional Activity Deficit; Sexual Dysfunction; Constipation; Diarrhea; Bowel Incontinence; Urinary Incontinence; Impaired Physical Mobility; Activity Intolerance; Sleep Pattern Disturbance; Knowledge Deficit; Sensory/Perceptual Alterations; Potential for Infection; Potential for Poisoning; Drug Toxicity; Altered Health Maintenance; Impaired Skin Integrity; Altered Nutrition: Less Than Body Requirements; Impaired Swallowing; Impaired Verbal Communication; and Altered Oral Mucous Membrane. The prevention and treatment of these problems are critical to the ability of elderly persons to be optimally independent in a variety of areas of daily living. Rehabilitation is the approach that is most appropriate, although it has not been a high-priority service for the elderly in our society (Brody, 1985). Nurses could do much to make rehabilitation a priority. Because the nursing diagnoses just mentioned represent phenomena that nurses are expected to treat, it is important that knowledge about the diagnoses be more fully developed. The work of Hoskins et al (1986) on the validation of nursing diagnoses in the chronically ill is the only published study found describing the nursing diagnoses among this population. The 169 subjects in the study ranged in age from 25 to 90 years. The fact that the median age was 68 years and that the majority of subjects were women makes the findings of this study somewhat generalizable to the chronically ill elderly. Although no data on the frequency of the nursing diagnoses were reported by Hoskins et al and the labels were somewhat different than those found in the NANDA taxonomy, most of the 51 nursing diagnoses found in this sample of community-dwelling chronically ill persons are represented in the book. Among those that are especially relevant to this population are

Sexual Dysfunction, Fear, Body Image Disturbance, Social Isolation, Anxiety, and Knowledge Deficit.

From the chronic physical illnesses that commonly affect the dependent elderly (eg, chronic obstructive pulmonary disease, cerebral vascular accident, pneumonia, heart disease, diabetes, cancer, arteriosclerosis), several other important nursing diagnoses also emanate, including Fluid Volume Deficit; Decreased Cardiac Output; Ineffective Breathing Pattern; Altered Tissue Perfusion; and Pain. Because nurses are the principal case managers of health care in nursing homes, it is imperative that they are prepared to identify, intervene, and monitor the physiologic sequelae of common chronic illnesses. Prompt attention by nurses is essential for preventing acute exacerbation of the underlying pathology, for preventing unnecessary deterioration of the elderly person's physical condition, and for maintaining optimum mental and physical function.

Furthermore, treatment and care of illnesses and functional losses can be disruptive and may precipitate a number of adverse responses. The nursing diagnosis Translocation Syndrome is included in this book because it is a problem that often is undetected and may be manifested in a variety of behaviors that are misdiagnosed.

Although there are a limited number of reports of epidemiologic studies of the nursing diagnoses of elderly populations in the literature, Gordon and Sweeney (1987) have noted the need for this research in a variety of settings and populations for early identification of nursing diagnoses and initiation of treatment. This research is also expected to describe trends in the diagnoses that are treated by nurses, promote testing of the linkage of interventions and diagnoses, encourage the development of computerized information systems, and aid the development of cross-cultural and national studies and data bases.

Five studies have reported findings on the incidence of nursing diagnoses among elderly and long-term care patients. Hallal (1985) reported 536 diagnoses for a sample of hospitalized elderly. Leslie (1981) studied the nursing diagnoses for the elderly population in one long-term care institution, reporting a total of 1521 diagnoses. Rantz et al (1985) and Rantz and Miller (1987) studied the incidence of nursing diagnoses in elderly residents of a single long-term care institution. Hardy et al (1988) described the prevalence of nursing diagnoses in a sample of 121 elderly and long-term care residents of a state veterans care facility. Table 1 contrasts the methods and findings of the five studies. The table also shows diagnoses described in each of these studies that characterized at least 10% of the sample.

Twenty-six of the diagnoses reported by at least one of the studies are discussed in separate chapters of this book, including all of the diagnoses that were found to be prevalent in all of the five studies. Additional chapters were added to discuss in more detail diagnoses that are specific types of a more general nursing diagnoses, for example, Impaired Skin Integrity: Dry Skin and Impaired Skin Integrity: Decubitus Ulcer.

Table 1

Studies of Nursing Diagnoses Of Elderly and LTC Clients

	HALLAL 1985	LESLIE 1981	RANTZ ET AL. 1985	RANTZ & MILLER 1987	HARDY ET AL. 1988
Methods:					
Setting	Hospital	LTCF	LTCF	LTCF	LTCF
Sample size (N)	106	210	328	328	121
Males	40	—	—	—	104
Females	66	—	—	—	17
Average age (yr)	76.6	85	—	—	73.4
Average length of stay (yr)	—	—	—	—	6.5
Data Source	Student Care Plans	Problem-Oriented Records	Resident Care Plans		Client Record
Assessment of accuracy of Dx	Clinical Faculty	—	—		Geront. Nurse Experts
Findings:					
Average no. diagnoses per resident	5.06	11.5	4.6	5.4	3.6
Range no. diagnoses per resident	1-17	1-22	—	—	1-12
Diagnoses by frequency rank (1 = most frequent)					
Self-Care Deficit: Bathing/Hygiene	—	—	8	11	1
Self-Care Deficit: Total	7	4	2	2	1
Impaired Physical Mobility	1	1	1	1	2
Alteration in Thought Processes	11	3	3	3	3
Alteration in Urinary Elimination	4	7	—	13	4
Potential for Injury	—	2	6	8	5
Self-Care Deficit: Dressing/Grooming	—	—	—	—	6
Impaired Skin Integrity	5	9	12	6	7
Alteration in Comfort: Pain	2	6	14	12	8
Impaired Skin Integrity: Potential	—	—	5	5	8
Alteration in Health Maintenance	—	—	—	—	8
Ineffective Individual Coping	—	12	—	—	9
Alteration in Bowel Elimination: Constipation	4	8	11	9	10
Alteration in Nutrition: < Body Requires	2	13	9	7	11
Decreased Cardiac Output	12	—	4	4	—
Anxiety	—	5	—	—	—
Fear	3	—	—	—	—
Potential Altered Nutrition: > Body Requires	—	13	7	14	—
Disturbed Self-Concept	6	14	—	—	—
Sensory Perceptual Alteration	8	10	14	18	—
Sleep Pattern Disturbance	6	—	—	—	—
Potential for Infection	—	—	10	10	—
Ineffective Airway Clearance	9	—	—	19	—
Fluid Volume Deficit	10	—	—	—	—
Diversional Activity Deficit	—	—	13	15	—
Impaired Verbal Communication	—	11	—	—	—
Translocation Syndrome	—	—	—	16	—
Alteration in Nutrition: > Body Requires	—	12	—	17	—
Social Isolation	—	—	—	20	—
Alteration in Socialization	—	—	—	21	—

Table 2

Theories of Aging

BIOLOGIC THEORIES

Deliberate Biologic Programming

- entropic approach to aging
- cellular level theory of aging
- each cell holds a finite capacity for reproduction
- each cell contains preprogrammed capacity for termination
- aging is the result of intrinsic destiny
- decline of biologic, cognitive, motor fucntion is inevitable

The Wear-and-Tear Theory

- aging is viewed ontogenetically
- structural and functional changes may be accelerated by abuse and stress accumulation
- decremental model of aging

Stress-Adaptation

- emphasizes the effects of positive and negative effects of stress on aging
- perception influences stress response
- stress may deplete reserves predisposing person to illness
- stress may lead to more effective adaptation
- stress generally presumed to accelerate aging

INTERACTIONAL THEORIES

Disengagement

- controversial
- disengagement is a gradual, intrinsic, inevitable process
- characterized by mutually satisfying withdrawal between older adults and society
- cohorts prefer company of same-age groups exclusively
- no account for heterogeneity of the elderly

Activity Theory

- contrasts with disengagement theory
- activity is desired by the elderly
- older adults should (and desire to) remain active and involved

---

Finally, the editors, who have extensive knowledge and experience with institutionalized elderly, added a number of diagnoses to the volume. Reactive Depression; Activity Intolerance; Spiritual Distress; Altered Role Performance: Potential Loss of Right of Self-Determination; and Altered Family Processes are examples of diagnoses that the editors believe to be frequent among the dependent elderly. These diagnoses often are poorly assessed and independently treated. Many of these diagnoses are secondary to physical conditions and other losses that accompany aging. The content of the book has been designed to promote nurses' awareness of the potential occurrence of these diagnoses and to add to nurses' ability to recognize signs and symptoms, make the appropriate diagnosis, and initiate and evaluate treat-ment. Finally, the content is intended to promote conceptual development and clinical validation of diagnoses.

The elderly are a heterogeneous group varying in age, health, occupational status, activity, and therefore in how the aging process affects each of them. The chapters in this book deal with nursing diagnoses that are common to the elderly but not attributable to aging alone. What may be considered "normal aging" may depend on the theory of aging that is predominant in the discipline or practice of the reader. An outline of current selected theories of aging are provided in Table 2 as a reference for the reader in critiquing diagnoses and interventions and in reviewing the theories used by authors.

Table 2 (*continued*)

Activity Theory (*continued*)
- lost roles and pastimes should be replaced with meaningful substitutes
- assumes homogeneity
- lacks empirical validation

Life Review

- reminiscence is normal and universal
- return of past experiences to the conscious level
- reintegration of unresolved conflicts
- successful reintegration provides ego integrity and meaning
- may result in anxiety, fear, and depression related to unresolved issues

PERSONALITY THEORIES

Erikson

- developmental model, sequence of eight psychosocial stages
- each phase characterized by specific developmental tasks
- predetermined structural order to maturation
- assumes inborne coordination to average expected environment
    no allowance for individual differences
- eighth stage — Ego Integrity vs. Despair
- ego integrity requires successful negotiation of all life stages and meaningful integration of past

Continuity Theory

- stability of personality over time
- habits, preferences, associations, commitments are stable
- ". . . you are like you always were, only more so"
- acknowledges individual differences and uniqueness

Developmental Tasks in Later Maturity

- the "examination stage"
- desire control over living situation
- desire continuity of intimacy (including sexual activity)
- strive to maintain optimum level of health
- desire contact with family and extended family
- pursue former and new activities
- find meaning after retirement
- refinement of personal philosophy
- adjustment occurs to losses of significant others

References

American Association of Retired Persons: *A Profile of Older Americans.* Washington, DC, 1986.

Brody JA Life expectancy and the health of older people. *J Am Geriatr Soc* 1982; 30:681–683.

Brody SJ: Rehabilitation and nursing homes. Pages 147–156 in: *The Teaching Nursing Home.* Schneider EL (editor). Raven Press, 1985.

Davis K: Paying the health bills of an aging population. Pages 299–318 in: *Our Aging Society: Paradox and Promise.* Pifer A, Broute L (editors). Norton, 1986.

Gordon M, Sweeney M: Methodological problems and issues in identifying and standardizing nursing diagnoses. *ANS* 1987; 9(3): 1–15.

Hallal J: Nursing diagnosis: An essential step to quality care. *Gerontol Nurs* (Sept) 1985; 35–38.

Hardy MA, Maas ML, Akins J: The prevalence of nursing diagnosis among elderly and long-term residents: A descriptive comparison. *Rec Adv Nurs Sci* 1988; 21:144–158.

Hing E: Use of nursing homes by the elderly: Preliminary data from the 1985 Nation Nursing Home Survey. *NCHSD Advance Data* (May) 1987; 135:1–12.

Hoskins LA et al: Nursing diagnosis in the chronically ill: Methodology for clinical validation. *ANS* 1986; 8(3):80–89.

Leslie FM: Nursing diagnosis: Use in long-term care. *Am J Nurs* 1981; 81:1012–1014.

Liptzin B: Major mental disorders/problems in nursing homes: Implications for research and public policy. In: *Mental Illness in Nursing Homes: Agenda for Research.* Harper M (editor). U.S. Government Printing Office, 1986.

Rantz M, Miller T: How diagnoses are changing in long-term care. *Amer J Nurs* 1987; 87:360–361.

Rantz M, Miller T, Jacobs C: Nursing diagnosis in long-term care. *Am J Nurs* 1985; 85:916–926.

Roybal ER: Federal involvement in mental health care for the aged. *Amer Psychol* 1984; 39(2):163–166.

Rovner BW, Rabins PV: Mental illness among nursing home patients. *Hosp Community Psychiatry* 1985; 36(2):119–128.

NURSING DIAGNOSES
AND INTERVENTIONS
FOR THE ELDERLY

I

Health-Perception– Health-Management Pattern

MERIDEAN MAAS, PhD, RN, FAAN
KATHLEEN BUCKWALTER, PhD, RN, FAAN

Overview

THE NURSING DIAGNOSIS ALTERED HEALTH Maintenance is particularly relevant for the elderly as they adjust both to the normal changes associated with aging and to personal expectations and cultural values and norms. This diagnosis, set forth by Tackenburg in Chapter 2, examines health behaviors and the individual's perceptions of health that influence those behaviors. Tackenburg distinguishes between Altered Health Maintenance and Self-Care Deficit, noting that the elderly person's ability to maintain health independently is largely dependent on the ability to perform self-care within the context of cultural values and beliefs regarding health.

Falling is the most common accident as well as the leading cause of accidental death among the elderly. In Chapter 3, Potential for Trauma: Falls, Ross, Watson, Gyldenvand, and Reinboth note that falls can exact a serious toll, both physiologically and psychologically, for older persons. Most falls in the elderly result either from changes that accompany the aging process or from disease entities, although Chapter 3 highlights other contributing factors that increase the risk of falling. Ross et al also present the Risk Assessment for Fall Scales I & II (RAFS), an assessment tool developed by their colleagues, which can be used by nurses to determine the risk of falling. Exercise, elimination rounds, signage, warning devices, and patient and staff education are all presented as interventions to prevent falling.

It is well known that the elderly are vulnerable for overprescription and overuse of medications, making the diagnosis Potential for Poisoning: Drug Toxicity an important area for nursing assessment, diagnosis, and intervention. In Chapter 4, Weitzel discusses the pharmacodynamics and pharmacokinetics among the elderly, focusing on important variables in drug administration and polypharmacy. Weitzel developed a tool to monitor for digitalis toxicity that can serve as a prototype for identifying persons at risk for drug toxicty. Weitzel urges an interdisciplinary approach to the prevention of drug toxicity in the elderly, including careful monitoring and drug holidays.

Infections are an increasing problem for institutionalized elderly, with between 5% and 20% of patients residing in extended care facilities manifesting one or more infections. Infections, especially urinary tract, respiratory tract, and decubitus ulcers, contribute to nursing home admissions and increased mortality. In Chapter 5, Potential for Infection, Titler and Knipper enumerate a variety of predisposing factors to infection in the elderly that they have developed as an assessment tool. They propose interventions to maximize host resistance and to reduce the risk for common infections among the institutionalized elderly.

1

Normal Changes With Aging

MARITA TITLER, MA, RN

MARY A. HARDY, PhD, RN, C

Definition:

Describes the client's perceived pattern of health and well-being and how health is managed.

HEALTH PERCEPTION AND MANAGEMENT OF ONE'S health are not likely to change with age alone. However, life events that are common to persons as they age, such as loss of job, family members, independence, income, and physical ability, may alter one's attitude toward oneself (Eliopoulos, 1987). These physical and social changes may impede the elderly person's interaction with the environment and other people and thus potentially limit adaptive responses.

With aging, changes in skeletal muscle reduce muscle strength, endurance, and agility. Posture is also modified with a general forward flexion of the head and neck, kyphosis of the spine, bent upper limbs, and slight flexion of the hips and knees. This flexed posture is caused by deterioration in the vertebral column and intervertebral discs, ankylosis of ligaments, joint shrinkage, sclerosis of tendons and muscles, and degeneration of the extrapyramidal central nervous system. These alterations interfere with balance by shifting the center of gravity forward. When combined with a shuffling gait, hip and knee flexion, prolonged reflex time, and decreased proprioception, these factors create a strong disposition for falling (Carnevali and Patrick, 1986).

Waning immunity and changes in other defenses contribute significantly to infection and the resulting morbidity associated with aging (Fox, 1986). Changes in the body's first line of defense that accompany aging enhance colonization and invasion with pathogenic organisms and can lead to a clinical infection. The mucous membranes and skin act as natural physical barriers to infectious organisms. Secretory immunoglobulin (IgA), a deterrent to infection at various mucosal surfaces, decreases with age. Natural skin secretions such as perspiration and sebum create a hostile environment to bacteria. The continuous sloughing of skin ensures a degree of cleanliness and periodic removal of surface microorganisms. In contrast, breaks in skin integrity decrease the efficacy of the elderly's first line of defense mechanisms. Thinning of the skin layers, decrease in collagen strength, and a decline in elasticity of the skin make the skin more prone to tearing and subsequent skin breakdown. Accompanying decline in elasticity of vessels and decreased competency of venous valves further contribute to skin breakdown due to venous stasis.

The potential for drug toxicity in the elderly exemplifies the complexity of factors that may lead to altered maintenance of health for the elderly person with a chronic illness. Physical changes including altered absorption in the gastrointestinal tract, reduced glomerular filtration rate, and decreased metabolic functioning of the liver in addition to reduced total body water content and plasma albumin concentration increase the risk for cumulative effects, enhanced effects, and drug interactions. Coupled with these physical changes are vision, memory, and financial factors that put the elderly at risk for many inadvertent mistakes in medication administration (Nesbitt, 1988).

Normal aging is associated with multiple changes in mobility. Therefore, normal aging contributes greatly to altered physical mobility and with it, increased potential for injury. Visual acuity, critical to providing proprioceptive information important to activities involving the ankles and feet, begins to decline at age 60, and plays a key role in the tendency to fall. The pupil loses its ability to accommodate and the retina deteriorates. The loss of orbital fat with subsequent mechanical displacement of the globe limits the visual field (Eliopoulos, 1987).

Other changes associated with aging predispose the elderly to infections of the genitourinary tract, oropharynx, respiratory tract, and gastrointestinal tract. Oropharyngeal colonization increases with aging and increasing physical dependency (Fox, 1986). The frequency with which bacteria adhere to epithelial cells of the genitourinary tract increases with advancing age, suggesting some cellular changes of aging (Fox, 1986). Hormonal age-related changes also occur in vaginal epithelium. There is decreased vaginal glycogen and a slightly higher vaginal pH in elderly women. This promotes increased colonization of the periurethral zone with gram-negative bacteria (Kunin, 1987). Other conditions that promote urinary retention in the elderly predispose them to infections of the urinary tract. These include prostatic enlargement, urethral stricture, neurogenic bladder, pharmacologic agents such as antidepressants and anticholinergics, and relaxation of the pelvic floor muscles.

Pulmonary function declines with age and makes it more difficult to cough up debris. This is because of a loss of elastic tissue surrounding the alveoli and alveolar duct, decreased mucus production, impaired ciliary action, decreased respiratory excursion, and weakening of the respiratory muscles (Felser and Raff, 1983; Gardner, 1980). An increase in the prevalence of diseases that predispose the elderly to infection, neurologic deficits that enhance the chance of aspiration, and changes that occur in the pulmonary system with aging put them at risk for respiratory infection (Freeman, 1985).

Reduced gastric acid predisposes the elderly to various enteric infections such as cholera and shigella. Achlorhydria (absence of free hydrochloric acid in the stomach) is found in about one third of individuals over 60 years of age (Fox, 1986).

The body's nonspecific phagocytic system is the second line of defense against infection. There is some disagreement about the adequacy of functioning in the elderly of the two main types of cells involved in phagocytosis, the polymorphonuclear leukocyte (neutrophil) and monocyte/macrophage. Both types of cells are needed to defend against invasion of microorganisms. Although the effect of aging on phagocytic activity of neutrophils is unclear, it appears that macrophage functioning is adequate (Fox, 1986). The change in phagocytic activity of neutrophils may be a function of disease processes and accompanying pharmacologic treatment regimens rather than the process of aging. For example, the increased incidence and poor prognosis of recovery from *Staphylococcus aureus* bacteremia in the elderly may be due to an impairment in ability to produce or release neutrophils rather than to an actual change in phagocytic abilities (Felser and Raff, 1983; Fox, 1986).

The immune response is the third line of defense against an invading organism. The aging process is accompanied by a declining immune system. Aging is associated with involution of the thymus gland and decrease in the production of the thymopoietin, which influences maturation of T lymphocytes. Lymph nodes, spleen, and gut-associated lymphoid tissue also decrease in size with aging. The stem cells from the bone marrow in the elderly are less able to repair damaged DNA and to migrate to the thymus for maturation. Many changes that occur in the stem cells are probably an accumulation of genetic damage with aging (Fox, 1985). Aging causes changes in both the humoral and cellular limbs of the immune system (Felser and Raff, 1983; Schneider, 1983). Although the elderly are able to mount a humoral immune response, their response to vaccines differs from that of a younger person. Antibody production is impaired to a certain degree, but the exact changes that occur are unclear (Fox, 1986; Potter, 1984; Schneider, 1983). The impairment in antibody production is probably due to thymic involution, reduction in function of the T cell and T cell subpopulations, and subsequent changes in the ability of B cells to mature properly and produce sufficient amounts of antibodies (Felser and Raff, 1983; Fox, 1986). The exact mechanisms for decline in cell-mediated immunity are not clear but are probably due to a decrease in the number of responsive T lymphocytes as well as impaired ability of T lymphocytes to proliferate (Fox, 1985; Weksler, 1986). Most evidence shows a loss of suppressor cells that control production of autoantibodies and thus an increase in autoantibody production with advancing age (Fox, 1986). Aging may also have an adverse effect on production of interleukin 1 and interleukin 2, both necessary for T cell recruitment and stimulation (Fox, 1986).

References

Carnevali DL, Patrick M: *Nursing Management for the Elderly.* Lippincott, 1986.

Eliopoulos C: *Gerontological Nursing.* Lippincott, 1987.

Felser JM, Raff MJ: Infectious diseases and aging: Immunologic perspectives. *J Am Geriatr Soc* 1983; 31:802–807.

Fox RA: Immunology of aging. Chapter 5 in: *Textbook of Geriatric Medicine and Gerontology*, 3d ed. Brocklehurst JC (editor). Churchill Livingstone, 1985.

Fox RA: Infection and immunity in old age. In: *Infections in the Elderly*. Denham MJ (editor). MTD Press Limited, 1986.

Freeman E: The respiratory system. In: *Textbook of Geriatric Medicine and Gerontology*, 3d ed. Brocklehurst JC (editor). Churchill Livingstone, 1985.

Gardner ID: The effect of aging on susceptibility to infection. *Rev Infect Dis* 1980; 2:801-808.

Kunin CM: *Detection, Prevention and Management of Urinary Tract Infections*. Lea and Febiger, 1987.

Nesbitt B: Nursing diagnosis in age-related changes. *J Gerontol Nurs* 1988; 14(7):7-12.

Potter JF: Immunity in the elderly. In: *Infection Control in Long-Term Care Facilities*. Smith PW (editor). Wiley, 1984.

Schneider EL: Infectious diseases in the elderly. *Ann Intern Med* 1983; 98:395-400.

Weksler ME: Biologic basis and clinical significance of immune senescence. In: *Clinical Geriatrics*, 3d ed. Rossman I (editor). Lippincott, 1986.

2

Altered Health Maintenance

Julie Tackenburg, MA, RN

Orpha Glick, PhD, RN

Health of individuals and groups has been the focus of nursing practice throughout nursing history. It is not surprising, then, that health is a key component of many conceptual models of nursing. The construct of health, in addition to the constructs of person, environment, and nurse or nursing, is commonly referred to as the metaparadigm of the discipline of nursing (Fawcett, 1989). These four constructs have been used as an organizing framework for assessment and nursing diagnosis in practice settings such as home health care (Keating and Kelman, 1988).

The focus of this chapter is the diagnosis and treatment of Altered Health Maintenance in elderly clients. This nursing diagnosis is one of several new diagnoses accepted for clinical testing at the 1982 (Fifth) conference of the North American Nursing Diagnosis Association (NANDA) (Kim et al, 1984). It was defined as the "inability to identify, manage and/or seek out help to maintain health" (Kim et al, 1984;475). This definition implies that maintaining health is the personal responsibility of the individual (as client); however, the actions of identifying, managing, and seeking out help can also be applied to the client as family, aggregate, or total community.

Although the NANDA definition includes several behavioral categories directed toward health maintenance, it provides little conceptual clarity for the meaning of the term *health maintenance*. An examination of the term is relevant because use of the words *health* and *health maintenance* in the health and social science literature has varied. For example, health maintenance has been described as an outcome of self-care and professional health care, as shown, for example, in the goal statement "to promote and maintain health." Second, it is used as a category of interventions initiated and carried out by health caregivers—most frequently, those in public and community health nursing. Finally, as a nursing diagnosis label, the term *health maintenance* is being used to represent a class of health-related behaviors that are or should be performed by the client. Because the focus of the chapter is the diagnosis Altered Health Maintenance, the presumption is made that a problem exists in one or more of the behavioral dimensions that define the concept.

CONCEPTIONS OF HEALTH AND HEALTH MAINTENANCE

In order to conceptualize health maintenance, it may be useful to first examine meanings of the terms *health* and *maintenance*. The popular mean-

The contributions of Elizabeth Weitzel, MA, RN are acknowledged in the review and development of this chapter.

ings or uses of the word *maintenance* include "to keep in existing state; to preserve from failure or decline; to sustain against opposition or danger" (*Webster's Ninth New Collegiate Dictionary,* 1988;718). When conceptually linked to health, the word *maintenance* connotes activities that support or preserve health. Although the interpretation seems obvious, the term *health maintenance* has been used interchangeably or in conjunction with the term *health promotion.* Because promotion means "to advance; to contribute to the growth or prosperity of" (*Webster's Ninth New Collegiate Dictionary,* 1988;941), a different conception emerges. Because some health-related behaviors may support or preserve as well as advance or move forward, the distinction in the two concepts may be in the desired outcome rather than in the behavior itself. It is also possible that in some cases the distinction is based on the initial functional capacity of the individual. For example, exercise may be used to *maintain* joint flexibility but to advance or *promote* cardiovascular endurance.

In contrast to the word *maintenance,* conceptions of the word *health* are more complex. Moreover, there is wide variation in conceptions of health among social scientists as well as health care professionals. Laffrey (1986) states that these differences often lead to confusion and even conflict in health care. Further, discrepancies between the conceptions and perceptions of the caregiver and health care consumer compound communication and decision making regarding intervention strategies and goals. Rubenstein et al (1984), for example, found that elderly clients in their study tended to "overstate" their ability to function, whereas their significant others tended to underrate the clients' functional ability.

As previously noted, nurse theorists have incorporated health as a major component of their work. Although it is a common theme, there are differences in the language used to define health. For example, Roy (1984;28) defines health as "a state and a process of being and becoming an integrated and whole person." King (1981;5) views health as "dynamic life experiences of a human being, which implies continuous adjustment to stressors in the internal and external environment through optimum use of one's resources to achieve maximum potential for daily living." Orem (1985;179) distinguishes between the terms *health* and *well-being.* She states that health is "a state of a person that is characterized by soundness or wholeness of developed human structures and of bodily and mental functions." Well-being on the other hand is a:

> *. . . state characterized by experiences of contentment toward fulfillment of one's self-ideal, and by continuing personalization. Well-being is associated with health, with success in personal endeavors and with sufficiency in resources. However, individuals experience well-being and their human existence may be characterized by features of well-being even under conditions of adversity including disorders of human structure and function.*
>
> (Orem 1985)

Parse (1981;14) takes a more existential view; that is, health is "a process of becoming as experienced by a person."

Pender (1987;27) presents a comprehensive view of health and defines it as the "actualization of inherent and acquired human potential through goal directed behavior, competent self-care and satisfying relationships with others while adjustments are made as needed to maintain structural integrity and harmony with the environment." These definitions of health address the personal growth and actualizing component as well as the dynamic equilibrium or stability of the biologic and self systems. They also indicate that health is viewed as a state *and* a process.

Smith (1981) described a multidimensional view of health that includes a clinical component; a functional component, or role performance; and adaptive and eudaimonistic models of health. She defines the clinical dimension as focusing on absence of disease or symptoms. The functional component, or role performance, is the ability to carry out one's usual social roles. The adaptive model refers to health as flexibility in making adjustments to changing environmental circumstance, and the eudaimonistic model incorporates the self-actualization dimension.

The comprehensive conceptualization of health demonstrated in the preceding definitions and models is consistent with the complexity of human existence and function. It provides for individuals who may experience a reduction in functional status or health secondary to age-related biologic changes or to a specific disease process yet continue to carry out role functions, adapt to environmental changes, and achieve higher levels of health in other dimensions. This is a particularly useful conception for the elderly, since many of them have at least one chronic illness (Filner and Williams, 1979) and have experienced losses in their social network or material possessions (Stanwyck, 1983). A multidimensional view of health is reflected in the writings of several authors who advocate health promotion for the elderly. Filner and Williams (1979), for example, view health as the ability to live and function effectively in society and to exercise self-reliance and autonomy to the maximum extent feasible; they do not necessarily view health as total freedom from disease. Thus, a definition of health for the older person often includes successfully dealing with chronic illness to allow maximal functioning for that individual. This is also consistent with the notion that health behavior may be directed toward maintenance in one dimension and promotion in another.

Clearly, health is a highly personal concept and can be judged only in the context of the individual's personal and cultural or ethnic value system. Further, the effects of age-related changes on body image of the elderly and the effects of body image on health behavior in this population have not been studied. Although there are gaps in knowledge about health maintenance in the elderly, health professionals must consider "normal" aging in their evaluation of health behavior in this population. Failure to distinguish accurately between normal aging and pathology may result in diagnosis and treatment of normal aging as disease (eg, treatment of altered sleep patterns that are normal for many older persons as insomnia). Conversely, pathology may be erroneously defined as normal aging and may not have the appropriate intervention; for example, acute confusion and depression are two conditions that are frequently overlooked or misdiagnosed in this age group.

Individual perception of what health is and personal descriptions of health status are partially formed by a person's environment and the individuals in it. This means that knowledge of sociocultural influences is important when assessing the elderly's health perception and their behavior. In order to respect cultural differences and to work within the framework and value structures of the elderly client, it is advantageous for nurses to recognize their own values, which may oppose the elder's perception. Knowledge of health conceptions across population groups increases the ability to understand and predict other health-related variables such as health choices. Laffrey (1986) suggests that one's conception of health may be a more significant influence on health behavior than actual health status. She found, for example, that in a sample of healthy adults (n = 95), persons who held a more eudaimonistic health conception engaged in health behaviors to promote higher levels of health. On the other hand, persons whose health conception was more clinical engaged in behaviors primarily to prevent illness.

HEALTH BEHAVIORS

The crux of health maintenance as a client initiative and responsibility is health behavior or health practices. Health behaviors are those activities initiated and performed by the person in order to preserve and enhance health and well-being.

Health behaviors are deeply integrated into an individual's lifestyle patterns. As previously noted, they are influenced by environmental constraints or resources and by personal and cultural beliefs and values. The categories of health behavior that are commonly recognized as health maintaining are represented in a problem classification system developed by the Visiting Nurses Association of Omaha, Nebraska (Simmons, 1980). There are four broad categories—environmental, psychosocial, physiologic, and health behaviors—of client problem "domains." Each domain includes subcategories of areas for assessment. The domain health behaviors is defined as "activities which maintain or promote wellness, promote recovery or maximize rehabilitation" (Simmons, 1980;8). These activities or behaviors have the potential for improving the quality of a client's life. They include (1) nutrition, (2) sleep/rest, (3) physical activity, (4) personal hygiene, (5) substance misuse, (6) medical–dental supervision, (7) therapeutic. regimen noncompliance (eg, treatment, medication, diet) and (8) performance in technical procedures (Simmons, 1980). Several of these areas represent behaviors for health promotion as well as for health maintenance. Pender (1987), however, distinguishes between behaviors that are undertaken to protect health (disease prevention) and behaviors that are designed to promote health. She notes that health protection behavior is "directed towards decreasing the probability of experiencing illness by active protection of the body against pathological stressors or detection of illness in the asymptomatic stage" (Pender, 1987;57). Health promotion, on the other hand, is directed toward increasing the level of well-being and self-actualization. In this chapter, health maintenance behavior is defined as lifestyle choices as well as preventive actions directed at early detection and control of effects of chronic disease.

Improvement in health maintenance in the elderly is likely to involve actual change in behaviors that are already well established. This is in contrast to the need to overcome resistance to social pressure that often operates in the young adult or adolescent. Chronic illness and multiple organ failure may also complicate health practices. In addition, the elder's own view of the future becomes very important to health practices, since wellness behaviors require that the individual have the ability to perform the activity as well as be motivated to plan for the future based on the results of such practices. Elderly persons with positive developmental characteristics have participated in behaviors that support this aspect of their health status. Engle (1984) identifies these characteristics of the elderly as (1) the desire to leave a legacy or to make contributions to the next generation; (2) positive interactions with the younger generation; (3) attachment to familiar objects, which provides continuity in day-to-day living; (4) a sense of immediacy related to the elder's opportunities to experience sensory and emotional stimuli on a daily basis; (5) a sense of life cycle reflective of introspection of previously held values and new understanding of philosophic matters; (6) creativity, curiosity, and surprise, which can be found in a zest for life; and (7) a sense of fulfillment in life to include the opportunity to review life, resolve conflicts, and be proud of personal achievements.

DETERMINANTS OF HEALTH BEHAVIOR

Researchers in several disciplines (eg, sociology, public health) have attempted to identify factors that influence an individual to initiate and sustain health-related behavior. Cummings et al (1980) conducted a study of 14 conceptual models of health behavior developed by social scientists over a period of approximately 25 years. The purpose of their work was to lay the "groundwork" for a unified framework for explaining health action. Eight of 11 living authors of the health models participated in the study. Participants were asked to compare a set of 109 variables (obtained from a review of the 14 models of health behavior) and place them into categories on the basis of their similarities. The specific model from which the variables were drawn was not identified; however, the names and definitions of behaviors were given as they appeared in the literature describing the model.

Analysis of study findings revealed six "clusters" of variables. They are (1) perception of illness and threat of disease, (2) knowledge of disease, (3) social network, (4) demographic variables, (5) access to health care, and (6) attitude toward health care. These investigators also observed subgroupings of behaviors within several of the categories. For example, the accessibility (to health care) variables aggregated into two distinct subgroups—those related to financial cost of care and those related to availability of services. The spatial arrangement of the major clusters in their analyses is also of interest and suggests association among certain clusters of behaviors. For example, items pertaining to knowledge about the disease were situated in close proximity to items dealing with perception and evaluation of symptoms. Similarly, items related to individuals' attitudes toward health care and items on accessibility to health services suggest a relationship in which access factors are affected by one's evaluation of health care. Further, the proximity between demographic variables and access may be a function of social class. This analysis and summary of variables that influence health behavior further illustrates the complexity of the diagnostic and treatment processes that surround health maintenance.

THE DIAGNOSIS ALTERED HEALTH MAINTENANCE

Altered Health Maintenance is a diagnosis that is made when health is potentially or actually threatened by existing health behaviors. The definition, etiologies, and defining characteristics of Altered Health Maintenance as proposed by NANDA are listed in Table 2.1.

Table 2.1

Altered Health Maintenance: Etiologies/Related Factors, and Defining Characteristics

---

NANDA (CARROLL-JOHNSON 1989)

Definition: Inability to identify, manage and/or seek out help to maintain health.

Etiologies/Related Factors

Lack of, or significant alteration in, communication skills
  (written, verbal, or gestural)
Lack of ability to make deliberate and thoughtful judgments
Perceptual cognitive impairment (complete/partial lack of fine
  motor skills)
Ineffective individual coping
Dysfunctional grieving
Unachieved developmental tasks
Ineffective family coping
Disabling spiritual distress
Lack of material resources

Defining Characteristics

Demonstrated lack of knowledge regarding basic health practices
Demonstrated lack of adaptive behaviors to internal/external
  environmental changes
Reported or observed inability to take responsibility for meeting
  basic health practices in any or all functional pattern areas
History of lack of health-seeking behaviors
Expressed interest in improving health behaviors
Reported or observed lack of equipment, financial, or
  other resources
Reported or observed impairment of personal support systems

TACKENBURG

Etiologies/Related Factors

Loss of relatives/friends
Abrupt change of residence
Acute or chronic illness/disability
Injury
Lack of awareness of positive or negative health behaviors
Low value of health
Inability to perform health behaviors
Inability to monitor self or environment
Inability to communicate
Inability to make reasonable decisions

Defining Characteristics

Physical signs of poor health (eg, pedal edema, shortness of breath
  may indicate nonadherence to diet or medication prescription)
Social withdrawal
Inattention to personal appearance
Misperceives and performs behaviors that do not support health
  or that present hazards to health (eg, skipping meals or
  having poor nutritional intake, smoking, excess use of alcohol
  or other controlled substances, lack of exercise)

As shown, the concept of health maintenance is very broad and incorporates physical, psychosocial, and cultural domains. Because of this range, it is conceivable that the diagnosis may be based on a deficit in only one behavioral sphere or may incorporate several domains. Using Orem's model, Peret and Stachoviak (1984;363) conceptualize health maintenance as a continuum ranging from complete dependence on a "second party" for health needs (dysfunctional health maintenance) to a partial level of dependence or relative independence in health maintenance. These authors view health maintenance as a function of nursing when there are developmental disabilities, deficits in adaptive behavior, or inability to communicate health care needs. Moreover, a high level of independent nursing judgement can be exercised in diagnosing and treating alterations in health maintenance.

Because the scope of health maintenance is very broad, specifying the particular behavioral domain (eg, eating patterns, medication use) as a subtitle of the diagnosis is useful in delineating the specific behaviors to be targeted for intervention. This was done in a nurse-managed wellness center described by Fehring and Frenn (1986). Carpenito (1987; 302) also suggests that the area of health maintenance be specified when making the diagnosis.

When considering indications for the diagnosis it is important to differentiate Altered Health Maintenance from Self-Care Deficit (see Chapter 24) and from Impaired Home Maintenance Managment. These three diagnoses are related but distinct. Table 2.2 compares the definitions, etiologies, defining characteristics, immediacy of impact from the diagnosis, degree of individual participation, and the interrelationship between these diagnoses. Some degree of ability in each area is necessary to avoid the other two diagnoses.

Carpenito (1987;293) notes that Altered Health Maintenance should be used to describe (1) an asymptomatic person who is at risk, (2) a person having chronic disease to promote attaining a higher level of wellness, or (3) a person having an acute problem but also having other areas of health at risk. In comparison, persons diagnosed with self-care deficits have actual health or self-care alterations. Home Maintenance Management focuses on the immediate living environment.

The person with Altered Health Maintenance may not experience the full impact of this diagnosis for some time after it becomes apparent to health professionals, whereas the person with a Self-Care Deficit experiences the effects immediately. The person with Impaired Home Maintenance Management may experience the impact of neglected safety factors immediately but not notice the effects of poor hygiene for some time. It is possible for someone else to manage home maintenance (family, employees, staff at an institution) without the older person participating. Both self-care and health maintenance require the older person's participation.

ETIOLOGIES/RELATED FACTORS

Problems with communication obviously decrease the older person's ability to maintain health independently. Likewise, a number of cognitive-perceptual and psychosocial factors affect health. NANDA recognizes lack of ability to make deliberate and thoughtful judgments, perceptual-cognitive impairments, ineffective individual/family coping, dysfunctional grieving, unachieved developmental tasks, disabling spiritual distress, and lack of material resources as having a strong relationship to the onset of Altered Health Maintenance (McLane, 1987). These factors are similiar to those identified for Self-Care Deficit and Home Maintenance Management (Table 2.2). Other persons often are more at risk because of the number of these factors that accumulate and interact within their lives, ultimately influencing health status.

DEFINING CHARACTERISTICS

For Altered Health Maintenance to be an appropriate diagnosis, the nurse must be able to identify at least some of the following parameters when assessing the older person. The older person demonstrates a lack of knowledge regarding basic health practices or demonstrates a lack of adaptive behaviors to internal or external environmental changes. The older person reports or the health professional observes inability to take responsibility for meeting basic health practices in any or all functional health patterns. There also might be a history of lack of health-seeking behaviors, or the older person may verbalize an interest in improving health behaviors (McLane, 1987).

When comparing these characteristics with those that define Self-Care Deficit and Impaired Home Maintenance Management, it becomes easier to distinguish among these similar diagnoses.

ASSESSMENT

The nurse must perform an assessment from which to develop nursing diagnoses and interventions. Gordon (1982) presents assessment for health perception and health management as part of the nursing history and suggests deriving information from oral and written reports from the patient, family, or both. Interview questions are offered as a possible format. However, the suggested format deals primarily with health perception and offers little structure for seeking information related to those health behaviors found in the literature, such as diet, exercise, and alcohol moderation. To make this format pertinent to the health-perception—health-management

Table 2.2

Comparison of Three Diagnoses: Altered Health Maintenance, Self-Care Deficit, and Impaired Home Maintenance Management

ALTERED HEALTH MAINTENANCE	SELF-CARE DEFICIT	IMPAIRED HOME MAINTENANCE MANAGEMENT
Definition		
Inability to identify, manage, and/or seek out help to maintain health	A state in which the individual experiences a decreased ability to feed, bathe, dress, or toilet himself or herself	Inability to maintain a safe home environment
Etiologies		
Lack of, or significant alteration in, communication skills	Visual disorders	Injury to individual or family member
Lack of ability to make deliberate and thoughtful judgments	Pain, discomfort	Cognitive, motor, sensory deficit
Perceptual-cognitive impairment (complete/partial loss of fine motor skills)	Immobilization, impaired physical functioning	Chronic debilitating disease
Ineffective individual family coping	Trauma or surgical procedures	Inaquate support system
Dysfunctional grieving	Perceptual/cognitive impairment	Lack of knowledge
Unachieved developmental tasks	Musculoskeletal disorders	Insufficient finances
Disabling spiritual distress	Neuromuscular impairment	
Lack of material resources	Decreased strength and endurance	
Defining Characteristics		
Demonstrated lack of knowledge regarding basic health practices	Unable to feed self, cut food	Household members express problems with maintaining home
Demonstrated lack of adaptive behaviors to internal/external environmental changes	Unable to wash body/body parts, obtain water, regulate temperature	Poor hygienic practices including unwashed or unavailable cookware, clothing, linens; accumulation of dirt, food waste, or hygienic wastes
Reported or observed inability to take responsibility for meeting basic health practices in any or all functional pattern areas	Unable to put on or take off necessary items of clothing	Unavailable support systems
History of lack of health-seeking behaviors	Unable to bring food from container to mouth	Overtaxed family members
Expressed interest in improving health behaviors	Unable to get to toilet/commode	Repeated infections or infestations
Reported or observed lack of equipment, financial, or other resources	Unable to sit or rise independently	
Reported or observed impairment of personal support systems	Unable to manipulate clothing	
	Unable to clean oneself	
	Unable to flush or empty toilet/commode	
Focus		
Health status at risk	Dependent for some or all activities of daily living (ADLs)	Home environment at risk
Immediacy of Impact From Diagnosis		
Longer term	Immediate	Immediate (safety factors)
		Long-term (hygiene factors)
Participation Requirement		
Individual must have some involvement to avoid or overcome diagnosis	Individual must be able to carry out ADLs independently to avoid or overcome diagnosis	Individual need not be involved in activities to avoid or overcome if others are present

(Continues)

Table 2.2

Comparison of Three Diagnoses: Altered Health Maintenance, Self-Care Deficit, and Impaired Home Maintenance Management *(Continued)*

ALTERED HEALTH MAINTENANCE	SELF-CARE DEFICIT	IMPAIRED HOME MAINTENANCE MANAGEMENT
Interrelationships		
At least partial health maintenance necessary to maintain self-care and home maintenance	Some degree of self-care necessary for health and home maintenance	Some degree of home maintenance necessary for long-term *independent* health maintenance
Health maintenance very difficult without self-care abilities or home maintenance management	Difficult to maintain self-care without health and home maintenance	Not possible to maintain home independently without partial health maintenance and most self-care abilities

Sources: Carpenito L: *Nursing Diagnosis: Application to Clinical Practice.* Lippincott, 1983. Carroll-Johnson RM (editor): *Classification of Nursing Diagnoses: Proceedings of the Eighth Conference.* Lippincott, 1989.

needs of the elderly, more specificity is needed. For example, assessment questions should include:

1. How would you evaluate your current state of health?
2. What practices do you routinely perform that contribute to your health?
3. What do you do to manage common illnesses such as colds or the flu?
4. Describe your activity and sleep patterns for a typical day.
5. What kinds of things do you do to keep mentally healthy?
6. How would you describe your personal relationships with family? friends?

Although these questions are still relatively open-ended, they are also specific to general health behaviors of the elderly (see Assessment Guide 2.1).

ASSESSMENT TOOLS

A tool designed to elicit a more comprehensive data base for diagnosis of Altered Health Maintenance was developed by Johnson-Saylor et al (1982). These clinical specialists developed an eight-item assessment form that directs some of its questions to the goals of (1) raising the patient's health consciousness; (2) helping the patient identify health risks in terms of lifestyle and family history; and (3) helping the patient identify strengths and resources. The self-administered assessment form is applicable to the health behaviors of the elderly, although it may present some difficulties for the elder who has questions, poor eyesight, or motor difficulty and cannot fill out the form. Its strength is that it helps persons become aware of psychological health issues and health-

maintaining strategies that are available within their lifestyle, thereby reinforcing a sense of control.

The Detroit assessment tool begins with a checklist of overall self-perception. Items from the Assessment of Life Condition Scale (ALCS) were selected for evaluation of health perception—of strengths and resources as well as stressors. Of particular importance to the elderly are the items in this section that relate to role satisfaction and issues of control over environment, self, and lifestyle choices. This is especially important to the institutionalized elderly, given the regimentation frequently seen in health institutions and nurses' attitudes toward the elderly (Alexy, 1985). Because institutional care tends to be directed toward outcomes for the majority, it is often difficult to respect individual needs. Disregard for individuality and adulthood can lead to depresssion and compromise positive health behaviors (Taft, 1985). Resistance to the establishment's mode of operation may leave the elder open to retribution from the staff and peers (Taft, 1985).

Another tool that could be used to determine health perception of the elder is the Health Self Determinism Index (Deci, 1975, 1980). This tool measures the intrinsic constructs that motivate health behaviors. However, the tool focuses on a small aspect of the health maintenance issue. The Health Self Determinism Index (HSDI) is a 20-item Likert scale. Subcategories in this instrument are self-determined health judgments, self-determined health behaviors, and perceived sense of competency in health matters. Cox (1985) demonstrated overall reliability for the items of this index, emphasizing the multidimensionality of motivation. The advantage of the tool is that despite its brevity, a fair assessment of the individual's motivation regarding health may be obtained. It is a helpful tool for evaluating health maintenance in the elder if motivational factors are in question. The HSDI is a tool that could refine motivational components after an assessment of health behaviors has been made. It does not address preventive or maintenance activities.

Another tool that assesses the patient's basis for health is the Health Belief Model (HBM) (Becker and Rosenstock, 1984). After numerous revisions, the HBM contains items that assess an individual's (1) perceived susceptibility to a specific disease; (2) perceived association between severity of a health condition and health-related behaviors; (3) perceived benefits of a health recommendation; and (4) the perceived effects of barriers, for example, pain or cost, to the health-related behaviors. This tool deals with a specific component of health behavior—motivation. The HBM is helpful when evaluating health practices of the elderly because it does address the realistic barriers experienced by many elderly, such as cost, transportation, fatigue, and personal relations with health care providers. Because of the intricacies of motivation (eg, self-image, culture) the HBM does not recommend interventions based on assessment findings, but only identifies the motivational/perceptual problems. It helps to individualize nursing interventions with the elder within a relevant lifestyle framework.

An assessment tool that addresses both aspects of health perception and health management was developed by the Department of Health and Human Services (1985). Items in this tool collect data on general and specific preventive and health maintenance behaviors. The 56-item Likert scale includes some open-ended responses, is administered, and presents assessment categories of interest to the elderly (eg, home safety, stress, dental care) that cannot be found in other instruments. It also assesses the elder's knowledge base for specific health behaviors, for example, high blood pressure and diet. The tool helps nurses gain insight into the older adult's health perception and management behaviors. Although quite long, the tool assesses environmental problems of the elder living alone and many of the chronic health deviations to which the elderly are predisposed.

CASE STUDY

Altered Health Maintenance

Mr. James is a 72-year-old man who lives alone. He is under treatment for emphysema, which includes bronchodilators, antibiotics, fluid intake of at least 2000 cc and low-flow oxygen at home. Mrs. James died 18 months ago from colon cancer. Since then, Mr. James's health has deteriorated causing his daughters concern. His ability to care for himself at home has decreased. Indeed, his records show that he has missed several doctor's appointments or has not made them at the recommended intervals. Prior to his retirement he was a department manager in a local industry. According to his daughters, Mrs. James managed all health care behaviors such as health care appointments, diet, and exercise. According to Mr. James, he only did those things "when I finally got tired of her nagging," although he "never did quit smoking," and "it gave her something to do."

Mr. James stated that his health is "good," that the doctors are trying to "make him older than he is," and that many of his friends "are worse off" than he is because "they're in nursing homes." He disregards his daughters' reports of intermittent confusion and increased chest pain and dyspnea with "those girls think everyone over 65 belongs in an old-age home."

Mr. James adheres to his health care program intermittently. He rarely goes out to socialize except for coffee once a month with a "few buddies." His level of physical activity is quite compromised, and the nurse notices that he becomes short of breath walking across the room. Further, he needs to support himself by grabbing furniture as he moves about. He reports sleeping poorly but "catnaps" during the day. Mr. James says he refrains from taking his bronchodilators because "they taste so bad." His daughters report that he has had several colds within the last 6 months. They are fearful hospitalization will be required if his condition continues to deteriorate. Mr. James has lost 22 pounds the past year because he's "too tired to fix meals." From the data collected, it appears that Mr. James has many health care needs that are not being met because of Altered Health Maintenance related to role disturbance, poor health behaviors and health status, a negative perception of health for the elderly, loss of a significant other, and lack of faith in medical treatment (see Table 2.3). This diagnosis is supported by decline in physical status, inability to assume health behaviors once managed by spouse, social withdrawal, lack of knowledge regarding self-care, and barriers to medical regimens such as taste, fatigue, and continuance of life-long negative health habits as a means of control.

NURSING INTERVENTIONS

The diagnosis of Altered Health Maintenance indicates a dysfunction in one or more components that contribute to health maintenance: physical, psychologic, and social. Thus, several nursing interventions are appropriate depending on the specific etiologies and related factors, for example, knowledge deficit, loss of control.

Many of the interventions for Altered Health Maintenance are based on change theory, motivation theory, learning theory, and various educational principles. Few interventions that influence Altered Health Maintenance in the elderly have been examined from a research perspective. The following examples, however, are based on research that used adult and geriatric populations.

Goal Setting

Goal setting is an intervention based in educational theory that identifies the adult learner as a problem solver. In this approach, active participation is preferred to

Table 2.3

Profile on Case Study Client, Mr. James

HEALTH MAINTENANCE DOMAINS	ASSESSMENT FINDINGS	HEALTH BEHAVIOR
Oxygenation	Dyspnea Chest pain Confusion	Refrains from taking medication Continues to smoke Misses appointments with health professionals
Food and water intake	Thick secretions Frequent colds Weight loss	Irregular meals
Sleep and activity	Inadequate sleep patterns	Fatigue Catnaps
Social interaction	Disturbance of social bonds Loss of significant other Disturbance of role	Social isolation Negative feelings regarding concern of family

passive response. Goal setting is intended to improve participation in health care facilities over a period of time. Alexy (1985) found that goal setting was an effective intervention for selected behaviors and that totally managed provider goals made a significant change in risk-reduction health behaviors such as changes in alcohol intake, seat belt use, and exercise. Collaboratively determined goals were effective for weight reduction behaviors, exercise levels, and global measures of life expectancy. Because the control group also had increased exercise levels, Alexy speculates that media influence independent of the study contributed to increased exercise in all three groups. Overall, goal setting was found to be effective for development of risk-reduction behaviors.

Media-Intensive Instruction

Another study used media-intensive instruction as a means to bring about reasonably stable change in health behaviors. The Heart Disease Prevention Program (Maccoby et al, 1977) used media-intensive instruction to increase knowledge levels of heart disease and associated behaviors. This format was also effective for bringing about changes in dietary and smoking habits. A follow-up study by Meyer et al (1980) found that mass media alone (minus the intensive instruction) took longer to achieve a change in behavior that was maintained for a period of time.

Counseling

Individual and family counseling interventions have been effectively used by nurses. Morisky et al (1983) demonstrated the use of counseling in 5- to 10-minute sessions to affect behaviors related to management of high blood pressure. The result of this intervention was a reduction in the mortality rate for the sample studied.

Social Bonds

The importance of social relationships to physical health has been ascertained in the literature. This is of particular note when dealing with the elderly who may be experiencing a loss of persons with whom social bonds have been an important part of their life. Thomas and Hooper (1983) reviewed six provisions of social bonds, including attachment, social integration (eg, sharing ideas), opportunities for nurturance (to be needed by another), reliable alliance (able to depend on someone), and obtaining guidance and support (in times of stress). They found that by using these characteristics, satisfying social bonds were operational in their sample of 40 healthy elderly subjects.

Another form of social bonds is that of pet ownership. Suggested by Florence Nightingale in *Notes on Nursing* (reprinted 1969), the use of pets as a form of therapy has increasing use. Erickson (1985) reviews the literature that documents the importance of pets and health maintenance, especially for the older individual. A more detailed discussion of pet therapy is presented in Chapter 25.

CASE STUDY

Nursing Interventions

Mr. James has many universal self-care needs that are not being met because of noncompliance with treatment for chronic emphysema. However, according to him his health is "good," even better than that of his friends in nursing homes. The professional health care team as well as his family are quite concerned about his deteriorating condition, and hospitalization or institutionalization seems probable in the near future. The nurse believes that Mr. James does not have many positive health maintenance behaviors. Given the assessment findings, it has been determined that his negative health behaviors (Altered Health Maintenance) are related to role disturbance, knowledge deficit, a loss of control, and grieving over his wife's death. Further assessment would be necessary to determine if this is normal or dysfunctional grieving.

Although Mr. James was obviously a man of great control in his employment position, his spouse managed all his personal activities at home. Health behaviors are new to his self-image, and he is having difficulty managing them.

One of the first things for the nurse to determine is Mr. James's level of knowledge and readiness to learn regarding his condition and the recommended treatment. Counseling regarding his recent losses should also occur concurrently with knowledge assessment. This may be individual professional counseling or use of a personal resource who has shared a similar loss. Possible referrals to social services, to a psychologist, or to a mental health nurse are discussed. While recognizing his personal loss, the counseling strategy should enhance a positive self-image and personal control as Mr. James's role is reestablished. Establishing mutual goals with Mr. James is also necessary. The health care team will have to prioritize their goals carefully, as they may not be those desired by Mr. James. One goal that the team shares with Mr. James is the desire to keep the patient independent in his home. By explaining how compliance with the health care regimen can help to accomplish this goal, the required treatments may become more meaningful to Mr. James. It is hoped that working through the barriers to treatment, such as the bad taste of medications, will enhance compliance with treatment without a change in the lifestyle of the patient.

Although correcting Mr. James's current physiologic status may be possible through hospitalization, without changing his underlying health behaviors he would soon revert to the same condition. Changing those behaviors will likely take time and occur in small increments. Referral to other supportive services such as "Meals on Wheels" or home health care may be necessary depending on the mutual goals established and the desires of the patient. Particular attention needs to be paid to Mr. James' ethnic and cultural values regarding health behavior.

One of the goals of the nurse and team was to increase Mr. James's awareness of "feeling better" physically. Although documentation in a log or diary is a common method for this, the nurse felt Mr. James was not motivated for this activity. Instead they chose to monitor his progress through his activity levels in his home. This would also give Mr. James an immediate reward for having the physical stamina to complete a task.

The overall goals of the health team were to:

1. Change Mr. James's health perception to one more closely aligned with that of the health team while maintaining maximum control for Mr. James.
2. Change Mr. James's health behaviors to those that would adequately meet his physiologic and emotional needs while remaining consistent with his values.

OUTCOMES

To determine if their strategies are successful, the nursing staff would observe the following changes in Mr. James' behavior:

1. Consistent compliance with medical regimen.
2. Increase in body weight to appropriate range.
3. Establishment of sleep patterns normal for him before the loss of his wife.
4. Engagement in regular physical and social activities.
5. An increased awareness of health and the effect of self-health behaviors in order to prevent future declines in health.

Achievement of these goals indicates that Mr. James has changed his present health maintenance behaviors to more positive perceptions and activities. The nursing interventions that support these goals are based on the psychosocial concepts of motivation, self-image, self-control, loss, and developmental tasks of the elderly. Although nurses should be positive regarding the potential for change in clients such as Mr. James, the staff also needs to be realistic in accepting the fact that he may not wish to change all the behaviors they deem undesirable to his health. Any intervention that helps to bring his health perception more in line with that of the health care professionals can be considered successful. Patience and persistence is of the essence. Mr. James has maintained his health beliefs and role responsibilities for many years. Therefore, changing them will only occur over a period of time.

SUMMARY

Many of the interventions related to Altered Health Maintenance have been researched in populations of middle-aged adults. They have also dealt primarily with concrete, measurable interventions associated with Knowledge Deficit (see Chapter 33). Research related to the motivational components of health maintenance behaviors is lacking, as are studies that relate the perceptions and developmental tasks of the elderly to health maintenance behaviors. It is unwise to assume that interventions successful in the middle-aged adult will be equally successful in the elderly population without modification. Morrison (1980;135) also contends that it is possible to "neglect areas ripe for preventive intervention" if health care for the elderly focuses only on chronic disease that is present. Nursing must remain eclectic in its search for suitable interventions for this diagnosis, as well as creative in their application and diligent in research to test their efficacy.

ASSESSMENT GUIDE 2.1

Assessment Guide for Altered Health Maintenance

Given the many assessment tools we have reviewed, it is possible to construct an interview form that would address Altered Health Maintenance specifically in the elderly. The following is an attempt to provide comprehensive assessment of those factors pertinent to the elderly.

1. How would you rate your health at this time?
2. Do you feel you have control over the activities and events that affect your health?
3. What kinds of things do you do that prevent you from getting ill, which would interfere with desired activities?
4. Is there any person, circumstance, or event that prevents you from caring for yourself as you would like?
5. How do you normally manage a change in your health status?
6. What newly occurring changes in your health status would prompt you to see your doctor?
7. Describe what interests, persons, or events give your life purpose and meaning.
8. What personal or social relationships are important to you?
9. What are your personal plans for the immediate and distant future?
10. Do you feel your present illness is a threat to your well-being? (If appropriate)
11. Do you feel your current treatment is helping to manage your present illness?
12. Do you consistently perform the following health-related activities?
    - Use a seatbelt in the car?
    - Engage in exercise for 30 minutes at least three times per week?
    - Refrain from smoking?
    - Use alcoholic substances in moderation (less than three times per week)?
    - Include fruits and vegetables in your meals as well as lean meats?
    - Keep your doctors appointments for routine physical examinations?
    - Perform self-breast/testicular examinations between visits?

References

Alexy B: Goal setting and health risk reduction. *Nurs Res* (Sept/Oct) 1985; 34:283–288.

Becker MH, Rosenstock IM: Compliance with medical advice. In: *Health Care and Human Behavior.* Steptoe A, Matthews A (editors). Academic Press, 1984.

Carpenito L: *Nursing Diagnosis: Application to Clinical Practice.* Lippincott, 1983.

Carpenito LJ: *Nursing Diagnosis: Application to Clinical Practice,* 2d ed. Lippincott, 1987.

Carroll-Johnson RM (editor): *Classification of Nursing Diagnoses: Proceedings of the Eighth Conference.* Lippincott, 1989.

Cox C: The health self-determinism index. *Nurs Res* (May/June) 1985; 34(3):177–182.

Cummings KM, Becker MH, Maile MC: Bringing the models together: An empirical approach to combining variables used to explain health actions. *J Behav Med* 1980; 3(2):123–145.

Deci E: *Intrinsic Motivation.* Plenum, 1975.

Deci E: *THe Psychology of Self Determinism.* Lexington Books, 1980.

Department of Health and Human Services: *Health Promotion and Disease Prevention Survey.* U.S. Government Printing Office, 1985.

Engle VF: Newman's conceptual framework and the measurement of older adults' health. *ANS* (Oct) 1984; 3(1):24–33.

Erickson R: Companion animals and the elderly. *Geriatr Nurs* 1985; 6(2):92–96.

Fawcett J: *Analysis and Evaluation of Conceptual Models of Nursing,* 2d ed. Davis, 1989.

Fehring RJ, Frenn M: Nursing diagnoses in a nurse-managed wellness resource center. In: *Classification of Nursing Diagnoses: Proceedings of the Sixth National Conference.* Hurley ME (editor). Mosby, 1986.

Filner B, Williams TF: Health promotion for the elderly: Reducing functional dependency. *Healthy People.* U.S. Government Printing Office, 1979.

Gordon M: *Nursing Diagnosis: Concepts and Practices,* 2d ed. McGraw-Hill, 1982.

Johnson-Saylor MT, Pohl J, Lowe-Wickson B: An assessment form for determining patients' health status and coping responses. *Top Clin Nurs* (July) 1982; 6(2):20–27.

Keating S, Kelman G: *Home Health Care Nursing: Concepts and Practice.* Lippincott, 1988.

Kim MJ, McFarland G, McLane A (editors): *Classification of Nursing Diagnoses: Proceedings of the Fifth National Conference.* Mosby, 1984.

King I: *A Theory for Nursing: Systems, Concepts, Process.* Wiley, 1981.

Laffrey S: Development of a health conception scale. *Res Nurs Health* 1986; 9:107–113.

Maccoby N et al: Reducing the risk of cardiovascular disease. *J Comm Health* 1977; 3(2):100–114.

McLane A (editor): *Classification of Nursing Diagnoses: Proceedings of the Seventh Conference.* Mosby, 1987.

Meyer AJ et al: Skills training in cardiovascular health education campaign. *J Consult Clin Psychol* 1980; 48:129–142.

Morisky DE et al: Five year blood pressure control and mortality following health education for hypertensive patients. *Am J Public Health* 1983; 73:153–162.

Morrison J: Geriatric preventive health maintenance. *J Am Geriatr Soc* 1980; 28(3):133–135.

Nightingale F: *Notes on Nursing.* Dover, 1969 (originally published 1859).

Orem DE: *Nursing: Concepts and Practice,* 2d ed. McGraw-Hill, 1982.

Orem DE: *Nursing: Concepts of Practice,* 3d ed. McGraw-Hill, 1985.

Parse R: *Man–Living–Health: A Theory of Nursing.* Wiley, 1981.

Pender N: *Health Promotion in Nursing Practice,* 2d ed. Appleton and Lange, 1987.

Peret KK, Stachowiak B: Alteration in health maintenance: Conceptual base, etiology and defining characteristics. In: *Classification of Nursing Diagnoses: Proceedings of the Fifth National Conference.* Kim MJ, McFarland G, McLane A (editors). Mosby, 1984.

Roy C: *Introduction to Nursing: An Adaptation Model,* 2d ed. Prentice-Hall, 1984.

Rubenstein L et al: Systematic biases in functional status assessment of elderly adults: Effects of different data sources. *J Gerontol* 1984; 39(6):686–691.

Simmons DA: *A Classification Scheme for Client Problems in Community Health Nursing.* DHHS Publication No. HRA 80-16. U.S. Department of Health and Human Services, 1980.

Smith JA: The idea of health: A philosophical inquiry. *ANS* 1981; 3(3):43–50.

Stanwyck DJ: Self-esteem through the lifespan. *Fam Community Health* 1983; 11–27.

Taft LB: Self-esteem in later life: A nursing perspective. *ANS* (Oct) 1985; 8:77–84.

Thomas PD, Hooper EM: Healthy elderly: Social bonds and locus of control. *Res Nurs Health* 1983; 6:11–15.

Webster's Ninth New Collegiate Dictionary. Merriam-Webster, 1988.

3

Potential for Trauma: Falls

Jo Ellen R. Ross, MA, RN
Carol A. Watson, PhD, RN
Teresa A. Gyldenvand, MA, RN
JoAnn L. Reinboth, MA, RN

The North American Nursing Diagnosis Association (NANDA) (Carroll-Johnson, 1989;528) defines "Potential for Trauma" as "accentuated risk of accidental tissue injury (eg, wound, burn, fracture)." Falling is one type of Potential for Trauma that is particularly prevalent among the elderly.

To date, literature on falls of elderly persons has been abundant. However, research has focused primarily on the causes of falls and has been retrospective in nature. Thus far, no organizing framework has been proposed that can provide guidelines for nurses who care for elderly who are at risk to fall. Therefore, the purpose of this chapter is to develop the diagnosis of Potential for Trauma: Falls, focusing on etiologies of falls, defining characteristics for the elderly at risk, and presenting the interventions that health care professionals can use to prevent falls. There is no specific NANDA diagnosis for Potential for Trauma: Falls at present, but the diagnosis is in development.

SIGNIFICANCE FOR THE ELDERLY

Falls can exact a serious toll on any victim, but are often fatal for the elderly. In examining the epidemiology of injuries, three factors contribute to the high Potential for Trauma in the elderly (Baker and Harvey, 1985): (1) Susceptibility to falls increases as multiple body systems deteriorate; (2) aging creates a lower threshold for injury as osteoporosis causes bone fragility; and (3) with aging, injuries result in progressively poorer outcomes. With aging, seemingly minor injuries may cause increasingly greater mortality and morbidity.

For persons 65 years and older, traumatic falls are the sixth leading cause of death. Deaths from falls accounted for 50% of the fatalities due to accidental trauma, more deaths than from all other accidents combined (Chipman, 1981).

Mortality

For individuals who are 65 years of age and older, falls are the leading accident as well as the leading cause of accidental death (Foerster, 1981; Metropolitan Life Insurance Co., 1982). Although the elderly compose only 11% of the total population in the United States, falls by elderly represent 70% of all fatalities due to falls (Metropolitan Life Insurance Co., 1982).

The negative outcomes of falls increase as one grows older, especially after the seventh decade

(Louis, 1983). People over age 80 who fall have a mortality rate that is eight times greater than that of persons 60 years and younger.

Although many falls lead to no apparent injury, other falls result in fractures with prolonged invalidism or death (Wild et al, 1981b). When a person sustains significant trauma, hospitalization may be prolonged because of extended healing intervals (Ellis and Nowles, 1977; Rodstein, 1981). As the length of stay increases, the number and severity of complications that can precipitate and cause death also increase (Foerster, 1981; Rodstein, 1981).

Murphy and Isaacs (1982) described a "post-fall" syndrome in 36 elderly hospitalized patients who had fallen at home. A severe "post-fall" syndrome was defined as an exaggerated tendency to clutch and grab while walking and an inability to walk without assistance. Patients who could walk alone but exhibited the need to clutch were described as having this syndrome to a moderate degree. After a period of 4 months, death had occurred in 9 of 10 patients who had exhibited a severe "post-fall" syndrome and in 3 of 16 patients who had demonstrated the moderate form. Only 1 of 10 persons with no signs of the syndrome had died. The authors could not determine whether the fall caused the syndrome or the syndrome had caused the fall.

Studies of hospitalized elderly who have fallen have shown (1) that about 10% of patients who are age 60 years or older die before discharge and that mortality increased markedly with age (Lucht, 1971), and (2) that only 20% leave the hospital after treatment (Naylor and Rosen, 1970).

Margules et al (1970) surveyed 5 years of accidents resulting in injury among elderly people living in care facilities. They found that 95% of the injuries were due to falls, and 60.9% of those individuals who sustained fractures died shortly thereafter.

Morbidity

Physiologic Effects Falls can exact a serious toll both physiologically and psychologically for older persons. The increased risk of falling relates directly to the decline in physiologic and mental functions in senescence. As muscles weaken and reflexes slow, the elderly are less able to recover their balance once they start to fall. Other factors that add to the high susceptibility to falls in the elderly include impaired sight (eg, decreased peripheral vision, susceptibility to glare) and increased sway while walking and standing. These factors reduce the ability to compensate in situations that may result in falls (Sehested and Severin-Nielsen, 1977). The potential for physical injury is also enhanced by osteoporotic changes and greater fragility of tissue in the elderly. (For further discussion of physiologic problems of aging, see Chapters 22 and 23.)

Snipes (1982) estimates that 75% of older persons' falls occur at or near home. Many factors contribute to falls in the home, and environmental hazards often are cited. Poor lighting, especially poor lighting on stairs, prevents the elderly person from seeing household clutter. Despite the presence of environmental hazards, most falls at home indicate a deterioration of health, for example, cardiac arrhythmias, hypovolemia, or muscle weakness (Gordon, 1982; Rodstein and Camus, 1973; Snipes, 1982).

Lucht (1971) studied 472 people age 60 or older who were treated at a hospital after experiencing falls in the home. Two hundred eighty-six had a total of 294 fractures; 90 were fractures of the neck of the femur.

Wild et al (1981a) studied 125 people aged 65 and older who reported to their doctors that they had suffered falls at home. Eighty-four sustained injury. Of the 84, 18 experienced fractures and 66 suffered soft-tissue injuries.

Unfortunately, once the elderly person moves to institutional care, falls are not eliminated. Foerster's (1981) study of a 242-bed long-term care facility revealed that 25% of the residents had experienced falls. Sehested and Severin-Nielsen's (1977) 1-year study reported a similar incidence of falls (26%) in patients who were hospitalized in a 97-bed geriatric department. Morris and Isaacs (1980) noted that 20% of patients hospitalized on two 28-bed geriatric units fell during a 1-year period of study.

In a 3-year study of elderly persons in a long-term care facility, Pablo (1977) noted that 65% of falls resulted in no injuries. The other 35% of falls resulted in a combination of minor injuries. He reported no serious injuries or deaths. In a survey of 6 months of incident reports at a university hospital, Ross (1980) recorded only two serious injuries out of 289 falls; both injuries involved patients over 64 years of age.

In the 5-year prospective study by Gryfe and colleagues (1977) of active ambulatory institutionalized elderly over age 65, 45% of the subjects suffered at least one fall during the study period. Of the 651 total falls, 114 caused severe morbidity, with 40 fractures and 11.4% soft-tissue injuries that required sutures.

In a Canadian geriatric hospital where 1803 falls occurred over 3 years, 62% of elderly experienced no injury. However, 11.9% had injuries requiring treatment, and 58 falls (3.2%) resulted in fractures (Berry et al, 1981). No injury or only minor injury occurred in surveys from a teaching hospital (Gibbs, 1982) and on a geriatric ward (Odetunde, 1982). Kulikowski (1979), in a Veteran's hospital, Walshe and Rosen (1979) at a community hospital, and Lynn (1980) at a university metropolitan setting relate that only 2% to 3% of those who do fall in an acute care hospital will injure themselves seriously.

Thus the rate of falls varies greatly within similar types of institutions as well as between hospitals and long-term care facilities. Likewise the percentage of injuries differs. In both categories, comparisons are difficult because of inconsistent and varied reporting statistics. Identification of factors that predict physiologic morbidity has been impossible because of incomplete data regarding specific high-risk factors of injury.

Psychologic Effects Health care providers must remember that the experience of a fall can be just as frightening to the elderly client who falls without injury as to the elderly client who sustains injury (Chipman, 1981).

Apart from the risk of fractures, a client experiences loss of confidence. Odetunde (1982;33) writes, "Every fall does some harm; it makes some psychological dent in the patient and/or those helping him." Colling and Park (1983;175) state, "The occurrence of a fall, and particularly a series of falls, even if no physical trauma occurs, causes stress for family members as well as the elderly person."

An elderly client with a history of falling may develop a fear of falling (Bhala et al, 1982). To prevent further falls, many elderly isolate themselves (Foerster, 1981), thus establishing a pattern of immobility as well as social isolation. Following a report about a grant to study falls (published in the *Journal of the American Association of Retired Persons*), Tinetti received 200 letters describing self-imposed immobility that was prompted by the fear of falling (cited in Baker and Harvey, 1985).

Nurses should not underestimate the damage a fall causes to the confidence and morale of elderly patients and their relatives, whether or not the fall causes physical injury.

Multiple Falls

Several authors report that elderly individuals who fall are at risk to fall again (Campbell et al, 1981; Perry, 1982; Prudham and Evans, 1981).

As with repeated falls in the home, institutionalized individuals who have fallen once are at risk for additional falls. Long-term care facilities appear to have a much higher incidence because of the chronic conditions of the residents. Foerster's (1981) study of 158 residents in a 242-bed long-term care facility reported that 40 patients fell a total of 105 times during the 10-week study period; 53% of those who fell experienced more than one fall. In a Canadian Veterans' home, 51% of patients fell more than once during the 3-year data collection period (Berry et al, 1981).

Other authors have found a much lower percentage of repeat fallers. Lynn (1980), Morris and Isaacs (1980), and Gyldenvand and Reinboth (1982) reported that 1 in 10 who fall will fall again. A study conducted in an extended care facility found that 2 of 14 fallers had fallen more than once (Reinboth and Gyldenvand, 1982). Gyldenvand (1984) noted that 2 of 29 fallers experienced repeat falls in a community hospital setting.

Repeated falls create ethical dilemmas for health professionals. There is a desire to "protect" patients by limiting mobility. Conversely, there is the desire to rehabilitate patients, which further exposes them to the risk of repeated falls.

Health care providers, and in particular nurses, are responsible for providing a safe environment for institutionalized elderly. To some extent, falls can be managed by the use of restraints, both physical and chemical. However, this approach creates problems because it limits mobility and defeats the goal of maintaining an optimal level of activity and independence for the older person.

ETIOLOGIES/RELATED FACTORS

Most falls in the elderly result either from changes that accompany the aging process or from disease entities, although there are several other contributing factors that increase the risk of falling. Etiologies or contributing factors to falls can be categorized as either extrinsic or intrinsic. Extrinsic factors include environmental precipitators of falls such as poor lighting, clutter, and slick footwear. Intrinsic factors are patient oriented and may be age- or disease-related factors such as confusion, poor balance, and gait disturbance.

Extrinsic Factors

In the home, external factors such as throw rugs, electrical cords, and clutter are major hazards that may cause individuals to fall. These items cause problems especially for the elderly because of reduced visual acuity and changes in gait. Many elderly use throw rugs to prevent wear on carpets or to cover worn areas. For the elderly who have difficulty with ambulation, many will arrange needed items close to their favorite chair. This can easily become cluttered and be a potential cause for a fall.

The choice of footwear for support and balance is important. The construction of the soles must be considered as well as the type of surface where the individual does most of his or her walking. For example, soles made of crepe or certain types of rubber can cause tripping as the soles stick to the carpet, especially if clients have a shuffling gait.

Stairs can be quite hazardous, especially in older homes and in some health care settings. In many homes, stairs are narrow and may contain clutter on the sides of each step. Lighting, especially illumination on basement steps, may be poor. If individuals have poor vision and if stairs are carpeted, the difference in lighting as steps begin and end may be difficult to perceive. Putting clear visual indicators of where the steps begin and end will help to prevent accidents. Adding skid strips to uncarpeted stairs also will help to prevent slipping.

Intrinsic Factors

Three intrinsic factors are primary causes of falls in the elderly: (1) the aging process, principally changes in mobility and vision; (2) the presence of disease processes; and (3) the use of drugs, particularly cardiovascular drugs and central nervous system depressants. Additional factors are noted in Table 3.1, which also contains the etiologies and defining characteristics listed by NANDA for Potential for Trauma (Carroll-Johnson, 1989). As mentioned previously, the diagnosis Potential for Trauma: Falls has not been approved by NANDA.

Altered Physical Mobility General impairment of gait and locomotion due to the changes brought about by the aging process predisposes the elderly individual to falling.

Alterations in gait that accompany aging differ in that women develop a narrow walking and standing base and walk with more of a waddle, whereas men adopt a flexed posture, a wide walking and standing base, and a small-step gait (Azar and Lawton, 1964). With an abnormal gait, defective balancing may occur (Wild et al, 1981a). Overstall et al (1977) indicated that sway is greater in women than in men. Fernie et al (1982) found that sway was significantly greater in persons who fell than in those who did not fall.

Sensory/Perceptual Alteration: Vision Vision plays a key role in the tendency to fall. A combination of proprioceptive and visual impairment dramatically increases the risk of falling. Visual acuity is required for safe ambulation. As vision deteriorates, it deprives the elderly of an integral part of their safety mechanism (Fozard et al, 1977).

Disease Processes The diseases most commonly implicated are those of the nervous system, the circulatory system, the respiratory system, and those that result in debilitation, such as cancer. Rodstein (1964) also found that out of 190 accidents involving 189 elderly residents, a strong correlation existed between the number of chronic diseases and the frequency and severity of falls.

The neurologic disorders associated with falls in the elderly include cerebrovascular disorders, Parkinsonism, spinal degeneration, tabes dorsalis, and cerebellar atrophy (Naylor and Rosen, 1970). These disorders generally cause disturbances in gait and balance in their victims.

Many cardiovascular changes that are associated with aging cause arrhythmias. In turn, these arrhythmias induce transient cerebral dysfunction, syncope, and dizziness (Raffery and Cashman, 1976).

With aging, the efficient control of blood pressure diminishes during postural changes. Therefore, orthostatic hypotension may be experienced and may contribute to falls (Rodstein, 1981). Similarly, ischemia, and specifically vertebrobasilar ischemia, accounts for the majority of drop attacks that are prevalent in the elderly. Lipsitz (1983;617) defines drop attacks as "a symptom of a variety of pathophysiologic processes that ultimately result in sudden, unexpected falls without loss of consciousness."

Diminished oxygen levels create vascular changes throughout the body, the cumulative effect being an alteration in blood supply to the brain, heart, and skeletal muscles (Kohn, 1977). A decreased blood flow to these structures can precipitate falls.

Debilitating disorders compound the effects of the normal aging process to create a higher risk of falling. Lynn (1980) determined that debilitating diseases (eg, anemia, neoplasms, immunosuppression) and other stressful processes (such as invasive procedures, diagnostic preps, reduced caloric intake, and bed rest) contribute to falls. Colling and Park (1983) also identified alcohol and drug abuse as debilitative factors associated with falls. The use of certain types of medications precipitate falls among the elderly. Studies (Cook et al, 1982; Feist, 1978; Rodstein, 1964; Wild et al, 1981a) reveal that hospitalized elderly who fall are often given diuretics, sedatives, analgesics, pain medications, barbiturates and/or hypnotics or tranquilizers. The drugs most commonly used by fallers were analgesics and sedatives (Barbieri, 1983; MacDonald and MacDonald, 1977; Odetunde, 1982; Oliva, 1965; Swartzbeck, 1983; Walshe and Rosen, 1979). In general, reports on the contribution of medications to falls cite the same types of medicines—those that affect the cardiovascular system and those that affect the nervous system.

Other Contributing Factors

The literature reveals that mental status is related to falls among elderly, but many studies are contradictory. The concept of mental status includes such aspects as level of orientation, affective states (confusion and depression), slowing of performance, judgment, memory, and dementia.

In an extended care facility, Reinboth and Gyldenvand (1982) found that 93% of the fallers had mental status alteration ranging from confusion to agitation.

A study by Campbell et al (1981) revealed that impaired mental function was a predictor of falls in elderly men. Walshe and Rosen's (1979) study of 53 individuals who fell in a 300-bed community hospital reported that the mental status of the clients was altered for about one half of the fallers. Similarly, Swartzbeck's (1983) study found that 50% of 554 fallers in her sample of elderly had problems with mentation.

In contrast, Kalchthaler et al (1978) found that elderly persons whom the nursing staff had rated as alert were involved in the greatest number of falls. Several

Table 3.1

Comparison of NANDA* Defining Characteristics for Potential for Trauma With the Risk Assessment for Falls Scale[†]

POTENTIAL FOR TRAUMA

Definition: Accentuate risk of accidental tissue injury (eg, wound, burn, fracture)

Defining Characteristics

Internal (individual) factors
  Weakness
  Poor vision
  Balancing difficulties
  Reduced temperature and/or tactile sensation
  Reduced large- or small-muscle coordination
  Reduced hand–eye coordination
  Lack of safety education
  Lack of safety precautions
  Insufficient finances to purchase safety equipment or effect
    repairs
  Cognitive or emotional difficulties
  History of previous trauma

External (environmental) factors
  Slippery floors, eg, wet or highly waxed
  Snow or ice on stairs, walkways
  Unanchored rugs
  Bathtub without hand grip or antislip equipment
  Use of unsteady ladder or chairs
  Entering unlighted rooms
  Unsturdy or absent stair rails
  Unanchored electric wires
  Litter or liquid spills on floors or stairways
  High beds
  Children playing without gates at top of stairs
  Obstructed passageways
  Unsafe window protection in homes with young children
  Inappropriate call-for-aid mechanisms for bed-resting client
  Pot handles facing front of stove
  Bathing in very hot water, eg, unsupervised bathing of
    young children
  Potential igniting of gas leaks
  Delayed lighting of gas burner or oven
  Experimenting with chemicals or gasoline
  Unscreened fires or heaters
  Wearing of plastic aprons or flowing clothing around open
    flame
  Children playing with matches, candles, cigarettes
  Inadequately stored combustibles or corrosives, eg, matches,
    oily rags, lye
  Highly flammable children's toys or clothes
  Overloaded fuse boxes
  Contact with rapidly moving machinery, industrial belts, or
    pulleys
  Sliding on coarse bed linen or struggling within bed
    restraints
  Faulty electrical plugs, frayed wires, or defective appliances
  Contact with acids or alkalis
  Playing with fireworks or gunpowder

RISK ASSESSMENT FOR FALLS

Operational Definitions

Sensory/Perceptual Alterations
1. Vision corrected with use of glasses or monocular
2. Blurred vision, cataract, or glaucoma
3. Visual field cut

Altered Thought Processes
1. Oriented to person, place
2. Oriented to person
3. Disoriented

Agitation
1. Yells out, abrasive language
2. Frequent calls with threatening language
3. Combative, requires restraints

Depression
1. Poor appetite, sleep difficulties
2. Low self-esteem
3. Poor concentration

Anxiety
1. Restless, sleepless
2. Rapid speech, asks for reassurance on immediate concerns
3. Preoccupied, increased psychomotor behavior

Altered Physical Mobility
1. Ambulates with assistive device
2. Requires assistance + an assistive device or 2 assistants
3. Stands and pivots with assistance only

Age
1. 19–59 years of age
2. 60–75 years of age
3. >75 years of age

Disease Process
1. 1 disease
2. 2 diseases
3. 3 diseases or more

Medications
1. Cardiovascular effector
2. CNS effector
3. Both

Impaired Verbal Communication
1. Hearing loss
2. Speech disorder
3. Both

Alteration in Elimination
1. Nocturia
2. Urgency
3. Frequency

Table 3.1

Comparison of NANDA* Defining Characteristics for Potential for Trauma With the Risk Assessment for Falls Scale†
(*Continued*)

POTENTIAL FOR TRAUMA

Defining Characteristics

Contact with intense cold
Overexposure to sun, sun lamps, radiotherapy
Use of cracked dishware or glasses
Knives stored uncovered
Guns or ammunition stored unlocked
Large icicles hanging from roof
Exposure to dangerous machinery
Children playing with sharp-edged toys
High-crime neighborhood and vulnerable client
Driving a mechanically unsafe vehicle
Driving after partaking of alcoholic beverages or drugs
Driving at excessive speeds
Driving without necessary visual aids
Children riding in the front seat in car
Smoking in bed or near oxygen
Overloaded electrical outlets
Grease waste collected on stoves
Use of thin or worn pot holders or mitts
Unrestrained babies riding in car
Nonuse or misuse of seat restraints
Nonuse or misuse of necessary headgear for motorized
    cyclists or young children carried on adult bicycles
Unsafe road or road-crossing conditions
Play or work near vehicle pathways, eg, driveways, lanes,
    railroad tracks

*Source: Carroll-Johnson RM (editor): *Classification of Nursing Diagnoses: Proceedings of the Eighth Conference.* Lippincott, 1989.
†Source: Gyldenvand T, Reinboth J: *Intervention Protocol: Elimination Rounds.* University of Iowa, 1982a.

explanations for this phenomenon were given: Alert institutionalized elderly clients are more mobile; alert elderly take more chances; and elderly who had been perceived as alert actually showed significant defects in judgment on closer examination. Likewise, Rodstein (1964) reported a low (14%) incidence of mental confusion among residents involved in accidents.

According to Cook et al (1982), clients with dementia have a higher incidence of falls when compared with those who are mentally normal (as shown by the inverse linear correlation between score on a Mental Status Questionnaire and fall frequency). Overstall (1978) states that with both dementia and depression, a tendency for patients to fall exists because the person misperceives environmental dangers and makes errors in judgments. Isaacs (1978) explains the link between dementia and falls as both the tendency for these clients to place themselves in hazardous situations and their reduced ability to correct imbalance.

Despite some inconsistent findings, the consensus from the literature suggests altered thought processes; for

example, confusion and poor judgment are related to Potential for Injury: Falls.

Altered Emotional States   Altered emotional states such as depression, anxiety, and agitation contribute to falls. Hussian (1981) reported that depression in the elderly can be manifested as confusion or clouding of cognitive function. Because affect and intellectual functioning may be dulled, moderate levels of disorientation may occur. In addition, depressed individuals may become preoccupied with fear and thoughts of self. They are oblivious to their surroundings and the hazards of the environment.

According to Chipman (1981), depression can cause a person to take more chances, which may lead to other behaviors that could cause a fall. Not only do long periods of depression add to the potential for falling, but injury following a fall can exacerbate or cause depression. As noted earlier in the discussion of psychologic aspects, the fear of falling can become a major problem for the elderly because this fear leads them to become less independent and mobile. With decreased mobility and independence, elderly individuals often elect to be alone, which may add to their depression and/or mental confusion. (See Chapter 35 for further discussion of affective states in the elderly.)

Impaired Verbal Communication   Difficulty with language or communication is another factor contributing to falls among the elderly. Lynn (1980) defined a communication problem as either a language disorder or a situation in which a person speaks a language for which no interpreter is available. Lynn found that dysarthria (difficulty speaking due to impairment of speech organs) and dysphasia (inability to express oneself) contribute to falls. Hearing loss also contributes to communication problems. Lynn infers that the inability to make one's wishes known or the inability to understand causes patients to attempt ambulation when it may be inadvisable. (See Chapter 45 for further discussion of this topic.)

Altered Elimination Pattern   The body's need for elimination has been determined to be an important factor in falls among the elderly (Foerster, 1981; Sehested and Severin-Nielsen, 1977; Walshe and Rosen, 1979). Using the toilet requires several complex, potentially dangerous movements. The individual must ambulate to the toilet, adjust clothing, position himself or herself on the toilet, maintain balance, stand up, readjust clothing, and leave the bathroom.

Research related to urinary problems has focused on the activity of going to and from the bathroom. Wells (1975) described 76% of the clients in a 350-bed geriatric hospital as having some degree of incontinence. A number of studies (Barbieri, 1983; Foerster, 1981; Oliva, 1965; Sehested and Severin-Neilson, 1977) reveal that a relatively high percentage of falls occurred among clients who fell while going to, using, or returning from the bathroom. Perhaps the need to eliminate is the one urge that is strong enough to make even the most compliant elder get out of bed and risk a fall. (See Chapters 14 through 17 for further discussion of this topic.)

ASSESSMENT AND DEFINING CHARACTERISTICS

Using the Risk Assessment for Falls Scale (RAFS)

The ideal method of identifying elderly patients at risk of falling is to develop a high-risk profile. This can be done by use of a rating scale that incorporates factors most frequently identified with falls. Table 3.1 compares internal defining characteristics identified by NANDA with the Risk Assessment for Falls Scale (Gyldenvand and Rein-

both, 1982b). The initial tool developed for this purpose was the Risk Assessment for Falls Scale I (RAFS I), which incorporated several of Lynn's (1980) fall categories. The RAFS I was first used to assess two patient populations: neuroscience patients and residents in an extended care facility (Gyldenvand and Reinboth, 1982b; Reinboth and Glydenvand, 1982).

In the data analysis for both institutions, the RAFS I was 100% accurate in predicting which clients were susceptible to falls using the criterion of a high-risk score of 5 and above on the RAFS I. No one fell who had a score below 5.

The data from the RAFS I, although accurate in identifying those who fell, also identified patients at high risk for falling who did not fall. In fact, three times as many high-risk patients did not fall as those who did fall (84 of 104 did not fall). Some overidentification is necessary in order to include all potential fallers in established fall prevention protocols. However, the gross overidentification of the RAFS I was deemed unsatisfactory. Therefore, the RAFS I was revised. The Risk Assessment for Falls Scale II (RAFS II) (see Assessment Guide 3.1) incorporated the factors that were significantly related to falls in the initial two studies and also included factors that appeared to be related to falls during the study but were not part of the RAFS I.

The RAFS II was used to assess clients during three studies. The instrument was piloted in an extended care facility (Reinboth and Gyldenvand, 1982) and used in an acute care hospital (Gyldenvand, 1984) and in three extended care facilities (Reinboth, 1985).

The accuracy of the RAFS II was determined to be 84%. Three weeks after data were collected, six more clients fell who had been identified as at high risk to fall. This finding increased the RAFS II's accuracy of prediction to 90%.

The RAFS II has demonstrated the potential for identifying elderly patients at risk for falling. The RAFS II provides a concise way to analyze the myriad of factors that have been related to falls. A score of 14 or greater on the RAFS II delineates those patients with a potential for trauma by falling. Once the diagnosis of Potential for Trauma has been made by assessment with the RAFS II, nursing interventions to minimize the risk for falling can be introduced.

Scoring the Risk Assessment for Falls Scale

In the Risk Assessment for Falls Scale (RAFS), the degree of risk is directly proportional to the RAFS score; that is, the risk increases as the score increases. The critical score for the samples that have been tested has been 14 and above. However, this score should be determined for specific elderly groups by scoring the patients and then prospectively following them to determine if those with a score of less than 14 fall. If elderly persons with the lower scores fall, a decision must be made. Is the incidence frequent enough to reduce the critical score?

Based on the admission nursing assessment, the RAFS should be completed during the first 24 hours after admission and preferably during the first 8 hours. Early assessment is crucial because, for most individuals, the risk for falling is greatest during the first days of hospitalization or admission to an extended care facility. Review each category and, using the operational definitions, score each category 0–3 or 0–2 in the category of days since admission. If the score is 14 or more, the elderly patient is at high risk. If there is an area that needs to be assessed over a longer period of time—such as depression—this segment can be delayed, but the rest of the instrument should be completed in the event the elderly patient is at increased risk from the other categories and therefore should be on precautions.

Reassessment should occur at predetermined intervals, for example, if the elder's condition has deteriorated overall or in certain categories such as mental status. This elderly individual's score may have increased to a point of being at risk. Also, special precautions may be discontinued if the elderly patient's condition has improved and the risk is changed.

Once scoring has been completed, the elder also should be evaluated for risk of trauma if a fall should occur. Elderly persons who are at great risk of sustaining significant trauma should be carefully evaluated and basic measures should be taken despite a marginal RAFS score. For example, if the elderly person has some type of bleeding disorder, a fall may cause significant bleeding. Thus this individual should receive education about falls and should be instructed to request assistance when walking if the individual has any problems with ambulation.

NURSING INTERVENTIONS

Although the literature abounds with suggested interventions to decrease the incidence of falls, few clinical studies have systematically investigated their effectiveness. Therefore, this section deals with those interventions for which empirical evidence exists related to limiting falls. Additional interventions for which clinical studies are indicated will also be identified.

Identification of Individuals at High Risk to Fall

The initial intervention is the identification of elderly at risk for falling. The RAFS I and RAFS II,

discussed earlier, are succinct assessment tools that nurses can use to determine the client's risk of falling. Once those at high risk are identified, nurses can intervene with strategies directed toward eliminating/altering those factors that place the elderly individual at risk.

Identification of Individuals at High Risk for Trauma

A patient's actual Potential for Trauma must be assessed in the initial intervention process. Because a tool such as the RAFS cannot be totally accurate, nurses must consider an elderly individual's potential for serious injury. Although the elderly person's risk for injury increases with age, certain disease processes will greatly increase the likelihood of injury or death in the event of a fall. Blood dyscrasias can cause severe bleeding at the site of impact. If the site is the head, serious and permanent sequelae may occur.

Nurses should institute preventive measures for those clients who will most likely sustain an injury in a fall. Therefore elderly who could sustain serious injury and who have scores that are close to "high risk" on fall assessment tools should be included in any prevention program. Individuals with metastatic cancer (especially with bony metastasis), with osteoporosis, or with prior fractures as a result of falling, also are at high risk for injury.

Exercise

Gait and locomotion disturbance is related to the potential of falling. Roberts (1985) studied the effects of physical activity on balance and perceptions of balance and found that walking improved balance. Further study needs to be done with randomized samples. However, the influence of regular exercise on balance and, in turn, the relationship between balance and risk of fall, suggests that exercise may be a relatively simple intervention that can be implemented in a variety of settings. Exercise also benefits other body systems.

Elimination Rounds

The need to eliminate will motivate even the most incapacitated elderly person to attempt ambulation. Gyldenvand and Reinboth (1982a), using the RAFS I scale, studied elimination patterns among neuroscience patients at risk for falling. Those identified at high risk were placed on individualized elimination rounds based on their elimination patterns. Elimination rounds were scheduled times when the patient was asked if the bedpan or a trip to the toilet was needed. Usually rounds were scheduled when the patient awakened and after meals if the person could not identify specific times. Night elimination rounds were scheduled incorporating the person's normal elimination pattern. Then vitals and treatments were scheduled during the elimination rounds so the individual did not need to be awakened excessively.

Findings suggested that although elimination rounds can significantly decrease the incidence of falls, many interactive variables contribute to the incidence of falls among the elderly.

When implementing elimination rounds, staff must do more than just assist the patient to the bathroom and leave. Questions such as "Is the patient steady enough that I can leave him alone?" or "Is this patient's compliance such that she will use the bathroom call light and wait until I can return to assist her back to bed?" must be decided.

When instructing the client to seek assistance to the bathroom and during ambulation, include the spouse and family. Many patients' families cannot safely assist their family member. Frequently the client is 150 to 170 pounds, whereas the wife or daughter who try to assist him weigh much less. These types of issues must be addressed during the teaching session. By citing the worse scenario to the family—that is, "If the patient were to start to fall, could you catch him?"—the client and family can clearly see that waiting for assistance is the best way to proceed.

Warning Devices

Predicting when an elderly patient needs to void is inexact. As evidenced in the preceding intervention of elimination rounds, some elderly fall despite structured nursing interventions. Mental confusion and faulty judgment may contribute to falls. A device that can alert nursing staff to elderly who are unable to ambulate on their own and are attempting to rise could be used to summon help before a fall occurs. Widder (1985) reported an alarm device that is secured just above the knee with a fabric band. When the axis of the leg shifts from the horizontal to a dependent angle of 45 degrees, a mercury switch completes a circuit that results in the alarm being sounded.

The device was pilot tested with orthopedic and general medical patients of all ages in an acute care hospital (Widder, 1985). High-risk patients were identified. The alarm device was placed on 16 high-risk patients during the month-long data collection period, with no falls occurring among these patients during the study. Findings showed that when the alarm sounded, nurses could respond before patients got out of bed. In many instances the sound of the alarm itself appeared to halt a patient's attempt to get out of bed.

Following the pilot study, the alarm was made available to all medical-surgical units and critical care units within the same hospital. The fall rate for the 5-month period following introduction of the alarm decreased by 45% over the same period from the previous year.

Patient Education

Education is one of the most important interventions for both clients and staff. Patients are often naive about how an illness, invasive tests, and/or bed rest can weaken an individual. As described previously, most falls occur in the first week of hospitalization. Tinetti et al (1986) determined that several of the one-time fallers in their geriatric sample fell during an acute illness. This knowledge provides prescribed periods of time when clients are at greater risk to fall and, consequently, when nurses should assist them to a greater degree.

The elderly client's lack of knowledge about falling could be addressed in a one-page brochure on safety. In this material, specific issues could be covered such as the need to wear one's prescription glasses whenever out of bed, and the importance of calling for assistance during periods of high risk. Material should be printed in large type for easier reading and then reinforced verbally with the elderly client.

Staff Education and Accountability

The importance of proper staff education is paramount to prevention. Staff must be convinced that falls among the elderly can be reduced, and a staff member's accountability for the patient must be emphasized. Expectations of performance must include implementation of preventive measures, starting with identification of elderly at risk to fall and concluding with evaluative discussion of successes and failures.

Staff in an 88-bed skilled nursing facility were able to reduce accidents and incidents (not categorized by type of occurrence such as falls) by 36% during a 1-year period (Daley and Goldman, 1987). The changes implemented included an intensive inservice education program on accountability and leadership in prevention of accidents; weekly meetings between nurses' aides and nursing supervisors in which prevention, proper use of protective devices, and responsibility were discussed; a relabeling of "high risk" to include anyone who had had an incident in the prior 6 months; client assignments for nursing aides; immediate investigation of all incidents; and revision of incident forms to include the name of the aide assigned to the patient.

Signage

The use of signs has been advocated as a way to remind alert and compliant elderly of the need to ask for assistance and to remind staff of those who are at risk for falling. The effectiveness of this technique in decreasing falls has not been reported, but by merely increasing awareness about a problem, the undesirable behavior may be decreased. Further study in this area is indicated.

CASE STUDY

Potential for Trauma: Falls

Mr. Cagney, age 75, has been admitted to an acute care hospital for surgical treatment of lung cancer. His wife of 50 years has Alzheimer's dementia and experiences intermittent confusion. She does not accompany him to the hospital. Friends have reassured Mr. Cagney that they will look in on his wife, but he worries that some incident may cause her to become confused while they are apart.

Mr. Cagney has had frequency and nocturia due to benign hypertrophy of the prostate. He has a history of a peripheral vascular disease that has caused him to have little proprioceptive sensation in his legs. He has mild unsteadiness if he does not watch his feet while walking. Mr. Cagney reports that he can usually walk well alone but has difficulty at night when he is unable to see well.

SCORING OF MR. CAGNEY'S RISK FOR FALLING

Mr. Cagney's scores on the RAFS II are shown in Table 3.2. The score of 14 placed Mr. Cagney at high risk for fall and gave him a nursing diagnosis of Potential for Trauma: Falls. The outcome to be achieved is the absence of falls during hospitalization. Because he is alert and oriented, the initial nursing plan is one of education and assistance to the bathroom during the night. Mrs. Scofield,

the nurse assigned to Mr. Cagney, discusses with him the potential to fall while hospitalized. She provides a written discussion of the hazards and verbally reinforces this material with Mr. Cagney. He states that he understands the necessity of using good judgment when ambulating.

Mrs. Scofield notes that Mr. Cagney has benign prostatic hypertrophy, and through discussion with Mr. Cagney about the need to void at night, she discovers that he rises to void two or three times per night, usually around 2:00 A.M. and 5:30 A.M. Mrs. Scofield requests that Mr. Cagney call for assistance at night when ambulating to the bathroom and suggests that during the night rounds, the nursing assistant or registered nurse check Mr. Cagney at 2:00 A.M. and 5:30 A.M.

Preoperatively, Mr. Cagney sustains no falls. Following his thoracotomy on the third hospital day, Mr. Cagney becomes confused at night. Because of the chest tube and increased weakness, he requires two people to assist him in ambulation.

Because of Mr. Cagney's confusion and unsteadiness, his potential for falling is greatly increased. Mrs. Scofield reviews with Mr. Cagney the continued need for safe ambulation. He states that he will continue to call for assistance when he wants to get out of bed.

To safeguard Mr. Cagney at night, Mrs. Scofield applies a warning device that sounds when he attempts to get out of bed. She places him in the room across from the nurses' station for better visibility. Finally, because she knows when he usually arises to void during the night, she again institutes elimination rounds. She modifies the rounds to awaken Mr. Cagney at these hours to take him to the bathroom. He experiences no falls during the night. The overall outcome of "The patient experiences no falls while hospitalized" was achieved.

Table 3.2

Scores on the Risk Assessment for Falls Scale II: Mr. Cagney Case Study

CATEGORY	SCORE	DECISION STRATEGY
Length of stay	3	Completed on the day of admission
Age	3	75
Balance	1	Proprioceptive disturbance creates potential problems at night as a result of night vision problems
Mental status	0	Alert and oriented
Agitation	0	No indication of a problem
Depression	0	Currently no indication of a problem; however, this may change in the future based on surgical outcome or if a problem develops with Mrs. Cagney
Vision	2	Difficulty with night vision
Communication	0	No problems
Medications	0	Currently on no CNS or cardiovascular effectors
Chronic diseases	3	Carcinoma affecting the pulmonary system as well as peripheral vascular disease
Urinary problems	2	Nocturia and frequency

Because of Mr. Cagney's problems with proprioception and night vision, Mrs. Scofield recognized a potential for falls at home. She reinforces the need either to turn on lights when arising at night or to have a night light in the bathroom, bedroom, and hall. Mr. Cagney acknowledges this need and states he will increase the amount of lighting at home.

OUTCOMES

The optimal outcome in the nursing diagnosis Potential for Trauma is no injury, psychologic or physiologic. Thus, as a cause of trauma, falls must be reduced to a minimum. When evaluating a program of prevention, the incident report is the best source of data. When the client is assessed for risk, the risk score should be recorded in the nursing kardex. When a fall occurs, the nurse manager should investigate the incident and determine the variables involved. Was the client at high risk? Had the patient's condition changed so the initial low-risk score was inaccurate? Were prevention measures appropriate for the individual? Had these measures been consistently applied? Does the fall signal a deterioration of the client's condition? Was falling the result of intrinsic or environmental factors? Once questions such as these are answered, appropriate changes and interventions can take place. Specific outcomes are (1) the number of falls decreases; (2) fewer injuries due to falls are sustained; (3) individuals verbalize a reduced fear of falling; and (4) more clients ask for assistance to ambulate.

SUMMARY

Falls occur too frequently among the elderly. With falling comes the Potential for Trauma, which, in the elderly, can be particularly devastating. By using an assessment tool to identify high-risk elderly, planned interventions can be implemented for those who are most vulnerable. Unfortunately, the empirical basis for most interventions is limited. Intervention strategies are determined more commonly by tradition, by intuition, or as a last resort. However, assessment of risk factors, etiologies, and contributing factors can focus on interventions most likely to be beneficial. The need for clinical studies to determine the most appropriate fall prevention interventions based on the elderly's fall risk profile provides a fertile area for nursing research. The interventions presented in this chapter provide direction for clinical research, but a wealth of other strategies abound. The resulting information provided by such studies will decrease the Potential for Trauma in the elderly when the incidence of falls decreases.

ASSESSMENT GUIDE 3.1

Risk Assessment for Falls Scale II(RAFS II)

Total Score_____
High Risk–14 or more

Patient Name _____ Sex _____ Age _____

Admission Date _____ Diagnoses _____

Categories	0	1	2	3	Score
(1) Assessment completed_____ days since admission		≥15 days	8–14 days	Admission to day 7	
(2) Years of age	<19	20–60	61–74	≥75	
(3) History of fall	No fall in last year	Fell in past 6 months	Fell in past 1–5 months	Fell in past 4 weeks	
(4) Balance	Ambulates well alone	Ambulates alone with assistive device	Needs assist & assistive device OR help of 2 persons	Can stand & pivot only with help	
(5) Mental status	Oriented × 3	Oriented × 2 (person/place)	Oriented × 1 (person/self)	Disoriented	
(6) Agitation	No	Mild; uses abrasive language occasionally	Moderate; calls out & uses threatening language	Severe; combative; must be restrained	
(7) Depressed	No	Mild; feels blue, burned out; has poor appetite but no weight loss or sleep disturbances	Moderate; statements of low self-esteem; fatigue; sleep problems & poor appetite	Severe; poor concentration; preoccupied; poor appetite, with weight loss of ≥10 lb; apathy	
(8) Anxious	No	Mild; alert, motivated, restless, sleepless	Moderate; asks for reassurance; focuses on immediate concerns; has rapid speech; may repeat questions	Severe; very preoccupied; focuses on specific details; exhibits psychomotor behavior; c/o feelings of choking or paranoia	
(9) Vision	Normal	Corrected by glasses or monocular vision (blind in 1 eye/lazy eye)	Blurred/cataract/ glaucoma	Visual field cut (hemianopsia, scotoma, tunnel vision)	
(10) Communication	Normal	Hearing loss	Speech disorder: dysphasia/language barrier	Both hearing & speech disorder or language barrier	

(Continues)

ASSESSMENT GUIDE 3.1

Risk Assessment for Falls Scale II(RAFS II) *(Continued)*

Categories	0	1	2	3	Score
(11) Medications (Check category of medicine)	No effectors	CV effector	CNS effector	Both CV and CNS effectors prescribed	
CV MEDs —diuretic —beta blocker —digitalis prep —vasodilator —other (name)	CNS MEDs —tranquilizers —hypnotic/analgesic sedative —psychotropic (eg, Haldol). —Other (name)				
(12) Chronic diseases (Check) —Cardiovascular —CNS —Pulmonary —Cancer. —Other (Name)	None	1	2	3 or more	
(13) Urinary —Nocturia ≥2 per night —Urgency—sudden strong urge —Frequency ≥6 times per day	None	1	2	All 3	

Total:_____

References

Azar J, Lawton AH: Gait and stepping factors in the frequent falls of elderly women. *Gerontology* 1964; 4:83–84, 103.

Baker SP, Harvey AH: Fall injuries in the elderly. *Clin Geriatr Med* 1985; 1:501–512.

Barbieri E: Patient falls are not patient accidents. *J Gerontol Nurs* 1983; 9:165–173.

Berry G, Fisher RH, Lang S: Detrimental incidents, including falls, in an elderly institutional population. *J Am Geriatr Soc* 1981; 29:322–324.

Bhala R, O'Donnell J, Thoppil E: Phobic fear of falling and its clinical management. *Physical Ther* 1982; 62(2):187–190.

Campbell AJ et al: Falls in old age: A study of frequency and related clinical factors. *Age Ageing* 1981; 10(4):264–270.

Carroll-Johnson RM (editor): *Classification of Nursing Diagnoses: Proceedings of the Eighth Conference.* Lippincott, 1989.

Chipman C: What does it mean when a patient falls? Pinpointing the cause. *Geriatrics* (Sept) 1981; 36:83–85.

Colling J, Park D: Home, safe home. *J Gerontol Nurs* 1983; 9:175–192.

Cook PJ, Exton-Smith AN, Brockelhurst JC, Lampert-Barber SM: Fractured femurs, falls and bone disorders. *J R Coll Physicians Lond* 1982; 16(1):45–49.

Daley I, Goldman L: A closer look at institutional accidents. *Geriatr Nurs* (Mar–Apr) 1987; 64–67.

Ellis JR, Nowles EA: *Nursing—Human Needs Approach.* Houghton Mifflin, 1977.

Feist R: A survey of accidental falls in a small home for the aged. *J Gerontol Nurs* (June) 1978; 4:15–17.

Fernie GR et al: The relationship of postural sway in standing to the incident of falls in geriatric subjects. *Age Ageing* 1982; 11(1):11–16.

Foerster J: A study of falls: The elderly nursing home resident. *J NY State Nurses Assoc* (June) 1981; 12:9–17.

Fozard JL et al: Visual perception and communication. In: *Handbook of Psychology of Aging.* Birren JE, Schaie KW (editors). Van Nos Reinhold, 1977.

Gibbs J: Bed area falls: A recent report. *Aust Nurses J* (Nov) 1982; 11:35–37.

Gordon M: Falls in the elderly: More common, more dangerous. *Geriatrics* 1982; 37:117–120.

Gryfe CI, Amies A, Ashley MJ: A longitudinal study of falls in an elderly population: Incidence and morbidity. *Age Ageing* 1977; 6:201-210.

Gyldenvand T: *Falls: The Construction and Validation of the Risk Assessment for Fall Scale II (RAFS II).* (Thesis.) University of Iowa, Iowa City, IA, 1984.

Gyldenvand T, Reinboth J: *Intervention Protocol: Elimination Rounds.* University of Iowa, 1982a.

Gyldenvand T, Reinboth J: *Pilot Study on Patient Falls in a Neurological Unit of a University Hospital.* University of Iowa, 1982b.

Hussian RA: *Geriatric Psychology: A Behavioral Perspective.* Van Nos Reinhold, 1981.

Isaacs B: Are falls a manifestation of brain failure? *Age Ageing* 1978; 7:97-105.

Kalchthaler T, Bascom RA, Quintos V: Frequent falls in the institutionalized elderly. *J Am Geriatr Soc* 1978; 26:424-428.

Kohn RR: Heart and cardiovascular system. In: *Handbook of the Biology of Aging.* Finch CE, Hayflick L (editors). Van Nos Reinhold, 1977.

Kulikowski ES: A study of accidents in a hospital. *Superv Nurs* (July) 1979; 44-58.

Lipsitz LA: The drop attack: A common geriatric symptom. *J Am Geriatr Soc* 1983; 31:617-620.

Louis M: Falls and causes. *J Gerontol Nurs* 1983; 9:143-156.

Lucht U: A prospective study of accident falls and resulting injuries in the home among elderly people. *Acta Sociomed Scand* 1971; 3:105-120.

Lynn FH: Incidents: Need they be accidents? *Am J Nurs* 1980; 80:1098-2001.

MacDonald JB, MacDonald ET: Nocturnal femoral fracture and continuing widespread use of barbiturate hypnotics. *British Med J* (Aug 20) 1977; 483-485.

Margules I et al: Epidemiological study of accidents among residents of homes for aged. *J Gerontol* 1970; 25:342-346.

Metropolitan Life Insurance Co: *Mortality from Leading Types of Accidents.* Metropolitan Life Insurance Co., 1982.

Morris EV, Isaacs B: The prevention of falls in a geriatric hospital. *Age Ageing* 1980; 9:181-185.

Murphy J, Isaacs B: The post-fall syndrome. *Gerontology* 1982; 28:265-270.

Naylor R, Rosen AJ: Falling as a cause of admission to a geriatric unit. *Practitioner* 1970; 205:327-330.

Odetunde Z: Fell walking. *Nurs Mirror* (Feb) 1982; 33-36.

Oliva M: This study of patient falls describes who falls where, when. *Mod Hosp* 1965; 105:91-93.

Overstall PW: Falls in the elderly: Epidemiology, aetiology, and management. In: *Recent Advances in Geriatric Medicine.* Churchill Livingstone, 1978.

Overstall PW et al: Falls in the elderly related to postural imbalance. *British Med J* 1977; 1:261-264.

Pablo RY: Patient accidents in a long-term-care facility. *Canad J Publ Health* 1977; 68:237-247.

Perry BC: Falls among the elderly. *J Fam Pract* 1982; 14:1069-1073.

Prudham D, Evans J: Falls in the elderly: A community study. *Age Ageing* 1981; 10:141-146.

Raffery EB, Cashman PM: Long-term recording of the electro-cardiogram in a normal population. *Postgrad Med J* 1976; 52:32-37.

Reinboth JLV: *A Study to Investigate the Interrater Reliability of an Assessment Tool to Assess Risk for Falling in Elderly Clients.* (Thesis.) University of Iowa, Iowa City, IA, 1985.

Reinboth J, Gyldenvand T: *Pilot Study of Falls in an Extended Care Setting.* University of Iowa, 1982.

Roberts BL: Walking improves balance, reduces falls. *Am J Nurs* 1985; 85:1397.

Rodstein M: Accidents among the aged: Incidents, causes, and prevention. *J Chronic Dis* 1964; 17:515-526.

Rodstein M: Heat disease in the aged. In: *Clinical Geriatrics.* Rossman I (editor). Lippincott, 1979.

Rodstein M: Accidents among the aged. In: *Topics in Aging and Long-Term Care.* Reichel W (editor). Williams & Wilkins, 1981.

Rodstein M, Camus AS: Interrelations of heart disease and accidents. *Geriatrics* 1973; 28:87-91.

Ross JE: *Survey of Patient Falls in a University Hospital.* University of Iowa, 1980.

Sehested P, Severin-Nielsen T: Falls by hospitalized elderly patients: Cause, prevention. *Geriatrics* (Apr) 1977; 32:101-108.

Snipes GE: Accidents in the elderly. *Am Fam Physician* (July) 1982; 26:117-122.

Swartzbeck E: The problems of falls in the elderly. *Nurs Manage* (Dec) 1983; 14:34-38.

Tinetti ME, Williams RF, Mayewski R: Fall risk index for elderly patients based on number of chronic disabilities. *Am J Med* 1986; 80:430-434.

Walshe A, Rosen H: A study of patient falls from bed. *J Nurs Adm* 1979; 9:31-35.

Wells R: Promoting urinary continence in the elderly in the hospital. *Nurs Times* 1975; 71:1908-1909.

Widder B: A new device to decrease falls. *Geriatr Nurs* 1985; 287-288.

Wild D, Novak USL, Isaacs B: Description, classification, and prevention of falls in old people at home. *Rheumatol Rehabil* 1981a; 20(3):153-159.

Wild D, Novak USL, Isaacs B: How dangerous are falls in old people at home? *British Med J* 1981b; 282:266-268.

4

Potential for Poisoning: Drug Toxicity

Elizabeth Weitzel, MA, RN

"All substances are poison; there is none which is not a poison. The right dose differentiates a poison and a remedy."

(Paracelsus, 1493–1541)

Health professionals and clients tend to think of drugs as the solution to certain health problems. However, we sometimes fail to take into account the effect drugs have on the total body. In dealing with the elderly, we must also remember that medication can only cause the cell to respond to the extent it is capable of responding; the aging body has fewer functioning cells than the younger body.

The elderly are admitted to hospitals for drug-induced illnesses at a significantly higher rate than younger persons (Brady, 1978; Carnosos et al, 1974). Thus, potential for drug toxicity is an important area for nursing assessment, diagnosis, and management. Further, aging clients should expect the nurse to advocate in their behalf to prevent drug toxicity.

The effects of aging on pharmacokinetics, the fate of drugs in the body, and pharmacodynamics, the response of the body to a given drug, are important in identifying areas for drug monitoring. Health professionals can use this information to maximize the effectiveness of drugs administered to the elderly. Unfortunately, health professionals sometimes contribute to the problem of toxicity by having unrealistic expectations of what drugs will do for an individual. One problematic expectation is that the right drug or drugs, given in the correct dosages, will improve all the health problems an older person is experiencing.

This expectation is misleading for several reasons. Physiologically, cells can respond only to a certain level of maximum input. Aging diminishes most body cell populations and consequently decreases function. Also, many of the health problems of the aged are chronic and will not be cured even with extensive drug therapy. In some instances, further cell deterioration leads to a narrowed therapeutic range. When the heart has become damaged, the upper limits of therapeutic levels of digoxin become lower, and the level of toxicity is lowered. Giving more digoxin will not make the heart function better but will lead to toxicity.

Another unrealistic belief is that all diagnosed problems of the elderly should be treated with medication. It is often advisable to treat with medications only the one or two primary conditions causing the most problems and not attempt to administer medication for additional pathologies until the primary condition(s) is controlled. This helps to avoid the unfortunate situation of treating drug side effects with more drugs.

The belief that toxicity can be prevented by keeping blood levels within normal therapeutic levels is also misleading. The complete clinical picture, including the functioning of the individual, must be evaluated to determine the appropriate level of medication, regardless of the "normalcy" of the blood levels.

At times, social stress rather than physical illness is at the root of the problem an older person is experiencing. It is logical that the solution to these problems lies in dealing with the social factors rather than administering drugs (Davidson, 1975).

CONCEPT OF POTENTIAL FOR DRUG TOXICITY

Drug toxicity is the condition that exists when the amount of a given drug in a person's body exceeds the amount necessary to bring about therapeutic effect (therapeutic level), or it has become a harmful agent in that person's body, producing adverse effects.

Side effects are responses to the medication other than the intended therapeutic effect. If the side effects become harmful, they are called adverse effects and are part of the toxic response to the medication.

Interactions of drugs are changes in pharmacokinetics in the presence of another drug or certain foods. Drug interactions with other substances can result in subtherapeutic or toxic responses.

Allergic reactions are usually the result of the drug acting as a hapten, a low-molecular-weight substance (which would not usually cause an allergic reaction) combining with endogenous protein to form an antigenic complex, a substance that stimulates antibody formation. When the drug is again introduced into the body, it provokes allergic responses from skin rashes to exfoliative dermatitis, acute uticaria, or severe arteritis. Respiratory symptoms and anaphalactic shock are other allergic responses that can occur. Penicillin is a classic example of a drug that stimulates allergic response. Allergic response may be idiosyncratic in the aging person, in terms of both what stimulates an allergic response and the precise symptoms that are manifested (Klassen, 1980).

CURRENT STATUS OF THE DIAGNOSIS

The diagnosis Potential for Poisoning: Drug Toxicity is not on the accepted NANDA list (Carroll-Johnson, 1989). It is subsumed under the diagnosis Potential for Poisoning (see Table 4.1). However, the importance of the subdiagnosis to nurses who work with the elderly justifies developing it as a distinct diagnosis.

ETIOLOGIES/RELATED FACTORS

The risk factors that increase the probability that the aging person will develop a potential for drug toxicity include the effects of drugs in the aging body, the variables of drug administration, and the effects of polypharmacy (Table 4.1).

Effects of Aging on Pharmacodynamics and Pharmacokinetics

Pharmacodynamics and pharmacokinetics are processes that determine how a given drug responds within the body. Both of these processes are somewhat altered within the aging body because of tissue loss and diminished organ function.

Pharmacodynamics refers to the responses of body receptors to a given drug and the subsequent effects of that drug. The changes in body receptors caused by aging are particularly apparent with the increased effects of warfarin (Coumadin) and diazepam (Valium), even when serum drug concentrations are constant (Gromlin and Chapron, 1983; Lamy, 1980; Reidenberg, 1980). Altered sensitivity of central nervous system (CNS) receptors and beta-adrenergic receptors is postulated but not proven.

Pharmacokinetics refers to the absorption, distribution, metabolism (biotransformation), and excretion of drugs in the body, all of which determine the amount of active components of a drug available to body tissues at a given time. Of the two processes, pharmacokinetics is probably more important in producing the toxic effects of medication in the aging body.

Absorption of Drugs Most oral medications are absorbed by passive diffusion, a process that is minimally altered with aging. Areas in which oral absorption may be altered are (1) slowing in gastric emptying, especially when taking anticholinergics or antidepressants; (2) increased transit time through the bowel, which is influenced by altered dietary patterns and food intake and changes in dentition; and (3) drug–drug or drug–food interactions such as those previously described with tetracycline and calcium-rich foods or medications (Lamy, 1982; Rock, 1985).

Distribution of Drugs For drugs to be effective in the body, they must be delivered to their sites of action. Distribution of drugs taken orally begins in the portal circulation, which takes the drugs to the liver, where enzymes may change the chemistry of the drug or pass it on unchanged. From the liver, the drug enters the systemic circulation, where it may be in a free state or partially bound to blood proteins or tissues.

Table 4.1

Etiologies/Related Factors and Defining Characteristics of Potential for Poisoning: Drug Toxicity

NANDA'S (CARROLL-JOHNSON, 1989) DEFINING CHARACTERISTICS

Definition: Accentuated risk of accidental exposure to or ingestion of drugs or dangerous products in doses sufficient to cause poisoning

Defining Characteristics:

Internal (individual) factors
    Reduced vision
    Verbalization of occupational setting without adequate safeguards
    Lack of safety or drug education
    Lack of proper precautions
    Cognitive or emotional difficulties
    Insufficient finances

External (environmental) factors
    Large supplies of drugs in house
    Medicines stored in unlocked cabinets accessible to children or confused persons
    Dangerous products placed or stored within the reach of children or confused persons
    Availability of illicit drugs potentially contaminated by poisonous additives
    Flaking, peeling paint or plaster in presence of young children
    Chemical contamination of food and water
    Unprotected contact with heavy metals or chemicals
    Paint, lacquer, etc in poorly ventilated areas or without effective protection
    Presence of poisonous vegetation
    Presence of atmospheric pollutants

WEITZEL'S ETIOLOGIES AND DEFINING CHARACTERISTICS FOR DRUG TOXICITY

Definition: The condition that exists when the amount of a given drug in a person's body exceeds the amount necessary to bring about therapeutic effect (therapeutic level), or it has become a harmful agent in that person's body, producing adverse effects

Etiologies/Related Factors

Effects of drugs in the aging body
Variables of drug administration
Effects of polypharmacy

Defining Characteristics (Signs and Symptoms)

See Table 4.2

Muscle atrophy and other tissue decreases, along with a low-protein diet, are contributors to protein loss among the elderly.

When serum proteins decrease, drugs that are usually protein-bound are found free in the serum in increased amounts. This increases the drug's effects on all the tissues with which it comes in contact, making both the therapeutic level and the toxic level occur at lower doses.

Another factor that increases the amount of free drug in the serum of the elderly person is the increased number of drugs taken. This enhances the chance of displacement by a drug that is more highly protein-bound. In older persons, who are normally not as well hydrated as younger individuals, a decreased amount of body water further increases the concentration of drugs in the serum. Both of these factors are particularly problematic with drugs like aspirin, in which the therapeutic and toxic ranges are very close. The addition of a new drug that displaces some of the bound aspirin, or increased dehydration, may be sufficient change to make the person become aspirin toxic.

Distribution is also dependent on regional perfusion. Tissue perfusion and cardiac efficiency are often decreased in the elderly relative to changes in blood vessels. Thus, a number of factors influence the distribution of drugs in the older person, with most of them contributing to the likelihood that drug toxicity will occur.

Metabolism or Biotransformation of Drugs   Metabolism is primarily a function of the liver and depends heavily on enzymes, which decrease with normal aging. Drugs such as cimetidine (Tagamet), chloramphenicol (Chloromycetin), and phenobarbital in high concentrations suppress enzymatic function. Hepatic blood flow decreases with aging, and some drugs are dependent on the amount of blood flowing through the liver for efficient metabolism.

Some metabolism may also occur in the intestinal wall during the process of absorption. Metabolism may inactivate a drug or change it into a form that continues to be active. Decreased liver function may increase the circulating active levels of a drug like propranolol (Inderal), which is dependent on enzymatic action to inactivate it. That same decreased liver function may decrease the active level of tricyclic antidepressants, since they are dependent on enzymatic action to change them into more active form.

Excretion of Drugs   This process occurs primarily in the kidney, with small amounts of drugs being excreted through saliva, sweat, lung exhalation, or lactation. Changes in renal function are more consistent and measurable than changes in hepatic function. The normal kidney loses 30% to 50% of its functioning between the ages of 35 and 70 and at the same time is experiencing a considerable decrease in renal blood flow. This causes decreased clearance of drugs. If the aging person also has hypertension, dehydration, urinary retention, diabetic nephropathy, pyelonephritis, atherosclerosis, or congestive heart failure, renal function is further compromised (Lamy, 1982).

The loss of renal function is important when a drug reaches the kidney in an active state. If the drug is not removed at the expected rate, the serum concentration rises. Each drug has an expected half-life $(1/2t)$, the amount of time it takes for half the dosage given to be metabolized into an inactive form or to be excreted. When this does not happen in the expected amount of time, the half-life increases and, in effect, the dosage of the drug is increased. Digoxin, a commonly used drug among the elderly, reaches the kidney in an active state. Because the aging kidney does not excrete digoxin at the expected rate, it has an extended half-life. As a result, toxicity may occur when renal function is decreased and the dosage given is not also decreased. Certain drugs may further decrease renal clearance. Lithium, commonly used in the treatment of bipolar affective disorders, is a drug that may decrease renal function and thus reduce clearance of other drugs.

Variables in Drug Administration

Only 5% of persons 65 and older in the United States live in institutions. The remaining 95% live in the community, with most assuming responsibility for the medications they use. These medications include those prescribed by the physician or dentist, over-the-counter (OTC) or nonprescription medications, and folk remedies. Older persons are purchasing 25% of all medications prescribed in the United States, even though they constitute only 11% of the population. They also spend three times more money on drugs than the rest of the population. One study found the incidence of drug reactions to be about two and one-half times greater in persons over 60 than in those younger than 60 (Exton-Smith and Windsor, 1971).

Adverse drug reactions requiring medical attention are more likely to occur to elderly persons in the community than to institutionalized elderly, since part of the role of the institution is to monitor for problems and seek early intervention (Lamy, 1982). Several studies have documented drug-associated hospital admission being more prevalent in the elderly (Bergman and Wiholm, 1981; Grymonpre et al, 1988; Ives et al, 1987).

Self-Administration   There is considerable potential for error in self-administration of drugs by an elderly person. Some studies have found omission of doses to be the most common error. Confusion, forgetfulness, or misreading directions may lead to missed doses or to ingestion of more than the prescribed amount. An elderly individual may try to "make up" missed doses by taking several at once, which may promote toxicity. Also, a dose may not be taken because the person wishes to avoid the side effects, feels the medication is too strong, or feels better and thinks the medication is no longer needed. Another very real factor for the elderly is the cost of purchasing the medication.

Omission of doses does not usually lead to toxicity, but it can change the balance among the drugs being taken and may lead to an exacerbation of illness. If the physician is unaware the elderly person is omitting doses, he or she may increase the dosage or prescribe stronger medication, which could result in toxicity.

When the elderly person self-medicates with prescription drugs from a previous visit to the doctor, with someone else's prescription, with OTC medications, or with home remedies, drug interactions and toxicity are more likely.

The elderly institutionalized individual may be at risk when first admitted if this person has been functioning well on the dose prescribed by the physician only because doses have been omitted. When the staff begins to administer the medication as prescribed, the person may become toxic. Also, the stress of relocation may cause the newly admitted person to become toxic on a dose that was previously therapeutic (see Chapter 42). To avoid these problems, some long-term care facilities establish a "baseline" by removing most, if not all, of a client's medication on admission. The client is then carefully monitored to determine what medications are needed (Moss, 1978).

Much has been documented about the rate of medication errors in hospitals and long-term care facilities (Moss, 1977). Although these errors certainly need to be corrected, they rarely cause the client serious problems. Self-administration of medications by capable older persons in long-term care settings or in a hospital setting has not received as much attention. When monitored by the staff, this practice could have several benefits, including increased self-esteem and independence for the older person. In the hospital or long-term care facility, self-medication is good preparation for discharge, and it allows the nurse to assess the accuracy of self-administration of medications. Perhaps the least important reason for implementing this practice is decreasing the amount of staff time required to administer medications.

Whether medications are self-administered by the older person or are administered by a medication aide, LPN, or RN, it is the RN's responsibility to assess whether the client is receiving the medication as ordered, to know what actions are desired, and to document those that are and are not taking place. It is likewise the role of the RN to determine if side effects are occurring and to report these to the prescribing physician. At times, it may be necessary for the RN to advocate for the aging client by pursuing changes in dosage or medications so that the client may function at an optimal level.

Effects of Polypharmacy   By definition, *polypharmacy* is the administration of several drugs to the same client, sometimes using more than one with similar effects. It is not unusual for an elderly person to have seven or more drugs prescribed for continuous maintenance therapy. If the elderly person develops an acute condition, the number of drugs often increases.

This becomes problematic, since pharmacologically, it is difficult to know what chemicals are active within an elderly person who is taking several drugs at the same time. Drugs may interact with other drugs or cause body tissues to respond differently than expected.

DEFINING CHARACTERISTICS

The precise signs and symptoms of drug toxicity are somewhat dependent on the drugs that are being taken (see Table 4.2).

Todd (1985;231) suggests that "in older adults, the first sign of an adverse reaction is often a change in mental function." Confusion that develops after starting a medication or after a physical or psychologic stressor may be an early indicator of drug toxicity. Other CNS symptoms include gait changes, insomnia or drowsiness, visual changes, slurred speech, ototoxicity, seizures, tremors,

irritability, or problems with temperature control. Anticholinergic effects such as dry mouth, constipation, blurred vision, urinary retention, headache, and restlessness are also symptoms within the nervous system (see Table 4.3). Preexisting pathology in the dependent elderly may be exaggerated; for example, the man with benign prostate hypertrophy may already have some urinary retention, which will become problematic when increased by adverse effects of medications.

All body systems can show toxic effects. Cardiovascular signs and symptoms include arrhythmias, tachycardia, palpitations, hypotension, congestive heart failure, hypertension, and bone marrow depression resulting in leukopenia, thrombocytopenia, anemia, or agranulocytosis.

Hepatic changes may result in jaundice, clotting problem, and other symptoms of decreased liver function. Gastrointestinal (GI) signs and symptoms include anorexia, nausea, vomiting, diarrhea, GI bleeding, or pancreatitis.

Renal dysfunction from toxicity may result in electrolyte imbalances, polyuria, urinary retention, or fluid retention. Dyspnea and asthmatic reactions are respiratory signs and symptoms. Skin responses to toxicity include rashes, urticaria, pruritus, and photosensitivity.

The profile of the person most likely to develop drug toxicity is as follows: over 75 years old; small stature; female; history of an allergic illness or adverse reaction; multiple chronic illnesses; kidney or liver dysfunction; taking more than five medications; changes in overall condition including mental status; taking "high-risk" drugs.

Because of the diversity of these defining characteristics, it is important that the nurse suspect drugs as the cause of developing confusion until another cause can be found; be aware of common toxic symptoms of drugs being used by clients; and always regard drugs as potential poison.

ASSESSMENT

General Drug History

Mullen and Grandholm (1981) have developed a tool for gathering a comprehensive drug history, which could be used to identify potential for toxicity. This tool is divided into information on nonprescription and prescription drugs as well as general information related to medications and the client's health problems. The usual fluid and protein intake are also assessed to help determine levels of hydration and protein intake.

In the revised version of the tool, the use of alcoholic beverages is singled out and explored more completely than in the original, since alcohol interacts with many drugs. It is particularly problematic when taking benzodiazepines (Valium, Dalmane) or theophylline. Chronic

Table 4.2

Etiologies/Related Factors and Toxic Defining Characteristics of Specific Drugs Commonly Prescribed in the Elderly

DRUGS	SIGNS AND SYMPTOMS
BENZODIAZEPINES Diazepam (Valium) Flurazepam (Dalmane) Lorazepam (Atavan)	Ataxia, restlessness, agitation, confusion, depression, anticholinergic effect
CIMETIDINE (Tagamet)	Confusion, depression
DIGITALIS	Confusion, headache, anorexia, nausea, vomiting, arrhythmias, blurred vision, other visual changes (halos, frost on objects, color blindness), paresthesia
FUROSEMIDE (Lasix)	Electrolyte imbalance, hepatic changes, pancreatitis, leukopenia, thrombocytopenia
GENTAMYCIN (Garamycin)	Ototoxicity (impaired hearing and/or balance), nephrotoxicity
L-DOPA*	Muscle and eye twitching, disorientation, asterixis, hallucinations, dyskinetic movements, grimacing, depression, delirium, ataxia
LITHIUM (Eskalith, Lithane)	Confusion, diarrhea, drowsiness, anorexia, slurred speech, tremors, blurred vision, unsteadiness, polyuria, seizures, muscle weakness
METHYLDOPA (Aldomet)	Hepatic changes, mental depression, fever, bradycardia, nightmares, tremors, edema
NONSTEROIDAL ANTI-INFLAMMATORY AGENCY (NSAIA) Ibuprofen (Advil, Motrin, Nuprin, Rufin) Indomethacin (Indocin) Fenoprofen (Nalfon) Phenybutazone (Butazolodin)† Piroxican (Feldene) Sulindac (Clinoril) Tolinetin (Tolectin)	Photosensitivity, fluid retention, anemia, nephrotoxicity, visual changes Confusion, plus above
PHENOTHIAZIDE TRANQUILIZERS	Tachycardia, arrhythmias, dyspnea, hyperthermia, postural hypotension, anticholinergic effects, restlessness
PHENYTOIN (Dilantin)	Ataxia, slurred speech, confusion, nystagmus, diplopia, nausea, and vomiting
PROCAINAMIDE (Pronestyl, Procan, etc)	Arrhythmias, depression, hypotension, SLE syndrome, dyspnea, skin rash, nausea, and vomiting
RANITIDINE (Zantac)	Liver dysfunction, blood dyscrasias
SULFONYLUREAS—1st generation Chropropamide (Diabinese) Tolbutamide (Orinase)	Hypoglycemia, hepatic changes, CHF Bone marrow depression, jaundice
THEOPHYLLINE (Bronkotabs, Elixophyllin, Quinibron)	Anorexia, nausea, vomiting, GI bleeding, tachycardia, arrhythmias, irritability, insomnia, muscle twitching, seizures
TRICYCLIC ANTIDEPRESSANTS Amitriptyline (Elavil, Endep, Amitril) Doxepin (Sinequan, Adapin) Imipramine (Tofranil)	Confusion, arrhythmias, seizures, agitation, tachycardia, hallucinations, jaundice Anticholinergic effects, postural hypotension

*Dosage must be reduced cautiously
†Should be given 1 week or less for persons over 60 because of frequent toxic effect, especially aplastic anemia

Sources: Ford R (editor): *Mediquik Cards.* Springhouse Corp., 1986. Barnhart E: *Physicians' Desk Reference.* Medical Economics, 1986. Salzman C: Basic principles of psychotropic drug prescription for the elderly. *Hosp Comm Psychiatry* 1982; 33:133-136. Todd B: Identifying drug toxicity. *Geriatr Nurs* 1985; 4:231-234.

Table 4.3

General Defining Characteristics of Drug Toxicity

Cardiovascular

Arrhythmias
Tachycardia
Palpitations
Hypotension
Congestive heart failure
Hypertension
Bone marrow depression (leukopenia, thrombocytopenia,
    anemia, and agranulocytosis)

Central Nervous System

Confusion
Gait changes
Insomnia
Drowsiness
Blurred vision or other visual changes
Slurred speech
Ototoxicity
Seizures
Tremors
Irritability
Problems with temperature control
Anticholinergic effects

Hepatic Changes

Jaundice
Clotting problems
Decreased liver function

Gastrointestinal

Anorexia
Nausea and vomiting
Diarrhea
GI bleeding
Pancreatitis

Renal

Electrolyte imbalances
Polyuria
Urinary retention
Fluid retention

Respiratory

Dyspnea
Asthmatic reactions

Skin

Rashes
Urticaria
Pruritus
Photosensitivity

alcohol usage can change the action of many drugs that are metabolized in the liver.

With this addition, use of this tool should help identify what drugs the client is taking, what is known about them, future learning needs, and the potential for or current symptoms consistent with toxicity.

A Tool to Monitor for Digitalis Toxicity

Weitzel (1976) developed an instrument (Assessment Guide 4.1) as a data collection tool for a pilot study conducted several years ago to "explore the effectiveness of nursing observations and subjective changes reported by the older client as a means of monitoring digitalis levels for the onset of toxic symptoms." It was designed to be used as a follow-up to monthly nurse-administered cardiovascular clinics at the Iowa Veterans Home, a state-operated rehabilitation and long-term care agency serving about 700 residents. Following the pilot study, the tool was adopted for use in these clinics. The data collected by the tool were instrumental in identifying persons at risk for digitalis toxicity and monitoring monthly changes in that person. Its use, on several occasions, has led to diagnosis of early digitalis toxicity and subsequent revision of medical orders.

This instrument also illustrates how nurses can develop tools for assessing signs and symptoms based on information in the literature for drugs that often cause toxicity in the elderly client. It gathers the data on one sheet so signs and symptoms can be clustered, giving focus and direction to the monitoring activity.

CASE STUDY

Potential for Poisoning: Drug Toxicity

Mrs. Alberts is a 75-year-old woman living in a nursing home. She had a seizure episode after a cerebrovascular accident a year ago and was started on phenytoin (Dilantin) 100 mg t.i.d. She has recently been nauseated, has high abdominal pain, and has eaten poorly for 2 weeks. Following tests yesterday, her physician diagnosed a peptic ulcer. He prescribed cimetidine (Tagamet) 300 mg with meals and at bedtime, and diazepam (Valium) 2 mg q.i.d. for 1 week to decrease Mrs. Alberts's anxiety. The nurse notes, in reading a pocket drug reference, that phenytoin toxicity increases with decreased serum protein and also with the administration of either cimetidine or diazepam. The nurse also notes that Mrs. Alberts's protein intake has been minimal for several weeks, and her fluid intake has been poor for the past week. The nurse infers that Mrs. Alberts may have a lowered serum protein level and may be dehydrated.

Dehydration would further concentrate the phenytoin levels in Mrs. Alberts's blood.

The nurse makes the diagnosis of potential for phenytoin toxicity related to concurrent administration of Tagamet and Valium as well as probable dehydration and lowered serum protein. After reading about the manifestations for phenytoin toxicity, the nurse notes that common signs and symptoms of phenytoin toxicity include CNS effects of ataxia, slurred speech, confusion, nystagmus, and diplopia, and GI effects of nausea and vomiting (Ford, 1986). The goal is to prevent phenytoin toxicity. Interventions would include monitoring Mrs. Alberts for the common signs of toxicity and increasing fluid and protein intake to decrease the likelihood of development of toxicity.

CASE STUDY

Poisoning: Drug Toxicity

Mr. Bean is an active 80-year-old living with his wife in his own home. He developed complete urinary retention and general malaise. His family physician diagnosed a urinary infection and a heart arrhythmia and prescribed Bactrim and Procan. At his 2-week follow-up visit, his urine was free of infection, and his arrhythmia was converted to normal sinus rhythm. He was sent home and instructed to take half a Bactrim tablet each day and to continue the Procan. He was scheduled to return in 3 weeks to set a date for surgery for his benign prostatic hypertrophy. In a few days, he awoke with joint pain, chills, and fever. He and his wife had been told "flu symptoms" were reason to contact the doctor immediately. Mrs. Bean called the doctor's office and talked with the RN, who recognized the symptoms as consistent with Procan toxicity. She advised that Mr. Bean take no more Procan and said she would have the doctor call as soon as he was available. The doctor subsequently called, directing Mrs. Bean to discontinue the Procan but to continue the half tablet of Bactrim each day until Mr. Bean's return visit. On discontinuing the Procan, Mr. Bean's symptoms gradually disappeared.

The exact etiologies for Mr. Bean developing a toxicity to Procan are not readily evident, but the onset of symptoms while taking the medication was reason to discontinue the medication and to monitor him for future arrhythmia. This case study also demonstrates that the nurse's role in actual drug toxicity is primarily dependent on the physician, but the nurse can teach the patient and family about possible adverse effects for which to monitor and whom to call if they develop.

NURSING INTERVENTIONS

Using an Interdisciplinary Approach

The very nature of drug administration makes prevention of toxicity an interdisciplinary function. The physician prescribes the drug for a specific function. The pharmacist dispenses the drug and applies knowledge of clinical pharmacy to the directions provided. The RN takes responsibility for the administration of the medication, whether giving it personally, supervising other health personnel in giving it, or teaching the client and/or significant other how to give the medication. The nurse is often the first to help the client identify adverse effects as they develop, especially in a long-term care facility. At times the dietitian may also be involved, for example, if there are food interactions or the necessity for dietary adjustments.

Elderly clients are best protected from toxic reactions when health professionals work with them to teach, monitor, and promote those actions necessary to keep the drug from becoming toxic, or to treat the toxicity promptly should it occur.

Clarifying Goals of Medication Administration

Davidson (1975;633) stated: "In geriatric medicine the aim of treatment is usually the amelioration of disease to the extent that the elderly person can return, in reasonable comfort, to his normal way of life . . . or to a comfortable, dignified death." This statement implies that health professionals need to keep the response of the older person as the prime measure of effective treatment. This chapter has discussed how the aging person's body may respond differently than a younger person's and how psychosocial factors can affect the older person. All health care should be designed for the individual being served. With the elderly, this individualization becomes even more important.

Gerontologists agree on some basic tenets for prescribing medication for the aged (Davidson, 1975; Exton-Smith and Windsor, 1971; Rock, 1985; Tandberg, 1981). These are included in Table 4.4.

Monitoring

Monitoring is usually the most effective intervention to prevent or minimize the effects of drug toxicity. Monitoring the client for therapeutic versus toxic response has been indentified previously as an interdisciplinary function. The nurse's role is one of knowing what defining characteristics indicate toxicity, advocating for any appropriate laboratory tests, and presenting any evidence of toxic reaction to the physician for definitive

Table 4.4

Basic Tenets of Prescribing for the Aged

Diagnose the source of the symptoms as clearly as possible
Prescribe for the diagnosis that is primary at that time, not the symptoms
Prescribe the shortest half-life possible and the drug least likely to cause adverse effects
Keep the regimen simple—3 or 4 drugs if client is living at home
Keep instructions simple, clear, and written so the older person can read them
Consider stopping previously prescribed drug if a new drug is needed
Review the entire drug regimen on a regular basis
Provide support for correct administration of medication for clients taking their own
    medications (eg, a person coming into the home to monitor or assist with setting up
    the medications; use of memory devices, such as divided pill containers, egg cartons,
    etc; and use of alarm clocks to help with timing)
Provide an accurate, effective, and efficient system of administration when someone other
    than the client is responsible for giving the medication
Monitor blood levels when appropriate; compare with client's level of functioning
Treat mental illness without prejudice to age
Keep in mind that drugs can cause health problems as well as cure or ameliorate them

---

treatment. If a toxic response is suspected and the physician is not readily available, the nurse is justified in withholding a dose of the suspected drug until the physician can be apprised of the client's reaction and any pertinent laboratory results.

Rock (1985) of Johns Hopkins Hospital has identified the following drugs as those most commonly monitored by laboratory tests in the elderly: digoxin (Lanoxin); gentamycin (Garamycin); propranolol (Inderal, Inderide); phenobarbital; diazepam (Valium); amitriptyline (Elavil, Edep, Etrafon, Limbatrol, Triavil); warfarin (Coumadin, Panwarfarin); theophylline; lidocaine; quinidine; and tolbutamide (Orinase). Sometimes the monitoring will disclose subtherapeutic effects or, as mentioned earlier, sometimes lab tests report blood levels in the "therapeutic range" but the individual has developed toxicity. Therefore, monitoring must be more than simply the results of a given blood sample; it must include the clinical picture the person presents, including level of functioning. The cost of the lab test compared to the usefulness of the results should also be considered.

When blood levels are monitored, it is important to know if "peak" or "trough" effect is being measured. Medical technologists or physicians are usually responsible for determining the timing, but they rely on the nurse to verify the time at which the prescribed dose has been given to the client. Accurate timing of drawing the sample is important. It is also important that the drug has been taken as prescribed for 24 to 72 hours prior to the test.

Practicing Client Advocacy

The role of client advocate involves the nurse and the physician in gathering and processing information about the older client's overall level of functioning. Even though the nurse does not prescribe medication, nursing input often helps identify a health problem, expected outcomes of treatment, and changes in function. The nurse may also influence the plan of treatment the physician will prescribe by clarifying treatment goals and coordinating with the physician, pharmacist, medical technologist, dietitian, social worker, or other clinicians to keep focused on the goals of the client and family members.

If a client becomes toxic, the physician may decrease the drug dosage or stop the drug entirely, depending on the severity of the toxic reaction. After the drug has been withheld for at least the length of the half-life, it may be started again at a lower dosage. In some instances, other medications will be given to reverse life-threatening toxic responses, such as anti-arrhythmia drugs for the person with digitalis toxicity who is experiencing severe arrhythmias.

Scheduling Drug Holidays

A *drug holiday* is a planned omission of specific medications from the regimen of selected clients for one or more days each week (Keenan et al, 1983). Benefits of drug holidays identified by one 99-bed Skilled Nursing Facility (SNF) (Keenan et al, 1983;103) include increased alertness of residents; reduced medication use and consequently a reduction in medication costs; fewer restrictions in scheduling resident activities on the drug holiday; and better use of professional nursing time and effort. The facility reduced consumption of medications by 9% and saved residents $4600 annually over a 2-year period by implementing drug holidays one day a week.

However, the use of drug holidays is a controversial intervention. Many early attempts were not successful because the plan was not individualized for each resident based on known responses to drugs for that person, serum drug levels, and so on. Some plans put more emphasis on decreasing the time staff spent administering medications rather than on the individual needs of the resident. Others scheduled the drug holiday for Saturday and/or Sunday, days when there are traditionally fewer staff members to monitor for and intervene with untoward effects of withholding medications.

Elderly clients often indicate some initial concerns over the withholding of medications, but most seem to accept drug holidays after adjusting to the change. Many residents have appeared more alert, and for some, the omission of specific drugs one day a week has helped them to feel less dependent on the medications.

Professional nursing time can be structured to plan for the individual client, both in the process of establishing the drug holiday and by using time not spent in actual administration of medications. If ancillary staff are administering medication, time that had been spent dispensing medications can be used in planning other client-centered activities (Keenan et al, 1983).

Some physicians have questioned whether 24 hours is sufficient time to significantly decrease long-term drug accumulation in a patient's body store. Some facilities have successfully implemented two drug holidays per week. This is still a short amount of time to effect a significant decrease in drugs that are stored in the body's fat supply; it may take weeks to deplete these body stores. It could be argued that individual clients might benefit physically from a simple reduction of the daily dose of drugs administered, although this does not take into consideration either the psychosocial effects on a patient or staff time benefits. Perhaps both a decrease in the number of drugs given and the implementation of drug holidays would be advisable in some situations. The use of drug holidays is one intervention that can help prevent drug toxicity. Drug holidays are most effective if carefully planned for the individual client and appropriately administered to use the "free" time that occurs to benefit both the client and the staff.

CASE STUDY

Interventions to Prevent Drug Toxicity

Mrs. Carr is 72 years old. She has diabetes, has had triple coronary bypass surgery, and is diagnosed as having a hiatal hernia and diverticulitis. She is also hearing impaired and wears a hearing aid in her left ear. Mrs Carr lives in her own home and administers her own medications.

Mrs. Carr recently sought nursing advice in establishing a schedule for taking her medications following hospitalization. She had exhibited signs of early digitalis toxicity—increased nausea; a dull, persistent headache; and circumoral tingling—and was hospitalized when her physician made the diagnosis. She was discharged from the hospital on Xanax 0.5 mg t.i.d., Humulin 10U q. am, Procardia 10 mg b.i.d., Lasix 40 mg b.i.d., Isordil 10 mg q.i.d., Tagamet 300 mg ac and hs, Tonocard 40 mg q.i.d., Lanoxin 0.125 mg q. am, Mylanta II 1 oz pc and hs, Surfac i b.i.d., Valium 5 mg t.i.d., and Rufin 400 mg ii with meals.

Defining characteristics identified by the nurse were (1) client confusion about what medications should be taken and when; (2) a medication schedule on the discharge sheet that had the client taking medication almost hourly from 6 a.m. to 10 p.m.; (3) omission of a potassium supplement, which the client had been taking in the hospital, and a low potassium level; and (4) client lack of knowledge about what symptoms to report to the physician.

In a consultation with the nurse, the physician confirmed that she wanted Mrs. Carr to take the medications as noted on the discharge summary. The physician also added a potassium supplement. Mrs. Carr's administration schedule was consolidated from 14 to 9 times daily.

The nurse developed a chart (see Assessment Guide 4.2) for Mrs. Carr to follow, directing which medications to take at what time, until her return appointment with the physician. Mrs. Carr's condition had continued to deteriorate. The physician discontinued both the Tonocard and Xanax, and Mrs. Carr's condition began to improve slowly. Gradually some of her other medications were discontinued and dosages reduced on others. The nurse continued to advocate for Mrs. Carr.

This case study demonstrates monitoring, advocacy, attempts to clarify goals of therapy, and devices to assist the elderly in taking medications (the chart). It also demonstrates that patient advocacy can be an ongoing process.

SUMMARY

Potential for Poisoning: Drug Toxicity is a diagnosis that nurses should keep in mind as they deal with aging clients. The defining characteristics are not always easily recognized. The nurse must be alert to any change in function as possibly being related to medications the older person is taking and report these changes to the physician. The nurse may need to become the client's advocate and present information to the physician in such a way that the medications are reviewed systematically, dosages adjusted, or the medication discontinued. Decisions about medications should be based on knowledge of changes generally experienced by the elderly. Maintaining an optimal level of function for the dependent elder in question by administering the smallest number of medications at the lowest dosage possible is the goal. In some situations, drug holidays may be a way for institutions to decrease serum blood levels in selected residents and also to give more flexibility to residents and staff. By effectively monitoring the older client, the actuality of drug toxicity should be minimized, allowing the client to live a more healthy life.

ASSESSMENT GUIDE 4.1

Assessment Tool: Potential for Digitalis Toxicity

Name _____   Date _____

Date started on digoxin _____   Dosage _____

Baseline: Creatinine _____ K _____ Apical Rate _____ Rhythm _____

Current: Creatinine _____ K _____ Apical Rate _____ Rhythm _____

Name of clinician _____

Evidence of: Resident Report   Staff Observation

excessive fatigue _____

headache that persists _____

drowsiness _____

confusion _____

dizziness _____

numbness or tingling _____

blurred vision _____

changes of color perception _____

halo vision _____

seeing frost on objects _____

anorexia _____

nausea _____

vomiting _____

diarrhea _____

abdominal pain _____

Remarks:

ASSESSMENT GUIDE 4.2

Chart for Administering Drugs: Mrs. Carr Case Study

Month _____

Time/Drug	1	2	3	4	5	6	7	8	9	10	11	12	→	31
7 A.M. Xanax Procardia Lasix Tonocard														
8 A.M. Humulin Isordil Tagamet Valium Rufin														
9 A.M. Lanoxin Mylanta II Surfax Potassium														
11:30 A.M. Isordil Tagamet														
12:30 P.M. after lunch Tonocard Valium Rufin Mylanta II Potassium														
2:30 P.M. Xanax Procardia														
5 P.M. Lasix Isordil Tagamet														
6 P.M. Tonocard Mylanta II Surfax														
10:30 P.M. with a snack Xanax Procardia Isordil Tagamet Tonocard Mylanta II Potassium														

References

Barnhart E: *Physicians' Desk Reference.* Medical Economics, 1986.

Bergman V, Wiholm BE: Drug-related problems causing admission to medical clinic. *Eur J Clin Pharmacol* 1981; 20:193.

Brady ES: Drugs and the elderly. In: *Drugs and the Elderly* (revised). Hayne R (editor). University of Southern California Press, 1978.

Carnosos GJ, Stewart RB, Cluff LE: Drug induced illness leading to hospitalization. *JAMA* 1974; 228:713-717.

Carroll-Johnson RM (editor): *Classification of Nursing Diagnoses: Proceedings of the Eighth Conference.* Lippincott, 1989.

Davidson W: The hazards of drug treatment in old age. In: *Textbook of Geriatric Medicine and Gerontology.* Brockelhurst J (editor). Churchill Livingstone, 1975.

Exton-Smith AN, Windsor ACM: Principles of drug treatment in the aged. In: *Clinical Geriatrics.* Rossman I (editor). Lippincott, 1971.

Ford R (editor): *Mediquik Cards.* Springhouse Corp., 1986.

Gromlin IH, Chapron DJ: Rational drug therapy for the aged. *Comp Ther* 1983; 9:17.

Grymonpre R et al: Drug-associated hospital admissions in older medical patients. *J Am Geriatr Soc* 1988; 36:1092-1098.

Ives TJ, Bentz EJ, Gwythr RE: Drug-related admissions to a family medicine in-patient service. *Arch Intern Med* 1987; 147:1117.

Keenan R et al: The benefits of a drug holiday. *Geriatr Nurs* 1983; 2:103-104.

Klassen CD: Principles of toxicology. In: *The Pharmacological Basis of Therapeutics,* 6th ed. Goodman L, Gilman A (editors). Macmillan, 1980.

Lamy PP: *Prescribing for the Elderly.* PSG Pub. Co., 1980.

Lamy PP: Comparative pharmokinetic changes and drug therapy in an older population. *J Am Geriatr Soc* 1982; 30(Suppl):11-19.

Moss BB: Effective drug administration as viewed by a physician administrator. In: *Drugs and the Elderly* (revised). Kayne R (editor). University of Southern California Press, 1978.

Moss FF: *Too Old, Too Sick, Too Bad: Nursing Homes in America.* Aspen, 1977.

Mullen EM, Grandholm M: Drugs and the elderly patient. *J Gerontol Nurs* 1981; 7:108-113.

Reidenberg MM: Drugs in the elderly. *Bull N Y Med Soc* 1980; 56:703.

Rock RC: Monitoring therapeutic drug levels in older patients. *Geriatrics* 1985; 40:75-86.

Tandberg D: How to treat and prevent drug toxicity. *Geriatrics* 1981; 36:64-73.

Todd B: Identifying drug toxicity. *Geriatr Nurs* 1985; 4:231-234.

Weitzel EA: Client report and nursing observations as early indications of digitalis intoxication. Unpublished study, 1976.

5

Potential for Infection

Marita Titler, MA, RN
Janie Knipper, MA, RN

Potential for infection is defined by the North American Nursing Diagnosis Association (NANDA) as "the state in which an individual is at an increased risk for being invaded by pathogenic organisms" (Carroll-Johnson, 1989;518). However, pathogenic organisms can invade a host without an actual infection occurring. Therefore, Potential for Infection is more clearly defined as *increased* risk of being invaded by pathogenic organisms, resulting in an infectious process that causes change in tissue structure and/or function.

Approximately 5% of the elderly in the United States reside in nursing homes. Currently, 25% of those over age 65 spend at least 3 weeks in a nursing home, and it is estimated that about 50% of the people now 65 years of age and over will enter a nursing home sometime during their life (Palumbo et al, 1987). Infections contribute to institutionalization of the elderly, and the risk of infection is greater for elderly persons who live in institutions.

SIGNIFICANCE FOR THE ELDERLY

Between 5% and 20% of the patients in extended care facilities have infections, many of which are preventable (Garibaldi et al, 1981; Setia et al, 1985). Infections are among the most common reasons for admission of nursing home residents to acute care facilities and contribute significantly to increased mortality of elderly clients in long-term care institutions (Irvine et al, 1984). During a 12-month surveillance of institutionalized elderly men, infections were the primary cause of 7 of 19 deaths and a contributing cause in two more deaths (Nicolle et al, 1984). Residents with two or more infections were at a greater risk of dying during the year than residents with no infections or with a single infectious episode.

The most frequent types of infections in long-term care facilities are urinary tract (Cohen et al, 1979), respiratory tract (Franson et al, 1986), and skin or soft tissue infections such as infected decubitus ulcers (Farber et al, 1984; Franson et al, 1986; Jackson and Fierer, 1985; Magnussen and Robb, 1980; Nicolle et al, 1984). Conjunctivitis and gastroenteritis occur less frequently (Garibaldi et al, 1981; Nicolle et al, 1984). However, lack of standardized protocols for infection surveillance in long-term care, variances in methods used to calculate infection rates, and variability in study designs make it difficult to generalize research results to all institutions.

According to the Center for Disease Control (CDC), persons over the age of 49 represent 10% of all acquired immune deficiency syndrome (AIDS) cases, or approximately 5,715 persons (American Society on Aging, 1988). Despite the fact that there is no unified data base for the elderly, it is believed that more than 1% of persons with AIDS in public hospitals are over the age of 65. We don't know, however, whether the AIDS virus presents in the elderly as it does in younger persons, or whether there are unique patterns of presentation of the disease and opportunistic illness. More research is also needed to define the natural history of this devastating disease in the elderly, including survival patterns and life expectancy.

ETIOLOGIES/RELATED FACTORS

The ability of the host to defend against infection is a major determinant of whether the patient becomes infected or colonized with the organism. A variety of treatment regimens, underlying pathologic conditions, and functional limitations experienced by the elderly enhance their susceptibility to infection (see Table 5.1).

Environmental conditions can enhance transmission or serve as a reservoir for the growth of infecting agents. Respiratory therapy equipment, room humidifiers, sinks, flowers, and other equipment all have been documented as sites of organism growth and/or transmission. Exoge-

Table 5.1

Risk Factors/Etiologies: Potential for Infection

Definition: The state in which an individual is at increased risk for being invaded by pathogenic organisms

Risk Factors

Inadequate primary defenses (broken skin, traumatized tissue, decreased ciliary action, stasis of body fluids, change in pH of secretions, altered peristalsis)
Inadequate secondary defenses (decreased hemoglobin, leukopenia, suppressed inflammatory response, and immunosuppression)
Inadequate acquired immunity
Tissue destruction and increased environmental exposure
Chronic disease
Prolonged physical immobility
Inadequate self-care abilities for hygiene
Invasive procedures
Malnutrition
Pharmaceutical agents and trauma
Insufficient knowledge to avoid exposure to pathogens

Source: Revised from Carroll-Johnson RM (editor): *Classification of Nursing Diagnoses: Proceedings of the Eighth Conference.* Lippincott, 1989.

nous infections are spread from patient to patient, personnel to patient, or equipment to patient, with the hands being a final common pathway (Smith, 1984).

Thus, institutions that care for the elderly can be the source of a variety of infecting agents. For example, gram-negative bacteria and fungi have steadily increased in importance as causes of nosocomial infections over the last several years (Smith, 1984). Antibiotic-resistant bacterial infections are also a danger for the institutionalized elderly. Patients are reservoirs for endogenous infective organisms, whereas environments, including health care personnel, serve as transmitters and reservoirs of exogenous organisms.

PREDISPOSITION OF THE ELDERLY TO INFECTION

The increased susceptibility of the elderly to infection is probably multifactorial (Felser and Raff, 1983). Risk factors fall into two general categories: (1) host factors that alter normal defense mechanisms; and (2) environmental factors that increase exposure or susceptibility.

Host Factors

Age-related changes, chronic diseases, and treatment and diagnostic interventions for those diseases put the dependent elderly at risk for infection (Brockelhurst, 1985; Rossman, 1986).

Presence of Underlying Disease Processes Disease is not a normal part of aging. However, the elderly have an increased incidence of various diseases that interact with changes in the immune system and other defense mechanisms to predispose them to infection. Changes in local defense mechanisms represent alterations in first-line defenses.

Dahlsten and Shank (1979) found that 85% of the patients in rural nursing homes had two or more chronic illnesses, with the overall ratio being 4.2 chronic disorders per patient. Disorders of the circulatory system were most prevalent, followed by disorders of the nervous system and sense organs. Acute infection was found in 26% of the patients, with the most prevalent acute disorder being urinary track infection (15%). Other investigators have reported an average of 2.4 to 3.3 medical diagnoses per patient residing in long-term care facilities (Cohen et al, 1979; Garibaldi et al, 1981; Nicolle et al, 1984; Setia et al, 1985). Common chronic disease processes in the institutionalized elderly are organic brain syndrome, arteriosclerotic vascular disease, organic heart disease, cerebrovascular accident, and other central nervous system disorders (Cohen et al, 1979; Farber et al, 1984; Garibaldi et al,

1981; Nicolle et al, 1984; Setia et al, 1985). Setia et al (1985) noted a statistically significant difference in the average number of medical diagnoses per patient in the infected group (2.8) as compared to the noninfected group (1.8).

Seventy-five percent of people over age 75 have some cardiac abnormality, many of which predispose them to infections of the lower respiratory tract. The presence of calcium on the mitral and aortic valves alters normal blood flow through the heart and predisposes the elderly to bacterial endocarditis (Potter, 1984). Atherosclerosis predisposes the elderly to infection because of impairment in local blood flow. Nicolle et al (1984) found that residents with ischemic heart disease who were receiving diuretic therapy were more likely to experience infection than residents who did not have these two variables present. The presence of underlying lung pathology such as chronic obstructive lung disease also increases the chance of acquiring a respiratory infection (Pennington, 1984).

Elderly people have reduced renal reserves, and some are chronically uremic. Uremia depresses the number of circulating lymphocytes and interferes with the phagocytic function of polymorphonuclear leukocytes (Fox, 1985a; Gardner, 1980; Moore-Smith, 1986). Uremia is also associated with respiratory tract infection and infectious arthritis (Gardner, 1980).

Between 6% and 20% of persons over age 65 suffer from diabetes (Potter, 1984). The elderly person with diabetes has an increased incidence of infection, particularly *Candida vulvovaginitis*, gingivitis, urinary tract infection, septic shock and gas-forming infection, endocarditis, and infectious arthritis (Gardner, 1980; Moore-Smith, 1986). In part, alterations in the cell-mediated immunity and disturbed polymorphonuclear activity associated mainly with insulin-dependent diabetes promote increased incidence of infection in this population. Ketoacidosis impairs defense mechanisms, particularly the phagocytic function of polymorphonuclear leukocytes (Moore-Smith, 1986; Phair and Reisberg, 1984). In addition, high glucose levels promote bacterial growth. The accelerated atherosclerotic process associated with diabetes impairs blood flow and alters secondary defense mechanisms. There is an increased incidence of skin and soft tissue infections in the institutionalized elderly with diabetes (Garibaldi et al, 1981; Nicolle et al, 1984; Setia et al, 1985).

Alcoholism alone or in conjunction with serious hepatic disease impairs the function of polymorphonuclear leukocytes (Phair and Reisberg, 1984). This may account partially for the increased incidence of pneumonias in the alcoholic patient.

Sixty percent of all malignancies develop after 60 years of age (Potter, 1984). Lymphomas lead to altered cell-mediated immunity. Multiple myeloma produces defective B cells with decreased immunoglobulin production (Moore-Smith, 1986). Solid tumors often alter cell-mediated immunity, but the process does not seem to be a significant risk factor for infection (Moore-Smith, 1986). Obstruction of a hollow organ or erosion of the gastrointestinal tract with a solid tumor is associated with bacteremia (Phair and Reisberg, 1984).

Acute nonlymphocytic leukemia can alter both cell-mediated and humoral immunity (Moore-Smith, 1986). Neutropenia also represents a serious risk factor for infection. The frequency and mortality of bacteremia is increased in people with polymorphonuclear leukocyte counts below 1000/mm^3 (Phair and Reisberg, 1984).

A preexisting infection can damage tissues and organs through such mechanisms as autoimmune reactions, deposition of immune complexes, and inflammation without the ability for repair. These changes can predispose the individual to secondary bacterial and viral infections. Aged individuals with particular types of infections have an increased likelihood of getting another infection. For example, the elderly person with an infection of the respiratory tract has a significantly increased likelihood of getting meningitis and endocarditis. Urinary tract infections predispose elderly persons to endocarditis. Pneumonia, bacterial endocarditis, urinary tract infection, and skin infection predispose aged individuals to infectious arthritis (Gardner, 1980).

Therapeutic Treatment Regimens Drugs, invasive treatment modalities, and admission to an acute care facility all can predispose the elderly to infection. Corticosteroids, frequently prescribed for chronic disease such as arthritis, have many deleterious effects on function of the lymphocyte, neutrophil, and macrophage, thereby suppressing the inflammatory response. Cancer chemotherapeutic agents attack rapidly reproducing cells, lowering the numbers of active immunologic cells.

Treatment with broad-spectrum antibiotics or narrow-spectrum antibiotics in massive and prolonged doses alters the normal body flora. Franson et al (1986) found a statistically significant correlation between the use of antibiotics and subsequent development of infection. Antibiotic therapy can result in a transient colonization of the respiratory tract with enterobacilli. However, antibiotic-related alterations of the gut flora may remain for months or years. In addition, gram-negative bacteria have the ability to transmit "antibiotic resistance" to previously nonresistant organisms.

Indiscriminate use of antibiotics may convert a self-limiting infection to a more serious and fatal infectious process. Superinfections are most likely to occur on the fourth or fifth day of treatment, especially in individuals with other debilitating diseases. The organisms most involved in superinfections are gram-negative rods, fungi, and resistant staphylococci (Moore-Smith, 1986).

Garibaldi et al (1981) found an association between use of sedatives or tranquilizers and the presence of lower respiratory tract infection. These drugs may decrease responsiveness and increase risk of aspiration.

Many elderly persons do not consider themselves at risk for AIDS. Yet many surgical procedures common in the elderly, such as total hip and knee replacements, routinely require 6–12 units of transfused blood. One out of every 40,000 units will be tested incorrectly as negative because the testing mechanism is not 100% effective. Furthermore, more than 25,000 people, many of whom were aged, received infected blood between 1977 and 1985, the year the antibody test was developed. Of these infected persons, 15,000 have already died; another 10,000 are still alive and carrying the virus (American Society on Aging, 1988). The many elderly persons who are still sexually active, particularly the 10% of elderly men believed to be gay or bisexual, continue to be at risk for developing AIDS.

Use of invasive instruments also compromises the mechanical barriers that serve as first-line defense mechanisms. Use of Foley catheters, intravenous and arterial cannulas, and tracheal intubation is associated with an increased infection rate (Phair and Reisberg, 1984). Presence of nasogastric tubes can interfere with normal swallowing and lead to aspiration, thereby promoting respiratory tract infection. Urinary catheters or other urinary instrumentation significantly increases the risk of urinary tract infection (Franson et al, 1986; Magnussen and Robb, 1980; Setia et al, 1985). The presence of an indwelling urinary catheter greatly increases the chance of developing asymptomatic bacteruria (Farber et al, 1984; Setia et al, 1985). In contrast, proper use of condom catheters by men is not associated with an increased incidence of infection (Franson et al, 1986). However, Hirsch et al (1979) caution that use of condom catheters increases the risk of urinary tract infection when used for long-term drainage in uncooperative men who repeatedly pull on the device.

Hospitalization of the elderly increases their exposure to unfamiliar organisms. The likelihood of receiving one or several invasive treatments is increased. Being exposed to other infected patients increases the chance that the infection will be spread. A significant number of nursing home infections, especially those that occur shortly after admission, are associated with organisms that closely reflect hospital-acquired pathogens (Smith, 1984g). Franson et al (1986) found a statistically significant increased incidence of infection in elderly long-term care residents who had experienced acute care hospitalization within 28 days prior to the surveillance period. Thus, the elderly should not be admitted to the hospital unless it is absolutely necessary.

Malnutrition Malnutrition in the elderly may be a consequence of underlying disease processes or environmental and social factors associated with aging. A more complete discussion of inadequate nutrition in the elderly is presented in Chapter 9. Malnutrition impairs the immune response, increasing susceptibility to infection.

Excluding the normal aging of the immune system, malnutrition is probably the most common cause of impaired immunity in adults (Potter, 1984). Protein-calorie malnutrition results in (1) depressed cell-mediated immunity; (2) altered bactericidal function of neutrophils; and (3) changes in the complement system and secretary IgA response.

Cell-mediated immunity is depressed in the presence of malnutrition. Protein calorie malnutrition, iron deficiency, and vitamin C deficiency are associated with delayed hypersensitivity. Anergy is a sensitive indicator of malnutrition. The appropriate use of parenteral nutrition and enteral feedings can reverse the anergic state (Phair and Reisberg, 1984).

Evidence of malnutrition, as indicated by loss of 10% body weight, skin test anergy, and hypoalbuminemia, is associated with an increased incidence of bacteremia and polymorphonuclear leukocyte dysfunction, especially in people over age 50 (Phair and Reisberg, 1984).

Functional and Structural Changes Various structural and functional changes predispose the body to infection. Some of these have been discussed as part of the first-line defense against infection and are not repeated here. Dehydration decreases the amount of fluid excreted or secreted at various sites. The mucus secreted by the lungs becomes thick and tenacious during dehydration, making it more difficult to expectorate mucus that contains bacteria and other inspired particles. Dehydration decreases the amount of urine formation, which in turn decreases the amount of urine that freely flows from the bladder on micturition. This concentrates the urine and reduces the natural defense gained from flushing the urinary tract with more dilute urine. Stagnant urine is often more receptive to organism growth in elderly persons because an existing infection or other debilitating disease has resulted in a higher urine pH (alkaline). The parotid gland remains free of infection as long as it is free of obstruction and there is a free flow of saliva, which requires adequate hydration.

Magnussen and Robb (1980) found that about 40% of the residents they surveyed had impaired mobility; associated changes in the lungs, skin, and circulatory circuit increase risk of infection. Franson et al (1986) demonstrated a statistically significant correlation between immobility and nursing-home-acquired infection at a hospital-based nursing home care unit.

Increased colonization of the nasopharynx occurs more frequently in the aged, particularly in those with decreased mobility. Colonization, a prerequisite to invasive infection, is inversely related to physical activity and severity of underlying illness (Phair and Reisberg, 1984). The physiologic changes associated with aging affect various body surfaces or linings and enhance colonization (Fox, 1986). Gram-negative colonization of the respiratory and urinary systems increases with age, immobility, debility, chronic disease, and level of care required for the resident. There is an increase in the adherence of bacteria to mucosal cells of the upper respiratory and urogenital tracts in the elderly. This is, in part, secondary to decrease in secretory IgA (Weksler, 1986).

Immobility interferes with complete expansion of the lungs, which contributes to atelectasis and infection. Venous return is compromised, resulting in venous stasis, edema, and skin breakdown. And because immobility compromises blood flow to areas of prolonged pressure, nonambulatory residents are at an increased risk of developing skin infections (Garibaldi et al, 1981; Setia et al, 1985).

Incontinence of the bladder and bowel is associated with infection, particularly of the lower respiratory tract, skin, and soft tissues (Garibaldi et al, 1981; Nicolle et al, 1984; Setia et al, 1985). It is unclear whether urinary and fecal incontinence are indicators of the at-risk resident or whether these functional abnormalities actually promote infection (Nicolle et al, 1984).

Environmental Factors

Some studies have found that the elderly are at highest risk for infection within the first 6 to 12 months of institutionalization (Garibaldi et al, 1981; Setia et al, 1985). The longer individuals were in the institution, the less likely they were to become infected. However, other research indicates an increase in urinary tract, skin, and soft tissue infections as length of stay increases (Standfast et al, 1984).

The close proximity of nursing home residents to one another promotes transmission of infections. Shared group activities, eating in common dining facilities, and sharing of inanimate objects such as bathtubs, commodes, and other objects all increase transmission (Smith, 1984g). Residents with indwelling urinary catheters, who have a high incidence of asymptomatic bacteriuria (Garibaldi et al, 1980; Jackson et al, 1985), should not be sharing rooms with other catheterized or severely debilitated residents. Limiting transmission is difficult, particularly because infections in the elderly are at times difficult to detect (Deal, 1979).

Physicians tend to spend less time with aging patients and thereby delay early detection and treatment of infection. A significant number of patients are admitted to nursing homes with incorrect primary and secondary medical diagnoses (Jackson et al, 1985; Smith, 1984g), creating confusion about the appropriateness of interventions. Because of limited financial resources, services that would be helpful in the diagnosis and treatment of infections are often not available. Limited surveillance for infection, outdated practice policies, and limited attendance of personnel at infection control training programs contribute to the problem of infection transmission (Crossley et al, 1985; Smith, 1984g).

For a resident to acquire an infection, there must be (1) an environmental reservoir for the infectious agent; (2) a means of transmitting the agent to the resident; and (3) invasion of the host. Environmental reservoirs common in nursing homes include food, air cooling systems, thermometers, bath tubs, humidifiers, linens, dust, nursing home personnel, and nursing home residents. As a general rule, gram-negative bacteria such as *E. coli, Proteus, Pseudomonas,* and *Serratia* are the most significant organisms in the inanimate environment. Gram-positive organisms such as staphylococci and streptococci are found on personnel (Smith, 1984g).

Hands are primary transmitters of infection (Checko, 1980; Smith, 1984g). As nursing home personnel go from room to room, they serve as potential transmitters of infectious organisms. Appropriate facilities for handwashing should be available in each resident's room (Checko, 1980).

Cross infections in the nursing home environment have been documented (Smith, 1984a). Cluster cases of lower respiratory tract infections, conjunctivitis, upper respiratory tract infections, and diarrhea were found in four homes and accounted for 20% of all infections identified. In addition, clustering of bacterial isolates according to species was observed in urine specimens of catheterized residents (Garibaldi et al, 1981).

Prevention Practices to prevent transmission of infections among residents are essential but not always employed. A survey of 378 nursing homes showed that one third of the agencies had no policies for the care of some types of infections, and written materials on infection control were not readily available in 65% of the nursing homes surveyed (Crossley et al, 1985).

Early detection and intervention of infected residents is essential in preventing infection in other residents. This can be accomplished in part by planning and implementing a quality infection control program. Many of the formal infection control programs mandated by federal and state governments are limited in scope (Checko, 1980; Crossley et al, 1985; Garibaldi et al, 1981). It is common practice to assign the duties of infection control practitioner to personnel who have other primary responsibilities such as the director of nursing or the nursing inservice educator (Checko, 1980; Crossley et al, 1985). Most nursing homes do not have a physician with experience in infection control participating in their infection control program (Crossley et al, 1985; Garibaldi et al, 1981).

Crossley et al (1985) found that 74% of the nursing homes surveyed spent less than 5 hours per week on infection control and surveillance. About one third of the time was spent in collecting, analyzing, and interpreting data on infections. Teaching infection control practices occupied, on the average, 28% of the time, and the remaining 34% of the time was used for attending meetings, consulting, and developing policies and procedures. Surveillance techniques included chart review (66%), review of culture reports (78%), chart monitoring of patients with urinary catheters (86%), antibiotic utilization review (76%), and completion of infection report forms by nurses and doctors (61%).

Because nursing home personnel can be both reservoirs and transmitters of infection, it is important for long-term care facilities to have (1) employee health practices that protect the resident and staff against infection, and (2) a quality educational program to teach personnel about the epidemiology of infectious disease. Only 10.6% of the facilities surveyed by Crossley et al (1985) required an immunization record as part of the employment process, and less than 5% offered influenza immunization at the time of employment. Almost one third of the nursing homes surveyed by Garibaldi et al (1981) did not require any health history as a minimum condition of employment. Only 35.7% of the institutions required physical examinations of prospective employees, and less than 11% required employees to have periodic health screening. Personnel who handle food were screened for *Salmonella* and *Shigella* prior to employment in less than 3% of the institutions.

Policies for managing employees' exposure to a resident with viral hepatitis, meningococcal meningitis, or tuberculosis existed in less than half of the institutions. In general, employee health practices focused on record keeping and reacting to employee illnesses as required by regulating agencies (Crossley et al, 1985). Limited sick leave compensation encourages work attendance of employees while they have a communicable illness. Six of the seven homes surveyed by Garibaldi et al (1981) offered no financial compensation for the first 3 days of employee sick leave.

Education   A majority of the caregivers in long-term care settings are nursing aides and licensed practical nurses (LPNs) (Garibaldi et al, 1981; Setia et al, 1985). Their limited understanding of the epidemiology of disease is a major shortcoming in control of infection in long-term care (Checko, 1980). Lack of knowledge, combined with a high turnover of nonprofessional employees, makes it difficult to maintain personnel who have adequate knowledge and skill to implement infection prevention practices. Thus, infection may be spread more readily in long-term care because of the high percentage of nonprofessional staff, the high patient-to-staff ratio, and rapid turnover of nonprofessional employees.

Improper cleaning, maintenance, sanitation, and/or sterilization of the inanimate environment also can promote infection in long-term care facilities. Different levels of cleanliness are appropriate for each part of the inanimate environment. Intravenous devices, tracheostomy tubes, or other invasive equipment need to be properly sterilized. Bedpans, commodes, bathtubs, and bedside tables require adequate cleaning. Contaminated

airflow systems and inadequate ventilation can contribute to the spread of certain airborne microbes such as staphylococcus, streptococcus, viruses, and mycobacterium. These microbes attach to dust, lint, and other particles (Smith, 1984d).

ASSESSMENT

Potential for Infection is operationalized by the presence of a significant number of risk factors in the host, in the environment, or both. Risk factors are presented in Assessment Guide 5.1 in the form of an assessment tool. Because this diagnostic label uses the qualifier "potential for," the risk factors are both the defining characteristics and the etiologies of infection. The assessment tool, developed from a review of the literature, is designed to identify elderly persons at increased risk of becoming infected as they reside in a long-term care facility. Content validity was established by three infection control nurse specialists. Larger scores represent increased risk for infection. Analysis of the scores of each risk factor category will assist the nurse in identifying interventions to prevent infection. Other available assessment instruments fail to focus on the potential for infection in institutionalized elderly (Applegate, 1987); some have been designed for detecting risk factors in the acute care setting, and some include the young as well as the elderly (Haberstich, 1984; Meister, 1983; Titler and Knipper, 1986).

The nursing diagnosis Potential for Infection can be made more specific by identifying the type of infection the resident is at risk of acquiring, for example, Potential for Infection: Respiratory. Describing more specific types of the diagnosis will facilitate efforts to determine expected outcomes and effective interventions. Outcomes for the elderly person must be determined for each specific diagnosis, for example, Potential for Infection: Urinary Tract, as well as the identified etiologies or risk factors. Desired outcomes for a specific diagnosis can be defined from assessment data contained in Assessment Guide 5.1.

CASE STUDY

Potential for Infection

Mrs. Jones, age 79, was admitted one week ago to Longview Care Center following a 14-day hospitalization for a left-sided cerebral vascular accident complicated by pneumonia and respiratory failure. Her mobility is limited, but she is able to stand using a walker and the assistance of one person. She has decreased muscle strength on her right side and is unable to lift her right arm and leg. She is oriented to self and significant others. She opens her eyes to speech and occasionally opens her eyes spontaneously. She is not able to obey verbal commands but localizes pain. She is confused and is frequently found making inappropriate statements to the nurses and other residents. Mrs. Jones has a Foley catheter, which was present on admission to the extended care facility. She has a 3 cm decubitus ulcer on her right hip, but no other skin lesions are noted. Her skin is dry and turgor is poor. Her hair is thinning and falls out easily with combing. Her mucous membrances are dry, but no oral mucous membrane lesions are present. She wore dentures prior to this illness. Her weight is 100 pounds and her height is 5 feet 5 inches. She has a nasogastric tube in place and receives enteral feedings four times a day. She has a number 7 Shiley tracheostomy and receives aerosol per T piece with an FIO_2 at 30%. She is unable to cough to clear her airway, necessitating periodic tracheal suctioning to keep her airway clear of secretions.

Mrs. Jones is incontinent of stool four to five times per week. Her dorsalis pedal pulses are 1 +, and she has pitting edema of her lower extremities and sacrum. Her lungs frequently have crackles on auscultation. Her heart tones are strong but irregular.

Past medical history includes anterior lateral myocardial infarction 6 years ago, chronic congestive heart failure, arthritis, and type II diabetes mellitus. She has a 40-pack per year history of smoking.

Laboratory and pharmacologic data available on the day of transfer from the hospital to Longview Care Center were as follows:

White blood count 8,000/mm³	Prednisone 10 mg t.i.d.
Red blood cell count 3.8 million/mm³	Digoxin .125 mg daily
	Ampicillin 250 mg q.i.d.
Hemoglobin 10 g/100 mL	Theodur 200 mg every 12 hr
Serum albumin 2.9 g/100 mL	Orinase 1 g daily
	Lasix 40 mg b.i.d.
Total protein 5.0 g/100 mL	Inhalation treatment with metapril .3 cc to 1 cc normal saline q.i.d.

Mrs. Jones currently shares a room with Mrs. Smith, a severely debilitated 97-year-old resident who has been at the center for 3 years.

Longview Care Center is a private, for-profit, 100-bed facility that usually runs 100% occupancy. Written policies on infection control require that available private rooms be used to isolate known infected residents. Sinks and bathrooms are available in each room. Residents share bathtubs. Routine cleaning of bathtubs is required following each use.

The infection control practitioner inspects the kitchen and laundry at least once a quarter. The airflow system is routinely checked every quarter and is found to be adequate. Ventilation is adequate in resident rooms as well as in meeting rooms and dining areas. Residents are encouraged to attend group activities unless they have a known infection.

The staff of Longview Care Center consists of 75% nursing aides, 10% LPNs, and 15% RNs. The average resident-to-staff ratio is 12 to 1. Employees are required to complete a health history and provide a record of immunization prior to employment. Employees are expected to report, in writing, incidents of their exposure to a resident with a contagious disease. Employees are not compensated for the first 3 days of employee illness. Infection control practices and policies are taught to new employees. Current staff receive an update and review of infection control every quarter. The infection control policies and practices are readily available at each nurses' station.

The infection control practitioner has primary responsibility as the director of nursing. The major surveillance mechanism used to detect infection is periodic (once/month) review of residents' charts. If an infection is suspected, a form is filled out and the family practice physician who is responsible for the resident's medical care is notified. This same physician serves on the infection control committee of the center.

Using the assessment tool in Assessment Guide 5.1, Mrs. Jones's risk factor score is 46. She has altered first- and second-line defenses and several underlying disease processes, and she is receiving several treatments that increase her Potential for Infection. She has some indicators of malnutrition but needs further nursing assessment of this risk factor. Her functional limitations include dehydration, altered mobility, bowel incontinence, and decreased level of consciousness. Several environmental variables and her decubitus ulcer also increase her chance of infection.

Mrs. Jones's total risk score of 46 clearly points out the need for frequent surveillance rounds, not solely chart review. Environmental interventions undertaken by the primary nurse included moving Mrs. Jones or Mrs. Smith to a different room and discouraging Mrs. Jones's attendance at group activities at present.

Interventions that focused on the alterations in Mrs. Jones's health status included measurement of gastric pH and proper use of antacids; evaluation of Mrs. Jones's response to ampicillin and prednisone; and assessment of skin, particularly on the lower extremities and feet. Mobility was to be promoted to aid circulation and mobilization of pulmonary secretions. Adequate hydration and nutrition were restored and maintained.

The nurse assessed the need for the Foley catheter and ultimately removed it. Intermittent simple catheterization was ordered, if catheterization became necessary. Oral hygiene to decrease oropharyngeal colonization of pathogenic organisms was instituted. Proper positioning, particularly during enteral feedings, was necessary to guard against aspiration. Breathing exercises and chest physical therapy and aseptic and atraumatic suctioning speeded resolution of Mrs. Jones's pneumonia. Mrs. Jones's health record was reviewed, and it was determined that immunizations were up to date. Proper handwashing by the nursing home personnel was emphasized. Outcomes measured following implementation of interventions showed a reduction in Mrs. Jones's score on the potential for Infection Assessment Tool (see Assessment Guide 5.1).

Finally, agency administration reviewed the infection control program that was in effect at Longview Care Center. Formation of an infection control committee was used to develop and institute more extensive infection control policies and procedures. Because of the large number of nonprofessional staff, an educational program encompassing more than just infection control policies and procedures (eg, organism transmission, isolation technique) was initiated.

NURSING INTERVENTIONS

Nursing interventions to decrease the risk of infection in the institutionalized elderly are many, varied, and guided by identified risk factors. Interventions must be individualized for each resident, based on the positive risk indicators from the Potential for Infection Assessment Tool (see Assessment Guide 5.1).

The reader is referred to the text *Infection Control in Long-Term Care Facilities* (Smith, 1984) for a more extensive discussion of an infection control program for long-term care. Making environmental changes, supporting host defenses, and intervening to decrease the risk of urinary tract, respiratory tract, and skin and soft tissue infections are important elements of a quality infection control program (see Figure 5.1).

First-Line Defenses

Maintenance of the first line of protection can help to prevent skin and soft tissue, gastrointestinal, urinary, and respiratory tract infections. Elderly persons may have decreased amounts of gastric acid, which predisposes them to gastrointestinal infection. The resident with a nasogastric tube in place should have gastric pH monitored at regular intervals at least once every 8 hours. Antacids may need to be withheld for gastric pH greater than 7 (Smith, 1984e).

Second- and Third-Line Defenses

The presence of exisiting infection, acute hypoxemia or acidemia, or other medical problems must be quickly identified by the nurse in order to receive prompt medical evaluation and treatment. A comprehensive plan should include treatment of established infections; minimization of antibiotic use, as well as the use of other drugs; and administration of steroids in minimal doses and identification of specific immune problems. Providing balanced nutrition from the four basic food groups can also enhance the function of second- and third-line defenses.

Control of underlying chronic diseases, such as diabetes or atherosclerosis, also can improve the resistance of the host (Smith, 1984e). The nurse has an important role in assisting the resident to maintain control of the chronic disease, as well as in educating the resident to prevent infection. For example, teaching the resident with diabetes about foot care or the resident with chronic obstructive lung disease about bronchial hygiene may enhance host resistance to infection.

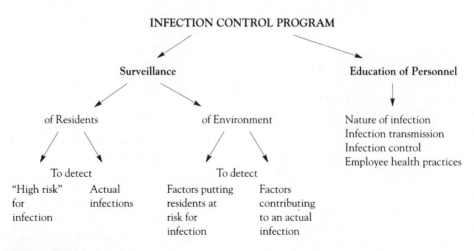

Figure 5.1

Elements of an infection control program.

Therapeutic Treatment Regimens

Use of antimicrobial therapy is appropriate for the resident with a known infection. However, such medications must be used judiciously because of the increasing resistance of organisms. Use of antibiotics prophylactically or in therapy often contributes to oropharyngeal colonization, which may result in superinfection. Microbiologic testing of organisms for their response to antibiotic therapy, as well as clinical evaluation of such variables as fever and sputum production, should guide antimicrobial therapy (Palmer, 1984). Cycling the type of antibiotic used to prevent desensitivity is also recommended along with improved hygiene in the environment and among health care personnel. Nevertheless, new antibiotics will have to be developed because of the ability of bacteria to alter their sensitivity to each new agent (Neu, 1984).

Invasive devices and treatments should be limited in order to decrease infection risk in nursing home residents. Policies regarding use of such devices must be instituted, using guidelines from the CDC.

Malnutrition and Functional/ Structural Changes

Nurses can make a significant contribution in minimizing additional risk factors such as malnutrition, dehydration, impaired physical mobility, bowel and/or bladder incontinence, and altered levels of consciousness. For a complete discussion of interventions for these risk factors see Units 2–4 and Unit 6.

Environmental Changes

Environmental control measures that decrease pathogens in the environment include sanitation, disinfection, sterilization, and handwashing. For a comprehensive discussion of these principles refer to *Infection Control in Long-Term Care Facilities* (Smith, 1984).

Residents with a urinary catheter should be separated from debilitated residents or from other residents with a urinary catheter. In addition, residents should be encouraged not to attend group activities when they are at high risk for infection or when they actually manifest signs of infection. Specific policies, based on guidelines from the CDC, must be established for isolation of infected residents. Staff of long-term care facilities should also have readily accessible infection control literature available for problem solving.

With some elderly patients, particularly those with AIDS, nurses should wear gloves when handling any body fluids such as blood, urine, feces, saliva, and airway secretions. For invasive procedures, nurses should wear masks or goggles.

Establishing employee health practices that protect residents against ill employees should be an integral part of environmental control to reduce the risk of infection. Surveillance of employees to ensure compliance with health practices may be necessary.

Finally, staff need to be educated about the predisposition to infection of institutionalized elderly and about environmental factors that increase their risk of infection. Clinicians also need to be educated that up to one third of all AIDS cases present first with central nervous system (CNS) symptoms and that all confusion in the elderly is not due to Alzheimer's disease.

Elderly persons with AIDS experience the same fears and anxieties as AIDS victims of any age: fear of death, discrimination, and desertion, and anxieties about an unstable social support network. A variety of epidemiologic, clinical, service, and educational issues must be addressed for elderly persons with AIDS. Finally, public education about AIDS and its transmission is as important in senior citizen centers as it is in elementary school classrooms.

Reducing the Risk of Common Infections in the Institutionalized Elderly

Urinary tract, respiratory tract, and skin/soft tissue infections are the three most frequent types of infection occurring in the institutionalized elderly. Table 5.2 indicates both manifestations of each type of infection and specific risk factors identified through a review of the literature. Further clinical testing is needed to establish the reliability and validity of these risk factors so that appropriate preventive measures can be instituted.

Infection Control Program

An infection control program is required for facilities participating in Medicare and Medicaid programs for Skilled Nursing Facilities (Smith, 1984f). An effective infection control program will provide guidelines for monitoring, preventing, diagnosing, and reporting infection, and may help to prevent legal liability. Programs initially establish an infection control committee with representatives from the medical and nursing staff, administration, pharmacy, housekeeping and dietary staffs, and the local Director of Health. The committee should have access to consultation services from a microbiology laboratory as well (Checko, 1980; Smith, 1984f). Such a committee may be required by state or local regulatory agencies and for voluntary accreditation by the Joint Commission on Accreditation of Hospitals (Smith, 1984).

The key committee member is the infection control practitioner (ICP). This person is generally a nurse, often

Table 5.2

Potential for Infection: Urinary Tract, Respiratory, Skin/Soft Tissue

Potential for Infection: Specific Type	Risk Factors	Interventions to Prevent Infection	Indicators for Actual Infection
Urinary	Dehydration Neurogenic bladder Urinary retention* Urinary stricture Prostate enlargement/ disease Presence of urinary catheters or other instrumentation* Long-term (more than 14 days) use of indwelling Foley catheters* (Kunin, 1987)	Maintain adequate hydration Use intermittent simple cath for residents with bladder emptying dysfunction Treat underlying cause of UT obstruction &/or disease Promote voiding on routine schedule Avoid unnecessary urethral catheterization & remove as soon as possible*(Kunin, 1987; Smith, 1984f) Discourage use of urinary catheters for specimen collection (Kunin, 1987) Evaluate source of incontinence (Ouslander, 1982) Use sterile closed urinary drainage system for indwelling urethral catheters* (Dukes, 1982) Insert urinary catheters using aseptic technique and sterile equipment* Refrain from opening the closed drainage system Promote handwashing immediately before and after any manipulation of catheter apparatus Avoid catheter irrigation unless obstruction is suspected When irrigation is necessary, use intermittent method If closed catheter system must be opened, disinfect catheter-tubing junction before disconnecting Obtain urine specimens from the sampling port, first cleaning the port with a disinfectant and aspirate urine with a sterile needle and syringe* (Kunin, 1987) Institute measures to maintain unobstructed flow of urine:* 1. Keep tubing from kinking and free of loops 2. Empty collecting bag regularly (every 8 hr) using a separate collecting container for each resident 3. Keep collecting bag below level of the bladder 4. Draining spigot and nonsterile collecting container should never come in contact 5. Change catheter when encrustation (sediment) is visible on sides of clear drainage tubing or when sandy sensation is felt as the catheter is rolled between examiner's fingers	Urine bacteria colony count greater than 1,000,000, plus one or more of the following: 1. Pyuria 2. Dysuria 3. Flank pain 4. Urgency 5. Frequency 6. Fever 7. Incontinence 8. Nocturia 9. Confusion with incontinence 10. Stress incontinence 11. Change in character of the stool 12. Foul smelling cloudy urine (Smith, 1984f; Kunin, 1987; Deal, 1979; Bently, 1986)

Table 5.2

Potential for Infection: Urinary Tract, Respiratory, Skin/Soft Tissue (*Continued*)

Potential for Infection: Specific Type	Risk Factors	Interventions to Prevent Infection	Indicators for Actual Infection
		Only persons with demonstrated knowledge and skill in aseptic insertion and maintenance of catheters should care for urinary catheters*	
		Use aseptic technique for irrigation. Materials should be discarded after use and sterile equipment and solution used for each irrigation*	
	Colonization of urinary tract with abnormal flora*	Secure catheter properly* (Kunin, 1987) Minimize use of antibiotics (Smith, 1984f) Refrain from use of antibiotic irrigations in catheterized residents Do not give antibiotics to prevent UTI (Smith, 1984f; Kunin, 1987; Britt et al, 1977; Butler & Kunin, 1968; Warren et al, 1983) Bathe urinary meatus with chlorhexidine-saturated sponges to decrease colonization of periurethral zone in females (Kunin, 1987)	
	Long-term use of condom catheters in confused males (Hirsch et al, 1979) Inability to clean perineum properly following voiding and defecation Length of stay in facility longer than one year	Remove daily, wash and dry penis and perineal area Change condom collectors daily (Kunin, 1987) Teach female residents to wipe perineum from front to back Residents with Foley catheters should not share rooms with other catheterized residents or severely debilitated residents (Maki et al, 1972; Kunin, 1987; Garibaldi et al, 1980)	
Respiratory	Intrinsic risk factors: Increased oropharyngeal colonization with abnormal flora* (Pennington, 1984) Antimicrobial therapy* Neurological deficit Malnutrition Neoplasia Diminished mucosal immunity (decreased secretory IgA level) Loss of cough and/or gag reflexes Decreased mucociliary clearance* Diminished pulmonary function Impaired surfactant production	Enhance lung defenses through immunization Meticulous oral hygiene Minimize aspiration of pharyngeal secretions by oropharyngeal suctioning, when indicated* Use of aseptic suctioning to decrease risk of transmission or organisms Judicious use of antimicrobial agents to reduce upper respiratory colonization Neurologic deficit may require intubation or tracheostomy to minimize aspiration (Johanson, 1984; Shell, 1980; Simmons & Wong, 1982; Smith, 1984d) Perform tracheostomy under aseptic conditions in an operating room, unless an emergency arises*	Fever Leukocytosis Pulmonary infiltrates seen radiographically Purulent tracheobronchial secretions (with or without pathogen on culture) Cough Pleuritic chest pain Any one or more of the following in combination with any of the above criteria: Positive blood culture Positive culture of pleural fluid Sputum culture and/or gram stain yielding pathogenic organisms

(Continues)

Table 5.2

Potential for Infection: Urinary Tract, Respiratory, Skin/Soft Tissue (*Continued*)

Potential for Infection: Specific Type	Risk Factors	Interventions to Prevent Infection	Indicators for Actual Infection
	Decreased lymphocyte numbers and function		
	Decreased neutrophils		
	Glucocorticosteroid and/ or cyclophosphamide		
	Presence of artificial airway	Wear sterile gloves on both hands for manipulation at tracheostomy site until wound has healed or granulation tissue has formed around the tube*	
	Sunctioning*	Use gloves on both hands and a sterile catheter for each series of suctioning*	
		Use sterile fluid for flushing catheter if necessary, then discard fluid*	
		Change suction collection tubing between residents	
		Change suction collection canisters between residents. If reusable, sterilize or provide high level disinfection	
		Use high-efficiency bacterial filters between collection bottle and vacuum source of portable suction devices that discharge contaminated aerosols (Simmons & Wong, 1982)	
	Diseases*	Deep breathing and coughing exercises*	
	COPD	Incentive spirometry, if tolerated	
	Chronic granulomatous disease	Ambulation*	
	AIDS	Frequent repositioning if bedridden*	
	Sarcoidosis	Chest percussion and postural drainage, as necessary*	
	Cardiovascular, thoracic or thoracoabdominal surgery	Discontinuance of smoking, or exposure to other toxins*	
	Radiation pneumonitis	Handwashing after contact with respiratory secretions* (Simmons & Wong, 1982; Shell, 1980)	
	Alcoholism		
	Splenectomy		
	Diabetes mellitus		
	Uremia		
	(Bradsher, 1983; Jay, 1983; Pennington, 1984; Simmons & Wong, 1982)		
	Extrinsic Risk Factors:	Use high-quality filters rated effective by American Society of Heating, Refrigerating, & Air Conditioning Engineers (ASHRAE)	
	Inadequate filtration of outside air by an air-handling system (Rhame et al., 1984)	Avoid draft (eg, open windows, open doors facing prevailing winds, elevator shaft draft) in rooms of high-risk residents to prevent subversion of air filter	
		Minimize dust disturbance during cleaning, repair and maintenance procedures	

Table 5.2

Potential for Infection: Urinary Tract, Respiratory, Skin/Soft Tissue (*Continued*)

Potential for Infection: Specific Type	Risk Factors	Interventions to Prevent Infection	Indicators for Actual Infection
	Use of nonhyperchlorinated water by immunosuppressed residents (Rhame et al, 1984)	Hyperchlorination of water used by immunocompromised residents Bathtub bathing by immunocompromised residents rather than showering If legionellosis becomes prevalent, all facility water should be treated using hyperchlorination Use of secretion precautions for residents with legionellosis (Rhame et al, 1984)	
	Transmission of airborne organisms through respiratory therapy equipment* (eg, oxygen devices, inhalation therapy equipment, mechanical ventilators, suction equipment (Simmons & Wong, 1982; Johanson, 1984)	Use of sterile fluids for nebulization or humidification* Once opened, discard container within 24 hrs Discard residual fluid in humidification device before refilling Discard condensation from respiratory therapy equipment* Replace Venturi and medication nebulizers and their reservoirs every 24 hr* Do not use room air humidifiers that create droplets to humidify* Clean, rinse, and dry reusable oxygen humidification reservoirs every 24 hr Change all oxygen tubing and masks between residents* Replace ventilator breathing circuits every 24 hr Change the breathing circuit on respiratory therapy machines between residents Sterilize or provide high-level disinfection on all hand-powered resuscitation bags between residents* Do not reuse any respiratory therapy equipment that is designed for single use* Sterilize or disinfect all reusable equipment after use* Sterilize or provide high-level disinfection of all respiratory therapy equipment between residents* Isolate residents with transmissible respiratory infections Do not allow personnel with respiratory infections to be assigned to direct care of high risk residents Institute a prevention program for all patient care personnel and high-risk residents if an influenza epidemic is anticipated.* This might include influenza vaccine and antiviral chemoprophylaxis (Simmons & Wong, 1982)	

(*Continues*)

Table 5.2

Potential for Infection: Urinary Tract, Respiratory, Skin/Soft Tissue (*Continued*)

Potential for Infection: Specific Type	Risk Factors	Interventions to Prevent Infection	Indicators for Actual Infection

Skin and soft tissue	Decreased mobility
	Dehydration
	Colonization with abnormal flora
	Diabetes*
	Atherosclerosis
	Decreased local tissue perfusion
	Malnutrition
	Bowel incontinence*
	Bladder incontinence*
	Immunocompromised*
	Presence of intravascular devices* (peripheral or central lines)
		Promote increased mobility (see Chapter 23)
		Promote fluid intake (see Chapter 12)
		Promote daily hygiene and bathing
		Educate residents about diabetes self-care; promote normoglycemia
		Promote tissue perfusion (see Chapter 20)
		Enhance nutritional intake (see Chapter 9)
		Promote bowel and bladder (see Chapters 16 & 17)
		Support host defenses
		Use intravenous (IV) therapy only for definite therapeutic or diagnostic indications*
		Handwashing before inserting IV cannula*
		Wear sterile gloves for insertion of central cannulas and cannulas requiring cutdown*
		Use upper extremity sites (or if necessary, subclavian and jugular sites) for insertion*
		Lower extremity sites should be changed as soon as satisfactory upper extremity site can be established*
		Scrub IV site with antiseptic prior to venipuncture*
		Do not use aqueous benzalkoniumlike compounds or hexachlorophene to scrub site*
		Secure cannula at insertion site*
		Apply a sterile dressing over insertion site. Tape should not cover the wound unless it is sterile*
		Record date of insertion in an easily found place* (eg, on the medical record and, if feasible, also on the dressing or tape)
		Evaluate resident daily for evidence of complications related to the cannula*
		Peripheral cannulas should be replaced every 48–72 hours. If complications are encountered prior to this time, the cannula should be replaced at that time*
		Insertion of central cannulas should be done aseptically with sterile equipment, eg, gloves and drape*
			Purulent drainage
			Isolation of pathogen via culture
			Signs and symptoms of inflammation:
			  erythema
			  edema
			  pain/tenderness
			  loss of function
			  heat
			Malodor
			Fever
			Lymphangitic

Table 5.2

Potential for Infection: Urinary Tract, Respiratory, Skin/Soft Tissue (*Continued*)

Potential for Infection: Specific Type	Risk Factors	Interventions to Prevent Infection	Indicators for Actual Infection
		Remove central cannulas as soon as they are no longer medically indicated or if they are strongly suspected of causing sepsis*	
		Routine changing of central cannulas inserted through a subclavian or jugular approach is not necessary*	
		IV administration tubing should be changed every 48 hr*	
		Maintain IV system as a closed system as much as possible; use injection ports that have been disinfected for entries into system*	
		Change entire IV system (cannula, administration set and fluid) if purulent thrombophlebitis, cellulitis, or IV-related bacteremia is noted or suspected*	
		Change cannula for phlebitis without signs of infection*	
		Culture fluid and save the bottle of an IV system suspected of being contaminated*	
		Record lot numbers of fluid and additives if fluid is confirmed as being contaminated.* Save remaining units from same lot	
		Notify local health authorities, CDC, and U.S. Food and Drug Administration immediately if contamination during manufacturing is suspected*	
		Handwashing before admixing parenterals*	
		Check all parenteral fluid for visible turbidity, leaks, cracks, and particulate matter; check manufacturer's expiration date before admixing and before use*	
		Label all admixed parenteral fluids stating the additives and their dosage, the date and time of compounding, the expiration time, and the person who did the compounding*	
		Use or discard all parenterals within 24 hr*	
		Complete or discard lipid emulsions within 12 hr of starting* (Simmons et al, 1981)	

* = Category I Center for Disease Control guidelines. Category I is strongly supported by clinical studies that show effectiveness in reducing risk of infection (Wong, 1982).

the director of nursing. However, nursing homes with greater than 150 beds should employ a full-time ICP. The role of the ICP or committee includes collection and evaluation of infection-related data; investigation of epidemics; education of staff; development of policies, procedures, and an employee health program; establishment of environmental and antibiotic monitors; and provision of a means for reporting activities and findings.

The Connecticut Public Health Code (Checko, 1980) mandates that an infection surveillance program include a system of reporting infections not only in patients but also in personnel. The code also states that the infection control committee will attempt to determine whether the infection was associated with the facility or personnel, and whether precautions were taken to prevent spread of the infection. This would appear to be a logical step for all states to take when reviewing their health codes.

Surveillance Traditionally, the major purpose of surveillance has been early detection and treatment of epidemics. Surveillance is "the activity that a health care institution employs in order to find, analyze, and control nosocomial infections" (Haberstich, 1984;157). It is the "collection, collation and analysis of data and the dissemination to those who need to know so that an action can result" (Thacker et al, 1983;1181).

Surveillance involves both behavioral and cognitive components. The behaviorial component is collecting information either directly, by physically observing and assessing the patient, or indirectly, through the use of equipment. The cognitive component involves the collection and evaluation of data to draw conclusions and make predictions. Surveillance not only assists in establishing baseline data but also provides a systematic method for continual data collection (Dougherty and Molen, 1985; Haberstich, 1984).

Surveillance is a two-fold process: (1) assessment of residents and their environment with subsequent analysis of collected data to identify residents at high risk for acquiring an infection; and (2) ongoing monitoring and data analysis, particularly of high-risk residents, for early detection and treatment of infection to prevent spread of infection among residents and personnel (see Figure 5.2).

Surveillance walks, or rounds, through resident care areas can provide clues to the presence of infection (Campbell, 1980; Haberstich, 1984). Rounds should focus on residents with specific risk factors such as an indwelling urinary catheter or antibiotic use, as well as on those with actual signs of infection, such as fever or abnormal radiology reports. Information can also be gleaned from residents' charts. However, chart review in nursing homes may be inaccurate because of the scant amount of recording that is done in the medical record (Checko, 1980; Haberstich, 1984; Jackson and Fierer, 1985). A survey of specific surveillance techniques (Crossley et al, 1985) revealed that residents' charts were reviewed by 53% of the homes with fewer than 50 beds and 68% with over 200 beds. These data, if combined with additional, more reliable sources, can be considered acceptable.

Other forms of surveillance include review of pharmacy records for antibiotic use; review of temperature records; reporting by nursing staff; the nursing kardex;

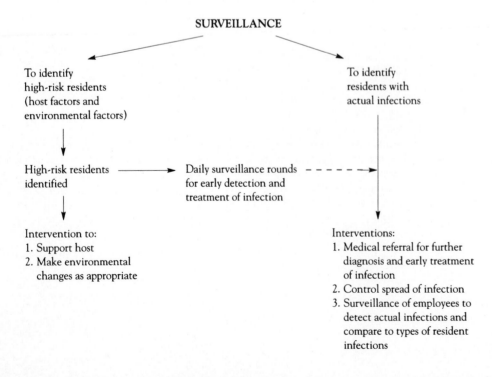

Figure 5.2

radiology reports; microbiology culture reports; admission records for diagnosis; hospital discharge summaries; physician's clinical notes; and direct observation of residents (Checko, 1980; Haberstich, 1984). The Crossley (1985; 2920) study found that 7% of homes with over 200 beds and 35% of homes of fewer than 50 beds indicated they "rarely or never" reviewed bacteriology culture reports. In extended care facilities antibiotics are often started without cultures being done; or if cultures are done, they are often done inappropriately. Specimen reports can be delayed, often for 2 weeks. Direct communication between the ICP and the laboratory is important because it shortens reporting time and facilitates the development of policies for collection and interpretation of specimens (Checko, 1980).

Physician reporting, when used alone, may lead to gross underestimation of nosocomial infection. National statistics indicated that 9.9% of all nursing home residents hadn't received two physician visits since entering the facility (Checko, 1980).

In lieu of these shortcomings, the nursing staff, those people most involved in direct resident care, are an extremely important source of information. Communication with the staff nurse who is familiar with each assigned resident may elicit enough information to detect "at-risk" as well as infected residents, thereby eliminating daily chart and kardex review (Checko, 1980).

A complete environmental surveillance should be carried out periodically to detect structure deficits in the facility that put residents at risk for infection. Periodic review of the facility's infection control program and employee health practices is also necessary. The Potential for Infection Assessment Tool (see Assessment Guide 5.1) should be completed within 24 hours of a resident's admission to the long-term care facility, on return of residents to the facility following hospitalization, and periodically throughout the resident's stay in the facility. Laboratory and nutritional data as well as other data may be more readily available on admission or readmission to long-term care. Those residents determined to be at high risk for developing an infection can then be monitored daily for early detection of infection. The assessment tool can be updated during rounds and when the ICP communicates with the nurse caring for that resident.

Research is needed to determine if identifying residents with Potential for Infection through routine surveillance would (1) lead to subsequent interventions to prevent infection, and (2) significantly decrease the number of admissions to acute care facilities, as well as morbidity and mortality related to infection.

Personnel caring for residents, particularly residents identified as at high risk for infection, must be astute in identifying signs and symptoms of actual infection. Vague complaints; an acute, unexplainable alteration in level of awareness; fever; vomiting; diarrhea; incontinency; or other changes in function should alert the nurse to a possible infection (Deal, 1979).

The CDC provides nosocomial criteria that can assist facility staff in diagnosing an actual infection. The criteria, however, are symptoms that persons of any age might display (Smith, 1984g). The elderly may not complain of these usual symptoms, may be asymptomatic, or may complain of only vague symptoms that might not normally cause one to suspect infection (Deal, 1979).

Complaints such as "I feel weak all over" or "I hurt all over" should not be quickly passed off as just part of the aging process or as being due to an arthritis flare-up. The resident should be carefully assessed to rule out an infectious process. "Just not feeling good" has often been associated with pneumonia, bacterial meningitis, or urinary tract infection. "I hurt all over" may indicate pneumonia, bacterial meningitis, furunculosis, appendicitis, or perirectal abscess. "I'm headachy and dizzy" may be an additional sign of bacterial meningitis or endocarditis (Deal, 1979).

The nurse also must observe for subtle changes in the elderly resident's sense of awareness. An altered sense of awareness that occurs over a period of days may be the only symptom of meningitis.

A loss of appetite may be caused by perirectal abscess, particularly in bedridden residents. Even if the resident does not complain of other symptoms, a rectal examination with digital palpation must be done to determine if tenderness is present (Deal, 1979).

The CDC has several surveillance forms that can be used to collect data on residents with actual infections. These can be obtained directly from the CDC or can be found in Chapter 9 of Smith's (1984) book, *Infection Control in Long-Term Care Facilities.*

Data collected on actual infections must be evaluated in order to determine if infection rates are deviating from normal, such as occurs in endemics or epidemics. The data can be used to look for clusters of infections that are occurring in the same body site or for infections of the same organisms, or it can be used to see if there are clusters of residents all having similar symptoms (Haberstich, 1984).

Surveillance data should be evaluated at the end of each week to assess for trends. The data should be reevaluated at the end of the month as well, followed by an assessment for seasonal trends. Surveillance data should be consistent enough to allow accurate comparisons. The comparisons should be done only within an institution, not with other institutions. The comparisons should examine any likenesses or differences with one month and the months previous to it, as well as with one month and the same month of the previous year. The evaluation should include the calculation of the infection rate as well as the prevalence rate. Infection rate is calculated based on the average daily census and the number of nosocomial infections in one month. For example:

$$\frac{15 \text{ nosocomial infections in 1 month}}{150 \text{ average daily census for same month}}$$

$$\times \ 100 \ = \ 10\% \text{ infection rate}$$

The prevalence rate examines the number of nosocomial infections present at any given time, For example, on one day, 7 of 150 residents had infections.

$$\frac{7}{150} \times 100 = 4.7\% \text{ prevalence rate}$$

These data should be shared with the medical and nursing staff, administration, and their employees (Haberstich, 1984).

A comparison also should be made to determine the number of infections occurring in residents that are the same as those identified in the employees. Data should be collected to determine the specific type of infections present in employees absent from work as well (Haberstich, 1984).

The ability to use surveillance effectively as an intervention to prevent and control infections will be influenced by the size of the facility and the level of care provided. Although 85.1% of all institutions surveyed by Crossley et al (1985) had infection control committees, 98.7% of all skilled nursing homes had such a program, but only 78% of other nursing homes with fewer than 50 beds had a committee. The nursing homes spending more than 20 hours a week on surveillance were also the larger facilities. The majority of all institutions, large and small, devoted less than 5 hours a week to surveillance. Written definitions related to nosocomial infection control activities existed in 55% of institutions with less than 50 beds and 79% with over 200 beds.

Factors that should be considered when implementing surveillance include the type and extent of information the institution expects to gain; the availability of resources and personnel to conduct surveillance; and the commitment from administration (Haberstich, 1984). Data surveyed by Crossley et al (1985) yielded statistics on residents having actual infections, but not on residents at risk for infection. Surveillance personnel usually were infection control nurses. Additional resources that might be helpful in surveillance include the CDC, city or county health departments, or the epidemiology section of the state health department (Checko, 1980).

Education   Education of personnel working in long-term care facilities should be an ongoing, integral part of infection control programs. The person performing the surveillance must have an understanding of the significance of the data collected or the value of close surveillance is lost (Dougherty and Molen, 1985). Many staff lack knowledge regarding transmission of microorganisms.

Campbell's (1980) survey of one long-term care facility showed that only 5% of 35 RNs and LPNs believed they were knowledgeable about the duties of the infection control committee. Only 2.5% believed they could relate laboratory and radiology results to the clinical situation of the resident. Only 24% believed they were knowledgeable about the sites of infections and the organisms involved. Long-term care facilities need to follow the pattern of acute care facilities and place more emphasis on education of their staff in regard to infection control (Crossley et al, 1985). Irvine et al (1984) also suggest that the number of hospitalizations of nursing home residents might be reduced if infection control policies were not only developed, but practiced.

Education of nurses employed in long-term care facilities must begin with changing attitudes and knowledge about the needs of the elderly (Campbell, 1980). Education and values clarification can assist the nurse in seeing the elderly as people with real health care needs and also as people who are at great risk for many chronic illnesses and acute infectious processes. Motivation of the staff to care and to learn is enhanced if they are included in plans and decision making and if they believe that their input matters. Brief audits of nursing care can help determine where infection problems are occurring, what residents are at greatest risk for infection, and therefore where the education needs to begin.

Team conferences that focus on a resident's problem can provide an opportunity to assess staff learning needs. Questions to ask might include: Which residents are at risk for infection and why?; How did the resident's infection start?; What kind of microorganisms are involved?; Where did they come from? Journal clubs, lectures, and workshops scheduled on a regular basis also can help staff meet their learning needs (Campbell, 1980). However, the most reliable source of information is often direct observation of infection control behaviors in the staff (Miller, 1984).

The educator must consider the educational background of the staff. The nursing staff may be an extremely diverse group in regard to education and experience. Often the majority of the nursing staff is made up of nursing assistants with little or no formal nursing education. Other facility staff, such as medical staff, food service, housekeeping, engineering, laundry, maintenance, and administration should be included in the educational process (Miller, 1984).

The educator may be anyone who observed an educational need and desires to offer an inservice, or may be the ICP who has observed deficiencies or has received input from staff members who have perceived deficiencies. For a complete discussion of the "how to" aspects of preparing and delivering an educational offering related to infection control, the reader is referred to Chapter 13 of the text *Infection Control in Long-Term Care Facilities* (Smith, 1984).

OUTCOMES

Outcomes that could be anticipated by implementing interventions as presented in this chapter are (1) an increase in the number of residents that are free of infection; (2) a decrease in the number of residents that receive a high score on the Potential for Infection Assessment Tool (see Assessment Guide 5.1); (3) a decline in the facility's infection rate; (4) a decline in mortality caused by infection; and (5) a decline in the number of residents requiring acute care hospitalization because of infectious process. The ability of the presented interventions to achieve the above outcomes is in need of further nursing research. Outcomes for the individual elderly person should be based on a specific type of diagnosis, for example, Potential for Infection: Respiratory. Analysis of scores for each category of the assessment tool will assist the nurse in identifying and implementing interventions that result in reducing risks and preventing infection in the dependent elderly person.

SUMMARY

The major factors that need assessment in determining potential for infection are (1) the host or resident and (2) the environment (both animate and inanimate).

Potential for Infection is a nursing diagnosis that can be treated by nurses. Two major components of a quality infection control program, surveillance and education, are major nursing interventions for this diagnostic label. Monitoring residents and their environment to detect residents at high risk for infection is one aspect of surveillance. Data analysis is important (1) to determine if the resident is at high risk for infection; (2) to select appropriate interventions to support host defenses in high-risk clients; and (3) to make appropriate changes in the environment as indicated by initial assessment data. Surveillance is also necessary for early detection of residents with actual infections, proper isolation, and a referral for medical diagnosis and treatment. Surveillance of employees to analyze the relationship between infections in residents and ill employees is helpful in isolating possible sources of infecting organisms.

ASSESSMENT GUIDE 5.1

Assessment Tool: Potential for Infection Using Mrs. Jones Case Study

Directions: If the risk factor indicator is present, put a 1 in the space following that indicator. If the risk factor indicator is not present, put a 0 in the space following the indicator. Put NA (not available) in the space following the indicator if that indicator is not available (eg, lab data). Add the numbers and put the total in the box for that risk assessment category. Sum the category sets to determine the score for altered host defenses and environmental factors. Sum the environmental factor score and altered host defense score to determine a total risk factor score.

HOST FACTORS

Altered First-Line Defenses

Break in the skin: 1 (total)
   decubiti 1
   burn 0
   trauma (eg, compound fx, injury from fall) 0
   surgical incision 0
   hypersensitivity reaction 0
   tear in the skin (not included above) 0
   other (not included above) 0
Poor oral hygiene: 0 (total)
   dental caries 0
   halitosis 0
   localized lesions of oral mucous membranes 0
   localized oral abscesses 0
Urethral stricture   NA
Prostate enlargement   0
Urinary retention   NA
Bowel constipation   0
Stasis of body fluids: 3
   bowel obstruction 0
   ascites 0
   tissue edema 1
   pulmonary edema 1
   venous stasis 1
Abnormal pH of body fluids   0
   (gut >7 ___ ; urine ___)
Decreased cough reflex   1
Colonization with abnormal flora: NA (total)
   urinary tract NA
   upper respiratory tract NA
   gastrointestinal tract NA
   genital tract NA
Total score for altered first-line defenses: 5

Altered Second-Line Defenses

Absolute granulocyte count <1000/mm3
   $\dfrac{\% \text{ granulocytes} \times \text{total WBC}}{100}$

      or   0
   Neutropenia (neutrophil count <1000/mm3)
Presence of preexisting infection   0
Hemoglobin <12.0 g/dL (female)   1
         <13.0 g/dL (male)
Acute hypoxemia   NA

ASSESSMENT GUIDE 5.1

Assessment Tool: Potential for Infection Using Mrs. Jones Case Study (Continued)

Acidemia	NA
Alkalemia	NA
Receiving corticosteroids	1
Decreased arterial circulation to body part	1
(eg, history of atherosclerosis plus pale, cool skin, decrease capillary	
refill, absence of peripheral pulses, pain)	
Total score for altered second-line defenses	3

Altered Third-Line Defenses

Anergy (eg, via skin testing)	NA
Currently or recently received immunosuppressive drugs	0
Currently or recently received radiation therapy	0
Total score for altered third-line defenses:	0

Disease Processes

Presence of 3 or more chronic health problems	1
History of smoking	1
History of alcohol abuse	0
Presence of	
peripheral arterial disease	1
venous insufficiency	1
peripheral neuropathies	NA
diabetes mellitus	1
diabetes ketoacidosis	0
central nervous system disease	
stroke	1
spinal cord injury	0
head trauma	0
chronic lung disease	1
renal insufficiency	0
uremia	0
chronic liver disease	0
leukemia	0
lymphoma	0
multiple myeloma	0
heart disease	
congestive heart failure	1
valvular heart disease	
Total score for disease processes:	8

Therapeutic Treatment Regimens

Drugs:	1 (total)
Antibiotics 1	
Sedatives ___	
Invasive devices/treatments:	6
urinary Foley catheter 1	
suprapubic catheter 0	
intermittent simple catheter 0	
nasogastric intubation 1	
enteral feeding through nasogastric tube 1	
peripheral intravenous catheter (#) 0	
central venous catheter 0	
Hickman/Broviac catheter 0	
dialysis catheter 0	
tracheostomy 1	
chest tube 0	

(Continues)

ASSESSMENT GUIDE 5.1

Assessment Tool: Potential for Infection Using Mrs. Jones Case Study (Continued)

receiving intermittent nasotrachael suctioning 0
receiving suctioning through a tracheostomy 1
uses a respiratory assist device 1
receiving dialysis 0
Recent hospitalization (within the last month)   1
Total score for therapeutic treatment regimens: 8

Malnutrition

Involuntary weight loss greater than
   10% of body weight   NA
20% above or below ideal body weight   1
Alcohol abuse   0
Ingesting little or nothing by mouth and not receiving other nutritional 0
   support
Anorexia   0
Recent history of nausea/vomiting   0
Easy pluckability of hair   1
Triceps skin fold (TSF) of 3 mm or less   NA
Midarm muscle circumference
   {(arm circumference – 0.314) × TSF} less than 15 cm   NA
Serum albumin 3.0 mg/dL or less   1
Serum transferrin 150 mg/dL or less   NA
Anergy (to skin testing)   NA
Total score for malnutrition: 3

Functional/Structural Changes

Dehydration   1
Impaired physical mobility (select one of the following and put the   3
   corresponding number in the blank)
   completely independent (0)
   requires use of equipment or device (1)
   requires help from another person for
      assistance, supervision, or teaching (2)
   requires help from another person and
      equipment or device (3)
   is dependent, does not participate in activity (4)
Bowel incontinence   1
Bladder incontinence   0
Decreased level of consciousness   1
   (score <12 on Glascow Coma Scale)
If total on Glascow Coma Scale is below 12 put a 1 in
   the blank next to decreased level of consciousness
Add numbers for Glascow Coma Scale rating −11

opens eyes (select one)	spontaneously	4
	to speech	3
	to pain	2
	nil	1

motor response (select one)	obeys commands	6
	localizes stimulus	5
	withdraws to stimulus	4
	abnormal flexion	3
	extends	2
	nil	1

ASSESSMENT GUIDE 5.1

Assessment Tool: Potential for Infection Using Mrs. Jones Case Study (Continued)

verbal response (select one)	orientated	5
	confused	4
	inappropriate words	3
	incomprehensible sounds	2
	nil	1

Total score for functional/structural changes: 6

Sum total score numbers to determine a score for altered Host Factors
   score   33

ENVIRONMENTAL FACTORS

Structural Deficits

Handwashing facilities not available in
   each resident's room   0

Inadequate ventilation   0

Inadequate/contaminated airflow system   0

No evidence of frequent routine cleaning of shared facilities (eg,   0
   commodes, tub, p.t. equipment)

Inadequate sterilization of invasive equipment

No evidence of routine voluntary inspection of critical areas (eg
   kitchen, laundry) physical therapy

Total score for structural deficits: 0

Management of Residents

Resident with foley catheters shares rooms with other catheterized   1
   residents or severely debilitated patients

Resident is encouraged to attend group activities when he/she is at   1
   high risk for or manifesting signs and symptoms of infection

Resident has been in facility less than 6 months   1

Written policies/guidelines for isolating infected residents are not   0
   available

Readily accessible infection control literature is not available   0

Total score for management of residents   3

Infection Control Program

Infection control practitioner has other primary responsibilities   1

Physician participating in the infection control program has limited   1
   experience in infection control

Limited time is spent on infection control surveillance   1

Written documents demonstrating routine surveillance for infection are   0
   absent

No evidence of routine monitoring of high-risk patients for presence of   0
   infection

No evidence of routine teaching of personnel on infection control
   practices (eg. handwashing, Foley care)

Chart review is the only surveillance technique used to detect   1
   infections

Total score for infection control program: 4

Nursing Home Personnel

Employee health practices do not require the following:

   preemployment immunization record   0

   preemployment health history   0

   preemployment physical examinations   1

   periodic health screening   1

   policies for managing employees' exposure
      to residents with contagious disease   0

   financial compensation for the first
      3 days of employee illness   1

(Continues)

ASSESSMENT GUIDE 5.1

Assessment Tool: Potential for Infection Using Mrs. Jones Case Study (Continued)

high percentage of nonprofessional staff giving direct patient care	1
high resident-to-staff ratio	1
high staff turnover	1
fewer than 2 employee inservices per year focus on infection-related topics	0
Total score for nursing home personnel:	6
Sum all total score numbers under ENVIRONMENTAL FACTORS to determine a score indicating the degree to which the environment is putting a resident at risk for infection	13
TOTAL RISK FACTOR SCORE (sum of altered host defenses and environmental factors)	46

References

American Society on Aging: Proceeding of Conference. San Diego, CA, March 1988.

Applegate WB: Use of assessment instruments in clinical settings. *J Am Geriatr Soc* 1987; 35:45–50.

Bently DW: Infectious diseases. Chapter 26 in: *Clinical Geriatrics*, 3d ed. Rossman I (editor). Lippincott, 1986.

Bradsher RW: Overwhelming pneumonia. *Postgrad Med* 1983; 74:201–217.

Britt MR et al: Antimicrobic prophylaxis for catheter-associated bacteriuria. *Antimicrobic Agents Chemother* 1977; 11:240–243.

Brockelhurst JC (editor): *Textbook of Geriatric Medicine and Gerontology*, 3d ed. Churchill Livingstone, 1985.

Butler HK, Kunin CM: Evaluation of polymyxin catheter lubricant and impregnated catheters. *J Urol* 1968; 100:560–566.

Campbell DG: Prevention of infection in extended care facilities. *Nurs Clin North Am* 1980; 15:857–868.

Carroll-Johnson RM (editor): *Classification of Nursing Diagnoses: Proceedings of the Eighth Conference*. Lippincott, 1989.

Checko PJ: Infection control in long-term care facilities: The state of the art. *Infect Control Urolog Care* 1980; 5:2–7.

Cohen ED et al: Nosocomial infections in skilled nursing facilities: A preliminary survey. *Public Health Rep* 1979; 94:162–165.

Crossley KB et al: Infection control practices in Minnesota nursing homes. *JAMA* 1985; 254:2918–2921.

Dahlsten J, Shank JC: Chronic and acute disease problems in rural nursing home patients. *J Am Geriatr Soc* 1979; 27:112–116.

Deal WB: Unusual manifestations of infectious diseases in the aging. *Geriatrics* 1979; 34:77–84.

Dougherty CM, Molen MT: Surveillance. Chapter 21 in *Nursing Interventions: Treatments for Nursing Diagnoses*, 1st ed. Bulechek GM, McClosky JC (editors). Saunders, 1985.

Dukes C: Urinary infections after excision of the rectum: Their cause and prevention. *Proc Royal Soc Med* 1982; 22:1–11.

Farber BF et al: A prospective study of nosocomial infections in a chronic care facility. *J Am Geriatr Soc* 1984; 32:499–502.

Felser JM, Raff MJ: Infectious diseases and aging: Immunologic perspectives. *J Am Geriatr Soc* 1983; 31:802–807.

Fox RA: The effect of aging on the immune response. Chapter 14 in: *Immunology and Infection in the Elderly*. Fox RA (editor). Churchill Livingstone, 1985a.

Fox RA: Immunology of aging. Chapter 5 in: *Textbook of Geriatric Medicine and Gerontology*, 3d ed. Brockelhurst JC (editor). Churchill Livingston, 1985b.

Fox RA: Infection and immunity in old age. Chapter 2 in: *Infections in the Elderly*. Deham MJ (editor). MTD Press, 1986.

Franson TR et al: Prevalence survey of infections and their predisposing factors at a hospital-based nursing home care unit. *J Am Geriatr Soc* 1986; 34:95–100.

Gardner ID: The effect of aging on susceptibility to infection. *Rev Infect Dis* 1980; 2:801–808.

Garibaldi RA, Brodine S, Matsumiya S: Infections among patients in nursing homes. *N Engl J Med* 1981; 305:731–735.

Garibaldi RA et al: Meatal Colonization and catheter-associated bacteriuria. *N Engl J Med* 1980; 303:216–218.

Haberstich MJ: Finding and analyzing infections in a nursing home. Chapter 9 in: *Infection Control in Long-Term Care Facilities*. Smith OW (editor). Wiley, 1984.

Hirsch DD, Fainstein V, Musher DM: Do condom catheter collecting systems cause urinary tract infection? *JAMA* 1979; 242:340–341.

Irvine PW, Van Buren N, Crossley K: Causes for hospitalization of nursing home residents: The role of infection. *J Am Geriatr Soc* 1984; 32:103–107.

Jackson MM, Fierer J: Infections and infection risk in residents of long-term care facilities: A review of the literature 1970–1984. *Am J Infect Control* 1985; 13:63–77.

Jay SJ: Nosocomial pneumonia: The challenge of a changing clinical spectrum. *Postgrad Med* 1983; 74:221–235.

Johanson WG: Prevention of respiratory tract infection. *JAMA* (May) 1984; 69–77.

Kunin CM: *Detection, Prevention and Management of Urinary Tract Infections.* Lea and Febiger, 1987.

Magnussen MH, Robb SS: Nosocomial infections in a long-term care facility. *Am J Infect Control* 1980; 8:12–17.

Maki DG, Hennekens CG, Bennett JV: Prevention of catheter-associated urinary tract infection. *JAMA* 1972; 221:1270–1271.

Meister S: *Development of an infection risk factors inventory.* (Essay.) Marquette University, Milwaukee, WI, 1983.

Miller SG: Infection control: Educational aspects. Chapter 13 in: *Infection Control in Long-Term Care Facilities.* Smith PW (editor). Wiley, 1984.

Moore-Smith B: Opportunistic infections. Chapter 11 in: *Infections in the Elderly.* Denham MJ (editor). MTP Press, 1986.

Neu HC: Current mechanisms of resistance to antimicrobial agents in microorganisms causing infection in the patient at risk for infection. *JAMA* (May) 1984; 11–17.

Nicolle LE et al: Twelve-month surveillance of infections in institutionalized elderly men. *J Am Geriatr Soc* 1984; 32:513–519.

Ouslander JG, Kane RL, Abrass IB: Urinary incontinence in elderly nursing home patients. *JAMA* 1982; 248:1194–1198.

Palmer DL: Microbiology of pneumonia in the patient at risk. *JAMA* (May) 1984; 53–60.

Palumbo FB et al: Recruitment of long-term care facilities for research. *J Am Geriatr Soc* 1987; 600–602.

Pennington JE: Respiratory tract infections: Instrinsic risk factors. *JAMA* (May) 1984; 34–41.

Phair JP, Reisberg BE: Nosocomial infections. Chapter 4 in: *Immunology and Infections in the Elderly.* Fox RA (editor). Churchill Livingstone, 1984.

Potter JF: Immunity in the elderly. Chapter 2 in: *Infection Control in Long-Term Care Facilities.* Smith PW (editor). Wiley, 1984.

Rhame FS et al: Extrinsic risk factors for pneumonia in the patient at high risk of infection. *JAMA* (May) 1984; 42–52.

Rossman I (editor): *Clinical Geriatric,* 3d ed. Lippincott, 1986.

Setia U, Serventi I, Lorenz P: Nosocomial infections among patients in a long-term care facility: Spectrum, prevalence and risk factors. *Am J Infect Control* 1985; 13:57–62.

Shell G: Upper and lower respiratory tract infections. *Nurs Clin North Am* 1980; 15:715–727.

Simmons BP, Wong ES: *Guidelines for Preventions of Nosocomial Pneumonia.* US Department of Health and Human Services, Centers for Disease Control, Atlanta, GA, 1982.

Smith IM: Infectious diseases of the geriatric patient. Chapter 3 in: *Infection Control in Long-Term Care Facilities.* Smith PW (editor). Wiley, 1984.

Smith PW: Epidemic investigation. Chapter 10 in: *Infection Control in Long-Term Care Facilities.* Smith PW (editor). Wiley, 1984a.

Smith PW (editor): Finding and analyzing infections in a nursing home. Chapter 9 in: *Infection Control in Long-Term Care Facilities.* Wiley, 1984b.

Smith PW (editor): Infection control: Educational aspects. Chapter 13 in: *Infection Control in Long-Term Care Facilities.* Wiley, 1984c.

Smith PW (editor): Infection control measures: The enviromental reservoir. Chapter 15 in: *Infection Control in Long-Term Care Facilities.* Wiley, 1984d.

Smith PW (editor): Infection control measures: The resident. Chapter 14 in: *Infection Control in Long-Term Care Facilities.* Wiley, 1984e.

Smith PW: Infection control program organization. Chapter 8 in: *Infection Control in Long-Term Care Facilities.* Smith PW (editor). Wiley 1984f.

Smith PW (editor): Nosocomial infections in nursing homes. Chapter 4 in: *Infection Control in Long-Term Care Facilities.* Wiley, 1984g.

Smith PW (editor): Urinary tract infection. Chapter 6 in: *Infection Control in Long-Term Care Facilities.* Wiley, 1984h.

Standfast SJ et al: A prevalence survey of infections in a combined acute and long-term care hospital. *Infect Control* 1984; 5:177–184.

Thacker SB, Keewhan C, Brachman PS: The surveillance of infectious disease. *JAMA* 1983; 249:1181–1185.

Titler MG, Knipper J: *Potential for infection: Respiratory.* (Paper.) University of Iowa, Iowa City, IA, 1986.

Viant AC, Linton KB, Gillespie WA: Improved method for preventing movement of indwelling catheters in female patients. *Lancet* 1971: 1:736–737.

Warren JW et al: Ineffectiveness of cephalexin in treatment of cephalexin-resistant bacteriuria in patients with chronic indwelling urethral catheters. *J Urol* 1983; 129:71–73.

Weksler ME: Biologic basis and clinical significance of immune senescence. Chapter 4 in: *Clinical Geriatrics,* 3d ed. Rossman I (editor). Lippincott, 1986.

Wong ES: *Guideline for Prevention of Catheter-Associated Urinary Tract Infections.* US Department of Health and Human Services, Centers for Disease Control, Atlanta, GA, 1982.

II

Nutritional–Metabolic Pattern

MERIDEAN MAAS, PhD, RN, FAAN

KATHLEEN BUCKWALTER, PhD, RN, FAAN

Overview

DECUBITUS ULCERS POSE A MAJOR THREAT TO the elderly, especially to those who are immobilized with chronic health problems. At present, the accepted NANDA diagnosis Impaired Skin Integrity includes no subdiagnostic categories. As Frantz notes in Chapter 7, Impaired Skin Integrity: Decubitus Ulcer, the complications of decubitus ulcers kill as many as 60,000 people annually, and the financial and human costs may be even greater. Frantz explores pressure as a primary etiologic factor in the development of decubitus ulcers. She presents an assessment tool for grading decubitus ulcers that is most useful to nurses in long-term care settings and describes interventions designed to promote circulation to ischemic tissue.

In Chapter 8, Hardy addresses another significant diagnosis for the elderly, Impaired Skin Integrity: Dry Skin, which at present is not among the list of accepted NANDA diagnoses. Although dry skin is a common problem among the elderly, the author notes that little systematic research has been done to identify etiologies or to test the efficacy of nursing interventions. Hardy reports her own research to test interventions related to this diagnosis, using a psychometrically sound assessment and evaluation tool.

Nutritional problems account for one third to one half of all health problems in the elderly, and many independently living elderly demonstrate nutritional deficiencies. In Chapter 9, Altered Nutrition: Less than Body Requirements, Rajcevich and Wakefield discuss risks of malnutrition, illnesses that interfere with nutrition, and psychosocial and economic factors that may influence nutritional intake. The important role of the nurse in assessment of nutritional status and diet history is emphasized as well as nutrition education and supplement feeding.

In Chapter 10, Impaired Swallowing, Ter Maat and Tandy take the complex process of swallowing and identify each stage of the swallow by specific signs and symptoms. In so doing, the authors expand the broader NANDA conceptualization and advance nursing care planning for specific aspects of dysphagia for elderly clients.

Oral complications and poor oral hygiene are often problems that accompany aging, particularly among the elderly who have chronic illnesses and functional losses. In Chapter 11, Eldredge, a dental hygienist, illuminates the diagnosis Altered Oral Mucous Membrane and sets forth plans for oral screening and care.

In Chapter 12, Reese explicates the NANDA diagnosis of Fluid Volume Deficit according to the most common causes among the elderly, an essential step toward systematically specifying interventions. Recognizing that the treatment for Fluid Volume Deficit is often medically controlled, Reese asserts that rehydration is the common nursing goal to treat all fluid deficits. She emphasizes that independent nursing interventions focus on prevention and notes that more research is needed to improve clinical assessment tools to detect fluid deficits and to test the effectiveness of preventive strategies.

6

Normal Changes With Aging

Mary A. Hardy, PhD, RN, C
Kathy Rajcevich, RN
Bonnie Wakefield, MA, RN

Definition:

Describes the pattern of food and fluid consumption relative to metabolic need and pattern indicators of local nutrient supply.

A THINNING AND LESS ELASTIC APPEARANCE TO THE skin is seen with aging. There are several reasons for these changes. Mitosis, or the creation of new epidermal cells, slows down. Collagen and subcutaneous fat decreases, and there is a diminished size, number, and functioning of sweat glands. Other functional changes that decline with age include growth rate or epidermal turnover, injury response, barrier function, chemical clearance rates, sensory perception, immunosurveillance, vascular responsiveness, thermoregulation, and sebum production (Calkins et al, 1986). Although it is commonly thought that decreased sebum secretion, fluid and nutritional status, and certain medications associated with the elderly contribute to skin dryness, Frantz and Kinney (1986) found that these factors were not substantiated.

Subcutaneous fat is lost on the limbs and face and increases over the abdomen and hips. Loss of subcutaneous fat and supportive tissue increases the evaporation of tissue fluids, thus contributing to decreased skin and subcutaneous hydration. Increased vascular fragility and thus vascularity, coupled with loss of supportive structures, make the capillaries, particularly of the limbs and face, more fragile. Nutritional deficits coupled with reduced circulation put the elderly at risk for irritations, injuries, and potentially serious skin breakdown (Nesbitt, 1988).

With normal aging, the systems that control the volume and concentration of body fluids exhibit a reduction both in reserve capacities and in ability to respond rapidly. The size of the kidney decreases with age, shrinking about 20% by the eighth decade. The number and mass of glomeruli, as well as the length and volume of the proximal tubules, decrease so that by age 70, approximately 30% to 50% of the glomeruli present at birth have disappeared. In addition, a reduction in renal blood flow accelerates after age 50, so that by age 70 renal blood flow is about half of its former peak. These changes in kidney perfusion produce a decline in glomerular filtration. The diluting ability of the kidney, or the ability to remove excess water, decreases and can result in a fluid volume excess. On the other hand, advancing age also reduces the concentrating ability of the kidney, resulting in a net loss of body fluids. For people over age 60, total body fluid composes about 46% and 52% of the body weight for females and males, respectively, compared to 52% and 60% in the young adult (Edelman, 1952). Total body water also decreases in relation to body weight as obesity increases.

Under usual circumstances, maintenance of adequate fluid volume is not a problem. However, the aged kidney's decreased ability to regulate fluid

Table 6.1

Key Nutrients Affected by Aging

Nutrient	Changes with Aging	Effect on Requirements
Calories	Decreased activity & BMR	Decreased
Calcium	Decreased absorption	Increased
Protein	Decreased absorption &/or metabolism	Increased
Vitamins*		
Folate	Impaired absorption	Increased
Iron	Impaired absorption	Increased
Thiamin	Impaired absorption	Increased
Vitamin B12	Impaired absorption	Increased
Vitamin C	Impaired absorption	Increased
Vitamin D	Decreased absorption	Increased

*Changes may occur because of aging and/or drug–nutrient action.

volume and the decrease in total body water combine to narrow the range of responses to fluid volume changes and the rate of response to abrupt changes. Abrupt alterations put the elderly at risk for cardiovascular, renal, and neurologic malfunctioning, thereby increasing morbidity and mortality in the aged.

Although many physiologic changes occur with aging, there has been little research to demonstrate the impact of alterations in physiology and metabolism on nutritional requirements in the aging population. There is a decrease in the basal metabolic rate, averaging 20% between the ages of 30 and 90 years (Watkin, 1982). There also tends to be a decrease in physical activity, leading to decreased energy needs. Additionally, reduction in energy requirements generally results in consumption of smaller amounts of nutrients.

Excretion of urinary creatinine, as measured by a 24-hour urine, decreases markedly, suggesting that the creatinine height index may be inaccurate in older individuals. Age-related immune and hematologic findings are identical to those found in malnutrition, and therefore it is difficult to ascribe host-defense abnormalities to altered nutritional states or to the aging process (Chernoff et al, 1984). In contrast, serum albumin is only minimally altered by aging; therefore, hypoalbuminemia is an excellent predictor of malnutrition in the elderly (Chernoff et al, 1984; Mitchell and Lipschitz, 1982).

Vitamin D and calcium absorption decline with age, and yet calcium requirements are higher, especially for postmenopausal women. Osteoporosis results from the prolonged negative calcium balance attributed to calcium loss from bones. This condition begins in the third decade for women and the fourth decade for men, but is more common in women. Although calcium supplementation may help, it will not cure the problem once it develops. Persons over age 70 may need to consume more protein per kilogram of body weight than younger people to avoid a negative nitrogen balance. This appears to be related to

changes in protein absorption and/or metabolism because lean body mass declines with age.

Changes in dentition, often due to periodontal disease, affect digestion in the aging population. Up to 50% of those over age 65 have lost their teeth (Watkin, 1982). Many cannot afford dentures, or they have ill-fitting dentures that are inefficient in mastication. The inability to chew food properly decreases the type and amount of food eaten and may inhibit proper digestion (Ebersole and Hess, 1985; Love, 1986; Rozovski, 1984).

Alterations in sensory perception of taste and smell, including decreased saliva production, number of taste buds, and olfactory fibers, have been identified as part of the normal aging process that may affect nutritional status; however, there is no agreement concerning the cause. These changes appear to decrease the satisfaction associated with eating, thus contributing to a decreased intake.

Changes in swallowing appear to be generalized, related to altered sensory and motor function; these changes may reduce the effectiveness of swallowing and chewing and may also influence the type and amount of food eaten. Other changes in physiology of the gastrointestinal tract that occur with aging are decreased peristalsis, decreased secretions, and decreased nerve transmission. Reduced gastric secretion of hydrochloric acid leads to impaired absorption of vitamins and minerals. Diminished saliva slows breakdown of starches. Hepatic insufficiency can lead to poor absorption of fat-soluble vitamins. Although the exact mechanism and extent of these changes are unknown (Thomson and Kulan, 1986), they may lead to digestion and absorption problems. Table 6.1 lists the nutrients that may be affected by the aging process.

References

Calkins E, Davis P, Ford A (editors): *The Practice of Geriatrics.* Saunders, 1986.

Chernoff R, Mitchell CO, Lipschitz DA: Assessment of the nutritional status of the geriatric patient. *Geriatr Med Today* 1984; 3:129–141.

Ebersole P, Hess P: *Toward Healthy Aging.* Mosby, 1985.

Edelman IS: Further observations on total body water I. Normal values throughout the life span. *Surg Gynecolog Obstet* 1952; 95:1–12.

Frantz RA, Kinney CN: Variables associated with skin dryness in the elderly. *Nurs Res* 1986; 35(2):98–100.

Love AE: Nutrition assessment guides resident well being. *Am Health Care Assoc J* 1986; 12:27–37.

Mitchell CO, Lipschitz DA: The effects of age and sex on routinely used measurements to assess the nutritional status of hospitalized patients. *Am J Clin Nutrition* 1982; 36:340–349.

Nesbitt B: Nursing diagnosis in age-related changes. *J Gerontol Nurs* 1988; 14(7):7–12.

Rozovski SJ: Nutrition for older Americans. *Caring* 1984; 3(11):11–17.

Thomson AB, Kulan M: The aging gut. *Canad J Physiol Pharmacol* 1986; 64:30–37.

Watkin DN: The physiology of aging. *Am J Clin Nutrition* (Oct) 1982; 750–756.

7

Impaired Skin Integrity: Decubitus Ulcer

RITA A. FRANTZ, PhD, RN

DECUBITUS ULCERS ARE LOCALIZED AREAS OF CELLULAR necrosis that occur over bony prominences exposed to pressure for a sufficient period of time to cause tissue ischemia. Normal tissue metabolism is dependent on a constant supply of nutrients and removal of waste products. Exposure of tissues to prolonged pressure in excess of capillary pressure inhibits circulation and limits normal exchange of metabolic substrates and waste products. If an inadequate level of circulation persists, cellular metabolism is disrupted and cell death ultimately occurs.

SIGNIFICANCE FOR THE ELDERLY

Decubitus ulcers pose a major threat to the elderly, especially those who are immobilized with chronic health problems. Although improvements in medical care and antibiotic therapy have extended life expectancy for the chronically ill elderly, these medical advances have simultaneously left a large group of patients at high risk for development of decubitus ulcers (Sather et al, 1977). As many as 60,000 people a year die from complications of decubitus ulcers (Kynes, 1986). Surveys indicate that from 3% to 4.5% of patients develop decubitus ulcers during hospitalization, and the occurrence is even more pronounced in long-term care (LTC) facilities, where the incidence rate increases to 11% to 33% of patients (Manley, 1978; Petersen and Bittman, 1971; Williams, 1972). In a survey of 10,000 patients in both hospital and home care settings, 8.8% of the patients were found to have at least one decubitus ulcer, and 70% of those ulcers occurred in individuals over the age of 70 (Barbenel et al, 1977). Similar findings of increased incidence in the elderly are reported by Lowthian (1979), who found that 13.8% of orthopedic patients over the age of 70 had decubitus ulcers. On a hospital unit devoted exclusively to geriatrics, 24% of the 250 patients admitted to the unit developed a decubitus ulcer (Norton et al, 1962). The high incidence level in the elderly was established further by Woodbine (1979), who reported that 24% of patients hospitalized on an orthopedic ward over a 3-month period developed a decubitus ulcer. Seventy-five percent of these ulcers occurred in patients over 78 years of age. A recent survey of a 1776-bed public health service area in Sweden confirms that this continues to persist (Ek and Boman, 1982).

The financial and human costs of decubitus ulcers are enormous. Hospital stays have been shown to increase from 13 days to 28 days for the patient with a decubitus ulcer (Gerson, 1975). The cost in dollars resulting from prolonged hospitalization to treat a single decubitus ulcer was estimated at $15,000 (Sather et al, 1977). Spiraling health care costs over the past 10 years have added dramatically to that amount. However, personal costs are highest for patients who must endure financial hardship, pain, and disability directly attributable to decubitus ulcers.

Although the occurrence of decubitus ulcers is not limited to the geriatric population, biophysiologic changes associated with the aging process increase the risk of skin breakdown in the elderly. As a consequence of aging, the elastin content of the soft tissue decreases, thereby limiting the weight-bearing capability of these structures. The body's mechanical load is shifted to the interstitial fluid and cells. Mechanical pressure squeezes the interstitial fluid out of the region, allowing cells to come in contact with each other. Having lost the cushioning protection of the interstitial fluid, cell membranes may rupture if the external pressure is high. Once the pressure is removed, interstitial fluid pressure may be sufficiently low to cause capillary bursting in the area affected by the external pressure. When such damage occurs, the lymphatic system is unable to clear the area of toxic intracellular debris. The cells in the area are poisoned, and a large area of necrosis will develop (Krouskop, 1983).

The aging process also alters collagen synthesis, which decreases the mechanical strength of soft tissue and renders it more fragile (Krouskop, 1983). Healing of a decubitus ulcer is compromised by decreased collagen synthesis, since collagen is the principal component of scar tissue.

In addition to the biophysiologic changes associated with aging, other contributing factors in decubitus ulcer development occur with greater frequency in the elderly. Chronic illness and the accompanying physical weakness and immobility limit the elderly person's ability to respond to stimuli arising from compressed tissue. Nutritional deficiencies reduce the subcutaneous tissue and muscle bulk, decreasing the mechanical padding between the skin and underlying bone. Hypoproteinemia predisposes the individual to edema formation, which decreases the elasticity, resiliency, and vitality of the skin and slows the rate of oxygen diffusion from the capillaries to the cells. Deficiencies of ascorbic acid, which commonly occur in the elderly, have been shown to accentuate the intensity and rate of tissue destruction that accompanies prolonged compression (Husain, 1953). Incontinence leads to a marked rise in static friction between the surface of the bed linen and the skin, intensifying the destruction of superficial tissue layers and increasing the potential for infection.

CURRENT STATUS OF THE DIAGNOSIS

Maintenance of the integument has been traditionally a primary responsibility of nursing. This is especially critical in the elderly population. Norton et al (1962) report clinical evidence indicating that if the continuity of nursing care lapses for only a brief period, it is sufficient for the immobilized geriatric patient to experience tissue damage. Clearly, the diagnosis and treatment of decubitus ulcers is an essential component of nursing practice.

Although decubitus ulcers have posed a long-standing problem, only recently has nursing attempted to define the problem and its etiologies and signs and symptoms more precisely. Although the lesions are generally understood to be areas of soft tissue necrosis resulting from pressure-induced ischemia, there continues to be controversy regarding proper terminology. Historically, the terms *decubitus ulcer* and *bedsore* were widely used to describe the lesions, since they were observed to occur most frequently in individuals who were confined to bed. Arising from the Latin word *decumbere*, which means "to lie down," the term *decubitus ulcer* implies that the lesion is caused solely by prolonged recumbence. More recent clinical observations have confirmed that the ulcer can occur in any position exposed to excessive pressure. The term *pressure ulcer* or *pressure sore* has evolved to reflect more accurately the etiology of the ulceration rather than the specific body position. The North American Nursing Diagnosis Association (NANDA) lists the diagnosis as Impaired Skin Integrity (Carroll-Johnson, 1989). The NANDA diagnosis is more general than the diagnosis set forth in this chapter, encompassing several types of impairment of skin integrity.

ETIOLOGIES/RELATED FACTORS

Although multiple factors are cited as variables in decubitus ulcer development, most authorities agree that the primary etiologic factor is pressure (Husain, 1953; Kenedi et al, 1976; Kosiak, 1959; Lindan et al, 1965; Reuler and Cooney, 1981; Scales, 1976). Defined as the perpendicular load or force exerted on a given area, the predominant effects of pressure on human tissue occur in the capillary bed (Bennett and Lee, 1985; DeLisa and Mikulic, 1985). The rate of blood flow through tissue capillaries is related to perfusion pressure (Burton and Yamada, 1951). When transmural pressure is reduced, blood flow decreases rapidly, with total cessation of capillary flow occurring at transmural pressures between 20 and 40 mm Hg. This level is considered the critical closing pressure and can be produced by increasing externally applied pressure or by decreasing intravascular hydrostatic pressure. Nichol et al (1951) demonstrated that capillary flow is unstable at low perfusion pressures and that low levels of positive pressure would result in either cessation or temporary reversal of flow.

An additional consideration in the etiology of decubitus ulcers is the duration of the pressure. Animal studies have determined that an inverse relationship exists between the amount of time and the amount of pressure needed to produce pathologic changes in tissue (Kosiak, 1959; Parish et al, 1983). Application of 60 to 70 mm Hg of pressure has been shown to produce pathologic changes in muscle tissue within 1 to 2 hours (Korsiak et al, 1958). Higher pressures can be tolerated for the same or longer periods if pressure is relieved intermittently for as little as 3 to 5 minutes. Husain (1953) noted that low pressure applied for long periods caused more tissue destruction than high pressure maintained for brief periods. He further determined that the degree of injury associated with tissue compression increases when a certain threshold is exceeded. This threshold is the product of pressure multiplied by time. Below a certain pressure–time threshold, release of the compression allows blood to flow back into the tissue, flooding the ischemic cells with nutrients and oxygen and producing a bright red flush called reactive hyperemia. This localized vasodilation has been shown to be a normal compensatory response to temporary ischemia (Lewis and Grant, 1925; Scales, 1976). However, when the pressure–time threshold is exceeded, ischemic injury will continue even with relief of the compression. The region develops interstitial edema, the blood vessels and lymphatic circulation become obstructed, and cellular destruction occurs.

Human tissue can tolerate a relatively high level of pressure as long as the stress or load is uniformly distributed over the whole body (Scales, 1976). However, when pressure is localized, as little as 1 pound per square inch is sufficient to cause tissue destruction, mechanical damage, and blockage of blood vessels (Chow and Odell, 1978). Local presure of greater than 1-1/2 pounds per square inch, or approximately 80 mm Hg, applied over a long period has been documented to cause skin necrosis (Trumble, 1930). Such excesses of pressure have been shown to occur when the body is being supported by a relatively small proportion of the total body surface area. Pressure measurements taken in the supine, prone, and side-lying positions produce readings in excess of the mean capillary pressure at the sacrum, heels, spine, hip, knees, costal margins, and occiput (Lindan et al, 1965; Kosiak, 1959). Movement from a supine to a sitting position increases the pressure over the ischial tuberosities from approximately 70 mm Hg to 300 mm Hg (Kosiak et al, 1958).

The close proximity of the bony prominences to the body surface results in the body's weight being supported by these small surfaces. The combination of pressure and time on bony prominences in excess of the critical pressure–time threshold is the primary etiology of decubitus ulcers.

Other factors have been implicated in the etiology of decubitus ulcers, although their role in producing tissue ischemia is less clear. Several authors cite shearing force as a causative agent in decubitus ulcer formation (Berecek,

1975; Brown et al, 1985; Reichel, 1958). They report clinical examples of sacral ulcers associated with elevation of the head of the bed and the accentuation of pressure on the posterior sacral tissues. As the patient's bony pelvic structure slides downward in bed, the sacral skin surface adheres by friction to the bed linen. The deeper fascia moves downward with the bone while the superficial fascia remains connected to the dermis. This results in stretching and distortion of the vessels that supply the skin from the underlying fascia and muscle. It is thought that if this state is allowed to persist for a sufficient period of time, a decubitus ulcer will result (Reichel, 1958). In the only empirical study of shearing force, Bennett and Lee (1985) report that in the presence of a high level of shear, vascular occlusion will occur with half the amount of pressure needed in the absence of shear. These findings suggest that although shearing force may accentuate the ischemic insult, pressure is the primary etiology of decubitus ulcers.

Friction is another frequently cited factor in the development of decubitus ulcers. Although not generally viewed as a primary factor in the etiology of decubitus ulcers, the force of skin rubbing against another surface strips away the protective stratum corneum and decreases the fibrinolytic reactions in the dermis. Having lost this protective layer, the skin that is subjected to pressure is at greater risk for necrosis. Loss of the stratum corneum is also accompanied by transepidermal water loss, which collects on the body surface. This causes the coefficient of friction to rise, increasing the adherence of the skin to its supporting surface (Lowthian, 1976). When combined with shearing force, the skin-adhering effects of friction tend to intensify the disruption of underlying fascia and blood supply.

Pressure, shearing force, and friction are all identified in the literature as factors that cause decubitus ulcers. However, close scrutiny of the pathologic events that lead to the ischemic injury suggest that the primary etiology is a combination of pressure and time on a bony prominence in excess of a critical pressure–time threshold. The presence of shearing force and friction can intervene and accentuate the effects of pressure, further limiting available circulation to tissues. Similarly, other factors such as nutritional deficiencies, impaired tissue perfusion and presence of infection can limit the pressure–time threshold by compromising the usual vitality of tissue and rendering it more susceptible to ischemic injury.

DEFINING CHARACTERISTICS

The clinical picture of a decubitus ulcer is tied directly to the underlying etiology. The primary location for decubitus ulcers to develop is over bony prominences on the lower half of the body. Sixty-seven percent of ulcers occur on the hips and buttocks and 29% occur on the lower extremities (Peterson and Bittman, 1971; Romm et al, 1982). The anatomic sites most frequently involved are the sacrum, the ischial tuberosities, the greater trochanter of the femur, the lateral malleolus and the heels. However, patients who are immobilized on the operating table for an extended period may exhibit ulceration on the posterior aspects of the scalp. Patients unable to move from a side-lying position may develop skin breakdown on the external ear. Elderly affected with kyphosis are prone to development of vertebral ulcerations. The specific location of a patient's decubitus ulcer will be determined by the position most frequently maintained by the individual (Seiler and Stahelin, 1986).

The defining characteristics of the ulcer itself are a function of the cutaneous changes associated with ischemic tissue injury. Pressure applied over a bony prominence compresses the tissue between the body surface and the underlying bone (Slater, 1985). Thus, the greatest pressure, and therefore the most extensive tissue destruction, occurs in the deep tissue proximal to the bone. Although the initial inflammatory response on the skin surface provides the first indication of ischemic injury, the destructive effects of impaired circulation have already progressed to necrosis of subcutaneous tissue, fat, and muscle (Slater, 1985; Vasconez et al, 1977).

The orderly progression of tissue changes associated with a decubitus ulcer has been most thoroughly described by Shea (1975). The earliest sign of a decubitus ulcer on the skin surface appears as an irregular, poorly defined area of erythema over a bony prominence that does not resolve within 30 minutes of pressure release. As a result of dilation of blood vessels and the accumulation of edema that characterizes the inflammatory response to ischemic injury, the area appears slightly raised, is excessively warm to the touch, and varies in color from pale pink to bright red. Digital compression creates total blanching of the area, which promptly returns to erythema when the finger is released. In normally innervated individuals, the area will be described as tender or painful. Because the epidermis remains intact, removal of the etiology, pressure, will result in disappearance of the erythema within 24 hours and total resolution of the reactive process within 5 to 10 days.

As the intense local pressure continues or repeated prolonged episodes of pressure occur, erythema becomes resistant to blanching with digital compression. The skin color varies from dark red to cyanotic. The acute inflammation extends to a fibroblastic response that disrupts connective tissue. The epidermal skin layer is destroyed, exposing the dermis. The ulcer may extend the full thickness of the dermis to the junction with the subcutaneous fat. Vesicles may be observed subepidermally, although these easily rupture and are rubbed off, leaving a glistening erythema. The edges of the ulcer become progressively more distinct. As the level of circulation in the area decreases, the skin temperature changes from warm to cool, and the area becomes indurated. With removal of the ischemia-producing pressure, the highly vascularized skin layers will heal in 2 to 4 weeks without permanent deformity.

Progression of the ischemia insult leads to reactive fibrosis, inflammation, and retraction of the dermis and subcutaneous fat. Extensive undermining occurs as avascular deep fascia resists penetration of the ischemic necrotic process into the underlying muscle. Bacterial contamination enters the wound, causing thrombosis of small vessels, compounding the ischemia, and creating a chronic inflammatory state. At this level of tissue destruction the ulcer appears as a draining, foul-smelling, irregular, full-thickness wound containing eschar and in some cases necrotic tissue. Extensive undermining of the skin creates a shallow crater that may develop sinus tracts. The wound base usually is not painful. The ulcer edge is distinctly outlined with rolled skin, alternating from dark to light pigmentation. The surrounding skin surface is erythematous, resistant to blanching, indurated, and warm to touch. The accompanying wound infection frequently stimulates a systemic inflammatory response with fever, dehydration, and leukocytosis.

When the ischemic tissue destruction continues unabated, the infectious, necrotic process penetrates the deep fascia, extending into the muscle, joint, and bone. There is rapid extension of the tissue undermining and development of osteomyelitis. Clinically, the ulcer presents as a deep crater with extensive undermining and sinus tract formation. Necrotic tissue is usually present, and foul-smelling drainage is profuse. The presence of bone can be identified at the base of the ulcer. In normally innervated individuals, pain is usually present at the base of the ulcer.

The signs and symptoms of decubitus ulcers are a direct reflection of the prolonged pressure that compromises blood supply to tissues. The changes in tissue morphology follow a predictable course of tissue destruction that can be clearly identified by the signs and symptoms. The integration of the identified etiology and signs and symptoms form the basis for defining the diagnosis.

STATUS OF THE DIAGNOSIS ACCORDING TO NANDA

NANDA's efforts to place the concept of decubitus ulcers within the accepted taxonomy of nursing diagnoses have produced confusing, ambiguous results. Taxonomy I contains two diagnoses that relate to the concept: Impaired Skin Integrity and Impaired Tissue Integrity (NANDA, 1989). Table 7.1 contains the etiologies (related

Table 7.1

Comparison of Etiologies and Signs and Symptoms for Three Nursing Diagnoses Related to Decubitus Ulcers

NURSING DIAGNOSIS	ETIOLOGIES (RELATED FACTORS)	SIGNS AND SYMPTOMS (DEFINING CHARACTERISTICS)
Impaired Skin Integrity*	*External (Environmental)* Hyper or hypothermia; chemical substance; mechanical factors (shearing forces, pressure, restraint); radiation; physical immobilization; humidity *Internal (Somatic)* Medication; altered nutritional state (obesity, emaciation); altered metabolic state; altered circulation; altered sensation; altered pigmentation; skeletal prominence; developmental factors; immunologic deficit; alterations in turgor (change in elasticity)	Disruption of skin surface Destruction of skin layers Invasion of body structure
Impaired Tissue Integrity*	Altered circulation; nutritional deficit/excess; knowledge deficit; impaired physical mobility; irritants; chemical (including body excretions, secretions, medications); thermal (temperature extremes); mechanical (pressure, shear, friction); radiation (including therapeutic radiation)	Damaged or destroyed tissue (cornea, mucous membrane, integumentary, or subcutaneous)
Impaired Skin Integrity: Decubitus Ulcer	Pressure × time Shearing force Friction	*Stage 1* Irregular, poorly defined area of erythema (slightly raised, warm to the touch, pale pink to red, tender or painful) over a bony prominence that persists over 30 minutes after pressure is relieved *Stage 2* Well-defined area of erythema that resists blanching with digital compression; dark red to cyanotic; extends full thickness of dermis; vesicles may be present; cool to the touch *Stage 3* Irregular full-thickness wound extending into underlying muscle; foul-smelling drainage and eschar on wound surface; may contain necrotic tissue, sinus tracts; ulcer edge outlined with rolled skin alternating dark to light pigmentation; surrounding skin appears erythematous, resistant to blanching, indurated, and warm to the touch; may have systemic inflammatory response: fever, dehydration, leukocytosis *Stage 4* Deep crater extending to muscle, joint, and bone; necrotic tissue; foul-smelling drainage; visible bone at base of ulcer; pain at base of ulcer

*Carroll-Johnson R: *Classification of Nursing Diagnoses: Proceedings of the Eighth Conference.* Lippincott, 1989.

factors) and signs and symptoms (defining characteristics) for these diagnoses contrasted with those described in this chapter.

Examination of the definitions for the NANDA diagnoses reveals a lack of specificity in delineating the phenomenon of decubitus ulcer. Both Impaired Skin Integrity and Impaired Tissue Integrity are defined as disruptions in the skin or integument. The defining characteristics are identified broadly as disruptions or destruction of skin tissue. Specific, measurable signs and symptoms have not been delineated, although preliminary work has attempted to operationalize the diagnosis of Impaired Skin Integrity. Cattaneo and Lackey (1987) analyzed open-ended responses given by 42 enterostomal therapy nurses to the statement, "When I see the nursing diagnosis, impaired skin integrity, to me it means..." Following validation by a panel of nurse experts, 28 terms or phrases were identified that define impaired skin integrity. Although this listing provides more specific descriptors of the diagnosis than the NANDA taxonomy, the terms are not conceptually distinct, with signs and symptoms, antecedents, and assessment factors collectively represented. The lack of a narrowly focused diagnosis with a specific underlying etiology further contributes to this state of conceptual confusion.

In this author's view, the diagnostic concept herein described as decubitus ulcer would more accurately be labeled as a pressure sore. This label is conceptually congruent with the well-established etiology of pressure over a bony prominence in excess of a critical pressure–time threshold. The documented pathologic events that occur in the presence of this etiology give rise to a cluster of observable, measurable changes in the skin and underlying tissue. The pattern of these changes would define the signs and symptoms of the diagnosis.

Several authors have attempted to develop a system for assessing and categorizing pressure sores using degree of tissue breakdown as an organizing framework. However, a great deal of disparity exists among the proposed approaches. The number of categories or grades of tissue breakdown varies from three to six (Blom, 1985; Edberg et al, 1973; Jones and Millman, 1986; Morrison, 1984). Some systems use illustrations or visual representations to distinguish characteristics of the various grades, whereas others rely on narrative descriptions. The assessment and classification system developed by Shea (1975), which combines pictorial examples with narrative descriptions, represents the most thorough assessment tool currently available. From this classification system an assessment tool can be devised that allows the nurse in the long-term care setting to grade the level of tissue destruction easily. The following classification scheme shows the assessment parameters for grading decubitus ulcers.

Grade 1: Erythema that persists over 30 minutes after pressure is relieved; no skin breakdown

Grade 2: Erythema that resists blanching with digital compression; skin breakdown involves epidermis to full thickness of dermis

Grade 3: Full thickness wound extends into subcutaneous fat, muscle, or deeper; presence of drainage; ulcer edge outlined with rolled skin; may contain necrotic tissue or sinus tracts

Grade 4: Deep crater extending to muscle, joint and exposed bone; presence of necrotic tissue and foul-smelling drainage

Although this tool provides a simple, easy-to-use method of quantifying level of tissue destruction, there is need to refine the assessment parameters further to allow for identification of discrete improvement or deterioration in the ulcer. To this end, additional research is needed to identify and clinically validate precise descriptors of tissue changes associated with the various stages of injury. These findings would provide the basis for development of an assessment and classification system for pressure sores containing stages; this system could be further divided into levels according to specific tissue characteristics. Such a system would allow clinicians to assess accurately the progression of ulcer healing or deterioration both within grades and between grades. Having defined the diagnosis to this level of precision, foci for nursing interventions can be delineated that are specific to each level of tissue injury.

CASE STUDY

Impaired Skin Integrity: Decubitus Ulcer

W.B. is a 75-year-old man with T_{4-5} paraplegia secondary to a ruptured thoracic aortic aneurysm 8 years ago. Since that time he has been unable to move his lower extremities and has been confined to bed or to a wheelchair. He requires assistance to shift positions and describes often lying on his left side for several hours at a time.

On admission to the hospital, W.B. had an open wound over the left trochanter that extended through the dermis to the subcutaneous tissue. The floor of the wound was moist and ruby red and contained a small amount of nonodoriferous serous drainage. There was an area of necrotic tissue approximately 1 cm in diameter located in the central portion of the wound. The edges of the wound were relatively distinct. Digitized tracings made of the wound edges revealed a circumference of 20.8 cm and a surface area of 30.3 sq cm. The ulcerated area had been present for 12 months and had been resistant to healing despite trials with several wound-treatment protocols. Wound cultures revealed the presence of a rare gram-negative rod and one colony of *Pseudomonas aeruginosa*. Peripheral tissue surrounding the wound was erythematous, indurated, and warm to the touch. The skin resisted blanching with digital pressure.

The Diagnosis Impairment of Skin Integrity: Decubitus Ulcer was inferred from the clinical data. The patient's report of lying on the left side for extended periods of time established the etiology of pressure over a bony prominence, that is, the greater trochanter. The observed indicators of tissue injury and inflammation in the area overlying the greater trochanter correspond with known signs of a decubitus ulcer.

NURSING INTERVENTIONS

The primary objective in the treatment of decubitus ulcer is the promotion of circulation to the ischemic tissue. Adequate circulation is a vital element in creating an optimum environment for decubitus ulcer healing, since the substrates essential to normal healing are carried by the blood (Hunt, 1980). Although a myriad of devices, techniques, and topical agents have been employed in the treatment of decubitus ulcers, no one form of therapy has been found to be totally effective. Miller and Sachs (1974) suggested that adjunctive therapies for decubitus ulcers are rarely beneficial unless pressure is reduced, allowing a return of adequate blood supply to the tissues. Until recently, there was no known means of enhancing blood supply to tissues by direct stimulation of cutaneous vasodilation. Kaada (1982) demonstrated that application of distant, low-frequency transcutaneous electrical nerve stimulation (TENS) produced marked and prolonged cutaneous vasolidation with patients diagnosed as having Raynaud's disease and diabetic polyneuropathy. Using skin temperature as a measure of peripheral vasodilation, he found a rise in the temperature of ischemic extremities from 22 to 24°C to 31 to 34°C. The latency from the stimulus onset to the abrupt rise in temperature averaged 15 to 30 minutes with a duration of response from 4 to 6 hours. Subsequently, Kaada briefly described three case studies of patients with decubitus ulcers, ranging in size from 115 to 750 sq mm, that were previously resistant to healing for 7 months to 2 years. When TENS was added to their existing modalities of treatment, the ulcers were healed in 8 to 10 weeks (Kaada, 1983).

More recently, enhanced decubitus ulcer healing was demonstrated in six geriatric patients confined to a long-term care facility who were treated with TENS as an adjunct to preexisting treatment (Barron et al, 1985). These ulcers had been treated by conventional methods for 1 to 11 months with minimal improvement. Treatments consisted of microelectro energy force administered percutaneously across the surface of the ulcer three times a week for 3 weeks. Results showed that two of the ulcers had healed before the third week. Of the remaining four decubitus ulcers, the total surface area of three decreased by more than 99%, and the remaining one decreased in size by 55%.

Low-voltage electric current also has been shown to promote wound healing of resistant skin burns (Fakhri and Amin, 1987). In a sample of 20 patients with burns ranging in size from 10 by 5 cm to involvement of most of the lower extremities, TENS was added to their burn care treatment twice weekly until complete healing was achieved. In 19 of 20 subjects, epithelialization was observed at the periphery of the ulcer 3 days after starting the electric therapy. Complete healing of the burn ulcer occurred in all study subjects except one, who was anemic. The time taken for complete healing varied from 2 weeks for the smallest ulcer to 3 months for an ulcer that involved extensive areas of the lower extremities.

Although wound cultures showed a quantitative decrease in the level of infective organisms present after TENS was initiated, epithelialization proceeded regardless of the level of organisms present.

Although these preliminary studies suggest beneficial effects from using TENS as an adjunct in decubitus ulcer treatment, the mechanism of action of electric therapy remains unknown. Kaada (1982) proposes that the beneficial effects of TENS on ulcer healing are likely due to activation of normal physiologic vasodilatory reflexes and neurohumoral agent release either in the brain or locally in the peripheral vessels, which is induced by cutaneous nerve stimulation. This response was found to be maximized when cutaneous stimulation was applied at a traditional Chinese acupuncture site (ho-ku), located in the web of the hand between the first and second metacarpal bones. It is speculated that stimulation of acupuncture points may activate sympathetic nerve fibers that lie parallel to the vascular structures beneath the acupuncture site (Mannheimer and Lampe, 1984). Vessels in the form of communicating veins that connect superficial and large veins have been located at some acupuncture points (Plummer, 1980). It is hypothesized that the acupuncture point may actually be a minute hole or opening within which neurovascular and/or lymphatic elements are located. Because sympathetic nerve fibers parallel vascular structures, these findings may point to the relationship of acupuncture and autonomic nervous system mediated vasodilation. The resulting vasodilation and increase in blood supply enhances the delivery of oxygen and nutrients to the ulcer for healing.

Fundamental to the treatment of decubitus ulcers is the provision of adequate circulation containing the elements essential to tissue regeneration. Preliminary clinical reports provide encouraging evidence of enhanced decubitus ulcer healing with TENS. Although controlled clinical trials are needed to test this nursing intervention further, application of TENS has the potential to promote ulcer healing by reversing the ischemia-producing effects of pressure.

Circulation to the ischemic ulcer can be further promoted by instituting measures to relieve pressure over the bony prominence. Recently there has been a proliferation of pressure-relieving devices designed to distribute the pressure more evenly over the entire body surface. Although this equipment has been widely adopted in an effort to control surface pressure, there have been few clinical trials to evaluate the relative effectiveness of various devices. Maklebust et al (1986) tested six surfaces purported to be pressure reducing and found only an air-filled bed, a low-air-loss bed, and a special three-layered air cushion that resulted in diminished tissue interface pressure below 32 mm Hg.

Although certain of these devices have been shown to reduce the pressure factor in the pressure–time threshold, primary reliance on such mechanical apparatus may create a false sense of security. At best, such devices will lengthen the time interval before ischemic injury occurs. In order to ensure that circulation is maintained in adequate amounts to preserve tissue integrity, repositioning by tilting the patient 20 to 30 degrees at least every 2 hours is essential (Shea, 1975). These small shifts in body weight reduce the pressure under bony prominences and allow the normal compensatory mechanism of reactive hyperemia to occur. Building on this physiologic principle, a protocol for using informal, unscheduled small shifts of body weight was designed as part of the Conduct and Utilization of Research in Nursing (CURN) project (Horsley, 1981). Clinical trial of the protocol in a long-term care facility demonstrated that small shifts in body weight were effective in reducing the number of decubitus ulcers (Brown et al, 1985). Regardless of the technologic devices used to reduce pressure, a consistently applied protocol of shifting body weight from bony prominences is essential to maintain tissue integrity.

Unscheduled small shifts in body weight can easily be incorporated in routine nursing care. Each time a staff member enters the patient's room he or she can reposition the patient's arm, hip, knee or other body part. This will change the site where a body part contacts a compressing surface. Similarly, body weight can be shifted by raising or lowering a leg or lifting the arms. When a patient is positioned on the right or left side with pillows supporting the back, simply loosening the pillows slightly will shift the patient's weight to a different point on the trochanter and iliac crest and allow circulation to be restored to the previous pressure point. Patients who are mentally alert and physically able can be taught to perform these small shifts in body weight during waking hours or to remind others to perform the shifts. To assist the patient in remembering to carry out these movements, a schedule can be devised that coordinates the needed movements with other regularly occurring stimuli such as daytime television programming.

OUTCOMES

Patient outcomes indicative of enhanced circulation to the ischemic tissue are a reflection of cellular regeneration and repair. In those ulcers in which the ischemic insult has resulted in disruption of the epidermis or deeper tissue layers, fleshy, beefy red projections or granules appear on the surface of the ulcer. This granulation tissue arises as an outgrowth of new capillaries and provides the vascular bed for scar tissue formation. The overall size of the ulcer decreases as the wound edges marginate. The erythema and edema on the skin surface gradually dissipate as adequate circulation returns. Ultimately, the skin surface is restored to a soft, pink, nonpainful state.

Evaluation tools to document the progression of decubitus ulcer healing are notably lacking in the literature. The previously discussed grading systems have the potential to document the progression of healing as well as deterioration. However, their assessment parameters would need to be broadened to include descriptive changes in tissue associated with healing at each level of injury. Additionally, an evaluation tool would need to include some measure of ulcer size. This could be obtained by tracing the ulcer onto a transparent film (Yucel and Basmajian, 1974) and then measuring the ulcer diameter by using a ruler (Lee et al, 1979) or by employing a graduated scale (Van Ort and Gerber, 1976). An evaluation tool that would precisely measure changes in tissue characteristics and ulcer size would provide the most comprehensive documentation of patient outcomes in response to nursing interventions.

CASE STUDY

Nursing Interventions

Nursing interventions to treat W.B.'s decubitus ulcer consisted of application of .25% acetic acid gauze packing to the wound three times a day, application of TENS treatment for 30 minutes three times a day, placement on a low-air-loss bed (Kin-Air-Beta) and shifting of body weight every 2 hours. TENS treatments were administered using a battery-powered dual channel (Medtronic Comfort Wave, Model 7721 UR) TENS that delivers constant square wave pulses by means of two pairs of surface electrodes. One set of electrodes was placed with the negative electrode situated between the first and second metacarpal bone of one hand and the positive electrode situated at the same site on the other hand (the ho-ku point of traditional Chinese acupuncture). A second set of surface electrodes was positioned with the positive and negative electrodes placed immediately superior and inferior to the ulcer edges. Shifting of body weight consisted of adjusting supporting pillows to tilt the patient 20 to 30 degrees from his or her previously assumed position.

Over the 3-week period that the patient was followed, the digitized tracings made of the wound edges showed notable decreases in the circumference and surface area. The circumference decreased from 20.8 cm to 13.2 cm, and the surface area diminished from 30.3 sq cm to 10.5 sq cm. The floor of the ulcer appeared beefy red and was filled with granulation tissue. The previously noted necrotic tissue had disappeared. The erythema and induration on the peripheral tissue surrounding the ulcer dissipated, leaving soft, flesh-toned skin.

SUMMARY

Although decubitus ulcers are a frequently encountered problem in the elderly population, their diagnosis and treatment remain poorly defined. Multiple labels are used to delineate the problem, and treatments consist of various concoctions. Assessment tools fail to document accurately the progression of tissue injury or healing. To resolve this theoretical confusion, future efforts to conceptualize the body of knowledge related to decubitus ulcers should be organized to articulate with the physiologic events known to be associated with their occurrence. Such an organization of knowledge would clearly define meaningful diagnostic labels based on measurable signs and symptoms and a conceptually congruent etiology. The systematic use of such a taxonomy would delineate the foci for nursing interventions and suggest a logical scientific rationale for their application.

References

Barbenal JC et al: Incidence of pressure-sores in the greater Glasgow Health Board Area. *Lancet* 1977; II(8037):548-550.

Barron JJ, Jacobson WE, Tidd G: Treatment of decubitus ulcers: A new approach. *Minn Med* 1985; 68:103-106.

Bennett L, Lee BY: Pressure versus shear in pressure sore causation. In: *Chronic Ulcers of the Skin.* McGraw-Hill, 1985.

Berecek KH: Etiology of decubitus ulcers. *Nurs Clin North Am* 1975; 10:157-170.

Blom MF: Dramatic decrease in decubitus ulcers. *Geriatr Nurs* (Mar/Apr) 1985; 84-87.

Brown MM et al: Nursing innovations for prevention of decubitus ulcers in long-term care facilities. *Plast Surg Nurs* 1985; 5:57-60.

Burton AC, Yamada S: Relation between blood pressure and flow in the human forearm. *J Applied Physiol* 1951; 4:329-339.

Carroll-Johnson R (editor): *Classification of Nursing Diagnoses: Proceedings of the Eighth Conference.* Lippincott, 1989.

Cattaneo CJ, Lackey NR: Impaired skin integrity. Pages 129-135 in: *Classification of Nursing Diagnoses: Proceedings of the Seventh Conference.* McLane AM (editor). Mosby, 1987.

Chow WW, Odell EI: Deformations and stress in soft body tissues of a sitting person. *Biomed Engineer* 1978; 100:79-82.

DeLisa JA, Mikulic MA: Pressure ulcers—what to do if prevention fails. *Postgrad Med* 1985; 77(6):209-220.

Edberg E et al: Prevention and treatment of pressure sores. *Phys Ther* 1973; 53:246-252.

Ek AC, Boman G: A descriptive study of pressure sores: The prevalence of pressure sores and the characteristics of patients. *J Adv Nurs* 1982; 7:51-56.

Fakhri O, Amin MA: The effect of low-voltage electric therapy on healing of resistant skin burns. *J Burn Care Rehab* 1987; 8:15-18.

Gerson LW: The incidence of pressure sores in active treatment hospitals. *Int J Nurs Stud* 1975; 12:201-204.

Horsley JA: *Preventing Decubitus Ulcers: CURN Project.* Grune and Stratton, 1981.

Hunt TK: *Wound Healing and Wound Infection: Theory and Surgical Practice.* Appleton-Century-Crofts, 1980.

Husain T: An experimental study of some pressure effects on tissues with reference to the bedsore problem. *J Pathol Bacteriol* 1953; 66:347-358.

Jones PL, Millman A: A three-part system to combat pressure sores. *Geriatr Nurs* (Mar/Apr) 1986; 78-83.

Kaada B: Vasodilation induced by transcutaneous nerve stimulation in peripheral ischemia (Raynaud's phenomenon and diabetic polyneuropathy). *Europ Heart J* 1982; 3:303-307.

Kaada B: Promoted healing of chronic ulceration by transcutaneous nerve stimulation (TNS). *VASA* 1983; 12:262-263.

Kenedi RM, Cowden JM, Scales JT (editors): *Bedsore Biomechanics.* University Park Press, 1976.

Korsiak M: Etiology and pathology of ischemic ulcers. *Arch Phys Med Rehab* 1959; 40:62-69.

Kosiak M et al: Evaluation of pressure as a factor in the production of ischial ulcers. *Arch Phys Med Rehab* 1958; 39:623-629.

Krouskop TA: A synthesis of the factors that contribute to pressure sore formation. *Med Hypoth* 1983; 11:255-267.

Kynes P: A new perspective on pressure sore prevention. *J Enterost Ther* 1986; 13:42-43.

Lee BY, Trainor FS, Thoden WR: Topical application of povidone iodine in the management of decubitus and stasis ulcers. *J Geriatr Soc* 1979; 27:302-306.

Lewis T, Grant RT: Observations upon reactive hyperemia in man. *Heart* 1925; 12:73-120.

Lindan O, Greenway RM, Piazza JM: Pressure distribution on the surface of the human body. *Arch Phys Med Rehab* 1965; 46:378-385.

Lowthian P: Underpads in the prevention of decubiti. In: *Bedsore Biomechanics.* Kenedi RM, Cowden JM, Scales JT (editors). University of Park Press, 1976.

Lowthian P: Pressure sore prevalence. *Nurs Times* 1979; 75:358-360.

Maklebust J, Mondoux L, Sieggreen M: Pressure relief characteristics of various support surfaces used in prevention and treatment of pressure ulcers. *J Enterost Ther* 1986; 14:85-89.

Manley MT: Incidence, contributing factors and costs of pressure sores. *S Afr Med J* 1978; 53:217-222.

Mannheimer J, Lampe G: *Clinical Transcutaneous Electrical Nerve Stimulation.* Davis, 1984.

Miller ME, Sachs ML: *About Bedsores: What You Need to Know to Help Prevent and Treat Them.* Lippincott, 1974.

Morrison S: Monitoring decubitus ulcers: A monthly survey method. *ORB* (Apr) 1984; 112–123.

NANDA: *Taxonomy I Revised–1989 With Official Diagnostic Categories.* NANDA, 1989.

Nichol J et al: Fundamental instability of small blood vessels and critical closing pressures in vascular beds. *Am J Physiol* 1951; 164:330–344.

Norton D, McLoren R, Exton-Smith AN: *An Investigation of Geriatric Nursing Problems in Hospitals.* London: National Corporation for the Care of Old People, 1962.

Parish LC, Witkowski JA, Crissey JT: *The Decubitus Ulcer.* Masson, 1983.

Petersen NC, Bittman S: The epidemiology of pressure sores. *Scand J Plast Reconstr Surg* 1971; 5:62–66.

Plummer JP: Anatomical findings at acupuncture loci. *Am J Chinese Med* 1980; 8:170.

Reichel SM: Shearing forces as a factor in decubitus ulcers in paraplegics. *JAMA* 1958; 166:172–175.

Reuler JB, Cooney TG: The pressure sore: Pathophysiology and principles of management. *Ann Intern Med* 1981; 94:661–666.

Romm S et al: Pressure sores: State of the art. *Tx Med* (Apr) 1982; 78:52–60.

Sather MR, Weber CE, George J: Pressure sores and the spinal cord injury patient. *Drug Intell Clin Pharm* 1977; 11:154–168.

Scales JT: Pressure on the patient. Pages 11–17 in: *Bedsore Biomechanics.* Kenedi RM, Cowden JM, Scales JT (editors). Macmillan, 1976.

Seiler WO, Stahelin HB: Recent findings on decubitus ulcer pathology: Implications for care. *Geriatrics* 1986; 41:47–57.

Shea JD: Pressure sores: Classification and management. *Clin Orthop* 1975; 112:89–100.

Slater H: *Pressure Sores in the Elderly.* Synapse, 1985.

Trumble HC: The skin tolerance for pressure and pressure sores. *Med J Aust* 1930; 2:724.

Van Ort SR, Gerber RM: Topical application of insulin in the treatment of decubitus ulcers. A pilot study. *Nurs Res* 1976; 25:9–12.

Vasconez L, Schneider WJ, Jurkiewicz MJ: Pressure sores. *Curr Prob Surg* 1977; 14(4):1–62.

Williams A: A study of factors contributing to skin breakdown. *Nurs Res* 1972; 21:238–243.

Woodbine A: A survey in McClesfield. *Nurs Times* 1979; 75: 1128–1132.

Yucel VF, Basmajian JM: Decubitus ulcers: Healing effect of an enzymatic spray. *Arch Phys Med Rehab* 1974; 55:517–519.

8

Impaired Skin Integrity: Dry Skin

MARY A. HARDY, PhD, RN, C

DRY SKIN, COMMONLY REFERRED TO AS XEROSIS, IS A problem frequently experienced by elderly persons (Eliopoulos, 1979; Parent, 1985), although the statistics vary somewhat between studies. In a study of 160 subjects over the age of 64, more than three fourths had dry, scaly skin (Tindall and Smith, 1963). Frantz and Kinney (1986) found that 59% of a sample of retirement center residents between the ages of 65 and 97 had dry skin. A recent study of 68 noninstitutionalized elderly found that pruritus was the most frequent complaint (29%), xerosis was present in 85%, and there was very little association between the objective finding of xerosis by a dermatologist and patient complaint (Beauregard and Gilchrest, 1987).

Care of the integument has been within the defined scope of nursing practice since Nightingale (1914). Nightingale defined skin care as "personal cleanliness," suggesting that the ideal bath incorporates soap, rubbing, and a large quantity of soft water that the skin will absorb. Assessment and treatment of the patient's skin has traditionally centered around cleanliness, the condition of the skin being a sign of overall health. More recently, nursing assessment has included a systematic measure of the condition of the skin and scalp, of which "dryness" is one factor (Luckmann and Sorensen, 1974;1252).

The treatment, or more accurately the care of the skin, was described quite extensively by Harmer and Henderson (1960;324–338). The nurse's responsibility in the care of the skin focused on bathing, lubricating, and massaging. Although Harmer and Henderson noted the decreased glandular and circulatory functioning of aging, the care needs of the elderly were not stated to vary from the treatment of others, except in the frequency of bathing and the application of oils. As problems associated with aging have gained more attention in the literature, however, nursing interventions specific to the elderly have been addressed (Burnside, 1976; Fitzsimmons, 1983; Hogstel, 1983).

The problem of dry skin causes primary discomforts such as itching, burning, scaling, and cracking (Atkins, 1977; DeLancey and North, 1983) and, if severe, may result in a compromised self-image and social isolation for elderly persons (Jowett and Ryan, 1985). It is important that nurses diagnose and treat the primary effects of dry skin as well as the disturbances in self-perception, self-concept, and role that may occur as a result. In addition, nurses must be aware that if primary effects are untreated, secondary effects such as infection and increased anxiety/agitation may further complicate the diagnosis and treatment of dry skin.

SIGNIFICANCE FOR THE ELDERLY

A significant amount of literature describes the major physiologic factors of aging that contribute to the problem of dry skin for the elderly: reduced activity of the sebaceous glands (Cornell, 1986; Dotz and Berman, 1984; Hogstel, 1983; Spoor, 1958); loss of supportive connective tissue (Cornell, 1986); and evaporation of moisture from the skin (Shelley and Shelley, 1982; Walther and Harber, 1984). In addition, the elderly are somewhat more at risk for dry skin because of its association with an inadequate diet (Atkins, 1977); with consumption of medications such as sulfonamides, thiazides, phenothiazines, and quinidine (Walther and Harber, 1984); with pathologies related to diseases such as diabetes and Parkinsonism (Sutton and Waisman, 1975); and with lack of humidity (Shelley and Shelley, 1982), which may occur in the environment of institutionalized and isolated persons.

A recent study, however, examined the association of dry skin in the elderly with many of the above variables and posed questions concerning the true nature and etiologies of dry skin. Frantz and Kinney (1986) used a sample of 76 elderly individuals between the ages of 65 and 97 in long-term care facilities or retirement homes to test the relationship between dry skin and sebum content. Although 59% of the subjects had dry skin, no significant relationships were found between age, gender, fluid and nutritional intake, bathing, medication history, or sebum content and the occurrence of dry skin. However, subjects within the sample who were defined as having dry skin experienced more severe dry skin if they had been more frequently exposed to the sun and if they were 80 years of age or older. Lastly, subjects with dry skin used significantly more lotions to treat their skin, and those with the more severe levels of dry skin bathed less frequently. This finding is not surprising in view of commonly held beliefs that the application of moistening agents and decreased bathing are effective treatments for dry skin. The findings of this study point out the prevalence of the problem, help in isolating contributing factors, and describe some of the treatment choices made by those who suffer from dry skin. Although dry skin can be a problem at all ages, the functional abilities of the elderly make nursing interventions to treat the problem of dry skin a much more complex process.

CURRENT STATUS OF THE DIAGNOSIS

Conceptual Considerations

The diagnoses Impaired Skin Integrity: Actual and Impaired Skin Integrity: Potential were accepted for testing by the North American Nursing Diagnosis Association (NANDA) in 1975 (Carpenito, 1987). Although Carpenito (1987;7) indicated that the two diagnoses were combined on NANDA's amended list as "Skin Integrity, Impairment of," both diagnoses appear in the Proceedings of the Eighth Conference (Carroll-Johnson, 1989). One clue to explain this apparent contradiction was a comment made by Kim and associates (1984;55) about the diagnosis Impaired Skin Integrity: Potential: "This diagnosis remains the same as that of 1978, but the group recommended further development." Between 1975 and 1989 little change has taken place in the conceptualization of the diagnosis except that etiologies have become risk factors.

However, the subdiagnosis Impaired Skin Integrity: Dry Skin is not on the list of diagnoses accepted for testing by NANDA (Carroll-Johnson, 1989). Kim and associates (1984) treat the diagnosis Impaired Skin Integrity: Actual in a similar way to the diagnosis published by NANDA (Carroll-Johnson, 1989). Etiologies and risk factors are categorized as external or internal. Major defining characteristics are (1) disruption of skin surface; (2) destruction of skin layers; and (3) invasion of body surface (Carroll-Johnson, 1989; Kim et a1, 1984).

Examination of the current conceptualization of the overall diagnosis Impaired Skin Integrity and of Carpenito's (1983) subdiagnosis Impaired Skin Integrity related to pruritus is important to a discussion of dry skin because of the appearance of etiologies, defining characteristics, and approaches commonly described in the literature as pertinent to dry skin. For instance, the etiologies for the diagnosis Impaired Skin Integrity related to pruritus include dehydration, lack of humidity, medication regimen, and aging. Furthermore, dry skin is one of the "causative and contributing factors" associated with the subdiagnosis Impaired Skin Integrity related to pruritus. Lastly, the interventions outlined for this etiology are some of those that are identified in the literature as specific to the treatment of dry skin: bathing, lubricating, and handling of linens.

Pruritus is often experienced by persons with anxiety, allergies, dry skin, or infection. The ineffective treatment of these etiologies may result in further impaired skin integrity in the form of skin breakdown and secondary complications. A more useful approach to the statement and conceptual development of the diagnosis Impaired Skin Integrity would be to consider pruritus as a defining characteristic: "Impaired Skin Integrity, Potential for, related to infection as evidenced by pruritus and expressed need to scratch." Or pruritus may be seen as an etiology of Impaired Skin Integrity in untreated skin dryness: "Impaired Skin Integrity related to dry skin as evidenced by pruritus, scratching, and ecchymosis in areas of scratching."

Some authors have viewed pruritus as a symptom. "Mild to severe pruritus is a predominant feature leading to scratching and subsequent excoriations. Without treatment, eczematoid changes may occur; secondary infections which can be confirmed by KOH prep or culture may develop" (Pearson and Kotthof, 1979;348). This approach is in keeping with the current dermatologic and nursing literature, which most often have treated pruritus as an accompanying symptom of dry skin (Parent, 1985; Parth and Kapke, 1983). The view of pruritus as a symptom of dry skin promotes further differentiation and refinement of the diagnosis Impaired Skin Integrity and the subdiagnosis Impaired Skin Integrity: Dry Skin and the relevant etiologies, defining characteristics, and interventions. The subdiagnosis statement may appear in this way: "Impaired Skin Integrity: Dry Skin related to inadequate hydration as evidenced by scaling, fissuring, and pruritus on lower legs and arms." Differences in the conceptualization of the diagnosis Impaired Skin Integrity by Kim and associates (1984) and Carpenito (1987) and the author's conceptualization of the diagnosis Impaired Skin Integrity: Dry Skin are illustrated in Table 8.1.

ETIOLOGIES/RELATED FACTORS

The treatment of skin dryness requires an examination of the etiologies/related factors. Carpenito (1987) has explicated the etiologic and contributing factors for impaired skin integrity into three categories: pathophysiologic, situational, and maturational. Within all three categories there are factors that have been associated with dry skin: too frequent bathing and use of soap (Gioiella and Bevil, 1985; Parent, 1985; Walther and Harber, 1984); excessive perspiration (Cornell, 1986); seasonal change and exposure to the sun (Arndt, 1983; Parth and Kapke, 1983); diabetes (Sutton and Waisman, 1975); dehydration (Parent, 1985); medications, steroid therapy (Atkins, 1977; Walther and Harber, 1984); smoking (Fitzsimmons, 1983); lack of humidity (Fenske, 1982; Gaul and Underwood, 1951; Hogstel, 1983; Parent, 1985); stress (Atkins, 1977); and maturation related to aging (Cornell, 1986; Spoor, 1958; Weiner et al, 1973). Carpenito identifies pruritus as a defining characteristic of impaired skin integrity as well as an etiology.

Table 8.1

Comparison of Conceptualization of Diagnoses, Etiologies, and Defining Characteristics

DIAGNOSIS	ETIOLOGIES	DEFINING CHARACTERISTICS
Impairment of Skin Integrity: Actual	Pathologic: Dehydration	Denuded skin
	Situational: Environmental Humidity	Erythema
		Lesions (primary and secondary)
	Maturational: Elderly: dryness	Pruritus
		Disruptions of skin layer (incision, pressure sores, etc)
Impairment of Skin Integrity	Pruritus	Subjective: reports itching
		Objective: scratch marks, rash, lesions, irritability
(Carpenito, 1987)		
Skin Integrity, Impairment of: Actual	External:	Disruption of skin
	Chemical substance	Destruction of skin layers
	Mechanical factors	Invasion of body structures
	shearing forces	
	pressure	
	restraint	
	Humidity	
	Internal:	
	Medication	
	Altered circulation	
	Developmental factors	
	Alternations in skin turgor	
(Kim et al, 1984)		
Impaired Skin Integrity:Dry Skin	Inadequate environmental humidity	Flaking skin
	Inadequate hydration of skin	Cracking
	Dehydration	Fissuring of skin
	Maturation of skin	Erythema
	Exposure to strong soaps	Scaling
(Hardy, 1987)		

The existence of confounding dermatoses, either primary or secondary to the skin dryness, make determination of the validity of the diagnosis of skin dryness difficult. Arndt (1983) and Epstein (1983) both note the difficulty of determining the differential diagnosis of the xerosis from other primary and secondary pathologies. Pellerano (1985;215) states, "Management of skin diseases thus proves a very thorny problem, primarily owing to the difficulty in detecting the etiological agent responsible for the disease, and secondarily because of the ever-present risk that a simple lesion may be liable to complications."

In addition to the confounding dermatoses that may occur concurrently with or as a result of untreated dry skin, there must be an examination of the other physiologic and psychosocial conditions that must be ruled out as potential etiologies. Interdisciplinary collaboration may be necessary in the assessment of skin condition and in ruling out of pathology requiring medical intervention.

DEFINING CHARACTERISTICS

Signs and symptoms most often identified in the literature for the diagnosis of dry skin are: (1) leathery feeling; (2) itching; (3) flakiness; (4) chapping; (5) inflammation on occasion; and (6) fissuring, particularly of anterior plantar surfaces and heels (Cornell, 1986; Gioiella and Bevil, 1985; Parent, 1985; Weiner et al, 1973). As illustrated in Assessment Guide 8.1, Hardy (1987) used a construct of dry skin that included redness, scaling, cracking, and flaking.

ASSESSMENT

An accurate and thorough assessment and history, including subjective and objective data, is necessary to determine which etiologies are operating in any specific situation. At this time attention will be focused on the assessment of the skin with an understanding that factors such as health and medical history may have a bearing on the conclusions drawn by the nurse as a result of the examination of all systems. It is important to note that the use of the term *skin* in this chapter refers to the face, neck, trunk, and extremities. Although the scalp is contiguous to the integument, it is not commonly included in the assessment or treatment of skin per se, but is seen as separate and related to the hair. Dry scalp and hair in the elderly are conditions that merit further investigation and refinement.

Skin assessment has received considerable attention in the nursing literature during the last decade. Hannigan (1978) outlined a thorough history and assessment process with an emphasis on the integumentary system. Hannigan included, as do most such guides, data collection related to

chronology, onset, duration, frequency, severity, environment in which symptoms occur, and evaluation of skin, hair, nail color, vascularity, lesions, edema, moisture, temperature, texture, thickness, mobility, and turgor. Malkiewicz (1981) later refined the assessment of the integumentary system by suggesting specific questions understood by the client as a mechanism for eliciting accurate, usable data and described common skin lesions and their assessment. Pearson and Kotthoff (1979) described clinical protocols for the geriatric client and provided a detailed history format, assessment method, and rationale, as well as common problems and treatments for the integumentary system. A system of documenting the location of skin lesions may incorporate an anatomic outline of the body with problem areas shaded on the outline and accompanied by detailed narrative descriptions (Urosevich, 1981). More recently, DeLancey and North (1983) described skin assessment in narrative terms, outlining physical and psychosocial examination guidelines. Hogstel (1983), Parth and Kapke (1983), and Gioiella and Bevil (1985) described skin assessment for the elderly and common skin changes that accompany aging.

The anatomic location of usual skin dryness varies by author. Parent (1985;49) states that "dry skin is usually seen on the extremities, although the trunk and face may be affected," whereas Arndt (1983) states that the anterior tibia, the dorsa of the hands, and the forearms are the most frequent sites. Dotz and Berman (1984) state that dry skin is most likely to appear as ill-defined patches all over the body but that it is most frequently seen on the hands and shins. The feet may be another source of dryness. Two studies outlined specific assessment of the feet of the elderly and may be particularly useful in developing the body of knowledge related to dry skin assessment and treatment (Brown et al, 1982; King, 1978). None of the assessment tools reported in the literature provide data about reliability or validity testing.

Frantz and Kinney (1986) reported a systematic assessment of dry skin, and although the tool was not outlined in detail in the report of the study and no reliability and validity measures were provided, the authors made a copy of the tool available. The Skin Condition Data Form (SCDF) included data collection on prescription and over-the-counter medications currently in use, interview questions regarding the occurrence of dry skin, including itching, and history related to endogenous and exogenous factors associated with dry skin and bathing practices (Frantz and Kinney, 1986).

Hardy (1987) determined the interrater reliability and the content and criterion validity of an adapted form of the SCDF tool (shown in Assessment Guide 8.1).

Percents agreement between the raters on history, current skin practices, and observed dryness were 87.3%, 62.5%, and 68% respectively. The fact that many of the subjects were cognitively impaired and much of the history and current practice information came from clinical records and nursing staff may have contributed to somewhat low interrater agreement.

CASE STUDY

Impaired Skin Integrity: Dry Skin

Bill is an 80-year-old black man who has been in a nursing home for 20 years. Bill was admitted following a cerebrovascular accident (CVA), which severely affected his left side. No family was available to care for him. Bill is currently taking Methyldopa 250 mg every morning and Reglan 10 mg b.i.d. because choking while eating is often followed by emesis. The Reglan has decreased these episodes. Bill also takes Diazide 2 caps every morning and K-lor 40 mEq every morning. Sebulex shampoo is prescribed for weekly shampoo, and although he is bathed weekly without soap, Lachydrin ointment is applied to areas of dry skin daily: legs, arms, face, and scalp.

Bill's dry skin is characterized as flaking and scaling. No seasonal differences have been observed. Although treated with Sebulex and Lachydrin, few benefits have been seen. Potential for Impaired Skin Integrity: Pressure Sores because of limited mobility and activity is treated with the application of lotion to and rubbing of reddened areas. Only one open skin area has occurred on the coccyx, and it was cleared with more frequent turning.

Bill is turned every 2 hours and is up in a wheelchair for about 2 hours each day. There is some limited use of his right side, and on good days he can wave, attempt to speak, and partially feed himself. Bill requires the assistance of two persons to pivot transfer. The environmental humidity of the unit on which he resides is measured monthly to be maintained at between 40% and 50%. When able to go out, Bill likes to fish and bowl and does so when he is able approximately every other month. In addition, in the summer Bill is outside for about 10 minutes twice a month.

Nutritionally, Bill suffers from periodic episodes of decreased alertness, choking, visual impairment, limited self-feeding and hyperextended neck, which interfere with ingestion of liquid and solid food. Bill ordinarily eats most of what is offered on a 2- to 4-gram sodium pureed diet, but he requires staff feeding. Fluid intake has, however, become a problem in the past year because of losses in functional abilities, increasing episodes of impaired alertness, and choking. The Reglan seems to have helped this, although fluids are still less than 2000 cc per day. Hospitalization for dehydration has occurred at least once in the past 10 months, and during that time Bill's weight dropped steadily from 158 to 150 pounds.

NURSING DIAGNOSIS

The nursing diagnosis for Bill is Impaired Skin Integrity: Dry Skin related to systemic dehydration; secondary to inadequate fluid intake, antihypertensive medication regimen, and inadequate external hydration secondary to average humidity of 45% and evaporation, as evidenced by flaking, scaling, and redness of face and scalp and flaking and scaling of skin on legs and arms.

NURSING INTERVENTIONS

Research Base

The diagnosis Impaired Skin Integrity: Dry Skin is not among NANDA's (Carroll-Johnson, 1989) list of accepted diagnoses. The research base for this diagnosis is in need of development and evaluation. Although there is considerable literature available to the nurse prescribing treatments for dry skin in the elderly, research in this area is minimal. Three studies were found in the literature, one in nursing, on the treatment of dry skin.

Spoor (1958;3299) analyzed the effects of a water-dispersible oil as an additive for the bath in the treatment of patients with "dry, itchy, scaly, lichenified skin." Spoor reported successful therapeutic effect and personal acceptance of the treatment in 10 of the 12 subjects described. Weiner et al (1973) reported limited success in the treatment of dry skin over a wide geographic area with a topical moisturizing and lubricating lotion. The Weiner sample consisted of 153 persons, most of whom were over the age of 50. The findings showed excellent results in 25 cases, good results in 81 cases, fair results in 35 cases and poor results in 12 cases. Lastly, Brown et al (1982) tested the use of 10-minute foot soaks followed by mineral oil application for the treatment of skin dryness of the feet in 31 long-term care residents. An analysis of the treatment, which was introduced three times per week for a total of 2 weeks, resulted in significant ($p < .01$) improvement in the skin condition of the feet when the Wilcoxon signed-rank statistical test was applied to pre- and posttest measures of skin dryness for all subjects.

Literature Review

Although there has been inconclusive evidence of the cause of many of the changes that take place in the skin of aging persons, loss of supportive connective tissue and inefficient output of secretory glands have received most of the blame for skin dryness in the elderly (Walther and Harber, 1984). Explication of these dermatologic changes associated with aging has received considerable attention in the dermatology literature. The overwhelming conclusion of this literature is that dry skin in the elderly can be treated. The specific measures used have one common theme—moisture retention. Moisture may be added to the skin through bathing, and its evaporation can be prevented by the application of an occluding agent.

Intervention Prescription

The literature review and the research base suggest that appropriate intervention for the treatment of dry skin is to maintain a systematic bathing procedure, a controlled environmental humidity at 60% (Arndt, 1983; Parth and Kapke, 1983) or more (Gaul and Underwood, 1951; Parent, 1985; Weiner et al, 1973), and limited sun exposure. Specifically, the bathing procedure should include:

1. Immersing affected areas into water that is 90–100° (Arndt, 1983; Dotz and Berman, 1984; Parth and Kapke, 1983; Pearson and Kotthof, 1979) in the form of a deep-water bath or shower for 10 to 15 minutes
2. Bathing at a frequency of between daily and twice weekly
3. Bathing with a superfatted, mild soap used for cleansing
4. Patting dry (Anderson, 1971) with cotton linen that has been rinsed adequately to prevent static and retention of detergents (Cornell, 1986; Fitzsimmons, 1983)
5. Applying an occluding agent immediately while the skin is still wet and the individual is still in the humidity of the bathing room
6. Dressing in loose-fitting cotton clothing (Arndt, 1983; Cornell, 1986)

The variables associated with the preceding treatment regimen that require individualization are those that relate to the feasibility of tub bathing for many elderly persons, the determination of the requisite frequency of effective treatment, and the selection of a mild bath soap and an after-bath occlusive agent. Although these may seem "routine" measures, systematic attention and a research base are needed to treat dry skin in the elderly effectively.

Bath Procedure

The use of a bedbath or partial bath in the treatment of dry skin is suggested by Walther and Harber (1984). This has not been tested, however, and would intuitively not allow for the absorption of significant amounts of water to moisturize the skin effectively. Spoor (1958) tested the use of a bathtub or total immersion of affected areas, and Brown et al (1982) tested the use of an immersion in the form of foot soaks with significant beneficial effects. In many cases, however, total immersion may not be practical. In these instances, a "porta-bath," illustrated in Figure 8.1, can be used.

The porta-bath is a litter with flexible vinyl sides that allow the patient to be transferred to and from the litter easily. The sides are raised to form the "tub" and to serve as a safety measure during transportation to the bathing room. The use of such a bathing device allows for immersion of most of the body and can incorporate a modified shower or rinse of the bath water over the nonimmersed areas. In cases in which such a modified bathtub is not possible, a shower, perhaps with some sort of assistive device, may be useful (Epstein, 1983). The nurse should use bathtubs that allow for safe total body immersion, for example, in the form of a whirlpool, for individuals for whom a traditional bath, porta-bath, or shower are not possible. Assistive devices such as lifts may be necessary for persons with certain debilitations; (eg, significant contractures or obesity).

Frequency of Bathing

Although there is agreement that too-frequent bathing should be avoided, there is little direction concerning what frequency is optimal. Arndt (1983) suggests bathing every 1 to 2 days; Hogstel (1983) suggests a full bath two to three times a week and a partial bath daily, Fenske (1982) makes no specific recommendation on frequency but suggests that the use of soap be restricted to malodorous areas. Walther and Harber (1984) note that the elderly often bathe too frequently; they recommend that sponge baths be substituted for tub bathing but recommend no specific frequency. Epstein (1983) suggests, however, that unless they are bathing more than once daily, there is no reason for those with dry skin to cut down on bathing. Pearson and Kotthof (1979) go somewhat further, suggesting the soaking or submerging of affected areas for 10 to 15 minutes but do not prescribe a frequency. Beauregard and Gilchrest (1987) found that subjects aged younger than 80 had a tendency to bathe somewhat more frequently (6.1 versus 5.4 baths or showers per week) and that subjects over 80 had a tendency to use either the tub or the shower exclusively, whereas those younger than 80 used both. Of the 68 community dwelling subjects aged younger than 80, 2.4% required assistance in bathing or showering, whereas 17.4% aged 80 or older required assistance.

The frequency of bathing, because of a lack of conclusive data on the effectiveness of specific choices, may be determined by the functional abilities of the resident and the related feasibility, ease, and safety associated with those choices. For instance, individuals who are not able to assist with their own baths or who require the use of a lift into the tub or shower may begin with a prescribed frequency of three times weekly. The effectiveness of this frequency may then be evaluated: The frequency may be determined to be appropriate or may need to be decreased or increased. In contrast, an

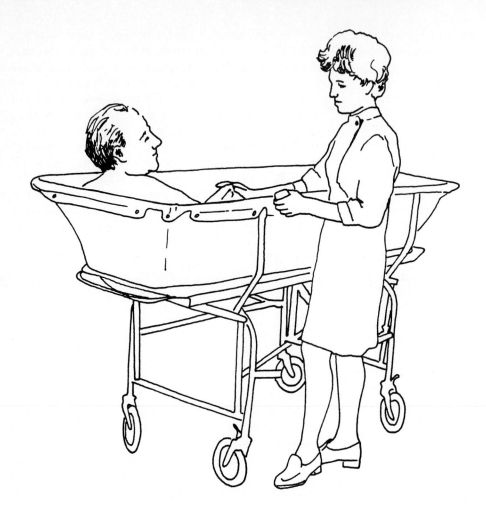

Figure 8.1
Portabath.

individual who is ambulatory and has stayed away from tub bathing because it was associated with dry skin may benefit and prefer daily bathing with the preceding protocol. This is an area that requires testing on an individual basis by the client and the nurse and on a broader basis through systematic research, in order to understand the empirical implications of bathing frequency.

Bath Soap

The characteristics of the desirable soap for use by the elderly are unanimous: mild, superfatted, nondetergent, nonperfumed, nonhexachlorophine (Anderson, 1971; Arndt, 1983; Atkins, 1977; Cornell, 1986; Fitzsimmons, 1983; Fenske, 1982; Hogstel, 1983; Parent, 1985; Pearson and Kotthof, 1979). The specific brands of such soaps include Basis, Dove, Tone, Caress (Walther and Harber, 1984), Neutrogena, and Emulave (Parth and Kapke, 1983). Only Dove was tested in a laboratory study and found to have been less "irritating" than other soaps

(Frosch and Kligman, 1979). This is another area of inquiry that requires attention by the nursing community.

After-Bath Occlusive Agent

There is considerable agreement that the use of high-potency corticosteroid ointments may lead to even further epidermal atrophy than is associated with aging (Cornell, 1986; Fenske, 1982; Parent, 1985). The application of creams containing urea or lactic acid may be of some benefit in maintaining moist, smooth skin (Pearson and Kotthof, 1979), but the continued use of such products may result in irritation (Epstein, 1983).

An oil base is consistently suggested as the primary ingredient or factor in the agent that is applied immediately after bathing when skin is hydrated (Arndt, 1983; Cornell, 1986; Epstein, 1983; Parent, 1985; Parth and Kapke, 1983; Pearson and Kotthof, 1979; Walther and Harber, 1984). In the study by Brown et al (1982), mineral oil was applied because of its economy and ability to hold water. Pearson and Kotthof (1979) suggest petrolatum,

Eucerin (water in oil agent), or vegetable oil and note that some debate exists about the efficacy of lanolin and mineral oil, the former because it may sensitize skin (Parent, 1985) and the latter because it may act as a drying agent. Epstein (1983) recommends the use of economical products such as petrolatum and mineral oil, noting that the use of vegetable oil may leave distasteful odors. Arndt (1983) also suggests that the elderly may "be best able to tolerate" petrolatum as an occlusive agent, but also mentions commercial brands such as Keri, Nivea, Aquaphor, and Eucerin. Mineral oil, petrolatum (Parth and Kapke, 1983), and lanolin are noted as effective agents for use as occlusive agents, but because of a "greasy" feeling, petrolatum may result in less compliance than oil-in-water or water-in-oil preparations (Dotz and Berman, 1984; Parent, 1985). Cornell (1986;33) suggested that the best occlusive agent to use following a bath and throughout the day for the treatment of dry skin in the elderly is a compound of equal parts water and "one of the greasier over-the-counter products." The study by Weiner et al (1973) used Dermo-Pedic Foot Lotion, a lotion containing "ethyoxylated" lanolin in an aqueous base and Allantoin. The Spoor (1958) study tested the effects of a water-dispersible bath oil, Sardo. This is contradictory to the argument that the use of oil in bathwater is hazardous (Hogstel, 1983; Parthe and Kapke, 1983) and that the oil becomes suspended rather than being absorbed (Epstein, 1983; Pearson and Kotthof, 1979). Lastly, Boisits (1986) reported that in a clinical trial of occlusive agents at a relative humidity of 20%, there was a 98% reduction in moisture loss with petrolatum, an 83% reduction with lanolin, and a 31% reduction with mineral oil. Other less commonly used products tested by Cheeseborough-Ponds, Inc., reported by Boisits (1986), resulted in reductions ranging from 59% with avocado oil to a negative 19% with anhydrous glycerin.

Lanolin is much more expensive than either mineral oil or petrolatum while baby oil is less expensive than mineral oil. Because of its economical nature, because of the repeated mention of its effectiveness in the literature, and because its use has been tested empirically by Brown et al (1982), mineral oil may be the agent of choice. Petrolatum, although potentially very effective as an occlusive agent, may be considered unappealing to the client who is concerned about staining clothing. Again, the nurse and client must evaluate the effectiveness and desirability of products, and a program of research to test the effects of such agents is needed.

Humidity

Although the maintenance of sufficient environmental humidity is repeated by nearly all persons addressing the subject of dry skin in the elderly, some variance in the ideal level is reported. The majority of authors state

that humidity should be maintained at over 60% (Gaul and Underwood, 1951; Parent, 1985). Tools to measure the humidity of an institutional or private home setting will aid in determining the need for intervention in increasing environmental humidity. In private homes the use of humidifiers or pans of water on radiators or, where possible, humidifiers installed in forced-air systems will increase humidity (Arndt, 1983; Walther and Harber, 1984). In institutional settings, central environmental controls may have such humidifying elements and may require adjustment. In other cases, such humidifying equipment may need to be added, or room humidifiers may be used.

Exposure to Sun

The skin's aging process is a combination of both longevity and the effects of ultraviolet light. This is why the skin that is least exposed to the sun, the skin under the chin or on the upper thigh and buttocks, for instance, tends to be less damaged or "aged." Skin that has been more exposed to ultraviolet light is also more vulnerable to epidermal thinning with age (Cornell, 1986). These actinic (ultraviolet) related skin changes can be controlled by decreasing direct exposure to the sun. Obviously, clothing may be worn to prevent exposure of most vulnerable areas: cotton shirts with long sleeves, brimmed hats, lightweight pants, or leg covering. In addition, individuals may be advised to make use of shaded areas when outdoors or to limit their outdoor activities to early morning and late afternoon (Cornell, 1986).

Evaluation

The most effective tool for evaluating the effectiveness of a treatment intervention for dry skin would be the systematic use of a post-hoc measure of the guide used for the assessment prior to intervention. Modification of the SCDF illustrated in Assessment Guide 8.1 to allow notation of signs and symptoms within a range of scores (ie, "1" for absent, "4" for severe) would provide the nurse with a tool to assess for both direction and magnitude of change following treatment.

A pilot study to evaluate the effectiveness of the bathing protocol outlined previously was conducted using 15 institutionalized residents ranging in age from 54 to 86. The modified SCDF (Assessment Guide 8.1) was used to assess skin condition every 2 weeks during the 18 weeks of the study: three times preintervention, three times during the 6 weeks of the intervention, and three times post-intervention. Multivariate analysis of variance (MANOVA) was used to analyze the repeated measures of total skin dryness and the four individual dimensions of skin dryness at nine data collection points. The intervention was found to reduce total skin dryness significantly (p = .031) as well as three of the four individual dimensions of the dryness construct: redness (p = .001), scaling (p = .007), and flaking (p = .002). When scores were averaged into three periods, before, during, and after, however, only scaling as an individual measure remained significant (p = .001); total dryness was not significant (p = .199). This is probably because residual effects were seen in the 2 weeks following the intervention, a finding that is consistent with the literature that indicates that clinicians may expect to see delayed responses in the elderly (Fenske, 1982). Cracking did not change significantly over time, perhaps because this dimension was difficult to assess or did not contribute significantly to dryness scores. Although the small sample size for the pilot study limits the generalizability of these findings, it provides beginning evidence of the empirical effects of a bathing intervention for treating dry skin in the elderly.

Another element of the assessment and treatment of impaired skin integrity in the elderly that is in need of testing is the timeframe of response on the part of the elderly client to the intervention. How long after the introduction of a treatment for dry skin should the client and the nurse expect a response? Fenske (1982;300) warned that delayed responses to allergens should be expected in the elderly because of "muffled immunocompetent cells, altered blood vessels, and less permeable dermis." Fenske suggested, therefore, that the elderly should be assessed for a delayed response up to 2 weeks after the use of a patch test, whereas younger persons should show a response within 48 to 72 hours, up to 1 week in time. This may have implications for the evaluation of the effects of many interventions for impaired skin integrity in the elderly and should be considered in evaluating treatments for dry skin.

It may be useful to incorporate the use of a body diagram, as was described by Urosevich (1981), on which areas of dryness are shaded on a chart showing an anterior and posterior view of the human body. This shading is done to match the approximate surface area of dryness and is accompanied by a narrative statement that describes the size, location, and nature of abnormalities. Urosevich suggests that this chart be attached to the assessment and used to determine changes that occur over time.

In addition to the interventions previously outlined, the nurse must evaluate the response of the client to the effects of these interventions while keeping in mind that the nature of knowledge about the myriad of etiologic factors associated with dry skin limits the predictability of outcomes for measures used to treat these etiologies. In the case presented, there is relevance for lack of adequate environmental humidity and inadequate fluid intake as etiologic factors. Most of the etiologic factors for which systematic evidence is lacking are treatable by the professional nurse. The isolation of potential etiologic factors and the evaluation of effective intervention(s) are crucial to the treatment of actual and potential responses to illness

and to the development of nursing science. For instance, the testing of interventions such as maintenance of an adequate fluid and nutritional intake may need to be explored if interventions used to treat more common etiologic factors, such as inadequate hydration of the skin, sun exposure, and inadequate environmental humidity, are ineffective.

OUTCOMES

The elderly person effectively treated for Impaired Skin Integrity: Dry Skin should

1. Experience a reversal of symptoms such as flaking, scaling, and fissuring
2. Experience decreased itching
3. Have signs of diminished or absent inflammation
4. Be able, if not cognitively impaired or aphasic, to describe the factors that may be contributing to his or her dry skin condition
5. Be able to describe the procedure and rationale for treatment

In the case study presented previously, the bathing intervention should be implemented in addition to careful attention to fluid intake. Although several weeks should be allowed to evaluate skin condition, improvement may be seen as a result of the bathing intervention. If skin condition becomes more dry when environmental humidity is lower or fluid intake decreases episodically, the nurse may have to manipulate variables one at a time in order to isolate the etiologies that are operating. If, however, the prescribed bathing intervention is in use and changes in humidity and episodic fluid deficits do not significantly change the skin dryness condition, then the nurse may infer that the intervention is effective and that moisture retention in the skin is the accurate etiology.

Bill has recently experienced losses in functional abilities that require different application of the intervention. He has been receiving bathing techniques that accommodate the outlined intervention, and he has been using Dove soap. No other soap is applied between baths. Bill may benefit from continuing to shower in order to maximize those weight-bearing and range-of-motion abilities he has currently.

Showering with the outlined intervention should be started at two times weekly and if no change is observed, increased to three or four times weekly, until the requisite frequency is met. Bathing frequency should be increased in the same manner. In addition, fluid intake must be closely observed. If, in consultation with the physician, there is agreement that withdrawal of ointments may not be harmful, such withdrawal would assist in determining the effectiveness of the intervention. Current daily hygiene should be continued, using only water for washing face and hands.

SUMMARY

Current knowledge about the nursing diagnosis Impaired Skin Integrity: Dry Skin has been presented. Very little nursing literature has been devoted to this diagnosis or to the systematic assessment, treatment, and evaluation of interventions for dry skin in any age group. As the taxonomy of nursing diagnoses evolves, this diagnosis may be added. Personal observation, however, has led to the conclusion that skin dryness is considered an accoutrement to aging and institutionalization. Although professional nurses can describe the problems their clients have with dry skin and the resulting treatment, explication of the diagnostic statement, isolation of etiologies, and evaluation of treatment methods are lacking. It is important that this area of gerontologic nursing practice be refined and tested.

ASSESSMENT GUIDE 8.1

Modified Skin Condition Data Form

Enter a number in each box: 1 = absent   3 = moderate
                           2 = mild   4 = severe

Body Site	Redness	Scaling	Cracking	Flaking
Face				
Neck				
Upper Arms Anterior				
Posterior				
Lateral				
Forearms Anterior				
Posterior				
Lateral				
Hands –Dorsal				
Trunk Anterior				
Posterior				
Lateral				
Thighs Anterior				
Posterior				
Lateral				
Lower Leg Anterior				
Posterior				
Lateral				
Feet Dorsal				
Plantar				
Heels				
Between Toes				

References

Anderson HC: *Newton's Geriatric Nursing.* Mosby, 1971.

Arndt KA: *Manual of Dermatologic Therapeutics,* 3d ed. Little, Brown, 1983.

Atkins J: Care of the hair and scalp. *Nurs Mirror* (Mar) 1977; 45-48.

Beauregard S, Gilchrest B: A survey of skin problems and skin care regimens in the elderly. *Arch Dermatol* 1987; 123:1638-1643.

Boisits EK: The evaluation of moisturizing products. *Cosmetics Toiletries* (May) 1986; 101:31-39.

Brown M et al: Nursing innovation for dry skin care of the feet in the elderly: A demonstration project. *J Gerontol Nurs* 1982; 8:393-395.

Burnside IM: *Nursing and the Aged.* McGraw-Hill, 1976.

Carpenito LJ: *Nursing Diagnosis Application to Clinical Practice.* Lippincott, 1987.

Carroll-Johnson R (editor): *Classification of Nursing Diagnoses: Proceedings of the Eighth Conference.* Lippincott, 1989.

Cornell RC: Aging and the skin. *Geriatr Med* 1986; 5:26-33.

DeLancey VL, North C: Skin assessment. *Top Clin Nurs* (July) 1983; 4:5-10.

Dotz WI, Berman B: Aids that preserve hydration and mitigate its loss. *Consultant* (Aug) 1984; 46-62.

Eliopoulos C: *Gerontological Nursing.* Harper and Row, 1979.

Epstein E: *Common Skin Disorders,* 2d ed. Medical Economics Books, 1983.

Fenske NA: Problems of aging skin. *Consultant* (Jan) 1982; 287-300.

Fitzsimmons VM: The aging integument: A sensitive and complex system. *Top Clin Nurs* 1983; 4:32-38.

Frantz RA, Kinney CN: Variables associated with skin dryness in the elderly. *Nurs Res* 1986; 35:98-100.

Frosch PJ, Kligman AM: The soap chamber test. *J Am Acad Dermatol* 1979; 1:35-41.

Gaul LE, Underwood GB: Relation of dew point and barometric pressure to chapping of normal skin. *J Investigative Dermatol* 1951; 19:9-19.

Gioiella E, Bevil C: *Nursing Care of the Aging Client.* Appleton-Century-Crofts, 1985.

Hannigan L: Nursing assessment of the integumentary system. *Occup Health Nurs* (Jan) 1978; 10:19-22.

Hardy M: A pilot study of the diagnosis and treatment of Impaired Skin Integrity. *Nursing Diagnosis* 1990; 1(2):57-63.

Harmer B, Henderson V: *Textbook of the Principles and Practice of Nursing.* Macmillan, 1960.

Hogstel MO: Skin care for the aged. *J Gerontol Nurs* 1983; 9:431-437.

Jowett S, Ryan T: Skin disease and handicap: An analysis of the impact of skin conditions. *Soc Sci Med* 1985; 20:425-429.

Kim M, McFarland GK, McLane AM (editors): *Pocket Guide to Nursing Diagnoses.* Mosby, 1984.

King PA: Foot assessment of the elderly. *J Gerontol Nurs* 1978; 4:47-52.

Luckmann J, Sorensen KC: *Medical-Surgical Nursing: A Psychophysiologic Approach.* Saunders, 1974.

Malkiewicz J: The integumentary system. *RN* (Dec) 1981; 44:55-60.

Nightingale F: *Notes on Nursing: What It Is, and What It Is Not.* Appleton, 1914.

Parent LS: Therapy of skin problems in the elderly. *U.S. Pharmacist* (Apr) 1985; 10:48-54.

Parth C, Kapke K: Aging and the skin. *Geriatr Nurs* (May-June) 1983; 158-162.

Pearson LJ, Kotthof MK: *Geriatric Clinical Protocols.* Lippincott, 1979.

Pellerano S: Use of a combination of an anti-inflammatory steroid, an antibacterial agent and an antifungal in dermatological practice. *Internat J Clin Pharmacol Ther Toxicol* 1985; 23:215-218.

Shelley WB, Shelley ED: The ten major problems of aging skin. *Geriatrics* 1982; 37:107-113.

Spoor HJ: Measurement and maintenance of natural skin oil. *NY State J Med* (Oct) 1958; 3292-3299.

Stead WL: Survey of skin conditions occurring in long-stay and psychogeriatric wards. *Nurs Times* (Aug) 1979; 1450-1452.

Sutton RL, Waisman M: *The Practitioner's Dermatology.* Dun-Donnelley, 1975.

Tindall J, Smith J: Skin lesions of the aged. *JAMA* 1963; 186:1039-1042.

Urosevich PR (editor): *Nursing Photobook.* Nursing 81 Books, Intermed Communications, 1981.

Walther RR, Harber LC: Expected skin complaints of the geriatric patient. *Geriatrics* 1984; 39:67-80.

Weiner EM et al: Treating the dry skin syndrome. *J Am Podiatry Assoc* 1973; 63:571-581.

9

Altered Nutrition: Less Than Body Requirements

KATHY RAJCEVICH, MSN, RN
BONNIE WAKEFIELD, MA, RN

NUTRITION IS THE SCIENCE OF THE RELATIONSHIP OF health, well-being, and disease to ingestion, absorption, and use of food and nutrients (Ebersole and Hess, 1985; Worthington, 1979). The ability to obtain and maintain proper nutrition depends on multiple influencing factors. Food and nutrients must be made available for ingestion in appropriate types and amounts and absorbed to maintain body structure and function.

SIGNIFICANCE FOR THE ELDERLY

It is estimated that between one third and one half of the health problems of the elderly relate directly to nutrition (Hendricks and Hendricks, 1981). As many as 50% of the independently living elderly demonstrate nutritional deficiencies (Goodwin et al, 1983). The elderly are also more likely to be in a marginal state of nutritional status on entry into the health care system.

The National Research Council (1989) publishes the Recommended Dietary Allowances (RDAs). The RDAs state the minimum levels of intake of essential nutrients to meet the known nutritional needs of healthy individuals adequately. The recent revision of RDAs has somewhat more specific information for the elderly than provided in the past. For adults over age 50 with light to moderate activity, 2300 kilocalories are recommended for men, and 1900 kilocalories are recommended for women. A normal variation of 20% is acceptable, as is true for younger adults. Requirements for persons beyond age 75 are said to be likely to be less because of reduced body size, reduced resting energy, expenditure, and reduced activity.

Nutritional requirements differ according to the age of the elderly person: For example, the nutritional requirements for a 51-year-old are different from those of a 95-year-old. There is a consensus that because of changes in metabolic rate and activity, caloric intake should be reduced as one ages by 5% per decade from ages 55 to 75, with a further reduction of 7% beyond age 75 (Ebersole and Hess, 1985; Kart et al, 1978; Worthington, 1979). The percent of body fat increases relative to lean muscle mass. Caloric ranges for elderly men are from 2000 to 2800 calories, and for elderly women from 1200 to 2200. The RDAs are established for caloric intake from ages 51 to 75 and then over age 75. However, there is no evidence that the need for nutrients decreases with age (Kart et al, 1978). This suggests that as one ages, the food ingested must be of better quality to fulfill nutrient needs and still decrease calories.

Lipschitz et al (1985) noted that the risk of malnutrition is highest in two groups: (1) hospitalized elderly and (2) persons of low socioeconomic status (which includes a significant proportion of elderly). Malnutrition in the elderly is influenced by multiple factors. These include (1) biologic changes associated with aging; (2) illness; (3) psychosocial influences; and (4) economic factors. Refer to overview for biologic changes associated with aging that influence malnutrition.

ETIOLOGIES/RELATED FACTORS

Illness

In addition to normal changes associated with aging that may interfere with nutrition, the elderly population has an increased frequency of chronic illnesses. Recommended treatments in chronic illnesses may limit food types and/or palatability. Examples are diabetes (carbohydrate intake), chronic heart failure (sodium intake), renal failure (potassium, sodium, protein intake), and hepatic disease (protein intake). Medications prescribed for chronic illnesses may be involved in many drug–nutrient interactions (see Table 9.1) and may induce nutritional deficiencies. Medications can influence the ingestion or absorption of nutrients in several ways.

Nutritional evaluation is essential for any elderly patient receiving one or more drugs that could interact with nutrient intake or absorption. Drug–nutrient interactions include (1) depression of drug absorption; (2) increases in drug absorption; and (3) nutrient depletion as an adverse drug reaction. Drug–nutrient interactions should be evaluated every 6 months (Roe, 1986).

Table 9.1

Drug-Induced Nutritional Deficiencies

CATEGORY	DRUGS	NUTRIENTS AFFECTED	POSSIBLE MANIFESTATIONS
Alcohol		Malabsorption of folate, thiamine	Neurologic Hematologic Compromised nutritional status
Antacid	Aluminum hydroxide Sodium bicarbonate	Phosphate depletion Iron, vitamin D, and folate malabsorption	Osteomalacia
Antibacterial	Broad spectrum	Decreased absorption related to diarrhea	Compromised nutritional status
Anticoagulant	Warfarin	Vitamin K antagonist	Hemorrhage
Anticonvulsant	Phenytoin Phenobarbital	Calcium Vitamins D & K Changes in metabolism Folate malabsorption	Osteomalacia anemia
Anti-inflammatory	Colchicine Salicylazo sulfapyridine	Decreased absorption of fat; sodium; vitamins K, B_{12}	Osteomalacia
Antituberculosis	Isoniazid INH	Vitamin B_6 Niacine malabsorption	Peripheral neuropathy Pellegra
Cardiac	Captopril Digoxin Hydralazine Procainamide	Sodium depletion Loss of zinc, potassium Vitamin B_6 malabsorption Decreased appetite	Electrolyte imbalances Electrolyte imbalances Compromised nutritional status Compromised nutritional status
Diuretics	Furosemide Ethacrynic acid Triamterene Hydrochlorothiazide	Reduced calcium, zinc, potassium, and magnesium reabsorption Sodium depletion Lower glucose tolerance	Electrolyte imbalance
Hypoglycemic	Metformin Phenformin	Malabsorption of vitamin B_{12}	Anemia
Hypolipemic	Sequestrant Cholestyramine	Decreased absorption of fat-soluble vitamins A, K, B_{12} Folate Iron	Osteomalacia

Sources: Roe DA: *Drug Induced Nutritional Deficiencies,* 2nd ed. AVI, 1985. Roe DA: Drug-nutrient interactions in the elderly. *Geriatrics* 1986; 41:57-74. Vitale JJ, Santos JI: Nutrition and the elderly. *Postgrad Med* 1985; 78(5):79-89.

In the elderly, protein–calorie malnutrition (PCM) is usually caused by decreased nutritional intake related to anorexia. Lipschitz (1982) identified three groups of patients with PCM. The largest group includes those hospitalized with a secondary diagnosis of PCM. The second group has a primary diagnosis of PCM. The third group are those who are institutionalized, and the PCM is related to inadequate nutrient intake. PCM is also associated with socioeconomic and psychologic factors in the elderly, such as depression, loneliness, poverty, and decreased ability to care for oneself.

PCM is expressed in two forms: marasmus and kwashiorkor. These two forms may not be clearly differentiated. Marasmus is caused by both calorie and protein deficiencies. These individuals show a lack of body fat and muscle wasting. Serum protein status and immune function may not be affected. Kwashiorkor is caused by a deficient protein intake along with catabolic stress. Kwashiorkor is characterized by hypoalbuminemia, edema, and depressed immunity (Lerman, 1986). PCM increases hospital stay and can increase mortality. When PCM is present, the body's defense mechanisms are interrupted.

Psychosocial Factors

Many of the factors that influence nutritional adequacy or inadequacy of the elderly lie in the psychosocial realm. These include life-long habits, role changes, loneliness, and increasing dependence on others.

The elderly have developed life-long eating habits based on tradition, religion, ethnicity, and economic backgrounds, which may not coincide with their nutritional needs (Ebersole and Hess, 1985). Modifying life-long habits may be a principal consideration when assisting the elderly person to improve nutritional status. Expectations that the elderly person will change these habits may have the opposite effect, however, resulting in stress, anger, and depression (Weber, 1980).

There may be a change in roles, as well as increased loneliness, because of the loss of a spouse or companions, and this may influence nutritional intake. Loneliness may also increase drinking among elderly alcoholics, which can have nutritional implications if the elderly person substitutes drinking for eating nourishing food (Feldman, 1983).

Thirty-six percent of elderly women and 15% of elderly men live alone, a statistic that tends to be related to poor nutritional status (Bowman and Rosenberg, 1982). Munro (1985) found that men from 65 to 69 years of age average 9.3 years of independent living, followed by 3.8 years of dependence. Women of the same age group have 10.6 years of independent living, but a lengthy 8.9 years of dependent living. Living alone can influence cooking and eating behaviors. Because mealtimes are a social activity as well as an eating activity, the elderly who are alone may lack motivation to cook and eat.

Failing motor abilities and eyesight may also make meal preparation impossible. Poor dentition due to lack of teeth or ill-fitting dentures may make chewing difficult. Regardless of setting, these losses of function may make an elderly individual dependent on others for meals or limit the choice of foods. The decision of when and what to eat may be made for the elder, thus decreasing their control and choices.

Economic Factors

It is estimated that 20% of the elderly have limits imposed on nutritional intake by poverty (Hendricks and Hendricks, 1981). Total income decreases by one half for retirees, and many elderly live on fixed incomes that do not keep up with inflation. The elderly pay, on the average, 50% more for food because they buy food in smaller quantities, eat in restaurants, and purchase convenience foods. They may also be forced to buy poorer quality food (Hendricks and Hendricks, 1981). All of these factors place them at risk for inferior dietary intake.

The number of people who own and are able to drive cars declines with each year over 65 years of age, and public transportation may be unavailable. The majority of grocery stores are now only accessible by car, as neighborhood grocery stores are disappearing. Although convenience stores may be available, the prices are extremely high, and the selection of fresh fruits, vegetables, and meats is limited.

In reviewing the National Health and Nutrition Examination Survey from 1971 to 1974, Davis et al (1985) found that a higher proportion of persons living alone were below poverty levels. Women living alone were the highest proportion below poverty (40%). Income levels below poverty had a substantial impact on nutrient intake, although women living alone tended to have better dietary intake than men living alone regardless of income level. Governmental and community-assisted programs, food stamps, meals-on-wheels, congregate meals, and shopping assistance may be available in various communities. Even when available, however, they may not be used. Poor housing necessitated by low income may lack adequate food storage and preparation areas. Health care may also be affected by low income, especially dental care, resulting in loss of teeth, inability to obtain dentures, and lack of maintenance of dentures. If the elderly person cannot chew effectively, the diet is more likely to be inadequate in protein and fresh fruits and vegetables.

CURRENT STATUS OF THE DIAGNOSIS

The etiologies and defining characteristics associated with Altered Nutrition: Less Than Body Requirements currently accepted for clinical testing by the North American Nursing Diagnosis Association (NANDA) are listed in Table 9.2 (Carroll-Johnson, 1989) and compared with Keithley (1979) and this chapter's authors, Rajcevich/Wakefield. No published studies or tools related to this diagnosis were located. One clinically oriented article (Price, 1979) applies the process of making this diagnosis to a case study. Carpenito (1985) also discusses this diagnosis as a collaborative problem with medicine, stating that in any event, it is one that requires complex nursing care. Much has been written related to the effect and treatment of inadequate nutrition; however, no studies have been done to validate this nursing diagnosis using an elderly population. The defining characteristics for this diagnosis need to be validated in all age groups.

DEFINING CHARACTERISTICS

Several nutritional deficiencies are manifested clinically; therefore, assessment should include a consideration of these signs. Clinical signs identified by Keithley (1979), related to possible nutritional deficiencies, are listed in Table 9.2. Chernoff et al (1984) identify confusion or recent alteration in mental status as the most common symptom of protein–calorie malnutrition and dehydration. In patients with protein–calorie malnutrition, fluid intake is often deficient, and confusion probably relates to dehydration. Chernoff et al (1984) go on to identify four key criteria in the identification of malnutrition in the elderly: (1) a history and a physical, which provide strong clues; (2) a history of significant weight loss; (3) a serum albumin level less than 3 g/dL in the absence of liver disease or evidence of excessive urinary or gastrointestinal losses; (4) the presence of anemia, lymphocytopenia, and anergy.

ASSESSMENT

Yen (1983a) identifies admission to a health care facility or program as one indication of the need to assess the nutritional status of older adults. The goal of assessment is to assist in identification of problems so that a plan to improve and maintain nutritional status can be developed. Specifically, nutritional assessment serves four functions:

1. It reveals information on the body's energy reserves, lean mass, visceral transport proteins, and the immune system
2. It identifies and characterizes the type of malnutrition present
3. It provides baseline values for serial monitoring

4. It permits realistic goals to be established for protein, energy, and other essential nutrients (Shuran and Nelson, 1986)

Various parameters have been suggested for assessment. Most commonly included areas are a diet history, anthropometric measurements, laboratory values and immunologic assessments, and clinical presentation.

Diet History

A thorough diet history is the first step in identifying patients with special nutritional needs. Keithley (1979) outlines 10 categories essential to a diet history, including appetite, weight, diet pattern, eating patterns, chewing and swallowing, physical activity, medication history, illnesses, sociocultural factors, and elimination practices. Others (Chernoff et al, 1984; Hickler and Wayne, 1984; Vitale and Santos, 1985; Yen, 1983b) have identified additional key questions to be included in the history. The diet history is summarized in Assessment Guide 9.1.

Anthropometric Measurements and Laboratory Values

According to Chernoff et al (1984), several known changes in stature and body composition in the elderly may be attributed to the aging process itself. These changes are similar to those observed in malnutrition at any age. Because of this, it can be difficult to interpret abnormal values observed in the elderly person. Anthropometric body measurements are frequently part of the nutritional assessment (Assessment Guide 9.2). These include triceps skinfold and arm circumference, which indicate measurements of fat and protein stores. Standards for these measurements are set for young adults. When standards are available for the elderly, these measurements may improve the prediction of malnutrition in the elderly. Because there is a marked reduction in lean muscle mass in the elderly and changes in the percentage of fat stores, these measurements may not be the best predictors of malnutrition; however, further study is needed. Other anthropometric measurements include height, weight, and usual weight compared to the ideal body weight. Body weight changes in the aging process, and therefore by itself is not a good predictor of malnutrition. For example, a person could be obese and still be severely malnourished. A history of weight loss may be a more important indicator of malnutrition in the elderly. Common laboratory measurements that are frequently used in nutritional assessment include serum albumin, total iron-binding capacity, serum transferrin, lymphocyte count, and 24-hour urinary creatinine. Serum transferrin is a poor predictor of malnutrition in the elderly, since the elderly

Table 9.2

Altered Nutrition: Less Than Body Requirements

CARROLL-JOHNSON (1989)

Definition. The state in which an individual experiences an intake of nutrients insufficient to meet metabolic needs

ETIOLOGIES/RELATED FACTORS

Inability to ingest or digest food or absorb nutrients because of biologic, psychologic, or economic factors

Defining Characteristics

Loss of weight with adequate food intake
Body weight 20% or more under ideal for height and frame
Reported inadequate food intake less than RDA
Weakness of muscles required for swallowing or mastication
Reported or evidence of lack of food
Lack of interest in food
Perceived inability to ingest food
Aversion to eating
Reported altered taste sensation
Satiety immediately after ingesting food
Abdominal pain with or without pathologic conditions
Sore, inflamed buccal cavity

RAJCEVICH/WAKEFIELD

Etiologies/Related Factors

Biologic changes associated with aging
Illness
Psychosocial influences
Economic factors

Defining Characteristics

Dehyration
Alteration in mental status
History of significant weight loss
Serum albumin < 3g/dL
Anemia
Lymphocytopenia
Anergy

KEITHLEY (1979)

Defining Characteristics

Hair dull, dry, thin, fine, straight, and easily plucked
Face swollen. Dark cheeks and dark areas under eyes. Skin on nose and mouth bumpy or flaky. Enlarged parotid glands
Eyes dull. Membranes dull and either too pale or too red. Eyelid corners red and fissured
Lips red and swollen, especially at corners of mouth
Tongue swollen, appears raw, purple, with swollen sores or abnormal papillae
Teeth missing or emerging abnormally. Cavities or dark spots showing. Gums spongy and bleed easily
Thyroid glands swollen
Skin dry, flaky, swollen, dark with lighter or darker spots, some resembling bruises. Skin appears tight and drawn
Nails spoon-shaped, brittle, and ridged
Muscles wasted, legs knock-kneed or bowed, bumps on ribs, joints swollen
Heart rate above 100, enlarged heart, abnormal rhythm, high BP. Enlarged liver and spleen. Musculoskeletal hemorrhages
Patient irritable and confused. Experiences burning and tingling of hands and feet. Loss of sense of position and decreased ankle and knee reflexes

have a reduced transferrin level that may be related to higher tissue iron stores and not malnutrition. Abnormalities in lymphocyte count and anemias are not uncommon in the well-nourished elderly, therefore making these tests poor predictors by themselves. Urinary creatinine is influenced by renal and liver dysfunction, common in the elderly. Serum albumin is only minimally altered by aging, and therefore hypoalbuminemia may be the best predictor of malnutrition in the elderly (Chernoff et al, 1984; Mitchell and Lipschitz, 1982; Seltzer et al, 1979).

CASE STUDY

Altered Nutrition: Less Than Body Requirements

Mrs W, a 71-year-old white woman, is being admitted to a local care facility following discharge from an acute care hospital. She is 5' 3" tall and weighs 105 lb after a weight loss of 7 lb during the recent hospitalization. She is able to walk short distances without assistance but has right side arm and leg weakness and spends most of the day sitting in a chair. She has poor muscle tone. Mrs. W wears full dentures. Her hemoglobin is 10 mg on admission, with pale conjunctiva observed. Her intake is less than 1000 calories each day. On physical examination the nurse noted a broken area of skin over the coccyx.

Mrs. W verbalizes that she has "little appetite," that she "doesn't really need to eat much," and that she "feels weak." She also states that she has lost 15 lb over the past year. From the history and interview the nurse determines that Mrs. W had a left hemispheric cerebrovascular accident (CVA) complicated with pneumonia prior to admission to the care facility. She has been widowed for 2 years and has lived alone since her husband's death. One son and daughter visit occasionally.

From these data the nurse makes the following nursing diagnosis: Altered Nutrition: Less Than Body Requirements, related to social isolation, anorexia, emotional stress, and inability to prepare/procure food as evidenced by verbalized little appetite, weight loss, pale conjunctiva, and poor muscle tone.

Mrs. W was at risk because of poor nutritional status. Her weight loss and skinfold measurements demonstrated a lack of muscle and fat reserve. Her skin was broken down over her coccyx, and her condition was complicated by pneumonia. She had not been cooking much since her husband's death, no longer felt the need or desire to cook complete meals, and missed the company of her husband at meal times. Without her husband to accompany her, she had decreased the amount of time she spent on social activities. Because of this diminished activity level, she felt that she needed to eat less to avoid weight gain.

NURSING INTERVENTIONS

Plans for providing adequate nutrient intake must be individualized, including food and supplement intake as well as the number and timing of meals. Proper nutrients must be made available. However, unless these nutrients are consumed, they are of little value.

Referrals may need to be made to occupational therapy or physical therapy to evaluate use of special utensils or exercises to improve the patient's ability and desire to eat. The ability to chew and swallow properly is essential to begin the process of ingestion. The speech therapist can assist with difficulties with dysphagia (see Chapter 10). Problems with dentition, fitting and use of dentures, and muscle difficulties in swallowing can influence ingestion and need to be corrected so that the patient is able to eat. Those individuals who are edentulous or who have ill-fitting dentures may limit the type of food selected and eaten. Inability to chew could severely decrease the amount of protein intake (Hogstel and Robinson, 1989).

If nausea and vomiting are present, the cause must be determined and steps taken to alleviate the problem. Nursing interventions should include reducing noxious stimuli, teaching techniques to alleviate nausea and vomiting, identifying foods and eating habits to reduce nausea, identifying foods that increase protein/calorie intake, and assisting with meal planning (Carpenito, 1985).

Environmental Structuring

Improving the setting and socialization at mealtime can improve nutrient intake. Making meal settings aesthetic and pleasant can improve an individual's will to eat (Irwin, 1987). Making mealtime a time of sharing and pleasant interchange can also improve the will to eat. Mealtime is traditionally the time for family sharing and socializing. Once families are gone, other socialization should be provided to return meaning to the mealtime. Even the socialization provided by the individual delivering the Meals on Wheels may provide positive socialization experiences for the elderly at home. Active senior citizen centers can also provide socialization.

Nutrition Education

Although the nurse should have a direct impact on nutritional status, a team approach to treating nutritional status seems optimal, and a collaborative effort is necessary between the nurse and the dietitian. Dugdale et al (1979) found that physicians and nurses generally know more about the theoretical basis of nutrition than the practical aspects. In order for patient education to be as beneficial as possible, the nurse must combine the theoretical knowledge of nutrition with practical, individual application. Efforts should be directed to assist the individual to substitute favorable eating habits for poor eating habits. Education should also encompass activity and exercise to improve appetite. Patients must have input into mutually agreed on goals. Knowing the type of food that is important to the patient is valuable information, particularly in ethnic populations. Food likes and dislikes are important to identify in order to prepare food that the elderly person will actually eat at mealtime and for supplemental nutrition. Family members must also be involved in the education process. Their attitudes and beliefs can influence the patient's response to teaching. Informed family members may be a useful source of supplemental nutrition.

Enteral Feeding

Enteral feeding is a method used to provide supplemental nutritional support when persons are unable to chew and ingest food for adequate nutritional food and fluid intake. Enteral feeding can be delivered by nasogastric tube or surgically placed gastrostomy or jejunostomy tubes. Cataldi-Betcher et al (1983) found the following complications in those patients receiving enteral feedings: 6.2% experienced gastrointestinal complications; 3.5% experienced mechanical complications; and 2% experienced metabolic complications. Gastrointestinal complications included diarrhea and inadequate gastric emptying. Refer to Chapter 15 and the CURN protocol (Horsley et al, 1981) for further discussion of prevention of diarrhea in tube-fed patients. Mechanical complications include fluid and electrolyte imbalance (Seltzer et al, 1984). When enteral feedings are used, the patient needs to be evaluated for tolerance to the feedings and nutritional benefit. Total parenteral nutrition can be used in the extremely malnourished individual when other methods are not appropriate (Starker et al, 1985).

CASE STUDY

Nursing Interventions

Collaboration between the nurse and the dietitian resulted in a nutritional plan for Mrs. W. Nutritional education was provided to Mrs. W and to her son and daughter. Improved nutritional intake was linked with increasing social contacts for Mrs. W. She was encouraged to eat with two of the other residents that she liked. Because Mrs. W enjoyed breakfast, increased amounts of food were provided at that meal. To improve both her appetite and her social contacts, Mrs. W was referred to an activity therapist for a plan of recreational activities. A referral was also made to physical therapy to determine if deficits related to the CVA had affected her ability to eat. Supplemental feeding was not indicated because Mrs. W was not extremely malnourished, was responsive to educational strategies, and was able to eat independently without difficulty.

Within a few months, Mrs. W had improved. Mobility and some swallowing difficulties detected by the physical therapist were being treated. She enjoyed her daily recreational activities. At times, she would still become somewhat depressed over the loss of her husband; however, these periods were brief. She was eating a good breakfast, and smaller meals for lunch and dinner, with occasional between-meal snacks. Mrs. W could also verbalize an understanding of the importance of good nutrition and its relationship to her physical and mental health status. A 5-lb weight gain was noted, along with improved muscle tone.

OUTCOMES

Ongoing, systematic assessment and evaluation are necessary to determine response to interventions. The goals of nursing interventions are to increase amounts of nutrients ingested; improve quality of nutrients ingested; achieve adequate nutrition based on identified needs; and promote client understanding of nutritional needs.

SUMMARY

This chapter addressed the changes and factors associated with nutrition in the elderly, the application of the nursing diagnosis Altered Nutrition: Less Than Body Requirements to an elderly client, and interventions used to treat this diagnosis. The need to establish age-specific standards for nutritional requirements are identified. Nurses also need to be knowledgeable about normal aging changes so that signs associated with malnutrition can be differentiated and not assumed to be a part of "getting old." In this way, undernutrition can be recognized early and appropriate treatment instituted.

ASSESSMENT GUIDE 9.1

Diet History

Appetite
Increased or decreased
Changes in food preferences

Weight
Increase or decrease
Rapid or slow changes
Recall of maximum/minimum weights

Diet Pattern
Typical day's eating pattern
Allergies
Special diet order by physician
Likes and dislikes

Eating Pattern
When and where does he or she eat
Time of day
Snacks

Chewing and Swallowing
Dentures
Caries
Sore gums
Mouth pain
Food of proper consistency

Physical Activity
Exercise pattern
Daily activity
Strong enough to open packages/set up meal/hold utensil
Tire while eating/self-feeding

Medication History
Current medications
Alcohol intake

Illnesses
History or illness requiring medications or surgical treatment
Chronic GI disease
Surgery on GI tract
Acute infection

Sociocultural
Finances
Five senses adequate/compensated (ie, eyeglasses)
Cultural habits/ethnic background
Depression
Mental status changes
Confusion
Recent loss of spouse

Elimination
Changes in bowel habits
Use of laxatives

ASSESSMENT GUIDE 9.2

Standard Anthropometric/ Biochemical Measurements

Anthropometrics
Height
Weight
  Actual
  As percentage of ideal weight
  Changes
Sex
Frame
Triceps skinfold
Arm circumference
Arm muscle circumference

Lab
Serum albumin
Total iron-binding capacity
Serum transferrin
Lymphocytes (TLC)
WBC
24° urine
Urine urea nitrogen
Urinary creatinine
Creatinine height index
Hemoglobin and hematocrit

Other
Protein intake
Calorie intake
Nitrogen balance
Obligatory nitrogen loss
Basal energy expenditure in K cal/day
Measure of cell-mediated immunity
  (skin testing)

References

Bowman BB, Rosenberg IH: Assessment of nutrition. *Am J Clin Nutrition* 1982; 35:1142–1151.

Carpenito LJ: Diagnosing nutrition problems. *Am J Nurs* 1985; 85:584–592.

Carroll-Johnson R (editor): *Classification of Nursing Diagnoses: Proceedings of the Eighth Conferences.* Lippincott, 1989.

Cataldi-Betcher E et al: Complications occurring during enteral nutrition support: A prospective study. *J Parenteral Enteral Nutrition* 1983; 7:546–552.

Chernoff R, Mitchell CO, Lipschitz DA: Assessment of the nutritional status of the geriatric patient. *Geriatr Med Today* 1984; 3:129–141.

Davis MA et al: Living arrangements and dietary patterns of older adults in the United States. *J Gerontol* 1985; 40:434–442.

Dugdale AE, Chandler D, Baghurst K: Knowledge and belief in nutrition. *Am J Clin Nutrition* 1979; 32:441–448.

Ebersole P, Hess P: *Toward Healthy Aging.* Mosby, 1985.

Feldman EB: *Nutrition in Middle and Later Years.* PSG, 1983.

Goodwin JS, Goodwin JM, Garry PJ: Association between nutritional status and cognitive functioning in healthy adult populations. JAMA 1983; 249:2917–2921.

Hendricks J, Hendricks CD: *Aging in Mass Society — Myths and Realities.* Winthrop, 1981.

Hickler RB, Wayne KS: Nutrition and the elderly. *Am Fam Physician* 1984; 29:137–145.

Hogstel MO, Robinson NB: Feeding the frail elderly. *J Gerontol Nurs* 1989; 15(4):16–20.

Horsley J, Crane J, Haler K: *Reducing Diarrhea in Tube-fed Patients: CURN Project.* Grune and Stratton, 1981.

Irwin M: Encourage oral intake—yes, but how? *Am J Nurse* 1987; 87:100,106.

Kart GS, Mestress ES, Mestress JF: *Aging and Health: Biologic and Social Perspectives.* Addison-Wesley, 1978.

Keithley JK: Proper nutritional assessment can prevent hospital malnutrition. *Nursing* 1979; 9(2):68–72.

Lerman R: Malnutrition in hospitalized patients. *Hosp Pract* 1986; 21(3A):22–31.

Lipschitz DA: Protein caloric malnutrition in the hospitalized elderly. *Primary Care* 1982; 9:531–542.

Lipschitz DA et al: Nutritional evaluation and supplementation of elderly subjects participating in a Meals on Wheels program. *J Parenteral Enteral Nutrition* 1985; 9(3):343–347.

Mitchell CO, Lipschitz DA: The effects of age and sex on the routinely used measurements to assess the nutritional status of hospitalized patients. *Am J Clin Nutrition* 1982; 36:340–349.

Munro HN: Nutrient needs and nutritional status in relation to aging. *Drug-Nutrient Interactions* 1985; 4:55–74.

National Research Council: *Recommended Dietary Allowances,* 10th ed. National Academy Press, 1989.

Price MR: The patient is starving . . . but why? RN (Nov) 1979; 45–48.

Roe DA: *Drug Induced Nutritional Deficiencies,* 2nd ed. AVI, 1985.

Roe DA: Drug-nutrient interactions in the elderly. *Geriatrics* 1986; 41:57–74.

Seltzer MH et al: Instant nutritional assessment. *J Parenteral Enteral Nutrition* 1979; 3:157–159.

Seltzer MH et al: Specialized nutrition support: Patterns of care. *J Parenteral Enteral Nutrition* 1984; 8(5):506–510.

Shuran M, Nelson RA: Updated nutritional assessment and support of the elderly. *Geriatrics* 1986; 41:48–70.

Starker PM et al: Response to total parenteral nutrition in the extremely malnourished patients. *J Parenteral Enteral Nutrition* 1985; 9:300–302.

Vitale JJ, Santos JI: Nutrition and the elderly. *Postgrad Med* 1985; 78(5):79–89.

Weber HI: *Nursing Care of the Elderly.* Reston, 1980.

Worthington B: *Nutrition in Nursing Management for the Elderly.* Carnevali DL, Patrick M (editors). Lippincott, 1979.

Yen PK: Nurse-dietitian teamwork. *Geriatr Nurs* 1983a; 4:49,57.

Yen PK: Special help for eating problems. *Geriatr Nurs* 1983b; 4:257–258.

10

Impaired Swallowing

Marilyn Ter Maat, MS, RN, C
Luann Tandy, BSN, RN

Impairment in uncompensated swallowing, or dysphagia, is a discomfort or a difficulty in swallowing. It may be seen in many geriatric patients with disorders such as cerebral vascular accidents (CVAs), Parkinson's disease, multiple sclerosis, lesions of the medulla, dysfunction of the tongue, head trauma, amyotrophic lateral sclerosis (ALS), and surgical treatment for oral, oral-pharyngeal, or laryngeal cancer (Hargrove, 1980; Sayles, 1981).

The nursing diagnosis Impaired Swallowing, approved by the North American Nursing Diagnosis Association (NANDA) in 1986, is broad and encompasses all stages of swallowing (McLane, 1987). The nursing diagnosis developed in this chapter separates each stage of the swallow with signs and symptoms specific to each stage. This separation by stage advances planning of the nursing care of the swallowing impaired elderly patient (see Table 10.1).

To understand the causes of dysphagia better, a brief overview of the anatomy and physiology of the normal swallowing process is provided.

ANATOMY AND PHYSIOLOGY OF SWALLOWING

Swallowing is a complex process and involves the oral cavity, pharynx, larynx, and esophagus (Cherney and O'Neill, 1986; Hargrove, 1980; Maloof, 1985). These anatomic structures are illustrated in Figure 10.1.

Swallowing occurs in stages (see Figure 10.2). A normal swallow takes 5 to 15 seconds: 1 to 2 seconds for the oral stage; 1 second for the pharyngeal stage; and 5 to 10 seconds for the esophageal stage (Cherney and O'Neill, 1986; Dobie, 1978). Table 10.2 presents the function of cranial nerves in the various stages of swallowing.

The anticipatory stage is the first phase of swallowing and occurs before any food reaches the mouth. It is during this stage that decisions are made concerning the quantity, the type of food, the setting, and the rate at which food is eaten (Cherney and O'Neill, 1986).

The second stage is the oral preparatory stage. A quantity of food is placed in the oral cavity, the lips close, and this begins the reflex action of swallowing. The tongue manipulates and controls the location of the food. The soft palate and uvula close off the nasopharynx to prevent reflux.

The third stage of swallowing is the oral stage. This stage begins when the bolus or mass of food passes the anterior fossa arches, and the swallow reflex is triggered. The tongue moves the food posteriorly in an anterior-to-posterior rolling action.

Table 10.1

Comparison of Conceptualization of Diagnosis

NURSING DIAGNOSIS: IMPAIRED SWALLOWING (NANDA)

Definition The state in which an individual has decreased ability to voluntarily pass fluids and/or solids from the mouth to the stomach (McLane, 1987)

Defining Characteristics Observed evidence of difficulty in swallowing (eg, stasis of food in oral cavity, coughing/choking). Evidence of aspiration. (Carroll-Johnson, 1989; Gettrust et al, 1984; Larsen, 1981; Tilton & Maloof, 1982; Welnetz, 1983)

Related Factors Neuromuscular impairment (eg, decreased or absent gag reflex, decreased strength or excursion of muscles involved in mastication, perceptual impairment, facial paralysis); mechanical obstruction (eg, edema, tracheostomy tube, tumor); fatigue; limited awareness; reddened, irritated oropharyngeal cavity

NURSING DIAGNOSIS: IMPAIRED SWALLOWING (TER MAAT & TANDY)

Definition The state in which an individual has decreased ability to voluntarily pass fluids and/or solids from the mouth to the stomach (Carroll-Johnson, 1989)

Signs and Symptoms	*Diagnosis*
Poor attention span; unable to initiate or finish task of eating; eats when fed; poor memory	Impaired Swallowing: Anticipatory Stage
Drooling; poor lip closure; facial muscle weakness; poor tongue strength; inability to chew; reduction of oral sensation	Impaired Swallowing: Oral Stage
Reduced gag reflex; ineffective or absent cough; frequent choking; nasal regurgitation; frequent pneumonias; recent weight loss; hoarse voice; gurgling breath sounds	Impaired Swallowing: Oral-Pharyngeal Stage
Frequent eructation; odorous breath; recent increase in dental problems; heartburn; coated tongue; gurgling voice	Impaired Swallowing: Esophageal Stage

---

This stage of the swallow, lasting approximately 1 second, is under voluntary control.

The fourth stage is the pharyngeal stage. It is the most essential stage, involving further movement of the bolus and protection of the airway. The triggering of the swallow reflex induces a number of physiologic activities simultaneously. The tongue prevents food from reentering the oral cavity; this is accomplished by closure of the velopharyngeal valve due to the elevation and contraction of the soft palate. This is facilitated by the superior pharyngeal constrictor muscle, which narrows the upper pharynx. Pharyngeal peristalsis is initiated, causing the downward squeeze of the bolus through the pharynx to the cricopharyngeal sphincter (Cherney and O'Neill, 1986; Hargrove, 1980; Maloof, 1985). At the same time, the larynx is elevated and brought forward by the suprahyoid and thyrohyoid muscles. This is observed as "bobbing of the Adam's Apple" (Dobie, 1978). The cricopharyngeus muscle then relaxes, allowing the material to pass from the pharynx into the esophagus, and respiration resumes. This fourth stage in the swallowing process is involuntary and reflexive and takes about 1 second.

The esophageal stage is the last stage of swallowing and takes 5 to 10 seconds to complete. This stage starts with the lowering of the larynx; the primary peristaltic wave propels the bolus to the lower esophageal sphincter, causing the contraction of the cricopharyngeal muscle to guard against reflux. If the first peristaltic wave does not complete the task, successive stronger waves will move the bolus into the stomach (Cherney and O'Neill, 1986; Dobie, 1978; Hargrove, 1980).

TYPES OF DYSPHAGIA

Several types of dysphagia have been described in the literature, including dysphagia mechanica, pseudobulbar dysphagia, dysphagia paralytica, and functional dysphagia (Kadas, 1983; Martin et al, 1981). Dysphagia mechanica patients experience difficulty swallowing because of the loss of sensory guidance of the structures needed to complete the process, which usually occurs with brain damage or pathology. There should be little difficulty in recognizing dysphagia mechanica because of the physical alteration of the swallowing mechanism, usually affecting the oral stage (Kadas, 1983; Martin et al, 1981).

Pseudobulbar dysphagia usually occurs because of upper motor neuron damage, especially to the right

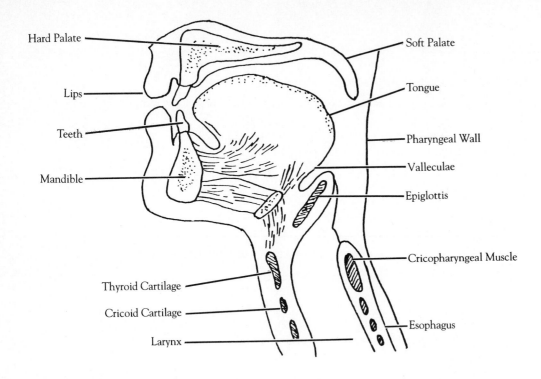

Pharynx
Uvula
Epiglottis
Valleculae
Tonsils
Pharyngeal constrictor muscles

Larynx
Single cartilages:
Thyroid
Cricoid
Epiglottis
Paired cartilages:
Arytenoid
Corniculate
Cuneiform

Oral Cavity
Lips
Teeth
Hard palate
Soft palate
Cheeks
Floor of mouth
Tongue
Fossal arches
Mandible

hemisphere. Because the patient frequently has upper motor neuron damage he or she may lose the cortical controls of swallowing and cognitive control over the swallowing process. This condition usually affects the oral and pharyngeal stages (Kadas, 1983; Martin et al, 1981).

The patient with dysphagia paralytica has paralysis caused by disease or trauma. This patient usually has lesions in the lower motor neuron system that can result in muscle weakness and impairment of oral reflexes. Once again, the oral and pharyngeal stages of swallowing are affected, and the patient with this condition usually is dysarthric (Kadas, 1983; Martin et al, 1981). Functional dysphagia results from an emotional or behavioral disturbance that can cause spasms in the throat or distortion of messages from the cerebral cortex (Kadas, 1983).

Griffin and Tollison (1980) describe dysphagia in three ways: as transfer dysphagia, transport dysphagia, and delivery dysphagia. Transfer dysphagia is caused by a disturbance in the process from the beginning of the swallow of the bolus from the oropharynx to the cervical esophagus. Transport dysphagia occurs when the bolus is interrupted during the esophageal stage by a lesion or disorder of the

esophageal muscle. Delivery dysphagia results when the bolus has difficulty entering the stomach because of a lesion or abnormal functioning of the sphincter.

ETIOLOGIES/RELATED FACTORS AND DEFINING CHARACTERISTICS

Impairment in uncompensated swallowing can take a number of forms because of the varied etiologies that can affect almost any stage of the swallowing process. In the anticipatory stage, the elderly person may be afraid to swallow or may not find the food appealing. As a patient progresses through the aging process, the elderly person may need intense amounts of stimulation to maintain adequate alertness through mealtime, or may need soft stimulation to avoid distraction at mealtime (Cherney and O'Neill, 1986).

Impairment in the oral stage can occur both neurologically and mechanically. A neurologic problem in this

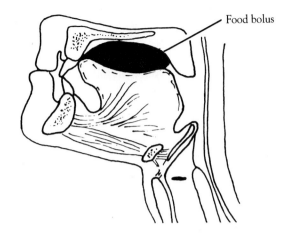

Food bolus

Oral Stage

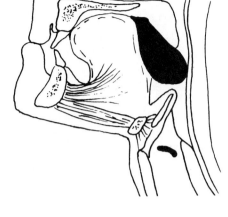

Oral Preparatory Stage

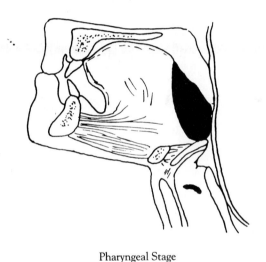

Pharyngeal Stage

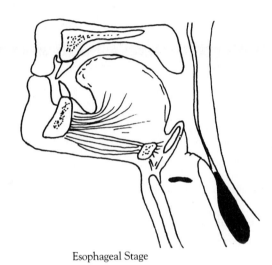

Esophageal Stage

Figure 10.2

Stages of swallowing.
(*Source:* Russell Tandy, BSN, RN.)

Credit: Russell Tandy, RN

stage will disrupt the grinding and shaping of food and the preparation of the bolus for the next stage.

The close association of the cranial nerves V, VII, IX, X, and XII used in the oral stage can produce certain generalizations. There may be decreased or reduced lip closure, and reductions in oral/facial sensation, which can cause drooling. A decrease in buccal tension may result in pocketing of food in the cheek. A reduction in mandibular movement may result in inadequately chewed food. Choking or coughing may be caused by decreased tongue movement that may interfere with bolus formation. Another problem frequently encountered in the elderly is the loss or reduction of sensations, including taste, temperature, touch, and texture (Cherney and O'Neill, 1986; Dobie, 1978). In general, patients who have had some type of oral surgery may have difficulty with mastication, formation, and transportation of the bolus.

The greatest concern with regard to managing swallowing impairment is during the pharyngeal stage. If there is an impairment during this stage there may be problems in interruption of respiration and protection of the airway. Symptoms during the pharyngeal stage are delayed or absent triggering of the swallowing reflex. This can be caused by food falling over the tongue into the vallecula, possibly causing aspiration. Another symptom is nasal regurgitation possibly caused by decreased velar elevation. Decreased closure of the glottis may also result in aspiration. Obstruction may also occur at the cricopharyngeal muscle due to a decreased opening. When the bolus is liquid, it pools in the vallecular and pyriform sinuses (Cherney and O'Neill, 1986; Dobie, 1978). Another cause of problems during this phase is surgical resection of the pharyngeal and laryngeal areas for control of a malignancy while maintaining vocal and swallowing functions.

Table 10.2

Cranial Nerves Involved in Swallowing Process

NERVE	ACTIVATES	STAGE
V (Trigeminal)	Swallowing reflex Separates oral and nasal cavity Controls bolus movement Stimulates salivation and chewing Provides sensations to the face, teeth, gums, tongue	Oral
Impairment:	Loss of sensation and inability to move mandible	
VII (Facial)	Provides sense of taste and control over muscles of face Swallowing reflex Separates oral and nasal cavity Controls movement of the bolus	Oral
Impairment:	Increased salivation and pouching of food and inability to pucker lips	
IX (Glossopharyngeal)	Transmits sensation to the soft palate, tonsils, pharynx Passage of air from nose to pharynx Influences the sense of taste Influences production of saliva Moves food inside mouth	Oral, pharyngeal, and esophageal
Impairment:	Decreases taste sensations, salivation and gag reflex	
XX (Vagus)	Sensation in the palate, base of tongue, pharynx, larynx Moves food inside the mouth Passage of air from nose to pharynx Passage of bolus to the esophagus Passage of bolus to the stomach	Oral, pharyngeal, and esophageal
Impairment:	Difficulty in swallowing, nasal regurgitation, decrease gag reflex	
XII (Hypoglossal)	Controls the muscles of the tongue Moves food inside mouth Passage of bolus to the esophagus	Pharyngeal
Impairment:	Inability to position food, pouching	

Other symptoms of impairment during this stage of the swallowing process are "gurgling" voice or breathing, reduced or absent sensation to the pharynx, dysarthria, and a delayed or absent gag reflex. During the esophageal stage a disruption in the bolus through the esophagus occurs. Esophageal dysphagia is a common disorder of the elderly. These disruptions can be caused by obstruction, possibly due to tumors, esophageal reflux, pain caused by nonperistaltic contractions, and a diverticulum caused by dysfunction in the cricopharyngeal muscle (Cherney and O'Neill, 1986; Dobie, 1978).

ASSESSMENT

There are several "red flags" that alert the nurse to the possibility of dysphagia. To begin the assessment, the nurse should sit with the patient and obtain a history of the current problem. If the patient is unable to communicate, the nurse should obtain the history from the medical record and/or a family member. To determine when the difficulty began, question the patient, if possible, to discover if she or he has experienced nasal regurgitation, hoarseness, or aspiration. While conversing with the patient, listen for abnormalities in speech pattern and tone. A hypernasal tone indicates a paralyzed palate and oropharynx; a hoarse voice may be a partial paralysis of the 10th cranial nerve (Larsen, 1981; Sayles, 1981).

The nurse should question patients about the consistency of food they are able to handle. If liquids are more difficult, this may indicate a neurologic disease, whereas difficulty with solids is more indicative of a stricture or obstruction (Dobie, 1978). The nurse should also visit and observe the elderly person eating during mealtime, assist the person with eating, and note how the elder handles and swallows a variety of foods and liquids.

Complaints of pain or comments such as "I feel like there's something stuck in my throat" warn the nurse that a patient is at risk for swallowing impairments. To determine the cause of discomfort, an indirect laryngeal examination should be done by a credentialed practitioner. A probable finding would be food debris in the valleculas or pyriform sinuses, indicating that the swallowing mechanism has failed to clear the bolus from the pharynx into the esophagus. This debris could potentially be aspirated into the trachea; the bolus should therefore be removed with suction.

It is also important to assess the patient's saliva production. Saliva assists with bolus formation. If the patient has a dry mouth, he or she may choke easily because the food cannot be formed into a bolus and may crumble in the mouth. Thick, ropey secretions also interfere with eating (Loustau and Lee, 1985). During the assessment interview, observe the patient for drooling, poor lip closure, and facial muscle weakness. These symptoms indicate a possible problem with the oral stage of swallowing once the bolus is formed.

The nurse should also observe for facial weakness by noting if the face is symmetrical, and test for muscle weakness by asking patients to put their lips together. If they cannot maintain the closure, weakness is present (Loustau and Lee, 1985).

Tongue strength may be assessed laterally by asking the patient to press his tongue to the sides of the mouth against the assessor's hand. To check strength in the midline position, the patient should push her tongue against a tongue blade. Poor coordination or inability to use the tongue interferes with formation of the bolus in the oral stage (Loustau and Lee, 1985).

Physical assessment also includes checking three reflexes: the swallowing reflex, the cough reflex, and the gag reflex (Loustau and Lee, 1985). To assess the swallowing reflex, palpate the larynx by placing a finger on the thyroid cartilage when the patient swallows. The larynx should elevate, displacing the finger downward.

Laryngeal elevation can also be evaluated by giving the patient a small sip of water or ice chips and observing the swallow. Patients who cough are exhibiting the cough reflex that protects the trachea from aspiration. If the patient does not cough ask him or her to try to cough. If the patient cannot cough voluntarily, do not feed him or her until further testing can be done because there is potential for aspiration.

Be particularly alert to the elderly patient who has experienced a recent unintentional weight loss or exhibits signs of dehydration. This patient may fear choking and has thus restricted dietary intake voluntarily. Also be aware of any indications of lung aspiration such as increased temperature and adventitious lung sounds (Groher, 1984; Martin et al, 1981).

Throughout the interview and assessment the patient's mental status should also be noted (see Chapter 29). Look for poor short-term memory, distractibility, and inappropriate conversation from the patient. Eating requires a great degree of attention and planning, and the patient who appears to have poor judgment, perceptual impairments, or motor planning is at risk for uncompensated swallowing (Groher, 1984).

CASE STUDY

Anticipatory Stage Dysphagia

A 69-year-old man with Alzheimer's disease is evaluated for inability to eat. The patient sits down to eat a meal, eats three to four bites, and then sits without eating. This elderly patient needs constant encouragement to eat; he is easily distracted by activities in the room or conversations with him. He eats only when fed by another person, has poor short-term memory, and is more confused toward evening. Table 10.3 summarizes this patient's signs and symptoms and lists the additional data needed.

Table 10.3

Data on Case Study—Anticipatory Stage Dysphagia

SIGNS & SYMPTOMS	DIAGNOSES RULED OUT	ADDITIONAL DATA NEEDED
Poor memory	Swallowing impairment	Neurologic assessment, including visual fields
Easily distracted	Esophageal stage	Weight history
Sits down at a meal but eats only 3–4 bites then leaves	Swallowing impairment Oral stage	Current weight Recent weight gain
Confusion	Swallowing impairment	Mental status
Eats when fed	Oral-pharyngeal stage	Orientation at mealtime
	Altered Nutrition:	c/o food sticking in throat
	More Than Body Requirements	Drooling
		Facial muscle weakness
		Pocketing of food

TENTATIVE DIAGNOSIS

Impaired Swallowing: Anticipatory stage as evidenced by inability to complete a meal.

NURSING INTERVENTIONS

Anticipatory Stage

To make feeding a success, the nurse must first evaluate the patient's mental status. A tired, confused, or lethargic patient does not create a successful feeding session. The session should be close to the patient's normal mealtime but not following a tiring trip to x-ray or therapy. Eating takes concentration, and the elderly patient must be as alert and fresh as possible (Groher, 1984). The meal should be eaten in a pleasant environment away from excess stimulation. When the patient first starts swallowing retraining, feeding should be done in a one-to-one situation close to suction equipment in case of choking. As patients progress and the nurse feels comfortable with their abilities, they may eat in a group situation. In some settings a speech pathologist may initiate the feeding process.

Elderly patients need to be in proper body alignment. They should be sitting upright with hips and knees at a 90° angle. The head should be flexed slightly forward to protect the airway. If a pillow is used to align the head, place the pillow behind the patient's shoulders. Having the pillow behind the head places the patient in an incorrect position and may cause an abnormal reflex pattern (Dobie, 1978; Groher, 1984; Loustau and Lee, 1985; Silverman and Elfant, 1979).

If at all possible, elderly patients should not be fed in bed. If they cannot sit in a chair, the head of the bed should be raised as high as possible. The nurse should remain unhurried and calm, as the eating situation may be fearful, especially for the elderly patient (Loustau and Lee, 1985). In the elderly, memory impairment is a frequent problem. Group situations are helpful because they provide someone for the patient to mimic. Elderly patients placed across from someone who eats well will be cued nonverbally and will tend to eat in a more timely fashion. Furthermore, the group environment gives an air of normality to the eating situation as if the patient were in a family situation.

CASE STUDY

Oral Stage Uncompensated Swallowing

A 78-year-old woman was admitted to the hospital with a right-sided CVA and presented with left facial droop, deviation of the tongue to the right and reduction of oral sensation. She refused oral intake because of drooling and inability to chew. After fluoroscopic evaluation it was determined that the patient was experiencing difficulty in the oral stage of swallowing. Table 10.4 summarizes this patient's signs and symptoms and lists the additional data needed.

TENTATIVE DIAGNOSIS

Impaired Swallowing: oral stage as evidenced by inability to form bolus.

Oral Stage

Many difficulties can occur in the oral stage. The elderly patient with oral and facial weakness has problems manipulating the bolus for swallowing. To strengthen the

Table 10.4

Data on Case Study—Oral Stage Uncompensated Swallowing

SIGNS & SYMPTOMS	DIAGNOSES RULED OUT	ADDITIONAL DATA NEEDED
Left facial droop	Impaired Tissue Integrity: Oral Mucous Membrane	Fluid intake
Deviation of tongue to the right	Negative side effects of prescribed treatment	Calorie count
Reduction of oral sensation		Medication regimen
Drooling		Monitor weight
Refusing oral intake		Skin turgor
Cannot chew		Hydration status
		Does patient have dentures?
		Mental status/memory
		Oral status
		Communication abnormalities in speech pattern and tone
		Food pouching
		Tongue strength

lips and facial muscles the nurse can prescribe that the elderly person practice the following exercises in front of a mirror (Groher, 1984;137–138). The nurse should also have the exercises rehearsed by any assisting staff or family caregivers to be sure the elderly person gets the appropriate assistance and actually does the exercises as prescribed.

1. Smile broadly with lips closed and open.
2. Frown tightly.
3. Alternate lip pursing and retraction.
4. Practice producing the letters u, m, b, p, w.
5. Puff out cheeks with air and hold.
6. Purse lips and blow.
7. Suck hard on a frozen popsicle.
8. Hide tip of tongue under top lip.

To strengthen the tongue have the elderly patient:

1. Pronounce "la, la, la," "ta, ta, ta," d, n, z, s.
2. Push against a tongue depressor.
3. Lick a lollipop.
4. Count the teeth with the tongue.
5. Push the tip of the tongue against the roof of the mouth and the lower teeth.
6. Lick jelly off the lips.

To feed elderly patients with oral stage difficulties, place one-fourth (1/4) to one-third (1/3) teaspoon of food on a teaspoon and present it to them to observe and smell. When the patient opens his mouth, place the spoon in the center of his tongue and allow him to remove the food with his lips. The pressure created by the spoon helps initiate mouth closure (Groher, 1984).

The pressure and placement of the spoon helps the elderly patient to keep her head lowered and in midline. Never present food above mouth level, as this encourages raising of the head. After the patient has removed the food from the spoon, withdraw the spoon with the same downward pressure and watch for the patient's larynx to rise, indicating she has swallowed (Groher, 1984). Make sure the patient has cleared her mouth from the first bite before serving her the second. Also observe for pocketing of food in the cheeks (Sayles, 1981).

While the patient is eating, observe for signs of hypersensitivity to hot or cold. Food temperature should be varied enough so that the patient is aware that something is in his or her mouth, but not so extreme as to cause discomfort. The nurse should observe for signs of fatigue and discontinue feeding if the elderly patient becomes tired, as a tired patient cannot concentrate on the eating task at hand.

Assisting the patient who has problems moving the bolus posteriorly may require adaptive equipment such as a glossectomy spoon (shown in Figure 10.3) or syringe (Groher, 1984; Martin et al, 1981). The glossectomy spoon is used to place the bolus at the back of the throat where

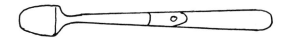

Figure 10.3

Glossectomy spoon.
(*Source:* Russell Tandy, BSN, RN.)

it may then be swallowed. The spoon has a plunger that pushes the food off the end of the spoon (Groher, 1984; Martin et al, 1981). Another useful item of equipment is a syringe with a tube attached that is of an equal distance from the lip to the uvula. A squeeze bottle used for drinking water at athletic events may also be used. The nurse can place pureed food in the bottle or syringe, then position the tube at the back of the throat. The bottle is squeezed so that the food is carefully deposited on the back of the tongue. The placement of the bolus on the back of the mouth prevents drooling and promotes swallowing. Elderly patients may be able to do this for themselves (Groher, 1984; Martin et al, 1981).

Another complication of the oral stage may be thick, ropey secretions that occur from infrequent swallowing. To manage this problem the nurse should have the patient lick his or her hand, sprinkle meat tenderizer on the hand, and then lick the tenderizer off. The tenderizer has a papain in it that thins the mucus. Chewable papaya tablets, which may be purchased at the drug store, have the same effect as the tenderizer. This treatment should be started 10 minutes before the patient eats (Martin et al, 1981).

CASE STUDY

Oral-Pharyngeal Stage Uncompensated Swallowing

An 82-year-old man was evaluated for easy fatigability, generalized weakness, and a recent weight loss of 15 pounds. His wife reported that while eating he experienced choking, predominantly with liquids, and nasal regurgitation. In the last 6 months he had been hospitalized for pneumonia three times. The physical examination revealed a reduced gag reflex and a poor cough. Fluoroscopic examination revealed difficulty in the oral-pharyngeal stage of swallowing. Table 10.5 summarizes this patient's signs and symptoms and lists additional data needed.

TENTATIVE DIAGNOSES

Impaired Swallowing: Oral-pharyngeal stage as evidenced by recent weight loss.

Impaired Swallowing: Oral-pharyngeal stage as evidenced by frequent pneumonias.

Table 10.5

Data on Case Study—Oral-Pharyngeal Stage Uncompensated Swallowing

SIGNS & SYMPTOMS	DIAGNOSES RULED OUT	ADDITIONAL DATA NEEDED
Fatigues easily	Respiratory insufficiency	Diet history
Generalized weakness	Self-care deficit	Facial muscle strength
Recent weight loss of 15 pounds	Inability to procure food	Oral condition
Chokes on liquids		Tongue strength
Nasal regurgitation		Respiratory care at home
Hospitalized for pneumonia three times in 6 months		Signs and symptoms of dehydration
Reduced gag reflex		
Poor cough		

Oral-Pharyngeal Stage

Aspiration is the major problem in the oral-pharyngeal stage. There are many elderly patients who aspirate, and the nursing staff is not always aware of it. A classic warning sign that a patient is choking is the protective cough. Patients may not always cough, however, even if they are aspirating, because of decreased innervation to the mouth and esophagus. If an elderly patient is aspirating over 10% of each bolus, she or he will probably develop aspiration pneumonia. The percentage of aspiration can be estimated by video fluoroscopy. Patients who aspirate may have a rapid heart rate and may suddenly turn gray. Gasping, choking, a hoarse voice, and gurgling sounds in the chest are other indicators (Groher, 1984).

The nurse should not give thin liquids to the elderly patient who aspirates because transit time from lips to esophagus is too rapid, and the liquid falls over the back of the tongue before the swallow is initiated. To thicken liquids, add gelatin to juice or add powdered milk to milk products and creamed soups. However, the nurse should try to avoid milk products unless they are baked into food, as they produce mucus (Groher, 1984). Baby cereal is another good thickening agent that can be used to improve the nutritional value of the meal. Thick liquids such as tomato juice and nectars can also be served. Thin liquids can be mixed with food or given in the form of slushes. Finally, straws are contraindicated for elderly patients with oral-pharyngeal problems because they cause the liquid to be propelled too quickly, and it pours over the back of the tongue.

A helpful device with problems in the oral-pharyngeal stage of swallowing is the nose-cut cup (Groher, 1984;144) (see Figure 10.4). These cups may be purchased or created by cutting a semi-circle one half the depth of the cup on one side. The elderly patient then drinks from the side that is intact, and the cutout allows the patient to drink without tipping his or her head back.

To decrease the chance of aspiration, nurses may teach elderly patients to supraglottic swallow. This technique is very simple. Instruct the patient to take a sip in his

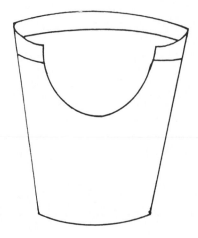

Figure 10.4

Nose cup.
(*Source:* Russell Tandy, BSN, RN.)

mouth, hold his breath, tip chin to chest, swallow, raise the chin, and cough twice or clear his throat. Tipping the head closes off the larynx and the trachea, preventing aspiration. Coughing clears the residue that may have accumulated around the opening to the trachea.

For the elderly patient who is found to be at risk for aspiration, the first feeding should be pudding or gelatin. These foods remain in a bolus and do not fall apart in the mouth. As the patient progresses, she or he may ingest pureed foods and thick liquids.

Besides aspiration, the dysphagic elderly patient may experience oral-pharyngeal residue and stasis. Stasis occurs when the food stays in the esophagus and pharynx, and residue occurs when food sticks to the side of the pharynx. Patients with these problems clear their throats frequently and may feel as though something is stuck. They also may experience a premature full feeling. The elderly patient with stasis residue is at risk for choking while eating, but not when drinking.

The elderly patient who has been on pureed feedings for an extended period of time may become tired of the consistency and taste. If acceptable to the patient, these foods may be spiced up by adding ketchup, spaghetti sauce, or spices. The nurse is cautioned to avoid sticky food such as peanut butter that may stay on the palate (Loustau and Lee, 1985). For elderly patients who cannot tolerate large meals, consider six small feedings rather than three meals per day (Groher, 1984).

Family members can provide support to the elderly patient and assist in the feeding process. They should therefore be included in the teaching/training process as much as possible (Groher, 1984).

Following the meal, the elderly patient should be kept upright for 15 to 30 minutes to prevent aspiration and provide good oral care. The patient with swallowing impairment is prone to dental problems as food pockets in her mouth. Because tongue movements are impaired, the patient is not able to sweep her mouth to remove food particles (Groher, 1984).

CASE STUDY

Esophageal Stage Uncompensated Swallowing

A 73-year-old man presented with complaints of heartburn, frequent eructation, odorous breath, and a recent increase in dental problems. He did not complain of difficulty swallowing solids or liquids, but stated that his heartburn was worse at night. Physical examination was normal for a man of this age. Diagnostic evaluation by radiology and speech pathology revealed esophageal reflux. Table 10.6 summarizes this patient's signs and symptoms and lists additional data needed.

TENTATIVE DIAGNOSIS

Impaired Swallowing: Esophageal stage—reflux as evidenced by pyrosis.

Esophageal Stage

In the esophageal stage of swallowing, esophageal reflux may be present. The elderly patient who exhibits a gurgling voice, odorous breath, coated tongue, heartburn while eating, frequent eructations, and a recent increase in dental problems may have esophageal reflux. To improve this situation, the nurse should instruct the patient not to lie down after a meal, as reflux is greater when lying down. Serving a small evening meal and giving 2 ounces of a cola beverage just prior to sleep may also be helpful. It is believed that the CO_2 in the cola creates pressure in the lower esophageal sphincter, which holds the food in the stomach. In addition, eating a high-protein diet and elevating the head of the bed 6 inches are recommended. Because these elderly may be prone to esophagitis, the nurse should be alert for this problem and the need for a referral to the physician or nurse practitioner for appropriate drug therapy.

OUTCOMES

The long-term outcome of dysphagia management is to return the patient to normal functioning. With the geriatric population, however, this goal is not always a reality because of their multiple and chronic medical problems.

Dysphagia treatment should be discontinued if no improvement is seen in 3 to 4 months. By this time the patient should be able to take in sufficient calories orally. If this is not the case, an alternative method of nutrition should be considered. Treatment is deemed successful if aspiration is less than 10% of the bolus and the oral-pharyngeal stage is less than 5 seconds.

INTERDISCIPLINARY MANAGEMENT OF IMPAIRED SWALLOWING

A swallowing retraining team (dysphagia team) consists of a nurse trained in dysphagia treatment, an occupational therapist, a dietitian, a speech pathologist, a physician, and a radiologist. Nurses who engage in swallowing retraining need specific education and training.

Table 10.6

Data on Case Study—Esophageal Stage Uncompensated Swallowing

SIGNS & SYMPTOMS	DIAGNOSES RULED OUT	ADDITIONAL DATA NEEDED
Heartburn	Airway Clearance: Ineffective	Normal diet
Frequent eructation	Impaired Tissue Integrity: Oral Mucous Membrane	Size of meals
Odorous breath	Ineffective breathing patterns	Eating patterns
Recent increase in dental problems		
Heartburn is worse at night		

Knowledge and understanding of the anatomy and physiology of the mouth, the neck, the esophagus, and the cranial nerves involved in the swallowing process is necessary to determine where the impairment is and how best to intervene with the elderly patient. The nurse on the team has direct responsibility for monitoring the elderly patient and reporting his or her status to the team. In some hospitals nurses serve as team leaders for the swallowing retraining team.

The nurse must be skilled with safety techniques, including CPR with blocked airway, suctioning, tracheostomy care, and how to use resuscitation equipment. In order to provide swallowing rehabilitation the nursing staff needs to learn specific oral exercises and feeding and swallowing techniques. They also must be familiar with different dietary selections and what textures are available in the diets provided.

SUMMARY

In the geriatric population, swallowing remains a critical survival function. A good knowledge base of anatomy and physiology of the head and neck and understanding of the stages of swallowing are essential for the nurse working with these patients. The nurse working with the geriatric patient has the opportunity to play an important role in dysphagia treatment alone or as part of a swallowing retraining team. Many of the interventions presented in this chapter are practical and can be used easily in any setting.

References

Carroll-Johnson R: *Classification of Nursing Diagnoses: Proceedings of the Eighth Conference.* Lippincott, 1989.

Cherney LR, O'Neill P: Swallowing disorders and the aged. *Top Geriatr Rehabil* 1986; 1;45–57.

Dobie R: Rehabilitation of swallowing disorders. *Am Fam Physician* 1978; 17:84–95.

Gettrust KV, Ryan SC, Engleman DS: *Applied Nursing Diagnosis: Guides for Comprehensive Care Planning.* Wiley, 1984, pp. 15–16.

Griffin J, Tollison J: Dysphagia. *Am Fam Physician* 1980; 22(5):154–160.

Groher M (editor): *Dysphagia.* Butterworth, 1984.

Hargrove R: Feeding the severely dysphagic patient. *J Neurosurg Nurs* 1980; 12:102–107.

Kadas N: The dysphagic patient: Everyday care really counts. *RN* 1983; 46:38–41.

Larsen GL: Chewing and swallowing. In: *Comprehensive Rehabilitative Nursing.* Martin N, Holt NB, Hicks DB (editors). McGraw-Hill, 1981.

Loustau A, Lee K: Dealing with the dangers of dysphagia. *Nursing* (Feb) 1985; 47–50.

Maloof M: Self feeding deficits. Application of rehabilitation concepts to nursing practice study guide. *Rehabil Nurs Institute* 1985; 115–118.

Martin N, Holt N, Hicks D: *Comprehensive Rehabilitation Nursing.* McGraw-Hill, 1981.

McLane A (editor): *Classification of Nursing Diagnoses: Proceedings of the Seventh Conference.* Mosby, 1987.

Sayles S (editor): *Rehabilitation Nursing: Concepts and Practice.* Rehabilitation Nursing Institute, 1981.

Silverman EH, Elfant IL: Dysphagia. *Am J Occupational Ther* 1979; 33:382–392.

Tilton CN, Maloof M: Diagnosing the problem in stroke. *Am J Nurs* 1982; 82:596–601.

Welnetz K: Maintaining adequate nutrition and hydration in the dysphagic ALS patient. *Canad Nurse* 1983; 79:30–34.

11

Altered Oral Mucous Membrane

JANIS B. ELDREDGE, MS, RDH

THE ELDERLY ARE AT HIGH RISK FOR ORAL COMPLICATIONS and disease. Throughout the aging process, physiologic changes of the mucous membranes can cause a loss of tissue integrity and protective properties, bringing oral discomfort and dysfunction to the elderly person. The mucosa of the alveolar ridges, the palate, the lips, the tongue, the sublingual areas, and the vestibule become thinner, smoother, less resilient, drier, and more susceptible to gingivitis, periodontitis, glossitis, angular cheilitis, hyperemia halitosis, xerostomia, fungal infections, and cancerous lesions (see Assessment Guide 11.1).

For these reasons it is important that nurses who care for the elderly are able to diagnose Altered Oral Mucous Membrane accurately. The diagnosis is defined by the North American Nursing Diagnosis Association (NANDA) as "the state in which an individual experiences disruptions in the tissue layers of the oral cavity" (Carroll-Johnson, 1989; 531).

ETIOLOGIES/RELATED FACTORS

Dental researchers and clinicians continue to clarify etiologic alterations in the oral mucosa (Miles, 1972; Squier et al, 1975). Table 11.1 contains the etiologies developed by NANDA and those described in this chapter.

Histologically, the epithelial surface atrophies, and the rete pegs become shorter, causing a reduction of interface with connective tissue and thinning of the oral epithelium, particularly in the mandibular residual ridge area (Garguilo et al, 1961; Graham, 1968; Loe and Karring, 1971; Marwah et al, 1960; Ryan et al, 1974; Shaklar, 1966; Zimmerman and Zimmerman, 1965). Loss of adipose and glandular tissue decreases the depth of the submucosa and reduces its cushioning effect, leaving the vessels and nerves vulnerable to pressure. Although the number of elastic fibers is thought to increase, their degeneration into thick clumps and the replacement of muscle fiber with loose, flabby, connective tissue causes a loss of tissue resiliency and firmness of shape (Graham, 1968; Loe and Karring, 1971; Shakler, 1966).

The diminished hormonal status of women contributes to oral mucosal changes such as pallor and atrophy after menopause. Mucosal atrophy may reflect nutritional deficiencies of iron or B vitamins in all elderly persons (Squier, 1982).

The gradual disappearance of glandular tissue, accelerated by the pressure of complete dentures, reduces salivary secretions and results in xerostomia

Table 11.1

Etiologies/Related Factors of Altered Oral Mucous Membrane

NANDA (CARROLL-JOHNSON, 1989)	ELDREDGE
Radiation to head/neck	Irradiation
Dehydration—NPO >24 hr	Dehydration
Mouth breathing	Fluid loss, eg, sweating, vomiting*
Lack of or decreased salivation	Diminished salivary gland function
Trauma—chemical, eg, acidic foods, drugs/alcohol*—mechanical, eg, ill-fitting dentures*	Mechanical trauma, eg, ill-fitting dentures*
	Chemical trauma, eg, acidic foods, alcohol*
Ineffective oral hygiene	Poor oral hygiene
Infection	Infection
Malnutrition	Vitamin deficiencies: B, C, iron, protein
Medication	Medication
	Depression
	Stress
	Local irritants
	Compromised immune system
	Disease: Sjögren's syndrome, obstruction, tumors, excision, aplasia
	Diminished hormones—women
	Atrophy of epithelial surface
	Decrease in cell division
	Loss of adipose/glandular tissue
	Degeneration of elastic fibers/replacement of muscle with loose connective tissues

* List of examples not complete

(dry mouth). Xerostomia does not result from the aging process alone, but is a side effect of stress, disease, and medications. Secretion of saliva is regulated by the autonomic nervous system and is stimulated by four basic factors (Mason and Glen, 1967). Factors regulating the salivary center are most often affected by depression, a common problem for the elderly. Factors affecting the autonomic outflow pathway are strongly influenced by over 250 drugs that have xerostomic potential. Factors affecting salivary gland function include Sjögren's syndrome, obstruction and infection, tumors, irradiation, excision, and aplasia. Factors affecting fluid or electrolyte balance include any condition that creates a loss of fluid, for example, vomiting, diarrhea, and sweating.

Burning sensations in the tongue are also common among the elderly and tend to be concurrent with vitamin B complex and estrogen deficiencies, anemia, and xerostomia from emotional upsets. When filiform and fungiform papillae are lost on the dorsal surface, the tongue becomes smooth, atrophic, and more sensitive. Loss of circumvallate papillae decreases the number of taste buds, reducing the ability to taste (Squier, 1982). "Normal-sized" sublingual varicosities on the ventral surface of the tongue appear enlarged in comparison with the atrophic glands and adipose tissue in that area. In addition, the tongue in the edentulous mouth flattens and broadens, increasing in size to fill the edentulous space.

Cellularity, vascularity, and water content of the mucosa decreases with age; intercellular substances increase. Vessel fragility may account for increased varicosities or hyperemia. Regeneration of tissues proceeds more slowly in the elderly, and wound healing can be delayed when vitamin C deficiency and protein deficiency are present (Squier, 1982) and when a source of infection is allowed to remain in the oral cavity. Intercurrent infections only prolong the healing process.

Reduced gingival stippling, increased fibrosis, and diminished keratinization are generally effects of aging, as is the apical migration of the gingival cuff surrounding the tooth, the dentogingival junction. Although not inevitable with age, and often intensified by periodontal disease, the dentogingival junction migrates from its attachment on the enamel crown of the tooth to the cemento-enamel junction, and eventually to the cemental root surface. This gingival recession involves attrition of the tooth surface with compensatory eruption of the tooth. When retraction of the gingival margin does not accompany tooth movement, the attached gingiva increases in width (Squier, 1982).

The periodontal ligament is affected by age-related decreases in cell division, vascularity and fibroplasia, and an increase in arteriosclerosis. Collagen fibers appear thicker and often become calcified to the point of ankylosis of the tooth.

Most changes in the oral mucous membranes and periodontium of the elderly result from non-age-related extraneous causes: (1) poor oral hygiene; (2) local irritants; (3) infection; (4) mechanical trauma from ill-fitting dentures or other dental appliances; (5) mechanical trauma from endotracheal or nasogastric tubes, coarse foods, or oral surgery; (6) chemical trauma from alcohol, medication, or acidic foods and beverages; (7) radiation therapy; (8) mouth breathing; and (9) dehydration. Tissue changes may also occur secondary to systemic factors such as altered hormonal status, malnutrition, or impaired cardiovascular function (Squier, 1982).

The development of oral cancer is not part of the aging process. However, the increasing number of alterations in physiologic functions of elderly persons may contribute to the development and progression of neoplasia (Hill and Rowe, 1982). Strong etiologic relationships exist between older persons, especially males, and different health care attitudes and environmental factors such as greater cumulative sunlight exposure, prolonged pipe smoking, tobacco chewing, and snuff-dipping (Hill, 1982; Kramer et al, 1978). Evidence linking Herpesvirus hominis type I (HSV I) and a compromised immune system in the elderly with oral squamous cell carcinoma is weak (Lehner et al, 1973).

Patients who have allergies to particular foods and/or drugs are apt to experience severe oral problems. Stroke and arthritis victims who no longer are able to manipulate a toothbrush are more susceptible to periodontal infections. Patients with Alzheimer's disease often present a problem because of confusion and lack of cognitive processing, making it very difficult for caregivers to provide adequate oral hygiene. Multiple sclerosis, Parkinson's disease, epilepsy, and cardiovascular disorders all can affect oral hygiene care and periodontal disease. Arthritis may restrict movement of the temporomandibular joint, making it difficult to open the mouth. Facial muscles may be affected by muscular dystrophy, making the wearing of dentures nearly impossible.

DEFINING CHARACTERISTICS

Defining characteristics for the diagnosis Altered Oral Mucous Membrane identified by NANDA and those discussed in this chapter are listed in Table 11.2. An early sign of an oral problem is halitosis, or bad breath. For many elderly, especially the institutionalized, halitosis results from inadequate oral hygiene due to arthritis or other physical limitations, disinterest, forgetfulness, lack of knowledge, or lack of supplies. Halitosis also can be a sign of ulcerations from ill-fitting dentures, leukoplakia, hemorrhagic gingivitis, severe periodontitis, oral cancerous lesions, or even more involved systemic complications. This symptom should not be treated by merely passing mouthwash.

Other signs of oral mucosa problems in older adults are unusual or poor eating habits and the deliberate selection

Table 11.2

Defining Characteristics of Altered Oral Mucous Membrane

NANDA (CARROLL-JOHNSON, 1989)	ELDREDGE
Oral pain/discomfort	Toothache, burning sensation in tongue
Coated tongue	Dry mouth (xerostomia)
Xerostomia (dry mouth)	
Lack of or decreased salivation	Coated tongue
	Smooth, atrophic, more sensitive tongue
Stomatitis	Enlarged varicosities on ventral surface of tongue
Oral lesions/ulcers	Leukoplakia, bright red palate
Leukoplakia	Hemorrhagic gingivitis
Hyperemia	Bleeding, inflamed, edematous, sensitive gums
Edema	Gingival recession
Desquamation	Flattened, broadened tongue in edentulous mouth
Vesicles	Delayed wound healing
Oral plaque	Frequent infections of oral mucosa
Carious teeth	Caries in teeth
Halitosis	Halitosis
	Distorted facial expression
	Loss of appetite or taste
	Difficulty swallowing
	Unusual or difficult speech/eating habits
	Attitudinal changes
	Mobility of natural teeth

of soft foods for meals and snacks. These practices may hide serious problems such as ulcers.

As noted earlier, xerostomia (dry mouth), the condition caused by decrease or lack of salivary secretions, may be associated with the following symptoms: general oral soreness, burning sensations, repeated denture sores, difficulty speaking and swallowing, abnormal taste sensations (usually sour or metallic), or trouble with denture retention (Ettinger, 1982). Routine screening examinations will often reveal additional signs: mucosal inflammation, mucosal atrophy, fissuring of the tongue, increased plaque formation, increased periodontal disease, increased dental caries (especially root caries), and infection by *Candida albicans.*

In the edentulous mouth, the tongue may flatten and broaden to fill the space once occupied by the teeth. The papillae of the tongue become atrophic, and many disappear completely, causing loss of taste. Occasionally, the dorsal surface will be coated with thick, ropey saliva, white in appearance and difficult to rinse away. White patches that are removable with mild scraping may be a form of leukoplakia, a precancerous condition. Lesions on the sides and posterior third of the tongue indicate the need for an oral cancer examination. On the ventral surface, otherwise "normal"-sized varicosities may appear oversized in the older adult when compared with other atrophic structures in that area.

Xerostomia may leave the lips taut, dry, and desquamated, and the elderly individual may be observed chewing or biting at loose pieces of tissue. Inflammation or chapping at the corners of the mouth (angular cheilitis) may be caused by drooling from ill-fitting dentures. Oral lesions, ulcerations, or leukoplakia on the lips can result from holding the barrel of a pipe in the same location, chewing the lips, or having an accumulation of excessive sun exposure.

Oral malignant neoplasms compose 2% to 5% of all malignant tumors in the United States; 90% of these tumors are squamous cell carcinomas, and the rest are predominantly tumors of the salivary glands (Hill and Rowe, 1982). The lips are the most frequent oral site of primary squamous cell carcinoma (eight times more common in men than in women). Tumors on the lateral borders of the tongue, the most common intraoral site, may present as a localized mucosal thickening, a persistent ulcer, or a deep, swollen mass. Putative premalignant lesions have high rates of malignant transformation on the floor of the mouth and appear as speckled leukoplakia or an erythroplakia. Carcinoma of the buccal mucosa is relatively uncommon in the United States, but verrucous carcinoma of the buccal sulcus and adjacent buccal mucosa is sometimes seen in elderly people who practice "snuff dipping" (Hill and Rowe, 1982). Lesions with the worst prognosis tend to be those with the most structural disorganization and dysplasia (Arthur and Farr, 1972). Although there is no conclusive evidence that age-related alterations in physiologic functioning contribute to the development of neoplasms, prognosis is more than likely influenced by diminished immune system functioning (Hill and Rowe, 1982).

Sores that do not heal in approximately 2 weeks should be examined by a dentist or a physician. Although delayed healing may be associated with vitamin and protein deficiencies, an active source of infection is the major impediment to recovery.

Nurses need to be more cognizant of the signs of oral disease and periodically explore the oral cavity for indications of change in their elderly patients or residents. Because the early lesion is usually unobtrusive and painless, patients are often unaware of the lesion and do not seek assistance. One might expect the aging oral epithelium to have a smoother, more satiny appearance; reduced stippling; and a thin or nonexistent keratinized layer. However, gingiva that appears edematous, inflamed, hemorrhagic, highly sensitive, or overly dry is a sure sign of an oral problem. A tongue coated with food and bacterial debris, white patches of leukoplakia, a blazing red palate from denture stomatitis, and the sloughing of necrotic, inflammatory tissue from the lining of the cheeks are not healthy indications. Nurses should be aware of and assess for all diseases, including those common to the oral cavity, that afflict the elderly.

ASSESSMENT

Dental needs of the elderly can be numerous and varied, especially for those individuals who reside in long-term care facilities. Often they are no longer able to perform adequate oral hygiene measures, or they suffer multiple diseases and complications, many of which affect the oral cavity. Elderly persons who have kept their teeth may face complex problems related to periodontal disease and rampant dental caries. Professional dental examinations every 6 months to a year are imperative to the oral health and sometimes to the life of the individual, whether dentate or edentulous. At least once a month nurses need to make "dental rounds" with their patients, discussing oral problems and performing a brief dental screening (see Assessment Guide 11.2).

Individuals who have been overexposed to the sun should be closely watched for evidence of squamous cell carcinoma of the lip. Distorted facial expressions, difficult or unusual speech patterns and eating habits, a sudden loss of appetite or taste, and difficult swallowing may reveal dentures that impinge on delicate mucosa, loose and ill-fitting appliances, "cotton mouth" (overall dryness), extreme mobility of natural teeth, chronic toothache, or burning tongue. Operant verbal and nonverbal behavior, attitudinal differences, and chronic depression may be secondary to oral irritations, just as complications of the oral cavity are often the result of systemic disease, radiation therapy, and medications.

Communication is one of the most important aspects of dental and oral screening. Take the time to listen to complaints and accounts of past dental experiences. Sit at eye level and look directly at the elderly patient while you converse. This exchange leads into extraoral and intraoral assessments.

A spot check dental examination is simple and inexpensive, requiring only a disposable mirror or tongue blade, a few squares of gauze, and a penlight. Nurses should be able to recognize and differentiate normal from abnormal conditions and notify a dentist if abnormalities fail to disappear in 2 weeks.

First, visually examine the face of the patient for balance of features (symmetry), uniformity of facial color, sun exposure, and raised areas. Examine the lips for color, texture, lumps, bumps, fissures, lesions, or corners that are cracked, red, or crusty. Standing behind the patient, gently palpate the gland areas as you move the pads of your fingers across the sides and front of the neck, under and around the ramus and chin. Ask the patient to remove any partials or dentures before your intraoral screening, and observe the physical condition and cleanliness of the appliance as well as the manner in which it is handled by the patient.

Pay particular attention to the palate for inflammation (denture stomatitis or infection by *Candida albicans*), a result of not removing dentures for 6 to 8 hours daily, preventing the palatal mucosa from breathing and relubricating. Check the bony ridges that support the dentures for red or white areas, ulcerations, lumps or bumps. Check the insides of the cheeks, the lips, and the throat for abnormal coloration, white patches, or sores. Examine all sides of the tongue by holding it with a gauze square and gently moving it from side to side. The varicose veins on the ventral side are "normal," unless found to be unusually large or hemorrhagic. Closely examine the floor of the mouth for speckled leukoplakia or erythroplakia, signs of oral cancer, but do not be alarmed by bony projections, known as tori, behind the mandibular anterior teeth.

Test the remaining teeth for movement; excessive mobility should be corrected as soon as possible. Loose teeth are uncomfortable, especially during mastication, and can be accidentally swallowed or aspirated. Look for large cavities or sharp, broken teeth, and ask the patient about oral discomfort. Edema, spontaneous bleeding, heavy calculus buildup, and tooth mobility are signs of severe periodontal problems. Dentures that appear loose and ill-fitting can usually be relined or adjusted to fit better for the health and comfort of the individual. A sure sign of a denture problem is the frequent use of denture creams and adhesives.

The nurse should also examine carefully for caries, excessive plaque and food debris, thick and ropey saliva, burning tongue, and an overall uncomfortable dryness and sensitivity of the mouth in order to identify xerostomia. It is also important to observe any reduction in salivary flow that results in a loss of cleansing action and a decrease in lubrication of the mouth, which may decrease the bacteriostatic power of the saliva (McLeran, 1982).

Gingival recession and exposed root surfaces contribute to oral hygiene problems. Exposed root surfaces are generally quite sensitive, difficult to brush, and more susceptible to dental decay (McLeran, 1982). The method and frequency of a patient's brushing need not be criticized. Rather, minor changes to enhance dexterity and overcome physical and mental limitations can be suggested. Partials and dentures should be examined for plaque and calculus deposits and for whether or not they have been labeled with the patient's name or initials.

Because eating habits often change in the elderly, the diet should be scrutinized for adequate nutrition. Elderly persons should also be instructed that certain foods and the absence of others contribute to dental caries.

CASE STUDY

Altered Oral Mucous Membrane

B.W., a 67-year-old black man with mental retardation, resided at Maplewood Care Facility. He was fully ambulatory, spoke with difficulty, and rarely made direct eye contact, but seemed to understand what was spoken to him and was usually cooperative. He had fairly normal neuromuscular coordination, but poor dexterity of his large hands. He refused to brush his teeth, wanted his remaining teeth extracted, and asked for complete upper and lower dentures.

B.W. had a history of sickle cell anemia, although no active or acute signs or symptoms were present. There were no definite contraindications for routine dental care, since blood counts, red cell morphology, and life span were normal.

An examination of extraoral soft tissue revealed no remarkable conditions. An intraoral examination revealed inflamed and hemorrhagic gingival tissue where teeth were present. All other tissues were unaffected. B.W. had seven remaining mandibular teeth and one tooth in the maxillary arch. Several of these teeth were grossly decayed, and severe periodontal disease was evident from extensive bone loss and severe mobility of the teeth. The nurse referred B.W. to the dentist for evaluation and treatment recommendations. Based on B.W.'s refusal to brush his teeth, inflamed and hemorrhagic gingival tissue, badly decayed remaining teeth, and the periodontal disease, the nursing diagnosis Altered Oral Mucous Membrane due to poor oral hygiene was made.

The dentist recommended two treatment options:

1. Extract #2, #19, #21, #28
   Do amalgam restoration on #20
   Complete upper denture
   Lower transitional partial denture, anticipating future loss of remaining four mandibular teeth due to periodontal disease
2. Extract all remaining teeth
   Evaluate in 6 to 8 weeks for complete upper and lower dentures

NURSING INTERVENTIONS

Once emergency referrals and treatment are complete, an oral hygiene plan of care should be developed for the elderly person (see Assessment Guide 11.3). These care plans benefit the individuals for whom they are designed and serve as an ongoing guide for nursing staff.

The first factor to be established is whether the elderly person is dentate or edentulous. Second, the medical condition (both mental and physical), drug history, and nutritional status should be evaluated. Soft tissue considerations include lesions or sore spots, gingival and periodontal conditions (including tooth mobility), and the amount of plaque and calculus present. Carious lesions, both coronal and root, may warrant special fluoride recommendations and dietary counseling.

While designing the care plan, keep in mind four categories of elderly dental patients: (1) the self-sufficient patient who is somewhat dextrous, mentally alert, and motivated to perform oral hygiene skills; (2) the semi-self-sufficient patient who is sometimes depressed, forgetful, and uninterested and needs some assistance to perform dental techniques adequately; (3) the patient who can cooperate with a caretaker, even though mentally unable to comprehend, communicate, or meet daily hygiene needs; and (4) the completely dependent, comatose patient (McLeran, 1982).

The individual oral hygiene care plan includes written instructions to the patient and/or assisting aide, a checklist of oral hygiene aids required, the amount of assistance needed, and specific recommendations. A copy of the plan should be included in the patient's medical record. Providing necessary dental aids and demonstrating improved oral hygiene techniques in a positive manner will prevent delays in implementation.

Cleansing the Oral Cavity

Self-sufficient elderly should cleanse their mouths with a soft, multibristled, small-headed toothbrush, replaced regularly, and clearly labeled with the person's name. Brushing once a day is adequate if done thoroughly. However, after meals brushing is highly recommended, since the elderly regularly experience xerostomia, halitosis, and rampant root caries. Elderly persons need to grow accustomed to the circular motion of the bristles at the gingival margin.

Although interproximal plaque is removable only with dental floss, flossing is not routinely suggested for elderly patients. Even the most self-sufficient elderly have some difficulty manipulating dental floss, and flossing can traumatize tissues. However, the highly motivated elder person might be encouraged to try wider dental tape, 3-ply nylon yard, or pipe cleaners for interproximal cleaning.

Older persons with any natural teeth, and especially those with carious lesions and sensitive root surfaces, should use a fluoridated toothpaste that has been screened and endorsed by the American Dental Association (ADA) for fluoride and abrasive content. Above all, elderly patients should be using a pleasant-tasting paste, or they may refuse to brush. The acutely ill or unconscious patient's teeth can be brushed with a dry toothbrush and wiped with a piece of gauze soaked in mouthrinse. Toothpowders are judged by their abrasiveness and should not be used on exposed root surfaces.

Mouthrinses are not to be substituted for other plaque-removal techniques, but they can be effective when used in conjunction with brushing. Fluoridated mouthrinses have a substantial positive effect on decalcification and carious lesions and reduce the sensitivity of exposed root surfaces.

Disclosing solution or tablets, though useful to the nursing staff in evaluating the presence of plaque, may not help the patient with visual deficiency or decreased manual dexterity. Therefore, they are seldom recommended for use by the geriatric patient.

When run on low power and used correctly, oral irrigating devices (eg, Water Piks) will rinse debris from the mouth. However, they will not remove plaque from the surfaces of the teeth and may cause tissue damage if used incorrectly. These devices are more cumbersome and difficult to use than a toothbrush, and definitely should not be used on an unconscious or critically ill patient.

The use of periodontal stimulators and toothpicks demands a degree of dexterity or tissue damage will result. An aide or family member can be trained to use the stimulators on an elderly patient if recommended by a professional.

A modified toothbrush handle will allow some elderly persons to clean their own teeth sufficiently. Rubber, styrofoam, or aluminum foil balls placed on the end of a toothbrush handle; a bicycle handle grip; elastic, velcro, or vinyl tubing; a handle of self-cured acrylic resin; or just plain gauze wrapped with adhesive tape will make the brush easier to hold and manipulate.

Electric toothbrushes come with an oversized handle, and the head vibrates to clean the teeth and gums without much effort on the part of the elderly patient. It is often easier for an aide or family member to use the electric brush when assisting the completely dependent patient.

Brushing the teeth of patients who can cooperate only by opening the mouth and rinsing must be done at the bedside or in a wheelchair. Begin by elevating and supporting the head and back with pillows or with the cradle of your arm. The wheelchair can be moved near a hand sink for rinsing, but a basin must be available for the bedridden patient to rinse. Place a towel over the patient's chest and shoulders and under the chin. A mouth prop made of several tongue blades wrapped in gauze may be necessary for access to the mouth. Position the head to one side and then to the other. Brush all surfaces of the teeth and gums, rinsing periodically for the patient's comfort and for the operator's visibility. When using the dry-brush method, diluted mouthrinse is more pleasant for the patient and freshens the mouth. On completion, wipe the mouth, cheeks, and chin clean.

Brushing the teeth of the unconscious or acutely ill patient must be done at the bedside with a few variations in procedure. Position the head to one side, drape the chest and shoulders with towels, and lubricate the lips with Vaseline or mineral oil, although care should be taken with use of oil-based products for unconscious or severely compromised elderly persons because of the dangers of aspiration and hypostatic pneumonia. Gently open the mouth with a tongue blade, and prop it open with several tongue blades wrapped in gauze. Clean all surfaces of the teeth, gums, tongue, and buccal mucosa with a soft brush, a damp washcloth, or a gauze square wrapped around the index finger. Then swab the mouth with a Q-tip or gauze square saturated with fresh-tasting mouthrinse. Dry the lips, outer cheeks, and chin and relubricate the lips with Vaseline or mineral oil.

Oral hygiene for persons with either partial or complete removable dentures should include daily brushing of the appliance and nightly removal and soaking in a cup of lukewarm water, a white vinegar solution, or a commercial denture cleaner. Each person should have a denture cup with a foam cushion insert to break the fall of a dropped appliance. Food, stains, and calculus should be thoroughly removed from the artificial appliances immediately after meals and snacks. Food debris that accumulates under prosthetic appliances is degraded by enzymes and causes inflammation of the oral mucosa. The elderly should be taught and encouraged to clean their own appliances on a daily basis. Those who are physically unable to do this will need a dedicated nurse or aide who will make this a daily commitment.

The most effective way to clean complete and partial dentures is first to scrub the appliance with soap and water over a sink or basin half filled with water. (The water will act as a cushion and prevent breakage if the appliance is accidentally dropped.) Harsh, abrasive cleansers will scratch the pink acrylic; hot water will warp the acrylic denture material; and bleaches will completely change the color of the denture. Concentrate on cleaning the wire clasps with clasp brushes. In an ultrasonic cleaning unit, agitate the appliance for 5 to 10 minutes. During this time, the oral mucosa and tongue can be thoroughly cleaned with a soft toothbrush or a soft, terry washcloth. Using the thumb and forefinger, gently massage all tissues covered by the dentures. Rinse the oral cavity with warm salt water or mouthrinse and return the clean appliances to the patient for reinsertion. Broken or ill-fitting dentures should be reported to a dentist immediately. Denture reline and adhesive products can harm the oral mucosa and should not be used. In institutions, each elder's dentures should be marked with the patient's name to avoid being lost or placing dentures in the wrong person's mouth.

Promoting Wellness of Oral Mucous Membrane

The state of natural teeth and dentures of institutionalized elderly people has been found to be extremely poor. Many elderly are unable to perform oral hygiene procedures without a great deal of assistance; others consider oral health a low priority compared to other health problems. Decreasing physical ability and diminished concern encourage an unclean and unhealthy mouth. Promotion of cleanliness, maintenance of the highest degree of oral health, and preservation of the oral apparatus and its functions have a profound psychologic effect on most individuals and foster the development of a strong, positive approach to life. The maintenance of that self-image should be encouraged in every individual, regardless of age.

Oral discomfort can be eased through the following suggestions:

Dietary: Avoid dry and bulky, spicy, or acidic foods; alcoholic and carbonated beverages; and tobacco. Provide adequate nutrition and fluids.

Environmental: Keep air humid, especially during sleep; use lubricant to protect the lips from drying and cracking.

Oral Hygiene and Prevention: Maintain daily hygiene, routine screenings, and regular checkups by a dental professional; give reminders to brush or rinse after meals and snacks (natural *and* artificial teeth); give mouthrinses as needed (warm salt water for infection or fluoride for the caries prone).

Saliva Stimulation: Use artificial saliva or drug therapy if not medically inadvisable. Sugarless gum or sugarless candies also may be used.

Physician and Nurse Awareness: Know the oral side effects of prescribed drugs; confer with dentist on drug dosage adjustment or change.

CASE STUDY

Nursing Interventions

B.W. had no medical conditions that contraindicated tooth extraction. The benefit gained from elimination of the grossly carious sources of potential infection was much improved oral and overall health. B.W.'s sister and all those involved in his care agreed that he would be happier with all remaining teeth extracted. They felt that he could adjust to complete dentures if given encouragement and appropriate oral care by his nurse and dental care providers.

B.W.'s primary nurse prescribed regular assessment of soft tissues (including condition of dentures, diet, environment, and drugs), cleansing of the oral cavity, and promotion of wellness of oral mucous membranes as described previously. Special attention was given to appliance design so that B.W. could more easily perform his own oral care and inspect his own dentures. The handles of the very soft bristled brush used to cleanse his oral cavity and the brush used to clean his dentures were built up with gauze and adhesive tape to allow easier grasp. A cup with a large handle was provided, and the handle was further thickened to aid in rinsing. The nurse evaluated B.W.'s ability and readiness to learn and developed a specific teaching plan.

OUTCOMES

It is a common misconception that the elderly, especially those in institutions, no longer require dental care. Most dental problems in geriatric persons result from neglect, not aging. The more we know about the mouth and how it is affected by internal and external conditions, the easier it will be to help elderly patients prevent oral problems and to relieve their discomfort. The intent of the nursing staff should be to eliminate pain and emergency situations through prevention and control of oral infection and disease and to assist in restoring and maintaining the optimum condition of the oral mucosa through patient education, encouragement, and prescription and implementation of daily oral hygiene regimens. Clearly, the nurse's ability to assess and diagnose Impaired Tissue Integrity: Oral Mucous Membranes, to prescribe appropriate interventions, and to evaluate the attainment of desired outcomes are crucial to the well-being of elderly persons.

The expected outcomes of the interventions prescribed for B.W. were restoration and maintenance of the oral mucosa to the optimal condition possible, prevention or resolution of infection and pain, diminished influence from contributing factors, and self-care in oral cleansing and appliance surveillance.

Three months after institution of the interventions, B.W. was cleansing his own mouth and dentures as prescribed by the nurse. The adaptations of the brushes and drinking cup appeared to make the difference in B.W.'s willingness to perform this aspect of his self-care. B.W. was also free of infection and pain. No emergencies had occurred. Although he was not attentive to the inspection of his dentures, he allowed staff to assess the condition of his oral mucosa and dentures.

SUMMARY

Because the elderly are at risk for loss of tissue integrity, oral discomfort, and oral dysfunction, it is important that nurses are able to diagnose Altered Oral Mucous Membrane and prescribe an oral hygiene plan of care. Halitosis, unusual or poor eating habits, and selection of soft foods are early signs of impaired oral mucous membranes that should alert the nurse to the need for a thorough assessment to specify the diagnosis and etiology(s). The design of nursing oral hygiene interventions depend on the etiologies that are identified. Expected outcomes of the interventions for the elderly are optimal restoration and maintenance of the oral mucosa, maximizing self-care and oral function.

ASSESSMENT GUIDE 11.1

Glossary of Dental Terms

Acanthosis A diffuse hyperplasia and thickening of the prickle cell layer of the epidermis

Alveolar ridges (1) Alveolar bone or alveolar process is the bone of the maxilla (upper jaw) and mandible (lower jaw) that surrounds and supports the teeth; (2) alveolar ridge refers to the crestal portion of the alveolar bone

Angular cheilitis A condition characterized by redness, fissuring, and dry scaling at the angles of the mouth

Buccal Referring to the inner portion of the cheek or oral structures directed toward the cheek (derived from buccinator muscle)

Circumvallate papillae Circumvallate papillae are the largest of the four types of papillae and fewest in numbers; located on the dorsal surface in the posterior one third of the tongue. They have a large circular shape with a flattened top that extends above the other papillae, and they help to perceive taste

Disclosing solution A solution or chewable tablet that discolors deposits and stains but not clean tooth surfaces, revealing state of oral hygiene

Gingiva The part of the oral mucous membrane that covers the alveolar processes and the cervical portions of the teeth (commonly referred to as gums)

Gingivitis Inflammation of the gingival tissues; characterized by a color change from coral pink to red or bluish-red; may be soft, enlarged, and shiny with reduced stippling due to swelling; bleeds easily

Glossitis Inflammation of the tongue

Hyperemia Excess of blood in a part

Keratinization Formation of microscopic fibrils of keratin (horny tissue)

Palatin glands Minor salivary glands in the palate

Parakeratosis Any condition of the skin characterized by the formation of horny growths or excessive development of the horny growth

Periodontitis A disease characterized by inflammation and destruction of the periodontium with the possible sequelae of pocket formation, tooth mobility, recession of the gingiva, and alveolar bone loss

Periodontium Periodontal tissues surrounding and supporting the teeth, including the cementum (tissue that covers the root of the tooth), the periodontal ligament (attaches the tooth to the jaw), the gingiva (gum tissue), and the alveolar bone (a supporting bone)

Plaque Dense, organized bacterial system embedded in an intermicrobial matrix that adheres closely to the teeth, calculus, and other firm surfaces in the oral cavity

Prickle cell layer The innermost layer of the epidermis; rod-shaped processes with intercellular bridges connecting with similar adjoining cells

Rete pegs Inward projections of the epithelium into submucosal or connective tissue

Sjögren's syndrome A condition usually seen in middle-aged and elderly females in which total glandular secretions are reduced, eg, dry eyes, xerostomia (dry mouth), and enlargement of parotid glands

Stomatitis Generalized inflammation of the oral mucosa

Vestibule The portion of the oral cavity bounded on one side by teeth and gingiva or residual alveolar ridges and on the other by the lips and cheeks

Source: Compiled by Sheila Donahue, RDH, The University of Iowa.

ASSESSMENT GUIDE 11.2

Oral Mucous Membranes

Name _____ Room _____ Age _____

Address _____

Natural Teeth — Max. _____   Full Dentures — Max. _____

                        Mand. _____   Mand. _____

Partial Dentures — Max. _____   None — Max. _____

                        Mand. _____   Mand. _____

Denture Usage:

All Day _____

Night & Day _____

Occasionally _____

Never _____

Medical Problems:

CNS _____

Cardiovascular _____

Pulmonary _____

GI _____

Renal _____

Malignant disease _____

Arthritis _____

Other diseases limiting use of hands and arms _____

Prosthetic devices (ie, pacemaker, valve or hip replacement) Specify _____

Mental Status: 1. Alert   2. Semi-alert
                        3. Noncommunicative   4. Comatose

Physical Status: 1. Ambulatory   2. Walk with aid
                        3. Transport   4. Bedfast

Drug History: (current drugs and dosage) _____

_____

_____

Condition of Soft Tissue:
   Soft Tissue Examination (Site, Description)

Lip _____

Maxilla _____

Mandible _____

Buccal mucosa _____

Tongue _____

ASSESSMENT GUIDE 11.2

Oral Mucous Membranes (Continued)

Floor of mouth _____

Palate _____

Periodontal Condition:

Absence of gingivitis   _____

Gingivitis only   _____

Periodontal disease   _____

Condition of Natural Teeth:

No carious lesions   _____

No lesions, but extensive decalcification _____

Some carious lesions   _____

Extensive destruction from dental caries _____

Root caries   _____

No mobility   _____

Some mobility   _____

Very mobile teeth   _____

Calculus:	Right	Anteriors	Left
Max.	_____	_____	_____
Mand.	_____	_____	_____

Plaque:	Right	Anteriors	Left
Max.	_____	_____	_____
Mand.	_____	_____	_____

Dietary Evaluation:

_____ Eats regular meals

_____ Eats regular meals, but only soft foods

_____ Snacks frequently on sweet foods

_____ Has very little appetite; does not eat regular meals

_____ Sucks on hard candy (not sugarless) to lubricate mouth

_____ Frequently drinks coffee or tea with sugar

Brushing:
Number of times oral structures of the mouth are cleaned daily _____

	Good	Needs new one	Doesn't have
Condition of toothbrush	_____	_____	_____
denture brush	_____	_____	_____
clasp brush	_____	_____	_____

(Continues)

ASSESSMENT GUIDE 11.2

Oral Mucous Membranes (Continued)

Condition of dentures:

Good _____   Needs repair _____   Needs cleaning _____

Needs adjusting _____   Needs labeling _____

Soft debris _____ minimal _____ gross

Hard deposit _____ minimal _____ gross

Ability to carry out own oral hygiene? _____

(1) _____ completely self-sufficient

(2) _____ completely self-sufficient, but limited ability to perform oral hygiene procedures due to limited use of hands and/or arms

(3) _____ unable to care for daily needs; can cooperate, but dependent on others

(4) _____ comatose patient

Complaints made by patient: _____

_____

Examiner _____

Date _____

ASSESSMENT GUIDE 11.3

Individual Oral Hygiene Care Plan

Name _____

Oral hygiene maintenance recommendations:

_____ Requires complete assistance and care

_____ Requires some physical assistance

_____ Needs encouragement/periodic supervision

_____ Can maintain oral hygiene adequately

Oral hygiene aids: Description:

_____ Soft toothbrush   _____

_____ Modified toothbrush   _____

_____ Electric toothbrush   _____

_____ Denture brush   _____

_____ Clasp brush   _____

_____ Dental floss/tape   _____

_____ 3-ply nylon yarn   _____

_____ Pipe cleaners   _____

_____ Desensitizing toothpaste _____

_____ Fluoride toothpaste   _____

_____ Toothpowder   _____

_____ Fluoride mouthrinse   _____

_____ Warm salt water rinse   _____

_____ Mouthwash   _____

_____ Hydrogen peroxide rinse _____

_____ Glycerin swabs   _____

_____ Disclosing tablets/solution _____

_____ Oral irrigating device   _____

_____ Periodontal stimulators _____

_____ Denture cleaner   _____

_____ Dietary analysis   _____

_____ Specific others   _____

Additional comments: _____

_____

_____

Examiner _____

Date _____

References

Arthur K, Farr HW: Prognostic significance of histologic grade in epidermoid carcinomas of the mouth and pharynx. *Am J Surg* 1972; 124:489–492.

Carroll-Johnson R (editor): *Classification of Nursing Diagnoses: Proceedings of the Eighth Conference.* Lippincott, 1989.

Ettinger RL: Xerostomia. *Geriatric Curriculum Series.* Module 7. University of Iowa College of Dentistry, 1982.

Garguilo AW, Wentz EM, Orban BJ: Mitotic activity of human oral epithelium exposed to 30 percent hydrogen peroxide. *Oral Surg* (Apr) 1961; 14:474–492.

Graham CM: Mucosal tissues of aging patients. *Ann Aust Col Dent Surg* (Dec) 1968; 1:53–59.

Hill MW: Oral cancer and aging. *Geriatric Curriculum Series.* Module 6. University of Iowa College of Dentistry, 1982.

Hill MW, Rowe DJ: Influence of aging on oral cancer. *Dent Hyg* (Aug) 1982; 56:8.

Kramer IRH, El-Labban N, Lee KW: The clinical features and risk of malignant transformation in sublingual keratosis. *British Dent J* 1978; 144:171–180.

Lehner T et al: Cell mediated immunity to herpes virus Type 1 in carcinoma and precancerous lesions. *British J Cancer* 1973; 28 (Suppl 1):128–184.

Loe H, Karring T: The three dimensional morphology of the epithelium-connective tissue interface of the gingiva as related to age and sex. *Scand J Dent Res* 1971; 79:315–326.

Marwah AS, Weinmann JP, Meyer J: Effect of chronic inflammation on the epithelial turnover of the human gingiva. *Arch Pathol* (Feb) 1960; 69:147–153.

Mason DK, Glen AIM: The aetiology of xerostomia (dry mouth). *Dent Mag* (Dec) 1967; 84(6):235–238.

McLeran H: Oral hygiene care for the elderly. *Geriatric Curriculum Series.* Module 13. University of Iowa College of Dentistry, 1982.

Miles AEW: "Sans teeth": Changes in the oral tissues with advanced age. *Proc Roy Soc Med* (Sept) 1972; 65:801–806.

Ryan EJ, Toto PD, Garguilo AW: Aging in human attached gingival epithelium. *J Dent Res* (Jan–Feb) 1974; 53:74–76.

Shakler G: The effects of aging upon oral mucosa. *J Invest Dermatol* (Aug) 1966; 47:115–120.

Squier CA: Age changes in the oral mucosa. *Geriatric Curriculum Series.* Module 3. University of Iowa College of Dentistry, 1982.

Squier CA, Johnson NW, Hackeman M: Structure and function of normal oral mucosa. Pages 1–95 in: *Oral Mucosa in Health and Disease.* Dolby AE (editor). Blackwell Scientific, 1975.

Zimmerman ER, Zimmerman AL: Effects of race, age, smoking habits, oral and systemic disease in oral exfoliative cytology. *J Dent Res* (July–Aug) 1965; 44:627–631.

12

Fluid Volume Deficit: (1) and (2)

JEAN REESE, PhD, RN

THE TERM *FLUID VOLUME DEFICIT* DENOTES A DECREASE in body fluids. The loss may involve only the extracellular compartment or both the extracellular and the intracellular compartments of the body. The deficit can result from excessive loss of fluids, decreased intake of fluids, or both. The many conditions and disease states affecting the fluid volume of the body require differing interventions. Because of age-related changes in vital organ functions, the elderly are particularly prone to develop not only initial fluid imbalances, but serious sequelae as well.

SIGNIFICANCE FOR THE ELDERLY

With normal aging, the systems that control the volume and concentration of body fluids exhibit both a reduction of reserve capacities and an inability to respond rapidly. These restrictions can create both excess and deficit problems for the elderly. Under usual circumstances, maintenance of adequate fluid volume is not a problem of normal aging. However, abrupt alterations in fluid volume put the elderly person at high risk for imbalances. It is very important for nurses to recognize that variations in fluid balance, from which younger people recover easily, often cause serious illness for the elderly.

Epstein (1979) has asserted that the most dramatic age-related changes occur in the kidney. The aged kidney's decreased ability to regulate fluid volume and the decrease in total body water combine to narrow the range of responses to fluid volume changes. This diminished control of fluid volume can lead to cardiovascular, renal, and neurologic malfunctioning, thereby increasing morbidity and mortality in the aged. For more information regarding normal aging the reader should refer to Chapter 6.

CURRENT STATUS OF THE DIAGNOSIS

The present definition by NANDA (Carroll-Johnson, 1989) of Fluid Volume Deficit (1) and Fluid Volume Deficit (2) names three sites for dehydration to occur: vascular, cellular, and intracellular. The last two terms are redundant. A more accurate replacement for the term *cellular* would be *interstitial*.

The present nursing diagnosis of Fluid Volume Deficit is subdivided by the two related factors: (1) failure of regulatory mechanisms and (2) active loss

(Carroll-Johnson, 1989) (see Table 12.1). Potential categorizing by cause is an important and necessary step toward systematically specifying interventions (see Table 12.1). However, the isotonic, hypotonic, and hypertonic body fluids that arise from various types of fluid losses or inadequate intake also require differing treatments. The present categorization, therefore, blurs a rigorous specification of definitive treatments.

As with any intervention, the need for pacing according to the severity of the deficit also requires consideration.

Terms denoting fluid imbalances have been assigned various meanings in both medical and nursing literature (Carpenito, 1983; Lindeman, 1983; Metheney, 1987; Pestana, 1985). In order to interpret the present literature on fluid imbalance, one needs to understand the concept of tonicity, its effect on fluid movement between compartments, and the causes and results of these compartment fluid changes.

FLUID COMPARTMENT CHARACTERISTICS

The concept of how fluids are dispersed between body compartments is basic to understanding the effects of fluid volume disturbances. The body contains two fluid compartments—the intracellular (IC) and the extracellular (EC). The EC fluid compartment is further divided into the interstitial compartment (fluid between the cells) and the vascular compartment. These two compartments of EC fluid act essentially as a unit, with relatively unencumbered water and solute exchange occurring between them. The presence of red blood cells and the greater concentration of proteins differentiate the vascular fluid from the interstitial fluid. In contrast, for fluids to flow into or out of the cells, the extracellular compartment must be either hypotonic or hypertonic, respectively, to the intracellular compartment.

Sodium constitutes the major electrolyte contributing to the tonicity of the EC fluid compartment. Normal serum sodium ranges from 135 to 145 mEq/L, and serum osmolality, which closely follows serum sodium concentrations, ranges from 280 to 295 mOsm/L. The range of urinary osmolality is usually 500 to 800 mOsm/L, which is approximately 1.5 to 3 times greater than the serum osmolality.

DEFINING CHARACTERISTICS OF FLUID VOLUME DEFICIT

Fluid Volume Deficit exhibits certain common characteristics regardless of tonicity. One of these is rapid

weight loss, which directly reflects a decrease in fluid volume. Any weight loss greater than 500 g per day should be attributed to a loss of fluid volume. An exception to this rapid weight loss characteristic is "third spacing," in which fluid volume is lost from the vascular compartment yet retained in the body. Pleural and abdominal cavities, as well as the interstitium, can collect fluid. The phrase "more output than intake" is also not useful to characterize a fluid deficit in this instance.

Hypotension can occur with isotonic, hypotonic (hyponatremic), and hypertonic (hypernatremic) Fluid Volume Deficit. Hypotension develops later in hypertonic (hypernatremic) fluid deficit because the tonicity of the EC fluids draws water from the cells, thus maintaining vascular volume. Only when the EC volume losses continue with no replacement and the cells can no longer release water does hypotension appear. The development of hypotension may also be delayed with hyponatremic deficits if another substance such as glucose provides enough osmotic pull to maintain vascular volume.

A common characteristic of vascular plasma volume deficit is an increase in the hematocrit—as plasma volume decreases, the hematocrit rises. An elevated hematocrit will occur later in hypertonic losses, when the intracellular compartment can no longer supply fluids for the vascular volume.

Urine output varies depending on the causative factors for the Fluid Volume Deficit. If the cause for the volume depletion is active loss, such as from the gastrointestinal tract, and there is no renal disease, then the urine will be concentrated and in small amounts, but with low sodium concentration of less than 10 mEq/L. With alterations in renal functioning, the urine output may be dilute and in normal or large amounts, but with sodium concentration of more than 10 mEq/L.

ASSESSMENT

Several fundamental assessment and scheduled monitoring activities are commonly warranted for patients at risk for fluid imbalances. Initially, dependent elderly who come under a nurse's care should undergo a careful physical assessment and health history to establish a baseline of usual functioning.

Vital signs should be taken at intervals as warranted by the condition of the patient. An increase in heart rate and a decrease in pulse pressure reflect a decrease in vascular volume. An increase in temperature may signal dehydration.

Weighing the patient at the same time each day under the same circumstances yields a reliable record of rapid changes in body weight.

An accurate record of intake and output is of paramount importance, requiring that staff know the amount

Table 12.1

Fluid Volume Deficit: (1) and (2)

NANDA (CARROLL-JOHNSON, 1989)
FLUID VOLUME DEFICIT: (1)

Definition: A state in which an individual experiences vascular, cellular, or intracellular dehydration related to failure of regulatory mechanisms

Related Factor/Etiology	*Defining Characteristics*

Failure of regulatory mechanisms	**Major**
	  Dilute urine
	  Increased urine output
	  Sudden weight loss
	
	Other Possible Defining Characteristics
	
	Minor
	  Possible weight gain
	  Hypotension
	  Decreased venous filling
	  Increased pulse rate
	  Decreased skin turgor
	  Decreased pulse volume/pressure
	  Increased body temperature
	  Dry skin
	  Dry mucous membranes
	  Hemoconcentration
	  Weakness
	  Edema
	  Thirst

FLUID VOLUME DEFICIT: (2)

Definition: A state in which an individual experiences vascular, cellular, or intracellular dehydration related to active loss

Related Factor/Etiology	*Defining Characteristics*

Active loss	**Major**
	  Decreased urine output
	  Concentrated urine
	  Output greater than intake
	  Sudden weight loss
	  Decreased venous filling
	  Hemoconcentration
	  Increased serum sodium
	Minor
	  Hypotension
	  Thirst
	  Increased pulse rate
	  Decreased skin turgor
	  Decreased pulse volume/pressure
	  Change in mental state
	  Increased body temperature
	  Dry skin
	  Dry mucous membranes
	  Weakness

(Continues)

Table 12.1

Fluid Volume Deficit: (1) and (2) (*Continued*)

REESE

FLUID VOLUME DEFICIT: Dehydration (hypernatremia)

Related Factors/Etiologies

Diabetes insipidus
Hypercalcemia
Hypokalemia
Excess diuretic therapy
Decreased fluid intake
Loss of renal concentrating ability
Lack of thirst
Inability to obtain water
NPO for tests
Mental incapacity
High-protein tube feedings without sufficient water

Defining Characteristics

Common
  Rapid weight loss
  Hypotension
  Thirst
  Dry mucous membranes

Other Possible Defining Characteristics

Increase in heart rate
Decrease in pulse pressure
Low volume, concentrated urine
Diminished foot vein filling
Decrease in intensity of heart sounds
Decreased energy level
Decreased mental alertness
Fever
Flushing
Loss of sweating
Personality changes
Hallucinations
Delirium
Manic behavior
Coma
Convulsions

FLUID VOLUME DEFICIT: Isotonic

Related Factors/Etiologies

Hemorrhage
Burns
Vomiting and diarrhea
Elevated environmental temperature
Intestinal obstruction
Physical activity during hot weather

Defining Characteristics

Common
  Thirst
  Hypotension
  Tachycardia
  Weakness
  Decrease in venous filling
  Dry mouth
  Decrease in skin turgor
  Weight loss (except for intestinal obstruction)

Other Possible Defining Characteristics

Scanty, concentrated urine
Increased hematocrit
Low urinary sodium

Table 12.1

Fluid Volume Deficit: (1) and (2) *(Continued)*

FLUID VOLUME DEFICIT: Hyponatremia

Related Factors/Etiologies	*Defining Characteristics*
Same as for isotonic FVD	Common
In addition:	Supine tachycardia
Diuretic therapy	Hypotension that worsens on rising
Adrenal or pituitary insufficiency	Poor skin turgor
End-stage renal disease	Elevated BUN to greater degree than serum creatinine
Salt-losing nephritis	Dry mucous membranes
Renal tubular acidosis	Weight loss
Acute emotional distress	*Other Possible Defining Characteristics*
Tube feedings with low sodium content	Lethargy
Excessive sweating	Weakness
Anorexia	Confusion
Nausea	Convulsions
Intermittent or persistent vomiting	Decorticate posturing
	Coma
	Paralysis
	Hypertonic reflexes
	Low urinary sodium
	Low volume, concentrated urine

of fluid held by different containers. See Table 12.2 for an assessment tool for fluid deficit. A history of the elder's usual pattern of intake and output is useful both for comparison purposes and for specification of nursing care.

Telfer and Persoff (1965) found small foot vein filling to be the most reliable physical sign in monitoring dehydration states. The filling of a small foot vein diminished early in dehydration, often before the blood urea nitrogen (BUN) rose significantly. However, peripheral vascular disease may obliterate this sign in the elderly.

The second physical sign Telfer and Persoff (1965) found indicative of dehydration was a decrease in the intensity of heart sounds, notably a decrease of P2 when compared to A2. The changes occurring for both these assessment parameters reflect decreases in the amount of vascular volume.

The energy level of a dehydrated person is lowered, and complaints of tiredness or vague discomfort may be elicited. Mental alertness also decreases with worsening dehydration, and a stuporous state may be reached if no intervention is undertaken.

COMMON GOAL

The common goal for treating all fluid deficits is rehydration. This goal is accomplished by administering fluids with the necessary tonicity. These fluids may be water, isotonic solutions, or saline solutions. Rehydration may be accomplished with both oral and parenteral fluids, depending on the patient's ability to ingest fluids and on the severity of the deficit. On rehydration, the signs and symptoms of the deficit fade as a balanced fluid state returns.

ISOTONIC FLUID VOLUME DEFICIT

Losses of isotonic fluids decrease the volume of the extracellular fluid compartment but not the volume of the intracellular compartment. The vascular compartment, which constitutes about 7% of the body weight in the normal adult, is affected first. If the loss is rapid and large enough, shock develops from hypovolemia. If the loss is slow, the interstitium, which acts as a reservoir, will have time to contribute fluid to the vascular compartment. This movement of fluid moderates the effects of vascular volume loss. However, even a slow loss of 6 liters of isotonic fluid will produce shock (Pestana, 1985). A 2% reduction of body weight because of fluid loss causes thirst and oliguria; a 5% to 10% weight loss produces tachycardia and hypotension; and a 10% to 20% reduction can result in stupor and shock (Carroll and Oh, 1978).

Table 12.2

Assessment for Fluid Deficit

| Date |
| Weight |
| Blood pressure
Temperature
Pulse
Respiratory rate |
| Intake
  Oral
  IV
  Tube feeding
  Formula/water |
| Output
  Urine—amount
    specific gravity/Osm
    sodium
  Stool
  Emesis
  Drains
  GI tubes |
| Venous filling
  0–4 scale |
| Skin turgor
  (return time) |
| Blood values
  Sodium
  BUN
Osmolality |
| Mental alertness
  0–4 scale |
| Energy level
  0–4 scale |
| Thirst
  Y/N |

ETIOLOGIES/RELATED FACTORS OF ISOTONIC FLUID VOLUME DEFICIT

Vascular fluid losses of 1 to 2 liters, as in hemorrhage or burns, require immediate attention with packed red blood cells and isotonic fluids. A loss of 500 mL of blood by a healthy adult may cause short-lived lightheadedness, which disappears with fluid replacement. Vasoconstriction prevents major changes in hemodynamics, as evidenced by the rapid adjustment made by blood donors. In an elderly person with the same amount of blood loss, arteriosclerosis may slow the vascular compensation, and indicators of hypovolemia may appear.

Vomiting and diarrhea frequently cause isotonic EC fluid losses in the elderly. Gastrointestinal infections can spread very easily between residents of a nursing home. Marrie et al (1982), summarizing four studies of rotavirus infections in geriatric populations, reported that of 395 persons at risk, 153 became ill and 4 died. In the one study conducted by Marrie et al, most elderly persons had less than or equal to five diarrheal stools per day for a mean duration of 2.6 days. The investigators reported a wide range in number of stools per day, citing one elderly person who had 27 stools in one day! Of the two elderly in the Marrie study who died, one had nine diarrheal stools per day, and one had continual diarrheal incontinence. Clearly, hypermotility of the bowel decreases the time needed for absorption of intestinal fluids.

Elevated environmental temperatures affect the elderly more than they affect younger people because of the elderly's sluggish circulatory adaptive responses and their reduced total body fluids. In addition, decreases in the concentrating ability of the kidney and in the sensation of thirst increase the risk for fluid loss and dehydration in the elderly in hot weather. Excessive sweating can lead to hyponatremic volume depletion if replacement is with water only. These factors may have been responsible for the 81.2% increase in the death rate among geriatric admissions to two Great Britain hospitals during a summer heatwave, compared to the same time period the previous year when temperatures were typical (Fish et al, 1985). Hart et al (1982) and Applegate et al (1981) reported that the economically depressed elderly were being more affected by heat waves than were elderly with a higher economic status. Not having access to air-conditioned living quarters was cited as a factor in the occurrence of heat stroke. Cooling measures and volume replacement constituted the basic treatment modalities.

Engaging in physical activity during hot weather raises added concern about dehydration and heat stroke in the elderly. In a study by Irion et al (1984), older men did not dissipate as much heat as younger men during exercise, apparently because of decreased skin blood flow associated with reduced cardiac output.

Intestinal obstruction causes sequestering of fluids in the gut, reducing the circulating blood volume but not the body weight. Increased abdominal girth and discomfort with nausea and vomiting are indicators of fluid collecting in the gut. Fluid shifts to extravascular spaces, such as the peritoneal or pleural cavities, can lead to a low vascular volume as well.

DEFINING CHARACTERISTICS OF ISOTONIC FLUID VOLUME DEFICIT

Hypotension, tachycardia, weakness, a decrease in venous filling, dry mouth, and a decrease in skin turgor are typical signs and symptoms of an isotonic fluid deficit. Skin turgor in the elderly, however, is extremely hard to assess. In the healthy adult the skin, after being pinched in a fold, returns to its original shape within 1 second, whereas in the well-hydrated elderly its return may take 20 seconds. The time it takes for the return of the pinched fold of skin to its original position increases both with the severity of the fluid loss and with increasing age (Dorrington, 1981). Metheney (1987) suggested testing skin turgor over the sternum or inner aspect of the thigh in older patients to obtain a more valid assessment.

Persons with isotonic fluid losses will exhibit normal sodium levels, since an equal ratio of sodium and water has been lost. A scanty, concentrated urine with low urinary sodium reflects the saving of water and sodium by the kidneys—provided the lack of tubule reabsorption is not the cause of the deficit. Hematocrit, which reflects the ratio of red blood cells to plasma, will rise in proportion to the plasma deficit. However, if the person is losing whole blood, the hematocrit will not increase.

NURSING INTERVENTIONS

Isotonic fluid losses are treated by replacement of the lost fluid with fluid of like tonicity. Oral fluids, given frequently in small amounts, can be sufficient to replace a small deficit. Severe deficits require intravenous fluid therapy so that immediate and controlled replacement occurs. With rehydration, urinary output should increase toward 40 mL/hour with lessening concentration, and hypotension and dizziness on standing decrease. Pestana (1985) stated that the low side of volume replacement can be judged from the hourly urinary output but cautioned that urinary output is less reliable as an indication of overhydration, as pulmonary edema may occur before the kidneys can react. Blood pressure should rise if the compensatory mechanisms of vasoconstriction had been unable to adjust to the amount of volume loss. Previous energy levels should return.

For gastrointestinal losses, the administration of intravenous fluids depends on the severity of the diarrhea and the presence of nausea and vomiting. Parceling fluids throughout the day is necessary to prevent gastric distention while replacing lost fluids. The often-suggested intervention of providing the elderly person with preferred fluids is aimed at increasing fluid intake. Ingredients of ingested fluids are also important, with electrolytes such as sodium, potassium, and calories being vital. Gatorade, milk, and weak beef broth are examples of fluids with sodium and potassium for replacement. Treatment is also aimed at reducing bowel hypermotility and reducing the severity of the nausea and vomiting.

Eisenman (1986) suggested several preventive measures for physically active elders during hot weather: exercise during cooler times of the day and in the shade; wear light, porous, and white clothing; drink 16 to 32 ounces of fluid a half hour before starting exercise; and continue drinking 6 to 8 ounces every 15 minutes during the physical activity regardless of absent thirst. Another caution is to avoid large meals during hot weather to reduce the metabolic production of heat.

CASE STUDY

Isotonic Fluid Volume Deficit

Mrs. T, a 76-year-old retired anthropologist, lived in a retirement village apartment. She informed Ms. G, the village nurse, that she had had two large diarrhea stools during the night, was feeling somewhat tired, but had no nausea. Ms. G called on her within the hour and discovered that Mrs. T had returned the day before from an intercity tour. On this tour she drank water and ate at gourmet restaurants in various cities. She had no other health problems and took no medications except supplemental calcium.

She had abdominal cramping with the diarrheic stools and hyperactive bowel sounds, but no abdominal tenderness on palpation. Her temperature was normal, as were her other vital signs. She had drunk milk, weak tea, and broth totaling about "a quart and a half" in the early morning. She was "somewhat thirsty" but not hungry. She reported her urine as being "a darker yellow than usual." Ms. G reinforced Mrs. T's efforts for maintaining fluid volume and drew a blood sample for a complete blood count and electrolytes. Ms. G left after making certain fluids were readily available and that Mrs. T understood that she should continue drinking small glasses (150 mL) of fluids at least every hour. In 3 hours, Ms. G checked back after informing the village physician of the laboratory results. Mrs. T's electrolytes were within normal range, but her hemoglobin was 0.5 g/dL above her usual value, indicating a slight volume deficit. She had had two more diarrheal stools. The physician wrote an order for Lomotil, which Mrs. T did not want to use unless absolutely necessary. Instead, Mrs. T decided to eat some cooked white rice, which was a standard treatment used by the people she studied in the Mediterranean area. She had a diarrheal stool 2 hours later and a small formed stool 3 hours later. Ms. G called in the early evening for an update and advised Mrs. T to continue taking fluids even though her diarrhea had lessened.

The physical and mental functioning of this elderly woman were factors that helped her to avoid a situation that could have become critical. She had not lost a lot of fluid before she requested help and had replaced the deficit with enough isotonic fluids to maintain vascular volume.

Continuance of oral fluids would eventually lower her hemoglobin. In view of the age-related changes that reduced her compensatory range, continued monitoring was indicated.

FLUID VOLUME DEFICIT WITH HYPONATREMIA

The loss of sodium in excess of water from body tissue results in a hyponatremic fluid deficit. According to Pestana (1985) there is no mechanism whereby hypertonic fluid can be lost from the body. Rather, hyponatremic deficits occur when an initial loss of isotonic fluid is partially replaced by hypotonic fluid. Specifically, the loss of isotonic fluid results in a contraction of the extracellular volume. The kidneys respond to this change in volume by saving water. Retention of water, in turn, dilutes the extracellular fluid creating hyponatremia or sodium dilution. Thus, the kidneys correct for volume at the expense of tonicity.

ETIOLOGIES/RELATED FACTORS OF FLUID VOLUME DEFICIT WITH HYPONATREMIA

Any of the diseases or situations described in the isotonic fluid deficit can lead to hypotonic fluid deficit as long as the kidneys are responsive to vascular volume deficits. In addition, diuretic therapy frequently reduces fluid volume and causes hyponatremia. Ashouri (1986) reported on a group of eight elderly patients who had severe diuretic-induced hyponatremia. Clinical manifestations included coma, seizures, confusion, obtundation, and weakness. Hypovolemia was present, and no edema was observed. Of special significance in this group of patients was the occurrence of diuretic-induced hyponatremia among underweight elderly women. Other conditions, such as diarrhea, diabetes mellitus, and cerebrovascular accidents (CVAs), were suspect in potentiating the effect of the diuretic. The mean serum sodium level was $110 +/- 2$ mEq/L on admission.

Other excessive urinary losses of water and sodium occur with adrenal insufficiency and renal salt-wasting diseases. The lack of aldosterone caused by adrenal or pituitary insufficiency allows sodium loss by the renal tubules. Renal salt-losing diseases include end-stage renal disease, salt-losing nephritis, and renal tubular acidosis (Lindeman, 1983). Another causative factor cited by Lindeman was severe metabolic alkalosis due to vomiting, in which the kidneys excrete sodium bicarbonate in order to adjust the pH.

Booker (1984) cited three cases in which acute emotional stress was closely related to the onset of hyponatremic symptoms in previously healthy patients who were receiving diuretics. The stress-mediated release of antidiuretic hormone (ADH), which acts on the tubules to conserve water, was postulated as the factor that altered the electrolyte balance in these patients.

Rudman et al (1986) reported the occurrence of hyponatremia in tube-fed patients associated with the intake of 1 g sodium per 1700 calories. The deficit disappeared when sodium intake was elevated to 2 g per day. The investigators postulated that the elderly were less able to reduce urinary sodium excretion when sodium intake was decreased, as has been previously shown by Epstein and Hollenberg's 1976 study. Also, the loss of sodium may have resulted in a modest volume depletion, activating ADH-mediated retention of water, and leading to dilution of the serum sodium.

Ayus et al (1985) noted that hyponatremia resulted in less favorable outcomes among persons with alcoholism and/or severe malnourishment. A 53% difference in mortality occurred between alcoholic and nonalcoholic patients who had severe hyponatremia (serum sodium levels less than 120 mEq/L).

DEFINING CHARACTERISTICS OF FLUID VOLUME DEFICIT WITH HYPONATREMIA

Fundamental hemodynamic signs of hypovolemic hyponatremia are supine tachycardia and hypotension that worsen on rising (Narins et al, 1982). Poor skin turgor also accompanies the depletion.

BUN is elevated to a greater degree than is serum creatinine. If the kidneys are functioning normally, urine will have a low concentration of sodium but a high concentration of other waste products. However, renal disease and chronic partial urinary tract obstruction can cause excretion of isotonic urine with sodium. Adrenal insufficiency allows renal excretion of sodium and water (Narins et al, 1982). In these instances the urine concentration does not reflect the Fluid Volume Deficit.

Other signs and symptoms for hyponatremia include anorexia, nausea, intermittent or persistent vomiting, lethargy, weakness, confusion, grand mal seizures, coma with decorticate posture, bilateral rigidity, and extensor-plantar reflexes. Neurologic symptoms, such as paralysis, may persist even after correction of low serum sodium levels. A serum sodium level of about 110 mEq/L or lower is associated with confusion, coma, seizures, and obtundation. The signs of weakness, anorexia, nausea, and drowsiness can occur when the serum sodium level is around 125 mEq/L.

Cerebral edema may result from hyponatremia. As the extracellular compartment becomes less concentrated than the intracellular compartment, water moves into the cells (Rymer and Fishman, 1973). Hyponatremia may mimic a stroke with neurologic signs of confusion, drowsiness, hypertonic reflexes, seizures, and coma (Booker and Crimmins, 1984).

NURSING INTERVENTIONS

If hyponatremia is associated with neurologic symptoms, rapid correction with an intravenous hypertonic (3%) saline solution and a loop diuretic is warranted. The diuretic prevents vascular volume expansion in persons with a compromised cardiovascular system. Animal model studies have shown the development of extrapontine and central pontine demyelinating lesions with hypertonic saline correction to a normonatremic state (Ayus et al, 1985). Chronic hyponatremia seemed to be another factor in the development of demyelinating brain lesions.

Ayus et al (1985) recommended treatment within 12 to 24 hours of the hyponatremic onset with hypertonic saline to a mild hyponatremic state. Ayus et al (1985) also warned against correction to normonatremia or hypernatremia, indicating that a hyponatremic state of 125 to 130 mEq/L is satisfactory. Ashouri (1986) recommended early treatment of hyponatremia before structural changes occur and correction of the low serum sodium levels to a slightly hyponatremic level. These factors in the treatment of hyponatremia would appear to be least associated with morbidity and mortality. Descriptions of patients' demise even with correction of the serum sodium level have been recorded (Arieff and Witte, 1979). Administration of this regimen requires meticulous monitoring. Inadvertent rapid administration of a hypertonic saline solution can cause death. The brain shrinks and pulls away from the cranial vault, causing rupture of the cerebral vessels.

With less severe extracellular volume depletion, temporary withdrawal of the diuretic and volume repletion with an isotonic solution or oral fluids are indicated. Replacement for mildly hyponatremic states with volume depletion can be in the form of salty liquids or foods. Again, spacing and frequent small amounts should prevent gastric distention. Remember that nausea is a symptom of low serum sodium.

When diuretic therapy is initiated, awareness of the potential for hypovolemic hyponatremia is essential. Madias and Zelman (1982) suggested two ways to prevent volume depletion and hyponatremia with diuretic therapy: (1) a gradual increase in dosage accompanied by careful monitoring of weight and serum sodium levels, and (2) the use of alternate-day administration, which allows adequate diuresis but prevents volume depletion. Also, persons who are placed on low-sodium diets in conjunction with diuretics must be monitored even more closely for the development of hyponatremia and volume depletion.

Adrenal insufficiency is treated by means of hormonal replacement with adrenocorticotropic hormone (ACTH) and/or hydrocortisone along with a fluid intake that will replace both water and sodium losses. The amount and type of fluids for the fluid losses due to intrinsic renal disease are adjusted individually.

As a side note, the syndrome of inappropriate antidiuretic hormone (SIADH) results in hyponatremia but does not cause total body volume depletion as long as water is accessible. Indeed, absence of volume depletion is one criterion for diagnosing this disorder (Bartter and Schwartz, 1967). Another instance in which hyponatremia occurs with normal extracellular volume is with the age-related increase of vasopressin (ADH) release, resulting in impairment of urinary dilution.

CASE STUDY

Fluid Volume Deficit With Hyponatremia

Mr. H, age 78, is a resident in a nursing home. He was admitted to the emergency room because of newly developed coma associated with diarrhea. At the nursing home he received Isocal tube feedings (low sodium concentration of 23 mEq/L) diluted with water at a 1:1 ratio and given at a rate of 2500 mL/d because of dysphagia secondary to neuromuscular dysfunction. Hydrochlorothiazide 25 mg/d had been given for mild hypertension for several months. Serum sodium level was 112 mEq/L, serum osmolality was 235 mOsm/kg, and urine osmolality was 550 mOsm/kg on admission. Initial treatment was with 500 mL of 3% sodium chloride at a rate of 50 mL/hr. Mr. H began to respond to verbal stimulation within 3 hours. Intravenous fluids were continued with 5% dextrose and 0.45 saline at 25 mL/hr. After 24 hours the serum sodium rose to 130 mEq/L. By this time Mr. H was communicating with facial expressions and hand movements that equaled his preadmission level of performance. Fluid replacement continued until urinary output reached 40 mL/hr.

The associated factors leading to the low sodium levels included a decreased intake of sodium, an increased excretion of sodium, and, most likely, water retrieval from the glomerular filtrate caused by an antidiuretic response to the volume depletion brought on by the diarrhea. Fluid losses by the bowel tend to be isotonic.

Such rehydration and serum sodium adjustment demand frequent monitoring for level of mental alertness, focal neurologic signs, urinary output, vital signs, and breath sounds. Samples were drawn to follow serum sodium level. Adventitious breath sounds are of concern because the administration of hypertonic saline can lead to hypervolemia, resulting in pulmonary edema. If pulmonary edema does occur, a potent diuretic, such as furosemide, is administered. It is not unheard of for persons who experience low serum sodium levels to develop neurologic deficits.

Mr. H's diarrhea subsided without specific medication. It was surmised that the diarrhea upset the fluid and sodium balance, since Mr. H had no weakness or nausea to indicate a low serum sodium level prior to the diarrheic episode. However, another formula was selected that had a similar osmolality to the Isocal but a 10 mEq/L increase in sodium content. The agency transfer form to the nursing home contained information about hyponatremic states, as did a verbal report to the caregivers at the nursing home. Planned follow-up after Mr. H's return to the nursing home consisted of blood samples for serum sodium levels and recording of intake and output volumes.

FLUID VOLUME DEFICIT WITH HYPERNATREMIA

A decrease in water intake or an increase in water loss relative to sodium loss leads to a reduction in total body water and an increase in its concentration. The kidneys need a specific amount of water in order to remove solutes from the plasma. An increase in the solute load without a concomitant increase in water intake will result in the kidneys using body water to perform their functions.

ETIOLOGIES/RELATED FACTORS OF FLUID VOLUME DEFICIT WITH HYPERNATREMIA

The most common causes of hypernatremia in the elderly are mental incapacity and physical inability to obtain water even though thirst is present. However, Miller et al (1982) reported that a group of six elderly patients, whose mental status was considered normal and who lacked demonstrable hypothalamic or pituitary lesions, had no sensation of thirst with hypertonicity. Phillips et al (1984a) reported a decrease in thirst sensation in older men who experienced fluid volume depletion.

As noted previously, the elderly have a decline in water-conserving capacity or renal concentrating ability. However, this decrease does not become clinically significant unless fluid intake is limited.

Another situation that limits fluid intake and can create volume depletion for the elderly person is the nothing-by-mouth (NPO) preparation for diagnostic tests. An increase in risk arises with the simultaneous cleansing of the bowel.

A tube-feeding formula has been mentioned previously as a possible cause for hyponatremia. However, high-protein formulas can produce hypernatremic fluid deficits with azotemia (Gault et al, 1968). Tube feedings with high osmolality require water supplementation because of the increased solute load that is presented to the kidney.

In addition, diabetes insipidus, hypercalcemia, hypokalemia, or advanced renal disease may contribute to the development of dehydration. With each of these disorders, the kidneys lose their concentrating ability, thereby increasing the risk for hypernatremic fluid deficits if there is no water replacement.

DEFINING CHARACTERISTICS OF FLUID VOLUME DEFICIT WITH HYPERNATREMIA

Hypotension, which is a major indicator of isotonic and hypotonic dehydration, occurs later with fluid loss and hypertonicity because extracellular fluid volume is preserved by the outward movement of intracellular water. The pulse rate is affected by the same process. Urine volume may be low with maximal concentration. Conversely, if there is a high solute load being presented to the kidney, an increase in the volume of urine will occur. If loss of body water continues, fever, flushing, loss of sweating, and dryness of mucous membranes occurs with hemodynamic changes. Personality changes can progress to hallucinations, delirium, and manic behavior. Coma and convulsions can ultimately result.

NURSING INTERVENTIONS

Interventions are focused around providing water for intake. Caregivers need to provide fluids between meals for the dependent elderly. For elderly persons with a decreased thirst sensation, ingestion of 2 quarts of water a day may be prescribed. Setting in the refrigerator the amount of water to be drunk in one day can serve as a reminder. Health care providers need reminding to give an allotted amount of water to the elderly, particularly if the client is receiving high osmolar tube feedings. Scheduling the elderly early in the day for procedures that require them to be NPO after midnight can reduce the probability of a water deficit.

Increased water consumption is the usual treatment for volume depletion with hypernatremia. However, giving dextrose 5% in water intravenously for severe volume depletion can lead to cerebral edema. Phillips et al (1984b) suggested that treatment with isotonic saline initially rather than water alone might avoid the risks of cerebral edema. Hughes-Davies (1984) suggested that fluid replacement with a salty soup may be safer than tap water for those able to swallow. What must occur is administration of more water than sodium while preventing a fluid shift to the intracellular compartment.

During fluid replacement, attention must be directed to the patient's neurologic status: Level of alertness should increase, and a return to the predeficit personality should occur. Return of the vital signs to the predeficit level and an increase in urine output also indicate the desired response.

CASE STUDY

Fluid Volume Deficit With Hypernatremia

Mrs. G, an 81-year-old active woman, lived alone and maintained a garden. She generally worked in her garden in the mornings and continued doing so during a heat wave. She perspired but did not experience unusual thirst. She complained to her neighbors that she felt very tired and couldn't do her usual cleaning. Later that same day she called them because she became dizzy when she stood up. She was admitted to the hospital, where her blood pressure dropped from 142/88 to 110/66 on standing. She voided 100 cc of concentrated urine with a specific gravity of 1.026. She hadn't voided in 5 hours prior to admission. Her serum sodium was 160 mEq/L, and BUN was 58 mg/dL. She usually weighed 125 lb (56.8 kg) but on admission weighed just under 119 lb (54 kg).

She was treated with D5W in 0.45% saline intravenously at 100 mL/hr for 24 hours. Oral intake of water and fruit juices totaled 750 mL the first 24 hours of admission. Her energy levels improved, as did the hypotension. Urine output increased to 950 mL, and serum sodium dropped to 150 mEq/L in the first 24 hours of treatment. Oral intake increased to 2500 mL the second 24 hours. Intravenous fluids were discontinued. Urine output rose to 1250 mL the second 24 hours of treatment. She was discharged after 3 days with home care instructions.

Decreased sensitivity to thirst and active loss of fluids through perspiration combined to reduce this elderly woman's fluid volume. Her history, along with such signs as hypotension, oliguria, weight loss, and elevated BUN, indicated fluid volume deficit. The elevated serum sodium signaled hypernatremia.

The intervention of giving hypotonic saline rather than D5W reduced the likelihood of cerebral edema. The greater tonicity of the saline solution reduced the gradient for intracellular movement of water. Although the serum sodium level was elevated, the total body sodium was probably decreased. In this instance, more water than sodium was lost from the body. The rather cautious rate of intravenous fluid replacement was in consideration of the patient's age and the state of her cardiovascular system.

Oral administration of fluids was divided throughout the day, with increases being based on her tolerance for them. Improvement in the assessment parameters (BP, P, urine output, serum sodium levels, and energy levels) validated the intervention strategies. Before going home, she received instructions on what to do during hot weather. She was shown how adequate fluid intake can be assured by filling fluid containers in the morning from which she will drink during the day. In addition, a visiting nurse referral was acceptable to her until increased fluid consumption became habitual.

OUTCOMES

Outcome criteria are based on defining characteristics. Those defining characteristics that indicated the problem fade when the problem is receding. When decreased intake is the causative factor, having the person ingest 3000 mL per day should restore previous weight, decrease the urine specific gravity, increase urine output, allay thirst, wetten mucous membranes, and restore the energy level. When hemodynamic changes have occurred because of fluid loss, outcome criteria would include a rise in blood pressure, a decrease in pulse rate, and absence of dizziness on standing.

By judging the response against outcome criteria and interpreting its meaning, the nurse determines whether interventions should be continued, modified, or discontinued. Are the signs and symptoms lessening? Is the rate of change commensurate with expectations? Outcome criteria also serve as the basis for determining the types and frequencies of assessment/monitoring activities.

SUMMARY

The treatment for Fluid Volume Deficit is often medically determined. Consequently, independent nursing interventions focus on prevention, that is, educating the elderly about risk situations, modifying intake patterns, or altering the environment for those at risk. Research is needed to identify intake or eating regimens that prevent fluid imbalances and motivators that increase fluid intake. The improvement of clinical assessment tools to detect fluid deficits is another area to be explored by nurses.

References

Applegate WB et al: Analysis of the 1980 heat wave in Memphis. *J Am Geriatr Soc* 1981; 8:337–342.

Arieff AI, Witte JM: Death or permanent neurological disability despite correction of protracted hyponatremia. (Abstract.) *Kidney Internat* 1979; 16:955.

Ashouri OS: Severe diuretic-induced hyponatremia in the elderly: A series of 8 patients. *Arch Intern Med* (July) 1986; 146:1355–1357.

Ayus JC, Krothapalli RK, Arieff AI: Changing concepts in treatment of severe symptomatic hyponatremia: Rapid correction and possible relation to central pontine myelinolysis. *Am J Med* 1985; 78:897–901.

Bartter FC, Schwartz WB: The syndrome of inappropriate secretion of antidiuretic hormone. *Am J Med* 1967; 42:790–806.

Booker JA: Severe symptomatic hyponatremia in elderly outpatients: The role of thiazide therapy and stress. *J Am Geriatr Soc* (Feb) 1984; 108–113.

Booker JA, Crimmins J: Hyponatremia or stroke? (Letter.) *Med J Austra* (June) 1984; 799–800.

Carpenito L: *Nursing Diagnosis: Application to Clinical Nursing Practice.* Lippincott, 1983.

Carroll HJ, Oh MS: *Water, Electrolyte and Acid-Base Metabolism: Diagnosis and Management.* Lippincott, 1978.

Carroll-Johnson R (editor): *Classification of Nursing Diagnoses: Proceedings of the Seventh Conference.* Lippincott, 1989.

Dorrington KL: Skin turgor: Do we understand the clinical sign? *Lancet* (Jan 31) 1981; 264–266.

Eisenman PA: Hot weather, exercise, old age, and the kidneys. *Geriatrics* 1986; 41:108–114.

Epstein M: Effects of aging on the kidney. *Fed Proc* 1979; 38:168–172.

Epstein M, Hollenberg NK: Age as a determinant of renal sodium conservation in normal man. *J Lab Clin Med* 1976; 87:411–417.

Fish PD, Bennett GCJ, Millard PH: Heatwave morbidity and mortality in old age. *Age Ageing* 1985; 14:243–245.

Gault MH et al: Hypernatremia, azotemia and dehydration due to high protein tube feeding. *Ann Intern Med* 1968; 68:778–791.

Hart GR et al: Epidemic classical heat stroke: Clinical characteristics and course of 28 patients. *Medicine* 1982; 61:189–197.

Hughes-Davies TH: Thirst in the elderly. (Letter.) *N Engl J Med* 1984; 312:247.

Irion G et al: The effect of age on the hemodynamic responses to thermal stress during stress. In: *Modern Aging Research,* Vol 6. Cristofalo VJ et al (editors). Alan R. Liss, 1984.

Lindeman RD: Application of fluid and electrolyte balance principles to the older patient. In: *Clinical Aspects of Aging.* Reichel W (editor). Williams and Wilkins, 1983.

Madias NE, Zelman SJ: What are the metabolic complications of diuretic treatment? *Geriatrics* 1982; 37(2):93–96.

Marrie TJ et al: Rotavirus infection in a geriatric population. *Arch Intern Med* (Feb) 1982; 142:313–316.

Metheney NM: *Fluid and Electrolyte Balance: Nursing Considerations.* Lippincott, 1987.

Miller PD et al: Hypodipsia in geriatric patients. *Am J Med* (Sept) 1982; 73:354–356.

Narins RG et al: Diagnostic strategies in disorders of fluid, electrolyte and acid-base homeostasis. *Am J Med* (Mar) 1982; 72:496–519.

Pestana C: *Fluids and Electrolytes in the Surgical Patient,* 3d ed. Williams & Wilkins, 1985.

Phillips PA et al: Reduced thirst after water deprivation in healthy elderly men. *N Engl J Med* 1984a; 311:753–759.

Phillips PA et al: Thirst in the elderly. (Letter.) *N Engl J Med* 1984b; 312:247.

Rudman D et al: Hyponatremia in tube-fed elderly men. *J Chron Dis* 1986; 39:73–80.

Rymer MM, Fishman RA: Protective adaptation of brain to water intoxication. *Arch Neurol* 1973; 28:49–54.

Telfer N, Persoff M: The effect of tube feeding on the hydration of elderly patients. *J Gerontol* (Oct) 1965; 20:536–543.

III

Elimination Pattern

MERIDEAN MAAS, PhD, RN, FAAN
KATHLEEN BUCKWALTER, PhD, RN, FAAN

Overview

PROBLEMS WITH ELIMINATION CONSUME A large proportion of nursing resources. They also affect the psychologic well-being, body image, and physical and social status of many older adults, and are often related to the decision to institutionalize.

In Chapter 14, McLane and McShane consider the nursing diagnosis Constipation. This chapter reviews the types of constipation and stresses nursing interventions that develop health-related behaviors that contribute to healthy patterns of elimination. Numerous environmental and interactive variables related to this diagnosis are described, and data-based models of constipation are set forth, based in part on the authors' extensive research in this area. Interventions of health teaching, elimination repatterning, and diet management are examined according to subtype of constipation. Two new diagnoses—Colonic Constipation and Perceived Constipation—were approved at the 1988 NANDA conference.

In Chapter 15, Diarrhea, Wadle discusses the diagnosis from the perspective of both acute and chronic diarrhea and their multiple etiologies. Tube-feeding interventions as well as educational/ teaching interventions are highlighted to address this common and complex problem found among the institutionalized elderly.

In Chapter 16, Bowel Incontinence, Maas and Specht differentiate between normal defecation and bowel incontinence. The etiologies of this diagnosis are explicated, and the relationship to the problem of constipation is noted. Bowel programming and environmental structuring are identified as important nursing interventions to treat this diagnosis.

In Chapter 17, Urinary Incontinence, Specht, Tunink, Maas, and Bulechek elaborate the predisposing factors to this costly problem among the institutionalized elderly. They discuss the many types of urinary incontinence found in this population and interventions specific to these types. Specht et al discuss Stress Incontinence, Reflex Incontinence, Urge Incontinence, Functional Incontinence, and Total Incontinence which are approved NANDA diagnoses (Carroll-Johnson, 1989). The general label of Urinary Incontinence is not currently included in the NANDA taxonomy. However the approved Incontinence diagnoses are subsumed by the more general label. Specht et al also describe an additional diagnosis, Iatrogenic Incontinence, which is not an approved NANDA diagnosis. Finally, a decision tree is offered to assist nurses with differentiating specific types of incontinence.

13

Normal Changes With Aging

Mary A. Hardy, PhD, RN, C

Definition:

The elimination pattern describes patterns of excretory function (bowel, bladder, and skin) of individuals.

AGE-RELATED CHANGES IN THE GASTROINTESTINAL system include loss of elasticity in abdominal muscles and loss of muscle tone in the perineal floor and anal sphincter. These changes cause some older persons to have diarrhea. Other commonly occurring etiologic factors that put the elderly at risk for diarrhea include lactose intolerance, antibiotic therapy, and impaction.

Constipation, whether real or perceived, is also a common problem for the elderly. Decreased intestinal secretion of mucus reduces lubrication; slower peristalsis means more water is reabsorbed in the large intestine. In addition to the lack of fluid content in the bowel resulting from these changes, other factors that contribute to the prevalence of constipation among the elderly are an often inadequate fiber and fluid intake, decreased mobility, and a slower transit time (Gioiella and Bevil, 1985). As is true with most of the health patterns, medication consumption is a common risk factor among the elderly because of the number of medications they take as well as pharmacodynamic and pharmacokinetic changes. Anxiety and depression have also been cited as etiologic factors associated with constipation (Calkins et al, 1986).

The elderly are at high risk for incontinence, and frequently it is the deciding factor in whether elderly persons are institutionalized. The condition is symptomatic of a number of underlying changes in the anatomy and innervation of the lower urinary tract that have been found to occur in 11% to 70% of the elderly in the United States (Specht, 1986). Bladder capacity drops from approximately 500 milliliters to about 250 milliliters in elderly persons although no anatomic change has been observed. The ureters, bladder, and urethra lose muscle tone and elasticity, and periurethral structures atrophy. The sensation of needing to void is more variable. Delayed response time by sensory receptors may delay the urge to void until the bladder is full and can result in precipitancy, frequency, and increase in the volume of residual urine. Tissue changes associated with estrogen deficiency in women result in relaxed pelvic floor muscles and can result in stress incontinence. In men, prostatic enlargement can press the urethra closed and can cause retention, retention with overflow, or a weak urinary system. Autopsy data indicate that the incidence of benign prostatic hyperplasia is 95% in men dying at age 80 and over.

The risk for functional incontinence is even greater when changes associated with aging are accompanied by limited mobility and activity intolerance because these factors can tip the balance toward incontinence. Bed rest, acute infections, and increased dependence in activities of daily living have been associated with approximately 25% of the incidence of urinary incontinence. Iatrogenic incontinence resulting from treatment can occur as a result of drugs such as Valium and Sparine, locomotor defects such as distance to the bathroom, and environmental factors such as staff expectations that a resident will be incontinent.

The kidney is also affected by aging. In addition to renal mass, the glomerular filtration rate (GFR) and the tubular reabsorption rate, or the time required for the kidneys to concentrate urine, diminish. The histologic and physiologic changes thought to contribute to these declines include thickening of the tubular basement membrane, diverticuli of the distal nephron, sclerosis of the renal vessel walls, and reduction in the renal plasma flow (Calkins et al, 1986). It is important to point out that even though GFR decreases with normal aging, no concomitant increase is normally observed in creatinine blood levels. These changes put the elderly at risk for acid-base imbalances because of decreased ability of the kidney to filter hydrogen ions (Calkins et al, 1986; Nesbitt, 1988).

References

Calkins E, Davis P, Ford A (editors): *The Practice of Geriatrics.* Saunders, 1986.

Gioiella EC, Bevil CW: *Nursing Care of the Aging Client: Promoting Health Adaptation.* Appleton-Century-Crofts, 1985.

Nesbitt B: Nursing diagnosis in age-related changes. *J Gerontol Nurs* 1988; 14(7):7–12.

Specht J: Genitourinary problems. In: *Nursing Management for the Elderly,* 2d ed. Carnevali D, Patrick M (editors). Lippincott, 1986.

14

Constipation

AUDREY M. MCLANE, PhD, RN
RUTH E. MCSHANE, PhD, RN

THE LITERATURE IS REPLETE WITH DEFINITIONS OF constipation. The term constipation is used in various ways to include any or all of the following: character of stool; frequency of defecation; time required for passage of the stool through the intestinal tract (intestinal transit time); and difficulty expelling rectal contents through the anal sphincter. A constipated stool is generally described as excessively dry, hard, and of insufficient size. Normal stool frequencies vary from three times per day to once every 3 days. Persons are described as constipated when the interval between defecation is more than 3 days. The increased interval usually results in a hard, dry stool that is difficult to expel (Benson, 1975). Some definitions include the notion of a change in bowel habits precipitated by personal or environmental factors. Because health professionals are usually helping individuals during a life transition, the concept of change may be an important consideration. The notion of change was incorporated in the working definition of constipation proposed by the Diagnostic Review Committee (DRC) of the North American Nursing Diagnosis Association (NANDA) at the Seventh Conference on Classification of Nursing Diagnoses. Constipation is "a state in which an individual experiences a change in normal bowel habits characterized by a decrease in frequency and/or passage of hard dry stool" (Carroll-Johnson, 1989).

Classification of constipation into types based on defining characteristics, contributing factors, or interventions required has not occurred in nursing. Development of an empirical base for such a classification system is a high priority, given the number of persons who are treated or who treat themselves for constipation. Because some persons describe a lifetime of constipation, the notion of a "change in bowel elimination" may apply to all types. The characteristics of the constipated stool, usually described as dry, hard, and difficult to expel, may also vary. Difficulty in expelling rectal contents is not limited to hard, dry stools. Weak pelvic floor muscles and/or neuromuscular diseases make it impossible for some individuals to expel even a soft, semiformed stool. Given these and other variations (well-known to experienced clinicians), it becomes difficult to explain the state of the art of nursing diagnosis of patterns of bowel elimination.

The majority of studies of constipation have been conducted by researchers in health-related professions other than nursing. The purposes, theoretical frameworks, and, more important, the variables under study reflect the interests of those professions. For example, a nutrition researcher may be primarily interested in the effects of dietary changes; a physiologist, in factors influencing transit time;

and a physician, in the relationship between constipation and the onset/progression of disease, for example, colonic cancer. Although nurses are interested in all of these variables, the studies, taken individually and as a group, provide only minimal assistance in developing guidelines for professional nursing care.

Nurses view clients from a more holistic perspective, as individuals interacting with their environments in the pursuit of health. This perspective drives the conceptualization and selection of variables beyond the individual to the environment and to the interactions among individuals and their environments. The focus is on patterns of health-related behavior rather than on instances of health deviation.

Nursing's interest in environmental and interactive variables is practical as well as theoretical, since many environmental and interactive variables are amenable to nursing intervention. The methods, procedures, and norms for treatment of constipation have their historical roots in an earlier view of nursing as more art than science and in a field dominated by medical orders that varied from setting to setting. Moreover, the concentration of nurses and nursing care in hospitals led to the diagnosis and treatment of "instances" of constipation rather than "patterns" of elimination. Although laxatives and/or enemas may be appropriate treatments for short-term responses to the stress of surgery or use of constipating narcotic analgesics, such treatments do little to develop patterns of health-related behaviors that contribute to a healthy pattern of bowel elimination.

SIGNIFICANCE FOR THE ELDERLY

Despite the paucity of research about normal patterns of elimination of dietary wastes and about constipation as a specific problem of bowel elimination in older adults, there are subgroups of individuals who are known to be at increased risk of developing constipation. Among the well elderly, those at risk include persons who lead a sedentary lifestyle and individuals with problems of mobility. Among the elderly with chronic illnesses, the groups at risk include the homebound; geropsychiatric patients on long-term antidepressant medications; persons with limited mobility; individuals taking constipating medications, for example, narcotic analgesics for pain; and persons in long-term care facilities. Having insufficient financial resources to purchase well-balanced meals places both the well elderly and the chronically ill elderly at risk of developing constipation. A lifetime of poor eating habits, insufficient exercise, improper dentition to chew high-fiber fruits and vegetables, and inattention to the defecation reflex add to the vulnerability of groups already at risk.

These circumstances make the development and testing of models of constipation and the analysis of effects of interventions critical for nursing care of the elderly.

CURRENT STATUS: DEVELOPMENT OF MODELS OF BOWEL ELIMINATION

Initial conceptualization of the components in a model of constipation emerged from a qualitative study of older adults. Data from the study were used to elicit conceptual categories of diagnostic indicators (McLane et al, 1984). The usefulness of the categories for diagnosis was supported in a descriptive study of bowel elimination practices in 300 healthy adults who identified 22 defining characteristics and 10 contributing factors (McLane and McShane, 1986). Because participants in the study were healthy and managed their own bowel elimination problems, the limitations of the categories for understanding constipation in persons living with self-care deficits and chronic diseases were not studied. Obstacles to managing bowel elimination due to the unavailability of environmental resources were not sufficiently accounted for in the categories. For older adults, the availability of social support and financial resources, and access to health services may be critical variables affecting health practices and patterns of elimination. Self-care deficits (eg, altered mobility, impaired communication, impaired thought processes, the effects of chronic diseases on physiologic functioning, unfamiliar environments, and dependency, all common problems in institutionalized older adults) must also be fully accounted for in a model of constipation.

Two models were developed for this discussion of constipation in older adults (Figures 14.1 and 14.2). Figure 14.1 is a model of preventive health behavior, and Figure 14.2 is a model of factors contributing to three different types of constipation. Elements to include in the model were derived from the conceptual categories of diagnostic indicators (McLane et al, 1984) previously described, review of the literature, and examination of nursing care plans from a long-term care setting. Three types of constipation described by Benson (1975) were selected for inclusion in Figure 14.2 because of their compatibility with Contributing Factors I, which were derived, with few exceptions, from the conceptual categories of diagnostic indicators. Also included were descriptors of pathophysiologic process influencing bowel elimination (Contributing Factors II) (Benson, 1975). Other pathophysiologic descriptors were identified in the literature review and in the previously described study of bowel elimination practices of healthy adults (McLane and McShane, 1986).

Model of Preventive Health Behavior

The components of the model of preventive health behavior (Figure 14.1) include patterning; health behaviors; attending behaviors; self-care status; environmental resources; health status; and normal bowel elimination pattern. Researchers and clinicians agree that a normal bowel movement is regular, is easy to pass, and results in a complete passage of a formed stool (Battle and Hanna, 1980; Connell et al, 1965; Drossman et al, 1982; Martelli et al, 1978). Stool frequencies are considered to be normal when they vary within a fairly wide range, three times per day to once every third day. Although normal stool consistency is usually described as soft and formed, current research on the effects of fiber on stool consistency has led to the addition of more precise descriptions in terms of stool weight, with a normal stool weighing between 150 and 200 g/day (Godding, 1980;91).

Client appraisal, health beliefs, timing of evacuation, use of stimulus behaviors, and response to reflex are included in the model under the general heading of patterning. The term *patterning* refers to behaviors related to the production of a bowel movement (McLane et al, 1984). Client health beliefs influence expected frequency and expected time of day to have a bowel movement. Expectancies, in turn, influence timing, use of stimulus behaviors, and response to reflex, as well as all attending behaviors.

Attending behaviors (preventive and treatment) are defined as consistent use of a measure for preventing or alleviating constipation. Treatment attending behaviors are included in a model of prevention for older adults, since these behaviors may be required to mediate the influences of drugs, chronic diseases, and physiologic effects of aging and bowel elimination. The importance of teaching appropriate use of and avoidance of reliance on laxatives and enemas is highlighted by including treatment attending behaviors in the model. Further support for including treatments is based on the writings of expert nurses who care for the elderly. For example, Carnevali and Patrick (1979) exhort nurses to provide immediate relief for anyone who is constipated.

Health behaviors are defined as the use of measures to influence normal elimination. The health behaviors component of the model includes diet, fluid, and exercise. The effects of daily fiber and six to eight glasses of water per day are adequately supported in the literature (Godding, 1980; Pollman et al, 1978; Sklar, 1972). There is less empirical evidence to support the use of exercise, but indirect evidence, practice wisdom, and case reports support its efficacy. Poor mobility was significantly associated with more frequent complaints of constipation in a study of 201 elderly living at home (Donald et al, 1985). Indirect evidence for the beneficial effect of exercise on

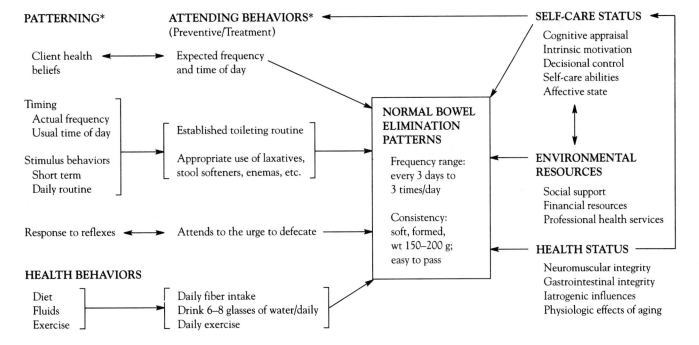

* McLane, A.M., McShane, R.E., & Sliefert, M. (1984)

Figure 14.1

Bowel elimination: A model of preventive health behavior.

bowel elimination was provided in one study of healthy older adults attending an exercise class who reported shorter periods of time between bowel movements than both healthy adolescents and healthy working adults (McLane and McShane, 1986). The delayed effects of aging when older adults are physically active and participate in physical fitness programs can be viewed as further indirect evidence supporting exercise as an important variable influencing bowel elimination. Examination of the model shows how the specific variables (attending behaviors)—daily fiber intake, fluid intake of six to eight glasses per day, and daily exercise—relate to the more abstract constructs composing health behaviors.

Environmental resources (social support, financial resources, and availability of professional health services) influence self-care status, which in turn influences all attending behaviors. Older adults may need assistance with frequent shopping for fresh fruits and vegetables. They must have sufficient financial resources to obtain fresh foods. An adequate social support network is also needed to enable the frail elderly to obtain preventive health care services.

In this model of preventive health behavior, self-care status includes cognitive appraisal, intrinsic motivation, decisional control, self-care abilities, and affective state. Orem's (1979) analysis of the 10 power components of self-care agency and Cox's (1986) interaction model of client health behavior provide the theoretical support for the selection of these variables.

Health status variables were conceptualized in physiologic terms to account for the frequent presence of pathophysiologic processes in the elderly without focusing on diseases. Health status areas of particular interest in the prevention of constipation (physiologic effects of aging, neuromuscular integrity, gastrointestinal integrity, and iatrogenic influences) are more abstract than other components of the model. However, clinicians and researchers will find them easy to operationalize for specific patients or populations. For example, iatrogenic influences refer to such variables as psychotropic drugs, narcotic analgesics, and overuse of laxatives, enemas, and suppositories. Psychotropic drugs may influence awareness of the defecation reflex, and narcotic analgesics slow the transit time of gastrointestinal contents.

The model of preventive health behavior is intended to provide clinicians with a more holistic view of factors contributing to bowel elimination. The model directs assessment and suggests specific variables derived from clinical practice, theory, and research that relate to the more abstract components of the model. The model may serve to guide researchers in the selection of concepts and constructs to be operationalized for a given study. The model does not illustrate the direction or magnitude of the relationships among the constructs and variables, nor are the relationships shown supported by sufficient empirical data.

ETIOLOGIES/RELATED FACTORS

Constipation: A Model of Contributing Factors

The model of factors contributing to constipation (Figure 14.2) shows the relationships between specific variables and the more abstract concepts/constructs described in Figure 14.1. Two categories of contributing factors, Contributing Factors I and Contributing Factors II, are shown to influence three types of constipation. Benson (1975) described the three types of constipation: imagined, rectal, and delayed. The first category, Contributing Factors I, shows the direct influence of the constructs patterning and health behaviors on the clustering of variables. On closer inspection, the variables suggested by self-care status and environmental influences can be identified. For example, low intrinsic motivation and decisional control (components of self-care status) are clustered with other variables that influence timing and stimulus behaviors. Environmental constraints and low social support (environmental factors) are clustered with variables influencing response to reflex. The relationships between the clusters and the types of constipation are suggested by the arrows.

The specific variables composing the second category of contributing factors, Contributing Factors II, were derived from clinical practice and the literature (Benson, 1965) to operationalize the health status areas. The variables were clustered to show their relationship to the types of constipation.

The expectation that a daily bowel movement is required for health leads some individuals to engage in treatment attending behaviors for imagined constipation. Persons with imagined constipation tend to overuse laxatives, enemas, and suppositories, which influence the physiologic integrity of the gastrointestinal tract (Contributing Factors II). Faulty appraisal based on inaccurate, out-of-date information and impaired thought processes (Contributing Factors I) also influence the development of imagined constipation.

Rectal constipation is characterized by normal stool consistency and delayed elimination. Three clusters of Contributing Factors I influence the development of rectal constipation. Most of these influences are mediated through their effect on following an established toileting routine and responding to the urge to defecate. Cluster one includes faulty appraisal and impaired thought processes; cluster two includes low intrinsic motivation, low decisional control, change in routine, emotional disturbances, and stress; and cluster three includes impaired communication, altered awareness, altered mobility, self-care deficits, environmental constraints, low or no social support, and weak pelvic floor musculature. Health status variables (Contributing Factors II) that influence the

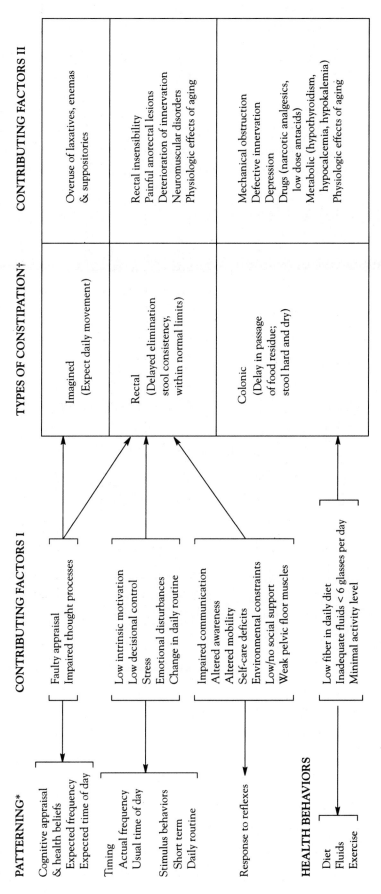

PATTERNING*

Cognitive appraisal
& health beliefs
Expected frequency
Expected time of day

Timing
Actual frequency
Usual time of day

Stimulus behaviors
Short term
Daily routine

Response to reflexes

HEALTH BEHAVIORS

Diet
Fluids
Exercise

CONTRIBUTING FACTORS I

Faulty appraisal
Impaired thought processes

Low intrinsic motivation
Low decisional control
Stress
Emotional disturbances
Change in daily routine

Impaired communication
Altered awareness
Altered mobility
Self-care deficits
Environmental constraints
Low/no social support
Weak pelvic floor muscles

Low fiber in daily diet
Inadequate fluids < 6 glasses per day
Minimal activity level

TYPES OF CONSTIPATION†

Imagined
(Expect daily movement)

Rectal
(Delayed elimination
stool consistency,
within normal limits)

Colonic
(Delay in passage
of food residue;
stool hard and dry)

CONTRIBUTING FACTORS II

Overuse of laxatives, enemas
& suppositories

Rectal insensibility
Painful anorectal lesions
Deterioration of innervation
Neuromuscular disorders
Physiologic effects of aging

Mechanical obstruction
Defective innervation
Depression
Drugs (narcotic analgesics,
low dose antacids)
Metabolic (hypothyroidism,
hypocalcemia, hypokalemia)
Physiologic effects of aging

* McLane, A.M., McShane, R.E., & Sliefert, M. (1984)
† Benson, J.A. (1975)

Figure 14.2

Constipation: A model of contributing factors.

development of colonic constipation are rectal insensitivity, painful anorectal lesions, deterioration of innervation, neuromuscular disorders, and physiologic effects of aging. Many of the physiologic effects of aging on delay in elimination have been accounted for under Contributing Factors I.

Colonic constipation is characterized by hard, dry stool and results from a delay in the passage of food residue in the gastrointestinal tract (increase in transit time). Health behavior variables, low fiber in daily diet, inadequate fluids (less than six glasses per day), and minimal activity (Contributing Factors I) delay the transit time of the products of digestion. Transit time may also be prolonged by health status variables: mechanical obstruction, defective innervation, depression, iatrogenic effects of drugs (eg, narcotic analgesics, low-dose antacids), metabolic disorders (eg, hypokalenia, hyocalcemia, hypothyroidism), and the physiologic effects of aging. Whether an increase in transit time in the entire large bowel or in particular parts of the bowel is a function of the normal aging process remains to be demonstrated. In one small study of 32 geriatric patients and 10 younger well adults, Melkersson et al (1983) did not find any difference in transit time pattern between old and young participants with normal bowel habits. In the geriatric patients (N = 32), transit time in the proximal parts of the colon did not differ when comparing constipated (N = 16) with nonconstipated (N = 16) patients. However, there was a significant difference in transit time in the rectosigmoid part of the bowel in constipated geriatric patients. Because wheat bran accelerates transit time through the rectosigmoid region of the colon (Melkersson et al, 1983), and because fiber is already accounted for as a variable (Contributing Factors I), perhaps including the construct physiologic effects of aging to generate health status variables introduces too much redundancy in the model.

The model of contributing factors is intended to capture the complexity of the phenomenon of constipation and to suggest the importance of clearer specification of etiologic variables in the diagnosis and treatment of constipation. The contributing factors assume even more importance when clinicians focus on establishing an improved pattern of elimination rather than on relieving an instance of constipation. Researchers may use the model to guide the selection of unique variables related to a population of interest. More empirical studies are needed to provide support for the relationships suggested in the model and to contribute to its refinement.

DEFINING CHARACTERISTICS

The nursing literature, the North American Nursing Diagnosis Association (NANDA), and the authors'

own research have contributed to the development of defining characteristics for constipation. The historical development of consensual and empirical validation for the diagnostic indicators of constipation is shown in Figure 14.3 (McLane and McShane, 1986;2061). From 1973 to 1984 the list expanded from 2 to 22 defining characteristics, but there was not a concomitant increase in empirical research.

The large number of defining characteristics puts a strain on clinicians and does not contribute to nursing's credibility as a scientific discipline. Researchers interested in the elderly may find different critical indicators than are found in other populations.

ASSESSMENT

An essential component of diagnosis is gathering clinical data to support the diagnosis. The emphasis in the nursing diagnosis literature on validating defining characteristics has resulted in a neglect of etiologic factors or related factors. Expert clinicians recognize the value of documenting the clinical evidence for the contributing factors when planning care for a client. Because diagnosis is not an end in itself but an intermediate step in designing treatment plans, and because the contributing or related factors guide the selection of treatments, it then becomes imperative for clinicians to assess and document the related factors. Ten factors (etiologies) contributing to the development of constipation were reported in a larger study of bowel elimination practices in healthy individuals, adolescents, middle-aged persons, and older adults (McLane and McShane, 1986). Being upset or worried and feeling sad or down were identified most often by respondents as precipitating an instance of constipation. Factors related to missed meals and usual foods not being available received the next highest frequency rating. Other factors reported include excessive sweating, medications (antacids and codeine), increase in body temperature, and vomiting.

In most cases of constipation in older adults, more than a single factor is responsible, making it difficult to pinpoint the cause. For example, an elderly patient may have defective innervation, inadequate intake of residue and water, mild depression, and a laxative habit. Thus, a detailed history with corroboration by relatives, home health aides, nurses, and physicians is essential. Drugs can be a major factor contributing to chronic constipation in the ill elderly. Opiates, particularly codeine, anticholinergic agents, ganglionic blockers used to treat hypertension, nonabsorbable antacids (eg, calcium carbonate and aluminium hydroxide gel), antidepressants, sedatives, and antiparkinsonian agents, contribute to hardening of the stool, impaired responsiveness to rectal distention,

1973 1st National Conference	1975 2nd National Conference	1978 3rd National Conference	1980 4th National Conference	1982 5th National Conference	1984 6th Conference
	Abdominal mass	Abdominal mass	Abdominal mass Abdominal pain	↓Bowel sounds Abdominal mass Abdominal pain ↑Abdominal pressure	Abdominal distention Δ Abdominal growling Abdominal mass Abdominal pain ↑Abdominal pressure Δ Abdominal size
	↓Appetite	↓Appetite	↓Appetite	↓Appetite	↓Appetite
	Hard, formed stool Frequency < 3 x week Headache	Hard, formed stool Frequency < 3 x week Headache	Hard, formed stool Frequency < usual patterns Headache	Hard, formed stool Frequency < usual patterns Headache Nausea	Blood with stool Dry, hard stool Δ Flatus Δ Frequency Headache Indigestion Mass in rectum Oozing liquid stool
	Rectal fullness	Rectal fullness	Rectal fullness	Rectal fullness	Rectal fullness
	Rectal pressure Straining at stool	Rectal pressure Straining at stool	Rectal pressure Straining at stool	Rectal pressure Less than usual amount of stool Straining at stool	Rectal pain with BM Rectal pressure Small volume of stool Straining at stool Swollen rectal veins
					Unable to pass stool
Infrequent or difficult evacuation of feces					

* McLane, A.M., McShane, R.E. Elimination. In J.M. Thompson, et al. *Clinical Nursing* (p. 2061). St. Louis, Mo: The C.V. Mosby Co., 1986.

Figure 14.3

Historical development of consensual and empirical validation—diagnostic indicators: Constipation.

reduced segmentation of the colon, and disruption of a complex, learned behavior (Benson, 1975). (See also Chapter 30.)

A common guide for client interview and physical assessment of bowel elimination patterns is viewed as a requisite for developing standards of care for persons with constipation. The two models shown in Figures 14.1 and 14.2 and the long list of defining characteristics make it evident that a detailed interview guide is needed to assess patterns of bowel elimination. No comprehensive guides were found in the literature. Manning et al (1976) suggest that bowel histories be interpreted with caution. In their study, one in six patients was wrong in predicting the number of bowel movements per week by as much as three movements.

Resnick (1985) described physical examination of geriatric clients for constipation. The examination includes inspection of the abdomen for distention, hernias, and scars; palpation of abdominal muscles for tone, tenderness, and abdominal masses; and palpation of liver and spleen. The rectal examination, viewed by Resnick as the most improtant step, included inspecting the perineum for hemorrhoids, fissures, scars, and strictures; checking for anal tone; detecting rectoceles; and exploring the rectum for stool masses. Rectoceles are detected by asking clients to bear down, and anal tone is evaluated by instructing the client to tighten anal muscles around the examiner's gloved finger. Exploration of the rectum provides the opportunity to detect masses or stool, determine stool consistency, obtain stool for occult blood, and rule out a fecal impaction. Mager-O'Connor (1984) described a step-by-step process for removal of fecal impactions in geriatric patients. Further examination by a physician may include sigmoidoscopy, barium enema, or colonoscopy.

Assessment of a bowel elimination pattern must be done in conjunction with a complete assessment and examination of the client, since untreated constipation and an inappropriate treatment plan may result in complications. Stitt (1983) described the proneness of elderly patients to complications from constipation. Cardiovascular changes, nonobstructive gastrointestinal side effects, and psychologic symptoms were viewed as the most common complications. Straining at stool raises intrathoracic pressure and increases risk of coronary insufficiency and arrhythmias. Straining may also aggravate symptoms of hiatal hernia by raising intra-abdominal pressure. Obstructive gastrointestinal effects include development of megacolon, impaction, and fecal incontinence. Psychologic symptoms common to the elderly with chronic constipation include restlessness and confusion. Stitt (1983) cautions against sedating patients with constipation, since the drug may further decrease awareness of a distended rectum.

CASE STUDY

Colonic Constipation

Mr. Rice, age 78, complained of constipation during an admission interview at a skilled care facility where he was admitted for rehabilitation following an above-the-knee amputation (auto accident). Data obtained from interview of the patient and his son included the following: uses Milk of Magnesia daily; strains to pass hard, dry stool every 2 to 3 days; has minimal intake of fruit, vegetables, and whole-grain cereals; drinks coffee with meals and wine before retiring; expresses dislike of institutional food. Prior to hospitalization Mr. Rice walked 2 miles daily, participated in exercise sessions at a senior citizen center twice weekly, and lived alone in his own home with the weekly assistance of a cleaning service. Physical examination revealed an alert, tall, slim man who appeared younger than his stated age. His abdomen was moderately distended; a mass was palpated in his left lower abdomen; and he had no tenderness or scars. Skin was dry with poor turgor. Rectal examination was negative except for the presence of a large mass of impacted stool.

TENTATIVE DIAGNOSIS

Colonic constipation (with impacted stool) related to low intake of fiber, moderate dehydration, long-term laxative use, inability to engage in usual activities (walking/exercise), and delayed response to urge to defecate related to altered mobility.

Goals	Treatments
Obtain relief from impacted stool	Instill warm mineral oil to soften stool in lower rectum (retain 20–30 minutes). Use well-lubricated gloved finger to break stool into smaller fragments and gradually remove. Monitor for cardiovascular side effects (eg, dizziness, chest pain) and local pain or bleeding.
Increase intake of fiber and fluids	Collaborate with dietitian to add bran (2–4 g initially) to diet, with gradual increases to 12–20 g. Provide six to eight glasses of water daily. Teach patient/son importance of fruits, vegetables, bran in diet. Monitor intake of fiber and fluids.

Establish a new pattern of activity

Collaborate with physical therapist to develop/implement desired level of daily exercises and activities. Coach/monitor daily exercises and activities. Teach/monitor daily exercises and activities.

Establish an acceptable toileting routine

Provide bedside commode (temporarily) to facilitate response to urge to defecate. Assist/monitor transfer to commode. Provide assistance to toilet as ability to ambulate improves. Teach importance of responding to urge to defecate. Monitor stool for frequency and consistency. Teach use of Dulcolax suppository as needed instead of daily laxative.

EXPECTED OUTCOMES

No further episodes of impaction; gradually increases fiber in diet (eats bran muffin daily) and fruit between meals; reports easy passage of formed stool and feelings of complete evacuation every 1–2 days; increases ambulation 5–10′ daily; drinks six glasses of water daily; and keeps record of activities and food/fluid intake.

CASE STUDY

Rectal Constipation

Responding to an urgent message from a client's daughter, the home health nurse visited Mrs. Johnson to evaluate the daughter's request to give her mother an enema. Mrs. Johnson, age 72, was recovering from a stroke (3 days posthospitalization) with residual weakness but no paralysis. Data obtained from interview of the client and her daughter included the following: inability to pass rectal contents for past 3 days; rectal and abdominal discomfort; feeling of rectal fullness; daily use of stool softener; abdominal distention; occasional rectal incontinence (one to two times weekly); generalized weakness; limited daily activity (gets up in chair for meals); loss of interest in usual activities; and a 5-year (posthemorrhoidectomy) history of frequent enema use to produce a bowel movement. Physical examination revealed a well-nourished elderly woman in obvious discomfort with a distended abdomen that was not

tender to the touch. A large mass of soft unformed stool and poor anal tone were found during rectal examination. Stool was negative for occult blood.

TENTATIVE DIAGNOSIS

Stool retention (rectal constipation) related to general weakness, weak abdominal muscles, poor anal tone, and moderate depression.

Goals

Obtain immediate relief from physical symptoms

Establish a regular pattern of bowel elimination

Strengthen abdominal and rectal muscles

Increase activity level within limits of exercise prescription from physician

Treatments

Use Dulcolax suppository and follow with Fleets enema if necessary.

Collaborate with client and caregiver to develop an acceptable toileting routine, including immediate response to urge to defecate; use of bedside commode; and use of stimulus behaviors (eg, drink warm liquid on arising).

Teach client abdominal and pelvic exercises. Teach caregiver to coach and evaluate exercise sessions.

Develop daily exercise plan including active range of motion; use of walker with assistance 2–3 times daily; use of exercise log.

EXPECTED OUTCOMES

Exercises abdominal and rectal muscles (with coaching) three times a day; engages in active range of motion without assistance three times daily; extends walking distance with walker 5′ daily; requests assistance to use toilet in response to urge to defecate; has stool frequency, color, and consistency within normal limits; uses Dulcolax suppository occasionally to facilitate defecation; has no incontinent episodes.

NURSING INTERVENTIONS

The discussion of nursing interventions in this section is based on the three types of constipation (imagined, rectal, and colonic) and their contributing factors as outlined in Figure 14.2. Health teaching with a goal of changing health beliefs is the intervention for imagined constipation. Rectal constipation is treated by repatterning, with the goal of establishing a toileting routine with regular passage of stool. Modification of health behaviors in the areas of diet, fluid, and exercise is the treatment of choice for colonic constipation, with particular attention to the provision of a high-fiber diet.

Perceived Constipation: Health Teaching

Prior to beginning a program of health teaching, the nurse monitors the health beliefs and health practices of the client and caregiver. Discussion of health beliefs and use of a daily log to record health practices can facilitate the design of a learning program. As client and caregiver begin to recognize an association between their beliefs about bowel elimination and their behaviors, the benefits of adopting alternate health practices can be emphasized. Hahn (1982) reported on use of the health belief model to gain a better understanding of constipation. She found that perceived benefits rather than cues were associated with adoption of health-oriented elimination practices. Selection of teaching strategies depends on the client's and caregiver's self-care status and contextual variables.

Rectal Constipation: Repatterning

The elements to consider in repatterning bowel elimination are outlined in the model of preventive health behavior (Figure 14.1) and the model of contributing factors (Figure 14.2). Attention to the mosaic of defining characteristics and contributing factors unique to a client are illustrated in the case study on rectal constipation (see page 156). The nurse collaborates with the client and caregiver to establish a toileting routine including immediate response to the urge to defecate; use of a bedside commode; and recognition and use of stimulus behaviors. Abdominal and pelvic muscles are strengthened through the use of exercise, and mobility is improved through active range of motion and assistance with walking. Client health status, self-care status, and environmental variables function as resources or constraints in the formulation of goals and measureable outcomes, which, in turn, provide a structure for selecting specific strategies to modify the contributing factors. It is clear from this example that repatterning is not viewed as an a priori cluster of activities that can be standardized on care plans. Instead, repatterning requires a unique configuration of activities and techniques derived from an analysis of all the variables contributing to the bowel elimination problem of an individual.

Colonic Constipation: High-Fiber Diet

Fiber, fluid, and exercise are considered the best remedies for constipation (Resnick, 1985). An increase in dietary fiber produces its effect on constipation by providing bulk, gentle laxative, and ease of elimination (Zimring, 1976). Physiologically, the added fiber absorbs water and shortens intestinal time (speed at which stool passes through the intestines). The shortened transit time also decreases water absorption in the large intestine. In the rectal area, the bulk serves as the primary mechanical factor to initiate evacuation.

Edible fiber includes dietary fiber from plant foods; partly synthetic polysaccharides (eg, methylcellulose); processed preparations not taken as foodstuffs; and fiberlike materials from animal tissues (Godding, 1980). Daily intake of fiber can be increased by use of whole-grain breads and cereals, leafy vegetables, and raw and cooked fruits. Some fruits have a laxative effect as well as being high in fiber (eg, bananas, prunes, dates, figs, and rhubarb). Bran, the end product of milling wheat, contains 20% indigestible cellulose and is a good source of bulk. Processed bran products contain variable amounts of fiber: 100% Bran, 7%; All Bran, 7.5%; Bran Buds, 7%; and Raisin Bran, 3%. In contrast, unprocessed bran contains 14% fiber (Hui, 1983).

The full effect of adding dietary fiber may not be evident for 3 weeks to 3 months. Because some individuals reject the additon of large amounts of dietary fiber, it may be prudent to add 2 to 4 g initially, with gradual increases to 20g, the recommended daily amount (see the case study on colonic constipation, page 155). Persons with a compromised nutritional status (undernourished) may not be good candidates for the addition of dietary fiber, since excessively high fiber could reduce the availability of essential nutrients and minerals.

Six to eight glasses of fluids per day are needed to maintain normal metabolic processes and prevent excessive reabsorption of fluid from gastrointestinal contents. Elderly individuals with mobility problems and/or their caregivers frequently limit fluid intake to avoid trips to the bathroom or increased risk of episodes of urinary incontinence. Ambulatory elderly may limit fluid intake to avoid using public facilities or to prevent interruption of sleep. Limitations of fluid intake are often compounded by extra fluid loss from diuretics used to control blood pressure or minimize fluid retention subsequent to chronic congestive heart failure. It may be necessary to prescribe 6 to 8 ounces of water at specified hours during the day to ensure an adequate intake. Individuals who are taking prescribed medications several times a day could be encouraged to drink a glass of water with the medication to prevent incomplete swallowing of tablets or capsules.

Exercise in some form is essential for total body functioning and well-being. Normal defecation depends on adequate abdominal and pelvic muscular strength as well as sufficient strength to use available toilet facilities. Persons with restricted mobility may require exercise to strengthen the upper arm muscles to transfer from bed to commode or from wheelchair to toilet. In order to increase pelvic floor muscle tone and sphincter function, pelvic floor strengthening exercises must be done correctly four times per hour for 3 months. Individuals can be taught to identify the pelvic floor muscles by telling them to stop and restart the flow during urination and tighten and relax the ring of muscle around the anus. Mandelstam (1980) suggests counting slowly from one to four while tightening the muscles from back to front. The pelvic tilt will also help strengthen pelvic floor muscles and abdominal muscles. Some individuals are able to do sit ups with knees bent and arms flexed behind the head to strengthen abdominal muscles. Walking briskly for 15 minutes daily is an excellent form of exercise. Many senior citizen centers provide guided exercise sessions several times a week for individuals with permission from their physicians. Goal setting and use of an exercise log that is reviewed jointly by the nurse and client are important elements of any exercise program. More data are needed to support the relationships suggested in the models of constipation and to determine their usefulness in guiding day-to-day practice. Older individuals who are active and exercise regularly are certainly at less risk of developing chronic constipation than persons with mobility restrictions. The effect of a program of exercise on preexisting constipation, however, needs to be studied. More data are also needed on the prophylactic administration of wheat bran in hospitalized or institutionalized older adults and the frail elderly. No discussion of diagnosis and treatment is complete without recognition and acknowledgment of the influence of a nurse's theoretical orientation on the diagnostic and treatment process. Because conceptual frameworks drive the assessment and goal selection steps of the nursing process (Joel, 1985), their influence on diagnosis and treatment may be viewed as indirect. However, because goal setting precedes and channels the selection of interventions, a nurse's theoretical orientation permeates the selection and design of interventions. The scientific content in a substantive area, for example, constipation, is open to selective interpretation and application in light of a particular view of a client interacting in an environment and seeking health, with health defined by the nurse, by the client, or by the nurse and client.

SUMMARY

In keeping with the format of this publication and space limitations, one intervention was discussed for each subtype of constipation. This in no way negates the earlier discussion of the multifaceted nature of constipation as illustrated in the models (Figures 14.1 and 14.2), case studies, and their associated care plans. Nursing assessment of the specific type of constipation is essential for prescribing interventions to achieve the desired outcomes for the elderly.

References

Battle EH, Hanna CE: Evaluation of a dietary regimen for chronic constipation: Report of a pilot study. *J Gerontol Nurs* 1980; 6(9):527–532.

Benson JA: Simple chronic constipation: Pathophysiology and management. *Postgrad Med* 1975; 57(1):55–60.

Carnevali DL, Patrick M: *Nursing Management for the Elderly.* Lippincott, 1979.

Carroll-Johnson R (editor): *Classification of Nursing Diagnoses: Proceedings of the Eighth Conference.* Lippincott, 1989.

Connell AM et al: Variation in bowel habit in two population samples. *British Med J* 1965; 2:1095–1099.

Cox CL: The interaction model of client health behavior: Application to the study of community-based elders. *ANS* 1986; 9(1):40–57.

Donald IP et al: A study of constipation in the elderly living at home. *Gerontology* 1985; 31:112–118.

Drossman DA et al: Bowel patterns among subjects not seeking health care. *Gerontology* 1982; 83:528–534.

Godding EW: Physiological yardsticks for bowel function and the rehabilitation of the constipated bowel. *Pharmacology* 1980; 20:88–103.

Hahn K: Constipation: Nursing diagnosis and the health belief model. Unpublished Master's research. The University of Wisconsin, 1982.

Hui YH: Diet and diseases of the gastrointestinal system. In: *Human Nutrition and Diet Therapy.* Hui YH (editor). Wadsworth, 1983.

Joel L: Nursing theory and nursing diagnosis. Paper presentation. Annual nursing diagnosis conference 1985. Wisconsin Nurses' Association Nursing Diagnosis Interest Group.

Mager-O'Connor E: How to identify and remove fecal impactions. *Geriatr Nurs* 1984; 5(3):158–161.

Mandelstam D: Special techniques: Strengthening pelvic floor muscles. *Geriatr Nurs* 1980; 1:251–252.

Manning AP, Wyman JB, Heaton KW: How trustworthy are bowel histories? Comparison of recalled and recorded information. *Brit Med J* 1976; 2:213–214.

Martelli H et al: Some parameters of normal bowel motility in normal man. *Gastroenterology* 1978; 75:612–618.

McLane AM, McShane RE: Empirical validation of defining characteristics of constipation: A study of bowel elimination practices of healthy adults. In: *Classification of Nursing Diagnoses: Proceedings of the Sixth National Conference.* Hurley ME (editor). Mosby, 1986.

McLane AM, McShane RE, Sliefert M: Constipation: Conceptual categories of diagnostic indicators. In: *Classification of Nursing Diagnoses: Proceedings of the Fifth National Conference.* Kim MJ, McFarland GK, McLane AM (editors). Mosby, 1984.

Melkersson M et al: Intestinal transit time in constipated and non-constipated geriatric patients. *Scand J Gastroenterol* 1983; 18(5):593–597.

Orem DE: *Concept Formalization in Nursing: Process and Product.* Little, Brown, 1979.

Pollman JW, Morris JJ, Rose P: Is fiber the answer to constipation problems in the elderly? A review of literature. *International J Nurs Studies* 1978; 15:107–114.

Resnick B: Constipation: Common but preventable. *Geriatr Nurs* (July/Aug) 1985; 213–215.

Sklar M: Functional bowel distress and constipation in the aged. *Geriatrics* (Sept) 1972; 79–85.

Stitt VJ: Constipation in the elderly. *J National Med Assoc* 1983; 75(9):908–912.

Zimring JG: High-fiber diet versus laxatives in geriatric patients. *NY State J Med* 1976; 18:2223–2224.

15

Diarrhea

KAREN WADLE, MA, RN

DIARRHEA IS ONE MANIFESTATION OF GASTROINTESTI-nal (GI) disturbance. "The word diarrhea originates from the Greek terms *dia* (through) and *rhein* (to flow)" (Krejs and Fordtran, 1983;257). Krejs and Fordtran (1983) define diarrhea as an abnormal increase in stool liquidity, daily stool weight greater than 200 grams, and stool frequency greater than three per day, although the authors admit this definition is subject to variation among individuals. Bond (1982) defines diarrhea as the passage of over 200 grams of stool per day (as compared with an average daily stool weight of 100 to 150 grams per day), with a stool content of 70% to 90% water (compared to a normal stool content of 60% to 80% water). Diarrhea may be defined as an acute problem lasting from 24 to 48 hours or as a chronic problem lasting continuously or intermittently for several weeks (McLane and McShane, 1986).

In aging individuals, the gastrointestinal system is subject to physiologic changes, as are other body systems. Changes include decreases in motility, gastric juice secretion, free acid content, total acid production, and pepsin content. Salivary and pancreatic digestive enzyme production also decreases. With aging, there is a decrease in the ability of the immune system to adapt to environmental stresses; thus, the elderly are more susceptible to infectious processes (Schmucker and Daniels, 1986). Lifestyle changes brought about by physiologic, economic, and sociologic factors such as nutritional habits and exercise patterns also are important considerations in assessing gastrointestinal function in the aged. The three key processes of the gastrointestinal tract are digestion, absorption, and metabolism (Broadwell, 1986). These factors are all subject to alterations that can predispose the individual to diarrhea as the elderly experience chronic illnesses, effects of the treatment of these illnesses, and decline of organ systems and their interdependent functioning. Specific prevalence rates in the elderly will be discussed with each etiology later in this chapter.

NURSING DIAGNOSIS

In 1988, the North American Nursing Diagnosis Association (NANDA) modified the label for Altered Bowel Elimination: Diarrhea to Diarrhea (Carroll-Johnson, 1989). Assessment, diagnosis, and planning of interventions are enhanced by distinguishing between acute and chronic etiologies.

Generally agreed on defining characteristics of the nursing diagnosis Diarrhea include abdominal pain; cramping; increased stool frequency; increased frequency of bowel sounds; loose, liquid stools; and urgency (McLane and McShane, 1986). Carpenito (1983) defines increased frequency of stools as meaning more than three stools per day. McLane and McShane (1986;2070) note that "several authors who contribute regularly to the nursing diagnosis literature formulated definitions of diarrhea, but there is no normative definition."

ETIOLOGIES/RELATED FACTORS AND DEFINING CHARACTERISTICS

It is useful to distinguish between large stool and small stool diarrhea. Table 15.1 is based on Krejs and Fordtran's (1983) discussion. The etiologies and defining characteristics for acute and chronic diarrhea discussed below are listed in Table 15.2 and compared with those identified by NANDA (Carroll-Johnson, 1989).

Acute Diarrhea

Acute diarrhea is associated with three main etiologies: (1) infection; (2) drug reactions; and (3) alterations in diet (McLane and McShane, 1986). Additional factors identified include heavy metal poisoning and fecal impaction (Krejs and Fordtran, 1983) (Table 15.2).

Infection Age-related changes in the mucosal surfaces, such as those of the respiratory and gastrointestinal tracts, are associated with increased susceptibility to infectious diseases (Schmucker and Daniels, 1986). Institutionalization creates additional risks of infection for the elderly because of close proximity to other persons who may have infections.

Infectious diseases pose a greater threat to life in the elderly than in younger patients (Vartian and Septimus, 1986). Statistics from the World Health Organization (1975) report a 400-fold increase in mortality associated with gastrointestinal infections in the elderly. Reduced motility and gastric acidity, which may accompany aging or may result from gastric surgery or the use of medication, can increase susceptibility to viral pathogens and bacterial agents such as *Shigella, Clostridium difficile, Salmonella,* and *Campylobacter* (McFarland and Stamm, 1986; Vartian and Septimus, 1986). Bacterial endotoxins such as clostridial and staphylococcal toxins may be present in food that is improperly prepared or refrigerated or may be formed in the gastrointestinal tract by organisms such as *Escherichia coli* (Bond, 1982). The elderly, particularly those living in rural areas where private and municipal water sources may become contaminated by infected animals, may be infected by intestinal parasites such as the protozoa *Giardia lamblia* or (less commonly in the United States) *Entamoeba histolytica* (Bond, 1982). Infectious diarrhea may occur following travel, especially to a foreign country where bacterial contamination of water supplies is common. Diverticula are saccular outpouchings occurring through defects in the circular muscle layer of the colon (Burakoff, 1981). Fecal material becomes trapped within these diverticula, resulting in

Table 15.1

Differentiation of Signs and Symptoms Commonly Associated With Small Stool and Large Stool Diarrhea

	SMALL STOOL DIARRHEA	LARGE STOOL DIARRHEA
Location of underlying disorder or disease	Left colon and rectum	Small bowel or proximal colon
Stool qualities	Dark in color Frequent small amounts Rarely foul smelling Flatus and mucus sometimes expelled without stool Stool, when passed, is mushy, mixed with visible mucus or blood	Light in color Large amounts Foul smelling Watery, soupy, or greasy Free of gross blood Contains undigested food particles
Pain location	When present, likely to be in hypogastrium, in left or right lower quadrant, or in sacral region	When present, likely to be periumbilical or in right lower quadrant
Pain quality	Griping, aching, or with tenesmus (ineffective, painful straining at stool)	Intermittent, cramplike, accompanied by borborygmus (gurgling splashing sound)

Source: Krejs C, Fordtran J: Diarrhea. Chapter 16 in: *Gastrointestinal Disease: Pathophysiology, Diagnosis, Management,* 3d ed. Sleisenger MH, Fordtran JS (editors). Saunders, 1983.

Table 15.2

Etiologies/Related Factors and Defining Characteristics of Diarrhea

NANDA (CARROLL-JOHNSON, 1989)

Definition: A state in which an individual experiences a change in normal bowel habits characterized by the frequent passage of loose, fluid, unformed stools

Defining Characteristics
Abdominal pain
Cramping
Increased frequency
Increased frequency of bowel sounds
Loose, liquid stools
Urgency

Change in color

WADLE

Etiologies/Related Factors: Acute	*Defining Characteristics*
Infection	Small bowel: nonbloody, watery stools, low-grade fever
	Absence fecal leukocytes
	Colon: Bloody mucous stools with fecal leukocytes; fever
Drug reactions	Watery stools after medication ingestion, eg, antibiotics, antihypertensives, digitalis preparations
Heavy metal poisoning (Krejs and Fordtran, 1983)	Watery stools of purging type with anorexia, abdominal pain, muscle cramps, and joint pain
Fecal impaction (Krejs and Fordtran, 1983)	Watery stools after a period of absence of bowel movement
	Digital identification of hard stool
Alteration in diet (McLane and McShane, 1986)	Change in diet pattern
	Increased fruit, vegetable, and lactose intake
	Tube feedings or formula
	Watery stools with cramping and flatulence
Chronic (McLane and McShane, 1986)	Alternating constipation and diarrhea
Irritable bowel syndrome	Abdominal pain
	Psychologic factors
	Stressful life situations
Lactose deficiency	Watery stools with gas and bloating
Cancer of the colon	Reported change in bowel habits
Inflammatory bowel disease—ulcerative colitis	Watery stools with abdominal cramps, rectal bleeding
	Fever
	Weakness
Chronic disease	Watery stools with abdominal cramps
	Fever
	Weakness
GI surgery	Stools that are murky, frothy, and contain oil
Malabsorptive disorders, eg, celiac sprue	
Laxative use	
Alcohol use	

inflammation. Symptoms include lower quadrant abdominal pain, fever, and frequent episodes of diarrhea or diarrhea followed by severe constipation. The elderly are especially prone to the development of diverticulitis, and the incidence increases with advancing age. It is estimated that as many as one half of adults over 70 years of age will have diverticular disease (Burakoff, 1981; Vartian and Septimus, 1986).

Assessment factors specific to infection as an etiology in acute diarrhea differ depending on whether the organisms involve the small bowel or the colon. Small bowel infection usually produces "nonbloody, watery diarrhea and low-grade fever" (Vartian and Septimus, 1986;55). Infection in the colon "can produce stools with blood, mucus, and fecal leukocytes, usually in association with fever" (Vartian and Septimus, 1986;56).

Drug Reactions Drugs may produce diarrhea as part of their intended effect, such as that produced by laxatives, or as a side effect other than the intended effect. Antibiotics are frequently accompanied by diarrhea because of alteration of normal flora or by inflammation of intestinal mucosa. Antibiotics most often implicated in producing diarrhea are ampicillin, cephalosporins, clindamycin, lincomycin, neomycin, and tetracyclines (Bond, 1982). In the elderly, the prevalence of infections commonly treated with antibiotics, such as pneumonia, cholecystitis, and urinary tract infections, increases the magnitude of the problem of diarrhea in this population.

The prevalence of chronic illnesses in the elderly also increases their exposure to medications used to treat these conditions. A number of medications can cause diarrhea in the elderly. Medications that are commonly prescribed for elderly persons are antacids, antibiotics, antihypertensives, cancer chemotherapeutic agents, colchicine, digitalis preparations, lactulose, potassium supplements, propanolol, and quinidine.

Obtaining a drug history is an important step in assessing the possibility of drug reaction as a cause of acute diarrhea. See Chapter 4 for further discussion of drugs that may cause diarrhea and GI irritation and for guidelines for the nurse's assessment. If the patient is unable to provide a reliable account of medications being taken, a record review or consultation with other health care professionals who have treated the patients is essential.

Diet Alterations Alterations in diet among the elderly may be brought about by a number of factors, including economic problems, inability to shop for food frequently, loss of teeth, and intolerance or inability to digest foods adequately. Ironically, changes in diet patterns may be brought about by institutionalization or dependence on mobile meal programs in which well-planned diets may be higher in fruit and vegetable products containing long-chain carbohydrates that are incompletely digested in the small intestine (Bond, 1982; McLane and McShane, 1986). Economic factors may restrict the elderly in the purchase of more expensive protein diet items and increase their consumption of carbohydrates or of lactose-containing foods such as milk sugars. Lactose intolerance is associated with cramping, flatulence, and diarrhea (McLane and McShane, 1986). Diarrhea associated tube feeding has been linked to milk-based formulas (Walike and Walike, 1973, 1977). Economic factors as well as physical limitations may inhibit the ability of the elderly to shop frequently for food items, limiting the types of foods they purchase and increasing the incidence of food spoilage due to lengthy storage. Drug–food interactions may suppress or stimulate appetite, alter nutrient digestion and absorption, and alter the metabolism and excretion of nutrients (Roe, 1986).

The use of formula feedings in the elderly also may be associated with diarrhea. Suggested causes include the composition, osmolarity, and temperature of the feeding and the method of infusion (Taylor, 1982). Most of the formulas have been altered to be low in lactose or lactose-free, and some have been adjusted to be more compatible with the body's osmolarity requirements. Temperature of feedings and methods of infusion will be discussed in the section on nursing interventions. Assessment of diet habits, with particular attention to recent changes in eating patterns and foods ingested, is important in determining the effects of diet on elimination patterns.

Other Factors Heavy metal poisoning is suggested as another possible cause of acute diarrhea (Krejs and Fordtran, 1983). Because of their living conditions, elderly persons might be exposed to such things as lead content in old paint. The use of favorite old dishes or utensils with crazed or cracked finishes has been associated with heavy metal poisoning from lead content in pottery materials. Diarrhea of a purging type, along with anorexia, vomiting, abdominal pain, muscle cramps, and joint pain, is suggestive of heavy metal poisoning.

Fecal impaction is defined as a large, firm, immovable mass of stool in the rectum or in some cases higher in the colon. Diarrhea is caused as liquid stool from the proximal colon is forced around the impaction (Krejs and Fordtran, 1983). This is a special risk factor for the elderly because of dietary changes, as previously discussed, as well as decreased exercise patterns and decreased GI function and circulation. The frequency of impaction is highest in the institutionalized elderly (Krejs and Fordtran, 1983). Assessment of fecal impaction is based on the presence of diarrhea after a period of absence of bowel movement and can be determined by digital examination of the lower bowel. X-ray examination is necessary to confirm fecal impaction high in the bowel.

Chronic Diarrhea

McLane and McShane (1986) identify several etiologies for chronic diarrhea. These include irritable bowel syndrome, lactase deficiency, cancer of the colon, inflammatory bowel disease, gastrointestinal surgery, radiation enterocolitis, malabsorption diseases, laxative abuse, alcohol abuse, and chemotherapeutic agents.

Irritable Bowel Syndrome Irritable bowel syndrome is a motor disorder that is manifested by alternating constipation and diarrhea, abdominal pain, and the absence of detectable organic pathology. Psychologic factors and stressful life situations are influential in the production of these symptoms (Schuster, 1983). The elderly experience many stressful life situations, such as retirement, loss of mate, chronic illness, and loss of independence, and may develop this syndrome as a response to these life losses. These factors should be assessed by interviewing the patient and family members familiar with significant life events.

Lactase Deficiency Lactase deficiency and the resultant lactose intolerance is associated with diarrhea, gas, and bloating following the ingestion of foods such as milk, cheese, ice cream, or puddings and sauces made with milk or milk products (Alpers, 1983). The elderly often include a high number of dairy items in their diet because they can be prepared quickly, can be more comfortably eaten by edentulous persons, and may be more economically feasible to purchase than other foods. Lactase deficiency may also exaggerate symptoms of other intestinal disorders such as irritable bowel syndrome or inflammatory bowel disease (Bond, 1982). A diet history can provide the nurse with useful assessment data. The incidence of lactose intolerance is highest among blacks, Native Americans, Mexican-Americans, and Jews (Englert and Guillory, 1986).

Colon Cancer Several factors are important for the nurse to assess in this possible etiology. Change in bowel habits is often the earliest sign of cancer of the large bowel (Bond, 1982). Occult blood in stools or frank rectal bleeding, alternating diarrhea and constipation, increased gaseousness, and abdominal pain are presenting symptoms. Diets high in fat, protein, and beef and deficient in dietary fiber have been suggested as etiologic factors. Heredity is also a predisposing factor, as is inflammatory bowel disease. Risk for colorectal cancer rises sharply at age 50, doubling each decade after 40 years of age (Winawer and Sherlock, 1983). In addition to cancer itself, measures used to treat the cancer such as gastrointestinal surgery, radiation therapy, and chemotherapy are all associated with diarrhea.

Inflammatory Bowel Disease Diseases of the gastrointestinal tract that are characterized by an inflammatory process are also causes of chronic diarrhea. Such diseases include ulcerative colitis and Crohn's disease. The diarrhea occurring in ulcerative colitis is accompanied by abdominal cramps, rectal bleeding, fever, and weakness (Bond, 1982). The cause is unknown, and, although the disease is often diagnosed in younger persons, the incidence of onset in persons over age 50 is almost equal to the incidence of onset in younger persons. Treatment of inflammatory bowel disease in the elderly is complicated by a high incidence of diabetes, arteriosclerosis, hypertension, emphysema, and diverticulosis in the elderly population (Cello, 1983). Crohn's disease is also of unknown etiology, and, although a more common problem in younger persons, it is increasingly diagnosed in persons over 60 years of age (Foxworthy and Wilson, 1985). Symptoms of Crohn's disease are similar to those in ulcerative colitis, but rectal bleeding is less common.

Perianal ulcerations, fistulas, and abscesses are associated with Crohn's disease (Bond, 1982).

Gastrointestinal Surgery Surgery to treat such conditions as ulcerative colitis, Crohn's disease, or, as previously mentioned, tumors of the gastrointestinal tract causes varying degrees of diarrhea and malabsorption, depending on the portion of the gastrointestinal system removed. Gastric surgery increases the rate of entry of osmotically active carbohydrates through the small bowel, resulting in diarrhea. Major small bowel resections result in severe diarrhea and malabsorption (Bond, 1982). This is due to the decrease in surface area of the small bowel normally used to absorb fluid and nutrients into the bloodstream. As a result, the contents of the bowel contain a higher percentage of water as they pass through the gastrointestinal system and are excreted. Record review, consultation with treating professionals, patient interview, and inspection for surgical scars are sources of assessment data for the nurse.

Malabsorption Disorders Celiac sprue is a disease of malabsorption of nutrients associated with lesions of the small intestine and related to gluten intolerance. Gluten is a substance found in cereal grains. First onset of symptoms is often in childhood, with a second onset in persons age 40 to 50 (Broadwell, 1986; Trier, 1983). The diarrhea of celiac sprue is related to increased volume and osmotic load introduced into the colon because it is malabsorbed by the small intestine and is aggravated by dietary fats and bile salts (Broadwell, 1986). Dietary habit assessment should include a review of specific foods associated with production of diarrhea. Stools of patients with malabsorption disorders are described as murky, frothy, and containing oil (Krejs and Fordtran, 1983).

Laxative Use Laxative use and abuse may be a problem in the elderly population. Concern for lessened frequency of bowel movements associated with decreased motility in the aging gastrointestinal tract and with decreased exercise may lead elderly persons to overuse laxatives to increase stool frequency. A drug history taken by the nurse should include a review of laxative use.

Alcohol Use Alcohol ingestion, an increasingly recognized problem in the elderly, is likely to cause malabsorption in the elderly patient (Roe, 1986). Other factors that link alcohol abuse to the production of diarrhea include exocrine pancreatic insufficiency, vitamin deficiencies, hypermotility, and inhibited jejunal water and electrolyte absorption (Martin et al, 1980; Van Theil et al, 1981). Patients' significant others should be interviewed to assess the use of alcohol as a factor contributing to diarrhea in the elderly.

Assessment Guide 15.1 presents an assessment tool for the nursing diagnosis of diarrhea, developed by this chapter's author.

CASE STUDY

Diarrhea

Mr. Anderson, a 75-year-old man with multi-infarct dementia, has resided in a long-term care facility for 4 years, since he has become increasingly confused and debilitated. He is unable to ambulate even with assistance, and sits up in a chair for several short periods throughout the day and evening. Mr. Anderson is edentulous and has recently been placed on nasogastric tube feedings because he was unable to swallow even soft foods without choking. (He had aspirated food on two occasions and had to be treated for aspiration pneumonia.) Mr. Anderson has been receiving a lactose-free, isotonic formula (osmolite) delivered by continuous drip infusion. After 1 week on this feeding regimen, Mr. Anderson began having watery stools four or five times a day for 2 days. (See Table 15.3 for differential diagnosis and assessment.)

NURSING INTERVENTIONS

Tube-Feeding Interventions

The major nursing interventions studied have been those associated with tube feedings. Anderson (1986) states that properly administered tube feedings do not cause diarrhea, but patients on tube feedings sometimes develop diarrhea from an underlying problem or from therapy. Malnutrition, osmolality, drug therapy, contaminated formula, and methods of administration may be associated with diarrhea in patients receiving tube feedings.

A research-based lactose-free tube-feeding protocol has been developed for clinical testing (Horsley et al, 1981). The research suggests that diarrhea, as well as other symptoms of gastrointestinal distress (eg, nausea, belching, flatulence) for lactose-intolerant individuals, will be reduced if lactose is removed from tube-feeding formulas (Walike and Walike, 1973, 1977; Walike et al, 1975). Improved nutrition is also expected to result. In general, it is recommended that all persons with tube feedings may be given lactose-free diets. Because of the special needs of elderly clients, lactose-free diets that are also low sodium, low residue, or low protein need to be available. Nurses, physicians, and dietitians need to be knowledgeable of the prevalence, the clinical significance, and the physiology of lactose intolerance among the elderly to implement and evaluate the protocol successfully.

Malnutrition, which may be a consequence of serious illness or of underfeeding, results in malabsorption of nutrients and in diarrhea. The diarrhea can in turn worsen the malnutrition (Anderson, 1986). Malabsorption can be treated with a chemically defined or free amino acid formula to improve nutritional status (Konstantinides and Shronts, 1983). Slowing the rate of feeding to 20–30 cc per hour can also aid absorption of nutrients (Anderson, 1986).

Tube-feeding formulas are frequently diluted with water to "offset the diarrhea that the osmotic load of full-strength formula is often assumed to cause" (Anderson, 1986;704). Anderson states that patients may be able to absorb undiluted, hyperosmotic loads unless "malnutrition, poor visceral protein status and depleted GI

Table 15.3

Case Study—Diarrhea: Differential Diagnosis and Assessment

NURSING ASSESSMENTS	DIAGNOSES RULED OUT	ADDITIONAL DATA NEEDED
Watery stools, negative for blood 4–5 times/day of 2 days' duration	Diarrhea associated with chronic bowel disease such as cancer, inflammatory bowel disease	Evidence of malabsorption
No history of chronic GI disease		
Lactose-free formula	Lactose intolerance	
Negative stool culture and feeding/tubing cultures	Infectious disease	Additional cultures of feeding/tubing to rule out contamination caused in administering
Absence of fever		
Normal WBC		
No recent change in significant life events	Irritable bowel syndrome	
Addition of potassium chloride elixir to drug regimen		Serum albumin level urine urea nitrogen concentration
		Evidence of malnutrition (muscle wasting, skin and hair changes, edema)

mucosa alter the osmotic gradient." "Most formulas are isosmotic (approximately 300 mOsm/Kg H_2O) . . . and need not be diluted" (Anderson, 1986). Malnourished patients with serum albumin levels below 3 may be assisted by giving hyperosmotic solutions at half strength at a slow (25 cc/hr) rate (Anderson, 1986; Konstantinides and Shronts, 1983).

Drug therapy with antibiotics or drugs such as potassium chloride, which change the osmolality of the formula, may be associated with diarrhea in tube-fed patients. Other drugs such as antacids, digitalis, and antiarrhythmic drugs also may cause diarrhea. Lactobacillus preparations may aid in slowing motility, to combat drug-induced diarrhea (Anderson, 1986; Konstantinides and Shronts, 1983).

Methods of administration of formula and the risk of possible contamination of feedings are closely related factors with the potential to produce diarrhea in tube-fed patients. Replacing an intermittent or bolus feeding procedure with a continuous drip procedure, either by gravity flow or by mechanical feeding pump, is suggested to reduce the risks of gastrointestinal side effects such as diarrhea. Taylor (1982), in a comparison of gravity flow and continuous infusion pump tube feeding in neurosurgical patients, found that diarrhea occurred in both methods of tube feeding. Another study of 80 patients found that use of an infusion pump controlled diarrhea in 10 of the patients who had serious gastrointestinal disorders, but was less successful in patients with poor gastric emptying or swallowing reflex impairment (Jones et al, 1980).

Temperature of the formula administered in tube feeding has been suggested as a cause of diarrhea, with reference to the need to give the feeding at room temperature or to heat it to body temperature (Griggs and Hoppe, 1979). However, a study of gastric motility in monkeys found that the temperature of the formula affected gastric motility for only 6 minutes. The gastric motility rate then returned to fasting baseline rate (Williams and Walike, 1975). Heating the formula may promote the growth of bacteria and, in itself, present a cause for diarrhea in debilitated patients (Bettice, 1971). Several studies of contamination of tube-feeding systems have found hands of caregivers to be the major source of contamination and support the need for meticulous handwashing procedures (Iannini et al, 1983; Schreiner et al, 1983; Schroeder et al, 1983). Additional measures to prevent contamination of tube-feeding systems include hanging a fresh feeding every 4 to 8 hours (never add new formula to formula that has been hanging) and changing feeding containers and tubing every day. Unnecessary handling or manipulation of the feeding system should be avoided (Konstantinides and Shronts, 1983).

The nurse can manage diarrhea associated with tube feedings by adjusting the type of tube feeding used, by monitoring the rate of infusion based on patient tolerance, and by preventing contamination of feedings by careful handwashing in preparing, administering, and monitoring the feeding (Carpenito, 1983; McLane and McShane, 1986). Because of the danger of greater dehydration, Anderson (1986) stresses that tube feedings should be continued while measures are instituted to treat the diarrhea, rather than stopped as has been recommended in the past.

Educational/Teaching Interventions

Another area of suggested nursing interventions in diarrhea involves health teaching regarding medication use and side effects, diet, stress reduction, and aseptic techniques (Carpenito, 1983; McLane and McShane, 1986). Patient teaching may present a special challenge to the nurse working with the elderly. Presence of illnesses such as Alzheimer's disease or other organic brain disorders affecting the elderly may limit the patient's ability to learn. Careful assessment of the patient's ability to learn is essential. The elderly may also not have an available support system wherein others can be taught to help the patient manage these aspects of their life. Teaching should definitely be used as an intervention for the elderly who can profit from it. If teaching is not feasible, referral to appropriate support systems may be necessary. For more detailed information regarding patient teaching, see Chapter 33.

Other Suggested Interventions

Proper food and fluid intake and exercise can prevent development of impaction-related diarrhea (McLane and McShane, 1986). Replacement of lost fluid is also suggested as a nursing intervention. Carpenito (1983) suggests increasing oral intake to maintain urine specific gravity at normal levels (1.003–1.030) and encouraging fluids high in potassium and sodium. Intravenous replacement of fluid and electrolytes may be required (McLane and McShane, 1986). Nurses can monitor body weight, skin condition, and laboratory findings to assess nutrition, hydration, and electrolyte levels.

Perirectal skin may be excoriated because of the acidity and digestive enzyme content of diarrheal stools (Carpenito, 1983; McLane and McShane, 1986). Measures suggested in the literature to treat skin problems associated with diarrhea include thorough cleansing with mild soap and warm water following each diarrheal stool. Applying soothing ointment or spray and exposing the irritated skin to the air are also suggested (Englert and Guillory, 1986).

CASE STUDY

Nursing Interventions

The nursing interventions instituted for Mr. Anderson, the 75-year-old resident with multi-infarct dementia who developed diarrhea one week after being placed on osmolite nasogastric feedings, included diluting the formula to half strength and slowing the rate of the continuous drip feeding to 25 cc/hr. An antidiarrheal agent was added to his drug regimen, to slow gastric motility and aid in absorption of nutrients in the feeding. The nurse did not mix any medications with the feeding. Rather, the feeding was stopped, the tubing was cleansed, and medications were given by feeding tube; and the feeding was then restarted in 30 minutes. Mr. Anderson's diarrhea subsided within 36 hours, and his stool consistency changed to a small, soft, formed stool after 48 hours. The antidiarrheal agent was stopped.

Throughout the period of diarrhea, Mr. Anderson's perirectal skin was cleansed with warm, soapy water; thoroughly rinsed with clean water; and allowed to air dry. Then the perirectal skin was lightly covered with a soothing, waterproof ointment to prevent further irritation and excoriation. This produced a gradual lessening of redness of the skin, and the area was healed within 3 days of the cessation of diarrhea.

Mr. Anderson's laboratory findings were monitored continuously, and the potassium chloride elixir was stopped based on these findings. The feeding was returned to full strength to deliver adequate calories to maintain adequate nutrition.

TENTATIVE DIAGNOSIS

Altered Bowel Elimination: Diarrhea related to effect of potassium supplement on osmolality of feeding, resulting in lessened absorption of nutrients.

OUTCOMES

Goals or expected outcomes for nursing interventions suggested include decrease in episodes of diarrheal stools and relief of associated symptoms (McLane and McShane, 1986); maintenance of nutritional, fluid, and electrolyte balances; and relief of irritation to the perianal area (Carpenito, 1983). In the case study previously cited, the nurse assessed that the addition of potassium chloride elixir had altered the osmolality of the feeding. Interventions are therefore needed to assist the patient in absorption of nutrients from the feeding, particularly in patients whose serum albumin level is below 3. Diluting the formula to one-half strength and infusing the feeding in a continuous drip at 25 cc/hr will aid absorption. The nurse may also assess the need for a drug to decrease gastric motility to aid absorption further (Anderson, 1986). Monitoring of intake and output of laboratory test results, and of skin, hair, and muscle quality will provide ongoing evaluation of the patient's fluid, electrolyte, and nutritional status.

SUMMARY

The elderly are subject to physiologic changes of the gastrointestinal system, which may be manifested by acute or chronic diarrhea. Etiologies and defining characteristics were discussed. An assessment tool developed by the author was presented. Nursing interventions for managing diarrhea associated with tube feedings were described, as well as health teaching for the elderly who can profit from it. Much research is needed into nursing interventions used to manage acute and chronic diarrhea. Skin-care methods, tube-feeding procedures, and the effectiveness of patient teaching need to be studied. Further studies on the effects of variables such as temperature, caffeine, tobacco products, and food substances on gastrointestinal motility are also required. Most current interventions are based on an understanding of the physiology of the gastrointestinal system. Feasibility and acceptability to the patient of various nursing interventions remains to be evaluated.

ASSESSMENT GUIDE 15.1

Assessment Tool for Nursing Diagnosis of Diarrhea

	Present	Absent

Signs and Symptoms:

Abdominal pain
Cramping
Stool frequency greater than 3/day
Increased frequency of bowel sounds
Loose, liquid stools
Urgency

Etiologies:

Infection:
    Stool culture + for bacteria
    Stool culture + for parasites
    Recent travel to foreign country
    Diverticular disease
    Small bowel infection signs
      Nonbloody, watery diarrhea
      Low-grade fever
      Absence of fecal leukocytes
    Colon infection signs
      Stools with blood, mucus
      Presence of fecal leukocytes
      Fever

Drug Reactions:

Drug regimen includes:
    Antacids
    Antibiotics
    Antihypertensives
    Chemotherapeutic agents
    Colchicine
    Digitalis preparations
    Lactulose
    Potassium supplements
    Propanolol
    Quinidine
    Other drugs known to cause diarrhea

Diet Alterations:

Recent history of diet changes
    Increased fruit and vegetable intake
    Increased lactose-containing foods
    Tube-feeding formula instituted or changed

Fecal Impaction:

Absence of bowel movements for several days
    prior to diarrhea onset

History of Chronic Bowel Disorder:

Irritable bowel disorder
Lactase deficiency
Cancer of colon
Gastrointestinal surgery
Malabsorption disease
Laxative use
Alcohol abuse
Antineoplastic therapy

References

Alpers D: Dietary management and vitamin-mineral replacement therapy. Chapter 109 in: *Gastrointestinal Disease: Pathophysiology, Diagnosis, Management*, 3d ed. Sleisenger MH, Fordtran JS (editors). Saunders, 1983.

Anderson BJ: Tube feeding: Is diarrhea inevitable? *Am J Nurs* (June) 1986; 704–706.

Bettice D: The case of vomiting of tube feedings by neurosurgical patients. *J Neurosurg Nurs* 1971; 3:93–111.

Bond JH: Office-based management of diarrhea. *Geriatrics* (Feb) 1982; 52–64.

Broadwell DC: Gastrointestinal system. Chapter 11 in: *Clinical Nursing*. Thompson et al (editors). Mosby, 1986.

Burakoff R: An updated look at diverticular disease. *Geriatrics* (Mar) 1981; 83–91.

Carpenito LJ: *Nursing Diagnosis—Application to Clinical Practice*. Lippincott, 1983.

Carroll-Johnson R (editor): *Classification of Nursing Diagnoses: Proceedings of the Eighth Conference*. Lippincott, 1989.

Cello J: Ulcerative colitis. Chapter 67 in: *Gastrointestinal Disease: Pathophysiology, Diagnosis, Management*, 3d ed. Sleisenger MH, Fordtran JS (editors). Saunders, 1983.

Englert DM, Guillory JA: For want of lactase. *Am J Nurs* (Aug) 1986; 902–906.

Foxworthy DM, Wilson JA: Crohn's disease in the elderly—prolonged delay in diagnosis. *J Am Geriatr Soc* 1985; 33:492–495.

Griggs BA, Hoppe MC: Nasogastric tube feeding. *Am J Nurs* 1979; 79:481–485.

Horsley J, Crane J, Haller K: *Reducing Diarrhea in Tube-Fed Patients: CURN Project*. Grune and Stratton, 1981.

Iannini PB, Mumford F, Buckalew F: Microbial contamination of enteral liquid nutritional systems. *Proceedings of the Ross Laboratories Workshop on Contamination of Feeding Products During Clinical Use*. Ross Laboratories, 1983.

Jones BLM, Payne S, Slik DBA: Indications for pump-assisted enteral feeding. *Lancet* (May 17) 1980; 1057–1058.

Konstantinides NN, Shronts E: Tube feeding—Managing the basics. *Am J Nurs* (Sept) 1983; 1312–1320.

Krejs C, Fordtran J: Diarrhea. Chapter 16 in: *Gastrointestinal Disease: Pathophysiology, Diagnosis, Management*, 3d ed. Sleisenger MH, Fordtran JS (editors). Saunders, 1983.

Martin JL, Justus PG, Mathias JR: Altered motility of the small intestine in response to ethanol (ETOH): An explanation for the diarrhea associated with the consumption of alcohol. *Gastroenterology* 1980; 78:1218.

McFarland LV, Stamm WE: Review of *Clostridium difficile* associated diseases. *Am J Infect Control* (June) 1986; 99–109.

McLane AM, McShane RE: Bowel elimination, alteration in: Diarrhea—Theory and etiology. Pages 2069–2072 in: *Clinical Nursing*. Thompson et al (editors). Mosby, 1986.

Roe DA: Drug-nutrient interactions in the elderly. *Geriatrics* (Mar) 1986; 57–74.

Schmucker DL, Daniels CK: Aging, gastrointestinal infections and mucosal immunity. *J Am Geriatr Soc* 1986; 34:377–384.

Schreiner RL, Lemons JA, Jansen RD: Microbial contamination of continous-drip feedings in the newborn intensive care unit. *Proceedings of the Ross Laboratories Workshop on Contamination of Enteral Feeding Products During Clinical Use*. Ross Laboratories, 1983.

Schroeder P et al: A survey of factors leading to microbial contamination of enteral feeding solutions in a community hospital. *Proceedings of the Ross Laboratories Workshop on Contamination of Enteral Feeding Products During Clinical Use*. Ross Laboratories, 1983.

Schuster M: Irritable bowel syndrome. Chapter 54 in: *Gastrointestinal Disease: Pathophysiology, Diagnosis, Management*, 3d ed. Sleisenger MH, Fordtran JS (editors). Saunders, 1983.

Taylor TT: A comparison of two methods of nasogastric tube feedings. *J Neurosurg Nurs* 1982; 14:49–55.

Trier J: Celiac sprue. Chapter 63 in: *Gastrointestinal Disease: Pathophysiology, Diagnosis, Management*, 3d ed. Sleisenger MH, Fordtran JS (editors). Saunders, 1983.

Van Thiel DH et al: Gastrointestinal and hepatic manifestations of chronic alcoholism. *Gastroenterology* 1981; 81:594.

Vartian CV, Septimus EJ: Intra-abdominal infections in the elderly: Diagnosis and management. *Geriatrics* (Feb) 1986; 51–56.

Walike B, Walike J: Lactose content of tube feeding diets as a cause of diarrhea. *The Laryngoscope* 1973; 83:1109–1115.

Walike B, Walike J: Relative lactose intolerance. *JAMA* 1977; 238:948–951.

Walike B et al: Patient problems related to tube feeding. *Communicating Nursing Research*, Vol 7. Bately MV (editor). WICHE, 1975.

Williams KR, Walike BC: Effect of the temperature of tube feeding on gastric motility in monkeys. *Nurs Res* 1975; 24:4–9.

Winawer S, Sherlock P: Malignant neoplasms of the small and large intestine. Chapter 72 in: *Gastrointestinal Disease: Pathophysiology, Diagnosis, Management*, 3d ed. Sleisenger MH, Fordtran JS (editors). Saunders, 1983.

World Health Statistics Annual: I. Vital Statistics and Cause of Death. World Health Organization, 1975.

16

Bowel Incontinence

Meridean Maas, PhD, RN, FAAN
Janet Specht, MA, RN, C

Bowel incontinence is a common problem for elderly persons, especially those who are institutionalized or who suffer from chronic illnesses. As many as 20% of hospitalized elderly have been estimated to have fecal incontinence (Brockelhurst, 1951), yet few articles in the nursing and medical literature focus on this problem. More attention has been given to constipation and diarrhea, which often are associated with bowel incontinence. However, incontinence can occur in the absence of these conditions. The focus on diarrhea and constipation limits comprehensive bowel management to achieve regularity and control of evacuation.

The nursing diagnosis Bowel Incontinence is defined as "involuntary passage of stool" (Gordon, 1982;82). The Eighth Conference defined bowel incontinence as "a state in which an individual experiences a change in normal bowel habits characterized by involuntary passage of stool" (Carroll-Johnson, 1989;522). The following related factors (etiologies) were added for the diagnosis: neuromuscular involvement, musculoskeletal involvement, depression/severe anxiety, and perception or cognitive impairment (Table 16.1). The lack of development of this diagnosis is a reflection of the inattention to the problem of incontinence. This chapter further details etiologies for bowel incontinence and elaborates the defining characteristics to be used to infer more specific types of the diagnosis.

NORMAL DEFECATION AND BOWEL CONTINENCE

Normal defecation includes the action of two reflexes (Jones and Godding, 1972). The mysenteric plexus in the large colon controls the intrinsic reflex. The second reflex is in the sacral segments of the spinal cord (see Figure 16.1). These reflexes are usually initiated after eating, especially after the first meal of the day, when a strong peristaltic wave pushes fecal matter into the rectum. The distention in the rectum stimulates a defecation reflex through the mysenteric plexus to initiate further peristaltic waves from the descending colon toward the anus. The internal anal sphincter relaxes as the waves reach it, and if the external anal sphincter is also relaxed, defecation will occur.

Defecation is weak and ineffective unless aided by the spinal reflex. Stimulation to the rectum initiates signals through nerves to the sacral segments (2, 3, and 4) of the spinal cord, which in turn send impulses to intensify the peristaltic waves. A person with normal control is able to feel the desire to defecate when the stool enters and distends the

Table 16.1

Bowel Incontinence

NANDA (CARROLL-JOHNSON, 1989)

Etiologies/Related Factors	Defining Characteristics
	*Involuntary passage of stool

MAAS/SPECHT

Etiologies/Related Factors	Defining Characteristics	Intervention
	*Involuntary passage of stool	
Cognitive impairment	Low score on mental status measurement	Bowel programming (BP)
	Unable to recognize, interpret, and act on rectal fullness	Habit training (BP)
	Inability to find bathroom	
	Inability to recognize and name toilet articles	Environmental structuring
	Normal rectal reservoir capacity	
	Normal rectal tightening with digital exam	
	Normal anal sphincter contraction	
Constipation	Fecal impaction	Habit training (BP)
	Diarrhea	Nondigital stimulation (BP)
	Normal sphincter tone	
	Normal reservior	
	Immobility	
	Low fiber and fluid intake	
	Delayed defecation with dependence on others for toileting assistance	
Rectal sphincter abnormalities	Poor or absent control	Biofeedback
	Diarrhea	
	Normal rectal reservoir capacity	Control of diarrhea (BP)
	History of diabetes mellitus	
	History of anal/rectal surgery/injury	
	History of rectal/vaginal tear from childbirth	
Impaired reservoir capacity	History of idiopathic inflammatory disease	Reduction of stool volume (BP)
	Radiation proctitis	
	Presence of chronic rectal ischemia	
	History of subtotal colectomy with ileoanal anastomosis	
Upper motor neuron damage Sensory bowel incontinence Uninhibited and reflex bowel incontinence	Damage to brain or spinal cord above 12th thoracic	Gastrocolic reflex stimulation (BP)
	Unable to feel rectal fullness or urge to defecate	
	Unable to control defecation reflex	
	Frequent fecal impactions	
Lower motor neuron damage Autonomic bowel and motor neuron bowel dysfunction	Flaccid anal sphincter	Regular planned evacuation (BP)
	Injury or disease of medullaris or cauda equini	Push with abdominal muscles/manual compression
	Absence of defecation reflex	
	Constant dribbling of soft stools	
	Inability to expel formed stool in rectum	

*Critical defining characteristic regardless of etiology.

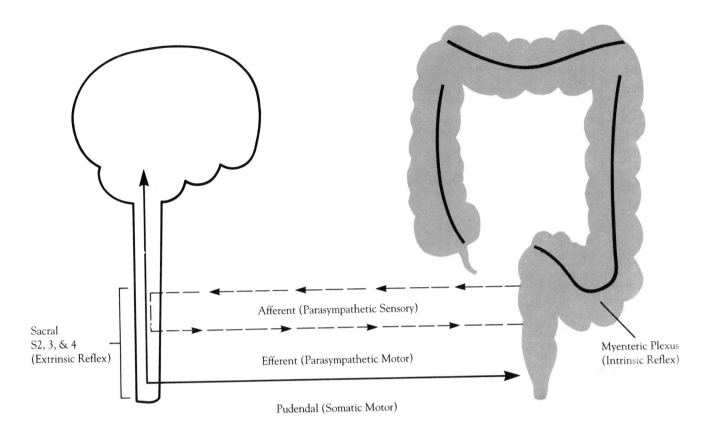

Sacral
S2, 3, & 4
(Extrinsic Reflex)

Afferent (Parasympathetic Sensory)

Efferent (Parasympathetic Motor)

Myenteric Plexus
(Intrinsic Reflex)

Pudendal (Somatic Motor)

rectum. The spinal reflex can be overridden by conscious inhibition from the brain, resulting in a contraction of the external sphincter. The defecation reflex will die out in a few minutes if the person prevents defecation. The reflex may not return for several hours. The reflex may be reinitiated by taking a deep breath or bearing down (increasing intra-abdominal pressure), but the reflex initiated in this way is not as effective as when it occurs naturally. Prolonged inhibition will result in progressive ineffectiveness of the defecation reflex.

Regular physical activity and exercise is also important for maintaining normal bowel function. Physical activity assists with muscle tonicity needed for fecal expulsion and increases circulation to the digestive system, which assists with the development of feces that are more easily evacuated and promotes peristalsis.

Anorectal continence refers to the ability to retain feces in order to evacuate at an appropriate time and place. Ordinarily the ability to control defecation is attained around 2 years of age. The loss of this ability by elderly persons is often a source of embarrassment, may deprive the person of social contacts, may affect self-esteem adversely, and is the cause of unpleasant caregiving tasks by family or other attendants. Even if control of feces can

be managed to avoid socially disruptive occurrences, the elderly person may not be able to control flatus, which may still lead to altered lifestyle and limited social interactions. Nurses who are sensitive to these consequences and who are equipped with knowledge of bowel physiology and the ability to diagnose and treat bowel incontinence can positively affect the quality of life for many elderly persons.

Bowel continence is dependent on four major factors (Wald, 1986). One factor, rectal sensation, was discussed previously. The second factor is the ability to contract the external anal sphincter and the puborectalis muscle. Henry (1983) describes the preservation of an angle between the lower rectum and the upper canal, the anorectal angle, as the most important factor in preserving continence. Figure 16.2 illustrates the angle that is created by the pull of the puborectalis muscle away from the rectum. The third factor is the motivation and the cognitive ability to make the appropriate decision to defecate or postpone defecation until a more appropriate time and place. The fourth factor is the ability of the rectum to accommodate the storage of feces. Hemorrhoids; inflammation due to colitis, infection, or irradiation; and surgical revisions are some of the causes of impaired reservoir capacity (Wald, 1986).

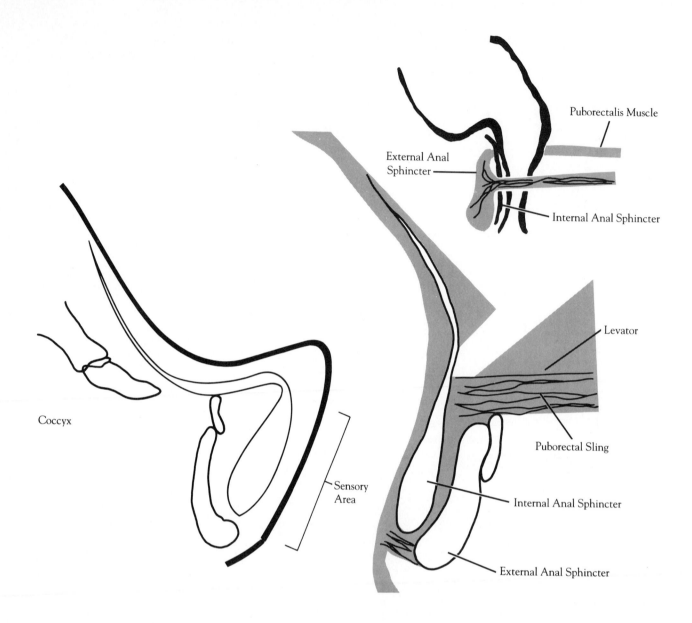

Coccyx

Sensory
Area

Puborectalis Muscle

External Anal
Sphincter

Internal Anal Sphincter

Levator

Puborectal Sling

Internal Anal Sphincter

External Anal Sphincter

SIGNIFICANCE FOR
THE ELDERLY

Along with urinary incontinence, fecal incontinence is a major problem experienced by institutionalized elderly persons (Brockelhurst, 1985). Although it is a less frequent problem than urinary incontinence, it is more unpleasant for the elderly person and for the caregivers. Fecal incontinence most frequently occurs with urinary incontinence among long-term institutionalized elderly (Brockelhurst, 1985).

There is a lack of documented information about age-related structure and function of the large intestine or changes in defecation. However, Goldman (1979) reports that studies of stool specimens in the elderly show little evidence of undigested nutrients. This is evidence that the digestive process is adequate in normal elderly persons (Goldman, 1979). Yet, many elderly have colon disorders. These disorders may result from a combination of factors such as dietary changes, environment, and medication and not necessarily from the aging process (Bhanthimnavis and Schuster, 1977).

The higher incidence of chronic illnesses and the functional losses with aging predispose the elderly to increased problems with bowel continence. The elderly not only are more apt to contract a disease that affects bowel function, but also are more apt to have mobility and cognitive impairments that make them unable to maintain bowel control. For instance, an elderly woman who has had colitis for a number of years can anticipate the frequent loose stools and plan trips to the toilet to avoid incontinence. If she becomes less mentally capable or less mobile, she will likely be incontinent. Bowel incontinence also is prevalent among elderly persons with diabetes mellitus, occurring in up to 20% of all persons with this disease (Wald, 1986). The probability of acquiring diabetes doubles each 10 years of a person's life, so the elderly are particularly predisposed to the illness (Blainey, 1986). More than 50% of elderly persons with diabetes have reduced rectal sensation, and many have rectosphincter abnormalities.

The main dietary changes that the elderly experience are a decrease in fiber intake, an increase in bulk, and an increase in intestinal motility. Because the elderly have an increased incidence of dentures, gum disease, and problems with swallowing, they often require foods that are easily chewed and swallowed. These foods are generally lower in fiber content. This is a problem because fiber intake is important for absorption of water in the bowel. The elderly are also often prone to dehydration because of inability to obtain fluids, lack of knowledge of the importance of adequate fluid intake, and use of diuretics in the management of chronic illness. Thus, the monitoring and provision of adequate fiber and fluid intake are important components of the nursing management of bowel programs for the elderly. Another dietary problem is lactose intolerance, which is frequently seen in the elderly as a cause of diarrhea and may cause bowel irritation and incontinence. This problem is explained in more detail in Chapter 15.

Environmental factors often contribute to bowel incontinence for the elderly. Lack of privacy can be a major deterrent to maintaining regular bowel evacuation and can lead to impaction or "accidents," especially when the elderly person is institutionalized. Examples of other environmental impediments to regular defecation or to the ability to toilet are inadequate assistance for toileting; inaccessibility of the toilet because of stairs, distance, or other architectural barriers; and lack of knowledge of transfer techniques from wheelchair to toilet. The nurse should thoroughly assess environmental factors that may prevent the elderly person from maintaining continence. Because of the positive influence that activity and exercise have on regular bowel function, the nurse should also pay careful attention to the elderly person's ability to remain active in his or her environment. The advantages of activity and exercise for optimizing the elderly person's functional abilities are more fully discussed in Chapter 23.

Many elderly are also on medications that may adversely affect bowel function and must be carefully assessed by the nurse. Narcotics, barbiturates, propoxyphene hydrochloride, tranquilizers, and antacids can cause constipation. Iron can result in constipation or diarrhea, and magnesium-based antacids and digitalis preparations can cause diarrhea. For more information about the adverse effects of medications on the elderly the reader is referred to Chapter 4.

ETIOLOGIES/RELATED FACTORS AND DEFINING CHARACTERISTICS

Brockelhurst (1985) discusses three major causes of bowel incontinence. The first is underlying disease of the colon, rectum, or anus, for example, diverticular disease, proctitis, cancer of the colon or rectum, hemorrhoids, prolapse, or colitis. Nurses should carefully observe and refer instances of fecal incontinence for further medical evaluation, since the underlying cause is often treatable, and more serious problems often can be prevented with prompt treatment.

Constipation of long standing, fecal impaction, is the second major cause of incontinence in the elderly (Brockelhurst, 1985). Incontinence may take the form either of diarrhea around the impaction or of "smearing" from having the rectum full and not emptied. This is evidenced by a study reported by Brockelhurst (1985) that found a larger percentage of elderly persons with bowel incontinence to have rectums with larger quantities of feces than persons without incontinence. It is important for nurses to be aware that the stool found in the rectum of constipated individuals is not always hard and dry, but is often soft and puttylike in consistency, even if transit time is as long as 7 days (Brockelhurst and Khan, 1969). This tends to negate the long-accepted belief that constipation can be eliminated by increased fluids and fiber alone. Henry (1983) asserts that overdistention of the rectum by feces causes a continuous stimulation of the reflex, resulting in reduced internal anal sphincter tone. If a client is constipated, nurses can monitor and intervene to prevent impactions (see Chapter 14).

The third major causes of bowel incontinence discussed by Brockelhurst (1985) is a neurogenic change in the rectum similar to the hyperreflexia found in the bladders of elderly persons with urge urinary incontinence (see Chapter 17). In a study comparing the toleration of a distended balloon in the rectum between incontinent elderly men and elderly men without bowel incontinence, the incontinent men expelled the inflated balloon in response to rectal contractions that they were unable to inhibit (Brockelhurst, 1985). On the other hand, the men who were not incontinent were able to retain the balloon by overriding the urge to defecate.

The most common etiologies of Bowel Incontinence in the elderly and the corresponding defining characteristics are displayed in Table 16.1 contrasted with those listed by the North American Nursing Diagnosis Association (NANDA) (Carroll-Johnson, 1989).

ASSESSMENT

Assessment of bowel incontinence in the elderly involves the consideration of several contributing factors. Davis et al (1986) describes five types of bowel dysfunction: (1) uninhibited bowel dysfunction, which occurs when there is an upper motor neuron lesion above cervical 1; (2) reflex bowel dysfunction, which is also upper motor neuron damage between cervical 1 and lumbar 1; (3) autonomic bowel dysfunction, which is due to lower motor neuron damage below L1; (4) sensory neurogenic bowel dysfunction in which there is damage to the sensory component of the reflex arc; and (5) motor neurogenic bowel dysfunction in which there is damage to the motor component of the central nervous system or the reflex arc.

With uninhibited and reflex bowel incontinence the rectal reflex is intact, but the voluntary control of the reflex is absent. In autonomic bowel incontinence the reflex arc may be partially or completely damaged. Sensory bowel incontinence is distinguished by the individual having no awareness of stool in the rectum. In contrast, the elderly person with motor neurogenic bowel incontinence is aware of the stool in the rectum but cannot evacuate it. Assessment of anal sphincter tone can determine the presence of an intact reflex arc. Wald (1986) reported poor correlation between digital evaluation of the internal rectal sphincter and objective tests in the laboratory. However, assessment for the presence of the reflex by sensing the internal rectal sphincter muscle tighten around a gloved finger inserted into the rectum is often recommended in general tests and provides some guidance for accurate diagnosis. An additional reason for digital rectal examination is to check for fecal impaction and other rectal abnormalities.

The evaluation for bowel incontinence should begin with a comprehensive history of the frequency, duration, and severity of the elderly client's bowel incontinence. The pattern of incontinence should be carefully determined. The client interview should also elicit any symptoms that accompany the bowel incontinence such as presence or absence of warning, time between sensation and defecation, amount of straining with defecation, and presence of constipation and diarrhea. It is important to determine whether or not the individual is incontinent of urine; has diabetes; has had any anal, rectal, or spinal surgery; has cognitive deficits, or has other neurologic and bowel diseases. If the client is a woman, note the number and character of vaginal deliveries. Finally, health management information, including fluid intake, dietary patterns and habits, usual activity and exercise, types and frequency of medications used, coping strategies and the client's knowledge of bowel physiology, and the process of defecation need to be ascertained. In order for the assessment to result in an accurate diagnosis and effective treatment, environmental factors such as privacy and access to toilet as well as the functional ability of the elder for toileting must be determined. (See Assessment Guide 16.1.)

The following case study illustrates the process of diagnosis, including the identification of additional data to be collected, which would be available to the nurse who used the tool in Assessment Guide 16.1.

CASE STUDY

Bowel Incontinence

Mr. B has lived at Get Rest nursing home for 6 months. He is 80 years old and married, but his spouse continues to live at home. Mr. B has been incontinent of both urine and feces since his admission to the nursing home. He is disoriented to time and place at all times. He has severe bilateral hearing loss and dense bilateral cataracts. He dislikes being touched; when he is touched, he strikes out. Mr. B receives a mechanical, soft, general diet with raw bran. He can feed himself about half of the time. Ordinarily he has a fluid intake of less than 1000 cc daily. He spends about 14 hours each day in bed and 10 hours each day in a wheelchair. He is able to walk about 5 feet with the assistance of 2 attendants. He suffered a hip fracture when he fell at home 3 years ago. The hip was pinned at the time of the fracture, and he has never regained independent ambulation. He complains of pain when ambulation is attempted.

A rectal examination at the time of his admission to the nursing home revealed an enlarged prostate and poor sphincter tone. Mr. B has a history of laxative abuse. His wife reports that he has been incontinent of feces for approximately 1 year prior to admission. At present, if his bowels do not move daily, he gets a bowel obstruction. Consequently he is on a vigorous bowel program of a daily Dulcolax suppository, followed by a Fleets enema if there are no results. In addition he receives Laculose and Senakot twice each day and Exlax p.r.n. His abdominal muscles are flaccid, and he is unable to expel feces. He gives no indication of urge to defecate and wears disposable briefs at all times. Table 16.2 summarizes the significant signs and symptoms and lists the additional data needed for Mr. B's assessment.

TENTATIVE DIAGNOSIS

Bowel incontinence related to upper motor neuron damage (sensory bowel incontinence) as evidenced by inability to feel rectal fullness, by inability to control defecation reflex, and by frequent impactions.

Table 16.2

Bowel Incontinence: Differential Diagnosis

SIGNIFICANT SIGNS AND SYMPTOMS	DIAGNOSES RULED OUT	ADDITIONAL DATA NEEDED
No expression of urge to defecate		Can identify rectal fullness?
Decreased rectal sphincter tone		Rectal reservoir capacity?
	Impaired reservoir capacity	Stool in rectal vault?
Unable to "bear down" to defecate	Cognitive impairment	Comprehensive mental status assessment
Disoriented to time and place		Can name toilet articles and use appropriately?
Soft, puttylike stools		Complete evacuation?
		Presence of diarrhea?
Poor food and fluid intake	Rectal sphincter abnormalities	
Minimal physical activity		Tolerance for increased activity?
		Injury below thoracic vertebra 12?
Frequent impactions	Constipation	Lower motor neuron damage?

NURSING INTERVENTIONS

The interventions for each of the etiologies of Bowel Incontinence are shown in Table 16.1. The desired outcome of interventions for bowel incontinence is to achieve a predictable pattern of defecation to avoid discomfort, embarrassment, and loss of self-esteem for the elderly person. The maintenance of social support and interaction systems is also a desired outcome. Unpleasant odor and embarrassment that can accompany fecal incontinence may cause family, friends, and other social contacts to avoid the elderly person who is incontinent. The maintenance of skin integrity is another important outcome. However, the interventions used to achieve the outcomes will differ depending on the specific etiology. Etiologies can also be mixed, so it is important to specify carefully all causes of the bowel incontinence for the elderly individual. Interventions for bowel incontinence to achieve regular, planned evacuation of the bowel include bowel programming and environmental structuring.

Bowel Programming

The aim of bowel programming is to provide regular evacuation at a time planned with the elderly individual, resulting in a minimum of bowel accidents. Bowel programs must be tailored to accommodate each elderly person's physiologic and psychosocial problems, the person's particular environment, and the individual's functional abilities. Habit training, control of diarrhea, digital and nondigital stimulation of the gastrocolic reflex, reduction of stool volume, and biofeedback are specific forms of bowel programming that are used to treat bowel incontinence, depending on the etiology of the problem.

Prior to beginning any type of bowel program the bowel must be empty. This can be accomplished by the use of enemas, suppositories, laxatives, or a combination of two or more. Brockelhurst (1985) recommends cleansing of the bowel with phosphate enemas for 7 to 10 days prior to initiation of bowel programming. He argues that this removes the etiology of constipation; however, most sources do not explicitly suggest such extreme cleansing. Bowel cleansing is also a measure that can be used to control diarrhea when the elderly person is not constipated. This is especially effective when the source of diarrhea is an irritant that has been ingested and when there is intraintestinal infection. Cleansing can soothe inflammation and provide opportunity for the bowel to heal and become less motile. However, nurses should cautiously prescribe enemas for the elderly because of the risk of contributing to fluid and electrolyte imbalance. The elderly can more easily experience fluid and electrolyte imbalance and become dehydrated, particularly if fluids intake is poor or restricted when enemas are given (Robinson, 1985).

Ordinarily there are at least four components to bowel programming. One component is appropriate diet and fluid. Fluid intake is usually recommended at 1500–2000 cc each 24 hours, excluding coffee, tea, and grapefruit juice because of their diuretic effects. Drinking a glass of warm or hot liquid prior to meals facilitates gastrocolic reflex. High-fiber foods are also important for nondigital stimulation of the gastrocolic reflex and habit training because they prevent hard stools and promote peristalsis (Bergstrom, 1975). Foods should be as fat free as possible to stimulate the gastrocolic reflex, since fats slow digestion and delay the reflex. When diarrhea is present but the elderly person is not constipated, the foods selected should be low in fiber. Any foods that produce a laxative effect, a great deal of gas, or an allergic reaction should be eliminated from the elder's diet. The reduction of stool volume is the form of bowel programming that is needed when impaired reservoir capacity is the etiology of bowel incontinence. Reduction of stool volume is accomplished primarily through fiber restriction and the use of medications to increase transit time and absorption (Wald, 1986).

The second component of bowel programming is increasing activity and exercise (Bergstrom, 1975). Physical activity increases body circulation, including circulation to the bowel, and promotes digestion and peristalsis. The exercise program can include abdominal exercise to increase muscle strength for expulsion of feces. The most effective form of exercise in many cases will be getting the elderly person to do whatever is possible, given the individual's physical and cognitive functional abilities.

Timing is the third aspect of bowel programming that is important to incorporate. A plan in which the elderly person defecates each day is usually the most successful. This involves establishing a regular time to sit on the toilet, usually 5 to 15 minutes, timed in such a way as to take advantage of the gastrocolic reflex. This reflex occurs in response to food intake and is strongest in the morning (Davis et al, 1986). Combined with appropriate food and fluid intake and regular exercise, the consistency and regularity of the timing are what can lead to the formation of habit and can make other less natural measures to promote bowel movements unnecessary.

Finally, the fourth component of bowel programming includes laxatives, suppositories, massage of the anal sphincter, and enemas to promote regular, planned bowel evacuation. These approaches are most appropriate when bowel cleansing is required and when there is a spinal cord injury. With upper motor cord lesions, digital stimulation of the gastrocolic reflex is effective because the reflex arc is intact. Suppositories are helpful to use early on in intiating a bowel program. Suppositories stimulate the gastrocolic reflex similar to digital stimulation and relax the anal sphincter. With lower motor cord lesions, enemas may be needed to evacuate the bowel. However, the nurse should attempt to establish regular evacuation by teaching the elder to bear down with abdominal muscles or to express manually by pushing on the lower abdomen if at all possible. For controlling incontinence with diarrhea for persons who were not constipated, Read et al (1982) found Imodium up to 4 milligrams as often as four times a day to be more effective than Lomotil.

Bowel programs must be established and maintained for at least 10 to 15 days (Sharpless, 1982). However, absence of defecation or frequent loose stools require immediate attention. For this reason, the maintenance of a daily bowel record, which assesses food and fluid intake, laxative used, time and type of bowel evacuation, and the facility used, is important for evaluating the effectiveness of the intervention and identifying when there are problems.

Biofeedback is an approach for bowel programming that has been investigated at the National Institute on Aging, Laboratory of Behavioral Sciences (McCormick and Burgio, 1984). The biofeedback procedure for fecal incontinence gives the patient sensory feedback of anal sphincter activity (Wald, 1986). McCormick and Burgio (1984;19) reported that out of 13 older persons treated with biofeedback for fecal incontinence, "Four became continent and seven experienced more than 50% improvement." One patient in the McCormick study was cognitively impaired and was not a candidate for biofeedback. This points out one disadvantage of biofeedback as an intervention to be used for the elderly who are incontinent of feces, since cognitive impairment is prevalent among institutionalized elderly and is a frequent etiology.

Environmental Structuring

Privacy, accessibility, comfort, functional positioning, and safety are the essential features of environmental structure to promote bowel continence. The elderly, especially if institutionalized, are often subjected to bowel elimination with minimal privacy. This can be particularly difficult for older persons who have been socialized to be modest. Most persons feel embarrassed when they must have bowel movements in the presence of another person. Thus, lack of privacy can cause elders to avoid defecation, which can lead to constipation and incontinence. Nurses should carefully prescribe and monitor approaches that will assure that the elderly person is able to defecate privately.

The nurse should also assess the elder's ability to ambulate to the bathroom, walking or in a wheelchair, as well as the person's ability to get to the bathroom in time to avoid an accident. If the elder is in a wheelchair, transfer ability must also be assessed and the appropriate interventions prescribed to correct or compensate for any lack of ability. In addition, architectural barriers must be assessed, and care should be taken to remove or rearrange furniture and equipment that will obstruct the ambulant elderly person.

Assistive devices should be provided in bathrooms so that the elderly person has the needed support for safe transfer, clothing adjustment, and hygiene. Fecal evacuation is more apt to be successful if the elder feels safe and not in danger of falling. Prescriptions should incorporate the principles that peristaltic activity is greater when the person is in an upright position, as gravity assists the expulsion of feces. It is also important for the prescribed intervention to include instructions to staff to be responsive to the timing of defecation, impressing on staff the importance of consistency with the plan of care. Finally, the nurse should provide emotional and social interventions (eg, relaxation therapy, social support) if depression or anxiety is judged to be the etiology of incontinence.

The need for all staff to be nonjudgmental when the elder requires assistance or when there is an incidence of incontinence is an essential, but often overlooked, aspect of the environment.

CASE STUDY

Nursing Interventions

Mr. B has most elements of bowel programming included in his plan of care. However, the outcome of regular bowel evacuation was not achieved until scheduled toileting was initiated and maintained for 10 days. Following implementation of the toileting schedule, which was prescribed after breakfast each day, Mr. B was continent except when his son visited each week and brought him chocolate bars. The nurse discussed with the son the importance of his father avoiding high-fat foods. The son then began to bring fresh fruit for Mr. B. Although some of the staff complained about the difficulty of the toileting schedule, they were very pleased when Mr. B no longer had "accidents" in bed and agreed that the schedule was worth the effort.

OUTCOMES

As mentioned previously, a bowel record is a useful tool for monitoring the effectiveness of the interventions for bowel incontinence. Mr. B had no skin impairment prior to the interventions for incontinence, and his skin integrity continued to be maintained. The outcome of avoiding embarrassment of Mr. B and his family was achieved by providing privacy and by achieving continence.

SUMMARY

Bowel Incontinence has been analyzed as a diagnostic concept with multiple etiologies for the elderly. Critical signs and symptoms were identified from a review of the literature and incorporated in a tool and process for assessment and diagnosis. Desired outcomes of treatment of bowel incontinence were described, and the interventions of bowel programming and environmental structuring were discussed. No research was found in the literature that validated the signs and symptoms of bowel incontinence, and few studies that tested interventions for the diagnosis were located. It is hoped that the conceptual development of the diagnosis will stimulate and assist researchers and clinicians to study and use the diagnosis and interventions. These activities are essential for the further development and validation of the diagnosis and effective interventions.

ASSESSMENT GUIDE 16.1

Assessment Tool for Bowel Incontinence

Name: _____ Sex: _____ Age: _____

Previous Bowel Pattern:

Frequency: Time: Amount: Consistency:

Present Bowel History:

Frequency: Time: Amount: Consistency:

Impactions:

Methods used to initiate defecation:

Recent Changes:

Color: Bleeding: Pain: Other:

Medical Diagnoses:

Relevant Bowel Disorders:

Rectal exam:

        Tone: Fissure: Fistula: Hemorrhoids:

        Other:

Loss of control:

        Partial/complete?

        Patient's reaction:

Medications:

ASSESSMENT GUIDE 16.1

Assessment Tool for Bowel Incontinence (Continued)

Physical Exercise/Activity:

Abdomen:

Scars/possible adhesions: Hardness:

Bloating: Ascites:

Diet and Eating Habits:

Consistency: Fiber: Schedule/Time:

Fluid intake: Type: Amount:

Laxative Use:

Frequency: Type: Amount:

Use of Enemas:

Frequency: Type: Amount:

Emotional/Mental Status:

Depression: Anxiety: Cognition:

Stressors:

Coping style/strategies:

Functional Abilities:

Manual dexterity in – removing clothing:

                    – handling equipment:

Ambulation:

Transfer: Toileting:

References

Bergstrom D: *Introduction to Bowel and Bladder Care.* Rehabilitation Publication Number 715. American Rehabilitation Foundation, 1975.

Bhanthimnavis K, Schuster M: Aging and gastrointestinal function. In: *Handbook of the Biology of Aging.* Finch C, Hayflick L (editors). Van Nos Reinhold, 1977.

Blainey C: Diabetes mellitus. Pages 403–422 in: *Nursing Management for the Elderly,* 2d ed. Carnevali D, Patrick M (editors). Lippincott, 1986.

Brockelhurst J: A study of the bladder, rectum and anal sphincter in senile incontinent patients. Page 46 in: *Incontinence in Old People.* Brockelhurst J (editor). Livingstone, 1951.

Brockelhurst J: *Textbook of Geriatric Medicine and Gerontology,* 3d ed. Livingstone, 1985.

Brockelhurst JC, Khan Y: A study of faecal stasis in old age and use of Dorbanex in its prevention. *Gerontol Clin* 1969; 11:293–300.

Carroll-Johnson R (editor): *Classification of Nursing Diagnoses: Proceedings of the Eighth Conference.* Lippincott, 1989.

Davis A et al: Bowel management: A quality assurance approach to upgrading programs. *J Gerontol Nurs* 1986; 12(5):13–17.

Goldman R: Decline in organ function with aging. In: *Clinical Gerontology,* 2d ed. Rossman I (editor). Lippincott, 1979.

Gordon M: *Nursing Diagnosis: Process and Application.* McGrawHill, 1982.

Henry M: Faecal incontinence. *Nurs Times* (Aug) 1983; 17:61–62.

Jones F, Godding E (editors): *Management of Constipation.* Blackwell Scientific, 1972.

McCormick K, Burgio K: Incontinence: An update on nursing care measures. *J Gerontol Nurs* 1984; 10(10):16–23.

McLane A: *Classification of Nursing Diagnoses: Proceedings of the Seventh Conference.* Mosby, 1987.

Read M et al: Effects of loperamide on anal sphincter function in patients complaining of chronic diarrhea with fecal incontinence and urgency. *Dig Dis Sci* 1982; 27(9):807–814.

Robinson SB, Demuth PL: Diagnostic studies for the aged: What are the dangers? *J Gerontol Nurs* 1985; 11(6):7–12.

Sharpless J: *A Problem-Oriented Approach to Stroke Rehabilitation.* Charles C. Thomas, 1982, pp. 410–421.

Wald A: Biofeedback therapy for fecal incontinence. *Ann Intern Med* 1986; 95(2):146–149.

17

Urinary Incontinence

JANET SPECHT, MA, RN

PATRICIA TUNINK, MA, RN

MERIDEAN MAAS, PhD, RN, FAAN

GLORIA BULECHEK, PhD, RN

URINARY INCONTINENCE IN THE ELDERLY POPULATION is a problem of considerable magnitude. Urinary incontinence is most simply defined as nonvoluntary voiding when the pressure in the bladder is greater than the resistance of the urethra. Urinary leakage that is objectively demonstrable and presents a social or hygienic problem is the definition accepted by the International Continence Society (Millard, 1981). Although these definitions oversimplify the complex processes that can occur with incontinence, they describe the essential nature of the problem for the person that experiences it. With normal urinary elimination the bladder stores urine that flows from the kidneys through the ureters into the bladder. As the bladder fills, it distends and sends a message along autonomic pathways to nerves in the spinal cord and cerebrum. Emptying of the bladder occurs when the parasympathetically innervated detrusor muscle relaxes concurrently with the bladder neck and urethral sphincters, which are innervated by sympathetic and somatic nerves. The distended detrusor muscle first gives the signal of a full bladder, which can be overridden with voluntary cortical control. Incontinence can result from the loss of voluntary control mechanisms, from deficits in neuromuscular function and urinary tract pathologies such as infection and obstruction, or from environmental and treatment-induced causes.

SIGNIFICANCE FOR THE ELDERLY

Although the incidence of incontinence in the elderly is known to be substantially higher than the 2% incidence identified in the general population, studies of prevalence vary widely in their findings. Williams (1983) identifies the limitations of available epidemiologic studies as inconsistent definitions; biases in patient selection; methodologic differences that make comparisons impossible; and deficient documentation of relevant information in existing records. Studies have documented that the incidence of incontinence in the elderly is from 14% to 40%. A survey of elderly persons age 62 to 90 in Edinburgh, Scotland reported the incidence of incontinence for men as 25% and for women as 42% (Milne et al, 1972). Yarnell and St. Leger (1979) reported that 11% to 17% of elderly persons living at home and 40% to 60% of elderly persons living in nursing homes in the United States were incontinent. It has been estimated that health care providers are aware of only half of the incontinent cases (Yarnell and St. Leger, 1979) because the elderly often are reluctant to report this intimate and embarrassing problem to physicians or nurses.

Although incontinence is a common problem for the elderly that has major impact on the quality of their lives, incontinence is not an inevitable or irreversible consequence of aging. There are a number of interventions that can be used to prevent or treat incontinence. Nursing interventions are discussed later in the chapter.

CONSEQUENCES OF INCONTINENCE

Incontinence presents many secondary complications for the elderly person including physiologic, social, psychologic, and economic effects. Physiologic effects include predisposition to impaired skin integrity, impaired skin hygiene, and a small hyperactive bladder. Social consequences are withdrawal from persons and activities, rejection by others, and, often, the need to leave home and move to a nursing home. Urinary incontinence is one of the major reasons for elderly persons being admitted to long-term care facilities (Specht, 1986). The embarrassment and shame that the incontinent elder feels, combined with social rejection by others, often results in depression, self-neglect, low self-regard, and reclusion. Urinary incontinence is a costly problem both for the incontinent person and for the health care system. Costs for equipment needed to manage the problem and for institutionalization accrue to the individual. It has been estimated that the management of incontinence accounts for one third of the costs of nursing home care in Great Britain (Ouslander, 1981). Ouslander and Kane (1982) report that in the United States $2000 to $4500 per year per person is spent to manage incontinent persons with disposable incontinence pads or catheters. The management of incontinence in institutions is labor intensive and accounts for a large portion of the cost of care.

ETIOLOGIES/RELATED FACTORS

The risk of urinary incontinence increases with age. This is not to say that growing older itself causes incontinence. There is nothing involved with the normal aging process that causes a loss of control of urine. Rather, older people are more apt to incur illnesses, injuries, and surgeries and are more vulnerable to urinary tract infections. In addition, the diminished efficiency of body systems and organs that often accompanies aging can predispose the elder to incontinence. Diminished sight and decreased mobility (flexibility, balance, strength) can increase the time taken to locate and reach the toilet. Chronic illnesses that often accompany aging (eg, cere-

brovascular accidents, Parkinsonism, arthritis, multiple sclerosis) have the greatest impact on mobility, and the neurogenic consequences of many of these diseases (eg, the neuropathy of diabetes mellitus) interfere with control of urine functions. Decreased facilitation and inhibition in cerebral function may make the control of urine unpredictable. James (1979) notes the association of mental impairment and incontinence in the elderly. With normal aging the kidneys become less able to concentrate urine, and the bladder has less capacity, becomes more irritable, and may hold residual urine. This leads to nocturia, frequency, urgency, and vulnerability to infection. The elderly person may not experience the sensation to void until the bladder is nearly full. Delayed sensation may lead to increased precipitancy and thus further compromise the time needed to reach a toilet. Decreased muscle tone in the pelvic floor and external sphincter can result in leakage due to stress (Wells, 1980). Further, when the elder is at rest or sleeping, the kidneys may function more efficiently and increase the risk of nocturia. In summary, although the changes that accompany aging do not in and of themselves necessarily cause incontinence, they make the balance between continence and incontinence for the elderly person more delicate so that other factors more easily precipitate incontinence.

Acute illness and hospitalization can also be predisposing factors that interfere temporarily with normal function. Quite often the acutely ill, hospitalized elder remains incontinent because of inappropriate assessment and treatment of the problem. Factors that predispose elderly persons to urinary incontinence are the prolonged use of indwelling catheters in elders who could have regained continence had the catheter been removed earlier; drug therapy such as diuretics, hypnotics, and tricyclic antidepressants that either increase the speed of urine production or dull sensations; environmental factors including physical obstacles and staff attitudes and expections that may make the elderly person incapable of continence either because of an inability to reach the toilet in time or because of a feeling of little use to try to be continent. Nurses must have knowledge of all of these predisposing factors in order to assess, diagnose, and treat incontinence in elderly persons. Each factor will be discussed in more detail as it relates to the more definitive types of urinary incontinence.

ASSESSMENT

The diagnosis and management of urinary incontinence in the elderly person has been constrained by the tendency to view incontinence as a single global diagnosis. This has been partly because of a lack of research to describe more specific types of incontinence. However nurses have also been slow to recognize their role in the diagnosis and treatment of incontinence and have lagged in the development and acquisition of the knowledge needed. As a result it has only been recently that the North American Nursing Diagnosis Association (NANDA) has added five more specific incontinence diagnoses to their taxonomy (McLane, 1987). These five diagnoses are Stress Incontinence, Urge Incontinence, Reflex Incontinence, Functional Incontinence, and Total/Continuous Incontinence. Although this is a step in the right direction, we believe there are seven distinct urinary incontinence diagnoses that fall within the general rubric of Urinary Incontinence. They are Urge Incontinence, Stress Incontinence, Reflex Incontinence, Overflow Incontinence, Functional Incontinence, Iatrogenic Incontinence, and Total/Continuous Incontinence. The seven definitive diagnoses can be divided into three general types: Incontinence due to problems with bladder filling, incontinence due to problems with bladder emptying, and incontinence due to spurious functional and environmental maintenance deficits.

Table 17.1 contains the etiologies and defining characteristics listed by NANDA (Carroll-Johnson, 1989) compared with those discussed by the authors. Griffin (1983) outlines the categorization of incontinence as transient versus established to highlight the need for assessment to identify reversible causes amenable to treatment. The differential diagnosis of a definitive urinary incontinence requires a careful and thorough assessment for the signs and symptoms that are associated with the specific etiologies for each of the seven incontinence diagnoses. Effective nursing intervention for incontinence is dependent on this critical first step because treatment must be directed at the underlying causes. Assessment Guide 17.1 presents a tool that nurses can use to gather assessment information.

Assessment information must be gathered through interviews with the elder, family member, or significant other; observation; physical examination; and consultation with other caregivers (Brink, 1980). Careful attention to establishment of rapport, privacy, and a comfortable unhurried environment will greatly influence the ability to gather accurate data about this sensitive area.

Medical literature usually recommends urodynamic studies as essential for assessment in order to make an accurate diagnosis (Griffin, 1983). Although cystometry and urethral pressure profiles can assist with the identification of signs, they should be used with caution for the elderly (Specht, 1986) because the elderly can often show abnormalities with urodynamic studies even when they are continent (Williams, 1983).

The data base that is gathered for making an accurate nursing diagnosis of incontinence must encompass the risk factors, physical causes, psychosocial causes, environmental causes, and information about how functional abilities are affecting continence for the elder (Brink, 1980; Brink et al, 1985; Specht, 1986; Wells and Brink, 1981).

These data categories are listed in Table 17.2. Assessment tools should be evaluated for adequacy by the extent that they guide the nurse to elicit these data. Nursing interventions that will assist with reestablishing continence cannot be determined without adequate and thorough assessment of the multiple factors contributing to specific types of incontinence (Rottkamp, 1985). In a pilot study to validate nursing diagnoses of urinary incontinence, Tunink (1988) found that 16 out of 17 elderly male subjects had more than one type of incontinence. A critical part of assessment is the Continence Specification Record (Assessment Guide 17.2). This helps to determine the number and pattern of incontinent episodes as well as the associated relevant events, such as activity level and fluid intake. Robb (1985) recommends a 3-day record of incontinence episodes.

Bladder-Filling Incontinence

The three bladder-filling incontinence diagnoses are Urge Incontinence, Reflex Incontinence, and Stress Incontinence.

Urge Incontinence Urge incontinence is involuntary urination that occurs soon after a strong sense of urgency to void (Carroll-Johnson, 1989). It has also been defined as "an uncontrollable loss of urine preceded by an urge to void but failure to hold urine long enough to reach a toilet" (Diokono, 1983;70). Heightened urgency results from bladder irritation, reduced bladder capacity, or overdistention of the bladder. The irritation of the bladder stretch receptors causes spasms and emptying. The bladder capacity stretched to its limits, because of either a severely reduced capacity or overdistention, also empties precipitously (Carroll-Johnson, 1989).

Urge incontinence is associated with cerebrovascular accidents (CVA), incomplete suprasacral spinal cord injury, pelvic injury/trauma, multiple sclerosis (MS), brain tumor, previous brain trauma, enlarged prostate, interstitial cystitis, and smaller bladder capacity. A problem with assessment and diagnosis of urge incontinence in the elderly is that the signs and symptoms usually associated with detrusor instability in younger persons (urgency, diurnal and nocturnal enuresis) are common in all diagnoses of incontinence for elders (Hilton and Stanton, 1981). The common signs and symptoms for urge incontinence regardless of the specific etiology are ability to identify the urge to void and precipitancy. Diokono (1983;72) says that the key question to ask is "Do you have a feeling of urge to void and leak urine before reaching the toilet?" The urine loss with urge incontinence is larger and more prolonged than with stress incontinence. With urge incontinence there is a tendency for urine loss to be greater in the morning than in the evening (Malvern, 1981). Urgency and precipitancy are

Table 17.1

Etiologies/Related Factors and Defining Characteristics of Urinary Incontinence

URGE INCONTINENCE. The state in which an individual experiences involuntary passage of urine occurring soon after a strong sense of urgency to void (Carroll-Johnson, 1989)

NANDA (MCLANE, 1987)

Etiologies/Related Factors	*Defining Characteristics*
Decreased bladder capacity	Urinary urgency
Irritation of bladder stretch receptors	Frequency
Alcohol	Bladder contractures/spasms
Caffeine	Nocturia >2 X per night
Increased fluids	Voiding small or large amounts
Increased urine concentration	Inability to reach toilet on time
Overdistention of bladder	

SPECHT, TUNINK, MAAS, BULECHEK

Etiologies/Related Factors	*Defining Characteristics*
Bladder irritation	Common to all etiologies: urgency, precipitancy
WBCs/bacteria/fungi in urine	Dysuria, frequency, lower abdominal discomfort, turbid urine, high alcohol or caffeine intake, and increased urine concentration as in dehydration
Reduced bladder capacity	Frequency with smaller amounts of urine, and recent history of indwelling catheter
Overdistention of bladder	Deep sleep undisturbed by urge to void; increased urine production due to diabetes, diuretics, alcohol, caffeine, increased fluid intake; loss of equal amounts of urine throughout 24 hours

REFLEX INCONTINENCE. The state in which an individual experiences an involuntary loss of urine, occurring at somewhat predictable intervals when a specific bladder volume is reached (Carroll-Johnson, 1989)

NANDA (CARROLL-JOHNSON, 1989)

Etiologies/Related Factors	*Defining Characteristics*
Neurologic impairment, eg, spinal cord lesion that interferes with conduction of cerebral messages above the level of the reflex arc	No awareness of bladder filling
	No urge to void or feelings of bladder fullness
	Uninhibited bladder contraction/spasm at regular intervals

SPECHT, TUNINK, MAAS, BULECHEK

Etiologies/Related Factors	*Defining Characteristics*
(Same as NANDA)	Predictable pattern of voiding (time and amount) with no sensation of urge, voiding, or bladder fullness
	Evidence of spinal cord lesion above the conus medullaris

STRESS INCONTINENCE. The state in which an individual experiences a loss of urine of less than 50 mL occurring with increased abdominal pressure (Carroll-Johnson, 1989)

NANDA (CARROLL-JOHNSON, 1989)

Etiologies/Related Factors	*Defining Characteristics*
Degenerative changes in pelvic muscles and structural supports associated with increased age	Reported or observed dribbling with increased abdominal pressure
High intra-abdominal pressure	Urinary urgency
Incompetent bladder outlet	Urinary frequency > every 2 hours
Overdistention between voidings	
Weak pelvic muscles and pelvic supports	

Table 17.1

Etiologies/Related Factors and Defining Characteristics of Urinary Incontinence (*Continued*)

SPECHT, TUNINK, MAAS, BULECHEK

Etiologies/Related Factors	*Defining Characteristics*
Weakened pelvic muscles and support structures	Common to all etiologies: frequent leakage of small amounts of urine with activity, not preceded by urgency; gradual onset of frequent leakage; low residual urine < 100 cc; leakage of urine when bladder is full that is worse when standing
	Incompetent levatores ani assessed by digital exam of vagina; stretched pelvic floor fascia assessed by digital exam; and ineffective muscle tone for bowel evacuation
High intra-abdominal pressure	Obesity; gaseous distention of abdomen with skin stretched smooth and tympani on percussion; ascites; abdominal pelvic tumor; and palpable funneling of the bladder neck
Incompetent bladder outlet	Difficulty stopping stream of urine and negative difference between urethral pressure and bladder pressure with urodynamic studies
Overdistention of the bladder	History of regularly postponing urination; pattern of large (> 400 cc) and infrequent voidings; and palpable distended bladder

OVERFLOW INCONTINENCE. The state in which the bladder becomes sufficiently overdistended that voiding attempts result in frequent small amounts of urine often in the form of dribbling

SPECHT, TUNINK, MAAS, BULECHEK

Etiologies/Related Factors	*Defining Characteristics*
	Common to all etiologies: high levels of residual hesitancy; slow stream, passage of infrequent small volumes of urine (dribbling); a feeling of incomplete bladder emptying; sudden leakage of urine related to bending or turning; dysuria; and a palpable, full bladder > 2 fingers above the symphysis pubis
Impaired bladder neuromusculature (weak detrusor, strong sphincter)	Evidence of absent or weak sensory and/or motor impulses to the detrusor; no evidence of weak musculature for bowel evacuation with absence of fecal impaction
Obstruction of the bladder outlet	Presence of fecal impaction; prostatic enlargement > +3; difficulty or inability to pass a urethral catheter; and documented obstructing tumor

TOTAL/CONTINUOUS INCONTINENCE. The state in which an individual experiences involuntary passage of urine occurring soon after a strong sense of urgency to void

NANDA (CARROLL-JOHNSON, 1989)

Etiologies/Related Factors	*Defining Characteristics*
Neuropathy preventing transmission of reflex indicating bladder fullness	Constant flow of urine occurs at unpredictable times without distension or uninhibited bladder contractions/spasms
Neurologic dysfunction causing triggering of micturition at unpredictable times	Unsuccessful incontinence refractory treatments
Independent contraction of detrusor reflex due to surgery	Nocturia
Trauma or disease affecting spinal cord nerves	Lack of perineal or bladder-filling awareness
Anatomic (fistula)	Awareness of incontinence

(*Continues*)

Table 17.1

Etiologies/Related Factors and Defining Characteristics of Urinary Incontinence (*Continued*)

SPECHT, TUNINK, MAAS, BULECHEK

Etiologies/Related Factors	*Defining Characteristics*
Total incontinence: interruption of the reflex arc	Large amounts of unpredictable voidings, lack of awareness of incontinence or any bladder activity, and documented spinal cord or peripheral nerve lesion at or below the urinary reflex arc (sacral 2, 3, 4)
Continuous incontinence: anatomic fistula, impaired or misplaced urinary anatomy	Constant loss (trickle) of urine without distention or bladder spasms; urine flow from an orifice other than the urethral orifice

FUNCTIONAL INCONTINENCE. The state in which an individual experiences an involuntary, unpredictable passage of urine (Carroll-Johnson, 1989). The inability to reach the toilet on time due to environmental barriers or disorientation

NANDA (CARROLL-JOHNSON, 1989)

Etiologies/Related Factors	*Defining Characteristics*
Altered environment Sensory, cognitive, or mobility deficits	Urge to void or bladder contractions sufficiently strong to result in loss of urine before reaching an appropriate receptacle

SPECHT, TUNINK, MAAS, BULECHEK

Etiologies/Related Factors	*Defining Characteristics*
Physical deficits interacting with the environment	Common to all etiologies: large voidings with complete emptying of the bladder Impaired ambulation (lack of endurance, flexibility, balance, strength) that lessens timely access to receptacle; impaired manual dexterity (inability to remove clothing, manipulate penis, handle equipment); impaired transfer ability; and weak pelvic floor musculature (bladder empties immediately on change from lying to standing position)
Cognitive/sensory perceptual deficits interacting with environment	Inability to recognize or use familiar articles (poor vision, dysgnosia) or find way to and from toilet; inability to perform familiar action (dyspraxia); loss of cortical concept of body and self; disorientation to time, place, and/or person; memory deficits; misinformation and stereotypes about incontinence and how to control it; inability to communicate need for assistance such as aphasic, catastrophic reaction, dysarthria, low voice volume, and misperception of sensory and physical cues
Psychosocial factors interacting with environment	Expressed helplessness, hopelessness, powerlessness, anger, and frustration associated with urination; more reward and attention received for incontinence than other behaviors; expressions of insecurity associated with recent change in environment; lack of motivators to be continent (low social support and social isolation); regression and isolation due to loss of role and role reversal—extrusion by continent peers (Willington, 1975); conditioned reflex disturbance-positive stimuli associated with continence and negative stimuli for voiding (clean clothing, bed) are reversed (person fails to void when toileted but voids as soon as dressed or put in bed) (Willington, 1975); and intermittent incontinence with no complaint of frequency and urgency (Lapides, 1971)

IATROGENIC INCONTINENCE. The state in which incontinence results from treatments controlled by the physician, nurse, or other health caregivers

Table 17.1

Etiologies/Related Factors and Defining Characteristics of Urinary Incontinence (*Continued*)

SPECHT, TUNINK, MAAS, BULECHEK

Etiologies/Related Factors	*Defining Characteristics*
Health caregiver prescriptions, eg, restraints, medications, fluid limitations, bed rest, IV fluids	Prescribed medications that affect urinary function: diuretics (furosemide [Lasix], caffeine) and central nervous system stimulants (methylphenidate hydrochoride [Ritalin]) that increase precipitancy; hyponotics, sedatives, tranquilizer (diazepam [Valium]), antidepressants (Amytriptylline [Elavil]), barbiturates, phenothiazines that cause sleep too deep for arousal from bladder sensation; opiates (codeine, morphine) that result in constipation with fecal impaction; anticholinergic drugs (benztropine mesylate [Cogentin]) that may result in urinary retention and overflow incontinence
	Prescribed increased and decreased fluid intake: fluid intake 500 cc > normal intake resulting in significantly greater output than usual to cope with; fluid restriction that concentrates urine resulting in bladder irritation and precipitancy
	Prescribed activity restriction: bed rest that results in poorly emptying bladder, restricted access to toilet, postponement of voiding, and/or lack of access to fluids; physical restraints leading to restricted movement, dependence on others for toileting assistance, agitation, powerlessness, and resignation to incontinence
	Prescribed continence aids: indwelling catheter resulting in reduced bladder tone and increased infection; incontinence pads resulting in expectations of incontinence and loss of staff and client desire to achieve client continence

indicators of urge incontinence that are common to all etiologies. More specific defining characteristics for each etiology are listed in Table 17.1.

Reflex Incontinence Reflex incontinence is the involuntary loss of urine caused by completion of the spinal cord reflex arc (bladder contraction) in the absence of higher neural control (Carroll-Johnson, 1989). Voiding will often occur as a specific and predictable volume is reached. This form of incontinence occurs with complete lesions of the spinal cord above the conus medullaris. "There is no sensation of urgency or voiding. A reflex bladder contraction occurs with bladder filling or response to perineal or lower abdominal stimuli" (Wheatley, 1982;77). One problem with this type of bladder is that the external sphincter as well as the detrusor muscle may be spastic, thereby preventing adequate emptying of the bladder. The person with reflex incontinence, upper motor neuron bladder, usually does not receive the message of the need to void, but there may be sensations associated with a full bladder such as sweating, restlessness, and abdominal discomfort that warn the person of the need to empty his or her bladder. The nurse can help this patient find "trigger areas" that initiate the voiding reflex when stimulated (Delehanty and Stravino, 1974).

Digital stimulation of the anus and rectum is usually the most effective stimulus, but tapping the abdomen or doing push-ups on the commode chair may also be effective in precipitating voiding.

Reflex incontinence and urge incontinence are often grouped together as neurogenic or uninhibited bladder. The distinction between reflex incontinence and urge incontinence is particularly difficult when the elderly person has an incomplete spinal cord lesion or damage to the cerebral cortex, as with dementia, CVA, or MS, which results in partial sensation of urge to void and partial bladder control. Some sensation of urgency is a distinguishing characteristic for urge incontinence and is a positive prognostic indicator for regaining continence. The critical signs and symptoms for reflex incontinence are listed in Table 17.1

Stress Incontinence Stress incontinence is the leakage of urine that occurs with increased intra-abdominal pressure, often occurring with coughing, sneezing, or lifting (Carroll-Johnson, 1989). The International Continence Society defines *stress incontinence* as "the involuntary loss of urine when the pressure in the bladder exceeds maximal urethral pressure in the absence of a detrusor contraction" (Harrison, 1983;144). It is characterized by a

Table 17.2

Data Base for Assessment of Urinary Incontinence

RISK FACTORS

Constipation and fecal impaction
Untreated vaginal infections
Untreated urinary tract infections
Slowed gait and insecure balance
Clothing that is difficult to remove
Poor nutrition, low fluid intake and weakness
Use of diuretics, tranquilizers, sedatives, or tricyclic antidepressants
A view of self as old, powerless, neglected
Lack of physical activity, flexibility, and perineal muscle tone
Staying in bed a great deal

PSYCHOSOCIAL ETIOLOGIES/RELATED FACTORS

Low self-concept and self-esteem
Negative attitude toward aging
Feelings of helplessness and powerlessness
Regression due to loss of role and role reversal
Lack of motivators to be continent (low social support and social isolation)

FUNCTIONAL ETIOLOGIES/RELATED FACTORS

Physical mobility, strength, and balance
Manual dexterity
Visual and other perceptual deficits
Communication deficits
Relationship among schedules of food and fluid intake, activities, sleep and voiding
Orientation, perception of bladder cues, memory, learning readiness and ability
Time between urge and voiding

PHYSICAL ETIOLOGIES/RELATED FACTORS

Fecal impaction, the leading cause of incontinence in the elderly (Willington, 1980)
Prostatic enlargement in men
Weakness of supporting pelvic muscles
Atrophic vaginitis and urethritis in women
Urethral sphincter weakness
Cystocele, rectocele, and uterine prolapse in women
Urinary tract infection
Dehydration
Effect of drug treatment
Effect of medical/nursing treatment: catheterization, surgeries, intravenous fluids, prescribed fluid restriction, immobilization
Neurologic deficits and impaired mental status

ENVIRONMENTAL ETIOLOGIES/RELATED FACTORS

Inaccessibility of toilet
Lack of privacy
Use of urinals, bedpans, cans
Lack of equipment to support mobility and balance
Poor lighting
No way to call for help
Lack of familiarity with physical environment
Unknowledgeable, disinterested, unresponsive, insensitive, and/or insufficient caregivers
Inappropriate type of clothing
Lack of sensory stimulation and environmental cues
Distance to toilet

---

sudden loss of urine associated with increased physical activity (coughing, laughing, lifting) and with no other voiding symptoms present (Diokono, 1983).

The etiologies for stress incontinence are weakened pelvic muscles and support structures, high intra-abdominal pressure, overdistention, and incompetent bladder outlet. The signs and symptoms that are seen for all etiologies of stress incontinence include frequent leakage of small amounts of urine with activity, not preceded by urgency; gradual onset; low residual urine (greater than 100 cc); and leakage when the bladder is full that is worse on standing. Wetting less at night than during the day is characteristic. Diokono (1983;70) suggests that the key question to ask the individual is "Do you lose urine when you cough or strain?" Although bladder prolapse and cystocele are reported in the literature as causes of stress incontinence in women, Diokono (1983) says there is no direct relationship.

When the etiology for stress incontinence is weakened pelvic muscles and support structures, the critical signs and symptoms, in addition to those that are common to all etiologies, are incompetent levatores ani, assessed by digital examination of the vagina; stretched pelvic floor fascia, assessed by digital examination; and ineffective muscle tone for bowel evacuation.

The patient lies in a crook position with knees apart. The gloved index and middle fingers of one hand are inserted into the patient's vagina. If there is stretching of the fascia, the downward thrust of "bearing down" will tend to push the fingers out of the vagina. When the fingers are withdrawn until the two distal phalanges are palpating the posterior vaginal wall, the strength of the levator ani muscles can be assessed. The patient is instructed, "Do not let me pull out my fingers." The levator ani muscles then act alone, and the strength of their action from a flicker to a firm squeeze can be assessed (Harrison, 1983).

Contributing factors to be assessed are obesity, multiple pregnancies and deliveries, history of an occupation that required bouncing or heavy lifting, and history of constipation with straining to defecate. Studies have shown that the number of children has an effect on the risk for incontinence if it is greater than two; the risk does not continue to increase after five children (Norton, 1984). Additional specific indicators for each etiology of stress incontinence are detailed in Table 17.1.

Bladder-Emptying Incontinence

Overflow incontinence and total/continuous incontinence are the incontinence diagnoses related to the bladder-emptying function.

Overflow Incontinence Overflow incontinence occurs when the bladder becomes sufficiently overdistended that voiding attempts result in frequent small amounts of urine, often in the form of dribbling. This type of incontinence is paradoxical because the inability to void occurs concurrently with incontinence. Overflow incontinence results from bladder hypotonia due to impaired bladder neuromusculature or from bladder outlet obstruction. Bladder hypotonia can be caused by diabetes mellitus, pelvic trauma, extensive pelvic surgery, lesions or injuries of the conus medullaris, herpes zoster, multiple sclerosis, tabes dorsalis, pernicious anemias, and poliomyelitis. The bladder reflex arc is lost, but parasympathetic innervation prevents vesicle hypersensitivity and hypertonicity. The external sphincter remains strong, but the detrusor loses its contractility. The bladder stores large volumes of urine at low pressure. Bladder outlet obstructions result from prostatic enlargement, bladder neck musculature hypertrophy, bladder neck contracture postsurgical, urethral stricture disease, and fecal impactions.

High levels of residual urine, hesitancy, slow stream, passage of infrequent small volumes of urine (dribbling), a feeling of incomplete bladder emptying, sudden leakage of urine related to bending or turning, dysuria, and a palpable full bladder more than two fingers above the symphysis pubis are common signs and symptoms seen with all etiologies of overflow incontinence.

Griffin (1983) reports that urodynamic studies are often necessary to distinguish obstruction from atonic causes of overflow incontinence. These studies are indicated if the critical signs and symptoms listed in Table 17.1 are not conclusive. The results of the studies would be used to guide specific treatment.

Total/Continuous Incontinence Total/continuous incontinence is an unpredictable or continuous loss of urine resulting from neuropathy of bladder stretch receptors, damage to cerebral neuron control of urination, spinal cord or peripheral nerve lesions below the reflex arc, or anatomic fistulas from surgery, accidental trauma, or malformations (Carroll-Johnson, 1989). Total/continuous incontinence is often diagnosed after stress, urge, reflex, or functional incontinence have been ruled out.

With total incontinence, neuropathy of the bladder stretch receptors and spinal cord or peripheral nerve lesions below the reflex arc that can occur with diabetes mellitus, Parkinson's disease, MS, and other degenerative neurologic diseases and from surgery or trauma interrupt the reflex arc and the brain does not receive the message that the bladder is full. Thus there is no reflex control of urination, and the voiding pattern is not predictable. This has been referred to as lower motor neuron bladder or autonomous bladder (Delehanty and Stravino, 1974). Controlled emptying occurs only from increased intraabdominal pressure by contracting the abdominal and diaphragmatic muscles or by external suprapubic pressure (Crede's method).

Continuous incontinent urine flow usually results from an anatomic fistula due to surgery or trauma or malformation such as ectopic urethral, bladder, or ureteral opening. With continuous incontinence the reflex control is intact, but urination cannot be controlled because the urinary anatomy is impaired or misplaced. Critical signs and symptoms for total and continuous incontinence are detailed in Table 17.1.

Incontinence Due to Spurious Factors

The two incontinence diagnoses related to spurious factors are Functional Incontinence and Iatrogenic Incontinence. These diagnoses are distinguished by the type of spurious factors that lead to incontinence.

Functional Incontinence Functional incontinence is the inability to reach the toilet on time due to environmental barriers or disorientation to place. "Functional incontinence refers to potentially continent individuals (frequently with compromised mobility) who cannot or will not reach the toilet in time to avoid an accident" (Williams, 1983). In general the etiologies for functional incontinence are physical, cognitive/perceptual, or psychosocial deficits interacting with the environment that limit the individual's mastery of continence. Thus involuntary loss of urine occurs even though there is normal bladder and urethral function. Large voidings with complete emptying of the bladder occur with all etiologies of functional incontinence. Ouslander (1981) suggests that functional incontinence may be the leading form of incontinence in nursing homes.

Environmental factors interact with physical, cognitive/perceptual, and psychosocial deficits to cause incontinence for the elderly. Much urinary incontinence results from the loss of the race between the bladder and legs. The following formula has been developed to assess the relationship between distance to the bathroom and bladder emptying (Fine, 1972).

T1 = time interval between onset of desire for urination and arrival of uncontrollable urination

T2 = rate of walking in feet per minute

D = distance to the bathroom

D/T2 = time taken by individual to reach toilet

If D/T2 > T1, incontinence will result

Environmental conditions such as lack of privacy, inaccessibility to toilet, poor lighting, inappropriate clothing, delay in answering "call lights," and use of equipment that tends not to promote normal voiding, as well as the attitudes and behavior of caregivers that may demean, punish, or accept incontinence as inevitable with aging, may impose incontinence on the elderly when they could be continent with a supportive environment. Delays in answering "call lights" in acute and long-term care settings are sometimes manifestations of staff attitudes that impose incontinence on elderly persons. The critical indicators for physical, cognitive/perceptual, and psychosocial etiologies of functional incontinence are listed in Table 17.1 and must be evaluated along with the specific environmental conditions for each elderly person.

Iatrogenic Incontinence Iatrogenic incontinence is incontinence that results from physician- and/or nurse-controlled factors, such as restraints, medications, fluid limitations, bed rest, and/or intravenous fluids. Without the treatment the elderly person would be continent. Although this diagnosis of incontinence is regrettable and we should seek to prevent its causes, iatrogenic incontinence is often easily reversed or compensated. The defining characteristics for iatrogenic etiologies are described in Table 17.1.

ASSESSMENT TOOLS

There are only a few tools in the literature for assessing urinary incontinence. Tools that are available contain a variety of weaknesses. Although some tools are very useful for collecting specific kinds of data, there are still none that are comprehensive or that allow the development of a data base that is adequate to make decisions about specific etiologies and interventions. Another major weakness of available tools is that the structure does not adequately assist the nurse with logical progression of diagnostic decision making. Assessment guidelines should include tools that help the nurse gather data to screen for etiologies and to focus and structure the search for more detailed information in specific areas that are crucial for the effective treatment of incontinence. For

example, the nurse needs to know both whether the elder is ambulatory and whether the speed of ambulation is adequate to reach the toilet facility after the urge and before urination. The authors designed the assessment tool in Assessment Guide 17.1 to overcome these weaknesses. Three gerontologic nursing specialists assessed the content validity of the tool. The tool has been used for assessment in a large long-term care facility for 3 years. The tool refers to other instruments that are available to measure specific characteristics that can be used to augment data collection. The assessment guide is not a questionnaire to be filled out. Rather it is a guide that the nurse can use to prompt the framing of questions to fit each client and situation and to remind him or her of data that are needed. It is important that the nurse use prompts to get the client (family) to describe subjective data and that the nurse follows patient cues for specific lines of questioning.

The Diagnostic Decision Process: Differential Diagnosis

In order to illustrate the process of assessment and diagnosis of specific types of urinary incontinence so that interventions can more precisely address the etiologies and result in more effective treatment of the client's problem, a flowchart for assessment and diagnosis, case studies, and tools for data collection are presented. Two case studies are presented. The cases are used to demonstrate how comprehensive and specific assessment tools are used and how the data that are collected are processed to distinguish specific incontinence diagnoses.

A flowchart for diagnosis of urinary incontinence is presented in Figure 17.1. The flowchart contains the seven specific diagnoses and the transient versus established dimensions as decision outcomes in the diagnostic process. Assessment Guide 17.1 and the flowchart (Figure 17.1) were pilot tested by Tunink (1986) with 17 (n = 17) elderly men with incontinence and modified to increase the usefulness of the tools.

CASE STUDY

Urinary Incontinence, Mr. S

Mr. S is an 80-year-old man, widowed for 10 years, who has been residing in a long-term care facility for the past 2 years. Mr. S had a cholecystectomy when he was 65 and a transurethral resection of the prostate for benign hypertrophy when he was 70. He has been treated for congestive heart failure for the past 5 years, and during the past 3 months he has been receiving 80 milligrams of Lasix each morning. Mr. S has had reduced activity because of his cardiac decompensation and has experienced

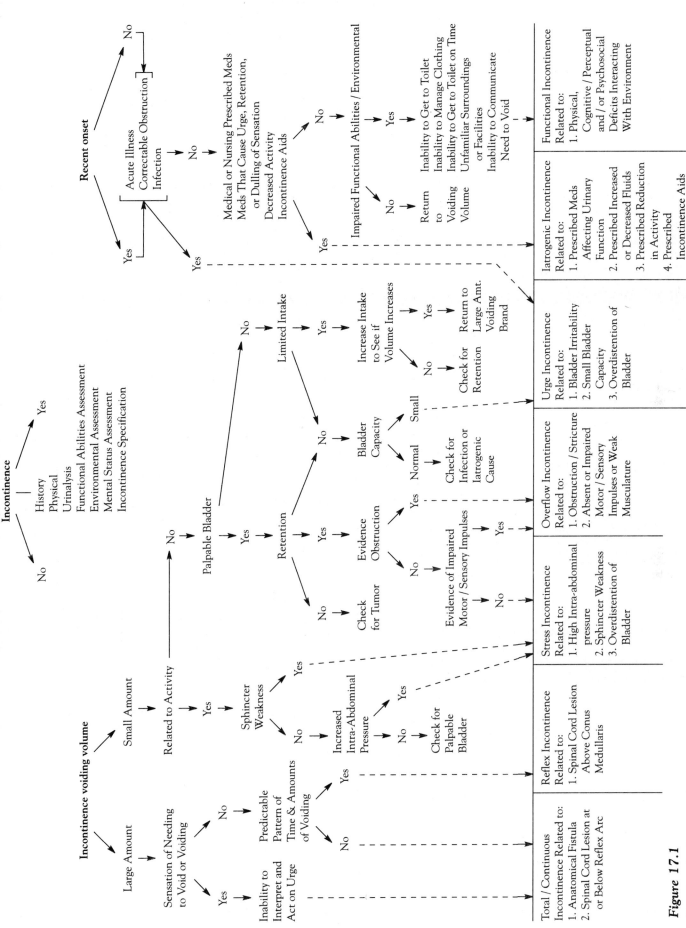

Figure 17.1
Flowchart for diagnosis of urinary incontinence.

Table 17.3

Significant Signs and Symptoms: Case Study, Mr. S

SIGNIFICANT SIGNS AND SYMPTOMS	DIAGNOSES RULED OUT	ADDITIONAL DATA NEEDED
Aware of need to void	Reflex incontinence	Time between urge/void
Voiding large amounts	Stress incontinence	Voiding pattern/schedule
Less intake/large amount coffee	Irritated bladder*	Intake pattern/amounts
History BHP/TURP	Obstruction	Relationship of medicine administration to incontinence episodes
Clear urine analysis	Infection	
Loss of strength/mobility	Functional incontinence*	Ability to manipulate clothing and get to toilet in time
Denial of wetness	Reflex incontinence*	Embarrassed or lack of sensation

*Not ruled out by additional data.

loss of strength and mobility for self-care activities. He has particular difficulty with small-motor tasks, including putting on and removing his clothing. He often does not remove his clothing at night and resists changing his clothing more than once or twice a week. Frequently, staff find his underwear and trousers wet with urine, which he denies. His voidings are usually in large amounts. He is a heavy coffee drinker and does not like decaffeinated coffee. Urinalysis revealed that the urine was clear of bacteria and fungi. Mr. S reports that he knows when he has to urinate but that emptying often comes before he has time to reach the toilet. He states that he has reduced his fluid intake other than coffee in an effort to reduce the need to urinate. Table 17.3 presents Mr. S's significant signs and symptoms, those diagnoses that can be ruled out, and the additional data needed.

TENTATIVE DIAGNOSES

General Types: Established Filling, Transient Spurious.

Urge Incontinence related to irritable bladder as evidenced by reduced fluid intake and coffee drinking.

Iatrogenic Incontinence related to prescribed medication as evidenced by Lasix therapy.

Functional Incontinence related to impaired mobility/dexterity as evidenced by inability to reach toilet and manipulate clothing after urge and prior to voiding.

CASE STUDY

Urinary Incontinence, Mrs. P

Mrs P, age 79, has been recently widowed and admitted to a nursing home. She has a history of diabetes mellitus for the last 20 years for which she takes daily insulin. For several years she has experienced neuropathy and pain in her legs and feet. She had a vaginal hysterectomy at age 55. She is very confused, which makes her dependent in all activities of daily living. Mrs. P is quite obese, with a large pendulous abdomen. Her bladder is palpable following urination. For the past 2 years she has been incontinent of bowel and bladder. With movement in bed or transfer she dribbles urine. Mrs. P entered the nursing home wearing disposable briefs. Urinalysis revealed a large amount of bacteria in the urine. She also has an inflamed vagina with purulent drainage. Her intake is usually 2000 cc each day, and she takes fluids whenever they are offered. She is not able to interpret urge or say when she has to go to the bathroom. Table 17.4 presents Mrs. P's significant signs and symptoms, those diagnoses that can be ruled out, and the additional data needed.

TENTATIVE DIAGNOSES

General Types: Established Emptying, Spurious; Transient Filling.

Overflow Incontinence related to impaired bladder neuromusculature as shown by no evidence of obstruction, evidence of weak musculature for bowel evacuation, absence of fecal impaction, high level of residual urine, and palpable bladder.

Functional Incontinence related to physical dependence and confusion as evidenced by inability to get to toilet facilities without help or to indicate need to void.

Urge Incontinence related to irritable bladder as evidenced by bacteria in urine, vaginitis/drainage.

NURSING INTERVENTIONS

Accurate diagnosis is essential to the treatment of urinary incontinence. Once the specific nursing diagnosis and etiology of urinary incontinence are identified, the appropriate intervention or interventions can be selected.

Table 17.4

Significant Signs and Symptoms: Case Study, Mrs. P

SIGNIFICANT SIGNS AND SYMPTOMS	DIAGNOSES RULED OUT	ADDITIONAL DATA NEEDED
Palpable bladder p̄ voiding	Obstruction	Check for prolapse/impaction
Voids small amounts	Stress incontinence	Check for sphincter/pelvic muscle weakness
Bacteria in urine/vaginitis	Irritated bladder*	Check onset of infection
Diabetes with neuropathy	Reflex incontinence	Amount of retention p̄ void
Incontinent of bowel	Stress incontinence	Check anal sphincter
Dependence in ADLs	Functional incontinence*	Voiding pattern/times/amount
Unable to interpret urge	Reflex incontinence	Voiding pattern/times/amount
		Any other indication of urge, eg, restlessness
Pendulous abdomen/obesity	Stress incontinence	Voiding pattern/times/amount
Leakage with movement	Stress incontinence	Types of activity leading to leakage

*Not ruled out by collecting additional data.

Treatments for urinary incontinence include the use of devices to collect or prevent the flow of urine, medications to influence bladder function, surgical procedures that relieve obstruction or correct some other bladder pathology, or training procedures that alter the patient behavior in some way (Ouslander et al, 1985).

It is beyond the scope of this chapter to discuss all of the treatments for incontinence. However, Table 17.5 contains a listing of primarily medical interventions for all types of incontinence. This chapter will focus on those treatments that are primarily nursing interventions (as opposed to medical interventions), some of which are not listed in Table 17.5. When successful, these nursing interventions result in the elimination or reduction in the number or frequency of incontinent episodes.

For most nurses, prescriptive authority still rests with their medical colleagues. For this reason, the medications used to treat urinary incontinence will be discussed only as they relate to nursing interventions, not to medical interventions. Similarly, although nurses will play a part in the accurate diagnosis of clients who require surgical intervention (either to correct bladder pathology or to insert devices that prevent urine flow), these treatments are essentially medical in nature and will not be discussed in this chapter. Devices used to collect urine (such as condom catheters, bedpans, or disposable pants) do not reduce the number or frequency of incontinent episodes, but merely manage urinary incontinence by keeping the client dry (McCormick and Burgio, 1984).

A number of interventions are available to nurses that do eliminate or control the number of incontinent episodes a client experiences. These include pelvic floor exercises; habit training; bladder training; and clean intermittent catheterization. Each of these interventions, along with any available research to support their use, will be presented. Additional interventions that have a less developed research base will also be briefly described.

Pelvic Floor Exercises

As discussed earlier in this chapter, the etiologies for stress incontinence are related to weakened pelvic muscles and support structures, or weakened bladder outlet. Pelvic floor exercises involve the repetitive contraction of the pubococcygeal muscle, the muscle that forms the support for the pelvis and surrounds the vaginal, urethral, and rectal outlets of the pelvis (Taylor and Henderson, 1986). Pelvic floor exercises, often called Kegel exercises, were named for the physician Arnold H. Kegel, who first described them as a treatment option for clients with stress incontinence (Kegel, 1948). The goal of this repetitive contraction is to strengthen the pubococcygeal muscle and decrease incontinent episodes. Associated exercises involve starting and stopping the urine stream while urinating, with a goal of strengthening the bladder outlet. Thus, pelvic floor exercises are instituted to treat clients with stress incontinence related to weakened pelvic muscles and/or weakened bladder outlet.

Pelvic floor raising exercises are also recommended for individuals who experience urge incontinence (Urinary Incontinence, 1986). By strengthening the muscles of the pelvic floor at the time the urge to void is experienced, the individual may be able to increase the bladder capacity and delay the incontinent episode. This intervention is often paired with a bladder-training regimen that also serves to increase bladder capacity (Burgio et al, 1985).

Researchers have used different exercise protocols in their studies. For instance, in one study, the clients were instructed to tighten the pubococcygeal muscle for 10 seconds and then relax it, repeating the exercise 100 times throughout the day (Taylor and Henderson, 1986). In another study, clients were instructed to practice 50 sphincter exercises daily in three positions—lying, sitting, and standing—and to contract their muscles after lifting or

Table 17.5

Treatments for Urinary Incontinence

TYPES OF TREATMENT	EXAMPLES	MECHANISM	USES
Drugs	Propantheline (Probanthine)	Diminish bladder contractions	Urge incontinence associated with bladder instability
	Imipramine (Tofranil)	Diminish bladder contractions	Urge incontinence associated with bladder instability
	Oxybutrin (Ditropan)	Diminish bladder contractions	Urge incontinence associated with bladder instability
	Flavoxate (Urispas)	Diminish bladder contractions	Urge incontinence associated with bladder instability
	Ephedrine (Sudafed)	Strengthen bladder outlet	Stress incontinence associated with sphincter weakness
	Phenylpropronolamine (Ornade)	Strengthen bladder outlet	Stress incontinence associated with sphincter weakness
	Estrogen (Premarin)	Increases supporting tissue around urethra	Stress incontinence
	Oral or topical Bethanechol (Urecholine)	Promotes bladder contraction	Overflow incontinence
Training procedures	Habit training	Caretaker determines individual's pattern of incontinence and gets him/her to toilet accordingly	Urge incontinence
	Bladder retraining	Caretaker establishes routine of fluid administration and toileting with progressive lengthening of toileting intervals to increase bladder capacity or reinitiate normal voiding	Urge incontinence After catheter use
	Pelvic floor exercises	Exercises to strengthen pelvic muscles	Overflow incontinence after overdistension injury
Stress	Biofeedback	With specialized equipment, patient is trained to inhibit bladder contractions or contract pelvic muscles	Mainly urge incontinence associated with bladder instability and stress incontinence associated with sphincter weakness
	Behavioral modification	Caretaker rewards incontinent individual for staying dry	Incontinence associated with underlying mental or emotional disorders; some forms of functional incontinence

Source: J. Ouslander and R. Kane, University of California at Los Angeles, 1984.

coughing (Burgio et al, 1985). Both studies recommended that clients also practice starting and stopping their urine stream, both highlighted the need for participating clients to be motivated and cognitively able to perform the exercises, and both required several repetitions of the exercises each day. The techniques were successfully used by elderly clients. Taylor and Henderson recommended that clients continue the exercises for the rest of their lives. Although Burgio et al did not include such a recommendation, they did note that two of three patients who reported fewer incontinent episodes at a 12-month posttreatment follow-up had continued their exercises while at home.

Although the use of Kegel exercises to treat stress incontinence does not require the use of equipment to measure the muscle contraction, many research studies include biofeedback as part of the intervention strategy (Burgio et al, 1985; Burns et al, 1985; Taylor and Henderson, 1986). Kegel measured the strength of pubococcygeal muscle contraction with a perineometer, a compressible air chamber inserted in the vagina and attached to a manometer. The client contracted vaginal muscles, and the perineometer recorded the strength of the contraction. The client practiced the exercises and was able to measure progress with the perineometer objectively. Further evaluation of the success of the exercise regimen was measured in a reduction in incontinent episodes (Kegel, 1948). Since Kegel's study, other biofeedback instruments have been designed, but the basic principle of measuring the strength of muscle contraction remains the same. Taylor and Henderson (1986) found that clients who received daily biofeedback while performing pelvic floor exercises achieved 100% continence, whereas the control group, who received biofeedback only at the beginning and end of the treatment period, achieved 67% continence. Other studies show that biofeedback-assisted exercise also yields more improvement in continence than exercise alone (Clinical News, 1986).

As indicated earlier, pelvic floor raising is also a useful treatment for urge incontinence. Burgio et al (1985) combined pelvic floor exercises with a program aimed at teaching clients more effective ways of handling bladder urgency. At a 6-month follow-up of eight clients treated with this regimen, five were totally continent and the remaining three showed, on average, an 84% improvement in frequency of incontinent episodes.

Implementing the Intervention Before the elderly can practice pelvic floor exercises, they must be aware of the muscles that are used in the exercises and then be able to tighten these muscles in a regularly scheduled exercise pattern. Written instructions are helpful. The following exercises will help identify the back portion of the pelvic floor:

- Sit or stand. Relax the muscles of legs, buttocks, and abdomen.
- Imagine you are trying to keep from passing a bowel movement by tightening the ring of muscle around the anus.

Awareness of the muscles in the front portion of the pelvic floor is enhanced by asking the oldster to stop, then restart, urine flow. Doing this with each urination is a way to have the exercises done regularly (Mandalstam, 1980). The exercises usually take 6 to 12 weeks to become effective (McCormick and Burgio, 1984). This means that the nurse will need to give feedback and encouragement to see that the exercises are carried out long enough to make a difference in incontinent episodes.

Habit Training and Bladder Training

Although the terms are frequently used synonymously, habit training and bladder training represent two separate interventions. The goals of the two interventions are different, and therefore, they are used in different circumstances. Habit training involves adjusting the toileting schedule to the client's responses. The aim is to avoid incontinent episodes. There is no attempt to restore

a normal pattern of voiding (Ouslander and Uman, 1985; Ouslander et al, 1985). Bladder training involves the gradual lengthening or shortening of periods between voidings, with the goal of restoring normal voiding patterns as well as continence (Ouslander and Uman, 1985; Ouslander et al, 1985). Another term frequently used is *scheduled toileting*. Scheduled toileting is similar to habit training except the toileting schedule is fixed and is not based on the client's pattern of incontinence (Greengold and Ouslander, 1986).

Bladder training, also referred to as a bladder drill or bladder reeducation, is a treatment of choice for clients with urge incontinence related either to overdistention or to reduced bladder capacity (Ouslander and Uman, 1985; Urinary Incontinence, 1986). When the bladder has a reduced capacity, the time between voidings is gradually extended until the client is able to void once every 2 to 4 hours without incontinence. When the bladder has been overdistended, possibly because of injury or medication use, the time between voidings is gradually reduced until a normal voiding pattern can be established. Candidates for bladder training must be mentally and physically capable of toileting themselves, and they must be motivated to do so (Greengold and Ouslander, 1986).

In a review of a number of research studies of bladder-training regimens, Hadley (1986) reported that cure rates ranged from 44% to 100%. Bladder-training protocols differed in a number of ways. Some allowed the clients to schedule their own voidings, whereas other studies had mandatory voiding schedules that ranged from 0.5 to 4 hours. When goal intervals were identified, they were 4-hour intervals. Most of the studies were clinical trials, although a few included untreated controls. Several of the protocols included additional interventions, such as the use of concomitant drug therapy or the use of self-charting of voiding/incontinence pattern (Hadley, 1986).

Several other interventions have also been identified as part of a bladder-training protocol. These include the careful timing of fluid intake, complete bladder emptying, the use of techniques to inhibit or stimulate voiding, and the use of reinforcement measures (Ouslander and Uman, 1985; Specht and Cordes, 1982). Fluid intake of approximately 2500 cc daily is recommended. Clients are instructed in the use of techniques to stimulate voiding (stroking the inner thigh or running water) or to inhibit voiding (Kegel exercises). Although these interventions have been identified as part of a bladder-training protocol, research studies that isolate and test these aspects are needed.

As indicated, habit training is used if the goal is to avoid incontinent episodes, but not to restore a normal voiding pattern. It is a technique that can be very successful with physically or mentally impaired clients because it generally depends on the motivation of the staff to toilet the client rather than on the motivation of the client (Ouslander and Uman, 1985; Ouslander et al, 1985). For this reason, habit training is a treatment option in clients with functional incontinence related to physical or cognitive/perceptual deficits (Ouslander and Uman, 1985; Urinary Incontinence, 1986). Habit training is an intervention frequently used in long-term care institutions, although many nursing homes used a fixed (as opposed to flexible) 2-hour scheduled toileting protocol (Ouslander and Uman, 1985).

There are fewer research studies available that have examined the effectiveness of habit training or scheduled toileting. Hadley (1986) reviewed three studies that showed cure rates of 26% to 68%. These studies also included other interventions such as staff reinforcement, aided toileting, scheduled fluids, or medication use. Long (1985) describes a study using habit training with elderly clients in a long-term care institution. The treatment included a flexible habit-training protocol, prescribed fluid intake, maintenance of an incontinence record, and prescribed (individualized) method of toileting. The author identified the most difficult part of the study as orienting/motivating the staff to the training protocol. Results of the study indicated that successful habit training was linked to mental status. The higher the degree of mental impairment, the less likely the client would be successful in attaining continence. Mental impairment was identified as a contributing factor to the incontinence (Long, 1985).

Implementing the Interventions

Increasing Fluids A regimen to increase fluids aims at increasing bladder capacity and decreasing detrusor activity. Older persons with incontinence normally reduce fluid intake, often up to 500 to 600 mL/day, in an effort to remain continent (Specht, 1981). A goal of 2400 mL is desirable. However, incontinence has been found to decrease when an intake of 1200 to 1800 mL/day is achieved and maintained (Specht, 1981). Certainly contraindications for increasing fluids need to be considered in planning a fluid regimen in which fluids are restricted because of a secondary medical problem (eg, congestive heart failure).

Planning daily living to increase fluid intake as a measure for improving continence would include the following elements:

1. Explain how the increasing of fluids can promote continence.
2. Negotiate with the person to maintain an intake and output record as well as recording continence and incontinence episodes.
3. Negotiate an acceptable, workable fluid intake schedule of both amounts and kinds of fluid that will gradually move toward the goal of the agreed-on intake goal.

4. Reward and support the older person's efforts (determine what constitutes reward and support for the given individual).
5. Work with spouses, family members, and companions so that their actions do not work against the plan.

Increased fluids need to be used in conjunction with a scheduled toileting program, particularly if there are factors such as functional impairments or mental clouding as additional causes or contributors to the incontinency.

Bladder Training and Habit Retraining Although these are two separate interventions, the methods of implementation for the two are similar, with the major difference being whether the staff/caregiver or oldster has major responsibility for implementing the intervention. Also, bladder training ends with improved bladder function, whereas habit retraining will be an ongoing process to monitor continence. However, with habit retraining the result is increased predictability and a workable schedule for caregivers and the elderly person.

When assessment indicates bladder training or habit retraining as the intervention of choice, the following plan is useful. Long (1985) and Specht (1981) used the protocol:

1. Gather data on fluid intake pattern, voiding patterns, sensation and awareness, underlying health problems, and potential for retraining (intact to mild cognitive impairment permits participation in the program) (Long, 1985).
2. Keep a Continence Specification Record for 3 days (see Assessment Guide 17.2).
3. Take or ask the person to go to the toilet, or have the elder use a bedpan on waking. The elder should remain on the toilet no longer than 5 minutes. If voiding is not occurring, try measures to encourage micturition, for example stroking inner aspect of thigh, deep breathing, bearing down, leaning forward at an acute angle, drinking water, and exerting manual pressure over the bladder area.
4. Repeat the previous step initially at 4-hour intervals and at bedtime. If incontinence occurs before 4 hours, reduce the interval to 3 hours (or less if incontinence reoccurs). Do not toilet more often than 1 to 2 hours because too-frequent voiding causes chronic low-volume voiding, leading to reduced bladder capacity, increased detrusor tone, and bladder wall thickening (Long, 1985).
5. Maintain the agreed-on fluid schedule (see Increasing Fluids section).
6. Keep a record of continence and incontinence episodes.
7. Reward success (determine what constitutes reward for this person); support and encourage the person when there are incontinent episodes.

In Long's (1985) study, the time required to establish a three to four toilet daily schedule without episodes of incontinence ranged from 4 days to 6 weeks, and at discharge 79% of the incontinent patients were continent.

Clean Intermittent Catheterization

Continuous indwelling catheterization is an appropriate management strategy for only a small number of incontinent clients: those with urinary retention that cannot be successfully treated by surgical or pharmacologic intervention, or by intermittent catheterization (Ouslander et al, 1985). Unfortunately, indwelling catheters are used in approximately 10% to 30% of incontinent individuals living in long-term care institutions (Ouslander et al, 1985). However, an alternative to the indwelling catheter is to use clean intermittent catheterization. Clean intermittent catheterization is a technique in which patients self-catheterize or are catheterized by caregivers at regular intervals. The technique may be recommended for use in clients with urinary retention related to a weak detrusor muscle (as in diabetic neuropathy) or blockage of the urethra (as in benign prostatic hypertrophy) and with reflex incontinence related to spinal cord injury (Lapides et al, 1976; Ouslander and Uman, 1985; Ouslander et al, 1985; Urinary Incontinence, 1986).

Intermittent catheterization was first introduced after World War II as a bladder-training technique for paraplegic and quadraplegic patients (Champion, 1976). At that time intermittent catheterization was conducted only under sterile conditions by a physician. Patients were catheterized at frequent intervals throughout the day. The procedure worked much as a bladder drill. Early studies showed that patients trained in such a manner for about 7 weeks were able to void at discharge from the hospital (Guttman and Frankel, 1966). Since that time, the procedure has been modified, and it is now taught as a clean, not sterile, self-catheterization. It is used for bladder training as well as for other clients for whom nerve supply to the bladder has been disrupted (Champion, 1976).

The rationale for clean intermittent catheterization is based on the assumption that the blood supply to the bladder must be maintained in order to promote the bladder's ability to fight infection. Bladder overdistention slows bladder circulation and predisposes the bladder to infection. Frequent catheterization of the bladder prevents overdistention and allows the bladder to fight infection (Horsley et al, 1982). This technique has been shown to reduce the incidence of complications associated with indwelling catheter use (Ouslander et al, 1985). The emphasis is not on maintaining sterility, but on frequent emptying of the bladder.

Clients, or their caregivers, are taught the basic principles of catheterization and the procedure for catheterizing using clean technique. Patients are frequently maintained on antibacterial medications for a period of 2 to 3 weeks, as well as on anticholinergic or cholinergic medications to assist bladder control (Horsley et al, 1982). A candidate for clean intermittent self-catheterization must have the manual dexterity to manipulate the catheter and must be motivated to perform the technique frequently throughout the day (usually when the bladder has distended with approximately 300 cc of fluid) and in any number of settings. Caregivers must possess these same qualities.

Lapides and colleagues (1976) reported a review of 218 patients who were taught clean intermittent catheterization. The subjects' ages ranged from 4 to 84 years, with 145 subjects between 21 and 84 years of age. The subjects had a number of different diagnoses related to voiding difficulties and incontinence. The results of this survey indicated that for clients experiencing incontinence related to reflex bladder contractions or overflow incontinence, clean intermittent catheterization combined with anticholinergic and alpha-adrenergic medication alleviated incontinence as well as chronic perineal dermatitis (Lapides et al, 1976).

Implementing the Intervention This is a clean, not a sterile, procedure. The emphasis is on frequency rather than sterility. The goal is to maintain a volume of urine in the bladder of 300 mL or less. This requires catheterization every 2 to 3 hours while the person is awake and one to two times during the night.

Candidates for the self-catheterization procedure should meet the following criteria:

1. Sufficient manual dexterity and mental ability to perform the procedure in its entirety at frequent intervals, or have another person to do it
2. A bladder capacity of 100 mL or more
3. A urethra that is intact and free from stricture

This routine has been used successfully at the Iowa Veterans Home with residents who had atonic bladders. Nurses had difficulty in moving to a clean rather than sterile approach and did complain about the frequency of the treatment. It is essential for nurses, family, and the older person to understand the principles of this method. Although this approach needs further testing, it holds promise and is preferable to indwelling catheters. It should be noted, however, that clean intermittent catheterization has been researched far more extensively in the child and young adult than in the elderly client. It is presently unclear, for instance, whether complications might be more common in a geriatric population (Ouslander et al, 1985). Although the theoretical principles supporting clean intermittent catheterization remain the same with elderly clients, further research with this intervention is needed to support its usefulness over time with older adults.

Other Treatment Options

Interventions for stress, urge, functional, retention, and reflex incontinence have all been discussed. Pelvic floor raising, bladder training and habit training, and clean intermittent catheterization have a research base at this time and can be recommended for treatment of specific types of urinary incontinence. It should be noted, however, that additional interventions may be indicated, depending on the client's type and etiology of urinary incontinence. For instance, a client experiencing functional incontinence related to physical deficits may benefit from a muscle-strengthening program and environmental modification to reduce the obstacles between the client and the commode. Similarly, the elimination of fecal impactions may eliminate overflow incontinence related to an obstructed bladder outlet (Specht and Cordes, 1982). Urge incontinence related to bladder irritation may be eliminated with a fluid intake of 2500 cc, if the irritation was due to highly concentrated urine in a dehydrated client (Specht and Cordes, 1982). Further research is needed for these and other interventions commonly used to treat urinary incontinence to determine which interventions are most useful and cost effective in elderly clients.

CASE STUDY

Nursing Interventions for Urinary Incontinence, Mr. S

The nurse discussed the urinary incontinence diagnoses with Mr. S, explaining the factors that contributed to each type of incontinence. Mr. S agreed that he desired to be continent. He and the nurse established a plan to achieve the goal of reducing his incidents of incontinence. After Mr. S understood the roles of caffeine and reduced fluid intake in causing his bladder to be irritated, he agreed to limit his coffee intake to 2-3 cups each day and to increase his total fluid intake to at least 1500 cc daily. He volunteered to try decaffeinated coffee and requested noncitric juices and a beer with his evening meal. With his approval, the nurse sent his trousers to have velcro fasteners placed on the fly instead of a zipper. Mr. S also agreed to toilet himself at least every 2 hours in an attempt to avoid urgency and precipitance of urination.

Mr. S and the nurse set up a weekly appointment to review his progress. At their third conference, Mr. S reported that he had only one incontinence episode during the past week and that it had occurred when he had not

been able to toilet for a period of 4 hours. He was having much better success with manipulating his clothing with the velcro fasteners, so the nurse had his other trousers altered. He also reported that he thought he could extend his toileting interval to 3 hours. He said he was able to tolerate the decaffeinated coffee and that he was pleased to no longer have the discomforts of urge to void and being wet.

CASE STUDY

Nursing Interventions for Urinary Incontinence, Mrs. P

Mrs. P's nurse acted first on the urinary and vaginal infection. She consulted with the physician, and Mrs. P was placed on medication to relieve the infections. In order to support the medication therapy and prevent overflow incontinence, intermittent catheterization was initiated every 3 hours. The plan was to increase the interval of time to 4 hours between catheterizations after the infection cleared. Intermittent catheterization was continued for 8 weeks, during which time the urine remained free of infection. Mrs. P was then placed on an every-3-hour voiding schedule and catheterized after each voiding. She continued to have residual urine of from 70 to 100 cc and was unable to cooperate with the voiding schedule because of her confusion. She was returned to an every-3-hour intermittent catheterization schedule. The nurse did not consider the use of pelvic floor exercises to strengthen supporting musculature because of Mrs. P's inability to understand and implement the exercises.

SUMMARY

Urinary Incontinence is a complex nursing diagnosis that requires detailed assessment data to differentiate the specific etiologies and type of incontinence. With the elderly, more than one etiology is often present and more than one type of incontinence must be treated. There are a number of interventions that nurses can use to treat incontinence successfully in elderly persons. However, the intervention chosen must be specific for the type of incontinence, and more than one may need to be tried before the desired outcomes of continence, increased comfort, and optimal independence are achieved. Nurses should anticipate that the elderly will need a considerable length of time to achieve success and that persistence and consistency of intervention strategies are essential. Including the elderly person and/or the family in determining desirable outcomes and strategies is fundamental to successful nursing intervention to resolve urinary incontinence.

ASSESSMENT GUIDE 17.1

Assessment Guide for Diagnosis of Urinary Incontinence

Date _____   Assessed by _____

Name _____   D.O.B. _____   Sex _____

Marital Status _____

I. History

A. Main Complaint _____

B. Urinary Symptoms

    1. Frequency: How often do you urinate during the day? _____

    2. Nocturia: How often do you urinate during the night? _____

    Do you awaken? _____ Number nights per week? _____

    3. Urgency: Once you are aware you need to urinate, how long can you wait? _____ Can you tell when your bladder is full? _____

    4. Stress: Do you ever lose urine when you laugh, cough, sneeze, or change position? _____ Do you lose a little or a lot? _____

    5. Reflex: Can you tell when you have passed urine? _____

    6. Hesitancy: Do you have difficulty starting to urinate? _____

    7. Stream: Has the size of the stream changed recently? _____

    Has the force of the stream changed recently? _____

    Can you start and stop the stream? _____

    8. Straining: Do you ever strain to urinate? _____

    Are you ever not able to urinate when you strain? _____

    Do you use manual expression to help urinate? _____

    9. Postmicturition Dribbling: Do you ever dribble urine after you have urinated? _____

    10. Dysuria: Do you have any pain or burning when you pass your urine? _____

    11. Turbidity: Is your urine clear? _____ Is it cloudy? _____

    Does it appear to contain mucus? _____

    12. Hematuria: What color is your urine? _____

    Does your urine ever have blood in it? _____

    13. Control: Do you ever have any problem controlling your urine?

    If so, when did this begin? _____

    How often does it occur? _____

    How much urine is lost? _____

    How do you manage this problem? _____

    Is this effective? _____

(Continues)

ASSESSMENT GUIDE 17.1

Assessment Guide for Diagnosis of Urinary Incontinence (Continued)

Do you take any precautions to protect your skin? _____

What precautions? _____

Do you have any skin breakdown? _____

How has your daily living been changed because you have difficulty controlling your urine? _____

_____

C. Fluid Intake

   1. Amount: How many cups of fluid do you drink in a day? _____

                  Do you restrict your fluids in any way? _____

   2. Kind: How much water do you drink daily? _____

                  Do you drink coffee? _____ Caffeinated? _____ Decaffeinated? _____

                  Tea? _____ Caffeinated? _____ Decaffeinated? _____

                  Cola? _____ Caffeinated? _____ Decaffeinated? _____

                  Chocolate drink? _____

                  Alcoholic beverages? _____

                  How much of each do you drink? _____

   3. Timing: Do you usually have fluids only with meals? _____

                  Do you drink fluids after supper or through the night? _____

D. Bladder Record

   The client (family member or significant other) is asked to fill out the Continence Specification Record, which is presented in Assessment Guide 17.2. If this is not possible, nursing staff institutions should fill it out. The record is filled out daily for one week.

E. Medical History

   1. Relevant past   Have you had any abdominal, genital, or gynecologic operations or treatments?
     health:

                  _____

                  Have you had any bladder or kidney infections? _____

                  Have you had any brain or spinal cord disease or injury of any kind? _____

      (Women)   Number of pregnancies? _____

                  Number of live births? _____

                  Have you reached menopause? _____

                  How old were you? _____

   2. Present health   What are your current health problems?
     status:

                  _____

   3. Medications: What medication are you taking? _____

ASSESSMENT GUIDE 17.1

Assessment Guide for Diagnosis of Urinary Incontinence (Continued)

F. Bowels

    1. Habits: How often do you have a bowel movement? _____

            Any difficulty? _____

            Constipation? _____ Incontinence? _____ Diarrhea? _____

    2. Treatment: Do you use any laxatives or other aids such as diet to assist with regularity? _____

G. Functional Abilities*

    1. Mobility: Any difficulty getting to the toilet? _____

            Any difficulty getting on and off the toilet? _____

            Any problems with balance that affect your ability to use the toilet? _____

    2. Manual dexterity: Do you experience any difficulty removing or adjusting clothing to go to the toilet?

            _____

            Do you have difficulty cleaning yourself following toileting? _____

    3. Vision: Can you see well enough to get to the toilet and use the facilities? _____

            Is your vision more of a problem at night? _____

H. Environment*   Is your bathroom or toilet located in a convenient place? _____

            Is it available to you any time you need it? _____

            Is there any problem with the physical layout of the toilet? _____

I. Psychologic State*   Describe your attitude and feelings about your incontinence _____

J. Social Relationships*   Has incontinence restricted your usual activities or relationships in any way? _____

II. Physical Exam

A. TPR _____ Weight _____

B. Abdomen

    1. Bowel sounds _____

    2. Scars _____

    3. Bladder distention $\bar{p}$ voiding _____

C. Genitalia

    1. Skin _____

    2. Urethral meatus _____

    Stress test (stand with full bladder and see if any urine leaks out)

    3. Women:

        a. Labia, vaginal mucosa _____ Dry _____ Moist _____

        b. Any protrusions from or in the vagina? _____

        c. Any objects in the vagina? _____

        d. Can the patient feel your finger in the vagina? _____

             Can she squeeze her vagina around it? _____

             Is the squeeze strong or weak? _____

(Continues)

ASSESSMENT GUIDE 17.1

Assessment Guide for Diagnosis of Urinary Incontinence (Continued)

4. Men:

   a. Penis circumcised? _____

   b. If not, is foreskin freely movable? _____

   c. Is the penis small and/or retracted? _____

   d. Is scrotum enlarged? _____ tender? _____ hard? _____

       hot? _____ inflamed? _____ other?_____

   e. Enlarged prostate? _____

D. Rectum

   1. Hemorrhoids? _____

   2. Anal tone firm? _____ weak? _____

   3. Stool soft? _____ hard? _____ none? _____

E. Mental Function:*

   1. Confused? _____ Oriented? _____ Forgetful? _____

   2. Ability to recognize toilet articles and how to toilet? _____

   3. Ability to perform familiar action, eg, push down to defecate? _____

   4. Is body perception intact? _____

       Test by touching contralateral buttock. _____

F. Urinalysis

   1. Bacteria or fungi? _____

       WBCs? _____ Specific gravity? _____

       Other abnormalities? _____

   2. Culture if significant bacteria? _____

G. Mobility*

   1. Ambulate by self? _____

   2. Transfer by self? _____

   3. Manipulation of clothing? _____

   4. Strength? _____ Endurance? _____

       Gait? _____ Balance? _____

   5. Time needed to get to toilet after urge and before voiding?

   _____

   6. Ability to get to toilet in time needed to avoid incontinence?

   _____

H. Urodynamic Studies _____

*Tools are available that expand the objective assessment of these items that should be used if there is reason to believe that the subjective indicators are not reliable or valid or need further measurement.

ASSESSMENT GUIDE 17.2

Urinary Continence Specification Record

Name _____ Date _____

Instructions:

1. In the first column, mark the time every time you void.
2. In the second or third column, mark every time you accidently leak urine.
3. In the fifth column, record your fluid intake for the hour.

Time Interval	Urinated in Toilet	Leaking or Large Accident		Reason for Accident	Fluids
6 A.M.					
7 A.M.					

References

Brink C: Assessing the problem. *Geriatr Nurs* (Nov/Dec) 1980; 1:241–275.

Brink C, Wells T, Diokono A: The continence clinic for the aged. *J Gerontol Nurs* (Dec) 1985; 9:651–655.

Burgio K, Whitehead W, Engel B: Urinary incontinence in the elderly. *Ann Intern Med* 1985; 104:507–515.

Burns P et al: Kegel exercises with biofeedback: Therapy for treatment of stress incontinence. *Nurse Pract* 1985; 10(2):28, 33–34, 46.

Carroll-Johnson R (editor): *Classification of Nursing Diagnoses: Proceedings of the Eighth Conference.* Lippincott, 1989.

Champion V: Clean technique for intermittent self-catheterization. *Nurs Res* 1976; 25(1):13–18.

Clinical News: Lowering the nation's incontinence bill. *Am J Nurs* 1986; 86:1215–1216.

Delehanty L, Stravino V: Achieving bladder control in Christofferson Va. In: *Rehabilitation Nursing: Perspective and Applications.* Coulter PP, Wolanin MO (editors). McGraw-Hill, 1974.

Diokono AC: Practical approach to the measurement of urinary incontinence in the elderly. *Comp Ther* 1983; 9:67–75.

Fine W: Geriatric ergonomics. *Gerontol Clin* 1972;14:322–332.

Greengold B, Ouslander J: Bladder retraining program for patients with post-indwelling catheterization. *J Gerontol Nurs* 1986; 12(6):31–35.

Griffin D: Urinary incontinence in the elderly. *Post Grad Med* (Feb) 1983; 7:143–156.

Guttman L, Frankel H: The value of intermittent catheterization in the early management of traumatic paraplegia and tetraplegia. *Paraplegia* 1966; 4:63–84.

Hadley E: Bladder training and related therapies for urinary incontinence in older people. *JAMA* 1986; 256(3):372–379.

Harrison SM: Stress incontinence and the physiotherapist. *Physiotherapy* (May) 1983; 69:144–147.

Hilton P, Stanton SL: Algorithmic method for assessing urinary incontinence in elderly women. *British Med J* (Mar) 1981; No. 282:940–942.

Horsley JA, Crane J, Haller KB: Intermittent catheterization: CURN Project, Michigan Nurses' Association. Grune and Stratton, 1982.

James MH: Disorders of micturition in the elderly. *Age Ageing* (Nov) 1979; 8:286.

Kegel AH: The nonsurgical treatment of genital relaxation. *Ann West Med Surg* 1948; 2(5):213–216.

Lapides J: Urinary incontinence. Pages 1629–1644 in: *Practice of Surgery.* Kendall AK, Korafin L (editors). Harper and Row, 1971.

Lapides J et al: Further observations on self-catheterization. *Transactions Amer Assoc Genito-Urinary Surg* 1976; 67:15–17.

Long M: Incontinence: Defining the nursing role. *J Gerontol Nurs* 1985; 11(1):30–35, 41.

Malvern J: Incontinence of urine in women. *British J Hosp Med* (Mar) 1981:224–231.

Mandelstom D: Special techniques: Strengthening pelvic floor muscles. *Geriatr Nurs* 1980; (4):251–252.

McCormick K, Burgio K: Incontinence: An update on nursing care measures. *J Gerontol Nurs* 1984; 10(10): 16–19, 22, 23.

McLane A (editor): *Classification of Nursing Diagnoses: Proceedings of the Seventh Conference.* Mosby, 1987.

Millard PH: The prevention of incontinence. *Practitioner* 1981, 225 (1362):1739–1743.

Milne JS et al: Urinary symptoms in older people. *Mod Geriat* 1972; 2:304–311.

Norton C: The promotion of continence. *Nurs Times* (Apr) 1984; 80 (Suppl)(14): 4, 6, 8.

Ouslander J: Urinary incontinence in the elderly. *West J Med* (Dec) 1981; 482–491.

Ouslander J, Kane R: The costs of urinary incontinence in nursing homes. Hyattsville, MD: *Report from the National Center for Health Services Research* (May) 1982.

Ouslander J, Uman G: Urinary incontinence: Opportunities for research, education, and improvements in medical care in the nursing home setting. In: *The Teaching Nursing Home.* Schneider EL (editor). Raven Press, 1985.

Ouslander J et al: *Technologies for Managing Urinary Incontinence.* Health Technology Case Study 33, OTA-HCS-33. U.S. Government Printing Office, 1985.

Robb S: Urinary incontinence verification on elderly men. *Nurs Res* 1985; 34:278–282.

Rottkamp BC: A holistic approach to identifying factors associated with an altered pattern of urinary elimination in stroke patients. *J Neurosurg Nurs* (Feb)1985; 17(1):37–43.

Specht J: *The Effects of Selected Nursing Interventions on Incidence of Incontinence of Institutionalized Elderly Men.* (Unpublished Master's Thesis.) University of Iowa, 1981.

Specht J: Genitourinary problems. In *Nursing Management for the Elderly*, 2d ed. Carnivelli D, Patrick M (editors). Lippincott, 1986.

Specht J, Cordes A: Incontinence. Pages 387–398 in: *Health Management of the Elderly.* Carnivelli D, Patrick M (editors). Lippincott, 1982.

Taylor K, Henderson J: Effects of biofeedback and urinary stress incontinence in older women. *J Gerontol Nurs* 1986; 12(9):25–30.

Tunink P: *Clinical Usefulness of an Assessment Guide, a Flowchart for Diagnosis of Urinary Incontinence and Critical Indicators: A Pilot Study.* (Unpublished Paper.) University of Iowa College of Nursing, 1986.

Tunink P: Alteration in urinary elimination. *J Gerontol Nurs* 1988; 14(4):25–31.

Urinary Incontinence. Proceedings of the 1986 NANDA conference. (Unpublished Report), 1986.

Wells T: Promoting urine control in older adults. *Geriatr Nurs* (Nov/Dec) 1980; 1:236–241.

Wells T, Brink CA: Urinary continence: Assessment and management. In: *Nursing and the Aged.* Burnside I (editor). McGraw-Hill, 1981.

Wheatley J: Bladder incontinence: Four types and their control. *Postgrad Med* (Jan) 1982; 7:75–82.

Williams M: A critical evaluation of the assessment technology for urinary continence in older persons. *J Am Geriatr Soc* 1983; 31:11.

Willington FL: Urinary incontinence: A practical approach. *Geriatrics* (June) 1980; 35:41–48.

Yarnell J, St. Leger A: The prevalence, severity and factors associated with urinary incontinence in a random sample of the elderly. *Age Ageing* 1979; 8(2):81–85.

IV

Activity–Exercise Pattern

MERIDEAN MAAS, Ph D, RN, FAAN

KATHLEEN C. BUCKWALTER, PhD, RN, FAAN

Overview

In Chapter 19, Dougherty provides an excellent overview of the diagnosis Decreased Cardiac Output. This diagnosis has stimulated controversy among proponents of the nursing diagnosis movement and among critical care nurses regarding whether nurses can independently treat actual and potential health problems related to this diagnosis, or whether they do so interdependently with medicine. Dougherty's chapter focuses on decreased cardiac output among the elderly and suggests that surveillance is an appropriate nursing intervention for this diagnosis in an older population.

Halm continues the discussion of respiration at the cellular level in Chapter 20, Altered Tissue Perfusion, noting that the elderly are predisposed to decreased perfusion because of changes that occur in the cardiovascular system with aging. Halm further notes that in spite of the prevalance of compromised tissue perfusion among the elderly, nursing studies of the incidence of diagnoses have not revealed Altered Tissue Perfusion to be a prevalent nursing diagnosis. Several assessment tools are reviewed and evaluated. Both independent and interdependent nursing interventions are detailed to treat specific etiologies of Altered Tissue Perfusion.

In Chapter 21, Ineffective Breathing Pattern, Wakefield reviews the respiratory problems most likely to be experienced by the elderly and notes the importance of distinguishing between problems that tend to be associated with the aging process and those that are due to disease. The need for nurses to assess elderly patients systematically in order to identify risk factors and etiologies to guide treatment is emphasized. Breathing retraining, exercise, and energy conservation are described as interventions that nurses can independently use to treat Ineffective Breathing in the elderly.

In Chapter 22, MacLean explicates the nursing diagnosis Activity Intolerance and identifies the most common risk factors for the elderly. She notes that there is a limited research base for causative factors and clinical cues related to this diagnosis in general, and virtually no research among the elderly or in long-term care settings. MacLean presents her own research on the reliability and validity of cues for diagnosing Activity Intolerance, and continues discussion of the exercise intervention, tailored to the elderly person experiencing Activity Intolerance. She recommends a highly individualized exercise program as the best approach to this pervasive problem.

In Chapter 23, Impaired Physical Mobility, Maas focuses on a nursing diagnosis that has a high incidence among the institutionalized elderly and that is often the reason for admission to long-term care settings. Consequences of impaired mobility in this population are elaborated, suggesting that problems with mobility are a common etiologic factor among many of the diagnoses set forth in this book. Additionally, eight etiologies for this diagnosis are discussed in terms of their signs and symptoms, and a case study highlighting differential diagnosis among these etiologies is presented. Exercise is the primary intervention recommended to treat impaired mobility among the elderly, and different types of exercise programs are suggested according to the specific etiology.

Lantz and Penn, in Chapter 24, using Orem's framework, discuss the diagnosis, Self-Care Deficit, among the elderly, noting the contrast in prevalence among both community and institutionalized elderly. Assessment tools are reviewed that are general as well as specific for various diseases. Stimulating dormant resources, strengthening of underused abilities, and establishing positive life patterns provide the rationale for interventions that are described. A tool for the evaluation of interventions to treat self-care deficits is also described.

Closely related to many of the other diagnoses discussed within this pattern, Rantz, in Chapter 25, discusses the diagnosis Diversional Activity Deficit, emphasizing that failure to treat this problem in the elderly leads to multiple adverse consequences. Likewise, she provides compelling empirical support for the notion that treatment of this deficit can improve cognitive, affective, and physiologic status; increase socialization; and, in general, contribute to an enhanced quality of life for the elderly individual. Reminiscence therapy is developed in some detail as the intervention of choice for this problem. Other rehabilitative therapies (eg, pets, music) are also discussed.

18

Normal Changes With Aging

MARY A. HARDY, PhD, RN, C

Definition:

The activity–exercise pattern describes the pattern of exercise, activity, leisure, and recreation.

THE RESPIRATORY, CARDIOVASCULAR, AND MUSCU-loskeletal systems work together; therefore, physiologic changes in each system affect the other systems. Changes in the pulmonary system associated with aging include loss of lung elasticity and slowed cough reflex due to reduced ciliary movement secondary to epithelial atrophy. Vital capacity decreases with age because the lungs become more fibrotic, the rib cage becomes less flexible, the alveoli enlarge and decrease in number, the bronchioles dilate, and the respiratory muscles decrease in strength. The resulting less efficient ventilation and decreased surface area mean less oxygen in the blood. This lower oxygenation may be compounded in persons with a low hemoglobin due to inadequate nutrition (Nesbitt, 1988).

The cardiovascular system also becomes less efficient with age. The cardiac muscle strength diminishes because of fibrosis and sclerosis of the endocardium, left ventricular wall thickening, increased fat infiltration in right atrium and ventricle, and stiffening of arterial walls due to declining baroreceptor response. These changes result in a drop in cardiac output, a decreased stroke volume, and a delay in the return to normal heart rate under stress conditions. Mitral and aortic valves develop calcifications and fibrosis; myocardial irritability develops with muscle loss and increase in fibers at the AV node, the SA node, and the bundle branches. Vascular resistance increases as a result of thickening and fibrosis of arterial intima. Arteries become rigid as elastin thins and calcium deposits are accumulated. Veins thicken, fibrose, dilate, and stretch. As renal blood flow lessens, decline in renal function can lead to sodium and water retention. These factors combine to increase the amount of energy required to do the heart's work and may cause characteristic signs of activity intolerance (Eliopoulos, 1987; Gioiella and Bevil, 1985).

The musculoskeletal system may also contribute to activity intolerance and impaired mobility, two closely related problems. With aging, there is a general slowing of nerve conduction and reaction time. The muscle cells become smaller and fewer, resulting in a gradual loss of muscle mass. Muscle strength may also decrease as a result of diminished protein synthesis in muscle cells, slower mobilization of glucose in response to exercise, and reduced glycogen stores that accompany reduced muscle mass. Risk of fractures, back pain, and tremors may occur because bones become more porous, vertical trabecular bone demineralizes, cortical bone atrophies, and intervertebral disks become dehydrated and narrow. Decreased range of motion and stiffness may result from generalized wear and tear on joints and changes in ligaments, tendons, and synovial membranes. These changes, coupled with an altered center of gravity and the subsequent fear of falling, often lead to intentional decreased mobility and eventual functional decline. A deconditioned status may occur from the combined problems of the respiratory, cardiovascular, and musculoskeletal systems (Nesbitt, 1988). Lifestyle is the source of many of the factors that lead to a diminished capacity for activity and exercise in the elderly. This fact is congruent with Williams's (1987) belief that age alone does not predispose the elderly to problems with activity.

References

Eliopoulos C: *Gerontological Nursing.* Lippincott, 1987.

Gioiella EC, Bevil CW: *Nursing Care of the Aging Client: Promoting Healthy Adaptation.* Appleton-Century-Crofts, 1985.

Nesbitt B: Nursing diagnosis in age-related changes. *J Gerontol Nurs* 1988; 14(7):7–12.

Williams TF: The future of aging. *Arch Physical Med Rehab* (June) 1987; 68:335–338.

19

Decreased Cardiac Output

CYNTHIA M. DOUGHERTY, PhD, RN

ALTHOUGH THE NURSING DIAGNOSIS DECREASED CARdiac Output was among those accepted in 1975 by the National Conference Group on the Classification of Nursing Diagnosis (Kim et al, 1982), it remains controversial as to whether or not it should be included on the list, since nurses do not independently provide treatment. However, this diagnosis is one frequently identified by staff nurses and clinical specialists in the critical care setting (Castles, 1982; Hubalik, 1981; Kim et al, 1982). Wessel (1981) and Dougherty (1985) have demonstrated that nursing interventions related to the nursing diagnosis Decreased Cardiac Output are both independent and collaborative.

For the diagnosis Decreased Cardiac Output, etiologies were not developed until the Fifth National Conference in 1982. Using a retrospective method, the defining characteristics for Decreased Cardiac Output were described by Kim et al (1984) and are currently those listed by the North American Nursing Diagnosis Association (NANDA) (Carroll-Johnson, 1989) (see Table 19.1). Validation of these etiologies and defining characteristics has been undertaken in a critically ill population (Dougherty, 1985).

This chapter focuses on the nursing diagnosis Decreased Cardiac Output for an elderly population. Cardiovascular changes associated with aging are discussed and a nursing intervention is proposed that can be used in the treatment of Decreased Cardiac Output. A case study provides an empirical illustration of Decreased Cardiac Output in an elderly person and demonstrates the linkage between the nursing diagnosis and interventions.

SIGNIFICANCE FOR THE ELDERLY

Cardiovascular disease is the major cause of death worldwide in persons over 65 years of age. In the United States alone, 72% of persons over age 65 have some type of cardiovascular (CV) disease (Rodstein, 1979), and 12,000 of these people die annually (U.S. Department of Health and Human Services, 1984). By the sixth decade of life, maximal coronary artery blood flow provides the CV system with 35% less blood than in previous years (Coyne and Hojlo, 1985). The reduction in work response of the left ventricle at rest is due to a decrease in stroke volume, a decrease in cardiac output, and a delay in contractile recovery. Under normal conditions the aged heart is able to maintain adequate function to sustain an active life, but sudden demands for more oxygen are poorly tolerated.

Table 19.1

Decreased Cardiac Output

NANDA (CARROLL-JOHNSON, 1989)

Definition: A state in which the blood pumped by an individual's heart is sufficiently reduced that it is inadequate to meet the need of the body's tissues

Etiologies/Related Factors

Mechanical
  Alteration in preload
  Alteration in afterload
  Alteration in inotropic changes in heart
Electrical
  Alterations in rate
  Alterations in rhythm
  Alteration in conduction
Structural

Defining Characteristics

Variations in hemodynamic readings
Arrhythmias; ECG changes
Fatigue
Jugular vein distention
Cyanosis; pallor of skin and
    mucous membranes
Oliguria; anuria
Decreased peripheral pulses
Cold, clammy skin
Rales
Dyspnea

DOUGHERTY

Definition: The inability of the heart to supply the amount of oxygenated blood needed for the body's metabolic requirements

Etiologies/Related Factors

Alterations in preload/filling pressure
  Decreased systemic venous return
  Decreased venous pressure or tone
  Decreased pulmonary venous volume
  Increased intrathoracic pressure
  Increased pericardial pressure
  Atrial arrnythmias
Alterations in ventricular contractility
  Increased myocardial oxygen consumption
  Decreased myocardial oxygen delivery
  Drugs affecting the contractile state of the left ventricle
Alteration in afterload/peripheral resistance
  Substances causing vasoconstriction or increasing systemic vas-
    cular resistance
  Aortic valvular disease
  High mean arterial pressure
  Pulmonary artery hypertension
  Pulmonary obstruction
  Increased pulmonary vascular resistance

Defining Characteristics

Cardiac arrhythmias	Cough	Weight gain of 10 or more pounds
Elevated serum enzymes	Hemoptysis	Lift or heave in the chest wall
Elevated BUN and creatinine	Rales	Fatigue, weakness
ECG changes (ST and T wave)	Chest pain	Confusion
Tachycardia	Heart murmurs	Decreased attention span or memory
S_3 and S_4	Jugular venous distention	lapse
Dyspnea	Enlarged liver and spleen	Anxiety
Orthopnea	Positive hepatojugular reflex	Insomnia
Paroxysmal nocturnal dyspnea	Ascites	Cold, clammy, diaphoretic, cyanotic skin
Wheezing	Nausea and vomiting	Slow capillary refill
Pleural effusion	Anorexia	Reduced peripheral skin temperature
Pulsus alterans	Abdominal distention	Decreased urine output
Chest film indicating congestion	Edema in dependent body parts	Cheyne–Stokes respirations

General risk factors that can cause stress and strain on the heart include obesity, smoking, emotional states, lack of exercise, constant intake of calories and animal fats, and other preexisting conditions (Ebersole and Hess, 1985). The poor response of cardiac function under stress in the elderly can be attributed to limited cardiac reserve (Syzek, 1976).

Significant changes that occur in the heart of an aged person are decreased cardiac output, a heart rate that remains unchanged or slower at rest, and an increase in time required for the heart rate to return to baseline level once it is elevated (Ebersole and Hess, 1985). Reduced efficiency and contractile strength of cardiac muscle are reflected in a cardiac output that decreases by 1% per year from the baseline of 5 liters/minute. Under resting situations or nonstressful conditions, lowered cardiac output is adequate for the older person because metabolic demands are minimal, basal metabolic rate has declined, and the body in general is smaller.

Decreased Cardiac Output becomes important when the elderly person is physically or mentally stressed by illness, activity, worry, or excitement. Catecholamines and other hormones that influence the force and speed of contractions decrease in amount, producing a longer interval between contractions, a decreased cardiac force, and a greater energy demand on the myocardium. Tachycardia is not as profound in an older person and takes longer to return to baseline. Lower contractile strength, decreased cardiac output, and reduced hormone stimulation together cause the heart to respond to increased oxygen demands with less efficiency and greater energy expenditure.

Normal sinus rhythm is the expected normal rhythm of the elderly person's heartbeart. Beginning at age 60 there is a significant decrease in the number of pacer cells, and by age 75, less than 10% remain. A heart rate of less than 50 is not uncommon. Arrhythmias are usually attributed to myocardial damage.

Changes in the CV system with advanced age include a reduced cardiac output, reduced stroke volume, and less capacity to adapt to environmental stressors with increases in heart rate. It is recognized that in an elderly population, Decreased Cardiac Output is most frequently a chronic problem or an acute exacerbation of a chronic problem. However, much more needs to be learned about cardiac output changes among elderly persons.

DEFINITION OF DECREASED CARDIAC OUTPUT

The function of viability of all body tissues is dependent on an adequate supply of oxygen and other nutrients from the circulating blood, and this supply is primarily determined by the cardiac output. The cardiac output must be great enough to deliver the amount of blood flow that is required to the tissues, no more and no less. Adaptation is the most remarkable of the characteristics of the heart; it alters its activity according to the requirements of the body as a whole (Starling, 1926). As indicated by the formula, cardiac output (CO) is equal to heart rate (HR) times stroke volume (SV).

$$CO = HR \times SV$$

When normal heart rate ranges from 60 to 100 beats/minute and is multiplied by a normal stroke volume of 60 to 130 cc, the product is a normal cardiac output of 4 to 8 liters/minute (Badeer, 1981; Guyton, 1976; Hurst, 1986).

Methods to measure cardiac output have been perfected in the last decade, so cardiac output now can be monitored with relative ease and safety. The development of the Swan-Ganz catheter has tremendously advanced the management and treatment of critically ill cardiac patients in the last decade. Cardiac output can be measured using the Fick principle, the indicator-dilution method, or thermodilution methods. The reader is referred to aphysiology text for in-depth explanations of these methods.

The inability of the heart to supply the amount of oxygenated blood needed for the body's metabolic requirements is termed pump failure or Decreased Cardiac Output. Decreased Cardiac Output has two major forms: congestive heart failure and cardiogenic shock (Loeb and Gunnar, 1981; Perloff, 1970; Weber and Janicki, 1979). Viewed on a continuum (Figure 19.1), congestive heart failure is a milder state of Decreased Cardiac Output, generally associated with a mortality rate of 40% and suggesting milder symptoms than cardiogenic shock or the other end of the continuum. Cardiogenic shock represents the most profound state of Decreased Cardiac Output, with mortality rates at 80% or higher and an array of symptoms involving all organ systems (Carey and Hughes, 1969; Foster and Canty, 1980; Loeb and Gunnar, 1981). The patient may stabilize at various points on the continuum as medical and nursing interventions are implemented. Progression from one state of Decreased Cardiac Output to another can occur rapidly and depends in part on the antecedent condition responsible for the decreased ability of the ventricles to pump blood to the body tissues.

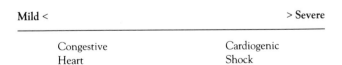

Figure 19.1

Decreased cardiac output continuum.

ETIOLOGIES/RELATED FACTORS

Humans are equipped with one heart composed of two distinct pumps. Each pump is separated by extremely complex vascular systems, which in turn are controlled by nervous and humoral systems (Burch, 1977; Guyton, 1976; Hurst, 1986). The regulation of cardiac output is determined by factors controlling heart rate and stroke volume.

The heart rate determinants of cardiac output are regulated by the rate of discharge from the sinoatrial node, change in pacemaker control by the sympathetic and parasympathetic nervous systems, local metabolic demands, and other neural control mechanisms (Badeer, 1981; Chapman, 1965; Harrison, 1977). Stimulation of the sympathetic nervous system will cause increases both in heart rate and in the strength of contraction by releasing norepinephrine at nerve-ending sites throughout the heart muscle (Guyton, 1981). Stimulation of the parasympathetic nervous system produces a decrease in heart rate only. An increase in heart rate alone can increase cardiac output three-fold within a limited time frame. Bradycardia does not always produce a decrease in cardiac output because stroke volume will increase to compensate for the drop. In patients with fixed stroke volume, decreases in heart rate will produce reductions in cardiac output, as in the patient who has suffered a myocardial infarction (Fowler, 1980; Segal, 1975; Shepard and Van Houtte, 1979). Tachycardia develops as a compensatory mechanism for decreased cardiac output. Increases in heart rate cause increases in myocardial oxygen consumption and decreases in coronary filling time, both of which may not be tolerated for extended periods of time in patients with already compromised cardiac reserve (Hurst, 1986; Kirklin and Rastelli, 1967; Loeb and Gunnar, 1981).

Stroke volume influences on cardiac output are determined by preload or filling pressure, myocardial contractility, and afterload or peripheral resistance (Haas, 1979; Harrison, 1977; Mueller, 1980) (see Table 19.1). Cardiac output under normal conditions is regulated primarily by the needs of various tissues for blood. Preload is the volume of blood that fills both ventricles during diastole, the right heart receiving blood from the systemic circulation. Factors affecting preload include systemic venous return, venous pressure or tone, pulmonary venous volume, intrathoracic pressure, pericardial pressure, and atrial contraction (Berne and Levy, 1981; Burch, 1977).

A decrease in venous return due to loss in intravascular volume, from hemorrhage, diuresis, or vomiting or a loss of fluid into the interstitial space due to burns, sepsis, or electrolyte imbalances, will decrease preload. Venous capacity or tone decreases with vasodilation of peripheral vessels and will in turn decrease preload. Pulmonary blood flow determines left ventricular preload and may be affected by right ventricular contractility or pulmonary embolism. During inspiration, intrathoracic pressure becomes slightly negative to enhance venous return, but with high inspiratory pressures as in mechanical ventilation, pulmonary hypertension, or tension pneumothorax, it will again decrease preload. Increases in pericardial pressure due to pericardial effusion, tamponade, or pericarditis prohibit blood from entering the right atrium and cause it to collapse. Venous return to the heart and preload are thus decreased.

Under normal conditions, atrial contraction occurring at the end of ventricular diastole contributes 30% of the volume of ventricular filling. If this atrial kick is lost or absent, as in atrial arrhythmias (atrial fibrillation, atrial flutter, paroxysmal atrial tachycardia), or is inappropriately timed, as in atrioventricular (AV) block, junctional rhythm, ventricular arrhythmias, or paced rhythm of the ventricles, cardiac output will fall. Thus, factors that cause a decrease in preload have the potential for causing decreases in cardiac output. The indicator of preload for the right ventricle is central venous pressure (CVP) and for the left ventricle is pulmonary artery wedge pressure (PAW) (Foster and Canty, 1980; Fowler, 1980; Swan et al, 1970) (see Table 19.1).

Ventricular contractility and distensibility is best explained by the Frank–Starling Law of the Heart, which states, "The energy of contraction is a function of the length of the muscle fiber" (Starling, 1926;261) (see Table 19.1). Within physiologic limits, the larger the volume the heart must pump, the greater the force of contraction.

The ability of the heart to contract is decreased by factors causing increased myocardial oxygen consumption, such as tachyarrhythmias, an enlarged ventricular diameter, high afterload, primary myocardial disease (cardiomyopathy), coronary artery disease, and myocardial infarction, all of which can cause myocardial ischemia with a secondary decrease in contractility. Ventricular contractility is also affected by factors that decrease myocardial oxygen delivery such as hypoxemia, acidosis, narrowing of the coronary arteries, and low arterial pressure. Drugs known to affect the contractile state of the ventricle include lidocaine, quinidine, propranolol, Pronestyl, and disopyramide (Kirklin and Rastelli, 1967; Loeb and Gunnar, 1981; Mueller, 1980; Sidd, 1978). Within certain limits, the heart will pump whatever amount of blood that flows into it without significant changes in cardiac output, unless contractility is severely affected (see Table 19.1).

Afterload is the resistance to blood flow and is determined by the diameter of arterioles in the pulmonary and systemic circulations (Haas, 1979; Levine, 1976) (see Table 19.1). Factors determining left ventricular afterload include cold temperatures or any substance that causes vasoconstriction and increases systemic vascular resistance; drugs such as Levophed, Aramine, epinephrine, and dopamine in high doses; pulmonary artery hypertension;

aortic valvular disease; or high mean arterial pressure (Badeer, 1981; Haas, 1979; Weber and Janicki, 1979).

Right ventricular afterload is determined by the pulmonary circulation. If pulmonary vessels constrict or obstruction to pulmonary blood flow is present, an increase in pulmonary vascular resistance occurs with subsequent increase in afterload of the right ventricle (RV). This will in turn decrease preload of the left heart (Berne and Levy, 1981; Foster and Canty, 1980). Factors affecting right ventricular afterload include any condition causing pulmonary constriction such as an increase in alveolar pO_2 or decrease in arterial pO_2, pulmonary embolism that causes obstruction to blood flow, pulmonary vascular defects, and vasoactive substances such as histamine, which will increase pulmonary vascular resistance.

Decreased Cardiac Ouput has been described as an inability of the heart to pump adequate amounts of blood to the tissues in order to meet the body's needs. The etiologic factors have been discussed in a framework of the determinants of cardiac output, namely heart rate and stroke volume. Although the mechanism of control differs for the heart rate and stroke volume, both are equally important in maintaining an adequate cardiac output to meet the body's demand. Intervening variables that may cause variances in cardiac output include age, sex, body size, and the 24-hour biologic rhythm cycle (Mattea, 1976; Miller and Helander, 1979). Next, defining characteristics of Decreased Cardiac Output are explored according to backward and forward effects of decreased blood flow to the tissue.

DEFINING CHARACTERISTICS

Under normal conditions, the ventricles of the heart are able to pump an amount of blood appropriate to the venous return and needs of the body. The indicators of Decreased Cardiac Output are a result of decreased blood flow to organs, redistribution of blood flow within organs, and congestion and edema of organs (Badeer, 1981). Clinical manifestations of decreased cardiac output represent an end stage when normal compensatory mechanisms are no longer adequate. It is important to realize that a disequilibrium has existed for an extended period of time before symptoms appear. Although there is overlap, indicators of heart function can be divided into left-sided and right-sided events. Failure frequently begins on one side before the other. The left ventricle is usually the first to fail. Therefore, left-sided dysfunction precedes right-sided dysfunction when the origin is cardiac. The defining characteristics of Decreased Cardiac Output are discussed according to left-sided and right-sided symptoms (Hurst, 1986; Kirklin and Rastelli, 1967).

A decreased pumping efficiency of the left ventricle (LV) causes both backward and forward effects. The forward effect is decreased tissue perfusion to organs, and the backward effect is increased volume and pressure in the pulmonary circulation. As the ventricle becomes less able to empty completely and effective cardiac output or cardiac index at rest falls, blood remains in the left ventricle at the end of systole. In an attempt to augment the amount of blood ejected from the left ventricle, the heart enlarges and increases its rate and force of contraction (Starling, 1926). This compensatory mechanism, primarily governed by the sympathetic nervous system, can maintain cardiac output for a time but eventually becomes ineffective and the heart decompensates. As decompensation progresses, more blood accumulates in the left ventricle and causes further dilation and hypertrophy (Burch, 1977; Guyton, 1981). Tachycardia and pulsus alterans (alternation of one strong beat with one weak beat during sinus rhythm) may be noted. Consequently, left ventricular end diastolic pressure (LVEDP) increases and a third heart sound (S3) appears. The third heart sound is produced by an imbalance between the volume of left ventricular inflow during the rapid filling phase of diastole and the inability of the left ventricle to accommodate the flow (Shepard and Van Houtte, 1979). These are early and classic signs of beginning failure of the heart. The fourth heart sound (S4) is produced late in diastole and is created when the atria contract with resistance to ventricular filling. It indicates decreased myocardial compliance and rising left ventricular pressure (Berne and Levy, 1981; Segal, 1975).

As pressure continues to increase in the left ventricle and blood backs up from the left ventricle to the left atrium (LA), a rise in LA pressure will be noted. Eventually pulmonary artery (PA) and venous pressures will increase, pulmonary artery wedge pressure will increase above plasma oncotic pressure in the lung, and signs of pulmonary vascular congestion develop. As fluid begins to accumulate in the lungs, more specific symptoms such as dyspnea, orthopnea, paroxysmal nocturnal dyspnea, and Cheyne-Stokes respirations will appear (Carey and Hughes, 1969; Shepard and Van Houtte, 1979).

A dry cough develops early in the failure phase of Decreased Cardiac Output as fluid acts as an irritant in the interstitial spaces. As the alveoli become filled with fluid, the cough will become productive, and occasionally pulmonary vessels will rupture, producing hemoptysis. Rales develop when pulmonary capillary pressure has exceeded normal plasma osmotic pressure, and fluid moves from the pulmonary capillary to the alveoli (Chapman and Mitchell, 1965; Mueller, 1980). Chest pain, wheezing, and pleural effusion may also be noted. Rales are first noted in dependent lobes of lung tissue. As pulmonary edema develops, they will gradually become diffuse and bilateral.

Increases in PA pressures will continue to affect the right heart, resulting in decreased output from the right heart. As pressure in the right heart rises, congestion in the venous system, abdominal organs, and capillary interstitial spaces occurs. This rising pressure causes an increase in right ventricular end diastolic pressure (RVEDP), increasing right atrium (RA) pressure, increasing CVP, and backup of blood from the right heart into the venous system (Foster and Canty, 1980; Perloff, 1970). Jugular venous distention (JVD) can be used to determine a general estimate of right heart venous return and RA pressure. An elevation of the JVD more than 1 to 2 cm above the Angle of Louis at 45 degrees signals increased RA pressure and may even produce observable venous pulsations (Berne and Levy, 1981; Burch, 1977). Increased pressure in the inferior vena cava causes the liver and spleen to become enlarged and congested. The patient may complain of abdominal pain, and the hepatojugular reflux may be positive. Ascites, edema of the bowel, nausea, vomiting, anorexia, and abdominal distention may also accompany venous congestion (Loeb and Gunnar, 1981; Mueller, 1980; Segal, 1975).

Venous system pressure continues to rise, causing edema in dependent body parts such as the sacrum and lower extremities. The patient may experience a weight gain of 10 pounds or more. With advancing decreases in cardiac output, fluid may accumulate in pericardial cavities. As the work and forcefulness of the RV decreases, a lifting or heave in the chest wall along the sternal border may be produced. In either RV or LV failure, rising pressure within the heart produces apposition of valves, resulting in murmurs (Perloff, 1970).

The forward effects of Decreased Cardiac Output are primarily the result of decreased blood flow to organs and tissues and usually appear early in the cycle. A decrease in blood flow to the musculoskeletal system produces complaints of fatigue, weakness, and restlessness. The patient may complain that his or her energy level is gone and may exhibit changes in posture, gait, and speech (Carey and Hughes, 1969). Blood flow to the heart and brain will be maintained by the sympathetic nervous system at the expense of the skin, kidneys, and muscle. Central nervous system signs of decreased perfusion are manifested by confusion, agitation, decreased attention span with memory lapse, and anxiety. The patient may complain of insomnia. As blood flow is decreased to the skin in response to vasoconstriction produced by the sympathetic nervous system, the skin becomes cold and clammy with slow capillary refill, diaphoretic, cyanotic, and pale. This redistribution of blood to the core organs will cause a decrease in skin temperature in peripheral areas, while the trunk remains warm (Fowler, 1980).

As vasoconstriction occurs in splanchnic, mesenteric, and renal vascular beds, a decrease in mean arterial pressure will decrease urine output. The glomerular filtration rate is decreased and is interpreted by the kidney as hypovolemia, which stimulates renin production, angiotensin, and further decreases in urine output. The kidney begins to conserve sodium and water via stimulation of the aldosterone and antidiuretic hormone mechanisms and will increase systemic blood volume (Perloff, 1970; Sidd, 1978).

As cardiac output becomes more severely decreased, the patient may begin to move toward the cardiogenic shock end of the continuum. Cardiogenic shock represents the most severe impairment of cardiac output. The exact cause is not known but can be predicted when greater than 40% of the heart muscle has become dysfunctional (Foster and Canty, 1980). There are usually profound decreases in stroke volume and arterial pressure; therefore, organs and tissues are severely deprived of oxygen. As a result, cells divert to anaerobic glycolysis, producing metabolic acidosis.

For survival, the sympathetic nervous system maintains perfusion to vital organs, with widespread arteriole and venule constriction, tachycardia, increased forcefulness of contraction, and dilation of coronary arteries. When cardiogenic shock is allowed to ensue and continue over an extended time period, compensatory mechanisms fail and death results (Foster and Canty, 1980).

Various biochemical and laboratory data also serve as indicators of decreased cardiac output. These include decreased ejection fraction below 40%, elevated serum enzymes (creatine phosphokinase [CPK], lactic dehydrogenase [LDH], asparate transferase [AST], and the isoenzymes of CPK and LDH), elevated blood urea nitrogen and creatinine, electrolyte imbalances, decreases in hemoglobin and hematocrit, electrocardiograph (ECG) changes (ST and T wave changes), and chest film findings indicating congestion (Perloff, 1970; Weber and Janicki, 1979).

ASSESSMENT

Tools for determining the severity of Decreased Cardiac Output based on clinical signs alone have not been developed. Critical defining characteristics for predicting cardiac output states also have not been identified. Assessment Guide 19.1 presents a cardiac output assessment tool developed by the author for research purposes. The cardiac output tool is divided into two parts. The first section focuses on assessing the etiology of the diagnosis Decreased Cardiac Output. The second portion focuses on the defining characteristics and consists of subjective, objective, and laboratory assessments. Many of the items on the initial tool were included for research purposes and do not have clinical relevance for making the diagnosis Decreased Cardiac Output. The tool presented here has not been adapted for use or tested in clinical settings or for an elderly population.

CASE STUDY

Decreased Cardiac Output

Mr. D is an 86-year-old widower who has become a resident of a long-term care facility after a recent hospitalization. His wife died over 10 years ago, and he has had repeated admissions to the hospital for congestive heart failure (CHF) over the past 2 years. At his last hospitalization, he was found to be in digoxin toxicity, and his serum potassium was 2.1. It was discovered after talking with Mr. D that he was not reliable in taking his medications or managing his finances. He has lost 44 pounds since his last medical appointment 1 year ago. Mr. D is alert, but he is oriented to place and time only occasionally. His short-term memory is very poor.

Mr. D's past medical history is significant for a myocardial infarction (MI) 5 years ago, which was complicated by cardiogenic shock. His last ejection fraction was 28%, and his ECGs continue to demonstrate ST and T wave abnormalities with frequent PVCs. His skin is warm and dry. Mr. D has smoked three packs per day for 28 years and occasionally drinks alcohol at night to induce sleep. He is able to ambulate 50 feet without dyspnea but cannot climb stairs without chest pain. He has frequent bouts of Decreased Cardiac Output when he overexerts himself or when he forgets to take his medication.

Currently Mr. D has a productive cough of white sputum in small amounts. His chest has course rales bilaterally in the bases. His vital signs are stable. Both ankles are edematous, and his feet turn dark purple when in a dependent position. His heart sounds are normal. He sleeps with three pillows at night and frequently awakens because of coughing. Mr D's priority nursing diagnosis is Decreased Cardiac Output related to myocardial destruction as evidenced by an ejection fraction less than 60%, cough, chest pain and dyspnea with minimal activity, rales in the chest, ankle edema, and three-pillow orthopnea.

NURSING INTERVENTIONS

Nursing intervention implies that a thorough assessment and accurate diagnosis have already been undertaken. Some nurses argue that independent nursing interventions do not exist for the diagnosis Decreased Cardiac Output. This discussion will introduce surveillance as one nursing intervention appropriate for the treatment of Decreased Cardiac Output in an elderly population.

Surveillance

The nursing intervention of surveillance is employed in many situations in which a particular health problem is developing or is likely to develop. *Webster's*

Dictionary defines *surveillance* as, "to watch over, a close watch, a vigil, to look over and examine closely, or to view or study as a whole." Surveillance is similar to observation and in nursing situations is called monitoring. For purposes of this discussion, surveillance is defined as the application of behavioral and cognitive processes in the systematic collection of information used to make judgments and predictions about an older individual's health status (Dougherty and Molen, 1985).

The behavioral component of surveillance involves the collection of information from both primary and secondary sources. Watching, listening, and measuring are basic behavioral activities of surveillance. In the nursing situation the behavioral component of surveillance involves direct observation of the elderly patient to survey mental and physical status, including inspection, palpation, percussion, and auscultation. Methods include taking vital signs, checking the color of skin and mucous membranes, auscultating heart and lung sounds, palpating pedal pulses, noting edema and temperature of extremities, recording reactions to medications, and monitoring the environment (Baldwin, 1983; Owen, 1982; Pool, 1976). All observations should be tailored to suit the individual patient, depending on the acuity and the nature of the health problems encountered.

The cognitive component of surveillance includes studying, interpreting, analyzing, evaluating, and intercepting data to indicate a range of probabilities and isolating those factors that are influencing a given situation (Dulles, 1963). In order to do this, the act of gathering information must be a reliable process. A theoretical knowledge base underlying the information collection is an essential part of the cognitive component.

Surveillance involves knowing both where to look and when to expect a change in response to a given treatment (Karch, 1976). Perception and the ability to relate sensory data to a relevant knowledge base are two important elements of surveillance. A basic understanding of normal and abnormal findings is essential because we see only what we know (Winslow, 1976). Establishing a baseline and preparing a systematic method for surveillance activities are essential components of this intervention. The essence of surveillance is piecing together tiny items of information, which, when taken by themselves, may appear to be unimportant. Surveillance is more than observation in that it includes the collection of vast amounts of information and encompasses a judgment or interpretation made about the data collected.

CASE STUDY

Nursing Interventions

When Mr. D was admitted to the nursing home after he recovered from his acute exacerbation with CHF, surveillance over his environment and physical symptoms was instituted with the goal of preventing further bouts of decreased cardiac output and subsequent hospitalizations. The following parameters of interest were monitored on a flow sheet by the primary nurse every 8 hours for the first 3 days after he returned to the long-term care unit: vital signs, lung and heart sounds, weight, cough and sputum production, jugular venous distention, ankle edema, activity tolerance, dyspnea, sleep patterns, number of cigarettes smoked, mental status, and reactions to medications. Serum potassium and digoxin levels were monitored when available.

Mr. D's living environment was also monitored and adjusted to reduce excessive activity and stair climbing. Mr. D moved from his current room to one that was across the hall from the dining room. He now is given a whirlpool bath instead of his regular shower. During the exercise class, Mr. D does mild arm and leg exercises while sitting in a chair. He has been asked to quit smoking. Siderails have been added to the walls of his room near his bed, in the bathroom around the stool and by the tub, and along the halls in the activity room. During planned exercise periods and walking, Mr. D's vital signs are monitored as well as the incidence of chest pain and dyspnea.

The patient outcome to be achieved is a cardiac output adequate to meet the oxygen demands of his body given the amount of functional myocardium that remains. Specific indicators that this goal has been achieved are vital signs within normal limits, absence of ankle edema, clear breath sounds, absence of chest pain and dyspnea, and performance of activities of daily living (ADLs).

Tools

Flow sheets are the tools used in most agencies for implementing the nursing intervention of surveillance. Two elements are essential to any surveillance tool: (1) a time frame, measured in minutes to hours; and (2) the parameter of interest, such as blood pressure or heart rate. The current health status of the elderly individual as well as the medical and nursing diagnoses determine the frequency of data collection and type of information needed. Successful surveillance for the older individual with chronic cardiovascular problems depends on the nurse's ability to diagnose the problem requiring the intervention of surveillance and then to choose theappropriate parameters of interest for monitoring. Successful integration of the data, making predictions based on the data, and taking actions that stem from this information are the goals of surveillance.

OUTCOMES

For the elderly individual with the nursing diagnosis Decreased Cardiac Output in the chronic state, one goal of nursing intervention is to assist the older person to conserve energy and balance oxygen demands with resources (Baldwin, 1983; Ebersole and Hess, 1985). Surveillance of the elderly individual's current living environment as well as physical symptoms would be the priority goal. The living environment can be examined and monitored for distances walked, energy expended on wasted activities, location of objects and other necessities frequently used for ADLs, stairs to be climbed, objects to be lifted, diet consumed, and utilities used to prepare meals (Ebersole and Hess, 1985). From efforts made at monitoring the environment, other suggested interventions directed toward balancing oxygen demand and supply may include consciously pacing daily activities and rest periods, rearranging the environment for easy accessibility to objects to reduce fatigue, assisting with meal preparation, placing articles of use at waist level, placing chairs along walkways to encourage rest periods when exercising, and combining standing with sitting exercises for those individuals with other chronic health problems. For specific surveillance parameters of physical symptoms see Table 19.2.

Surveillance of physical symptoms includes monitoring vital signs, checking pedal pulses, noting activities that result in chest pain or dyspnea,. monitoring cardiac rhythm and response to CV drugs, observing mental status and behavior, evaluating tolerance to activity, noting external jugular veins for distention, palpating for dependent edema and for temperature of the extremities, auscultating heart and lung sounds, and monitoring lab values (Baldwin, 1983; Owen, 1982).

The overall goal for an older person experiencing a chronic decrease in cardiac output is to balance oxygen demands and resources of the myocardium in order to achieve homeostasis while performing ADLs. The workload of the heart can also be reduced by modifying stress,

Table 19.2

Surveillance Parameters for Decreased Cardiac Output

Vital signs
Pedal pulses
Activities causing chest pain or dyspnea
Cardiac rhythm
Response to cardiovascular drugs
Mental status
Behavior
Activity tolerance
Jugular venous distention (JVD)
Dependent edema
Temperature of extremities
Heart and lung sounds
Lab values

Table 19.3

Outcome Criteria for Decreased
Cardiac Output Using the Nursing
Intervention of Surveillance

Vital signs within normal limits
Cardiac rhythm is normal sinus rhythm
Clear lungs
Normal heart sounds
No cough
Warm and pink extremities
No dependent edema
No JVD
Pupils equal and reactive to light
Normal mentation or behavior for that person
Minimal chest pain or dyspnea with activity
Activity tolerance remains stable
Normal lab values
No chest pain or dyspnea at rest

smoking, obesity, excessive activity, and fluid retention (Stier, 1986).

Evaluation

Evaluation is the ongoing measurement of goal attainment in relation to the stated nursing diagnosis. For the nursing diagnosis Decreased Cardiac Output in an elderly population, the overall goal is to balance the myocardial oxygen demands and resources in order to prevent acute exacerbations of Decreased Cardiac Output and, it is hoped, to prevent death. When physical symptoms and activity tolerance are carefully monitored, further decreases in cardiac output can be prevented. Table 19.3 outlines criteria that can serve as indicators that the nursing intervention of surveillance has been effective in aborting further advances in an already compromised cardiac output.

SUMMARY

Decreased Cardiac Output related to congestive heart failure and cardiogenic shock is a frequent problem for elderly persons. Cardiovascular changes associated with aging include decreased cardiac output, unchanged heart rate at rest, increased time for the heart rate to return to baseline once it is elevated, and decreased stroke volume. Defining characteristics are categorized according to left-sided and right-sided symptoms. A case study illustrates Decreased Cardiac Output, surveillance nursing intervention, and outcomes evaluation for an elderly man in a long-term care institution.

ASSESSMENT GUIDE 19.1

Cardiac Output Assessment Tool

Study number_____ Age_____

ID number_____ Sex_____

Time/Date_____

General appearance and medical history:

1. **Etiology:**	Yes	No	2. **Subjective symptoms:**	Yes	No
rheumatic fever	( )	( )	chest pain	( )	( )
heart murmur	( )	( )	shortness of breath	( )	( )
myocardial infarction	( )	( )	fatigue	( )	( )
pericarditis	( )	( )	palpations	( )	( )
pulmonary embolus	( )	( )	anorexia	( )	( )
phlebitis	( )	( )	nausea	( )	( )
stroke	( )	( )	anxiety	( )	( )
valvular disease	( )	( )	cough	( )	( )
arrhythmia	( )	( )	syncope	( )	( )
cardiomyopathy	( )	( )	orthopnea	( )	( )
fluid overload	( )	( )	PND	( )	( )
major trauma	( )	( )	edema	( )	( )
hypertension	( )	( )	weight gain	( )	( )
respiratory disorder	( )	( )	wheezing	( )	( )
other	( )	( )	other	( )	( )

*Total etiology*_____   *Total symptoms*_____

Signs: Key N = normal   A = abnormal   N/A = not applicable

			N	A	N/A
3. Temperature _____ °C oral, rectal, core N = 37°C			( )	( )	( )
4. Heart rate _____ /min.	N = 60–80/min.		( )	( )	( )
5. Respirations _____ /min.	N = 12–16/min.		( )	( )	( )
6. Heart rhythm _____			( )	( )	( )

N = sinus rhythm 60–80/minute *see also EKG

7. Arterial pressure   cuff _____ arterial line _____

			N	A	N/A
systolic _____ mmHg.	N = 90–140 mmHg.		( )	( )	( )
diastolic _____ mmHg.	N = 60–90 mmHg.		( )	( )	( )
mean _____ mmHg.	N = 70–90 mmHg.		( )	( )	( )

8. Pulmonary artery pressures

			N	A	N/A
systolic _____ mmHg.	N = 20–30 mmHg.		( )	( )	( )
diastolic _____ mmHg.	N = 5–16 mmHg.		( )	( )	( )
mean _____ mmHg.	N = 10–15 mmHg.		( )	( )	( )
wedge _____ mmHg.	N = 4–12 mmHg.		( )	( )	( )
cardiac output _____ L/min.	N = 4–8 L/minute		( )	( )	( )

			N	A	N/A
9. Skin color _____ N = pink			( )	( )	( )
A = pale, cyanotic, mottled, gray					
10. Skin temperature _____ N = warm/dry			( )	( )	( )
A = hot, cold, diaphoretic, cool, clammy					
11. Neck vein distension (JVD) external jugular _____ cm			( )	( )	( )
from angle of Louis at 45° elevation N = <1–2cm (below)					

ASSESSMENT GUIDE 19.1

Cardiac Output Assessment Tool (Continued)

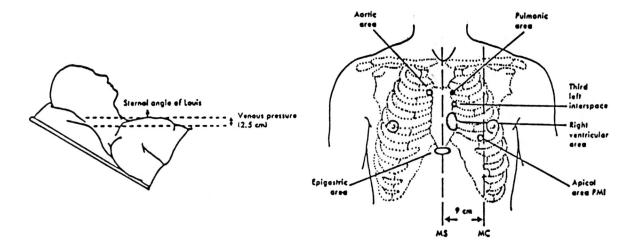

12. Heart sounds (above)

S$_1$ _____ split _____   N = S$_1$>S$_2$ apex   ( )   ( )   ( )

S$_2$ _____ split _____   N = S$_1$< S$_2$ base

A = S$_3$, S$_4$, friction rub, murmur, heaves, thrills, lifts

Describe _____

13. Peripheral pulses O = absent + 1 = abnormal + 2 = normal

carotid	R _____	L _____	R( )	( )	( )
			L( )	( )	( )
brachial	R _____	L _____	R( )	( )	( )
			L( )	( )	( )
radial	R _____	L _____	R( )	( )	( )
			L( )	( )	( )
femoral	R _____	L _____	R( )	( )	( )
			L( )	( )	( )
dorsalis pedis	R _____	L _____	R( )	( )	( )
			L( )	( )	( )
posterior tibial	R _____	L _____	R( )	( )	( )
			L( )	( )	( )

14. Edema

O = absent + 1 = slight indentation + 2 = indentation readily noticeable, disappears 10-15 seconds + 3 = deep indentation disappears 1-2 minutes + 4 = deep indentation present at 5 minutes. (Grade by pressure for 5 seconds)

	N	A	N/A
facial _____ N = O	( )	( )	( )
hand _____	( )	( )	( )
sacral _____	( )	( )	( )
ankle _____	( )	( )	( )
pretibial _____	( )	( )	( )

(Continues)

ASSESSMENT GUIDE 19.1

Cardiac Output Assessment Tool (Continued)

15. Urine output _____ cc/hr   N = average 30 cc/hr   ( )   ( )   ( )

16. Emesis _____   N = none   ( )   ( )   ( )

17. Respiratory pattern   N = inspiration = expiration   ( )   ( )   ( )
A = Kussmall(hyperventilation), Cheyne-Stokes, Biots (shallow with apnea), labored, shallow, ventilator control

Describe _____

18. Accessory muscles to breathe _____ yes _____ no N = none   ( )   ( )   ( )
A = abdominal, thoracic, intercostal, neck

19. Breath sounds N = clear vesicular anterior & posterior   R( )   ( )   ( )
A = rales, rhonchi, wheezes, rubs   L( )   ( )   ( )
R _____ L _____

20. Sputum _____ yes _____ no   color _____ N = none   ( )   ( )   ( )

21. Ascites _____ yes _____ no   Abd. girth _____ N = none   ( )   ( )   ( )
    ( )   ( )   ( )

22. Neurological N = oriented to time, place, and person
A = anxious, restless, confused, slurred speech
If abnormal, see Glasgow Coma Scale below

Total Glasgow Score (3-15) _____ N = 15   ( )   ( )   ( )

Pupils R size _____ reaction _____   R( )   ( )   ( )
    ( )   ( )   ( )
L size _____ reaction _____   L( )   ( )   ( )
    ( )   ( )   ( )

Best Verbal Response		**To Verbal Command Obeys**	6	**Open Eyes**		Pupils	Reactive +
Oriented and Converses	5	**To Painful Stimulus Best Motor**		Spontaneously	4		**Non Reactive −**
Disoriented and Converses	4	**Response**		To Verbal Command	3		**Closed C**
Inappropriate words	3	Localizes Pain	5	To Pain	2		● 5
Incomprehensible sounds	2	Flexion-Withdrawal	4	No Response	1	· 1	● 6
No Response	1	Flexion-Abnormal (Decorticate Rigidity)	3			◉ 2	● 7
		Extension (Decerebrate Rigidity)	2			● 3	● 8
		No Response	1			● 4	

23. Significant Lab Data   N   A   N/A
EKG N = sinus rhythm, PR .12–.20 QRS .06–.10 QT .36–.44, no ectopic beats, ST or T wave changes,   ( )   ( )   ( )
no Q waves, rate 60–80 minute, with + P & T waves.
Describe:

ASSESSMENT GUIDE 19.1

Cardiac Output Assessment Tool (Continued)

Enzymes CPK _____	N = 40–200 IU/L	( )	( )	( )
LDH _____	N = 100–225 IU/L	( )	( )	( )
AST _____	N = 7.5–40 IU/L	( )	( )	( )
CPK-MB _____	N = <2%	( )	( )	( )
LDH Isos 1 _____ 2 _____ 3 _____ 4 _____ 5 _____ N = 1<2		( )	( )	( )

ABG N = pH 7.35–7.45, pCO_2 35–45mm, pO_2 70–100mm HCO_3 22–26mm.   ( ) ( ) ( )

pH _____ pCO_2 _____ pO_2 _____ HCO_3 _____

Ejection Fraction _____ N = 60%		( )	( )	( )
Electrolytes Na _____ mEq/L	N = 136–142mEq/L	( )	( )	( )
K _____ mEq/L	N = 3.5–5 mEq/L	( )	( )	( )
Cl _____ mEq/L	N = 95–103mEq/L	( )	( )	( )
BUN _____ mg/dl	N = 8–18mg/dl	( )	( )	( )
Creatinine _____ mg/dl	N = .6–1.2mg/dl	( )	( )	( )
Hemoglobin _____ Gm/100cc	N = 13.5–18♂ 12–16♀	( )	( )	( )
Hematocrit _____ %	N = 40–54%♂ 38–47%♀	( )	( )	( )

Chest film N = normal heart size, clear lung fields, no pleural effusion, congestion, or interstitial edema.   ( ) ( ) ( )
Describe:

Total abnormal signs _____ Total signs & symptoms _____

References

Badeer HS: Cardiac output and venous return as interdependent and independent variables. *Cardiology* 1981; 67:65–72.

Baldwin PJ: Nursing care of the elderly person with an acute cardiovascular problem. *Nurs Clin North Am* 1983; 18:385–394.

Berne RM, Levy MN: *Cardiovascular Physiology*, 4th ed. Mosby, 1981.

Burch GE: Congestive heart failure is not due to low cardiac output per se. *Am Heart J* 1977; 94:269–273.

Carey JS, Hughes RK: Cardiac output—clinical monitoring and management. *Ann Thoracic Surg* 1969; 79:150–176.

Carroll-Johnson R (editor): *Classification of Nursing Diagnoses: Proceedings of the Eighth Conference.* Lippincott, 1989.

Castles MR: Interrater agreement in the use of nursing diagnosis. In: *Classification of Nursing Diagnosis*. Kim MJ, Mortitz DA (editors). McGraw-Hill, 1982.

Chapman CB, Mitchell JH: *Starling on the Heart*. Dawsons of Pall Mall, 1965.

Coyne M, Hojlo K: Physiologic aspects of aging. *Occup Health Nurs* 1985; 33:117–122.

Dougherty CM: The nursing diagnosis of decreased cardiac output. *Nurs Clin North Am* 1985; 20:287–299.

Dougherty CM, Molen MT: Surveillance. In: *Nursing Interventions: Treatments for Nursing Diagnoses*. Bulechek G, McCloskey JC (editors). Saunders, 1985.

Dulles A: *The Craft of Intelligence*. Harper and Row, 1963.

Ebersole P, Hess P: *Toward Healthy Aging: Human Needs and Nursing Response*. Mosby, 1985; 168–239.

Foster SB, Canty KA: Pump failure following myocardial infarction: An overview. *Heart Lung* 1980; 9:293–297.

Fowler N: *Cardiac Diagnosis and Treatment*. Harper and Row, 1980.

Guyton AC: Regulation of cardiac output. *N Eng J Med* 1976; 277:805–812.

Guyton AC: The relationship of cardiac output and arterial pressure control. *Circulation* 1981; 64(6):1079–1088.

Haas JM: Understanding hemodynamic monitoring: Concepts of preload and afterload. CCO (Sept) 1979; 2:1–8.

Harrison T: *Principles of Internal Medicine.* McGraw-Hill, 1977.

Hubalik KT: *Nursing Diagnosis Associated With Heart Failure in Critical Care Nursing.* (Unpublished Master's Thesis.) University of Chicago, Chicago, IL, 1981.

Hurst JW: *The Heart,* 7th ed. McGraw-Hill, 1986.

Karch AM: This assessment habit saves lives. *RN* (Oct) 1976; 76:42–44.

Kim MJ et al: Clinical use of nursing diagnosis in cardiovascular nursing. In: *Classification of Nursing Diagnosis.* Kim MJ, Moritz DA (editors). McGraw-Hill, 1982.

Kim MJ et al: Clinical validation of cardiovascular nursing diagnoses. In: *Classification of Nursing Diagnoses.* Kim MJ, McFarland GK, McLane A (editors). Mosby, 1984.

Kirklin JW, Rastelli GC: Low cardiac output after open thoracic operations. *Progr Cardiovasc Dis* 1967; 10:117–122.

Levine H: *Clinical Cardiovascular Physiology.* Grune and Stratton, 1976.

Loeb HS, Gunnar RM: Treatment of pump failure in acute myocardial infarction. *JAMA* 1981; 245:2093–2096.

Mattea EJ: Recognition and management of congestive heart failure. *Hosp Formulary* 1976; 11:447–482.

Miller JC, Helander M: The 24-hour cycle and nocturnal depression of human cardiac output. *Aviation Space Environmental Med* 1979; 50:1139–1144.

Mueller HS: Shock following acute myocardial infarction: Assessment, pathophysiology, and therapy. *CVP* 1980; 8:19–26.

Owen J: Patient observations: Caring for acute respiratory patients. *Nurs Mirror* (Apr) 1982; 154:7–10.

Perloff JK: The clinical manifestations of cardiac failure in adults. *Hosp Pract* (Sept) 1970; 5:43–50.

Pool M: STAT! How do you manage this patient. *J Emergency Nurs* 1976; 25–27.

Rodstein M: Heart disease in the aged. In: *Clinical Geriatrics,* 2d ed. Rossman I (editor). Lippincott, 1979.

Segal L: The heart that fails. *Emergency Med* (Nov) 1975; 7:211–214.

Shepard JT, Van Houtte PM: *The Human Cardiovascular System Facts and Concepts.* Raven Press, 1979.

Sidd JJ: Congestive heart failure. *Orthoped Clin North Am* 1978; 9:745–760.

Starling EH: Regulation of the energy output of the heart. *J Physiol* 1926; 62:243–261.

Stier FL: The nursing process for clients with heart and major blood vessel dysfunction. Pages 729–756 in: *Adult Health Nursing: A Biopsychosocial Approach.* Kneisl CR, Ames SW (editors). Addison-Wesley, 1986; 729–756.

Swan HJC et al: Catheterization of the heart in man with use of a flow-directed balloon-tipped catheter. *New Eng J Med* 1970; 283:451–477.

Syzek BJ: Cardiovascular changes with aging: Implications for nursing. *J Gerontol Nurs* 1976; 2:28.

U.S. Department of Health and Human Services. Advance report of final mortality statistics. *1982 Monthly Vital Statistics Report* 1986; 33:17.

Weber KT, Janicki JS: The heart as a muscle pump system and the concept of heart failure. *Am Heart J* 1979; 98:371–384.

Wessel SL: *Nursing Functions Related to the Nursing Diagnosis "Decreased Cardiac Output."* (Unpublished Master's Thesis.) University of Illinois, Chicago, IL, 1981.

Winslow EH: Visual inspection of the patient with cardiopulmonary disease. *Nurs Digest* (Winter) 1976; 4:20–23.

20

Altered Tissue Perfusion

Margo A. Halm, MA, RN, CCRN

CIRCULATION OF BLOOD IS VITAL FOR THE DELIVERY OF oxygen and nutrients to tissues and for the removal of metabolic waste products. The elderly are especially prone to Altered Tissue Perfusion because of changes that occur in the cardiovascular system during aging. Nurses in both acute and long-term care settings must assess elderly clients for defining characteristics of Altered Tissue Perfusion and institute a plan of care to modify the etiology. Health promotion interventions may help prevent Altered Tissue Perfusion, or, when alterations are already present, can help to maintain self-care abilities and functional health status among the elderly.

The North American Nursing Diagnosis Association (NANDA) provided a conceptual definition of Altered Tissue Perfusion: "The state in which an individual experiences a decrease in nutrition and oxygenation at the cellular level due to a deficit in capillary blood supply" (Carroll-Johnson, 1989;525). Altered Tissue Perfusion is categorized according to renal, cerebral, cardiopulmonary, gastrointestinal, or peripheral systems (Carroll-Johnson,1989). Similar definitions have been proposed by Carpenito (1983) and by Gordon (1982).

The term *ischemia* refers to reduced or absent tissue perfusion. This state may involve local, regional, or compartmental disruptions in circulation (Hart, 1981). This chapter will discuss only local reductions of blood flow and will not include the dynamics of systemic shock.

INCIDENCE OF ALTERED TISSUE PERFUSION IN THE ELDERLY

Cardiovascular problems are among the most common health alterations in the aging population (Wild, 1986). At least 40% of persons over age 65 will die from cardiac disease, 15% from cerebrovascular disease, and 5% secondary to other vascular impairments (Goldman, 1986). Yet, nurse researchers have rarely addressed the incidence of Altered Tissue Perfusion in elderly persons. Four studies that described the prevalence of nursing diagnoses among the elderly and long-term care residents (Hallal, 1985; Leslie, 1981; Hardy et al, 1988; Rantz et al, 1985), did not identify Altered Tissue Perfusion as one of the 30 most frequent nursing diagnoses. Decreased Cardiac Output ranked as the 4th (Rantz et al, 1985) and 12th (Hallal, 1985) most frequent diagnosis, and Fluid Volume Deficit ranked 10th in the Hallal (1985) study.

For 160 patients (Kim et al, 1984) from critical care and general medical-surgical populations (mean age of 60), Alteration in Coronary Circulation was the most frequently identified nursing diagnosis (47% of 160 patients), and Alteration in Peripheral Circulation ranked 7.5 (30% of 160 patients). For 169 chronically ill clients (Hoskins et al, 1986), 80% of whom were between the ages of 55 and 80, Altered Tissue Perfusion was diagnosed in 31% of the sample (49 subjects). Other diagnoses included Potential Decreased Tissue Oxygenation (28% or 44 subjects) and Impaired Circulation, Uncontrolled Hyptertension (15% or 23 subjects).

A number of physiologic changes associated with aging predispose the elderly to Altered Tissue Perfusion. Progressive loss of arterial elasticity occurs as fibers straighten, fragment, and split. This process is associated with increased calcium deposits. Fibrotic thickening of arterial walls increases peripheral vascular resistance and causes hypertension (Blake, 1976; Burggraf and Donlon, 1985; Goldman, 1986). The intima of veins becomes thickened, dilated, and stretched, and the collagenous capillary basement membrane thickens from childhood to old age. This thickening is believed to slow the exchange of nutrients and waste products across the capillary (Goldman, 1986). Increased capillary fragility may also be responsible for delayed wound healing (Burggraf and Donlon, 1985).

Slight variations in blood composition can have significant effects on tissue perfusion (see Table 20.1). The red blood cell count may be reduced from decreased production, decreased survival, or a change in the cell's enzymatic function. Platelets can exhibit increased adhesiveness and shortened life span as a result of reduced activity of the bone marrow (Jeppesen, 1986). These hematologic changes may predispose the elderly to anemia, increased thrombus formation, and prolonged bleeding. Elevated cholesterol levels are associated with the formation of atherosclerotic plaque, which affects systemic blood flow. Reductions in blood volume, not usually evident until at least age 80 (Jeppesen, 1986), may predispose the elderly client to fluid volume deficits and hypovolemia.

Cardiac output decreases 40% between the third and eighth decades as a result of calcification and fibrosis of the mitral and aortic valves, left ventricular wall thickening, and increased fat infiltration in the right atrium and ventricle. Decreases in cardiac output lead to proportionately greater reductions in renal pefusion than in coronary and cerebral perfusion (Burggraf and Donlon, 1985; Goldman, 1986). Myocardial hypertrophy, particularly in the left ventricular wall, may be the process that reduces coronary perfusion in humans. Cerebral blood flow and oxygen consumption rates show significant declines from age 17 to age 80, with a concomitant increase in cerebrovascular resistance (Goldman, 1986).

Glomerular filtration rate (GFR) and renal plasma flow decrease 46% and 53% respectively from age 20 to age 90 due to sclerosis of the glomeruli and atrophy of the afferent arterioles. Consequently, the filtration fraction (ratio of GFR to renal flow) progressively increases in the sixth or seventh decades. Splanchnic blood flow is also reduced, decreasing drug detoxification and small intestine absorption. In addition, arterial and venous varicosities in the gastrointestinal vasculature may be unrecognized sites of bleeding (Goldman, 1986).

The physiologic consequences of Altered Tissue Perfusion may include fluid and electrolyte imbalances,

Table 20.1

Changes in Selected Laboratory Values for the Elderly

LAB STUDY	NORMAL VALUES	CHANGES IN THE ELDERLY
Red blood cell count	3.6–5.0 million/cu mm (women) 4.2–5.4 million/cu mm (men)	Reduced (especially men)
Platelet count	150,000–350,000/cu mm	Unaffected
Hemoglobin	12–15 g/100 mL (women) 14–16.5 g/100 mL (men)	Reduced (especially men)
Hematocrit	37%–47% women 40%–54% men	Reduced (especially men)
Prothrombin time (PT)	11–16 seconds	Unaffected
Partial thromboplastin time (PTT)	30–45 seconds	Unaffected
Fibrinogen	200–400 mg/dL	Elevated (other clotting factors adequate)
Cholesterol	160–330 mg/dL	Elevated

Sources: Fischbach F: *A Manual of Laboratory Diagnostic Tests.* Lippincott, 1984. Goldman R: Aging changes in structure and function. Pages 73–101 in: *Nursing Management for the Elderly.* Carnevali D. Patrick M (editors). Lippincott, 1986. Jeppesen M: Laboratory values for the elderly. Pages 102–142 in: *Nursing Management for the Elderly.* Carnevali D, Patrick M (editors). Lippincott, 1986.

impaired gas exchange, altered nutrition, sleep deprivation, activity intolerance, impaired mobility, loss of a limb, and multiple system failure. These conditions often produce various degrees of pain and changes in functional health status, especially in the ability to perform activities of daily living (ADLs). Related psychosocial difficulties include anxiety, dependency, depression, powerlessness, social isolation, altered body image, ineffective coping, and health maintenance deficit (Herman, 1986; Linde, 1986; Wild, 1986).

Treatment of these alterations in the elderly has serious economic consequences, particularly because altered peripheral tissue perfusion often is associated with atherosclerotic changes in other areas of the body. Primary prevention is essential to reduce the predisposing factors of Altered Tissue Perfusion and thereby preserve quality of life for the elderly.

ETIOLOGIES/RELATED FACTORS AND DEFINING CHARACTERISTICS

Accurate diagnosis and management of Altered Tissue Perfusion in the elderly must be based on both physiologic and psychosocial factors. A complete database is essential, because age-related changes in the body's response to disease make diagnosis more difficult. Symptoms of illness vary in both quantity and quality and may include only a few or several of the following: fatigue, anorexia, confusion, incontinence, changes in ambulation, weight loss, or failure to thrive (Blake, 1976;410).

Specification of etiologies and defining characteristics for the renal, cerebral, gastrointestinal, cardiopulmonary, and peripheral categories of Altered Tissue Perfusion aids differential diagnosis and helps nurses determine whether independent nursing intervention or referral for medical treatment is appropriate. See Table 20.2 for the 1989 NANDA Eighth Conference defining characteristics of Altered Tissue Perfusion. Each general etiology and associated defining characteristics for Altered Tissue Perfusion are listed in greater detail in Table 20.2. The present discussion of etiologic factors will be limited to those conditions that most commonly affect tissue perfusion in the elderly.

Interruption of Arterial Flow

An interruption of arterial blood flow decreases the oxygenated blood supply to body tissues. The two major factors that influence the adequacy of circulation are the amount of blood delivered to a tissue and its metabolic demands. Cerebral and coronary vessels are particularly sensitive to hypoxemia and dilate to restore tissue perfu-

sion. Hypermetabolic states may precipitate ischemia when blood vessels cannot dilate or the cardiac pump cannot increase cardiac output to meet tissue needs. Redistribution of blood flow to meet tissue demands may also cause ischemia in regions where shunting occurs (Hart, 1981).

The patency of blood vessels may be compromised by conditions that obstruct vessel lumens, induce reflexive vasoconstriction, or produce mechanical pressure. Arterial blood flow in the elderly is most often obstructed by arteriosclerosis, a group of diseases characterized by thickening and loss of elasticity of the arterial wall (Fagin-Dubin, 1977). Atherosclerosis is a major type of arteriosclerosis that can affect any artery. The larger arteries such as the abdominal aorta and renal artery and vessels in the lower extremities are more commonly involved (Fagin-Dubin, 1977; Sexton, 1977; Wagner, 1986) (as illustrated in Figure 20.1).

The highest incidence of atherosclerosis occurs in postmenopausal women and men 50 to 70 years old (Jones et al, 1982; Wagner, 1986). Precursor lesions in the intimal layer appear in the first decade of life as reversible, fatty streaks in the aorta and coronary arteries. Plaques composed of fibrous scar tissue and lipid cores form in early adulthood. Accumulated lipids, cell debris, complex carbohydrates, blood, calcium deposits, and fibrous tissue characterize the complex lesion by middle age (Fagin-Dubin, 1977; Wagner, 1986). Severity of symptoms depends on the extent of the lesion, the degree of obstruction, and the presence of collateral circulation. Thinning of the medial layer can lead to aneurysm formation in the aorta and in the iliac and femoral arteries (Wagner, 1986).

Intimal degeneration may also precipitate ulceration and thrombosis of the plaque and cause partial or complete arterial occlusion. This obstruction increases vascular resistance and turbulent blood flow, further damaging vessel walls and triggering thromboembolism (Hart, 1981; Jones et al, 1982). Stenosis commonly occurs at the carotid bifurcation and origin of the internal carotid artery, providing a source of emboli and/or compromising flow to the cerebral arteries (Gorelick, 1986).

Vasospastic conditions that reduce patency usually affect vessels that are regulated by the sympathetic nervous system and by local substances such as histamine, prostaglandins, and catecholamines. Raynaud's disease, for example, is manifested by episodic and symmetrical vasoconstriction of small peripheral arteries and arterioles, particularly in the hands. The vasospasms, often precipitated by cold or emotional stress, produce blanching, cyanosis, and reactive hyperemia and, if severe, may lead to ulceration and gangrene of the affected parts (Hart, 1981; Jones et al, 1982; Wagner, 1986).

Internal obstructive pressure may be exerted by exudate and collagen formation of the inflammatory process, extracellular fluid accumulation (ascites or edema), and

Table 20.2

Etiologies/Related Factors and Defining Characteristics of Altered Tissue Perfusion

CARROLL-JOHNSON (1989)

Definition: The state in which an individual experiences a decrease in nutrition and oxygenation at the cellular level due to a deficit in capillary blood supply

Related Factors

Interruption of flow, arterial
Interruption of flow, venous
Exchange problems
Hypervolemia
Hypovolemia

Defining Characteristics

Skin temperature:
    Cold extremities
Skin color:
    Dependent, blue or purple
    *Pale on elevation, and color does not return on lowering leg
    *Diminished arterial pulsations
Skin quality: shining
Lack of lanugo
Round scars covered with atrophied skin
Gangrene
Slow-growing, dry, thick, brittle nails
Claudication
Blood pressure changes in extremities
Bruits
Slow healing of lesions

HALM (1989)

Etiologies
Interruption of Flow, Arterial

Renal
Hypovolemia
Sepsis
Congestive heart failure
Cardiac arrhythmias
Myocardial infarction
(Thompson et al, 1986)

Cerebral
Reduced patency to cerebral vessels and internal mechanical pressure
Orthostatis hypotension
(Carpenito, 1983)

Cardiopulmonary
Atherosclerotic coronary artery lesions
Pulmonary emboli or infarction
(Thompson et al, 1986)

Defining Characteristics

Renal
Decreased urine output
Hypertension
Edema
(Carpenito 1983; Thompson et al, 1986)

Cerebral
Altered level of consciousness
Restlessness
Altered thought processes
Memory losses
Confusion
Dizziness or faintness
Pupillary changes
Neurologic deficits
(Carpenito, 1983; Gorelick, 1986;
Taylor, 1985; Thompson et al, 1986)

Cardiopulmonary
Hypotension
Cold, clammy skin
Slow capillary refill
Tachycardia
Exertional angina
Tachypnea
Dyspnea and orthopnea
(Carpenito, 1983; Thompson et al, 1986)

Table 20.2

Etiologies/Related Factors and Defining Characteristics of Altered Tissue Perfusion (*Continued*)

HALM (1989)

Gastrointestinal	*Gastrointestinal*
Atherosclerosis	Abdominal distention
Postoperative complications that may occlude superior mesenteric	Positive guaiac findings of stool
vessels	Nausea or vomiting
(Thompson et al, 1986)	Thirst
	Elevated serum enzymes (SGOT, LDH, CPK)
	Constipation
	(Carpenito, 1983; Thompson et al, 1986)
Peripheral	*Peripheral*
Obstruction	Intermittent claudication
Inflammation	(at location of occlusion)
Vasoconstriction	Pain at rest
Vasospasm	Loss of motor and sensory function (pressure, temperature,
(Hart, 1981; Jones et al, 1982; Sexton, 1977)	trauma)
	Blood pressure changes in extremities
	Bruits
	Palpable pulsations
	Muscle weakness
	Paresthesias in affected part (numbness/tingling)
	Edema
	Decreased capillary refill
	Poor resistance to infection
	Nonhealing, painful ulcers; between or tips of toes, heels and
	above lateral malleolus. Deep, cavernous, and pale with even
	margins, necrotic or gangrenous tissue present—minimal gran-
	ulation
	(Carpenito, 1983; Herman, 1986;
	Jones et al, 1982; Kelly, 1985;
	Thompson et al, 1986; Wagner,
	1986; Wild, 1986)
Interruption of Flow, Venous	Ankle edema: asymmetry in limb circumference
	Calf pain on dorsiflexion: positive Homans' sign
	Cyanosis with dependency
	Brown pigmentation of skin around ankles and lower legs
	Skin temperature uniform (coolness or warmth)
	Numbness and tingling
	Leg heaviness and aching
	Superficial veins enlarged and tortuous
	Venous stasis ulcers: ankle/pretibial regions; moderately painful.
	Superficial with uneven edges, ruddy red granulated base; no
	gangrene
	(Doyle, 1986; Herman, 1986; Jones et al, 1982; Kelly, 1985;
	Thompson et al, 1986; Wagner, 1986)
Exchange Problems	Tachypnea
	Dyspnea
	Hypoxia
	Hypercapnia
	Pulmonary artery hypertension
	Cyanosis
	Apprehension
	Tachycardia
	Exertional angina
	(Roberts, 1987; Thompson et al, 1986)

(*Continues*)

Table 20.2

Etiologies/Related Factors and Defining Characteristics of Altered Tissue Perfusion (Continued)

HALM (1989)

Hypovolemia	Cold, clammy skin
	Ashen pallor to cyanosis
	Decreased skin turgor
	Normal serum sodium
	Hypothermia
	Weak rapid pulse
	Hypotension
	Arrhythmias
	Tachypnea or air hunger
	Decreased urine output
	Intense thirst
	Nausea/vomiting
	Weight loss
	Muscular weakness
	Restlessness
	Confusion
	Memory losses
	Altered levels of consciousness
	(Frantz, 1981; Kelly, 1985; Rice, 1981a)
Hypervolemia	Shortness of breath
	Dyspnea
	Moist crackles and rhonchi
	Productive cough—pink frothy sputum
	Puffy eyelids
	Acute weight gain
	Dependent pitting edema
	Ascites—abdomen dull to percussion
	Full bounding pulse
	Increased central venous pressure
	Reduced red blood cell count
	Reduced hemoglobin and hematocrit
	(Bruner and Suddarth, 1980; Kelly, 1985)

*Critical defining characteristics.

rapid cell proliferation (tumor growth). However, the degree of ischemia is related to the involved vessels and site. In chronic inflammation, blood vessels are compressed by fibroblastic proliferation and extensive scarring (Hart, 1981). The effects of external pressure on tissue perfusion are discussed in Chapter 7.

Renal

Altered renal perfusion may result from any systemic condition that produces ischemia to the kidney: hypovolemia, sepsis, congestive heart failure, cardiac arrhythmias, and myocardial infarction (Thompson et al, 1986). Vasoconstriction, the normal response of the kidney to decreased tissue perfusion, produces further ischemia and, if prolonged, may lead to tissue death and renal failure.

Cerebral

Altered cerebral perfusion may occur from reduced patency of the cerebral vessels and internal mechanical pressure. Orthostatic hypotension may be related to sudden position changes (especially from lying or sitting to standing), prolonged bed rest, impaired skeletal muscle function, aging, severe varicose veins, decreased blood volume or dehydration, and medications such as antihypertensives, diuretics, vasodilators, and neuroleptics, especially tricyclic antidepressants (Carpenito, 1983).

Atherosclerosis is primarily responsible for progressive compromise of the cerebral circulation. Plaques form cerebral thromboses and embolic debris, reducing blood flow to the areas of the brain supplied by the compromised artery. Signs and symptoms depend on the location and extent of the ischemic area. Neurologic impairment can be minimized if collateral circulation is adequate to

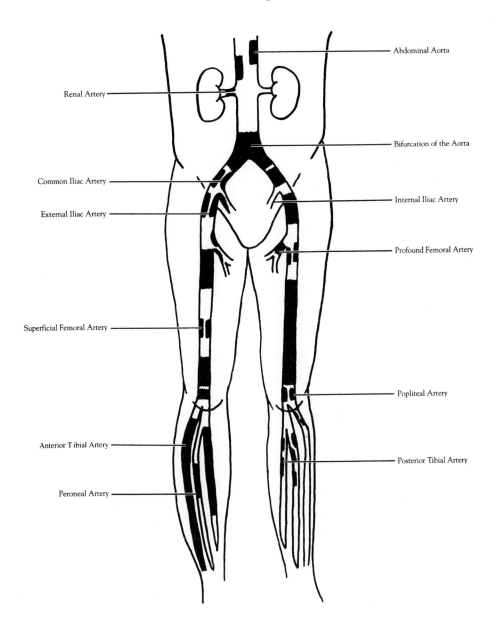

Renal Artery

Common Iliac Artery

External Iliac Artery

Superficial Femoral Artery

Anterior Tibial Artery

Peroneal Artery

Abdominal Aorta

Bifurcation of the Aorta

Internal Iliac Artery

Profound Femoral Artery

Popliteal Artery

Posterior Tibial Artery

Figure 20.1

Common locations of atherosclerotic lesions in peripheral blood vessel.

reestablish blood flow quickly after symptom onset (Gorelick, 1986).

Saccular and congenital aneurysms may spontaneously rupture into the subarachnoid space or brain parenchyma, trigger cerebral infarction due to underlying vasospasm or emboli, or exert internal pressure. Accumulated subarachnoid blood obstructs cerebrospinal fluid absorption pathways and causes hydrocephalus, which further compresses arteries, veins, and brain tissue (Gorelick, 1986).

Cardiopulmonary

Atherosclerotic coronary artery lesions restrict the blood supply to the myocardium, producing angina and tachycardia or myocardial infarction with reduced cardiac output. Pulmonary emboli or infarction may interrupt blood flow to the pulmonary capillary bed, impeding alveolar gas exchange. Tissue necrosis and hemorrhage occur at the site of infarction (Thompson et al, 1986). The mechanisms of altered pulmonary perfusion will be discussed with the etiology of exchange problems.

Gastrointestinal

Atherosclerosis or postoperative complications may occlude the superior mesenteric vessels to reduce intestinal blood flow. As peristalsis decreases in the distal segments of the bowel, the gastrointestinal tract rids its contents through vomiting (Thompson et al, 1986).

The liver is one of the first organs to deteriorate with profoundly altered systemic perfusion because of its high rate of metabolism and exposure to concentrated toxins.

The pancreas responds by activating pancreatic enzymes and releasing toxins such as myocardial toxic factor, which reduces myocardial contractility. Ischemia of the liver also elevates the serum enzymes of serum glutamic-oxaloacetic transaminase (SGOT), serum glutamic-pyruvic transaminase (SGPT), and lactate dehydrogenase (LDH). Yet, Jeppesen (1986) noted that these enzymes are normally higher in the elderly. Further tissue damage eventually decreases the liver's ability to detoxify materials (Thompson et al, 1986).

Peripheral

Emboli may occlude peripheral arteries, particularly vessels in the brain, kidneys, spleen, and lower extremities. Emboli commonly originate from the mitral and aortic valves or from mural thrombi associated with atrial fibrillation and myocardial infarction (Hart, 1981; Jones et al, 1982; Sexton, 1977).

Buerger's disease (thromboangiitis obliterans) is characterized by fibrotic thickening, segmental thrombi, and acute and chronic inflammatory responses in vessel walls. Gangrene may occur with significant occlusions (Hart, 1981; Jones et al, 1982; Thompson et al, 1986).

Interruption of Venous Flow

Interruption of venous blood flow reduces blood returned to the heart. Reduced vessel patency and changes in blood composition are the two primary factors that impair venous circulation. Valve leaflets that are overstretched from prolonged or excessive pressure cannot close properly and promote reverse flow, a condition known as venous insufficiency or stasis (Wagner, 1986). Venous stasis may also be precipitated by decreased skeletal muscle activity (Hart, 1981).

Venous stasis is a major factor affecting thrombus formation, but cannot individually precipitate thrombosis. Other predisposing factors such as vessel wall damage, venous inflammation, hypercoagulability, and immobility must be present for clot development (Carpenito, 1983; Doyle, 1986; Hart, 1981; Jones et al, 1982; Wagner, 1986). Thrombosis may occur in either superficial or deep veins and predominantly affects the lower extremities. The pulmonary arteries are common sites of emboli from venous origin (Doyle, 1986; Hart, 1981).

Conditions that increase the risk of thrombophlebitis in the aged client include major trauma, fractures of the long bones, severe burns, upper abdominal or pelvic surgery, congestive heart failure, varicose veins, cancer, prolonged bed rest, or immobilization of an affected part. Hypercoagulability and flow stasis are the major variables responsible for thrombosis in clients with these conditions (Hart, 1981).

Exchange Problems

Exchange problems occur when oxygen diffusion across the alveolar capillary membrane is impaired. Alterations in diffusion develop when either the distribution of air (ventilation) or the flow of pulmonary capillary blood (perfusion) to the alveolus is not adequate. The ventilation–perfusion (V/Q) ratio, normally 0.8, determines the alveolar gas composition (Thompson et al, 1986).

A low V/Q ratio (< 0.8) exists when there is less alveolar ventilation than perfusion. In contrast, high V/Q ratios (> 0.8) are directly related to shunting of blood from the pulmonary capillary bed. This condition, known as wasted ventilation, causes hypoxia and hypercapnia.

A high V/Q ratio may be caused by blockage or infarction of the pulmonary vasculature, compression or destruction of the pulmonary capillary bed, decreased blood pH, shock and decreased cardiac output resulting from cardiac arrhythmias, or a myocardial infarction (Roberts, 1987; Thompson et al, 1986).

Hypovolemia

Hypovolemia, a decrease in the intravascular blood volume in relation to the size of the intravascular compartment, is associated with a blood volume deficit of at least 15% to 25% (Rice, 1981a). Internal losses may result from the sequestration of fluid into third spaces, leakage of fluid from capillaries into the intestinal lumen, long bone fractures, extravascular pooling of blood, and impaired venous return. Fluids lost externally may include (1) whole blood from trauma, bleeding disorders, and surgery; (2) plasma from burn injuries; and (3) body fluid from the gastrointestinal tract or diuresis (Frantz, 1981; Kelly, 1985; Rice, 1981a).

Reduction of intravascular volume produces a decrease in venous return, ventricular filling pressures, stroke volume, cardiac output, and blood pressure. Ultimately, hypovolemic shock results in decreased perfusion to body tissues and organs (Rice, 1981a). The tissue type and its metabolic needs determine the length of time tissues can survive with inadequate prefusion (Carpenito, 1983; Jones et al, 1982).

Hypervolemia

Hypervolemia (circulatory overload) is an excessive increase in the intravascular blood volume that produces overload of all fluid compartments including the intracellular space. Volume overload may occur when isotonic solutions are administered too rapidly, especially in the very young or old. Patients with renal, cardiac, or hepatic disease may retain body fluid with normal or reduced intake. Long-term use of corticosteroids may also result in the retention of water and sodium (Bruner and Suddarth, 1980; Kelly, 1985).

ASSESSMENT

Of the few assessment tools available to guide the diagnosis of Altered Tissue Perfusion in the elderly (Carnevali and Enloe, 1986; Carpenito, 1983; Goetter, 1986; Herman, 1986; Quinless, 1986), most are broad in scope, are disease-based, and focus primarily on general physiologic indicators of tissue perfusion. Topical outlines frequently include subjective data related to past health history, risk factors and pertinent symptoms, and objective data focused on the review of biologic systems (Carnevali and Enloe, 1986; Carpenito, 1983). In addition, the tools often rely on the clinician's subjective interpretation of physiologic data collected by inspection, auscultation, palpation, and percussion. Specific assessment guides available for altered cerebral, cardiopulmonary, and peripheral tissue perfusion (Carpenito, 1983; Goetter, 1986; Herman, 1986; Quinless, 1986) are designed for a certain patient population or disease process and lack a conceptual focus.

Assessment and diagnosis of Altered Tissue Perfusion may also be based on a typology of 11 functional health patterns. Gordon's (1982) health assessment guide provides a holistic approach for the collection of basic patient data that is appropriate for individuals, families, and communities across age groups and nursing specialties.

Herman (1986) identified activity-exercise as the primary functional health pattern affected by Altered Peripheral Tissue Perfusion. Yet, the assessment tool identified specific cues to assess the impact of altered peripheral blood flow on other patterns such as health-perception–health-management, nutritional-metabolic, and self-perception–self-concept. Focused cue searches were also provided to assess client problems related to social isolation, pain self-management, and ineffective individual coping.

The assessment tool in Assessment Guide 20.1 identifies the critical assessment cues for each category of Altered Tissue Perfusion. Further classification of the five categories of Altered Tissue Perfusion with Gordon's functional health patterns would enable nurses to investigate the impact of Altered Tissue Perfusion on functional health status among the elderly.

CASE STUDY

Altered Tissue Perfusion, Mrs. R

Mrs. R, a 92-year-old white woman, has been a long-term care resident for 5 years. She has a 15-year history of progressive confusion and several falls with fractures of the humerus, femur, acetabulum, and pelvis. Mrs. R previously lived at home with her husband on the family farm. She was able to maintain her self-care during the first 6 years of confusion, then required continual assistance from family and homemaker health aides. The client received periodic health screening from public health nurses and medical intervention only for the injuries she sustained from falls. Mrs. R has experienced progressive memory loss and disorientation to time, place, and other persons. She rarely verbalizes a complete word or sentence but rather mutters incomprehensible sounds and sings what are believed to be religious songs. Infrequently, she briefly recognizes immediate family members and acknowledges them with smiles or comments such as "I haven't seen you in a long time." During the last 2 years, her profound state of confusion has required total nursing care. She is incontinent and unable to walk or feed herself. Table 20.3 presents the etiology, defining characteristics, and additional data needed for this case study.

NURSING DIAGNOSIS

Altered Tissue Perfusion related to interruption in arterial flow: cerebral, as evidenced by altered thought processes, restlessness, confusion, and memory loss.

Table 20.3

Nursing Diagnosis for Case Study, Mrs. R

ETIOLOGY	DEFINING CHARACTERISTICS	ADDITIONAL DATA NEEDED
Interruption in Arterial Flow* Cerebral	Altered thought processes Restlessness Confusion Memory losses	Cerebral flow studies Computerized Axial Tomography (CAT) Scan Neurologic exam Cholesterol levels Psychiatric nursing evaluation

*Unable to rule out.

CASE STUDY

Altered Tissue Perfusion, Mr. F

MR. F, a 76-year-old white married man, presented to the emergency room with complaints of acute lower abdominal pain, nausea, vomiting, and diarrhea. Severe, constant, and diffuse pain ascended to the epigastric region but did not radiate to his back or lower extremities. His abdomen was quiet, distended, firm, diffusely tender with guarding on light palpation, dull to percussion, and 120 cm in circumference. Stool was negative for occult blood. No rebound tenderness or palpable abdominal masses were present. The client has no previous surgeries or history of gastrointestinal health problems. Past medical history included hypertension, chronic obstructive pulmonary disease, and coronary artery disease. Mr. F also reported a moderate intake of alcohol, a two-pack per day history of smoking for 58 years, and dyspnea on exertion.

Physical examination revealed a 10-cm palpable pulsation over the aorta. Computerized axial tomography confirmed a 7.5-cm aortic aneurysm below the level of the kidney with no evidence of dissection or rupture, with fluid collections around the liver and stomach, and with no pancreatic abscess. On the basis of serum amylase levels (see Table 20.1), the tentative medical diagnosis was diffuse pancreatitis. Triple abdominal aortic aneurysm repair was postponed because surgery would pose a high risk of mortality.

After 3 weeks of medical management for pancreatitis, Mr. F's hemodynamic status was as follows: sinus tachycardia 134 beats per minute (BPM) without ectopy, blood pressure 90/54, pulmonary capillary wedge pressure 5 to 8 mm Hg, oxygen saturation 94%, and core temperature $38^1°C$. Mr F. had been intubated for mechanical ventilation because he had respiratory acidosis. Ventilator settings were 45% FiO2, tidal volume 1000 mL, assist-control mode with a rate of 16 and 5 cm positive end-expiratory pressure. Arterial blood gases were pH 7.40, PaO$_2$ 70, pCO$_2$ 34, and bicarbonate 22. Other laboratory results are shown in Table 20.4.

Chest expansion was equal and symmetrical with no evidence of air hunger. Coarse rhonchi were audible in all lung fields with crackles auscultated bibasilarly. Mr. F's skin was warm, pale, and diaphoretic with sluggish capillary refill. Radial and femoral pulses were full (2 +), whereas the pedal and posterior tibial pulses were diminished (1 +). Lower extremities were mottled, with nonpitting edema in the pretibial regions. Pitting edema was observed in the flank and upper thighs. No carotid bruits were auscultated, and heart sounds were distant without an S3 or gallop. Urine output averaged 20 cc per hour. Mr. F became progressively lethargic and opened his eyes only to noxious stimuli. Cough and gag reflexes were intact, and Babinski reflexes were absent. Corneal reflexes were weak, and pupils were equal and round but reacted sluggishly with direct and consensual light responses. Mr. F localized with his left upper extremity and withdrew all four extremities to central and peripheral noxious stimuli. Table 20.5 presents the etiologies, defining characteristics, and additional data needed for this case study.

NURSING DIAGNOSES

1. Altered Tissue Perfusion: renal, cerebral, cardiopulmonary, peripheral related to interruption in arterial flow as evidenced by decreased urine output, BUN 77/creatinine 3.3, altered level of consciousness, hypotension, tachycardia, and diminished pedal and posterior tibial pulses.
2. Altered Tissue Perfusion related to interruption in venous flow as evidenced by mottling and coolness of lower extremities, nonpitting edema of lower extremities, pitting edema of flank and upper thighs, abdominal distention, and fluid collection around the liver and stomach.
3. Altered Tissue Perfusion related to hypovolemia as evidenced by pallor, altered level of consciousness, confusion, restlessness, hypotension, sinus tachycardia without ectopy, tachypnea, distended firm abdomen, nausea and vomiting, and decreased urine output.

Table 20.4

Laboratory Results

Platelets	195/cu mm	Sodium	155 mEq/liter
White blood cells	20.4 cu mm	Potassium	6.3 mEq/liter
Red blood cells	3.35 million/cu mm	Chloride	113 mEq/liter
Hemoglobin	9.8 g/100 mL	BUN	77 mg/100 mL
Hematocrit	30%	Creatinine	3.3 mg/dL
PT	13 sec	Amylase	2420 Somogyi U/100 mL
PTT	22 sec	Glucose	416 mg/dL
Calcium	3.3 mEq/liter		

Table 20.5

Nursing Diagnoses for Case Study, Mr. F

ETIOLOGY	DEFINING CHARACTERISTICS	ADDITIONAL DATA NEEDED
*Interruption of Arterial Flow**		
Renal	Decreased urine output	
	BUN 77; Creatinine 3.3	
Cerebral	Altered levels of consciousness	Bruits?
Cardiopulmonary	Hypotension	Blood pressure changes of upper extremities
	Tachycardia	Trophic changes/ulcers?
Peripheral	Diminished pedal and posterior tibial pulses bilaterally	Color changes with position of lower extremities?
*Interruption of Venous Flow**	Mottling and coolness of lower extremities	Ulcers? Cyanosis with dependent position?
	Nonpitting edema of lower extremities	Serum enzyme levels
	Pitting edema of flank and upper thighs	
	Fluid collection around liver and stomach (potential for infection)	
	Abdominal distention	
*Hypovolemia**	Pallor	Weight?
	Altered level of consciousness	
	Confusion	
	Restlessness	
	Hypotension (90/54)	
	Sinus tachycardia; no ectopy	
	Tachypnea	
	Distended, firm abdomen	
	Nausea and vomiting	
	Decreased urine output	

*Unable to rule out.

NURSING INTERVENTIONS

The overall goals of nursing therapies for Altered Tissue Perfusion are (1) to maintain tissue perfusion and cellular oxygenation; (2) to reduce metabolic demands; and (3) to relieve ischemic pain (Hart, 1981; Thompson et al, 1986). Both independent and dependent nursing interventions for Altered Tissue Perfusion are outlined in Table 20.6. A variety of other nursing interventions are also appropriate to treat Altered Tissue Perfusion in the elderly, including surveillance, exercise, nutrition counseling, patient contracting, relaxation therapy, and values clarification.

Nursing therapies are most successful when the etiology of the health problem can be modified. However, changing the etiologies of Altered Tissue Perfusion may not be possible in the elderly client because the alterations are often due to the interaction of pathologic processes and progressive physiologic changes associated with aging. Therefore, patient teaching is often the intervention of choice to treat the defining characteristics of Altered Tissue Perfusion. The effectiveness of treatment can be evaluated by changes observed in the client's signs and symptoms, such as amount of walking prior to the onset of pain, nutritional status, well-being, and ability to maintain personal care and engage in ADLs, as well as by the duration that desired outcomes were achieved (Wild, 1986).

Patient Teaching

Ventura et al (1984) described the effects of mutual goal setting on modifying the risk factors of poor foot care, lack of exercise, and tobacco use for 34 male clients (mean age of 61) with peripheral vascular disease (PVD). Patient teaching booklets were used to assist those subjects engaged in mutual goal setting to select goals and activities for the behavior changes they desired. Of these clients, 71% decreased their amount of smoking, 34% increased the frequency of foot care, and 89% showed greater increases in the frequency, distance, and duration of walking, as well as PVD-therapy exercises. In addition, these clients tended to experience greater improvement in self-reports of pain and well-being. Generally 90% of patients who adhere to recommended exercise and risk factor modification programs show improvement in PVD symptoms (Doyle, 1986).

Table 20.6

Nursing Therapies for the Etiologies of Altered Tissue Perfusion: Renal, Cerebral, Cardiopulmonary, Gastrointestinal, Peripheral

ETIOLOGIES	NURSING INTERVENTIONS
Maintenance of Tissue Perfusion and Cellular Oxygenation	
Positioning	
Arterial flow	Extremities dependent or supine position
Venous flow	Elevation of affected lower extremities
	Avoid prolonged sitting or standing with extremities dependent
Hypovolemia	Elevation of lower extremities
Structural Support	
Arterial and venous flow	Moderate exercise program
	Buerger-Allen exercises
Venous flow	Active and passive exercises
	Elastic stockings (Ted hose)
Reduction of External Pressure	
Arterial flow	Turn or change positions every 1–2 hours
	Restrict modified Fowler's with patients on bed rest
	Support extremities with pillows
	Waterbeds, bed cradles, footboards
Reduction of Internal Pressure	
Arterial and venous flow	Bed rest
	Avoid massage of affected part
	Administration of anticoagulants
Venous flow	Elevate affected part 6 inches above heart
	Warm compresses to affected part
	Active exercise and ambulation after threat of embolism
Promotion of Vasodilation	
Arterial flow	Provide warm environment
	Encourage clients to wear warm clothes
	Moderate exercise program
	Intermittent heat applications
	Administration of vasodilators
Arterial and venous flow	Discourage smoking
Exchange problems	
Maintenance of Intravascular Volume	
Hypovolemia	Administration of whole blood, plasma, dextran
	Intravenous fluid replacement
Hypervolemia	Sodium restriction
	Administration of diuretics
Reduction of Metabolic Demands	
Arterial flow	Alternate periods of rest and activity
	Stress reduction strategies (visual imagery; relaxation therapy)
Cardiopulmonary	Monitor resting pulse and recovery rates with exercise
Cerebral	Administration of barbiturates
	Hypothermia
Arterial and venous flow	Prevent trauma and infection to extremities
Relief of Ischemic Pain	
Arterial	Rest affected part with pain
Cardiopulmonary	Administration of nitrates
Arterial and venous flow	Administration of analgesics
Venous	Application of moist heat to affected area

Sources: Doyle J: Treatment modalities in peripheral vascular disease. *Nurs Clin North Am* 1986; 21(2): 241–253. Hart L: Ischemia. Pages 293–318 in: *Concepts Common to Acute Illness.* Hart L, Reese J, Fearing M (editors). Mosby, 1981. Thompson J et al: *Clinical Nursing.* Mosby, 1986.

Because PVD usually occurs in persons over the age of 50, health habits are well established and difficult to change (Beaver, 1986; Sexton, 1977; Ventura et al, 1984). The elderly client can be provided with information on risk factor modification and preventive measures to improve tissue perfusion. Yet patient knowledge by itself is not sufficient to achieve required lifestyle changes (Ventura et al, 1984). Patient teaching that encourages active patient participation in self-care can best promote achievement of desired outcomes.

Teaching plans must be individualized to the readiness of the learner, the needs of the client, and the etiology of Altered Tissue Perfusion (see Figure 20.2). In addition, involvement of the family in patient teaching interventions is essential to ensure quality care.

CASE STUDY

Nursing Intervention, Mrs. R

Mrs. R's family should be taught that her progressive state of confusion resulted, at least in part, from plaque formation in the major blood vessels supplying the brain.

Family members should be encouraged to communicate with Mrs. R and to provide personal belongings to help familiarize her surroundings. Nurses must also support the family as they mourn the loss of the person they once knew (see Chapter 29).

Risk Factor Modification

Atherosclerosis is the most common pathologic process that affects peripheral tissue perfusion in the elderly. Primary risk factors are cigarette smoking, hypertension, and hyperlipidemia. Less influential factors include age, sex, obesity, diabetes, family history, sedentary lifestyle, and stress (Doyle, 1986; Fagin-Dubin, 1977; Herman, 1986; Turner, 1986; Wagner, 1986).

Cigarette smoking has been identified as the single independent factor most closely associated with atherosclerosis (Doyle, 1986). Low oxygen tension and high carbon monoxide levels are believed to accelerate the development of arterial lesions. Oxygen transport is impaired because carbon monoxide has a stronger affinity

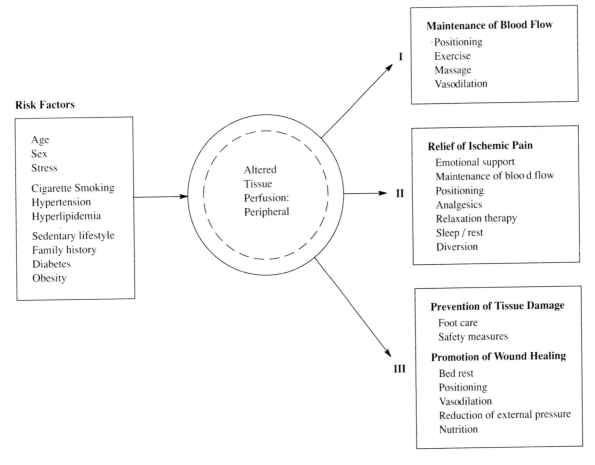

Figure 20.2

Patient teaching plan for altered peripheral perfusion.

to combine with hemoglobin than oxygen. As the intimal lining is subjected to hypoxic damage, it becomes more permeable to lipids and other constituents of plaque (Doyle, 1986; Fagin-Dubin, 1977). Nicotine also has vasoconstrictive effects that reduce peripheral blood flow and skin temperature and increase platelet adhesiveness for thrombus formation. Clients who quit smoking have improved exercise tolerance, increased graft patency after arterial reconstructive surgery, and lower amputation rates (Turner, 1986). Nursing interventions designed to help clients quit smoking may be successful only when the client has learned to value this goal. Patient education can assist the client to understand why smoking is harmful and how it contributes to PVD (Turner, 1986).

Hyperlipidemia is characterized by elevated levels of serum cholesterol, triglyceride, and low-density lipoproteins. Dietary measures and pharmacologic agents have not been shown consistently to reduce atherosclerosis and its complications in people over age 55 (Fagin-Dubin, 1977). Some individuals can achieve a 10% to 30% reduction in serum cholesterol in 2 weeks with a diet that provides (1) 30% of calories from fats and less than 10% from saturated fats; (2) cholesterol limited to 200 milligrams per day; and (3) a higher ratio of polyunsaturated fats (Doyle, 1986; Fagin-Dubin, 1977; Turner, 1986).

Exercising regularly, maintaining ideal body weight, and limiting alcohol intake may also help control elevated serum cholesterol and triglyceride levels. When dietary measures are ineffective, medications such as Lorelco (probucol) and Atromid-S (clofibrate) may be used to control hypercholesterolemia. However, clients must be cautioned that these drugs are not curative, and long-term use will be required to control cholesterol levels (Turner, 1986).

Over the age of 40, hypertension becomes a greater risk factor than hyperlipidemia (Fagin-Dubin, 1977). High arterial pressure damages the intimal lining and increases lipid permeability with the development of plaque. Plaque formation at arterial bifurcations may also be due to the increased turbulence and blood pressure at these locations (Doyle, 1986). Patient teaching should emphasize a reduced sodium intake and adjustment of total calories to prevent obesity (Turner, 1986). The purpose, frequency, dosage, and side effects of diuretics and antihypertensives must be explained to enhance the client's understanding and compliance.

Special instructions are necessary to promote adherence of hypertensive patients to medication regimens. Becker and Maiman (1980) found a direct relationship between understanding instructions and the degree of compliance. Fifty percent of these clients could not recall how long to take the medication, 26% did not know the dosage, 17% did not know the frequency, 16% misinterpreted "p.r.n.," and 23% could not identify the need for the medication. Of those clients who received intense instructions, 62% understood and 54% complied. In

contrast, 40% of the patients who did not receive instructions understood, but only 29% complied. Similarly, McKenney (1973) reported that patients who attended monthly medication classes and consulted with their physicians on a regular basis demonstrated increased compliance rates from 25% to 79%. However, patient teaching produced only a temporary effect on compliance rates, which returned to baseline after the study.

Preventive and Supportive Measures

Elderly clients must also be provided with information related to specific treatment goals, thereby enabling them to incorporate appropriate regimens into their health maintenance pattern.

Maintenance of Blood Flow Clients who have altered arterial flow should position their lower extremities at a level lower than their heart (Hart, 1981; Sexton, 1977; Turner, 1986). The head of the bed may be elevated on 6- to 8-inch blocks, or the client may be instructed to sit with the feet resting on the floor (Sexton, 1977; Wild, 1986). Persons with venous insufficiency should elevate their lower extremities approximately 6 inches above the level of the heart to promote venous return (Carpenito, 1983; Doyle, 1986; Eddy, 1977; Hart, 1981; Sexton, 1977; Turner, 1986; Wild, 1986). Prolonged standing or sitting with the lower extremities dependent should also be avoided. Elderly clients with venous insufficiency should be instructed to alternate short periods of sitting with walking, elevate the foot of the bed, and avoid using pillows behind the knees (Carpenito, 1983; Hart, 1981; Sexton, 1977; Turner, 1986).

The skeletal muscle pump is the primary mechanism that promotes venous return. During exercise, skeletal muscles contract and compress veins in the lower extremities, thereby increasing venous blood flow. Structural support of venous circulation may also be augmented by elastic stockings and/or positive pressure pneumatic devices, which exert even pressure on the lower extremities (Carpenito, 1983; Doyle, 1986; Hart, 1981; Wild, 1986). In addition, Buerger-Allen exercises facilitate arterial and venous flow by gravity and active muscle movement (Eddy, 1977; Hart, 1981).

The elderly client with intermittent claudication should walk several times per day to the point of discomfort, rest, and repeat walking. This regimen promotes the development of collateral circulation and increases the distance the client can walk without pain (Doyle, 1986; Sexton, 1977; Turner, 1986; Wild, 1986). Exercise should be stopped if angina, dizziness, shortness of breath, lightheadedness, nausea, or loss of muscle control is experienced (Carpenito, 1983). Exercise is contraindicated for persons with arterial or venous thrombosis. Rather, bed rest and restricted movement of the affected extremity are indicated until the thrombus attaches to the vessel wall (Hart, 1981; Turner, 1986).

Manual massage may also improve peripheral blood flow as pressure is exerted on deep veins, arteries, and capillaries and vasomotor nerves are stimulated to facilitate reflexive vasodilation. Massage also causes the release of acetylcholine and histamine, which produce local vasodilation (Hart, 1981).

Tobacco and exposure to cold should be avoided because these factors stimulate the sympathetic centers of the hypothalamus to reduce peripheral blood flow. Other measures that promote vasodilation include a warm (70° to 72°) environment, warm clothes, cotton or wool socks, warm baths, and electric blankets. Clients should also be advised to reduce emotional stress and to avoid crossing their legs and wearing garters or tight clothing (Carpenito, 1983; Eddy, 1977; Hart, 1981; Sexton, 1977; Turner, 1986; Wild, 1986). Vasodilators such as Pavabid, Priscoline, and Dibenzyline have limited effectiveness because atherosclerotic lesions impede the ability of arteries to dilate (Doyle, 1986; Hart, 1981; Turner, 1986). Vasodilators also reduce systolic blood pressure, which may further impair tissue perfusion (Doyle, 1986).

CASE STUDY

Nursing Interventions, Mr. F

Mr. F would normally be instructed on body positioning for interrupted arterial flow as previously described. However, tissue perfusion in this client was also compromised by the etiology of hypovolemia. Mr. F and his family should be informed that this hypovolemic state occurred from extravascular pooling associated with pancreatitis and impaired venous return due to his aortic aneurysm. Mr. F should be placed in a supine position with his lower extremities elevated to a 45-degree angle to maximize venous return (Rice, 1981b). Mr. F would also require intravenous fluid replacement, whole blood, and other blood products to maintain intravascular volume for adequate tissue perfusion.

Relief of Ischemic Pain Clients with Altered Peripheral Tissue Perfusion may experience different types of pain (Sexton, 1977; Turner, 1986). Intermittent claudication occurs during exercise in muscles distal to the obstruction and is relieved by rest. Rest pain occurs with severe arterial occlusions. Pain associated with ulcerations is often described as severe and relentless (Eddy, 1977; Sexton, 1977; Ventura et al, 1984).

Anxiety and powerlessness are common affective responses to acute or chronic pain or to threatened loss of an extremity. Nurses must explore the meaning of the patient's pain and encourage the expression of feelings and fears

to reduce the impact that emotional stress can have on the ischemic problem. Clients may regain feelings of control if they are provided with information on a variety of pain-relief techniques (Herman, 1986; Turner, 1986).

Although all of the methods previously identified to maintain tissue perfusion help relieve ischemic pain, rest of the affected extremity and appropriate use of positioning are most effective. Analgesics may be necessary, especially when ischemia is due to an infarct (Hart, 1981; Wild, 1986). The client should be informed that these medications are more effective when taken before the pain becomes intense. Other pain-relief measures include relaxation therapy, sleep or rest, and distraction (Beaver, 1986; Turner, 1986).

Prevention of Tissue Damage and Promotion of Wound Healing A diminished blood supply provides insufficient oxygen, nutrients, and leukocytes to control infection and promote wound healing. Consequently, minor trauma, burns, and infections may lead to ulcers, gangrene, and delayed wound healing. Tissue damage may be prevented by educating the patient about daily foot care and safety measures that may protect threatened areas from thermal, mechanical, or chemical trauma.

Meticulous foot care is of utmost importance to prevent tissue breakdown. Patients are advised to wear shoes and socks that are well-fitting, comfortable, and supportive. Mild soap must be used for daily washing of the legs and feet. The skin should be thoroughly rinsed, dried with gentle patting, and lubricated with lanolin or petroleum to prevent drying or cracking. Clients who have ulcers between their toes may be instructed to use cotton or Lamb's wool between their toes to absorb moisture and prevent infection and skin breakdown (Doyle, 1986; Eddy, 1977; Sexton, 1977; Turner, 1986; Wild, 1986). Patients should also be taught to inspect their legs and feet daily for dryness, cracks, redness, and maceration and to trim their nails after bathing. Nails must be trimmed straight across to prevent trauma and ingrown nails. Clients with thick toenails, corns, and calluses, and impaired vision or mobility should be referred to a podiatrist (Doyle, 1986; Eddy, 1977; Hart, 1981; Sexton, 1977).

Patients should be instructed to handle their lower extremities gently and to avoid scratching their legs and feet. Calamine lotion may be used to relieve pruritus. Clients should also be cautioned against exposure to extreme hot or cold temperatures. Although warmth promotes vasodilation, excessive heat increases local metabolic demands. Decreased sensitivity of the affected part to heat may allow the patient to be burned without realizing it. The temperature of bath water should be checked with a thermometer (105° to 110°) or wrist instead of the client's hand or toes. Heating pads and hot water bottles must be avoided on the lower extremities (Doyle, 1986; Hart, 1981; Sexton, 1977).

Clients with infected or slow-healing ulcers should be placed on bed rest, since resting tissues have lower metabolic needs (Sexton, 1977; Wild, 1986). Nurses must reinforce appropriate body positioning, promotion of vasodilation, and prevention of external pressure. For instance, bed cradles might be used to keep the weight of linens off the affected extremity. Elderly clients also require diet teaching to ensure adequate intake of protein and vitamins B_{12} and C to maintain tissue integrity and promote wound healing (Sexton, 1977).

OUTCOMES

An essential task in the planning phase of the nursing process is the identification of desired client outcomes or goals. The fundamental outcome desired for clients with Altered Tissue Perfusion is to reestablish adequate blood flow to meet metabolic tissue needs and promote functional health status. Desired outcomes for the etiologies of Altered Tissue Perfusion in the elderly are found in Table 20.7. These outcomes guide the selection of nursing interventions and also provide evaluation criteria for the effectiveness of treatments.

SUMMARY

The physiologic changes related to aging may predispose the elderly to Altered Tissue Perfusion. This state may be due to a number of etiologic factors: interruption of arterial flow, interruption of venous flow, exchange problems, hypovolemia, or hypervolemia. Nurses must critically analyze assessment data to accurately identify defining characteristics of altered renal, cerebral, cardiopulmonary, gastrointestinal, or peripheral tissue perfusion as well as indicators that signify two or more systems ar involved. This process of differential diagnosis was illu trated in two case studies that involved altered cerebr and gastrointestinal perfusion.

Nurses may use a variety of interventions to treat 1 response of the elderly to Altered Tissue Perfusion. T chapter discussed a health promotion interventic patient teaching—for the client with Altered Periph Tissue Perfusion. This teaching model focused on factor modification and the following preventive or portive measures: maintenance of blood flow, reli ischemic pain, and prevention of tissue damage promotion of wound healing.

Table 20.7

Desired Outcomes for the Etiologies of Altered Tissue Perfusion

ETIOLOGIES	OUTCOMES
Interruption of arterial flow	
Renal	Urine output equal to intake (1500–3000 cc) Blood pressure with normal limits Decreased edema
Cerebral	Increased level of consciousness Reduced restlessness Decreased altered thought processes Improved recent and remote memory
Cardiopulmonary	Normal blood pressure Warm, dry skin; brisk capillary refill Normal heart rate (660–100 BPM) Decreased angina Normal respiratory rate (12–24 breaths/min)
Gastrointestinal	Decreased abdominal distention Stool negative for occult blood Decreased nausea and vomiting Decreased thirst Normal serum enzymes: CPK: 0–4 IU/L, LDH: 115–225 IU/L, SGOT: 8–42 IU/L
Peripheral	Extremities warm with normal color Pulses palpable or doppled: Radial, femoral, popliteal, dorsalis pedis, posterior tibial Decreased intermittent claudication Improved sensory and motor function Decreased muscle weakness Diminished numbness and tingling

Table 20.7

Desired Outcomes for the Etiologies of Altered Tissue Perfusion (*Continued*)

ETIOLOGIES	OUTCOMES
	Decreased edema
	Brisk capillary refill
	Improved resistance to infection
	Ulcers granulating; no gangrene
Interruption of venous flow	Decreased ankle edema
	Negative Homans' sign
	Warm skin temperature of lower extremities
	Decreased numbness and tingling
	Decreased leg aches or heaviness
	Ulcers healing with granulation tissue
Exchange problems	Normal heart rate (60–100 BPM)
	Decreased angina with desired activity
	Decreased respiratory rate
	Decreased dyspnea or shortness of breath
	Arterial blood gases within normal limits: ph 7.35–7.45, pO_2 80–95, pCO_2 35–45
	Oxygen saturation 95%–99%
Hypovolemia	Reduced restlessness
	Increased orientation to time, place, person
	Improved memory
	Increased level of consciousness
	Blood pressure within normal limits
	Strong apical pulse with normal rate
	Decreased cardiac arrhythmias
	Normal body temperature
	Warm, dry, pink skin; normal skin turgor
	Moist mucous membranes
	Decreased respiratory rate; no air hunger
	Decreased muscle weakness
	Weight gain (client without altered nutrition: more than body requirements)
	Urine output 1500–3000 cc or equal to intake
	Absence of nausea and vomiting
	Normal thirst
Hypervolemia	Normal pulse quality
	CVP within normal limits (5–15 mm Hg)
	RBCs normal (3.5–4.5 million/cu mm)
	Hemoglobin 12–16 g/100 mL)
	Hematocrit 35%–45%
	No shortness of breath or dyspnea
	Clear breath sounds all lung fields
	Decreased productive cough
	Decreased periorbital edema
	Weight loss (for clients with altered nutrition: less than body requirements)
	Decreased dependent pitting edema
	Abdomen tympanic to percussion

ASSESSMENT GUIDE 20.1

Health Assessment Guide: Altered Tissue Perfusion

Identification Data

Name _____ Date _____

Phone _____ Relative _____

Age _____ Sex _____ Address _____

Occupation _____

Reason for Visit _____

General Appearance _____

HEALTH HISTORY

Allergies: Medications? _____ Foods? _____

Hospitalizations: Illnesses and surgeries

Reason   Date   Hospital/physician

Prescription/Nonprescription Medications

Name of medication   Dose   Frequency/reason

Habits

Use of alcohol?   Amount and frequency _____

Use of cigarettes?   Number packs/day _____ Number of years

If appropriate, number of years since quit _____

Family History

Identify family members with following health problems; include parents, grandparents, siblings, spouse, and children.

Diabetes _____

Kidney disease _____

Heart disease _____

Ulcers _____

Hypertension _____

Asthma _____

Arthritis _____

Allergies _____

Cancer _____

Bleeding/clotting disorders _____

Peripheral vascular disease _____

ASSESSMENT GUIDE 20.1

Health Assessment Guide: Altered Tissue Perfusion (Continued)

Emphysema _____

Cerebrovascular disease _____

Epilepsy _____

PHYSICAL ASSESSMENT

Renal Function
Urine output (cc/hr) _____ Blood pressure _____

BUN _____ Creatinine _____ Pitting or nonpitting edema?

Cerebrovascular
Level of consciousness?
Orientation to time, place, and person? Memory: Recent/past events
Pupil size, equality, reaction to light
Altered thought processes?
Alteration in sensory-perceptual abilities? Headaches? Dizziness?
Loss of motor function?

Cardiopulmonary Status
Skin color, temperature, capillary refill?

Apical rate? _____ ECG rhythm _____

Blood pressure: Lying _____ Sitting _____ Standing _____ Pulse pressure _____

Respiratory rate? _____ Dyspnea/shortness of breath?

Arterial blood gases _____
Angina? (frequency/precipitating factors/relief measures)
Sufficient energy for desired and required activities?
Self-care functions client able to perform:

Feeding   Grooming   Dressing   Bed mobility   Home maintenance
Cooking   Bathing   Toileting   General mobility   Shopping
General exercise patterns (type/regularity)

Gastrointestinal Function
How does client rate appetite? Anorexia?
Recent weight loss/gain? Amount? _____ Healing difficulties?
Nausea or vomiting? Abnormal thirst? Jaundice?
Change in bowel habits: Diarrhea? Constipation?
Presence of blood in stools? Last bowel movement _____
Quality and location of bowel sounds
Abdominal contour? Distention? Girth _____ (cm)
Abdominal pain? Hemorrhoids? Rectal bleeding?

Hemoglobin _____ Hematocrit _____ LDH _____ SGOT _____ CPK _____

Peripheral Vascular System
Skin color, temperature, turgor, capillary refill
Color changes with elevated and dependent extremity positions?
Pulse quality: Radial, brachial, femoral, popliteal, pedal, posterior tibial
Bruits? (location) Blood pressure changes in extremities?
Pitting/nonpitting edema? (location)
Loss of sensory/motor function? Numbness or tingling?
Intermittent claudication? (location and duration of exercise) Rest pain?
Homans' sign? Muscle weakness/leg heaviness?
Loss of hair on ankle or foot region? Thick brittle nails?
Ulcers?—Location, granulation tissue, infection, gangrene?

References

Beaver B: Health education and the patient with peripheral vascular disease. *Nurs Clin North Am* 1986; 21(2):265–271.

Becker M, Maiman L: Strategies for enhancing patient compliance. *J Comm Health* 1980; 6:113–135.

Blake D: Physical assessment of the aged: Differentiating normal and abnormal change. Pages 409–421 in: *Nursing and the Aged.* Burnside I (editor). McGraw-Hill, 1976.

Bruner L, Suddarth D: *Textbook of Medical-Surgical Nursing.* Lippincott, 1980.

Burggraf C, Donlon B: Assessing the elderly: Part one. System by system. *Am J Nurs* 1985; 85(9):974–984.

Carnevali D, Enloe C: Assessment in the elderly. Pages 26–52 in: *Nursing Management for the Elderly.* Carnevali M, Patrick M (editors). Lippincott, 1986.

Carpenito L: *Nursing Diagnosis: Application to Clinical Practice.* Lippincott, 1983.

Carroll-Johnson R (editor): *Classification of Nursing Diagnoses: Proceedings of the Eighth Conference.* Lippincott, 1989.

Doyle J: Treatment modalities in peripheral vascular disease. *Nurs Clin North Am* 1986; 21(2):241–253.

Eddy M: Teaching patients with peripheral vascular disease. *Nurs Clin North Am* 1977; 12(1):151–159.

Fagin-Dubin L: Atherosclerosis: A major cause of peripheral vascular disease. *Nurs Clin North Am* 1977; 12(1):101–108.

Fischbach F: *A Manual of Laboratory Diagnostic Tests.* Lippincott, 1984.

Frantz R: Shock. Pages 320–339 in: *Concepts Common to Acute Illness.* Hart L, Reese J, Fearing M (editors). Mosby, 1981.

Goetter W: Nursing diagnosis and interventions with the acute stroke patient. *Nurs Clin North Am* 1986; 21(2):309–319.

Goldman R: Aging changes in structure and function. Pages 73–101 in: *Nursing Management for the Elderly.* Carnevali D, Patrick M (editors). Lippincott, 1986.

Gordon M: *Nursing Diagnosis: Process and Application.* McGraw-Hill, 1982.

Gorelick P: Cerebrovascular disease: Pathophysiology and diagnosis. *Nurs Clin North Am* 1986; 21(2):275–287.

Hallal J: Nursing diagnosis: An essential step to quality care. *J Gerontol Nurs* 1985; 11(9):35–38.

Hardy M, Maas M, Akins J: The prevalence of nursing diagnoses among elderly and long term care residents: A descriptive comparison. *Advances Nurs* 1988:(21):144–158.

Hart L: Ischemia. Pages 293–318 in: *Concepts Common to Acute Illness.* Hart L, Reese J, Fearing M (editors). Mosby, 1981.

Herman J: Nursing assessment and nursing diagnosis in patients with peripheral vascular disease. *Nurs Clin North Am* 1986; 21(2):219–231.

Hoskins L et al: Nursing diagnoses in the chronically ill. Pages 319–329 in: *Classification of Nursing Diagnoses: Proceedings of the Sixth National Conference.* Hurley M (editor). Mosby, 1986.

Jeppesen M: Laboratory values for the elderly. Pages 102–142 in: *Nursing Management for the Elderly.* Carnevali, D, Patrick M (editors). Lippincott, 1986.

Jones D, Dunbar C, Jirovec M: *Medical-Surgical Nursing: A Conceptual Approach.* McGraw-Hill, 1982.

Kelly M: *Nursing Diagnosis Sourcebook: Guidelines for Clinical Application.* Appleton-Century-Crofts, 1985.

Kim M: Without collaboration, what's left? *Am J Nurs* 1985; 85(3):281, 284.

Kim M et al: Clinical validation of cardiovascular nursing diagnoses. Pages 128–138 in: *Classification of Nursing Diagnoses: Proceedings of the Fifth National Conference.* Kim M, McFarland G, McLane A (editors). Mosby, 1984.

Leslie F: Nursing diagnosis: Use in long term care. *Am J Nurs* 1981; 81(5):1012–1014.

Linde M: Cerebrovascular accidents. Pages 379–420 in: *Nursing Management for the Elderly.* Carnevali D, Patrick M (editors). Lippincott, 1986.

McKenney J: The effect of clinical pharmacy services on patients with essential hypertension. *Circulation* 1973; 48:1104–1111.

Quinless F: Assessing the client with acute cardiovascular dysfunction. *Top Clin Nurs* 1986; 8(1):45–56.

Rantz M, Miller T, Jacobs C: Nursing diagnosis in long-term care. *Am J Nurs* 1985; 85(8):916–926.

Rice V: Shock, a clinical syndrome. Part I: Definition, etiology, and pathophysiology. *Crit Care Nurse* 1981a; 44–49.

Rice V: Shock, a clinical syndrome. Part IV: Nursing intervention. *Crit Care Nurse* 1981b; 34–42.

Roberts S: Pulmonary tissue perfusion altered: Emboli. *Heart Lung* 1987; 16(2):128–137.

Sexton D: The patient with peripheral arterial occlusive disease. *Nurs Clin North Am* 1977; 12(1):89–99.

Thompson J et al: *Clinical Nursing.* Mosby, 1986.

Turner J: Nursing interventions in patients with peripheral vascular disease. *Nurs Clin North Am* 1986; 21(2):233–240.

Ventura M et al: Effectiveness of health promotion interventions. *Nurs Res* 1984; 33(3):162–167.

Wagner M: Pathophysiology related to peripheral vascular disease. *Nurs Clin North Am* 1986; 21(2):195–205.

Wild L: Cardiovascular problems. Pages 361–378 in: *Nursing Management for the Elderly.* Carnevali D, Patrick M (editors). Lippincott, 1986.

21

Ineffective Breathing Pattern

BONNIE McDONALD WAKEFIELD,
MA, RN

INEFFECTIVE BREATHING PATTERN IS "THE STATE IN which an inhalation and/or exhalation pattern does not enable adequate pulmonary inflation or emptying" (Carroll-Johnson, 1989;527). The specific relevance of this diagnosis for the elderly has rarely been examined. This chapter discusses what has been done in relation to the diagnosis in the elderly, with an eye toward future work to be accomplished.

SIGNIFICANCE FOR THE ELDERLY

Maximum levels of pulmonary function are reached between age 20 and 25, then decline progressively (Levitzky, 1984). The effects of aging, however, are difficult to separate from the effects of chronic exposure to air pollution, smoking, respiratory infections, and differences in lifestyle. The passage of time alone changes anatomy and the physiologic response to various stimuli. Normal loss may impede functional ability so that the results of aging may be additive or may complicate existing pathology. Attributing signs and symptoms such as dyspnea or fatigue solely to the aging process leads to progressive worsening of pathology due to lack of treatment.

Chronic obstructive pulmonary disease (COPD) is responsible for 7% of all disability payments made by the U.S. Social Security Administration (Zadai, 1986). Septicemia, COPD, pneumonia, and the flu are among the leading causes of death for those over age 70 (Winga, 1983; Zadai, 1986). Pneumonia is the leading cause of death from infectious disease in people over the age of 65 years. Signs and symptoms are often diminished, vague, or absent, preventing early and accurate diagnosis (Winga, 1983). This increased vulnerability to pneumonia is due to a progressive age-related impairment of lung defense mechanisms.

Risk factors for pneumonia and the flu include chronic lung disease, debilitation, residence in a nursing home or other chronic care facility, or age greater than 50 years (American Lung Association, 1986). Cigarette smokers are at particular risk because inhaled tobacco smoke blunts the effectiveness of both phagocytic and immunologic defense mechanisms (Morris, 1984). Inhaled particulates and agents other than tobacco smoke also suppress defense mechanisms, particularly when exposure is prolonged. Chronic disease states, more common in elderly persons, are also associated with an increased susceptibility to lower respiratory infections (Morris, 1984). Finally, the incidence of emphysema increases with age so that by age 90, almost all individuals have some degree of obstructive lung disease (Petty, 1983).

Nurses need to understand the basic changes associated with aging in order to make a differential diagnosis. Nurses are in a position to assess functional ability and the effects of normal and pathologic changes on activities of daily living (ADLs). Determination of the patient's motivation and abilities for rehabilitation aids in the development of comprehensive and coordinated intervention efforts.

ETIOLOGIES/RELATED FACTORS

Physiologic Changes With Aging

Two major functions of the respiratory system are ventilation and gas exchange. Other functions that may be affected by aging are neural control of breathing and defense mechanisms. Brandstetter and Kazemi (1983), Levitzky (1984), and Wahba (1983) provide excellent reviews of the effects of aging on respiratory system function.

Ventilation   The amount of effort required for ventilation is determined by compliance, airway resistance, and alveolar surface tension. Age-related changes occur in compliance and airway resistance, but not in the surface tension of the alveoli.

Compliance Ventilatory lung function deteriorates about two times faster after age 50 (Jedrychowski, 1983). Changes in lung volumes and mechanics are due to a decrease in the elastic recoil of the lung and a progressive stiffening of the chest wall (Brandstetter and Kazemi, 1983; Horvath and Borgia, 1984; Levitzky, 1984; Wahba, 1983). Collagen becomes more rigid, and cross linkage and rearrangement of collagen fibrils and elastin contribute to the loss of elastic recoil (Brandstetter and Kazemi, 1983; Levitzky, 1984; Wahba, 1983). Less pressure is required for lung expansion, and in conjunction with alveolar dilation, an increased static pulmonary compliance results (Brandstetter and Kazemi, 1983; Wahba, 1983). Dynamic lung compliance (measured during active breathing) decreases and becomes frequency dependent with age, probably due to the increased resistance to airflow in the small airways. In fact, most dynamic measurements of lung volume decrease with age (Levitzky, 1984; Wahba, 1983).

Whereas static pulmonary compliance increases, chest wall compliance decreases, resulting in a greater negative pleural pressure. Therefore, elastic recoil of the chest wall shifts from outward to inward at a much lower volume. The closing volume or closing capacity (the lung volume at which small airways begin to close during forced expiration) increases from about 30% of total lung capacity at age 20 to about 55% at age 70. These two changes result in premature

airway closure and poorly ventilated or unventilated alveoli at resting lung volumes. Small airways are more likely to collapse in the lower regions because of diminished elastic recoil and a higher gravity dependent intrapleural pressure. These conditions may result in less efficient matching of ventilation and perfusion and decreased arterial oxygen tension in the elderly (Levitzky, 1984).

Airway Resistance   Decreased diameter of the small airways, decreased stability, and increased closing capacity contribute to premature closure on expiration. These small airway effects are exacerbated when the lungs are in the supine position. A coincident increase in diameter of the larger and more central airways increases anatomic and physiologic dead space (Wahba, 1983). Dilation of the large airways concomitant with small-airway constriction and closure results in gas trapping and increased dead space, leading to ventilation–perfusion imbalances.

Perception of airflow resistance is blunted in elderly adults (Altose and Leitner, 1985), making small changes in respiratory resistance more difficult to detect (Rubin et al, 1982). Older individuals are less able to maintain a constant tidal volume (Altose and Leitner, 1985). Prolonged airway obstruction, as is experienced with lung disease, decreases the ability to sense changes in resistance (Rubin et al, 1982), as does cigarette smoke (Morris, 1984). Closing volumes also increase disproportionately to age in smokers (Wahba, 1983).

Gas Exchange   Arterial oxygen tension decreases each decade, whereas alveolar pO_2 remains constant or increases slightly (Horvath and Borgia, 1984). This results in a decrease in arterial pO_2 of 20% from age 20 to age 70 (Levitzky, 1984). This age-dependent widening of alveolar–arterial oxygen differences results from functional alterations in ventilation–perfusion dynamics (Horvath and Borgia, 1984). A physiologic shunt of alveolar ventilation becomes less uniform with age. Upper lung regions receive preferential ventilation without a corresponding increase of blood flow. The resulting alveolar dead space leads to underventilated pulmonary capillaries. Pulmonary diffusing capacity decreases 20% over the course of adult life because of a decreased alveolar surface area and decreased pulmonary capillary blood volume (Levitzky, 1984). The end result is a decrease in the effective pulmonary-capillary area (Brandstetter and Kazemi, 1983). Although these changes affect the pO_2, arterial CO_2 tension does not change with age (Levitzky, 1984).

Neural Regulation   Increased ventilation in response to hypoxia and hypercapnia is blunted, decreasing by one half by age 70 as compared to the response of a 25 year old (Brandstetter and Kazemi, 1983; Levitzky, 1984; Rubin et al, 1982; Wahba 1983). Hypothesized causes for this decrease in response include diminished neural output to the respiratory muscle (Brandstetter and Kazemi, 1983), diminished sensitivity of the central and arterial chemoreceptors (Levitzky, 1984; Rubin et al, 1982), or changes in central respiratory control (Levitzky, 1984).

Observed differences in respiratory patterns may be caused as much by changes in the mechanics of the respiratory system as by changes in chemoreceptor sensitivity or the central nervous system (CNS) (Brandstetter and Kazemi, 1983; Levitzky, 1984; Rubin et al, 1982). Blunted perception of airflow resistance is probably a result of impaired CNS processing (Altose and Leitner, 1985). Patients with COPD, when compared to age-matched controls, have exhibited significantly less variable rhythm and depth of breathing, suggesting neural adjustments in breathing control (Loveridge et al, 1984).

Defense Mechanisms Decreased numbers of cilia lead to a diminished efficiency of the mucociliary elevator. The reflex response to mechanical or chemical stimulation of the upper airway is decreased, and coughing is less efficient in terms of volume, force, and flow rate because of decreased respiratory muscle strength and altered mechanics of the lung and chest wall (Levitzky, 1984).

Structural Changes The alveolar ducts and respiratory bronchioles enlarge at the expense of the alveoli, leading to a decreased alveolar surface area. The number and size of interalveolar fenestrae increase with concomitant degeneration of adjacent elastic fibers. These changes appear to be the source of increased lung compliance and diminished pulmonary elastic recoil.

Pulmonary vasculature is less distensible, but resting mean pulmonary arterial pressure and pulmonary vascular resistance change little with age. There is an increased thickness of the larger pulmonary arteries.

The bronchial cartilage tends to calcify, leading to diminished chest wall compliance and increased dead space. Costal cartilages calcify, decreasing the mobility and compliance of the rib cage. Intervertebral spaces diminish in size and kyphosis increases, resulting in a shorter thorax, increased anterior–posterior diameter, and reduced total lung capacity. Increased deposition of abdominal and thoracic adipose tissue may also contribute to decreased chest wall compliance. Strength of the muscles of breathing is also lessened (Levitzky, 1984).

DEFINING CHARACTERISTICS

The three respiratory nursing diagnoses currently accepted by the North American Nursing Diagnosis Association (NANDA) are Ineffective Airway Clearance; Ineffective Breathing Pattern; and Impaired Gas Exchange. Although these diagnoses have existed for over a decade, little research has been conducted to investigate their validity.

The American Thoracic Society (1981) published Standards for Nursing Care of Patients wtih COPD. The nursing diagnoses in the standards were limited to areas requiring independent nursing action and are those with the most significant impact on the person with COPD. One diagnosis was Ineffective Breathing Pattern. Outcome criteria were listed, and evaluation focused on whether or not nursing care made a difference.

A few theoretical and clinically focused articles have been published on diagnoses related to respiratory problems. Humbrecht and Van Parys (1982) differentiated the three respiratory nursing diagnoses on the basis of medical diagnosis and symptoms. The defining characteristics listed for Ineffective Breathing Pattern were hyperventilation, Kussmaul's respiration or air hunger, orthopnea, prolonged expiratory phase, and paradoxical breathing. Only one of these, prolonged expiratory phase, is included in the NANDA listing of defining characteristics.

Sjoberg (1983) discussed the application of nursing diagnoses common to the COPD patient, including Activity Intolerance, Sleep Pattern Disturbance, Noncompliance, and Ineffective Coping. Ineffective Breathing Pattern was not identified as a specific diagnosis, but the defining charactertistics of this diagnosis were discussed as etiologies of Activity Intolerance, Sleep Pattern Disturbance, Noncompliance, and Ineffective Coping.

Carpenito (1983) grouped the three respiratory diagnoses under the broad diagnosis Alteration in Respiratory Function. She stated that some contributing factors affect the entire system, and therefore it is incorrect to use a specific diagnostic category. Interventions were directed at assessing, removing, or reducing the causative factors of fear, pain, and exercise/activity.

York (1985) presented a model for clinical validation of the nursing diagnoses Ineffective Airway Clearance and Ineffective Breathing Pattern. Clinical experts rated the appropriateness of the defining characteristics for each diagnosis, and clinical records were reviewed to identify the presence of the defining characteristics. The nurses surveyed agreed with the defining characteristics as proposed by NANDA; they also agreed that abnormal respiratory mechanics were associated with Ineffective Breathing Pattern. McDonald (1985) measured the frequency of the defining characteristics of the three respiratory nursing diagnoses in 41 care plans and identified interventions used to treat these diagnoses. Suggested changes in the defining characteristics are given in Table 21.1.

ASSESSMENT

No available assessment tools exist specifically for Ineffective Breathing Pattern. Research data collection tools developed by York (1985) and McDonald (1985)

Table 21.1

Etiologies/Related Factors and Defining Characteristics for Ineffective Breathing Pattern

NANDA (CARROLL-JOHNSON, 1989;527)	McDONALD WAKEFIELD (McDONALD, 1985)

Definition: A state in which an individual's inhalation and/or exhalation pattern does not enable adequate ventilation

Etiologies/Related Factors	*Etiologies/Related Factors*
Neuromuscular impairment	Obstructive lung disease
Pain	Infectious upper/lower respiratory disease
Musculoskeletal impairment	Physiologic changes of normal aging, eg, changes in ventilation, gas
Anxiety	exchange, neural control of breathing, defense mechanisms, structural
	changes
Decreased energy and fatigue	
Perception/cognitive impairment	

Defining Characteristics	*Defining Characteristics*
Dyspnea	Dyspnea/shortness of breath
Tachypnea	Tachypnea or bradypnea
Cyanosis	Cyanosis
Cough	Cough
Respiratory depth changes	Labored or shallow breathing
Shortness of breath	Abnormal ABGs
Fremitus	Assumption of 3-point position*
Abnormal ABGs	Pursed-lip breathing/prolonged expiratory phase*
Nasal flaring	Increased anterior–posterior diameter*
Assumption of 3-point position	Use of accessory muscles*
Pursed-lip breathing/prolonged expiratory phase	Fremitus
Increased anterior–posterior diameter	Nasal flaring
Use of accessory muscles	Altered chest excursion
Altered chest excursion	Hyperventilation
	Air hunger
	Orthopnea
	Paradoxical breathing

*Noncritical characteristics: It is not necessary for these characteristics to be present in order to make the diagnosis of ineffective breathing pattern.

were used to review care plans written for patients with respiratory problems. Both are essentially checklists that identify defining characteristics that would support a respiratory nursing diagnosis.

Guzzetta et al (1989) have published a collection of clinical assessment tools. Three of these tools may be useful when assessing patients with Ineffective Breathing Patterns: Pulmonary Assessment. Tool, Medical-Surgical Assessment Tool, and Gerontologic Assessment Tool. Within each of these tools is a section addressing oxygenation/pulmonary function. A compilation of the assessment parameters that address Ineffective Breathing Patterns is presented in Assessment Guide 21.1.

The etiologies/related factors and defining characteristics for the diagnosis Ineffective Breathing Pattern as approved by the North American Nursing Diagnosis Association are listed in Table 21.1.

CASE STUDY

Ineffective Breathing Pattern

Mr. K, a 70-year-old white man, had frequent, shallow respirations and could not finish a sentence without significant shortness of breath. Further examination revealed the following findings:

OBJECTIVE DATA

Vital signs: pulse 96, respiratory rate 28 at rest, BP 138/ 82
Increased anterior–posterior diameter of chest
Clubbing of fingers with moderate cyanosis of nailbeds
Height 6″, weight 170 pounds
Oriented to time, place, and person

SUBJECTIVE DATA

Verbalized fear of activity and fatigue: "I just can't get around like I used to. I just can't get enough air. Most of the time, I just sit around watching TV."

HISTORY

Smoked for 40 years (quit 5 years ago because of increased breathing difficulty). Decreased appetite is due to difficulty breathing while eating.

DIAGNOSES

Medical diagnosis: emphysema

Nursing diagnosis: Ineffective Breathing Pattern related to decreased energy and fatigue, decreased lung expansion, and anxiety, evidenced by dyspnea, shortness of breath, tachypnea, cyanosis, respiratory depth changes, and increased anterior-posterior diameter.

The assessment parameters for the diagnosis Activity Intolerance are similar to Ineffective Breathing Pattern; the key differences are in cardiac function. Mr. K did not experience abnormal heart rate or blood pressure in response to activity. When planning interventions, however, the nurse should be cognizant of the effect of ineffective breathing on Mr. K's activity level.

NURSING INTERVENTIONS

Often the disease states associated with Ineffective Breathing Patterns are not reversible. Education in self-care is critical for stabilizing and preventing symptoms and for promoting optimal functional capacity. Pulmonary rehabilitation programs typically have the following goals: reduce symptoms; reestablish independence; slow or arrest progress of disease; reduce hospitalization; increase exercise tolerance, appetite and well-being; improve psychologic status; and prevent complications and decline in function (Bradley, 1983).

It is valuable for all patients to understand the disease process and treatments, when to seek medical assistance, and how to accomplish activities of daily living. The greatest benefit of structured pulmonary rehabilitation programs, however, seems to be the improvement in subjective well-being (Bebout et al, 1983; Bradley, 1983; McCord, 1985; Shenkman, 1985; Wright et al, 1983). Other benefits include increased exercise tolerance and decreased number of hospital days (Wright et al, 1983). However, the usefulness of rehabilitation programs for the elderly has not been addressed.

Education Programs

Prior to the initiation of teaching, it is important to identify psychologic and social situations that contribute to disability and insufficiency (Dudley et al, 1980). Providing patients and family or friends with an opportunity to talk about particular problems and priorities is a significant first step in the process of mutual goal setting. It is also important to consider the patient's age, sex, education level, cultural background, and prior experience with the disease. Values clarification and behavior modification also may be useful in an education program (Hopp and Gerken, 1983).

The McLean et al (1983) Self-Administration of Medical Modalities (SAMM) program taught hospitalized patients about pulmonary disease and treatment through three progressive levels of self-care. The aim of the program was to foster independence through education. Although patients reported that SAMM helped prepare them for self-care at home, the age range of patients who participated in the program was not reported.

Education is often considered more effective if offered in a group setting, and indeed patients have reported benefits from the social support of a group (McCord, 1985). However, group classes are neither convenient nor accessible to all patients. Brough et al (1982) found no significant differences between group teaching and self-learning.

Response to rehabilitative efforts has been greater for patients with strong psychosocial assets, such as a vital interest in life, adequate financial resources and housing, social support, ability to cope with environmental modifications, freedom from oversensitivity, geniality, flexibility, reliability, a sense of good judgment, and a willingness to shoulder reasonable responsibility (Dudley et al, 1980). Patients assigned to either a pulmonary rehabilitation group or a self-help support group when compared with a control group had fewer hospital days and exhibited a higher level of physical and emotional well-being (Jensen, 1983). Prigatano et al (1984) found the degree of physical limitation measured by hypoxemia to be related to the degree of pulmonary disease. However, patients with mild hypoxemia had marked psychosocial limitations related to social interaction and recreation activities that were comparable to psychosocial limitations experienced by severely hypoxemic patients.

Shenkman (1985) found that patients who were most incapacitated by the disease were more likely to fail to complete a rehabilitation program. Furthermore, individuals who failed to complete the program had higher scores related to anxiety and depression. A vicious cycle ensues as persons who are in greater need of the psychosocial benefits tend not to complete rehabilitation programs. Identifying high-risk patients and increasing supports through activities aimed at reducing anxiety and enhancing coping skills may offset this pattern (Jensen, 1983; Prigatano et al, 1984). The patient needs to be educated about the following components of pulmonary rehabilitation programs: breathing retraining, exercise, energy conservation, and general health maintenance, including adequate nutrition, smoking cessation, and stress management. Two of these components, breathing retraining and exercise, are discussed in more detail.

Breathing Retraining Breathing retraining (BR) consists of education about COPD, chest wall muscle relaxation and movement synchronization, and pursed-lip breathing. Resistive breathing training (RBT) consists of breathing continuously against a resistance several times a day (Ambrosino et al, 1984). Breathing exercises (abdominal breathing, pursed-lip breathing, and resistive breathing training) improve emptying of air from alveoli through coordinated use of the diaphragm and abdominal muscles. Use of pursed-lip breathing may be beneficial during periods of excitement or shortness of breath because it slows the respiratory rate and decreases the work of breathing. Respiratory muscle weakness can be a major factor limiting exercise and the ability to perform activities of daily living (Martin, 1984).

Signs and symptoms of respiratory muscle fatigue include dyspnea, tachypnea, paradoxical chest wall and abdominal motion, altered chest excursion, and eventually elevated $PaCO_2$. Treatment includes increasing the energy supply through administration of oxygen or adequate nutrition, decreasing the work of breathing by decreasing airway resistance or congestion, decreasing energy requirements, or resting the respiratory muscles by mechanical ventilation (Braun, 1984). Breathing training can be an important aspect of therapy for elderly patients with compromised respiratory muscle function (Rochester, 1984).

Ambrosino et al (1984) concluded that RBT did not improve pulmonary function tests, blood gas analysis, or exercise tolerance in patients who received no benefit from previous programs of BR. Chen et al (1985) found that resistive breathing training for a 4-week period dramatically improved inspiratory muscle endurance but only slightly improved strength. The training program had no effect on pulmonary function exercise performance. In a review of fatigue and endurance and training of ventilatory muscles, Belman and Sieck (1982;765) stated:

> In general, improved ventilatory muscle endurance can be attained by resistive or hyperpneic training. In patients with lung disease, this training confers benefits with respect to exercise capacity, although it does not appear to be essential for improved exercise performance. Whether or not this training should receive widespread use is still unclear in view of the fact that exercise alone achieves similar benefits.

Ambrosino et al (1984) also questioned the relationship of rehabilitative techniques to dyspnea, as dyspnea seemed to correlate better with posture than muscle training. However, Martin (1984) found that individuals who received instruction in abdominal breathing, pursed-lip expiration, coordination of breathing, exercise, and the incentive spirometry exhibited improved inspiratory and expiratory muscle strength compared to persons receiving instructions in all techniques except incentive spirometry. Those with the most severe weakness benefited from the program most, and subjects in the incentive spirometry group reported informally an increased ability to perform ADLs.

Larson and Kim (1984) reported significant increases in muscle strength and sputum expectoration ability after training with an incentive spirometer resistive breathing device. Exercise performance diminished, but was measured under different environmental conditions, the initial measurement being taken in the spring and the second measurement in the summer. No changes were found in shortness of breath, coughing ability, or ADLs. Subjects liked visualizing the extent of their lung inflation with the spirometer. This positive effect may have contributed to the high compliance rate (98%) found in this study.

Zack et al (1984) recommended both ventilatory and nonventilatory muscle exercise in rehabilitation programs. Their 2-week program incorporated whole-body exercise (walking), inspiratory resistive loading, and use of supplemental oxygen. Although heart rate and oxygen uptake did not improve, endurance time and exercise capacity did. Most important, patients felt the program had been extremely useful and requested to continue to attend sessions. Studies pertaining to exercise prescription components for respiratory muscle training have found that respiratory skeletal muscles were responsive to training for improvement in strength and endurance. However, ingredients for successful training are unclear because of interstudy variations of several parameters (Sobush et al, 1985). Further studies are needed, particularly with the elderly, to produce safe and consistent guidelines for respiratory muscle training prescriptions.

Exercise Patients with breathing difficulties frequently limit activities for fear of inducing dyspnea. The deconditioning produced by activity results in dyspnea being induced at even lower intensity activities. With some limitations, improvement in exercise tolerance following exercise training programs in patients with COPD is fairly well established (Hughes and Davison, 1983). Specific physiologic correlates of enhanced exercise tolerance are not well defined. Studies consistently report, however, an enhanced sense of well-being following exercise training. The inability to exercise can have far-reaching negative consequences for physical independence and morale (Bradley, 1983).

Mohsenifar et al (1983) found significant changes in resting pulmonary function following exercise training, and small but significant reductions in exercise heart rate and blood lactate levels. All patients in the study experienced a subjective enhancement of exercise tolerance, and general sense of well-being and endurance time at least doubled for every patient. Both respiratory and non-respiratory (whole-body) muscle training have effected changes in resting pulmonary function, gas exchange, exercise-induced hypoxemia, or VO_2max (Zack and Palange, 1985). A significant increase was noted in maximum workload, 12-minute walk distance, and endurance time, which, the cohort reported, translated into substantial improvements in quality of life. Tydeman et al (1984) found no improvement in physiologic parameters, but exercise tolerance improved as measured by the 12-minute walk test. Program participants were able to walk 1600 meters in their own time without stopping, a distance that should enable them to perform most social activities. The group took 26 to 51 weeks to reach peak performance, but the greatest improvement in peformance occurred after approximately 4 weeks in the program. The exercises were easily tied to the home setting, and the improved level of functioning could be maintained at home. Because the patients improved in the absence of changes in physiologic parameters, it was hypothesized that improvement was due to increased confidence and positive attitude and the value of a group activity and support. Patients studied by Booker (1984) and Niinimaa and Shephard (1978) also reported after training that they could do more, felt better, and were less afraid of becoming breathless, despite lack of clinically significant objective changes. The long-term hazards of exercise in COPD patients and all older subjects remain unclear and potentially include cardiac arrythmias, systemic hypotension, transient blood abnormalities, fatigue of the diaphragm, and right ventricular failure. Unresolved questions remain regarding exercise level, intensity, duration, frequency, and type. However, properly supervised exercise appears to carry little immediate risk when tailored to the patient's impairment and can substantially improve most participants' quality of life and level of social and recreational activity (Huges and Davison, 1983; Zack and Palange, 1985). Improvements in social functioning could have far-reaching positive outcomes for the elderly.

Energy Conservation Avoidance of dyspnea helps the elderly person to carry out ADLs as independently as possible. Patients can be taught to simplify their daily routine and conserve energy by sitting for as many activities as possible, resting frequently during activities, alternating heavy and light tasks, breathing slowly with the diaphragm, carrying articles close to the body, and delegating tasks when possible (D'Agostina, 1983; American Lung Association, 1982).

OUTCOMES

Expected outcomes for these interventions include the following:

Breathing retraining:

- ability to slow respiratory rate during dyspneic periods
- subjective feelings of improved ability to perform ADLs
- improved sputum expectoration ability

Exercise:

- enhanced sense of well-being
- increased endurance time
- improved tolerance for exercise (specific physiologic correlates not well defined)

Energy conservation:

- avoidance of dyspnea

CASE STUDY

Nursing Interventions

Breathing exercises and an exercise program were prescribed for Mr. K. These interventions were directed at increasing his energy level, promoting adequate emptying of his lungs, and ultimately reducing his anxiety level. Mr. K was also informed of the rationale for the interventions, of the need for adequate nutrition, and of techniques for energy conservation.

The nurse instructed Mr. K in pursed-lip breathing techniques, first while sitting and then while walking. He learned how to pace himself with this breathing technique while walking, taking two steps on inspiration and four steps on expiration. He also used a hand-held incentive spirometer four times a day for visual positive reinforcement. Mr. K's exercise program began with walking the length of the room and progressed to the length of the hallway four times per day. Another client who enjoyed taking short walks began to walk with Mr. K and the two would often play cards after the walking sessions.

Six months later, Mr. K was able to walk the length of the hallway without shortness of breath, stopped his activity when dyspneic, and deliberately used the pursed-lip breathing maneuver. Although Mr. K's activity was still limited, he was less anxious about ambulating. He socialized more because he was able to converse without severe shortness of breath. A 5-pound weight gain was noted. Mr. K verbalized that he had not felt better in a long time.

SUMMARY

Nurses need to evaluate approaches to care in light of the increasing population of elderly and the concomitant changes that occur with aging. Lack of awareness of these changes may lead to the assumption that pathologic changes are a small part of aging and vice versa. Without an adequate knowledge base, assessment, diagnosis, and treatments may be unnecessary or inappropriate. Both practicing nurses and nursing students should receive education about the normal and pathologic changes that occur in the elderly. In addition, existing treatments used in pulmonary rehabilitation programs need to be tested for efficacy with the elderly.

ASSESSMENT GUIDE 21.1

Ineffective Breathing Pattern Assessment Parameters

Thoracic examination: Barrell _____ Scoliosis _____

Other _____

Complaints of dyspnea (yes/no) _____ Precipitated by _____

Orthopnea (yes/no) _____
Respirations:

Rate _____ Rhythm _____ Depth _____
Labored/Unlabored (circle)
Use of accessory muscles (yes/no) _____

Chest expansion (describe) _____

Pursed-lip breathing (yes/no) _____ Nasal flaring (yes/no) _____

Cough: productive/nonproductive (describe cough; frequency, etc.) _____

_____

Sputum: Color _____ Amount _____ Consistency _____ Character _____

Splinting (yes/no) _____

_____

Oxygen: percent and device _____

Breath sounds (describe) _____

_____

Arterial blood gases: pH _____ pO_2 _____ pCO_2 _____

O_2 saturation _____ Bicarbonate _____

Hemoglobin _____ Hematocrit _____

Heart rate _____ Skin color _____

Pulmonary function values _____

Mental status _____

References

Altose MD, Leitner J, Cherniack NS: Effects of age and respiratory efforts on the perception of resistive ventilatory loads. *J Gerontol* 1985; 40(2):147–153.

Ambrosino N et al: Failure of resistive breathing training to improve pulmonary function tests in patients with chronic obstructive pulmonary disease. *Respiration* 1984; 45:455–459.

American Lung Association: *Help Yourself to Better Breathing.* 1982.

American Lung Association: *Pneumonia: The Facts About Your Lungs.* 1986.

American Thoracic Society: Standards for nursing care of patients with COPD. *ATS News* (Summer) 1981; 31–38.

Bebout DE et al: Clinical and physiological outcomes of a university-hospital pulmonary rehabilitation program. *Resp Care* 1983; 28(11):1468–1473.

Belman MJ, Sieck GC: The ventilatory muscles: Fatigue, endurance and training. *Chest* 1982; 6:761–766.

Booker HA: Exercise training and breathing control in patients with chronic airflow limitation. *Physiotherapy* 1984; 70(7):258–260.

Bradley BL: Rehabilitation of patients with chronic respiratory disease. *Resp Ther* 1983; 13(4):15–21.

Brandstetter RD, Kazemi H: Aging and the respiratory system. *Med Clin North Am* 1983; 67(2):419–431.

Braun N: Respiratory muscle dysfunction. *Heart Lung* 1984; 13(4):327–332.

Brough FK et al: Comparison of two teaching methods for self-care training for patients with chronic obstructive pulmonary disease. *Patient Couns Health Ed* 1982; 4(2):111–116.

Carpenito LJ: *Nursing Diagnosis: Application to Clinical Practice.* Lippincott, 1983.

Carroll-Johnson R (editor): *Classification of Nursing Diagnoses: Proceedings of the Eighth Conference.* Lippincott, 1989.

Chen H, Dukes R, Martin BJ: Inspiratory muscle training in patients with chronic obstructive pulmonary disease. *Am Rev Resp Dis* 1985; 131(2):252–255.

D'Agostina JS: You can breathe new life into your COPD patients. *Nursing* (Sept) 1983; 72–77.

Dudley DL et al: Psychosocial concomitants to rehabilitation in chronic obstructive pulmonary disease. *Chest* 1980; 77(3):413–420.

Guzzetta CE et al: *Clinical Assessment Tools for Use With Nursing Diagnoses.* Mosby, 1989.

Hopp JW, Gerken CM: Making an educational diagnosis to improve patient education. *Resp Care* 1983; 28(11):1456–1461.

Horvath SM, Borgia JF: Cardiopulmonary gas transport and aging. *Am Rev Resp Dis* 1984; 129 (Suppl S68–S71).

Hughes RL, Davison R: Limitations of exercise reconditioning in COPD. *Chest* 1983; 83(2):241–249.

Humbrecht B, Vanparys E: From assessment to intervention: How to use heart and breath sounds as part of your nursing care plan. *Nursing* 1982; 12(4):34–41.

Jedrychowski W: Biological meaning of the prospective epidemiological study on chronic obstructive lung disease and aging. *Arch Gerontol Geriatr* 1983; 2:237–248.

Jensen PS: Risk, protective factors and supportive interventions in chronic airway obstruction. *Arch Gen Psychiatry* 1983; 40:1203–1207.

Larson M, Kim MJ: Respiratory muscle training with the incentive spirometer resistive breathing device. *Heart Lung* 1984; 13(4):342–345.

Levitzky MG: Effects of aging on the respiratory system. *The Physiologist* 1984; 27(2):102–107.

Loveridge B et al: Breathing patterns in patients with chronic obstructive pulmonary disease. *Am Rev Resp Dis* 1984; 130(5):730–733.

Martin LL: Respiratory muscle function: A clinical study. *Heart Lung* 1984; 13(4):346–348.

McCord M: Nursing management of pulmonary health care services within a community hospital. *Nurs Admin Q* 1985; 9(4):32–37.

McDonald BR: Validation of three respiratory nursing diagnoses. *Nurs Clin North Am* 1985; 20(4):697–709.

McLean DL et al: Self-administration of medical modalities (SAMM): Another method of rehabilitation education. *Resp Care* 1983; 28(11):1462–1467.

Mohsenifar Z et al: Sensitive indices of improvement in a pulmonary rehabilitation program. *Chest* 1983; 83(2):189–192.

Morris JF: Geriatric medicine, Vol 1. In: *Pulmonary Diseases.* Cassel CK, Walsh JR (editors). Springer-Verlag, 1984.

Niinimaa V, Shephard RJ: Training and oxygen conductance in the elderly. *J Gerontol* 1978; 33(3):354–361..

Petty TL: Respiratory diseases. In: *Care of the Geriatric Patient,* 6th ed. Steinberg FU (editor). Mosby, 1983.

Prigatano GP, Wright EC, Levin D: Quality of life and its predictors in patients with mild hypoemia and chronic obstructive pulmonary disease. *Arch Intern Med* 1984; 144:1613–1619.

Rochester DF: Respiratory muscle function in health. *Heart Lung* 1984; 13(4):349–354.

Rubin S, Tack M, Cherniack NS: Effect of aging on respiratory responses to CO_2 and inspiratory resistive loads. *J Gerontol* 1982; 37:306–312.

Shenkman B: Factors contributing to attrition rates in a pulmonary rehabilitation program. *Heart Lung* 1985; 14(1):53–58.

Sjoberg EL: Nursing diagnosis and the COPD patient. *Am J Nurs* 1983; 83(2):245–248.

Sobush D, Dunning M, McDonald K: Exercise prescription components for respiratory muscle training: Past, present and future. *Resp Care* 1985; 30(1):34–41.

Tydeman DE et al: An investigation into the effects of exercise training on patients with chronic airways obstruction. *Physiotherapy* 1984; 70(7):261–264.

Wahba WM: Influence of aging on lung function—clinical significance of changes from age twenty. *Anesthesia Analgesia* 1983; 62:764–776.

Winga ER: Pulmonary diseases of the aged. *Wisconsin Med J* 1983; 82:23–25.

Wright RW et al: Benefits of a community-hospital pulmonary rehabilitation program. *Resp Care* 1983; 28(11):1474–1479.

York K: Clinical validation of two respiratory nursing diagnoses and their defining characteristics. *Nurs Clin North Am* 1985; 20(4):657–668.

Zack MB, Palange AV: Oxygen supplement exercise of ventilatory and nonventilatory muscles in pulmonary rehabilitation. *Chest* 1985; 88(5):669–675.

Zack MB et al: Ventilatory and nonventilatory muscle exercise in COPD rehabilitation. *Resp Ther* 1984; 14(5):41–45.

Zadai CC: Cardiopulmonary issues in the geriatric population: Implications for rehabilitation. *Top Geriatr Rehab* 1986; 2(1):1–9.

22

Activity Intolerance

Susan MacLean, PhD, RN

Activity Intolerance is defined as "a state in which an individual has insufficient physiological or psychological energy to endure or complete required or desired daily activity (Carroll-Johnson 1989;543). Thus, the frequency, intensity, and duration of activity is dependent on a balance between the available energy (supply) and the energy needed for activity (demand). For the elderly in long-term care settings, the energy demand often exceeds the energy supply. Factors that may deplete available and potential energy include (1) physical conditions such as disease, chronic disabilities, pain, fatigue, and deconditioning; (2) psychologic conditions such as anxiety, depression, grief, and confusion; (3) poor or altered lifestyle behaviors such as smoking, obesity, poor nutrition, lack of regular exercise, and a sedentary lifestyle; and (4) personal–social factors such as stress from financial concerns, increased dependence on others, loss of freedom to come and go as desired, and institutionalization. These variables may deplete available energy, particularly when several conditions are present and interacting. Activity Intolerance often occurs because of this energy imbalance.

Activity Intolerance is an important concern for the elderly because of the hazards of inactivity that often occur with increased and earlier disability, decreased quality of life, and increased cost of care. Yet, nursing decisions regarding this frequent and serious problem have not been based on clinical studies. Currently, there is limited research and dissemination of information on cues for diagnosing Activity Intolerance, with no research on etiologic factors, assessment tools, interventions, outcome criteria, or prevention. Consequently, nurses have little or no information on which to base decisions concerning this health problem. The purposes of this chapter are to (1) describe the significance of Activity Intolerance for the elderly; (2) describe the current state of knowledge concerning Activity Intolerance; (3) present case studies to illustrate possible decision-making strategies concerning this nursing diagnosis; (4) review interventions that are relevent for treatment of the diagnosis; and (5) suggest research directions to stimulate the continued development of knowledge about diagnosis and management of Activity Intolerance in the elderly.

SIGNIFICANCE FOR THE ELDERLY

Physical activity has been cited as a factor influencing successful aging (Rowe and Kahn, 1987). Conversely, lack of physical activity is associated with increased morbidity and mortality and decreased quality of life (Chirikos and Nestel, 1985; Hofeldt, 1987; Masoro, 1987; Sowers, 1987; Walsh, 1987; Williams, 1987).

Some of the consequences of inactivity in the elderly include increased and earlier disability; increased cardiovascular and respiratory disease; increased loss of bone density; increased falls and fractures; increased confusion; decreased role performance; decreased independence and self-esteem; increased depression, grief, anxiety, guilt, and stress; and decreased satisfaction with life.

Because the elderly are living longer but with increased disability, the costs of care and treatment have increased. For example, problems with mobility (Williams, 1987) and the inability to maintain an independent lifestyle are leading causes of nursing home placement. Thus, Activity Intolerance is contributing to the escalating costs of home and institutional care. For the elderly, their families, and society, Actual and Potential Activity Intolerance are significant concerns.

NURSING DIAGNOSTIC CONCEPT: ACTIVITY INTOLERANCE

If nurses are to assume leadership in decreasing and eliminating Activity Intolerance, what information is available to them for decision making? Activity Intolerance has been identified as a frequent and important concern for patients in both acute care and rehabilitative settings (Creason et al, 1985; Kim et al, 1984). In addition, the physiologic and psychologic hazards of inactivity have been well documented (Lampman, 1987, Larson and Bruce, 1986; Masoro, 1987; Rowe and Kahn, 1987; Williams, 1987). Although there has been some awareness and concern about patients with Activity Intolerance and for those at risk, there is little research concerning causative factors and the efficient and accurate diagnosis of this health problem.

There is no standardized set of cues (signs and symptoms or defining characteristics) for diagnosing a patient's tolerance to activity. Thus, judgments about activity levels are based, at best, on the prior experiences of the nurse in similar situations. Because expertise varies considerably from nurse to nurse, especially in the long-term setting, patients may be misdiagnosed and may not receive appropriate interventions. Some patients may receive suboptimal levels of activity because the nurse overestimates the risk of activity and does not know the cues that indicate that more activity could be tolerated and beneficial. Or, patients may be stressed beyond their energy endurance because the nurse did not know the critical cues for terminating or decreasing activity intensity, frequency, or duration. Thus, Activity Intolerance often is incorrectly or suboptimally diagnosed. If the diagnosis is inaccurate, then the patient may not receive

the appropriate interventions to achieve such optimal outcomes as increased physical endurance, decreased disability, and improved quality of life.

Nurses can make an important contribution to health care by assuming responsibility and leadership in diagnosing, treating, and preventing Activity Intolerance in the elderly. As practitioners, educators, researchers, and administrators in long-term care settings, nurses with advanced gerontologic preparation can coordinate collaborative research and treatment teams; intervene with patients on a daily basis concerning a slowly changing long-term problem; educate patients, family, and staff about the problem and interventions; develop institutional long-range plans and standards concerning activity issues, programs, and care; and influence health care policy concerning the elderly.

ETIOLOGIES/RELATED FACTORS

Risk Factors

Williams (1987) states that no inevitable age declines are experienced by the elderly. Thus, age alone does not predispose them to problems with activity. There are many physical, psychosocial, and environmental variables that influence the development of intolerance to activity. The two major risk factors are chronic disease and prior lifestyle behaviors (Williams, 1987).

Chronic Disease Health professionals have been successful at treating many illnesses and injuries that previously resulted in death. They also are decreasing the infant mortality rate and extending the median age of death (Masoro, 1987; Walsh, 1987). Today, both an increasing number of healthy individuals and an increasing population of elderly with chronic, costly, disabling, and disheartening diseases reach senescence. The elderly with chronic diseases are admitted to long-term care facilities because they can no longer cope with the chronic illness and the consequences and can no longer maintain an independent lifestyle. One of the serious consequences of chronic illness is a decrease in energy and physical activity. Additionally, the decrease in activity level frequently exacerbates the chronic illness and further decreases the availability of energy for activity.

According to McCarthy (1975), energy is responsible for all life, movement, and activity. Energy must be available for the body to function at the required activity intensity, frequency, and duration. Even with light activities, large amounts of energy are needed because of the complexity of the body's response to activity. This response is dependent on the effectiveness of the cardiac, respiratory, and tissue systems to supply and use oxygen for energy transformation (MacLean, 1987). Nutrients also must be supplied to the cells for energy transformation, and waste products must be removed via intact gastrointestinal, circulatory, and renal systems. Although there are age-associated changes in these systems that may influence the supply of energy, it is pathology that disrupts the maximum functional capacity of these systems.

The cardiovascular system is a good example of a system that is altered by age-associated changes but continues to maintain adequate cardiac output into the 8th decade (Williams, 1987). However, when disease interferes with structural integrity of the heart, function is compromised. In individuals over 65 years of age, 30% to 60% are hypertensive, and 75% to 100% have coronary stenosis (Gerstenblith et al, 1987; Hagberg, 1987; Sowers, 1987). Cardiovascular disease is responsible for 50% of the mortality and the majority of hospitalizations in the elderly (Walsh, 1987). Thus, chronic cardiovascular disease may contribute significantly to deconditioning and an imbalance in oxygen supply and demand, factors that decrease energy supply (see Chapter 19). Other factors associated with the treatment of cardiovascular disease also alter available energy and subsequent activity. As discussed in Chapter 4, drug side effects, toxicities, and interactions also often cause fatigue, dizziness, orthostatic falls, and sleep disturbances (Nail and King, 1987; Sowers, 1987; Thomas, 1987). Deconditioning due to bed rest during hospitalization also causes intolerance to activity (see Chapter 23). Thus, with chronic disease, adaptation is necessary to ensure survival (Levine, 1966). The conservation of energy (eg, reduction in activity) is one of the body's natural defenses against disease processes (Levine, 1967).

Lifestyle Behaviors In addition to age-related changes and chronic disease, risk for Activity Intolerance also is influenced by lifestyle behaviors. For example, sedentary living, weight gain or loss, poor nutrition, inadequate stress management, smoking, and alcohol consumption increase pathology and may be responsible in part for the changes associated with aging (Buskirk and Hodgson, 1987; Gerstenblith et al, 1987; Hagberg, 1987; Larson and Bruce, 1986, 1987; Masoro, 1987; Rowe and Kahn, 1987; Sowers, 1987; Walsh, 1987).

Psychosocial Factors Lifestyle behaviors are influenced by the attitudes and beliefs of the individual, family members, and peers. Often the physically fit active elderly are considered deviant and the less physically fit elderly more the accepted norm. Thus, low energy levels and Activity Intolerance may be considered an acceptable norm for the elderly, and they may receive little or no support for changing to a more active lifestyle. To be able to sit and not work is considered one of the rewards of retirement and old age. With increasing consumer education and awareness of health and wellness, these stereotypic beliefs concerning the right to and the acceptance of inactivity may change.

Other psychosocial variables that place the elderly at greater risk for Activity Intolerance are anxiety and fear concerning falls; lack of companions to share activities; depression, hopelessness, loneliness, and withdrawal; and loss of autonomy and control. Rowe and Kahn (1987) cited several studies in which social support and increased control produced improvements in affect, activity level, and general health status.

The attitudes, biases, and influence of health professionals, politicians, and news media also increase the risk of Activity Intolerance in the elderly. The elderly often are not considered "good investments." It is considered useless to spend money for exercise facilities and programs, stress testing, collaborative health care teams, professional nurses, research, education, and rehabilitation when the elderly can't change, won't change, or don't need to change their health status.

The combination of lack of interest, financial support, and qualified health professionals also may explain the absence of creative, interesting interventions for treating and preventing Activity Intolerance in the elderly. The elderly in long-term care settings need the same close supervision, monitoring of progress, and variation of activities as their young, healthy, physically fit children and grandchildren. If the general attitude of the public and the elderly themselves is that Activity Intolerance is acceptable as part of old age, then little change will occur to improve their health or the quality of their lives or to reduce the costs of care.

DEFINING CHARACTERISTICS

Research on Diagnosing Activity Intolerance

The research concerning this health problem is limited to three studies and the data generated by the participants at the 1984 North American Nursing Diagnosis Association (NANDA) Conference (Kim et al, 1984). Kim et al (1984) and the NANDA participants focused on identifying etiologies and defining characteristics. Fitzmaurice (1986) concentrated on validating the NANDA defining characteristics, and MacLean (1987, 1989) identified and refined critical cues for diagnosing moderate Activity Intolerance related to an imbalance between oxygen supply and demand. In the three studies, the nurses' clinical background was cardiac nursing in acute care settings. No studies have been done in which Activity Intolerance in the elderly or in long-term care settings was the focus. Although some knowledge has been gained about Activity Intolerance from the studies that have been done, a reliable and valid list of cues for clinical use in diagnosing Activity Intolerance has not been identified as yet. As can be seen in the following review of the current research on diagnosing Activity Intolerance, much work remains to be done.

In 1984, the nursing diagnosis Activity Intolerance was accepted for clinical testing at the Fifth National Conference for the Classification of Nursing Diagnoses. At that time, four etiologies and eight defining characteristics were proposed (Kim et al, 1984) and are still those listed by NANDA (Carroll-Johnson, 1989) (Table 22.1).

During the Fifth National NANDA Conference, Kim et al (1984) reported that Decreased Activity Tolerance was one of the 10 most frequently identified nursing diagnoses by 18 staff nurses for 158 cardiovascular patients. Two defining characteristics, each with multiple indicators, were identified: inability to perform activities of daily living and indicators of inadequate gas exchange (Table 22.1).

Fitzmaurice (1986) conducted a second study concerning Activity Intolerance using 25 Masters-prepared nurses who had knowledge and experience working with cardiac patients. Fitzmaurice attempted to validate the NANDA cues for Activity Intolerance using a linear regression model and six of the eight cues. Electrocardiographic changes for arrhythmias and ischemia were not used (see Table 22.1). The four cues providing significant information were discomfort, blood pressure, dyspnea, and fatigue. Heart rate and weakness did not contribute significant information for making the diagnosis.

Because the reliability and validity of the cues from the previous studies were questionable, MacLean (1987, 1989) conducted an extensive literature review to identify other possible cues for diagnosing Activity Intolerance. Levine's (1966, 1967) principles concerning the conservation of structural integrity and energy provided a framework for identifying cues from the physiology, research, and practice literature. A list of 210 cues initially was identified. The list was reduced to 127 cues by eliminating cues that were vague, imprecise, wordy, redundant, or lay terminology. A randomly selected national panel (n = 122) of nurse experts refined and reduced the list of cues to a limited number of critical cues for diagnosing moderate Activity Intolerance related to an imbalance between oxygen supply and demand.

After three rounds of rating 127 cues using a Delphi survey, 19 cues were identified as the most important for making the diagnosis (Table 22.1). However, estimates by the nurse experts of the frequency of cue occurrence for these important cues indicated that the cues occurred infrequently. The sensitivity of the cues was low; only three cues occur more than 50% of the time a patient experiences Activity Intolerance. The specificity was good in that the cues are not observed when there is no Activity Intolerance. MacLean (1987, 1989) stated that until additional investigation is conducted to identify cues that are more reliable and discriminating, the use of cues from this and other studies for clinical diagnosis of Activity Intolerance is premature.

MacLean (1987, 1989) also compared lists of cues from studies on Activity Intolerance to identify consistencies in the findings. As seen on Table 22.1, dyspnea is the only cue listed across studies. The inclusion of dyspnea in all studies provides some evidence of its importance for diagnosing Activity Intolerance. Some categories of cues—for example, abnormal blood pressure and ECG responses—also were found in several studies; however, the specification of the cues varied. For example, in MacLean's study, cues had greater precision and indicated the expected quantity or quality of the cue. At this point in the development of nursing diagnosis, cues should be defined as precisely as possible so that efficient and effective assessment guidelines can be developed.

Inconsistencies across studies on the use of heart rate cues for diagnosing Activity Intolerance was an interesting finding. Heart rate cues were included on the NANDA list (Kim et al, 1984) and considered important by subjects in Fitzmaurice's study (1986), although subjects in this study did not use these cues. These cues were not considered important by the subjects in the studies by Kim et al (1984) and MacLean (1987, 1989). It is surprising that heart rate was not used considering it is quick, easy to perform, and readily available in all settings. Also, several authors (Harrington et al, 1981; Johnson, 1984; Winslow et al, 1985) reported significant changes in heart rate in cardiac patients engaged in low-level exercise.

Perhaps the differences in heart rate changes induced by normal and abnormal activity are not defined to the extent that they can be useful for making judgments. The heart rate cue also may not be helpful in discriminating Activity Intolerance from other diagnoses such as Fear or Pain. Further research on heart rate cues should produce interesting and useful information.

Other defining characteristics that were not consistently identified as important across studies were ADL performance (Kim et al, 1985) and syncope, cyanosis, and diaphoresis (MacLean, 1987, 1989). MacLean suggested that the defining characteristics identified as most important in her study may be influenced by both the diagnostic label and the identified etiology. Further investigations are needed to identify indicators for the diagnostic label, the etiology, and the combination of both in order to obtain a reliable, valid, and manageable set of defining characteristics for each nursing diagnosis.

Although important information has been obtained from past studies about the defining characteristics for diagnosing Activity Intolerance, the findings are insufficient for validation. At this time, the complexity of the nursing diagnosis framework concerning Activity Intolerance presents both a challenge to researchers and frustration to clinicians who do not have the assessment guidelines needed to make clinical judgments about this health problem. Continued investigation is needed in order to provide the diagnostic data that nurses can use to make efficient, accurate, and optimal decisions concerning Activity Intolerance.

Table 22.1

Comparison of Related Factors/Etiologies and Defining Characteristics (Cues): Activity Intolerance

KIM et al (1984)	NANDA (CARROLL-JOHNSON, 1989)	FITZMAURICE (1986)*	MACLEAN (1987, 1989)†
Related Factors/Etiologies			
	Bed rest/immobility Generalized weakness Sedentary lifestyle Imbalance between oxygen supply and demand		Imbalance between oxygen supply and demand
Defining Characteristics			
Indicators of inadequate gas exchange: dyspnea on exertion shortness of breath shallow respirations tachypnea orthopnea accessory muscle use labored breathing Cheyne-Stokes respiration Kussmaul's respirations pulmonary congestion adventitious breath sounds	Exertional dyspnea	Dyspnea (S + 0)†	Dyspnea Severe dyspnea Shortness of breath Labored breathing
Indicators of inability to perform ADLs: lethargy weakness self-management deficit requires assistance with care decreased activity tolerance decreased ADL performance frequent naps	Verbal report of fatigue or weakness	Fatigue (S + 0) Weakness (S)	Severe fatigue
	Abnormal heart rate Abnormal blood pressure	Abnormal heart rate (S) Abnormal blood pressure (S + O)	Systolic blood pressure greater than 250 mm Hg Diastolic blood pressure greater than 120 mm Hg
	Exertional discomfort ECG changes reflecting arrhythmias ECG changes reflecting ischemia	Discomfort (S + O)	Moderate to severe angina Ventricular arrhythmias Ventricular fibrillation Ventricular tachycardia: more than 3 consecutive beats Coupled premature ventricular contractions: 3 to 4 during exercise Premature ventricular contractions greater than 10% to 20% of beats Multifocal premature ventricular beats Second- or third-degree heart block ST segment depression greater than 2.0 mm Cyanosis Syncope Profuse diaphoresis

*ECG cues were excluded in this study.

†The etiology an imbalance between oxygen supply and demand was used in this study.

†S = subjective model; 0 = objective regression model.

ASSESSMENT

Once researchers identify and validate the critical cues for both the diagnosis and the etiologies, then the development and testing of accurate and efficient tools or guidelines for assessing and/or predicting patients' tolerance to activity can proceed. Until valid assessment tools and guidelines are developed, nurses must still make judgments about activity tolerance/intolerance. Some data about possible cues for diagnosing Activity Intolerance are available from the previously described studies (Table 22.1). The nurse can use this information, keeping in mind that the defining characteristics need further testing. As nurses work with patients, they can observe and record whether the cues (eg, blood pressure and heart rate changes) assist them with judgments about Activity Intolerance. This will enable nurses to build clinical evidence regarding validity of the cues.

Nurses can also collaborate with one another and other disciplines to improve decision making about Activity Intolerance. Accurate and precise documentation of the defining characteristics that nurses judge to be indicators of Activity Intolerance can be used as guidelines by nurses and other health professionals. Nurses' documentation should include the cues and the quantity or quality value observed before, during, and after activity; the type of activity; the intensity and duration of activity; the severity of the response to activity; the activity pattern for the period of care (ie, frequency and types of activity and inactivity observed during the nurse's time with the patient); and the patient's responses at rest. Information will then be available concerning the frequency of occurrence of cues when Activity Intolerance is present and when it is absent, thus capturing the sensitivity and specificity of the cues. Also, documentation will demonstrate which cues are helpful to the nurse working with a specific population.

As nurses generate a data base concerning Activity Intolerance, the reliable cues can be retained and the unreliable cues discarded. Through the use and refinement of what is currently known, assessment tools and guidelines can be developed. Nurses caring for the elderly in long-term care settings have an exciting opportunity to help in the development of these tools.

CASE STUDY

Activity Intolerance Diagnostic Process

In the previous section concerning the state of knowledge about Activity Intolerance, the limited research base for diagnostic decision making was described. Consequently, the following case study is not based on validated cues but rather on principles of decision making in combination with the current, available, possibly unreliable clinical cues. Thus, the case study illustrates a process that a nurse in the long-term care setting might use to gather information and make a judgment about Activity Intolerance.

Mr. T has been a resident in a long-term care facility for 5 months. He was admitted 1 month after his wife died because he was unable to care for himself and his apartment. Mr. T stated that he just did not have the energy. He stated that without his wife, he was alone, lonely, and helpless. His limited vision and other health problems also made it unsafe for him to live alone. His medical diagnoses include hypertension, congestive heart failure, diabetes mellitus (NIDDM) type II, and moderate diabetic retinopathy. His current medical regimen includes Diabinese 200 mg q.d., hydrochlorothiazide 25 mg q.d., and digoxin 0.125 mg q.d.

Mr. T's nurse is concerned about him because he appears depressed, and over the past 2 months he has been having increased difficulty caring for himself. Mr. T has told his nurse just to let him sit in his chair. He naps in his chair every morning and afternoon for at least an hour and states he is still exhausted most of the time.

The nurse began investigating the cause of Mr. T's behavior by listing possible nursing diagnoses that might explain what was observed (see Table 22.2): Decreased Cardiac Output, Sleep Pattern Disturbance, Activity Intolerance, Dysfunctional Grieving, and Fluid or Electrolyte Imbalances.

As seen in Table 22.2, the nurse gathered information to estimate the likelihood of each of the nursing diagnoses. Because decreased cardiac output and fluid and electrolyte imbalances were the greatest risk to Mr. T, the nurse closely monitored his physical status. The nurse documented orthostatic hypotension: lying 144/88, 86 and after 2 minutes standing, 124/78, 96 with dizziness; shortness of breath when bathing or dressing; moderate to severe dyspnea when walking 200 yards to the dining room; no angina; no mental confusion; no leg cramping; and slight edema below the ankles. Mr. T's vital signs at rest were BP 144/88, HR 86/reg, R 22; after walking 200 yards, BP 190/108, HR 118/reg, R 34 shallow; and after resting in a chair for 3 minutes, BP 160/95, HR 106/reg, R 28. The physician's progress note from the previous week stated there were no changes in Mr. T's medical status. There were no recent laboratory reports. The nurses' physical assessment showed no acute clinical manifestations of hypoglycemia, hyperglycemia, or digoxin, Diabinese, or hydrochlorothiazide toxicity. Fatigue and muscle weakness were present, but these were not new symptoms.

Because of lack of confirming evidence, the nurse ruled out Decreased Cardiac Output and Fluid Volume Deficit as nursing diagnoses. Dysfunctional Grieving also was ruled out because of the physical changes that were noted with activity. Grief, however, may be a contributing factor; therefore, the nurse decided to continue her assessment of

Table 22.2

Differential Diagnosis: Case Study for Activity Intolerance
Presenting Data: Exhaustion, difficulty with ADL's and self-care, naps frequently, depressed, inactivity
Hypothesized Diagnoses: Decreased Cardiac Output, Fluid or Electrolyte Imbalances, Drug Toxicities, Sleep Pattern
   Disturbance, Dysfunctional Grieving, Activity Intolerance

SIGNS AND SYMPTOMS (CUES)	DIAGNOSES RULED OUT	ADDITIONAL DATA NEEDED
Fatigue/exhaustion		Lab data on potassium, cardiac
Weakness		enzymes, blood gases, ECG not available
Difficulty with ADLs & self-care		
Mild orthostatic hypotension 140/88; 128/78 (standing)		
Shortness of breath on mild exertion		
Moderate to severe dyspnea on moderate exertion		
Slight edema below ankles		
VS 144/88-86R; 190/108-118R; 160/95-106R		
(resting, sitting) (activity) (after 3 min rest, sitting)		
No angina		
No confusion		
No leg cramping		
Normal heart and lung sounds		
No changes in medical status 1 week ago per MD	Decreased Cardiac Output	Data on electrolyte status & drug
	Fluid Imbalance	toxicity; continue assessment of grief
	Dysfunctional Grieving	as a contributing factor
Fatigue		
Muscle weakness		
No hypo- or hyperkalemia		
Acuchek blood glucose = 120	Electrolyte Imbalance	Lab data on glucose, potassium, and
		digoxin levels not available
No digoxin, Diabinese, or hydrochlorothiazide toxicity	Drug Toxicity	
Naps frequently		
Inactivity		
Sleep pattern continuous 6 to 8 hours per night	Sleep Pattern Disturbance	Data from night nurse on quantity &
Poor coping skills		quality of sleep
Able to express sadness and anger over wife's death	Dysfunctional Grieving	Data on grief status
Pallor, diaphoresis, dizziness with moderate exertion		Additional data concerning activity
Anxious about walking		intolerance
Uses supportive devices		
Avoids activity		

Mr. T's grieving status after other priority or high-risk diagnoses were evaluated. Although supporting laboratory data were not available, the nurses' physical assessment revealed no abnormalities supporting electrolyte imbalances or drug toxicities other than the long-standing nonspecific fatigue and muscle weakness. After consulting with the night nurse concerning Mr. T's sleep patterns, Sleep Pattern Disturbance also was eliminated because there was evidence of continuous sleep for 6 to 8 hours per night. A dysfunctional grieving status also was unlikely because of the lack of sleep pattern disturbances. In talking with Mr. T, he was able to express sadness and anger over his wife's death but appeared to be at a loss on how to proceed with his life without her. Although his coping skills were limited, the nurse concluded that Mr. T's grief was not dysfunctional at this time.

The remaining diagnosis the nurse considered was Activity Intolerance. Several data items gathered earlier supported the likelihood of this diagnosis: that is, abnormal changes in heart rate, blood pressure, and respirations with mild to moderate activity; orthostatic hypotension; pallor, dizziness, and mild diaphoresis with activity; decreased activity levels and self-care; frequent napping and inactivity; anxiety; and use of supportive devices with movement. Cues that were not observed but that are associated with this diagnosis are angina and arrhythmias. Therefore, the nurse made a tentative diagnosis of Activity Intolerance and continued to validate the diagnosis.

The nurse considered the following possible etiologies for the Activity Intolerance: deconditioning, imbalance between oxygen supply and demand, and ineffective individual coping. Given Mr. T's physical and psychologic state, the nurse hypothesized that all factors probably were contributing to his Activity Intolerance. During the previous 6 months, Mr. T participated in no programmed activity because of his feelings of loneliness, helplessness, anxiety over safety; his increasing fatigue, weakness, and exhaustion; and his placement in a nursing home where he sits quietly in his chair most of the day. The nurse concluded that he was in a deconditioned health state. Mr. T's difficulties in recovering emotionally following his wife's death, in coping with changes in social role and self-esteem, and in adjusting to institutionalization were contributing to his decreased activity and deconditioning. Although his cardiac condition is stable in an inactive physical state, with increasing activity levels, Mr. T experiences a decrease in available oxygen in the tissues for energy transformation. Therefore, the nurse concluded that an imbalance between oxygen supply and demand also may be contributing to Mr. T's Activity Intolerance. The next phase of the nurse's decision making was to develop with the patient and the physician (1) patient outcomes that were relevant, timely, measurable, and realistic for Mr. T; (2) interventions to achieve the desired outcomes; and (3) criteria to evaluate the effectiveness of the plan for improving Mr. T's activity tolerance and quality of life.

NURSING INTERVENTIONS

Although the research on diagnosing Activity Intolerance has been started, there currently are no reported studies on nursing intervention for treatment or prevention of Activity Intolerance. The linkage between the interventions and the diagnosis has not been established. In addition, no research data have been reported on desired, expected, and actual outcomes, nor on criteria or tools for evaluating the effectiveness of the interventions to minimize risks and achieve optimal outcomes. Research findings from the exercise physiology literature provide some evidence of the efficacy of exercise in the elderly. This information may be useful in developing nursing interventions for Activity Intolerance. However, these reports are limited in number and in generalizability, since the subjects frequently were healthy, independent elders and not disabled or institutionalized elders (see Chapter 23).

The benefits of life-long, high-level physical activity programs clearly are supported by research (Hagberg, 1987; Lampman, 1987; Larson and Bruce, 1986, 1987). In addition, Hagberg (1987) summarized several studies that demonstrated increases in aerobic capacity following endurance exercise programs for sedentary individuals up to 70 years of age. Hagberg described the adaptive capacity of 60- to 70-year-olds as similar to that of young men and women, and Larson and Bruce (1987) stated that achieving the benefits of exercise was not dependent on prior training in the younger years.

Several authors recommend exercise programs of low to moderate intensity to achieve a training effect in unconditioned elderly individuals. Larson and Bruce (1986;784) suggest exercise such as brisk, regular walking, 20 to 30 minutes, three to five times a week, at 70% to 85% of the maximum heart rate, a level that produces mild fatigue and dyspnea. They further advise that the exercise should be "dynamic, interesting, fun, varied, easily accessible, and without sequelae if it is to be habitual."

Lampman's (1987) exercise prescription includes a lower intensity level, 65% to 75% of maximum heart rate and more emphasis on duration, about 30 to 60 minutes with alternating vigorous and reduced intensity activity until peak intensity training can be maintained for 30 to 60 minutes after approximately 17 to 24 weeks of training. Total workout time is increased gradually over several weeks. The frequency of recommended exercise is three to five times a week to achieve a training effect with daily workouts, if desired, alternating high- and moderate-intensity days. Daily vigorous exercise is advised only after months of muscle conditioning.

Because of the variability in physical status of elderly persons, individualized exercise programs are recommended (Lampman, 1987; Larson and Bruce, 1986). These programs should include activities that use large muscle groups—for example, walking, swimming, dancing, cycling, and jogging (Lampman, 1987; Larson and Bruce, 1986)—and may include strengthening exercises using weights or exercise machines (Lampman, 1987).

A complete medical evaluation, including an exercise stress test, should be obtained before developing and undertaking an exercise program. The evaluation is important for identifying any risk to the individual. Larson and Bruce (1986) reported no evidence that the elderly in moderate exercise programs were at greater risk for injury. However, individuals taking certain drugs such as insulin, beta blockers, and calcium channel blockers may need close monitoring and dosage adjustment to prevent hypoglycemia and hypotension (Lampman, 1987). Lampman (1987) also notes that hypotension may result if nitroglycerin is taken just before exercising and that exercise-induced arrhythmias may occur if the individual's potassium level is low. Although many physical problems such as anemia, nutritional deficiencies, neuropathies, sensory impairments, respiratory and cardiovascular diseases, and musculoskeletal problems may alter the exercise prescription and increase risk management, they should not prevent the elderly from exercising (Lampman, 1987). Because most exercise programs for the elderly have been based on common sense (Larson and Bruce, 1987) rather than on scientific study, close supervision and safety monitoring should be an integral part of the program.

Risk/benefit management is even more essential for the frail elderly, for those over 70 years of age, or for those with multiple health care problems. Research on exercise for these individuals has not been done, nor have exercise programs been developed. Because residents of long-term care settings frequently are members of this population, cautious development of exercise programs, particularly as an intervention for Activity Intolerance, would seem logical. A collaborative approach using the expertise of the nurse, physician, exercise physiologist, nutritionist, and psychologist may produce a highly individualized, safe, effective exercise program to decrease Activity Intolerance and enhance fitness. Based on collaborative research, the cost-benefit, cost-effectiveness of these exercise programs could be demonstrated. Thus, in the future, instead of passively sitting in their chairs, these clients may be receiving and/or demanding their morning workout in the gym, their afternoon dance or yoga therapy, or their evening walk. The long-term care setting may no longer be perceived as the terminal point in an individual's life but rather as a place for rehabilitation, recovery, and new independence.

CASE STUDY

Nursing Interventions

This intervention case study illustrates a process that the nurse could use in developing a plan of action for Mr. T. It describes possible, but not clinically validated, interventions for Activity Intolerance.

Mr. T's diagnosis was Activity Intolerance related to deconditioning, an imbalance in oxygen supply and demand, and ineffective individual coping. He presented with signs and symptoms of both physiologic and psychologic inability to complete required and/or desired activities. He lacked energy, strength, and endurance. Therefore, the nurse identified the lack of physical activity and exercise as the focus of the plan of action because of the benefits of activity for deconditioned states, decreased energy, chronic fatigue, and depression.

Considering the multidimensional nature of the activity intolerance problem for Mr. T and the lack of scientific data and/or standardized protocols to aid decision making, the nurse decided to use a decision analysis model. Decision analysis is a useful technique for making rational decisions leading to optimum outcomes. Using this technique, the utility or value of each outcome is considered, the risks and benefits of each intervention are assessed, and a quantitative comparison of desirability of alternatives is done. These numerical evaluations lead to the rational selection of the best alternative for the individual patient (Kassirer, 1976; Schwartz et al, 1973).

Based on the history, clinical cues, and etiologies, Mr. T's nurse began a plan for initial intervention by listing by priority the desired outcomes and selecting criteria for measuring accomplishments of those goals (see Table 22.3).

Because Mr. T experiences moderate Activity Intolerance and has a history of diabetes, cardiac disease, and reduced vision, safety is considered a priority outcome and assigned the highest utility. Goals that address his deconditioned state and energy imbalance also are considered important. Because Mr. T's Activity Intolerance is influenced by his emotional status, goals of improvement in his mental health are sufficiently important to include in the plan of action. The outcomes in priority order include:

1. Safety as measured by no sequelae for activity, particularly angina, arrhythmias, respiratory distress, hypotension, hypoglycemia, falls, and musculoskeletal injuries
2. Increased energy level as measured by decreased vocalizations of fatigue and exhaustion; increased

---

Table 22.3

Analysis of Alternative Actions: Case Study for Activity Intolerance

INTERVENTIONS	DESIRED OUTCOMES					EXPECTED VALUE*
	Safety (5)†	Energy (4)	Conditioning (3)	Socialization (2)	Autonomy (1)	
Aerobic class	5†	10	60	20	5	290
Dance therapy	10	15	30	35	10	280
Active ROM	55	10	10	5	20	375
Progressive walking	30	20	20	15	15	335

*Expected value is a number indicating the desirability of the alternative. It is calculated by multiplying the utility value times the probability value and summed for each alternative. The greater the number, the more desirable the alternative for achieving the outcomes.
†Utility is the number indicating the value of the outcome; 5 = priority outcome; 1 = least valued outcome.
†Probability is the likelihood of the alternative achieving the outcome. It is calculated by dividing 100 points across the outcomes for each intervention. The larger the number the greater probability that the outcome will be achieved.

participation in activities of daily living and lifestyle activities; and increased physical movement

3. Increased physical conditioning as measured by an increase in duration, frequency, and intensity of participation in a progressive exercise program; decreased orthostatic hypotension; increased muscle strength; no shortness of breath or dyspnea on mild and moderate exertion; no exhaustion; and decreased fatigue

4. Increased effective coping as measured by decreased vocalizations of loneliness, hopelessness, and helplessness; increased socialization with family, friends, and other residents and staff; increased verbalization concerning acceptance of and adaptation to his wife's death, the long-term care setting, and his health status

5. Increased autonomy as measured by verbalizations of increased self-esteem; increased participation in self-care; increased decision making concerning daily and long-range planning; increased responsibility and control of daily schedule

Several exercise interventions are available to Mr. T for achieving the desired outcomes: aerobics class, two times a week for 30 minutes; movement or dance therapy, two times a week for 45 minutes; active range-of-motion exercise as desired; and a progressive walking program including group walking each evening for 30 minutes.

As seen in Table 22.3, the nurse evaluated the probability of each intervention achieving the desired outcomes during the initial phases of rehabilitation. The nurse assigned 100 points to each intervention and distributed them for each outcome based on the likelihood of the outcome being achieved by that intervention. The nurse next multiplied the utility or value of the outcome by the probability and summed the scores for each intervention to determine the expected value of each choice of action. Based on this decision analysis technique, the nurse determined that active range-of-motion exercises had the greatest expected value and were probably the best intervention to begin Mr. T's rehabilitation program. Introducing the beginning phase of a walking program also was a good choice of action to achieve the desired goals. The walking program also appeared, overall, the best alternative for achieving all the outcomes and not just some of the outcomes. Also, from the analysis of the interventions, the nurse could anticipate changes in the plan of action as utility values for outcomes change (eg, decreased concern for safety and more emphasis on conditioning).

Next, the nurse initiated a meeting with the physician, and later with Mr. T, to discuss the problem and plan of action. The physician and the nurse developed a plan to have Mr. T's endurance level evaluated using a low-intensity exercise stress test. An exercise prescription was based on the results. A low-intensity, low-duration exercise program was developed. Mr. T agreed to try active range-of-motion exercises each day and begin a walking program three times a week. He stated he preferred to walk on Monday, Wednesday and Friday at 4:00 P.M. after his afternoon rest. When able to walk without assistance, Mr. T said he would try the residents' walking group. His goal for himself was to be able to walk outside for 30 minutes, three times a week, in 5 months. When asked if a relative could bring him shoes made especially for walking and a comfortable jogging-type outfit, Mr. T said he felt like he was getting ready for the Olympics.

The initial rehabilitation plan is for Mr. T to walk slowly and rest when mild fatigue or dyspnea occurs and to stop if signs and symptoms of intolerance develop. As Mr. T achieves some of the goals, the plan of action will be reviewed and new goals and interventions added.

SUMMARY

From this chapter, two conclusions can be drawn. First, Activity Intolerance is a significant, multidimensional health problem for the elderly. The problem significantly affects the individuals and their families and consumes health resources. In addition, the consequences of Activity Intolerance contribute to many other health problems. Some of the health problems that have Activity Intolerance as an etiology are decreased independence, autonomy, and self-esteem; decreased self-care and home maintenance management; altered family processes; social isolation; problems with anxiety, depression, and coping; changes in mental status and/or confusion; problems with altered skin integrity, mobility, cardiac output, bowel and urinary elimination, and tissue perfusion; and injury.

Activity Intolerance often is accepted as a "normal" consequence of aging; therefore, it is not prevented or treated, even when causing other health problems. The concept of programmed exercise or activity may be undervalued by the elderly themselves who grew up in an era of vigorous lifestyle activity versus today's programmed activity, and who have an attitude of "I deserve to rest in my old age." Thus, the biases concerning activity in the elderly also contribute to the inadequate diagnosis and treatment of this health problem.

The second conclusion that can be drawn from this chapter is that the current state of knowledge about Activity Intolerance is grossly inadequate. Although some beginning research has been done on identifying clinical cues and etiologies, there is little or no reliable and valid information on which nurses can base their decision making concerning diagnosis, treatment, and prevention of Activity Intolerance. A few exercise studies have been done with healthy elders, but research with frail, institutionalized, and disabled elders over age 70 has been neglected. Thus, decisions concerning activity for the elderly in long-term care settings, when addressed, continue to be based on "common sense" rather than on sound scientific rationale.

It is clear that major research programs focusing on Activity Intolerance are needed. Some areas for new and continued research efforts include (1) identifying critical cues, etiologies, levels of severity, and differential diagnostic strategies; (2) identifying and evaluating desired and actual outcomes; (3) identifying and evaluating interventions and developing decison analysis strategies to enhance choice of action behaviors; (4) developing and evaluating assessment and evaluation guidelines/tools; (5) identifying and predicting individuals at risk; and (6) developing prevention programs.

In addition to the previous research areas concerning Activity Intolerance, nurses working with the elderly in long-term care settings also might focus their research efforts on the following areas: (1) the multidimensional nature of the problem—that is, identification of the physical, personal, and psychosocial variables that contribute significantly to Activity Intolerance in this population; (2) variations in clinical diagnostic parameters due to age; (3) the influence of attitudes and beliefs by family, health professionals, and the individual on diagnosis and treatment protocols for the elderly; (4) longitudinal studies examining the influence of lifestyle behaviors on Activity Intolerance and subsequent institutionalization; (5) the cost-benefit, cost-effectiveness of activity interventions in the long-term care setting; (6) measurement of quality of care; and (7) quality of life issues for the institutionalized elderly.

Nurses have an exciting opportunity to lead the research in this area, to influence health care policy concerning resources and quality of care for the elderly, and to head the collaborative teams working with this health problem. With increased recognition of the impact of Activity Intolerance for the elderly and increased knowledge concerning identification, treatment, and prevention, nurses will contribute significantly to the "successful aging" versus "usual aging" (Rowe and Kahn, 1987;143) of individuals in today's increasingly older society.

References

Buskirk ER, Hodgson JL: Age and aerobic power: The rate of change in men and women. *Fed Proceed* (Apr) 1987; 46:1824–1829.

Carroll-Johnson R (editor): *Classification of Nursing Diagnoses: Proceedings of the Eighth Conference.* Lippincott, 1989.

Chirikos TN, Nestel G: Longitudinal analyses of functional disabilities in older men. *J Gerontol* 1985; 40:426–433.

Creason NS et al: Validating the nursing diagnosis of Impaired Physical Mobility. *Nurs Clin North Am* 1985; 20:669–683.

Fitzmaurice JB: *Utilization of Cues in Judgments of Activity Intolerance: A Methodological Approach to the Validation of Nursing Diagnoses.* (Doctoral dissertation.) Boston College, Boston, MA, 1986.

Gerstenblith G, Renlund DG, Lakatta EG: Cardiovascular response to exercise in younger and older men. *Fed Proceed* (Apr) 1987; 46:1834–1839.

Hagberg JM: Effect of training on the decline of VO_2max with aging. *Fed Proceed* (Apr) 1987; 46:1830–1833.

Harrington KA et al: Cardiac rehabilitation: Evaluation and intervention less than 6 weeks after myocardial infarction. *Arch Phy Med Rehabil* 1981; 62:151–155.

Hofeldt F: Proximal femoral fractures. *Clin Orthopaed Related Res* (May) 1987; 218:12–18.

Johnson BL: Exercise testing for patients after myocardial infarction and coronary bypass surgery: Emphasis on predischarge phase. *Heart Lung* 1984; 13:18–27.

Kassirer JP: The principles of clinical decison making: An introduction to decision analyses. *Yale J Biol Med* 1976; 49:149–164.

Kim MJ, McFarland GK, McLane AM: *Classification of Nursing Diagnoses.* Mosby, 1984.

Kim MJ et al: Clinical Validation of cardiovascular nursing diagnoses. In: *Classification of Nursing Diagnoses: Proceedings of the Fifth National Conference.* Kim MJ, McFarland GK, McLane AM (editors). Mosby, 1984.

Lampman RM: Evaluating and prescribing exercise in elderly patients. *Geriatrics* (Aug) 1987; 42:63–76.

Larson EB, Bruce RA: Exercise and aging. *Ann Intern Med* (Nov) 1986; 105:783–785.

Larson EB, Bruce RA: Health benefits of exercise in an aging society. *Arch Intern Med* (Feb) 1987; 147:353–356.

Levine ME: Adaptation and assessment: a rationale for nursing intervention. *Am J Nurs* 1966; 11:2450–2453.

Levine ME: The four principles of nursing. *Nurs Forum* 1967; 6:45–59.

MacLean SL: *Description of Cues Nurses Use for Diagnosing Activity Intolerance.* (Doctoral dissertation.) University of Illinois, Chicago, IL, 1987.

MacLean SL: Activity intolerance: Cues for diagnosis. In: *Classification of Nursing Diagnoses: Proceedings of the Eighth Conference.* Carroll-Johnson R (editor). Lippincott, 1989.

Masoro EJ: Biology of aging: Current state of knowledge. *Arch Intern Med* (Jan) 1987; 147:166–169.

McCarthy RT: Heart rate, perceived exertion, and energy expenditure during range of motion exercise of the extremities: A nursing assessment. *Military Med* (Jan) 1975; 9–16.

Nail LM, King KB: Fatigue. *Sem Oncol Nurs* (Nov) 1987; 3:257–262.

Rowe JW, Kahn RL: Human aging: Usual and successful. *Science* (July) 1987; 237:143–149.

Schwartz WB et al: Decison analysis and clinical judgement. *Am J Med* (Oct) 1973; 55:459–471.

Sowers JR: Hypertension in the elderly. *Am J Med* (Jan) 1987; 82:1–8.

Thomas CD: Insomnia: Identification and management. *Sem Oncol Nurs* (Nov) 1987; 3:263–266.

Walsh RA: Cardiovascular effects of the aging process. *Am J Med* (Jan) 1987; 82:34–40.

Williams TF: The future of aging. *Arch Phys Med Rehabil* (June) 1987; 68:335–338.

Winslow EK, Lane LD, Gaffney FA: Oxygen uptake and cardiovascular responses in control adults and acute myocardial infarction patients during bathing. *Nurs Res* 1985; 34:164–169.

23

Impaired Physical Mobility

MERIDEAN L. MAAS, PhD, RN, FAAN

PHYSICAL MOBILITY IS CRITICAL FOR THE MAINTENANCE of health and quality of life of all persons and is especially important for the elderly. According to Milde (1981) mobility enables persons to move away from danger, to move to experiences that are enjoyable, and to maintain homeostasis. Mobility, care of one's person, and the performance of instrumental tasks to cope with the environment are behaviors that compose functional health (Hogue, 1985). When an elderly person is institutionalized, physical mobility may be impaired because of the effects of problems that have led to the elder's institutionalization and because of factors associated with the physical environment that further constrain mobility (Hogue, 1985). Thus the nursing diagnosis Impaired Physical Mobility has a high incidence among institutionalized elderly, ranking along with falls, incontinence, and mental confusion as the most common problems of elderly long-term care patients (Kane and Kane, 1981).

Impaired Physical Mobility is the "limitation of ability for independent movement within the environment" (Carroll-Johnson, 1989; Gordon, 1982) or the "decreased ability to move from one place or position to another" (Kelly, 1985). The diagnosis Impaired Physical Mobility is distinguished from physical immobilization, which is a total inability to move the body or any of its parts from place to place, to move from one body position to another, or to manipulate any physical environmental elements. When physical immobilization is present, nursing care will not eliminate it. Rather, nursing will then focus on the diagnosis and management of problems that are probable sequelae (eg, impaired skin integrity or constipation). Impaired Physical Mobility can vary in the extent of restricted movement, in the scope of affected body parts, in the length of time that movement is restricted, and in the amount of control the elderly individual has over the mobility impairment. Nursing intervention for Impaired Physical Mobility seeks to correct, compensate, or ameliorate the mobility impairment; to prevent further impairment; and to prevent or minimize physiologic, psychologic, and socioeconomic consequences of impaired mobility.

SIGNIFICANCE FOR THE ELDERLY

Few studies have been reported that document the incidence of Impaired Physical Mobility in specific populations of institutionalized elderly. Hardy et al (1988) conducted a descriptive study of the nursing diagnoses of long-term care residents in

263

a State Veterans Home and found Impaired Physical Mobility to be the second most frequent nursing diagnosis both in 1983 (35% of a sample of 99 residents) and in 1985 (26% of a sample of 121 residents). Other studies have shown this nursing diagnosis to be the most frequently used in long-term care facilities and hospitals for the elderly (Hallal, 1985; Leslie, 1981; Rantz et al, 1985).

A number of factors associated with aging predispose the elderly to Impaired Physical Mobility. There is a general decrease in muscle strength, endurance, and agility. Muscle strength declines steadily after young adulthood (Bosco and Komi, 1980), particularly in the legs (McDonagh et al, 1984). In general, muscle endurance is affected less than strength (Sato et al, 1986). Muscles atrophy, joints become less flexible and more flexed, and the individual generally becomes more frail.

Chronic illnesses are more common, thus the elderly person has greater potential for treatments that restrict activity and mobility. Reduced visual acuity, hearing impairments, arthritis, osteoporosis (especially in elderly women), less strength, poorer balance, and mental confusion make the elderly more at risk for falls, which often result in injuries that further reduce mobility. Even if the elderly individual does not fall, he or she tends to curtail mobility to avoid accidents.

The elderly also often experience changes in their social support systems that predispose them to impaired mobility. The loss of spouse, friends, and work role can eliminate many of the reasons to remain active and mobile. If the elder is also chronically ill, activity may become even less desirable and more difficult. If the person is institutionalized, chronic illness and functional losses often interact with the physical and social environment to restrict mobility further.

CONSEQUENCES OF IMPAIRED PHYSICAL MOBILITY

When physical mobility is viewed as an aspect of functional health, the consequences of impairment are broad, including physiologic, psychologic, and socioeconomic results (Table 23.1). These consequences are not inevitable, even though they are associated with the increased probability of physiologic decline with aging. The increment in functional dependence that accompanies Impaired Physical Mobility and its consequences can very often be avoided, corrected, or minimized by astute nursing diagnosis and management. This makes the problem of Impaired Physical Mobility among the elderly a high priority for care, teaching, and research.

Falls

The elderly with mobility limitations are prone to falls from gait changes, weakness, and diminished reflexes. If they fall once, they are more apt to fall again. Mobility limitations may also accompany chronic illnesses, which are more common among the elderly, and may be exacerbated by medical treatments and medications. In addition, old people are more apt to sustain fractures

---

Table 23.1

NANDA Related Factors and Defining Characteristics (Carroll-Johnson, 1989)

MOBILITY, IMPAIRED PHYSICAL

Definition:

A state in which the individual experiences a limitation of ability for independent physical movement

Related Factors

Intolerance to activity; decreased strength and endurance
Pain and discomfort
Perceptual or cognitive impairment
Neuromuscular impairment
Musculoskeletal impairment
Depression; severe anxiety

Defining Characteristics

Inability to move purposefully within the physical environment, including bed mobility, transfer, and ambulation
Reluctance to attempt movement
Limited range of motion
Decreased muscle strength, control, and/or mass
Imposed restrictions of movement, including mechanical; medical protocol
Impaired coordination

when they fall than younger people because of the higher incidence of osteoporosis, particularly in elderly women. One half or more of the elderly who could walk prior to hip fracture cannot walk afterward (Melton and Riggs, 1983). These circumstances, perhaps more than any others, are most responsible for high degrees of impaired mobility of the elderly leading to further physiologic, psychologic, and socioeconomic consequences. Chapter 3 provides further discussion of the relationship of falls and impaired mobility in the elderly.

Physiologic Consequences

In certain situations decreased physical mobility is beneficial. The workload of the heart is reduced when an individual is at rest because of lowered metabolism and oxygen consumption. Pain, tension, and venous pooling are often reduced when the musculoskeletal system relaxes with the body in a supine position. Many illnesses (eg, congestive heart failure, fractures) require degrees of decreased mobility for effective treatment. The ability of a part of the body to function is decreased when it is injured or diseased. The physiologic requirements on the body part may be greater than its ability to respond. Thus rest may be necessary to maintain homeostasis and to prevent further injury. Rest may be functional in these cases because it equalizes metabolic capacity and demand and promotes healing. However, the body and its organs will function optimally and the capacity to function will progress if demand is increased as ability and metabolic reserve increase. "The basis of the development of functional ability by any organ of the body is use" (Kottke, 1965;437). Thus, lack of use leads to a deterioration of functional ability. This is true for all body systems and organs.

The greater the impairment of physical mobility, the greater the probability that physiologic problems will result. The common kinds of physiologic deterioration that occur with Impaired Physical Mobility are reduced range of motion (ROM) of joints, loss of muscular strength and endurance, loss of skeletal strength, cardiovascular deterioration, metabolic imbalances, ischemic ulcers, deterioration of urinary function, decreased gastrointestinal function, and respiratory deterioration.

Reduced Range of Motion of Joints Reduced range of motion occurs with Impaired Physical Mobility because connective tissues around joint capsules and in muscle planes become dense (Kottke, 1965). The fibers of the involved muscles shorten and atrophy because they do not regularly shorten and lengthen through their full range. Trauma, inflammation, and poor circulation interact with impaired mobility to accelerate the formation of dense connective tissue. Initially the joint loses flexibility and the effective range of motion is constrained. Then, if the

process continues, range of motion is further curtailed and joints become more stiff and finally experience degenerative changes of contracture and ankylosis. The hip, knee, and ankle are most susceptible, although all joints can be affected. Restricted extension of joints is most apt to occur because of the greater strength of flexor muscles, the effects of gravity, and the difficulty in obtaining a full range of motion of joints while lying down or sitting.

Loss of Muscle Strength and Endurance Reduced strength and endurance result when muscle contraction is less than 20% of maximum tension each day (Kottke, 1965). Maintenance of muscle strength and endurance is dependent on frequent maximum tension contractions. A few strong contractions each day are sufficient to maintain muscle mass and strength if protein nutrition is adequate. However, a completely resting muscle will lose 10% to 15% of strength each week and can lose as much as 5.5% per day, with the most rapid loss occurring in the early phase of immobility (Muller, 1970). Endurance of muscle is largely a function of the circulation, nutrition, and removal of waste for the muscle. Immobilized muscles' venous pumps are more inactive, which leads to poorer circulation (Kottke, 1971). As circulation fails to meet the muscle's needs, endurance, strength, and muscle mass will decrease. The muscles most affected by immobilization are the gastrocnemius-soleus group, quadriceps, glutei, and erector spinae (Milde, 1981).

Loss of Skeletal Strength Loss of strength results from the increase in the reabsorption of bone that accompanies impaired mobility. Normally the skeletal structures are continually renewing with absorption and replacement of bone, which is dependent on muscle contraction and stress to promote bone deposit. Osteoporosis is the condition of greater bone destruction and reabsorption than production. The greater the degree of impaired mobility, the greater the loss of bone matrix and minerals, especially calcium and phosphorous. The long bones of the lower extremities, the os calcis, and the vertebrae are most susceptible to mineral loss. Loss of calcium increases rapidly from the first to the third week of immobility, reaches a peak at the fifth or sixth week, and then plateaus at a lower level, preventing further bone porosity (Deitrick et al, 1948; Dunning and Plum, 1957). The elderly are at increased risk for pathologic fractures as the bone becomes increasingly fragile.

Cardiovascular Deterioration Deterioration of the cardiovascular system is especially dramatic if the impairment of mobility is sufficient to cause extended confinement in bed or chair. The deteriorating effect is more pronounced if fever, injury, or disease are also present. Adaptability of circulation to an upright position deteriorates rapidly when the individual is in bed for extended periods. The normal sympathetic response of vasoconstriction to compensate for decreased arterial pressure and increased heart rate when the position is changed from supine to upright is not as effective. Rather, vasodilation and venous pooling occur, resulting in reduced circulating volume, decreased venous return, decreased cardiac output, increased pulse rate, and decreased blood pressure (Browse, 1965; Lamb, 1964; Pentecost et al, 1963; Stead and Ebert, 1941). After 21 days of bed rest, healthy young men in Taylor's (1949) study took more than 5 weeks after resumption of activity to regain cardiovascular response to the upright position. The elderly may deteriorate more rapidly and take more time to recover with activity.

The longer the period of bed rest, the greater the risk of venous thrombosis (Milde, 1981). The pumping action of muscles and vessels when body movement occurs is no longer operable, which decreases the emptying of vessels and increases stasis, especially in the calf where the largest percent of thrombi originate (Clark et al, 1974). In addition, the heart must work harder to achieve circulation when the body is recumbent because of altered distribution of blood in the body, increased cardiac output, and increased stroke volume.

Metabolic Imbalances In addition to the loss of calcium and phosphorous, other metabolic imbalances can occur with the breakdown of protein and excretion of nitrogen with reduced mobility. Other electrolytes (eg, potassium) have also been reported to go into a negative balance with immobility (Kottke, 1965). These assaults deprive the body of the energy that is necessary to fuel movement and maintain homeostasis. Hypercalcemia from disuse osteoporosis can cause a number of serious problems for the elderly including anorexia, malaise, nausea, vomiting, abdominal cramps, constipation, weight loss, and lethargy.

Ischemic Ulcers Ulcers of the skin and muscle can be a major consequence of Impaired Physical Mobility. Ischemic ulcers develop over body prominences (pressure points) where pressure prevents the flow of blood required to nourish cells. Ischemic ulcers can occur when the individual is in any position long enough to create sufficient pressure for cell necrosis. In addition the circulation of blood, which is to some extent facilitated by the movement of muscles, is reduced when mobility is impaired. Impaired Skin Integrity: Decubitus Ulcer is discussed in more detail in Chapter 7.

Deterioration of Urinary Function Decreased urinary function is most pronounced when impaired mobility results in the individual's confinement in a recumbent position. In an upright position, gravity assists the drainage of urine from the renal pelvis. In the recumbent position urine flow from the kidney into the ureter is against gravity. Because peristalsis is not sufficient to overcome the force of gravity, the renal pelvis may

completely fill before urine flows into the ureter. Thus urinary stasis results, predisposing the individual to renal calculi or infection.

The inability to relax the perineal muscles and external sphincter easily during recumbency creates futher urinary complications. Because of this difficulty, reflex action to micturate is not initiated even though the sensation to void is present. If voiding does not occur, the bladder becomes distended and the sensation to void may no longer be felt. Bladder distention can lead to overflow incontinence, pressure damage to the kidney, and infection.

If adequate drainage of urine from the kidney and bladder is maintained, the kidney nephron ordinarily is not damaged by prolonged confinement in a supine position (Olson, 1967). Therefore it continues to remove excess materials from the blood plasma. Because of the metabolic changes that accompany immobility (protein breakdown and decalcification of bone), the kidney excretes large amounts of minerals and salts. The excretion and precipitation of larger amounts of calcium salts create increased renal calculi in persons who are recumbent for long periods of time. Precipitation of calcium salts is encourged by impaired urine drainage, which increases the time for precipitates to form; by the alkalinization of urine due to the absence of acidic by-products of muscle metabolism; and from dehydration, which concentrates urine solids and increased stasis (Milde, 1981).

Decreased Gastrointestinal Function Gastrointestinal problems associated with impaired mobility involve ingestion, digestion, and elimination. Prolonged immobility leads to a negative nitrogen balance after about 6 days (Deitrick et al, 1948). Persons in negative nitrogen balance often are anorexic, which contributes to malnutrition and compounds other existing health problems. Lack of adequate nutrients along with impaired circulation and exchange of nutrients in the cells interferes with the ability to digest and use food. Reduced ingestion of fiber and fluid, impaired digestion, and muscle weakness are the major reasons that constipation is often a problem for persons with impaired mobility. The muscles of fecal expulsion (abdominals, diaphragm, levator ani) atrophy with prolonged immobility, rendering the person less able to evacuate the lower bowel. Opiate and anticholinergic medications, lack of privacy, failure to heed the defecation reflex, and failure to provide the optimal defecation position (sitting erect or squatting) can also contribute to constipation. A more detailed discussion of constipation in the elderly is presented in Chapter 14.

Respiratory Deterioration Respiratory deterioration from impaired mobility is caused primarily by reduced ventilation and inability to remove secretions. Full expansion of alveoli occurs with physical activity in the upright position, which is compromised when mobility is impaired. Optimum gaseous exchange can take place only when the alveoli are full of air, in close proximity with circulating blood, and when the air in the alveoli is being exchanged continuously (Olson, 1967). When a person is in a supine position, vital capacity is reduced by about 4% (Browse, 1965) by elevation of the diaphragm, changed contour of the chest, constraint on chest expansion, and redistribution of blood from the lower periphery.

Secretions become more difficult for the recumbent person to remove because of increased viscosity of mucus, dilated bronchi, reduced inspirational air volume and pressure, ineffective ciliary activity, reduced stimulation of the cough reflex from activity, and weakness of the muscles that aid coughing. If there is any degree of alveolar collapse, the problem of removing secretions is compounded further, since secretions continue to form, increasing the likelihood of stasis, tracheitis, bronchitis, and pneumonia.

Psychologic Consequences

Physical mobility influences the human being's self-concept, self-esteem, and ability to cope emotionally. The ability to interact physically with elements in the environment in order to meet human needs is closely allied with self-concept and feelings of worth. As discussed in Chapter 36, Body Image, a part of self-concept and esteem, includes the ability to move about at will. Impaired mobility alters these aspects of personality. As a result, immobility often leads to lack of interest and lack of motivation to learn and to solve problems. Drives and expectancies are diminished, and emotions may find expression in a variety of exaggerated or inappropriate ways such as apathy, anger, aggression, or regression (Olson, 1967).

Forced isolation and dependency deprive the person of intellectual and sensory stimulation that is needed for optimal perceptual behavior. As the quality and quantity of sensory information available to the elderly individual are reduced, the ability to interact with the environment is altered (see Chapter 44). Sensory deprivation often leads to distortions of time, form, pattern, space, mass, and temperature. These aberrations affect the relevance that activities such as sleeping, working, having sex, eating, and playing have for the elderly person who has a mobility impairment. If the threats to the ego and self are sufficiently overpowering, if high anxiety precipitates a turning inward of psychologic energy to protect the self, and if energy is withheld from interaction with people and realities in the environment, the elderly individual will be psychologically immobilized (Friedrich and Lively, 1981) and unable to cope effectively.

Socioeconomic Consequences

For the elder, socioeconomic consequences of impaired mobility are often severe. The mobility impairment often changes an individual's role activities as spouse, parent, employee, friend, and member of social groups and the community. Social responsibility usually requires physical activity and psychologic stability. With impaired mobility, social support networks are interrupted, leaving the elder with limited opportunity to maintain optimally functional social interactions and relationships. Impairment of mobility often is linked to the need for institutionalization in acute and long-term care settings. The chronic illnesses that tend to accompany aging further predispose the elderly to mobility impairments and interact with the impairment to continue a progressive cycle of physical, psychologic, and socioeconomic deterioration. The descent into functional dependence with loss of work roles and income, loss of control of monetary assets, and the need for health care can be devastating for the elderly person. The cost of health care for the elder can be staggering even if mobility is not impaired and institutionalization is not required. Impaired mobility can initiate a cycle of events involving injuries and physiologic, psychologic, and social deterioration that adds greatly to an already substantial economic burden for the individual and society. In 1977 the annual costs of hospital treatment for hip fracture alone were estimated to be one billion dollars (Owen et al, 1980).

ASSESSMENT

Assessment of the elderly person for the diagnosis and management of Impaired Physical Mobility requires that data be collected regarding the individual's physiologic and psychologic capabilities, the individual's physical and social environment, and the individual's interface with the environment. This is because mobility (also functional health) is affected by a composite of factors, and the specific composite is different for each elderly person. A comprehensive and detailed data base developed around these dimensions will allow the nurse to identify the specific factors that are associated with the client's mobility impairment and infer the extent, degree of control, and probable duration of the impairment. With these judgments the nurse can then proceed to the prescription of specific actions to treat the impaired mobility.

The etiologies (related factors) and signs and symptoms discussed can be compared with those listed by the Eighth Conference of the North American Nursing Diagnosis Association (NANDA) in Table 23.1 (Carroll-Johnson, 1989). In practice it will be necessary for the nurse to distinguish specific etiologies and to describe the extent, probable duration, and degree of control of the impairment in order to intervene effectively.

ETIOLOGIES/RELATED FACTORS

In general, the nurse can identify Impaired Physical Mobility by observing the client's limited activity and independent movement regardless of the specific etiology. The identification of signs and symptoms from which the nurse can infer the specific etiology(s) for decreased mobility allows the prescription of interventions that are more targeted and thus more effective. Table 23.2 summarizes the indicators (signs and symptoms) for each of the general etiologies and for more specific types of these etiologies.

Impaired Physical Mobility Related to Activity Intolerance

Activity intolerance is a decrease in energy due to loss of muscle mass and tone or to an alteration in cellular activity. The elderly sustain loss of muscle mass and tone with normal aging, but are also at risk for further weakness from disuse because of an increased prevalence of chronic illness and the tendency for less activity and movement. The elderly often experience social isolation, which removes much of the motivation to be active. The increased prevalence of chronic illness in the elderly also predisposes them to conditions that inhibit the production of energy by cells. Cells use energy for growth, muscle contraction, transport of electrolytes and nutrients across cell membrances, and initiation of nerve impulses (Guyton, 1986). The body will seek to keep its activity within the limits of its demand for energy relative to its ability to produce energy (Kottke, 1965). Table 23.2 shows the signs and symptoms of mobility impairment related to activity intolerance that are common to both loss of muscle mass and altered cellular function and that are specific to each.

Impaired Physical Mobility Related to Pain

Pain is a generalized or localized sensation of severe discomfort. The elderly are predisposed to chronic and acute pain, both somatopathic and psychogenic, because of the higher incidence of chronic illnesses and their treatment, increased trauma from falls and fractures, and susceptibility to infections. The elderly, like all individuals, respond to pain in a variety of ways. Responses are both physiologic and psychologic and are highly individual, which makes it difficult to identify a set of valid indicators that the nurse can assess for a differential diagnosis of pain for all persons. Chapter 30 presents additional information about pain.

Impaired Physical Mobility Related to Cognitive and Perceptual Deficits

Cognitive and perceptual deficits are the loss of ability to process sensory inputs mentally and/or the loss of sensations. The elderly, more than any other age group, experience diminished ability to receive sensory input. These deficits tend to accompany normal aging and also are secondary to illnesses that the elderly more often incur. The elderly also are more often subjected to environments that are socially and/or therapeutically restricted. These environments reduce sensory inputs. Because sensory feedback is essential for optimum mobility (eg, time and space orientation, reasons for movement and activity), restricted environments contribute to mobility impairment. Cognitive deficits are also common among the elderly and are mostly due to reversible and irreversible dementias, transient cerebral ischemias, and cardiovascular accidents. Without adequate cognitive abilities elders may not know how to move or why they should move, and may be unable to relearn movement. The signs and symptoms that are common to both cognitive and perceptual deficit etiologies of impaired mobility and those critical for decreased cognition and perceptual deficits are in Table 23.2.

Impaired Physical Mobility Related to Neuromusculature Impairment

Neuromuscular impairment is the loss of muscle movement due to interrupted central nervous system or peripheral innervation (Creason et al, 1985). The nervous system controls innervation and the functions of all body parts; thus, muscle contraction and reflexes are dependent on an intact neurologic system. Many conditions that the elderly are prone to develop can result in impaired neurologic function. Some of the more common conditions are degenerative diseases, demyelinating diseases, vascular diseases, trauma, tumors, and drug treatment. Paralysis with flaccidity or spasticity and paresis of muscles are not uncommon. Defining characteristics for impaired mobility related to neuromuscular impairment are in Table 23.2.

Impaired Physical Mobility Related to Musculoskeletal Disorders

Musculoskeletal disorders are losses or decreases of function of muscles and skeletal support systems that may be mechanical or structural in origin (Creason et al, 1985). Mechanical origins are external devices that restrict movement. Structural origins are physiologic limitations

Table 23.2

Etiologies/Related Factors and Indicators of Impaired Physical Mobility (Maas, 1988)

ETIOLOGIES/RELATED FACTORS	INDICATORS
Activity Intolerance Muscle Weakness	Decrease in graded muscle strength/resistance from baseline Decrease in muscle size/circumference from baseline Decrease in muscle tone/tautness when relaxed from baseline Complaints of muscle heaviness
Altered Cellular Function	Hypoxemia Decrease in tissue perfusion Dyspnea ECG—ischemia arrhythmias Fluid/electrolyte imbalance Acid/base imbalance
Shared Indicators	Complaints of fatigue or weakness Decreased endurance Tremors Reluctance to engage in activity or to move Abnormal rise in heart rate, blood pressure, and respiratory rate with activity
Pain	Verbal complaints of pain/discomfort with movement Protective changes in posture/gait Reluctance to move Expressed feelings of helplessness/depression Moaning, crying, irritability with movement Facial grimace with movement Diaphoresis; change in blood pressure, heart rate, and respiratory rate with movement
Cognitive Defects	Confusion Starts to move, forgets why or how Forgotten names/meaning or environmental stimuli for movement Cannot choose among one or more movements Cannot remember or follow instructions Aphasia (receptive) for language stimuli and descriptors of movement
Perceptual Deficits	Reduced ability to hear stimuli for movement Reduced ability to see stimuli for movement, eg, hemianopsia Reduced ability to feel stimuli for movement Reduced ability to smell stimuli for movement Reduced ability to identify extent, direction, or weight of movement of body or body part
Neuromuscular Impairment	Diminished balance Loss of coordination Decrease (weakness) or loss of muscular function Stiffness or rigidity of extremities Pain Tremors
Musculoskeletal Disorders	*Structural:* Limited range of motion Hypercalcinuria Hypercalcemia Decreased density of bone Amputation Contractures Dislocation of joints *Mechanical:* Presence of any external device (eg, brace, splint) that limits movement of any body part

(Continues)

Table 23.2

Etiologies/Related Factors and Indicators of Impaired Physical Mobility (Maas, 1988) (*Continued*)

ETIOLOGIES/RELATED FACTORS	INDICATORS
Psychologic Impairment	Anxiety
	Helplessness
	Hopelessness
	Depression
	Alienation
	Isolation
	Decreased eye contact
	Lack of attention to danger stimuli
	Muscular rigidity
	Smaller scope of perceptions
	(Friedrich and Lively, 1981)
Iatrogenic Factors	Use of physical or chemical restraints
	Use of drugs that sedate, analgese, anesthetize
	Bed rest without in-bed exercise, without regular change of position, or that is longer than an uninterrupted 24-hour period
	IV fluids, gastric suction, closed system urinary catheter, chest tubes or other treatments that keep the person in bed
	Failure to prescribe interventions to maintain mobility or prevent further immobility
Environmental Impediments	
Sociocultural	Inconsistent role expectations
	Lack of social relationships
	Altered power relationships, eg, parent/child; husband/wife; caregiver/client
	Conflicting cultural values, eg, elder/younger age groups
Physical	Presence of architectural barriers
	Long distance to services, family, friends, activities
	Lack of transportation
	Inadequate lighting
	Absence/misplacement of railings on stairs or in bathroom
	Lack of or ill-fitting assistive devices for ambulation
	Slippery surfaces
	Obstructions—cords, rugs, furniture in walkways, clutter
	Lack of assistive devices for self-care—clothing, utensils, furniture, appliances
Lack of Knowledge	Expression of inaccurate facts about movement and exercise for functioning health
	Inability to cite alternatives to and consequences of immobility
	Nonadherence to prescribed interventions for mobility impairment
	Stated admission of lack of knowledge
	Lack of recall of instructions

of movement. As with other factors related to impaired mobility, the elderly are often victims of chronic illnesses (eg, osteoporosis, fractures, arthritis, tumors, and edema) that interfere with the structural stability or flexibility of the skeleton, which is necessary for optimum movement. Further, external devices including casts, splints, traction, slings, wheelchairs, walkers, and canes are commonly used to aid ambulation, comfort, and anatomic alignment. Table 23.2 contains indicators for impaired mobility related to musculoskeletal disorders.

Impaired Physical Mobility Related to Psychologic Impairment

Psychologic impairment is an emotional response that occurs when stress overwhelms an individual's ability to cope effectively (Carnevali and Brueckner, 1970). Fear and grief from the many losses sustained with aging can be immobilizing for the elderly, who must often adjust to changes in lifestyle and environment without the benefit of their health and familiar support systems. The elderly are especially vulnerable to losses that weaken their control over aspects of living that ordinarily are taken for granted by younger persons. These circumstances can be so overwhelming that they are psychologically immobilizing, which in turn promotes physical immobility. The indicators to be observed for impaired mobility related to psychologic impairment are in Table 23.2.

Impaired Physical Mobility Related to Iatrogenic Factors

Iatrogenic factors that are associated with mobility impairment are medical regimens that affect an elderly individual's movement. These include bed rest, pharmaceutic agents (sedatives, tranquilizers, analgesics, anesthetics), restrictive and unfamiliar health care environments, surgery, restraints, and other treatments that restrict activity such as IV fluids, suction, and catheters. Although these circumstances are usually necessary for treatment of disease and injury, they can lead to serious problems, particularly for elders who have multiple predispositions to immobility and its consequences. Nurses should be vigilant about preventing or minimizing the effects of iatrogenic sources of immobility so that the elderly person is not compromised beyond what is absolutely necessary. Table 23.2 summarizes indicators for impaired mobility related to iatrogenic factors.

Impaired Physical Mobility Related to Impediments in the Sociocultural or Physical Environment

Impediments in the sociocultural or physical environment are social structures, processes, and/or cultural values and physical structures that limit activity and movement. Examples of sociocultural impediments are role conflicts and incongruencies, unbalanced power relationships, lack of social relationships, incompatible relationships, and incompatible cultural values. As mentioned previously, the elderly are at risk both for loss of social relationships and for role change. Role conflicts and incongruencies are apt to result when role changes occur. Further, power relationships of parents and children often reverse, with the elder parent becoming dependent and having diminished control. These constraints on mobility are usually present to some degree when the elderly enter institutions.

Caregivers are ordinarily younger and tend to have role expectations of elders and themselves that are not consistent with those held by the elders. Likewise, values are often divergent, and the caregivers hold a definite power advantage over the elderly. Incompatibilities in cultural values evolve from age-segregated subcultures. Ageism, prejudiced and negative stereotyping of older persons held by society, not only is expressed by younger generations but is internalized by older persons as well, making a self-fulfilling prophecy of such myths as "Old people should rest" or "Old people have had their day for involvement and activity." These circumstances tend to discourage mobility beyond immediate living quarters for many elderly persons who fear venturing out or who choose to avoid contacts that are uncomfortable. Physical constraints include stairs, distance, and lack of transportation. Older persons may not have the energy or ability to navigate stairs or walk long distances and may not be able to drive a car. Desired mobility is thus inhibited.

The defining characteristics for impaired mobility related to sociocultural and physical impediments in the environment are summarized in Table 23.2.

Impaired Physical Mobility Related to Lack of Knowledge

It is not uncommon for persons to be unable to deal effectively with disease or injury because they lack knowledge about what to do (Carnevali and Brueckner, 1970). In addition the elderly are more apt to have cognitive deficits due to illnesses such as cardiovascular accidents and dementia. Many myths about how to deal with illness also constitute a lack of knowledge. The roles of exercise and movement to maintain function and health may be less familiar to elderly persons who grew up believing, along with many in the health care community, that bed rest was always necessary and beneficial for the treatment of illness or discomfort. Thus elders may restrict their mobility because they are unaware of the need to maintain movement, of how to restore mobility, and of the resources that are available to assist them in order to prevent further impairment and the consequences that compromise their health and functioning. When elderly persons are knowledgeable, their involvement in decision making and their compliance are enhanced (Millar, 1983).

Table 23.2 contains indicators for impaired mobility related to lack of knowledge.

ASSESSMENT TOOLS

A variety of tools for assessing mobility in the elderly are available (Katz et al, 1963; Shanas et al, 1968; Wolanin, 1976); however, none is entirely satisfactory (Hogue, 1985). Assessment of mobility is often a part of functional assessment. Measures reviewed by Kane and Kane (1981) include assessment of transfer, mobility, walking, bed activities, locomotion, ability to propel wheelchair, and physical condition of lower limbs. Some tools are broad in scope but have less detail for assessing specific aspects of mobility. Some require instrumentation, whereas others do not. Most depend on the clinician's subjective conclusions from observation of patient performance. Many focus almost entirely on dimensions of the physical act of movement and ignore or neglect psychosocial and environmental factors that are associated with impaired mobility. Some focus on the extent the impaired mobility interferes with capability to perform activities of daily living (ADLs) and do not provide the detailed assessment needed to identify etiologies and focus interventions. The tool in Assessment Guide 23.1 is designed to be broad enough to encompass the data needed to identify causes of impaired mobility comprehensively and to be detailed enough to specify nursing interventions.

DIFFERENTIAL DIAGNOSIS OF IMPAIRED PHYSICAL MOBILITY

Differential diagnosis is a skill that needs to be developed further to distinguish among the nursing diagnoses that have been accepted by NANDA and to discriminate among diagnoses, where appropriate, that are subtypes of the accepted diagnoses. Two cases studies are presented to illustrate the process of differential diagnosis of more specific causes of mobility impairment in the elderly.

CASE STUDY

Impaired Physical Mobility, Mr. D.L.

Mr. D.L. is a 73-year-old married man who has resided for the past 5 years in a long-term care facility. He experienced a left cerebrovascular accident (CVA) with resultant expressive aphasia 3 months prior to his admission. He is alert, follows simple commands, makes choices about his life situation through nonverbal nods of his head and facial expressions, and yells when upset or when his needs are blocked. Since his admission he has attended and enjoyed many agency programs and activities, including dances, bingo, and cookie socials. He is selective about the unit activities he attends, but he does participate in music group and pet visits. Recently he has begun attending wheelchair bowling, but he watches and does not participate actively. He often comes and goes at activities and becomes upset and yells if hindered.

Mr. D. L. has right hemiparesis as a result of the stroke and ambulates independently in a wheelchair. The range of motion in his right shoulder is 45 degrees (normal = 180 degrees), and the shoulder is slightly internally rotated. His right elbow flexes to 45 degrees; right wrist is fixed and flexed; fingers extend 90 degrees; right hip has full flexion and 45-degree abduction and is slightly internally rotated;

knee has 90 to 100 degrees extension. The right ankle has only 10 degrees of motion in any direction. All joints on the right side are stiffened, and passive range of motion causes a moderate amount of pain, which Mr. D.L. indicates by grimacing, yelling if motion is continued, or refusing treatment. Muscles on the right side are slightly atrophied. Muscles on the left side are strong with full range of motion. After a reminder, Mr. D.L. is able to turn himself about in bed with the help of the trapeze or siderail. He is able to remain in a chosen position without assistance. He is unable to walk. He uses a pivot transfer to the wheelchair with one staff person assisting. He has a stable sitting balance. Once he is in the wheelchair, he is able to propel himself about with his left arm and leg. His right leg is supported on the leg rest. In the last 6 months he has had difficulty keeping his right leg on the foot pedal, which has hindered his mobility and upsets him a great deal. He is able to wheel himself approximately two city blocks and up and down ramps without cardiac or respiratory difficulty.

Mr. D.L. awakens between 7:00 and 8:00 A.M., leaves the unit when he chooses, and returns for lunch. He lies down for a nap in the afternoon and leaves the unit before supper or watches TV. After supper he goes to agency activities or watches TV and goes to bed between 8:00 and 9:00 P.M. He needs some assistance with dressing, grooming, bathing, hygiene, and eating. He is able to wash his own face and axillae, comb his hair, shave, brush dentures, and insert them. Given a lot of time he is able to put on his own shirt and button it. He feeds himself after his milk is open and his meat is cut. He uses a plate guard, a large tablespoon, and often his fingers. He is completely dependent in toileting, requiring staff to care for his indwelling catheter and involuntary stools. Table 23.3 presents the significant signs and symptoms and the additional data needed for this case study.

TENTATIVE DIAGNOSES

1. Impaired Physical Mobility related to pain as evidenced by pain and discomfort with range of motion and occasional refusal to do range of motion.
2. Impaired Physical Mobility related to musculoskeletal impairment as evidenced by stiffness in right upper extremity and limited range of motion in right shoulder, elbow, wrist, hip, ankle, and knee.

CASE STUDY

Impaired Physical Mobility, Mrs. P.N.

Mrs. P.N. is an 89-year-old widow who lives alone in her apartment in a housing complex for the elderly. She has an enlarged heart with frequent symptoms of shortness of breath, dizziness, occasional chest pain, and she tires

Table 23.3

Differential Diagnosis, Mr. D.L.

SIGNIFICANT SIGNS AND SYMPTOMS	DIAGNOSES RULED OUT	ADDITIONAL DATA NEEDED
Sufficient muscle strength to propel wheelchair Endurance (wheelchair) 2 blocks, up ramps	Activity Intolerance	Muscle resistance
Pain and discomfort with ROM Occasional refusal of ROM	Pain*	Frequency of refusing ROM
Able to move about in environment	Cognitive/Perceptual	Effect of expressive aphasia on communicating response to ROM Evidence of receptive deficits
Stiffness in R upper extremity Limited ROM: R shoulder, elbow, wrist, hip, ankle, knee	Musculoskeletal Impairment*	Potential to increase ROM
		Spasticity present?

*Unable to rule out.

easily with minimal activity. Mrs. P.N. has osteoarthritis in the shoulders, elbows, wrists, hands, and knees. She can no longer feed herself with her right hand, and her ROM in the right shoulder is about 90 degrees. She can manage to get her clothes on, but she cannot get them off unless they are very loose or have snaps or large buttons (1 inch or larger) clear down the front. She can no longer comb her hair, so she uses wigs. She has the most severe pain in her knees, which causes difficulty in going up and down stairs and in getting in and out of a chair.

Mrs. P.N. is absolutely convinced that she has cancer, even though she has been examined repeatedly with negative results. She doesn't believe that arthritis could cause so much pain. She believes everything that she hears on the radio and nothing that health personnel tell her in person. For example, she will not take any aspirin because she has heard that it is bad for you. In addition to her limited range she also has extreme weakness in her hands. She cannot open milk cartons, tightly screwed jar lids, or safety lid medicine containers. Mrs. P.N. has a wide-based gait and loses her balance easily. She refuses to use a cane or walker but often needs the support of another person or rail to go distances. She has fallen a number of times around the apartment and has become increasingly frightened to venture out. Most of the time she sits alone with the TV or radio or sleeps in her apartment.

Mrs. P.N. has been treated for hypertension for the past 20 years. Her blood pressure normally runs about 180/90, and if it falls below 160/80 she is so weak she can hardly move about at all. Her vision has deteriorated markedly, and she can only see shadows, which increases her fright of walking around in unfamiliar surroundings. Her hearing is impaired, so she cannot participate in group social situations, which further restricts her activity. She can hear the telephone ring and can hear fairly well to converse over the phone, which is her major means of socialization. She is fully oriented and listens regularly to

current events on the TV and radio. Much of the time she is depressed and often says, "I can't figure out why I am still alive." Mrs. P.N. has two sons and three grandchildren. One son lives a long distance away, but the other son lives in the same community, and he and his wife and daughter are very attentive. The son in town has power of attorney because of her visual problems and her inability to sign checks. Her relationship with her son has almost completely reversed. She appreciates the help he provides, but at the same time she resents being told what to do and often misinterprets his attempts to help as attempts to run her life. Table 23.4 presents the signs and symptoms and the additional data needed for this case study.

TENTATIVE DIAGNOSES

1. Impaired Physical Mobility related to activity intolerance as evidenced by shortness of breath with activity, weakness, and lack of endurance.
2. Impaired Physical Mobility related to pain as evidenced by verbal complaints of joint pain on movement, especially climbing stairs and getting in and out of a chair, and reluctance to move.
3. Impaired Physical Mobility related to psychologic impairment as evidenced by statements of hopelessness and fear of falling, moving, and venturing out.
4. Impaired Physical Mobility related to cognitive/perceptual deficit as evidenced by poor vision and hearing, poor balance, and reluctance to venture out.

NURSING INTERVENTIONS

For persons with Impaired Physical Mobility the ultimate desired outcome is increased activity and mobil-

Table 23.4

Differential Diagnosis, Mrs. P.N.

SIGNIFICANT SIGNS AND SYMPTOMS	DIAGNOSES RULED OUT	ADDITIONAL DATA NEEDED
Weakness and lack of endurance	Activity Intolerance	*Does regular exercise increase strength and endurance?
Shortness of breath (SOB) with activity		Amt of time required for SOB to abate
Weakness when BP <160/80	Iatrogenic Factors	Does antihypertensive med need to be reduced?
Limited range of motion in shoulders, wrists, hands, knees	Musculoskeletal Impairment	Effect of limited ROM on ambulation
Wide-based, unsteady gait; frequent falls, poor balance		Reason for refusing ambulation aids? Will ROM increase with exercise?
Joint pain in shoulders, hands, knees	Pain*	Extent pain limits mobility Explore methods of pain relief
Refuses aspirin or other analgesic	Lack of knowledge	Explore acceptance of short-term trial with medication
Poor vision and hearing	Cognitive/Perceptual Deficits*	Vision and hearing examination; are deficits correctable?
Reluctance to move and venture out	Psychologic Impairments*	Bases of fear
Fear of falling		When does she feel secure?
Expressions of hopelessness	Depression	Evaluation for depression?
Difficulty with stairs	Impediments in Physical/Social Environment	Location of barriers What overcomes difficulty with stairs?
Role conflict with son		Is mobility affected?

*Not ruled out.

ity. However, the elderly person's ability to be mobile is often complicated by several etiologies that make mobility too painful or too much effort. The elder may perceive mobility without purpose or to be unattainable. Although some form of active exercise is the only intervention that will restore or maintain muscle tone and strength for optimum activity and mobility, the nurse may need to intervene with other etiologies of impaired mobility before the elderly person can or will engage in active exercise. Or the nurse will have to supply the exercise for the elderly person when there are deficits that prevent the person from engaging in any active exercise.

OUTCOMES

The most meaningful evaluation of the effectiveness of a nursing intervention is whether the desired outcome(s) for the client is achieved. The desired outcomes for the etiologies of impaired mobility are summarized in Table 23.5.

The nurse's decision concerning the interventions that should be used to treat impaired mobility rests on the delineation of all etiologies and the determination of priorities for treatment. Based on the etiology and prognosis, the nurse may determine that active exercise will

never be possible at all. In this case the nurse will need to plan for exercise and activity that requires no voluntary muscle movement on the part of the patient. A number of the interventions that are appropriate for treating elderly persons with Impaired Physical Mobility related to the specific etiologies outlined here are described in other chapters in this book (eg, Chapter 7, 22, 30, 44). Because the overall desired outcomes of interventions for Impaired Physical Mobility are to maintain or increase mobility and to prevent or minimize consequences of immobility, neither of which can be achieved without some form of exercise, we have selected exercise as the intervention of choice for Impaired Physical Mobility. Table 23.6 lists other useful interventions that the nurse will likely need to use in the comprehensive treatment of elderly persons with mobility impairments. Some form of exercise for the elderly patient is necessary in addition to the use of all of these other interventions if mobility is to be increased or the consequences of immobility prevented.

Exercise Prescriptions

In a study of adults who had an average age of 75 and who lived in a high-rise apartment, 37% claimed to have no exercise, and a majority claimed only limited or brief episodes of exercise (Perry, 1982). Harris et al (1978)

Table 23.5

Desired Outcomes Associated With Etiologies/Related Factors of Impaired Physical Mobility

ETIOLOGIES/RELATED FACTORS	OUTCOMES*
Activity intolerance	Decreased fatigue Increased strength Increased endurance Increased willingness to move Normal increase in heart rate, blood pressure, or respiratory rate with activity Decreased tremors Increased muscle tone Decreased shortness of breath Ability to identify and perform activities that are most important to the person
Pain	Decreased pain on movement Increased willingness to move Decreased expressions of helplessness, depression Increased ability to move despite pain
Cognitive/perceptual deficits	Increased orientation Increased response to environmental stimuli with movement Pattern established for activity that does not rely on memory/decision Compensation for sensory/perceptual deficit established
Neuromuscular impairment	Improved or compensated balance/coordination Delayed loss of (or increased) muscle function/strength Decreased pain with movement Increased movement despite tremors
Musculoskeletal disorders	Increased/maintained range of motion Decreased bone calcium loss No dislocation of joints
Psychologic impairment	Decreased expressions of anxiety, helplessness, hopelessness Increased eye contact Increased social and environmental contacts Reduced muscular rigidity Larger scope of perceptions and attention to environmental stimuli
Iatrogenic factors	Maintenance of activity/mobility despite restrictive regimens Reduced use of physical/chemical restraints
Impediments in the social/ physical environment	Increased social relationships Adaptation to change in role expectations and power relationships Acceptance of cultural value conflicts Movement with environmental adaptations (safe and barrier free)
Lack of knowledge	Recall and expression of accurate information about relationship of activity and mobility to health Adherence to prescribed interventions

*Milde (1988) offers important help with measurement of muscle tone, strength, size, endurance, and range of motion as outcomes of interventions for impaired mobility.

found a 30% rate of participation in regular exercise in a study of persons age 50 or older, whereas the Surgeon General's Office reported that only 25% of noninstitutionalized adults age 65 and older exercise regularly (Healthy People, 1979). No study was found that documented the incidence of active exercise among institutionalized elderly; however, it can be assumed to be quite low because of environmental and physical constraints on chronically ill, elderly persons in these settings.

The outcomes of exercise are both physiologic and psychosocial. The benefits of regular physical exercise for the elderly have been documented (Dustman et al, 1984). Benefits included a slower rate of physical and cognitive decline, increased energy, improved sleep, better appetite, less pain, and less stress. Other benefits are strengthening and toning of muscles, enhanced range of motion and flexibility, and decreased boredom and social isolation. Exercise can also reduce the risk of venous stasis,

Table 23.6

Interventions for the Treatment of Impaired Mobility

INTERVENTIONS	ETIOLOGIES/RELATED FACTORS

Exercise
  Passive
  Active
    Aerobic
    Isometric
    Energy conservation
    Resistive exercise
    Transfer training
    Balance/coordination training
    Gait training
	Activity intolerance
	Cognitive/perceptual deficits
	Neuromuscular impairment
	Musculoskeletal impairment
	Iatrogenic factors
	Psychologic impairment
	Pain

Positioning	Activity intolerance Pain Neuromuscular impairment Musculoskeletal disorders Iatrogenic factors
Relaxation training	Activity intolerance Pain Musculoskeletal disorders Psychologic impairment

Environmental modification
  Environmental structuring
    memory aids
  Sensory stimulation
  Social support groups—Reminiscence
  Role supplementation
	Cognitive/perceptual deficits
	Psychologic impairment
	Environmental factors
	Lack of knowledge

Values clarification groups—Reminiscence	Environmental factors Psychologic impairment
Monitoring/surveillance	Iatrogenic factors Activity intolerance

thrombosis, and embolism. However, these benefits are often not realized by elderly persons because of the fear of injury, lack of resources and opportunity, low motivation, and lack of knowledge on the part of the client and/or the caregiver. Although a number of studies (Agre et al, 1988; Benestad, 1965; DeVries, 1970; Regensteiner, 1987; Seals et al, 1984) have demonstrated benefits of exercise for elderly subjects, public perceptions persist that the elderly will not benefit and that elderly persons desire to be sedentary. Because family members may hold these attitudes, nurses should include the family in teaching and planning exercise interventions so family members will support and encourage the elderly person. Exercise is therapeutic when it reduces muscle pain; increases strength, endurance, and flexibility; creates relaxation; and improves circulation. It is not therapeutic when it increases discomfort, causes anxiety, or taxes the heart (Kamentz, 1971). Therefore, preexercise screening and assessment are vital to the successful use of exercise. The elderly may be more prone to avoid preexercise screening

by a physician than younger persons because of the cost of examination and because of an orientation that physician visits are for illness (Simpson, 1986). This makes it imperative that nurses be able to assess the need for exercise, screen for risk, and prescribe and evaluate an exercise program.

Prescriptions for exercise use both active and passive exercise. Active exercise involves muscle contraction for movement and includes aerobic and endurance exercise, flexibility exercise, and resistive and isometric exercise. Passive exercise, the movement of joints with energy supplied by an external force (machine or therapist) that does not involve muscle contraction, is used to maintain flexibility of joint movement. Forms of exercise that require energy conservation or that are needed to regain balance or gait will involve one or more of the forms of active exercise. Their success often depends on the appropriate use of passive exercise during illnesses in order to maintain range of joint motion. All of these exercises can be used for individuals alone or in groups.

Exercise can be prescribed for persons who are ambulatory, in bed, in a chair, or on a stretcher. However, any form of exercise, passive or active, must be prescribed following a careful assessment of the etiology(s) of impaired mobility, including an evaluation of musculoskeletal and cardiovascular pathology. This discussion of exercise interventions focuses on rationale for using specific forms of exercise to treat impaired mobility in the elderly. The scope of the chapter does not allow a comprehensive discussion of exercise interventions. A list of resources for further study of the interventions is provided in Assessment Guide 23.2.

Exercise for Strength and Endurance The goals of exercise must also be individualized based on the elderly person's assessed strengths, weaknesses, and interests. Ordinarily active exercise prescription will be to approach an increased activity level gradually (DeVries, 1979).

Active exercise for elderly persons should begin with a "warm-up" period to prepare joints and muscles. "Warm-up" exercise usually employs range of motion and flexibility exercise but may also include a period of gradual increase of the intensity of exercise. The warm-up for aerobic and endurance exercise includes gentle stretching of muscles and avoids quick, forceful movements of all kinds. Warm-up is also used to reinforce and establish breathing patterns that maximize ventilation. Warm-up prepares the body for sustained activity and increased workload on the heart. If there is pain, the exercise should begin with motions of body parts where there is the least discomfort and move gradually, with the elder's willingness, to areas of the body where discomfort is greater. When specific motions are painful, it is usually helpful to hold the position following contraction and extension at the end points of available active range and then relax. Often it will be helpful to the client and will increase his or her willingness to perform if the therapist provides some physical support for the joint and body part during the active motion. It is important to taper off activity rather than abruptly stop. The "cool-down" period following vigorous exercise should be 5 to 10 minutes. During the cool-down, the individual exercises at a slower pace, using large muscle groups and ending with range of motion, stretching, contracting, and relaxing to prevent syncope that results from a sudden decrease in the supply of blood to large muscle groups.

Any chest, arm, neck, or jaw pain; light-headedness; pallor; or irregular or too rapid heart rate should be signals to cease exercise immediately and evaluate for the need to notify a physician. If breathlessness or rapid pulse persists for more than 10 minutes postexercise, if joint pain persists for more than 2 hours, or if there is prolonged fatigue or lethargy, there is need to reevaluate the exercise program.

Cardiovascular fitness is the primary aim of aerobic exercise. Running, walking, and jogging are most effective for fitness training with the most efficient cardiac output. Running and jogging, however, will be deleterious for many elderly persons. Thus, walking may be the most likely form of aerobic exercise to be used. Swimming may also be an option for some elderly who have access. Because more strenuous exercise may be contraindicated and because some elderly will also not be able to walk or swim, Simpson (1986) suggests "jarming," jogging with the arms, as an alternative. It is important to emphasize that aerobic exercise is a desirable intervention for many elderly persons and often can be prescribed for institutionalized elderly as well as for elderly persons in the community.

The aim of active exercise is to achieve an energy expenditure of 1000 to 2000 calories per week (Simpson, 1986). Thirty minutes of aerobic exercise can be expected to use about 300 calories when the heart rate is advanced to 70% of maximum. Target zones of 70% and 85% for heart rate have been established to guide the conduction of safe aerobic exercise. Active exercise for the elderly will often never reach the aerobic point; however, these values for obtaining maximum training effects should be used to set goals, identify high-risk elderly, and evaluate the effectiveness of interventions.

A fitness training program using aerobic exercise must be specified for each elderly person. Type of activity, intensity of activity, duration, frequency, warm-up and cool-down exercises, reasons to stop or modify the program, and the method for monitoring intensity need to be specifically outlined (Fair et al, 1979). For elderly persons, who may be receiving a number of medications, a drug history should be taken for accurate interpretation of heart rate response (see Chapter 4). Beta blockers are probably the most common cause of diminished heart rate response to exercise, and hypotensive effects of antihypertensive medications, antidepressants, and neuroleptics may be potentiated by exercise (Simpson, 1986). As noted previously, the description of aerobic exercise programs for fitness training in sufficient detail to guide their use by nurse clinicians is not possible within the scope of this chapter. The reader is referred to Allan's (1985) chapter "Exercise Program," as well as to other sources listed in Assessment Guide 23.2, for an excellent, detailed discussion of aerobic exercise prescription.

Exercise for Flexibility Flexibility exercises aim to increase or maintain the range of movement of a joint or joints. Active flexibility exercises are usually called calisthenics or active range-of-motion exercises. Passive flexibility exercises are the same as passive range-of-motion exercises. These exercises commonly include stretching to increase the range of joint and muscle movements. The idea is to achieve maximum joint range, flexion, contraction, inversion, eversion, rotation, adduction, and abduction where appropriate. Calisthenics of arm swings, neck rotation, hip and torso bending, leg swings, thigh abduction, and knee bends in concert with a breathing pattern of deep inhalation and exhalation are performed rhythmically, often to music.

Usually a method of last resort, passive exercise, along with splinting, is used to prevent contractures that deform and deprive the client of joint movement, flexibility, and alignment. These joint functions are required for comfortable positioning, for the ability to perform activities of daily living, and for the potential to increase activity, regain self-care abilities, and engage in active exercise for increased fitness. Elderly persons, especially those who are dependent on others for basic activities of daily living and who have few other reasons for movement, will develop contractures of joints in the positions that are maintained for long periods of time. This often makes upper extremities at high risk because even in sitting positions the arms and hands are often not moved. Neck flexion contractures are also common among elderly persons who sit for long periods or who use too large a pillow while in bed. These contractures interfere with swallowing and social interaction. Joint contractures can occur within 3 to 7 days, so the nurse should be vigilant with exercise to prevent all forms. Passive exercise should not be prescribed when the elderly person can cooperate in a form of active exercise, because of the risk of causing microtears in tissues that are already damaged and inelastic. Moreover, it is ordinarily a more painful form of exercise and has no effect on maintaining or increasing muscle tone and strength (Matson, 1985). Elderly persons in any circumstances, in bed or otherwise, need both active exercise to maintain physiologic integrity and passive exercise, judiciously prescribed, to prevent unnecessary loss of functional abilities.

Because there is a risk of tissue damage that can result in scar formation from increased fibrosis and thickening, a physical therapist or professional nurse who has a thorough knowledge of the anatomy and physiology of the neuromusculature and joints should always assess the client and prescribe the needed passive exercise intervention. One of these professionals should also perform the passive exercise until both the client and the therapist are assured that it can be carried out without undue discomfort and without tissue damage. Then it may be appropriate to delegate the implementation of the prescribed passive exercise to ancillary nursing personnel or to the family. In some instances, such as hemiplegia following stroke or paraplegia due to spinal cord injury, the client may be able to perform passive range-of-motion exercises on the affected extremities by using the unaffected ones.

When the potential exists to regain active exercise, the nurse should encourage the client to attempt to perform the range-of-motion exercises. Then, as the elderly person regains the ability for active movement, the therapist can move from passive exercises to active-assistive exercises and then to active range-of-motion exercise by providing the amount of support and assistance that is necessary to complete the movements. Finally, resistive exercises can be prescribed for strengthening of muscles. The advancement from passive to active movement and exercise can often be facilitated by exercising two or more joints simultaneously. This method invokes proprioceptive neuromuscular facilitation principles, which also reduces pain, decreases the chance of tissue damage, contributes to muscle tone, and reduces demands on the elderly person's endurance, as well as on the therapist's time.

The nurse should pay careful attention to the particular etiology and underlying disease that necessitates passive exercise. The prescription must be tailored to individual circumstances, as well as to other characteristics of the elderly client such as motivation, cognitive abilities, and condition of joints and muscles. For example, inflammation of the arthritic person's joints requires special attention to pain and possible trauma that movement will cause. Special attention should be given to the scheduling of analgesics and anti-inflammatory medications prior to manipulations of the joints. Stroke victims with hemiplegia need special attention given to the affected arm, which is more vulnerable to contractures, and to the shoulder, which may subluxate easily because of gravitational pull of the arm on weakened muscles that support the shoulder joint. The nurse should recognize that joint integrity is always at risk when the supporting musculature for the joint is weakened as a result of disease or immobility.

Passive range-of-motion exercise has been shown to have some positive effects on limited movement contractures in the elderly that result from extra-articular physiologic joint restriction secondary to neuromuscular dysfunction (Medeiros et al, 1977; Tanigawa, 1972). When contracted joints are the object of intervention, the aim is to stretch and lengthen the shortened muscles and move the joint through its range before ankylosed or permanently "frozen" joints result. The method of passive exercise used has traditionally been high-load brief stretch (Light et al, 1984). The elderly are predisposed to limited movement contractures of many joints, and chronic knee flexion contractures are especially common because of inactivity and prolonged periods of sitting. In a study of nonambulatory residents of a nursing home who demonstrated gradually progressive bilateral knee contractures, low-load prolonged stretch using extension by skin traction was shown to be more effective than the traditional high-load brief stretch in reducing the knee contractures (Light et at, 1984). Nurses should consider this intervention for use with the elderly, especially for knee, hip, and neck flexion contractures that occur so often in this population.

Byers (1985) studied the effects of non-weight-bearing, active evening and morning exercise on measures of joint stiffness with 30 patients who had rheumatoid arthritis. Stiffness decreased and mobility increased significantly after performance of evening exercises, particularly for finger joints. Although the findings of the study are not conclusive for all joints and perceived stiffness did not always correlate with objective measures of stiffness, these results are encouraging for the use of evening exercise by nurses to treat impaired mobility associated with inflamed and arthritic joints.

Continuous passive range-of-motion machines have been developed within the last several years. There are a number of different models of these machines, but they all consist of a motorized frame and a control that is used to turn the machine on and off and regulate the speed. When the machine is on and the client's limb is placed on it, the limb is flexed and extended continuously. Machines are available to exercise hand, shoulder, hip, knee, and ankle joints. They have essentially the same benefits as passive exercise performed by a therapist—that is, they prevent contractures, venous stasis, and thromboembolism—and are most often used for total joint replacements, ligament reconstructions, fixations following joint fractures, and synovectomies. They are contraindicated for patients with arthritis, contracted joints, or muscle paralysis, and for patients who are not competent mentally to turn the machine off when needed. Pain, potential injury to joints and muscles, and skin breakdown make the use of continuous passive motion hazardous (Johnson, 1983). The machines can be a useful adjunct for human energy to perform passive range-of-motion exercise, but the nurse must be selective regarding their use and vigilant in surveillance when they are in use.

CASE STUDY

Nursing Interventions, Mr. D.L.

Active flexibility exercise is prescribed for Mr. D.L. twice daily with the nurse's assistance to increase the range of motion in his right shoulder, elbow, wrist, hip, knee, and ankle and to maintain the range of motion in his other joints. Because he experiences considerable pain during range-of-motion exercise, which makes him unwilling to do the exercises part of the time, the use of an analgesic and a muscle relaxant administered before each exercise session was discussed with the physician and ordered for the patient. Mr. D.L. is encouraged to perform active range of motion on the joints that have limited range one additional time during the day. He is able to do this by using his unaffected upper and lower extremities to assist the affected side. Relaxation therapy is also used to reduce Mr. D.L.'s anxiety and to minimize further tightening due to muscle tension. Resistive exercise is also prescribed for Mr. D.L. to strengthen the muscle in his right leg. This is accomplished by having him complete the full range of motion of his right leg against some resistance provided by the therapist. When he is in bed Mr. D.L. performs isometric exercises against the footboard and the bed for strengthening. Because Mr. D.L. propels his

wheelchair considerable distance without difficulty, additional strengthening exercises for his left arm and leg are not prescribed.

CASE STUDY

Nursing Interventions, Mrs. P.N.

Mrs. P.N. has a prescription for active range-of-motion exercise once daily to maintain the flexibility of shoulders, wrists, hands, and knees. Because she refuses any analgesic and her pain is due to osteoarthritis, increased flexibility of the affected joints is not a realistic outcome. Rather the prescription is intended to prevent further loss of functional range of motion. To promote strengthening, a small amount of resistance during active range-of-motion exercises is also prescribed. Small weights (5 lb each), strapped to the upper and lower extremities, are worn while exercising. The weights can be gradually increased, if tolerated, to advance strengthening. After 4 weeks of exercise, improvement was noted in Mrs. P.N.'s balance and gait, and she has experienced no falls.

Isometric and Resistive Exercise Isometric exercise is exercise where muscles contract or tense without shortening or joint movement. Isometric exercises are used for strengthening a muscle group. For the exercise to be most effective, the muscle should exert as much effort as possible against resistance for a prescribed period of 5 to 15 seconds (Sorenson and Ulrich, 1966). This form of exercise is used to prevent loss of muscle strength when persons are immobilized because of surgical procedures, such as orthopedic procedures, or injuries that require casting or traction. The exercises are useful when the individual can participate in active exercise but for some reason cannot exercise in more normal activities. The exercises are also useful for muscles such as sphincters or perineal muscles that have more limited active movement during normal living.

Isometric exercises may be contraindicated for persons with abnormal cardiac function, although the effects are increased systolic and diastolic blood pressure during exercise rather than increased cardiovascular load (Nutter et al, 1972). Lavin (1973) reported that isometric exercise accentuated left ventricular function in patients with abnormal cardiac function. Patients should be encouraged to breathe through their mouths to avoid the Valsalva maneuver—increased intrathoracic pressure from forced exhalation against a closed glottis. Isometric exercises are, however, convenient to use with cooperative clients, and can be used to augment other active exercises periodically throughout the day. The client can implement these exercises without supervision or assistance by the nurse if the purpose, plan, and technique for the exercises are understood. Kegel exercises can help strengthen perineal musculature for relief of stress incontinence (Mandelstom, 1980). Isometric exercises have been used to treat other problems experienced by the elderly, including strengthening abdominal muscles to treat constipation, strengthening leg muscles prior to weight bearing following hip fracture, and strengthening the quadriceps in the person with arthritis who has knee involvement and finds weight bearing or other active joint movement too painful (Wolff, 1986). Isometric exercises are especially useful for strengthening abdominal, leg, and gluteal muscles to support an upright posture.

Resistive exercise is used to strengthen muscles. Resistance can be added to isometric exercise by having the client push against something like the bed, footboard, or resistance provided by the therapist. Resistive exercise can vary from isometric resistance exercise; to having an elderly person who has had a stroke begin to lift small leg and arm weights in preparation for learning to balance, stand, transfer, and walk; to high resistance weight lifting. Resistance is gradually increased as muscles acquire strength. Nurses can easily combine resistance exercise with active range-of-motion exercise. A small sandbag strapped to the foot or grasped in the elderly person's hand is a simple example. The nurse can also supply resistance by pushing against the body part that is being exercised. The important point is that a plan be developed to strengthen muscle groups that are needed for regaining or preventing the loss of functional abilities.

It is particularly important for the elderly person to participate in resistive exercise for strengthening, since muscles lose tone and mass with normal aging. If the elderly person is institutionalized or suffers chronic illness that inhibits mobility, the loss of muscle strength will be even more pronounced. Loss of strength leads to problems with balance, coordination, and gait, which predispose the elderly person to falls and injury.

The nurse should always be working to assist the elderly person to move to the highest level of functional ability. For maximum mobility, ambulation is the desired outcome. Although the maximum level of physical functional ability possible may not be ambulation, lesser levels of ability are still important achievements for maintaining mobility. A sequence of abilities leading to ambulation is required when illness, disability, and disuse have led to loss of the ability to ambulate. The first emphasis is on maintaining or regaining sufficient muscle strength and range of motion. Next, attention is focused on the development of sitting balance. Then standing balance and transfer ability are developed. Training in shifting body weight and in achieving a specific gait pattern are the final steps. Often ambulation includes training in the use of walkers, canes, or crutches.

Common problems of exercise programs for all adults are motivation and consistency. Exercise groups are used to overcome these problems for elderly persons. Group exercise adds psychsocial benefits to exercise, which in turn increases the motivation of individuals to exercise. Group exercise has been used successfully with the elderly in the community and in institutions. There comes a time in rehabilitation programs when the person is no longer progressing from individual exercises. At this stage, group treatment is a valuable accessory to individual treatment. The person still receives a certain amount of individual attention but learns to take some individual responsibility while working with others. One explanation may be that the elder is part of a group and not set apart because of disability. As a group, elders may also overcome belief in the myth that old people don't exercise or that it is childish. Active exercises must be tailored to the particular population of elderly persons as well as to individual capabilities. Exercises have to be designed for sitting positions if the person is confined to a chair or has difficulty with balance. Mr. D.L. is encouraged to attend group exercise sessions for persons in wheelchairs. Since he began attending, his participation in the exercise prescription has increased. Exercises should also be designed for persons who are in bed or who cannot achieve sitting balance. Reference to motions in more familiar words, such as "picking cherries" instead of "reaching up," can assist elders who are too cognitively impaired to participate.

SUMMARY

Impaired Physical Mobility is a nursing diagnosis for many elderly persons in the community and in institutions. Because of the number of etiologies, the process of diagnosis, intervention, and evaluation of the efficacy of treatment is complex. This chapter separated the several etiologies that can result in impaired mobility and analyzed the signs and symptoms that indicate specific types of impaired mobility. Case studies were used to illustrate the collection of client data with synthesis of the signs and symptoms into clusters that indicate specific types of impaired mobility. The aim is to promote the identification of types of impaired mobility so that nursing interventions can be prescribed that focus on specific etiologic factors and that are designed to achieve desired outcomes based on valid client data. Focused interventions that have clearly defined expected effects are needed for clinical nursing research.

Exercise was discussed as an intervention. Active and passive forms of exercise for strengthening muscles, for increasing endurance, for increasing and maintaining flexibility, and for retraining mobility were defined. Rationale for the use of these exercise prescriptions and their expected outcomes were presented. The use of exercise prescription was illustrated with the case studies.

ASSESSMENT GUIDE 23.1

Nursing Assessment: Impaired Physical Mobility

Name _____ Age _____ Date initial test _____

Address _____ Vocation _____ Sex _____

Reason for seeking care _____

General appearance _____

    Ambulant: with assistance, without assistance
    Chairbound: with assistance, without assistance
    Bedbound
    Body build
    Skin condition
    Skin coloration
    Hair and nails condition

General impression of mental attitude to condition, activity, exercise

_____

_____

_____

Client's view of physical abilities and drawbacks _____

_____

_____

What does the client want to be able to do? _____

_____

Family and social support system _____

_____

_____

Activities of Daily Living (cross-reference Self-Care Deficit)

    Bed activities
    Wheelchair activities
    Self-care activities
    Miscellaneous hand activities
    Walking activities
    Standing and sitting down
    Climbing and traveling activities

Cardiovascular Status (cross-reference Decreased Cardiac
Output)
    (See Allan J: Exercise program. Pages 203–206 in: *Nursing
    Interventions: Treatments for Nursing Diagnoses.* Bulechek
    G, McCloskey J (editors). Saunders, 1985. Simpson W:
    Exercise: Prescriptions for the elderly. Geriatrics (Jan) 1986;
    41:96 for preexercise assessment parameters.)

Neurologic Integrity
    Reflexes
    Control: voluntary/conscious/purposeful?
      Are automatic position changes made?
    Proprioception/Perceptual (cross-reference Sensory
    Deprivation)

Skin sensation: different types (blunt-sharp, hot-cold,
    hard-soft, two-point discrimination)
    Joint position?
    Stereognosis?
Vibration
    Muscle contraction response?
Vision/Hearing
    Can hear ordinary speech volume?
    Can hear/see own feet on floor, body moving against
      bed, chair?
    Visual fields? Can be roughly tested by holding two
      different colored pencils different distances apart and
      asking the client to describe
    Pupil reaction?
    Incoordinate eye movements (nystagmus)?
    Double vision?
Cognitive/Mental Status
    Orientation?
    Short-term memory?
Communication/Speech/Language (cross-reference Impaired
    Communication)
    Can use language to express needs, understand
      directions?

(Continues)

ASSESSMENT GUIDE 23.1

Nursing Assessment: Impaired Physical Mobility (Continued)

Laboratory Results
  Urine calcium?
  Blood calcium and other electrolytes?
  Hemoglobin?
  Blood gases?
  Serum phosphotase?

Joint Function and Range/Flexibility
  Imposed restrictions?
  Passive range?
  Active range?
    Every joint
  Reason for limitation, if any?
  Fixed deformities?
  Habitual posturing?

Muscle Activity/Strength/Tone/Mass
  Self-care abilities (see Chapter 24)
  Grip? (Use Grip Dynometer)
  How much weight can be lifted?
  Lift to standing position?
  Wheelchair?
  Flaccid, spastic, normal tone?
  Spastic when stimulated by touch or activity? Constant?
  Superficial and tendon reflexes?
  Fluctuation of tone?

Endurance
  Distance; can walk and/or use wheelchair?
  Time; can maintain sitting balance?
  Heart rate, respiration, and blood pressure; response to activity?

Pain
  Reluctance to attempt movement?
  Quality?
  Location?

Balance and Coordination
  Help needed to maintain posture?
  Response to balance disturbance with eyes open and closed?
  Ability to stop and start movement?
  Eye–hand coordination?
  General posture and stance?
  Gait?
  Frequency, type, precipitating factor of falls?

Feet and Footwear
  Any foot problems?
  Type of shoes worn?

Psychosocial Status
  Social Interaction?
  Depression?
  Expressed feelings, outlook (hopelessness, powerlessness)?
  Role relationships? Social support?

Medications/Treatments
  Physical or chemical restraints?
  Sedatives, analgesics, psychotropics?
  Prolonged bed rest?
  Braces, prosthesis, splints?

Environmental Barriers
  Stairs?
  Curbs?
  Available assistive devices?

ASSESSMENT GUIDE 23.2

Selected Resources for Exercise Prescription

Barbach L, Pardo A: *Exercises Can Be Fun.* New York: Potentials Development for Health and Aging Services, 1981.

Bulechek G, McCloskey J: *Nursing Interventions: Treatments for Nursing Diagnosis.* Saunders, 1985.

Lamb L: Stretching and flexibility. *The Health Letter* 1982; 29(10). Communications, Inc.

Leoper J: *Range of Motion Exercise.* Sister Kinney Institute, Division of Abbott NW Hospital, 1985.

Paillard M, Nowak K: Use exercise to help older adults. *Gerontol Nurs* 1985; 11(7):36–39.

Pep Up Your Life: A Fitness Book for Seniors. Designed by Richard O'Keeler, PhD, Program Director for the President's Council on Physical Fitness and Sports. Prepared and distributed by The Travelers Insurance Companies in cooperation with the AARP. PF3248 (1287) D549 The Travelers.

References

Agre J et al: Light resistance and stretching exercises in elderly women: Effect upon strength. *Arch Phys Med Rehabil* 1988; 69:273–276.

Allan J: Exercise program. In: *Nursing Interventions: Treatments for Diagnoses.* Bulechek G, McCloskey J (editors). Saunders, 1985.

Benestad AM: Trainability of old men. *Acta Med Scandinavica* 1965; 178:321–327.

Bosco C, Komi P: Influence of aging on the mechanical behavior of leg extensor muscles. *European J Applied Physiol* 1980; 45(2):209–219.

Browse N: *The Physiology and Pathology of Bedrest.* Charles C. Thomas, 1965.

Byers PH: Effect of exercise on morning stiffness and mobility in patients with rheumatoid arthritis. *Res Nurs Health* 1985; 8(3):275–281.

Carnevali D, Brueckner S: Immobilization: Reassessment of a concept. *Am J Nurs* 1970; 70:1502–1507.

Carroll-Johnson R (editor): *Classification of Nursing Diagnoses: Proceedings of the Eighth Conference.* Lippincott, 1989.

Clark W et al: Pneumatic compression of the calf and postoperative deep-vein thrombosis. *Lancet* 1974; 2:5.

Creason NS et al: Validating the nursing diagnosis of impaired physical mobility. *Nurs Clin North Am* (Dec) 1985; 20(4):669–683.

Deitrick J, Whedon G, Shorr E: Effects of immobilization upon various metabolic and physiologic functions of normal men. *Am J Med* 1948; 4:3.

DeVries H: Physiological effects of an exercise training regimen upon men aged 52–82. *J Gerontol* 1970; 25:325–336.

DeVries H: Tips on prescribing exercise regimens for your older patient. *Geriatrics* (Apr) 1979; 34:76–80.

Dunning M, Plum M: Hypercalciuria following poliomyelitis: Its relationship to site and degree of paralysis. *Arch Intern Med* 1957; 99:716.

Dustman RE et al: Aerobic exercise training and improved neuropsychological function of older individuals. *Neurobiol Aging* 1984; 5(1):32–42.

Fair J, Allan-Rosenaur J, Thurston E: Exercise management. *Nurse Pract* (May-June) 1979; 13–18.

Friedrich M, Lively S: Psychological immobilization. In: *Concepts Common to Acute Illness.* Hart L, Fehring M, Reece J (editors). Mosby, 1981.

Gordon M: *Nursing Diagnosis: Process and Application.* McGraw-Hill, 1982.

Guyton A: *Textbook of Medical Physiology.* Saunders, 1986.

Hallal JC: Nursing diagnosis: An essential step to quality care. *J Gerontol Nurs* 1985; 11:35–38.

Hardy M, Maas M, Akins J: The prevalence of nursing diagnoses among elderly and long term care residents: A descriptive comparison. *Recent Adv Nurs* 1988; 21:144–158.

Harris L et al: *Health Maintenance.* Mutual Pacific Life Insurance, 1978.

Healthy People: The Surgeon General's Report on Health Promotion and Disease Prevention Background Papers. DPHEW/PHH, U.S. Government Printing Office, Washington, DC, 1979.

Hogue CC: Mobility. In: *The Teaching Nursing Home.* Schneider EL et al (editors). Raven Press, 1985.

Johnson E: Continuous passive motion. *JAMA* 1983; 250–539.

Kamentz H: *Exercises for the Elderly.* American Pharmaceutical, 1971.

Kane RA, Kane RL: *Assessing the Elderly: A Practical Guide to Measurement.* Rand Corp., Heath and Co., 1981.

Katz S et al: Studies of illness in the aged. The index of ADL: A standardized measure of biological and psychosocial function. *J Am Med Assoc* 1963; 185:94ff.

Kelly M: *Nursing Diagnosis Sourcebook: Guidelines for Clinical Application.* Appleton-Century-Crofts, 1985.

Kottke F: Deterioration of the bedfast patient, causes and effects. *Public Health Rep* 1965; 80:437.

Kottke F: Therapeutic exercise. In: *Handbook of Physical Medicine and Rehabilitation,* 2d ed. Krusen F, Kottke F, Ellwood P (editors). Saunders, 1971.

Lamb L: An assessment of the circulatory problem of weightlessness in prolonged space flight. *Aerosp Med* 1964; 35:413.

Lavin M: Bed exercises for acute cardiac patients. *Am J Nurs* 1973; 73:1226–1227.

Leslie FM: Nursing diagnosis: Use in long term care. *Am J Nurs* 1981; 81:1012–1014.

Light K et al: Low-load prolonged stretch vs. high-load brief stretch in treating knee contractures. *Phys Ther* (Mar) 1984; 64(3):330–333.

Mandelstom D: Special techniques: strengthening pelvic floor muscles. *Geriatr Nurs* 1980; 1:251–252.

Matson K: Prevention of contracture deformities. *Clin Management* 1985; 2:37–40.

McDonagh M, White M, Davies C: Different effects of aging on the mechanical properties of human arm and leg muscles. *Gerontology* 1984; 30:49–54.

Medeiros J et al: Influence of isometric exercise and passive stretch on hip joint motion. *Phys Ther* 1977; 57:518–523.

Melton LJ, Riggs BL: Epidemiology of age-related fractures. In: *The Osteoporotic Syndrome.* Avioli LV (editor). Grune and Stratton, 1983.

Milde F: Physiological immobilization. In: *Concepts Common to Acute Illness.* Hart L, Fehring M, Reece J (editors). Mosby, 1981.

Milde F: Impaired physical mobility. *J Gerontol Nurs* 1988; 14(3):20–25.

Millar A: Exercise for the elderly. *Aust Fam Physician* 1983; 13:592–593.

Muller E: Influence of training and of inactivity on muscle strength. *Arch Phys Med Rehabil* 1970; 37:449.

Nutter D, Schlant R, Hurst J: Isometric exercise and the cardiovascular system. *Mod Concepts Cardiovasc Dis* 1972; 41:11–15.

Olson EV: The hazards of immobility. *Am J Nurs* 1967; 70:779–797.

Owen RA et al: The national cost of acute care of hip fractures associated with osteoporosis. *Clin Orthoped* 1980; 152:172–176.

Pentecost BL, Irving DW, Shillingford JP: The effects of posture on the blood flow in the inferior vena cava. *Clin Science* 1963; 24:149.

Perry B: Exercise patterns of an elderly population. *J Fam Med* 1982; 15:545–546.

Rantz M, Miller T, Jacobs C: Nursing diagnosis in long-term care. *Am J Nurs* 1985; 85:916–917, 926.

Regensteiner J: Conditioning for elders. *Generations* 1987; 12(1):50–53.

Sato T et al: Age changes in myofibrils of human pectoral muscle. *Mechanisms Aging Devel* 1986; 34:297–304.

Seals DR et al: Endurance training in older men and women. Cardiovascular responses to exercise. *J Appl Physiol* 1984; 57:1024–1029.

Shanas E et al: *Old People in Three Industrial Societies.* Atherton Press, 1968.

Simpson W: Exercise: Prescriptions for the elderly. *Geriatrics* (Jan) 1986; 41:95–100.

Sorenson L, Ulrich P: *Ambulation: A Manual for Nurses.* American Rehabilitation Foundation, 1966.

Stead E, Ebert R: Postural hypotension: A disease of the sympathetic nervous system. *Arch Intern Med* 1941; 67:546.

Taylor HL et al: Effects of bedrest on cardiovascular function and work performance. *J Appl Physiol* 1985; 2:223–239.

Tanigawa M: Comparison of the hold-relax procedure and passive mobilization on increasing muscle length. *Phys Ther* 1972; 52:725–735.

Wolanin MO: Nursing assessment. In: *Nursing and the Aged.* Burnside I (editor). McGraw-Hill, 1976.

Wolff H: Musculoskeletal problems. In *Nursing Management for the Elderly,* 2d ed. Carnevali D, Patrick M (editors). Lippincott, 1986.

24

Self-Care Deficit

JOHN LANTZ, PhD, RN
CATHY PENN, BSN, RN
JERRY STAMPER, EdD, RN
PEDRO NATIVIDAD, BSN, RN, CNP

OREM (1985) HAS DEFINED *SELF-CARE* AS ACTIONS PERsons perform on their own behalf in maintaining life, health, and well-being. When an individual's abilities to perform self-care are less than those required to meet specific health care demands, a self-care deficit exists. Nursing interventions are then required to assist the individual in meeting self-care needs or to prevent loss of self-care capabilities.

Self-care abilities and the demands of self-care vary over the life span. Young individuals have a developing self-care potential but are unable to assume responsibility for it. Adults have the potential to function fully in self-care roles. Elderly individuals, however, are seen as clinging to their self-care behaviors but becoming less able to fulfill them (Sullivan, 1980;59). The degree of direct nursing assistance required is determined by efficacy of the elder client's current actions taken to meet the self-care demands. Sullivan (1980) describes a continuum of self-care ability in the aged. From highest level of self-care ability to lowest, the levels are (1) the independents; (2) the independents-threatened; (3) the independents-delegators; and (4) the dependents (Sullivan, 1980;64). The nurse applies the most appropriate level of assistance, being careful not to exceed the degree of assistance required. In Sullivan's model, one would act as a consultant, developing possibilities and promoting continued growth of the independent elder. The independent-threatened client requires a therapeutic alliance, with the nurse complementing elder self-care actions for completeness. A delegated, partially protective approach is used by the nurse to provide supplementary means to achieve complete self-care with the independent-delegator client. The dependent client requires a fully protective approach by the nurse to compensate for relinquished self-care skills (Sullivan, 1980).

These levels of assistance are similar to Orem's (1985) systems of nursing assistance, which are (1) supportive-educative, in which the client can and should learn to perform the requirements of self-care but is unable without nursing assistance; (2) partly compensatory, in which both the client and the nurse perform tasks, depending on limitations in the client's physical condition, knowledge, or readiness to learn the required activities; and (3) wholly compensatory, in which the nurse acts for the client who is unable to participate in any manner. When acute exacerbations of chronic conditions resolve, or as the client's self-care ability increases, the intensity of nursing assistance is modified and gradually eliminated (Orem, 1985).

SIGNIFICANCE FOR THE ELDERLY

All of these approaches are appropriate to use with institutionalized elder persons; however, environmental barriers may prevent full exercise of the elder's self-care abilities. Institutional living, which is highly restricted in space boundaries, enhances limitations in self-care by limiting activities that the elder may have engaged in outside the institution (Wright, 1980).

Other barriers may exist in the long-term care facility. Institutional facilities may take a bureaucratic approach to meeting the residents' needs (Wright, 1980). Caregivers may see themselves as the predominant decision makers, possibly because they see residents as incapable of making decisions, and making decisions for the elder may seem easier for the staff (Ryden, 1985). Other caregivers may be unaware of how to use limited available time to promote self-care; institutions often have inflexible routines and time schedules for care activities. A philosophy of rehabilitation refocuses the care in long-term care facilities to maximize the elder's self-care abilities.

Maximizing Self-Care Potential With Rehabilitation

Principles of rehabilitation nursing promote self-care of the elder by motivating attempts toward independence. These principles include helping the individual to "(1) discover dormant resources, (2) enhance underutilized abilities, (3) establish positive life patterns, and (4) grow within existing limitations" (Murray and Kijek, 1979;15).

During periods of altered health, social, situational, and maturational factors may cloud the elder's awareness of self-care behaviors. The nurse acts as "discoverer" to help awaken the client to dormant resources. Strengthening underused resources when the client has low energy reserves, marked physical dependence, and impaired cognitive function becomes a great challenge in motivation (Ryden, 1985). Establishment of positive life patterns and continued growth in existing self-care limitations require learning new health activities and practicing these activities until they are integrated into one's daily life (Murray and Kijek, 1979).

It is appropriate to address these learning needs of the elderly individual over a lengthy period of time. The long-term care facility often has contact with an individual for an extended period of time. This facilitates a rehabilitation plan paced for the individual and repeated assessment to track progress. The long-term care facility also provides a safe environment that relieves the frail elderly from the burdens of home maintenance (housekeeping, cooking, obtaining transportation, managing money, (Lekan-Rutledge, 1988). Skillful nursing care prevents the development of complications and monitors for early detection of health care problems. Incorporation of rehabilitation principles emphasizes therapeutic goals rather than custodial care, focusing on remaining strengths and interventions to minimize functional disability (Lekan-Rutledge, 1988).

Self-Care Deficit

Orem (1985) identified self-care deficit in a broad context, as being all the actions an individual requires to maintain life, health, and well-being. The nursing diagnosis Self-Care Deficit was identified early in the conferences of nursing diagnoses (Kim and Moritz, 1982) and has evolved toward a narrower focus of personal care (feeding, bathing, dressing, and toileting). The development of the nursing diagnosis Self-Care Deficit reflects nursing contributions to multidisciplinary rehabilitation research. Functional performance may be described in terms of activities of daily living (ADLs) (basic aspects of personal care) and instrumental activities of daily living (requirements for maintaining a home and managing one's health care requirements). These functional categories are similar to the labels of alterations in activities of daily living (home maintenance management and health management) and self-care deficits (feeding, impaired swallowing, bathing/hygiene, dressing/grooming, toileting) found in the North American Nursing Diagnosis Association (NANDA) nursing diagnosis taxonomy (Carroll-Johnson, 1989).

The nursing diagnosis Self-Care Deficit is prevalent in institutionalized elders (Hardy et al, 1988; Leslie, 1981; Metzger and Hiltunen, 1987). Self-care abilities differ between elders who reside in the community and elders who reside in institutions. In a review of three large epidemiologic studies, Yurick et al (1984) describe the abilities of elders to perform self-care. Of community-residing elders, 94% to 99% could bathe independently, dress and groom themselves, and eat without assistance. This picture of independence changes markedly when one looks at degree of self-care ability for elders residing in institutions. The 1977 National Health Interview Survey (Yurick et al, 1984) found prevalence rates for independence in self-care as follows: 11.4% independent in bathing, 28.3% independent in dressing, 54.8% independent in toileting, and 66.4% independent in eating.

ETIOLOGIES/RELATED FACTORS

In the elderly, a number of etiologic and contributing factors to self-care deficit are identifiable. These factors are pathophysiologic, situational, or maturational. Pathophysiologic conditions are usually associated with chronic illness. Over 85% of all individuals over age 65 suffer from one or more chronic conditions (Lewis, 1984), which compound the degree of functional impairment. The three leading chronic medical conditions are heart conditions, arthritis/rheumatism, and visual impairments. Other pathophysiologic conditions include Alzheimer's disease and other dementias, diabetes, Laennec's cirrhosis, cardiovascular diseases, and neuromuscular and muscloskeletal disorders. An added dimension of these pathophysiologic conditions is a continued susceptibility to acute illness such as pneumonia and urinary tract infections. Pain and discomfort contribute to disuse and functional impairment (Carpenito, 1987). Finally, medications prescribed to treat chronic medical conditions may have unexpected side effects (eg, sedation, orthostatic hypotension) in the elderly. Multiple conditions may result in polypharmacology with potent drug interactions that may also affect functional ability. Assessment of self-care ability must be done with the individual's medical history in mind.

Situational conditions are those circumstances associated with trauma, surgical procedures, or impairment caused by other prescribed treatments, such as casts or braces (Carpenito, 1987). A major situational condition seen frequently in the elderly is injury from falls. People over age 60 make up almost 25% of all hospital admissions due to fall injuries (Butler and Lewis, 1982) (see Chapter 3).

Maturational conditions associated with self-care deficit are those continuous, ongoing changes that occur as one ages. Etiologies listed by NANDA (Carroll-Johnson, 1989) and those described here are listed in Table 24.1. Evaluatively, they are neither good nor bad but denote progressive changes with appropriate adaptive adjustment. Three areas commonly noted are decreased sensory ability, decreased motor ability, and muscle weakness. These conditions become a self-care deficit if an inverse relationship develops between the individual self-care capacity and the demand (Orem, 1980). Elderly clients in this situation feel that they cannot positively or negatively influence their destiny. Changes are seen as irreversible and increasing in nature. Role behaviors frequently associated with these feelings are passivity and dependency.

To a certain degree, allowing others to take control of most aspects of one's life temporarily is sometimes necessary and beneficial, especially in the sick role. The key to this state of being is its time-limited nature. Even in the case of serious illness, the elderly client should be given some choices, as there is a clear-cut positive association between a sense of control and a sense of well-being (Ryden, 1985). Lack of control over the myriad of everyday activities of daily living can precipitate a demoralizing sense of powerlessness and dependency (Pohl and Fuller, 1980).

The nursing diagnosis Impaired Physical Mobility also occurs frequently in institutionalized elders (Metzger and Hiltunen, 1987). Impaired Physical Mobility overlaps Self-Care Deficit, and Creason et al (1985) suggest that Self-Care Deficit may be the underlying nursing diagnosis when the intervention for Impaired Physical Mobility is to compensate in order to improve or maximize functional abilities.

ASSESSMENT

Just as there is diversity in the breadth of defining *self-care deficit*, so there exists a broad range of tools to assess self-care, functional performance, and self-care deficit. Considering self-care in its broadest terms, there are tools available to assess self-care ability. The Exercise of Self-Care Agency Scale (Kearney and Fleischer, 1979) measures the individual's perception of ability to perform self-care, based on subconstructs of active versus passive responses to situations, motivation, knowledge, and a sense of self-worth. Originally tested with college-age students, this tool has been tested with community-dwelling elders (Lantz, 1985), correlating a high degree of self-actualization to a high degree of exercise of self-care agency.

Self-care agency has also been described using 10 power components (Nursing Development Conference Group, 1979). Briefly, these power components are (1) be attentive and vigilant; (2) control the use of physical energy; (3) use direct body movement; (4) reason within a self-care framework; (5) be motivated to care for oneself; (6) make decisions and act on them; (7) learn, remember, and use self-care knowledge; (8) draw on cognitive, perceptual and communication skills; (9) prioritize self-care actions; and (10) integrate self-care actions with oneself, family, and community. Hanson and Bickel (1985) examined these power components in the construction of their questionnaire on the perception of self-care agency, providing a more inclusive theoretical basis of self-care. Tested with adults from various age groups (mean age 37.9, standard deviation 14.6) (Bickel, 1982), this tool requires further testing to establish validity and reliability with elderly populations.

Evers and Isenberg (1987) used an Appraisal of Self-Care Agency Scale to examine perception of self-care ability. This tool demonstrated significant reliability and validity for institutionalized and community-residing elders for self-appraisal and appraisal by independent nurse raters.

These tools include many items that appear to measure not only self-care ability (as defined by NANDA) but also ability to maintain health and home management.

Self-care agency has also been the basis of assessment tools for specific disease conditions, for example, hospitalized clients with chronic obstructive pulmonary disease (COPD) (Michaels, 1985) or community-dwelling

Table 24.1

Etiologies/Related Factors and Defining Characteristics of Self-Care Deficit

NANDA (CARROLL-JOHNSON 1989)

Feeding

Defining Characteristic:
  Inability to bring food from a receptacle to the mouth

Bathing/Hygiene

Defining Characteristics:
  *Inability to wash body or body parts
  Inability to obtain or get to water source
  Inability to regulate temperature or flow

Dressing/Grooming

Defining Characteristics:
  *Impaired ability to put on or take off necessary items
    of clothing
  Impaired ability to obtain or replace articles of clothing
  Impaired ability to fasten clothing
  Inability to maintain appearance at a satisfactory level

Toileting

Etiologies/Related Factors:
  Impaired transfer ability
  Impaired mobility status
  Intolerance to activity; decreased strength and endurance
  Pain, discomfort
  Perceptual or cognitive impairment
  Neuromuscular impairment
  Musculoskeletal impairment
  Depression, severe anxiety
Defining Characteristics:
  *Unable to get to toilet or commode
  *Unable to manipulate clothing for toileting
  *Unable to carry out proper toilet hygiene
  Unable to flush toilet or empty commode

PENN

Etiologies/Related Factors:
  Pathophysiologic
    Neuromuscular impairments
    Musculoskeletal impairments
    Uncompensated perceptual cognitive factors
    Visual disorders
  Situational
    Immobility
    Prescribed treatments
    Trauma or surgical procedure
    Changes in social support or availability of resources
    Limited health practice knowledge, experience, or skills
  Emotional
    Anxiety
    Depression
    Hopelessness
  Maturational
    Age-related physical constraints (Carpenito, 1983;
      Eliopoulos, 1983; Gordon, 1982; Kim & Moritz, 1982)

Self-Feeding

Defining Characteristic:
  Unable or unwilling to bring food from a receptacle
    to the mouth

Self-Bathing

Defining Characteristics:
  Unable or unwilling to:
  *Wash body or body parts
  Obtain water or get to water source
  Obtain water or get to water source
  Regulate water temperature or flow

Self-Dressing

Defining Characteristics:
  Unable or unwilling to:
  *Put on or take off clothing
  Obtain or replace articles of clothing
  Fasten regular or adatped clothing
  Maintain appearance at a satisfactory level

Self-Toileting

Defining Characteristics:
  Unable or unwilling to:
  *Get to toilet or commode
  *Transfer to and from toilet or commode
  *Manipulate clothing
  *Cleanse self after elimination
  Flush toilet or commode

*Critical defining characteristics.

psychiatric clients (Loveland-Cherry et al, 1985). One source of information for other current tool development is the self-care deficit theory network newsletter (Taylor, 1988), which can acquaint nurses with other contributions to research, theory, and practice advances in the self-care deficit theory. As with any assessment tool, reliability and validity must be established for different populations in different settings. This is a rich area for continued research.

Self-care may be defined in terms of functional ability, and various assessment tools are available to describe subcategories of functional self-care. In an excellent review of measures for physical functioning, Kane and Kane (1981) identify three general categories of items: (1) general physical health; (2) basic self-care activities of daily living (eg, dressing, bathing, toileting, feeding, mobility); and (3) instrumental activities of daily living (IADL) (eg, cooking, cleaning). Well-studied measures of physical functioning include the Katz Index of ADL (Katz et al, 1963), Bathel Self-Care Ratings (Sherwood et al, 1977), and the OARS: IADL section (Duke University, 1978). These global dimensions of self-care are insensitive to slight changes in functioning, making them more useful for large epidemiologic studies than for clinical assessment. The amount of detail required depends on the setting in which the assessment is done (acute care versus long-term care facility) and the purpose of distinguishing between levels of disability (description for research, screening, or planning care). Tools that include instrumental activities of daily living present some difficulty in use within environments that do not provide opportunities for these activities (Kane and Kane, 1981). When assessing community-residing elders, IADL tools should also address social support and environmental barriers. Feinstein (1982) stresses the importance of assessing not only the current level of function but also the probable etiology (effects of the medical condition versus prescribed limitations versus depression or fears about prognosis).

Self-care behaviors may be defined even more discretely as activities of basic personal care, the approach taken by NANDA (Carroll-Johnson, 1989). Deficits in self-care may occur in any of the subcategories of feeding, bathing/hygiene, dressing/grooming, and toileting. In a review of gerontologic nursing research, Adams (1986) found few nursing studies focusing on these subcategories. Defining characteristics of these subcategories (see Table 24.1) guide the assessment of the elderly for Self-Care Deficit.

Being able to discriminate among levels of disability is especially important when assessing elderly clients (Kane and Kane, 1981). Various scales are available to rank the performance of self-care on a continuum of dependent to independent. The scale suggested by NANDA is presented in Table 24.2. Further development of this scale (see Table 24.3) describes more completely the degree of assistance required from another person (McCourt, 1987) and is more sensitive to even small changes in function

Table 24.2

Suggested Scale for Functional Level (NANDA)*

0 =	Completely independent
1 =	Requires use of equipment or device
2 =	Requires help from another person for assistance, supervision, or teaching
3 =	Requires help from another person and equipment, device
4 =	Dependent, does not participate in activity

*Approved nursing diagnoses classified by human response patterns. Pages 542–543 in: *Classification of Nursing Diagnoses: Proceedings of the Eighth Conference.* Carroll-Johnson R (editor). Lippincott, 1989, with permission.

over time (deterioration or progress). Pairing this scale with precise behavioral criteria for feeding, bathing/hygiene, dressing/grooming, and toileting allows a systematic way of assessing the degree of self-care deficit.

Baer et al (1984) report initial testing of a rating system using McCourt's Index of Functional Ability. Assessing rehabilitation clients with spinal cord injuries (ages 21 to 65), the investigators assigned numeric values with behaviors observed (eg, dressing: 0 = independent; 1 = uses device such as dressing stick; 2.4 = client does 75% of the work, needs assistance with buttons, zippers; 2.6 = client does 50% of work, needs help with shoes or pants; 3 = required help from another person and device; 4 = dependent). Interrater reliability ranged from 40% to 100%, reflecting a need to define the tasks in more detail (eg, what 2.2 or 2.8 would represent) and to agree to evaluate only observed behaviors, not estimated ability (eg, dressing skills for those clients not dressing routinely). Further research is necessary to establish a reliable and valid tool for assessing self-care deficit.

Ideally, this will lead to one tool that could be used regardless of the etiology of the self-care deficit. The Self-Care Deficit Assessment Form (see Assessment Guide 24.1), developed by this chapter's author, is undergoing pilot testing (Penn, 1988) and requires further testing for reliability and validity for institutionalized elders.

These assessment data are directly observable during natural patient encounters such as mealtime or bath time. For the most reliable identification of the self-care deficit and evaluation of intervention effectiveness, the nurse should record the performance of the elder's self-care during or immediately after the observation of performance.

Because elders may experience "testing anxiety," the nurse should explain how this assessment will help individualize their care. Each subcategory (eg, feeding, bathing, dressing, grooming, toileting) should be assessed in separate encounters to reduce the effect of fatigue on the results. Generally, elderly persons perform best in the morning, so the rater may want to assess the person's ability at various times of the day to identify the time of

Table 24.3

McCourt Index of Functional Ability in Long-Term Care*

0 = Independent
1 = Requires use of equipment/assistive device
2 = Requires help from another person for supervision, assistance, or teaching
    2.2 Supervision or contact guarding
    2.4 Minimal assistance: patient does 75% of the work
    2.6 Moderate assistance: patient does 50% of the work
    2.8 Maximum assistance: patient does 25% of the work
3 = Requires help from another person *plus* equipment/assistive device
    3.2 Supervision or contact guarding in addition to equipment/assistive device
    3.4 Minimal assistance in addition to equipment/assistive device
    3.6 Moderate assistance in addition to equipment/assistive device
    3.8 Maximum assistance in addition to equipment/assistive device
4 = Dependent—does not participate in activity

*McCourt A: *Functional Assessment Tracking System*. New England Sinai Hospital, Stoughton, MA, with permission.

the day the elder is most likely to require self-care assistance.

The Self-Care Deficit Assessment Form uses the time intervals set by the short-term goal and long-term goal for reevaluation dates. More frequent evaluation may be required as determined by the short-term evaluation results.

Once the diagnosis Self-Care Deficit has been established, goals must be formulated. Traditionally, self-care has been viewed as the client's responsibility, whereas the nurse is accountable for teaching, guiding, and supporting self-care–oriented behaviors. In situations where self-care is not feasible, the nurse is then accountable for the maintenance of what was self-care until recovery or death occurs (Caley, 1980). However, with rapid developments in technical and skilled health care delivery, nurses are faced with a decrease in care time available to nurture self-care activities. It is simply quicker and more cost-effective to comb clients' hair than to motivate them to comb their own hair. To help deter this phenomenon, goals should be directed toward motivating, guiding, and supporting the elderly client toward self-care.

CASE STUDY

Self-Care Deficit

Mrs. J, age 73, recently moved to the long-term care facility because she could no longer keep up her home. Her son, who lives 200 miles away, was also concerned that she was not eating well or maintaining her personal care. Mrs. J has COPD, which limits her activity tolerance. She also has rheumatoid arthritis, involving her hands, wrists, and feet. She experiences early morning stiffness,

hand and wrist discomfort with fine motor movement, and easy fatigability, which is most noticeable early in the afternoon.

The admission assessment of Mrs. J's self-care abilities reveals independence in feeding, toileting, and oral care, but a desire to wear her housecoat all day and a reluctance to bathe.

NURSING INTERVENTIONS

Murray and Kijek (1979) identified goals in rehabilitation nursing based on the need for their clients not only to accomplish specific tasks but also to foster the desire to engage in such behaviors. These goals are directly associated with a self-care deficit in that motivation for care is essential rather than simply a focus on the tasks themselves. These goals are as follows:

1. Stimulation of dormant resources
2. Strengthening of underused abilities
3. Establishment of positive life patterns
4. Continued growth within existing life patterns

Each goal (described in more detail below) is broad based and universal, allowing for individualized interventions based on the elderly client's uniqueness.

Stimulation of Dormant Resources

Each individual is responsible for his or her own self-care and has an innate ability to carry out self-care tasks. Social, situational, and maturational factors may cloud or mask these abilities beyond awareness, such that elderly individuals may not be fully aware they are capable of carrying out self-care behaviors during periods of altered health. Regardless of the causes of the self-care deficit, the most beneficial role the nurse can play is one of "discoverer" to help awaken dormant resources and instruct elderly clients on their optimal use.

Strengthening of Underused Abilities

In a society where time is money and efficacy is a constant determinant, taking the time to strengthen dampened self-care behaviors can be viewed as ineffective and time consuming. Nursing goals are often reflected as narrow in scope, covering only the expeditious completion of activities of daily living without consideration for long-term behaviors or even future tasks. Ryden (1985) states that one of the greatest challenges facing caregivers is encouraging elderly persons to maintain control over themselves in the face of decreased energy, physical dependency, and altered cognitive functioning. Maintaining broad-based nursing goals that reinforce self-care behaviors not only encourages autonomy but has future positive effects on time management.

Tools for Independence

Nursing interventions are carefully selected so as not to exceed the degree of self-care assistance required. Interventions well suited to self-care deficit include use of assistive devices, client reeducation, self-monitoring, contracting, self-help groups, and reminiscence therapy (Penn, 1988).

Assistive Devices When planning interventions for self-care deficits, assistive devices are often some of the first considered interventions. Numerous adaptive aids are available, some through rehabilitation services, others through home health catalogues (such as specialty catalogues from JC Penney's or Sears).

The primary purpose of the assistive device is to maximize existing function and compensate for specific disabilities due to trauma or disease. These assistive, or self-help, devices differ from orthotic and prosthetic devices. Orthotic devices substitute for lost function. For example, an ankle–foot orthesis (AFO) supports the weight of the foot and the shoe for clients having foot drop. Prosthetic devices substitute for missing body parts, following amputation or enucleation. Assistive devices are prescribed for specific functions, such as dressing or eating. Specially made clothing with fasteners that can be manipulated by elderly persons who have limited dexterity or loss of the use of one arm,

hand, or leg can be very useful for helping the elder maintain maximum self-care.

Numerous assistive devices are available, each for a very specific disability. Proper selection of an assistive device requires specialized knowledge of the etiology of the self-care deficit and the best device to fit the patient's requirements; thus, consultation with an occupational therapist is recommended. Describing specific assistive devices is outside the scope of this chapter; the reader is encouraged to review other sources for more information. Excellent overviews of assistive devices for the elderly (Helm, 1987; Redford, 1986) are available.

Not every patient is able to use assistive devices. Several factors are worth considering before prescribing assistive devices. First, is the client mentally capable of learning to use the device? Some neurologic conditions result in "apraxia," or the inability to execute a planned motor act in the absence of muscle paralysis. The idea of the required movement is confused. For example, the elder may try to comb her hair with a pen. Or the individual may grasp the idea but be unable to carry out the intended action. The client may unbutton his cuff automatically to roll up his sleeves but may be unable to unbutton on request during dressing practice. The prescription of assistive devices for this client would not be beneficial.

Second, will the device provide significant improvement in self-care independence? If the client feels she can perform the required self-care without the device, or if she is opposed to the use of a device, she will not be motivated to use the device (Redford, 1986). Correct use of the device requires learning new skills. Knowledge of the client's values, attitudes toward the disability, and desired lifestyle can aid in motivating the learner.

Third, does the assistive device call for more physical endurance or muscle strength than the individual has? Many assistive devices are designed for a younger age group. For example, a young paraplegic adult may retain adequate upper extremity strength for sliding board transfers and grab bars that an older adult, who is experiencing gradual loss of muscle mass, will not possess (Faletti, 1985). Simplification of the task and energy conservation techniques are other possible approaches the elderly may use to adapt to a gradual decline in muscle strength and endurance (Maguire, 1985).

Reeducation Inherent in a rehabilitation approach to self-care deficits is reeducation in skills that maximize self-care in feeding, bathing, dressing, grooming and toileting. Short, structured practice sessions should focus on the specific skill the client must learn to overcome the unique characteristics of the self-care deficit (Penn, 1988).

Self-Monitoring Self-monitoring may be combined with a reeducation intervention. Self-monitoring involves the client in recording in a diary or chart factors that interfere with self-care, the degree of independence in self-care, and the application of the intervention. Self-monitoring then becomes one method to evaluate the effectiveness of the interventions and to identify areas for improving the plan (Penn, 1988).

Contracting Contracting also works well with a re-education intervention; it reinforces the client's role as an active participant in self-care. A contract identifies the desired behavior (eg, independence in oral care) in measurable terms that are acceptable to both the client and the nurse (Steckel, 1982). The desired behavior is then broken down into smaller steps, each building toward the end goal. The client then identifies rewards or reinforcers for successful completion of specific behaviors. Progress is recorded in a diary or chart (using the self-monitoring intervention). Reevaluation dates are determined at the initiation of the contract. The development of contracts dovetails with the nursing process and can be used for a health promotion focus or restorative focus (Steckel, 1982). Penn (1988) described the use of this intervention to treat self-care deficit of an elderly woman who had suffered a stroke and had moved in with her daughter following hospitalization.

Self-Help Groups Individuals may gather together to satisfy a common need or find mutual assistance to overcome a handicap. The philosophy of self-help groups is that an individual can best be helped by another person experiencing similar events. Important functions of self-help groups include providing information, giving emotional support, and role modeling (Kinney et al, 1985).

Reminiscence Therapy Reminiscence therapy is sharing life experiences, stimulating the recall of memories to assist the client to meet specific objectives (Hamilton, 1985). Often used to treat psychosocial nursing diagnoses, reminiscence therapy was found in one experimental study to affect self-care. Using this intervention to reduce depression in aged institutionalized clients, Hiebel (cited in Hamilton, 1985) found a concomitant increase in self-care activities and in the desire to socialize. Reminiscence therapy is an appropriate intervention for self-care deficit, particularly when the etiology is depression. See Chapter 25 for further discussion of reminiscence therapy.

Other Interventions For elders who remain totally dependent on the nurse for self-care assistance, a wholly compensatory system of nursing care becomes necessary. The primary interventions for a total-dependence self-care deficit would be the provision of bathing, skin care, positioning, feeding, oral care, and bowel and bladder

retraining (Bulechek and McCloskey, 1985). Research studies for effectiveness of ADL interventions are found in occupational therapy literature. There has been a lack of nursing research of the functioning of older persons in activities of daily living (Adams, 1986).

CASE STUDY

Nursing Interventions

The nurse and Mrs. J agreed to focus on bathing skills first, as using a warm shower could reduce early morning stiffness and aid in maintaining joint function. Restricted range of movement and pain with hand movement require assistive devices to ease the energy requirements of dressing and bathing.

Mrs. J was concerned that she might "overdo it." "I can't do very much for myself because I get short of breath." Contracting was used as an intervention so that Mrs. J could see that she controlled the pace of each day's goal. The nurse provided a checklist of the steps of bathing, and Mrs. J selected daily goals for the week, with the understanding that if she had difficulty achieving a goal, she could remain at that goal for an additional day. She was hesitant to select a reward for successful achievement of her weekly goal, but with encouragement she opted to get her hair styled.

Specific skills Mrs. J needed to learn included use of a wheelchair shower or bath bench and hand-held shower to simplify bathing and to conserve energy. Consultation with occupational therapy identified assistive devices to overcome limited movement. A wash mitt and built-up handles on grooming equipment allowed Mrs. J to perform bathing with a limited hand grasp. Mrs. J was encouraged to put all her bathing equipment in a basin and to carry the basin with her arms rather than with her hands.

By the first week, Mrs. J's self-care ability with bathing was 3.2; she used the assistive devices easily but required reminders for pacing activities. Further goals were set to achieve a rating of 1—independent with use of assistive devices. Mrs J enjoyed selecting her "treats" for completing a contract and verbalized feeling better about how she looked.

OUTCOMES

Self-care deficits are objectively measured using an assessment scale to obtain a baseline, and then after the intervention, to ascertain where improvement has been achieved. Using the evaluation data, the nurse and client set new goals or design a new plan.

Outcome criteria for the resolution of self-care deficit follow. The client:

Makes mutually agreeable plans with the nurse for rehabilitation goals

Demonstrates the ability to feed, bathe, dress/groom, and toilet oneself

Demonstrates correct use of adaptive equipment

Minimizes the potential for injury by demonstrating safety steps necessary for one's own residual disability

Maintains adequate nutritional and hydration status

Maintains clean, dry skin without body odor

Maintains groomed appearance in keeping with predeficit preferences

Wears clothes appropriate to weather/occasion

Maintains a pattern of fluid intake and voiding

Maintains predeficit defecation schedule

Verbalizes degree of adjustment to etiology of self-care deficit

Verbalizes degree of satisfaction with alternate ways of doing self-care tasks

SUMMARY

Self-Care Deficit is an activity-focused nursing diagnosis based on the assumption that self-control and self-determination are important components of nursing practice. For the elderly, who are experiencing a number of changes and losses, such control and self-determination are vital to maintaining human dignity and a feeling of "personhood." Self-Care Deficit as a nursing diagnosis responds to these needs and changes by providing care supportive to or restorative of life. The focus of action is on the client and his or her potential. Nursing implementation strategies facilitate the client to move toward involvement in his or her care. The nurse has the opportunity to influence both the objective extent of self-determination and the client's sense of situational control (Ryden, 1985). Self-Care Deficit as a diagnosis helps the nurse focus on what nursing can do to assist the client to achieve control and self-determination.

ASSESSMENT GUIDE 24.1

Self-Care Deficit Assessment Form

Client: Mrs. J

1. Admission Assessment Date: 3/29/88
2. Short-Term Evaluation Date: 3/29/88
3. Long-Term Evaluation Date: 4/29/88

Subjective Data: "I can't do much for myself because I get short of breath. I'm afraid I might overdo it. You don't have time to wait for me to do all this."

Objective Data:
General appearance—cleanliness, grooming, clothing, hair, nutritional status
Clean, unstyled hair; dry skin with slight odor; dressed in rumpled, soiled housecoat, slip, underwear, and slippers; dentures clean

Etiologies/Contributing Factors:
Physical—Arthritis, COPD
Mental—sl. anxious
Educational
Life experiences
Motivational—limits self-care to prevent dyspnea; senses attempts at self-care take too long
Socioeconomic—admitted to LTCF 3/17/89; Son lives out of state; One visit from neighbor since admission

Code: (see Table 24.3)

0 = Independent
1 = Requires equipment, assistive device
2 = Requires help from another person for supervision, assistance, teaching
    2.2 Supervision
    2.4 Minimal - 75 %
    2.6 Moderate - 50 %
    2.8 Maximum - 25 %
3 = Requires help from another person *plus* equipment/assistive device
    3.2 Supervision + device
    3.4 Minimal assist + device
    3.6 Moderate assist + device
    3.8 Maximum assist + device
4 = Dependent
N/O—Not Observed

SELF-CARE PERFORMANCE CHECKLIST

Dates	(1) 3/22/88	(2) 3/29/89	(3) 4/29/88
Rater's Name	CP	CP	
Feeding		Rating	
Opens cartons/sets up tray	2.8	2.2	
Uses fork/spoon	0	0	
Uses knife to cut meat	0	0	
Butters bread	0	0	
Drinks from cup/glass	0	0	
Chews solid food	0	0	
Swallows solids and liquids (if more than zero, refer to Impaired Swallowing diagnosis)	0	0	

Comments: none

Bathing			
Gets to water source, bath	0	0	
Obtains soap/towels	0	0	

ASSESSMENT GUIDE 24.1

Self-Care Deficit Assessment Form (Continued)

Regulates water flow/temperature	2.8	0
Undresses to bathe (if more than one, specify garments requiring assistance)	see "drsg"	see "drsg"
Washes and dries:		
face and hands	0	0
arms	3.6	2.2
trunk, genitalia	3.6	2.4
back	3.6	2.6
legs	3.8	2.4
feet	3.8	2.6
Shampoos and dries hair	N/O	3.4

Comments: 3/22—observed in patient bathroom, basin bath
3/29—observed in shower, with chair & hand-held shower head, wash mitt

Dressing:		ON	OFF	ON	OFF	ON	OFF
Puts on/takes off:							
underwear		0	0	0	0		
pantyhose		N/O	N/O	N/A			
slacks or skirt	(slacks)	N/O	N/O	2.4	2.4		
bra		4	4	2.6			
slip or undershirt		0	0	N/A			
blouse or shirt 3/22—hscoat; 3/29—blouse		2.4	2.4	2.4	2.4		
velcro		N/O	N/O	N/O			
snaps		2.6	2.6	2.4	2.4		
buttons		4	4	2.4	2.4		
zipper		N/O	N/O	N/O			
belt or suspenders		N/O	N/O	N/O			
hook and eye		N/O	N/O	2.6	2.8		
stockings or hose		3.2	3.2	1	1		
braces/splints		N/A	N/A	N/A	N/A		
shoes		3.2	3.2	1	1		
ties shoelaces		N/O	N/O	2.8	2.8		
sweater		2.6	2.6	2.2	2.2		
coat		N/O	N/O	2.4	2.4		
overshoes		N/O	N/O	2.6	2.6		
mittens/gloves		N/O	N/O	0	0		
Obtains/replaces articles of clothing		2.2	2.2	0	0		
Selects appropriate clothing (for weather, occasion)		2.6	2.6	0	0		

Comments: 3/22—dresses while seated in chair; 3/29—never wears pantyhose, needs velcro bra fastener

(Continues)

ASSESSMENT GUIDE 24.1

Self-Care Deficit Assessment Form (Continued)

Grooming

Brush/comb hair	2.2	1
Style hair	N/O	2.8
Brush teeth/dentures	0	0
Shave face, underarms, or legs	N/O	N/O
Apply makeup	N/O	1
(if part of predisability routine)		(lipstick, rouge)
Apply deodorant	2.2	1
Clean/trim fingernails	N/O	2.6
Turn faucet	0	0
Obtain and replace articles	0	0
Plug in cord	N/O	2.8 (hairdryer)
Blow nose	0	0

Comments: 3/29—using built-up handled grooming equipment

Toileting

Uses toilet substitute (urinal, bedpan) only	N/A	N/A
Transfers to commode/toilet (if more than two, refer to impaired physical mobility dx)	0	0
Undresses	0	0
Sits on toilet/commode	0	0
Cleanses self	0	0
Flushes toilet	0	0
Rises from toilet	0	0
Redresses	0	0
Washes hands	0	0
Uses tampon or sanitary napkin	N/O	N/O

Comments:

Nursing Diagnoses:

Label: Self-care deficit in bathing (level 3.6)
Etiology: limited ROM and decreased activity tolerance
Defining Characteristics: assistance required to regulate water flow and to reach body parts
Label: Self-care deficit in dressing (level 2.6)
Etiology: limited ROM and decreased activity tolerance, decreased motivation
Defining Characteristics: assistance required to put on, take off, and fasten clothing; recent option to stay dressed in sleepwear

Nurse/Client Goals:

To complete assessment of full dressing by 3/29
To be 75% independent with bathing and dressing (with or without assistive devices) by 4/29
To select daily goals from bathing checklist
To get hair cut and styled on 3/29 if daily goals for 5 days are reached

References

Adams M: Aging: Gerontological nursing reasearch. *Ann Nurs Res* 1986; 4:77–103.

Baer CA, Delorey M, Fitzmaurice JB: A study to evaluate the validity of the rating system for self-care deficit. Pages 185–191 in: *Classification of Nursing Diagnoses: Proceedings of the Fifth National Conference.* Kim MJ, McFarland GK, McLane AM (editors). Mosby, 1984.

Bickel L: *A Study to Assess the Factorial Structure of the Perception of Self-Care Agency Questionnaire.* (Thesis.) University of Missouri, 1982.

Bulechek GM, McCloskey JC (editors): Future directions. Chapter 28 in: *Nursing Interventions: Treatment for Nursing Diagnoses.* Saunders, 1985.

Butler RN, Lewis MI: *Aging and Mental Health,* 3d ed. Mosby, 1982.

Caley JM: The Orem self-care nursing model. Pages 302–314 in: *Conceptual Models for Nursing.* Caley JM, Rickle L Sr., Roy C (editors). Appleton-Century-Crofts, 1980.

Carpenito LJ: *Nursing Diagnosis: Application to Clinical Practice,* 2d ed. Lippincott, 1987.

Carroll-Johnson R (editor): *Classification of Nursing Diagnoses: Proceedings of the Eighth Conference.* Lippincott, 1989.

Creason N et al: Validating the nursing diagnosis of impaired physical mobility. *Nurs Clin North Am* 1985; 20(4):801–808.

Duke University Center for the Study of Aging and Human Development: *Multidimensional Functional Assessment: The OARS Methodology.* Duke University, 1978.

Eliopoulos C: A self-care model for gerontological nursing. *Geriatr Nurs* 1984; 5(8):366–369.

Evers GC, Isenberg MA: Reliability and validity of the appraisal of self-care agency (ASA) scale. *International Nursing Research Conference Abstracts: Nursing Advances in Health: Models, Methods, and Applications.* American Nurses' Association, 1987.

Faletti MV: From can openers to computers: Technology can enhance functional ability and independence for the aged. *Caring* 1985; 14(1):56–58.

Feinstein AR: The Jones criteria and the challenges of clinimetrics. *Circulation* 1982; 66(1):1–5.

Gordon M: *Nursing Diagnosis: Process and Application.* McGraw-Hill, 1982.

Hamilton DB: Reminiscence therapy. Chapter 10 in: *Nursing Interventions: Treatments for Nursing Diagnoses.* Bulechek GM, McCloskey JC (editors). Saunders, 1985.

Hanson BR, Bickel L: Development and testing of the questionnaire on perception of self-care agency. Chapter 27 in: *The Science and Art of Self-Care.* Riehl-Sisca J (editor). Appleton-Century-Crofts, 1985.

Hardy M, Maas M, Akin J: The prevalence of nursing diagnoses among elderly and long term care residents: A descriptive comparison. *Rec Adv Nurs* 1988; 21:144–158.

Helm M: *Occupational Therapy with the Elderly.* Churchill Livingstone, 1987.

Kane RA, Kane RL: *Assessing the Elderly: A Practical Guide to Measurement.* Lexington, 1981.

Katz S et al: Studies of illness in the aged: The Index of ADL: A standardized measure of biological and psychosocial function. *JAMA* 1963; 185:94ff.

Kearney BY, Fleischer BJ: Development of an instrument to measure exercise of self-care agency. *Res Nurs Health* 1979; 2:25–34.

Kim MJ, Moritz DA: *Classification of Nursing Diagnosis: Proceedings of the Third and Fourth National Conferences.* McGraw-Hill, 1982.

Kinney CKD, Mannetter R, Carpenter M: Support groups. Chapter 14 in: *Nursing Interventions: Treatments for Nursing Diagnoses.* Bulechek GM, McCloskey JC (editors). Saunders, 1985.

Lantz JM: In search of agents for self-care. *J Gerontol Nurs* 1985; 11(7):10–14.

Lekan-Rutledge D: Gerontological nursing in long-term care facilities. Chapter 25 in: *Gerontological Nursing: Concepts and Practices.* Matteson MA, McConnell ES (editors). Saunders, 1988.

Leslie FM: Nursing diagnosis: Use in long-term care. *Am J Nurs* 1981; 81(5):1012–1014.

Lewis CB: Rehabilitation of the older person: A psychosocial focus. *Physical Ther* (Apr) 1984; 64(4):517–522.

Loveland-Cherry C et al: A nursing protocol based on Orem's self-care model: Application with aftercare clients. Chapter 29 in: *The Science and Art of Self-Care.* Riehl-Sisca J (editor). Appleton-Century-Crofts, 1985.

Maguire GH: Activities of daily living. Chapter 3 in: *Aging: The Health Care Challenge.* Lewis CB (editor). Davis, 1985.

McCourt AE: Implementing nursing diagnosis through integration with quality assurance. *Nurs Clin North Am* 1987; 22(4):899–904.

Metzger KL, Hiltunen EF: Diagnostic content validation of ten frequently reported nursing diagnoses. Pages 144–153 in: *Classification of Nursing Diagnoses: Proceedings of the Seventh Conference.* McLane AM (editor). Mosby, 1987.

Michaels C: Clinical specialist consultation to assess self-care agency among hospitalized COPD patients. Chapter 28 in: *The Science and Art of Self-Care.* Riehl-Sisca J (editor). Appleton-Century-Crofts, 1985.

Murray R, Kijek JC: *Current Perspectives in Rehabilitation Nursing.* Mosby, 1979.

Nursing Development Conference Group: *Concept Formalization in Nursing: Process and Product,* 2d ed. Little, Brown, 1979.

Orem DE: *Nursing: Concepts of Practice,* 2d ed. McGraw-Hill, 1980.

Orem DE: *Nursing: Concepts of Practice,* 3d ed. McGraw-Hill, 1985.

Penn CE: Self-care deficit: Promoting independence. *J Gerontol Nurs* 1988; 14(3):14–19.

Pohl J, Fuller S: Perceived, choice, social interaction, and dimensions of morale of residents in a home for the aged. *Res Nurs Health* 1980; 3:147–157.

Redford JB: Assistive devices for the elderly. Chapter 15 in: *The Practice of Geriatrics.* Calkins E, Davis PJ, Ford AB (editors). Saunders, 1986.

Ryden MB: Environmental support for autonomy in the institutionalized elderly. *Res Nurs Health* 1985; 8:363–371.

Sherwood ST et al: *Compendium of Measures for Describing and Assessing Long Term Care Populations.* Hebrew Rehabilitation Center for Aged, Boston, 1977.

Steckel SB: *Patient Contracting.* Appleton-Century-Crofts, 1982.

Sullivan TJ: Self-care model for nursing. *New Directions for Nursing in the 80's.* ANA Publication 1980; 57–68.

Taylor SG: *Self-Care Deficit Theory Curriculum Network Newsletter.* University of Missouri, 1988.

Wright GN: Functional limitations. Chapter 5 in: *Total Rehabilitation.* Little, Brown, 1980.

Yurick AG et al: *The Aged Person and the Nursing Process,* 2d ed. Appleton-Century-Crofts, 1984.

25

Diversional Activity Deficit

MARILYN RANTZ, MSN, RN

THE DEFINITION OF *DIVERSIONAL ACTIVITY* FOCUSES ON the ideas of change and deviation or on the ideas of enjoyment and pleasure. Diversion as change simply means activities that are different from one's usual activities. Diversion as enjoyment or pleasure means activities that are recreational and pursued during leisure time for the purpose of personal amusement or satisfaction. Leisure time is time that is free from obligations (Rubenfeld, 1986). A refinement of the North American Nursing Diagnosis Association's (NANDA) definition of Diversional Activity Deficit is "the state in which an individual experiences decreased environmental stimulation from, and/or decreased interest or engagement in, recreational/ leisure activities."

SIGNIFICANCE FOR THE ELDERLY

The growth of community-based therapeutic recreational programming for the elderly in independent living arrangements illustrates a recognition of the need to address Diversional Activity Deficit and counteract its potentially harmful outcomes. The elderly in independent living arrangements frequently experience chronic illnesses, limited finances, lack of transportation, social isolation, impaired mobility, impaired sensory functions (deafness, blindness), fear of neighborhood crime, and/or exertional physical limitations that contribute to their vulnerability to Diversional Activity Deficit (Ebersole and Hess, 1985; Lawton et al, 1984; Rubenfeld, 1986). The institutionalized elderly have many of these same factors impeding their involvement in diversional activities. Other factors include interfering institutional care delivery routines, space constraints, accessibility to resources, availability of staff to provide individualized assistance with learning new activities, lack of peer group with similar interests or cognitive capability, and/or lack of staff encouragement for residents' involvement in therapeutic recreational programming.

The negative outcomes of failure to diagnose and treat Diversional Activity Deficit in the elderly include social isolation, withdrawal, depression, poor self-esteem, decreased life satisfaction, further declines in physical endurance and coordination, and/or further decline in mental cognition.

Empirically supported positive outcomes such as improved cognitive function (Hamilton, 1985; Hughston and Merriam, 1982); improved learning capacity (Yesavage, 1984); increased alertness, awareness, receptiveness, and interaction; and focused discussion with peers (Baker, 1985; Beck, 1982;

Cook, 1984; Lesser and Lazarus, 1981) warrant serious attention to treatment of Diversional Activity Deficit in the elderly. Reduced anxiety (Schuster, 1985), decreased depression (Andrysco, 1982; Parent and Whall, 1984), improved self-esteem (Brickel, 1980–1981; Parent and Whall, 1984), and improved morale (Goldberg and Fitzpatrick, 1980) have been measured. Increased socialization (Brennan and Steinberg, 1983–1984; Parsons, 1984; Walker, 1984), decreased hostility (Robb and Stegman, 1983; Robb et al, 1980), and increased engagement, psychosocial well-being, and psychologic health (Greene and Monahan, 1982; McCormack and Whitehead, 1981) have resulted from successful interventions. Positive physical outcomes that have been measured include improved sleep patterns (Kaye, 1985), improved survival independent of health status, and lowered blood pressure (Baun et al, 1984). Specific positive physical results retard the progress of degenerative conditions/diseases and increase muscle strength, endurance, and joint flexibility (Allen, 1985; Ebersole and Hess, 1985; Johnson-Pawlson and Koshes, 1985). These are impressive outcomes of importance to nurses caring for the elderly.

The magnitude of the negative outcomes if the diagnosis is left unrecognized and untreated, as well as the magnitude of the positive outcomes if the diagnosis is identified and treated, establishes Diversional Activity Deficit as a significant nursing diagnosis in the care of the elderly. Elderly in both institutional and independent living arrangements are vulnerable to this condition; the incidence is projected as high-frequency.

CURRENT STATUS OF THE DIAGNOSIS

At the 1986 Sixth Conference a definition of Diversional Activity Deficit was accepted: the state in which an individual experiences a decreased stimulation from or interest or engagement in recreational or leisure activities. Within NANDA's taxonomic structure, Diversional Activity Deficit was placed within the Level I concept "Human Response Pattern" of "Moving" and as a subhead under the Level II concept subcategory of "Alteration in Recreation" (NANDA Diagnosis Review Committee, 1986).

The roots of the diagnosis Diversional Activity Deficit in the elderly can be traced to the aging theories proposed in the 1950s and 1960s and the subsequent proliferation of studies attempting to support or refute the theories. An important by-product of these efforts was the identification of negative outcomes of withdrawal from society and the positive outcomes that could be demonstrated through strategically planned interventions. These theories include the activity theory (Havighurst and Albrecht,

1953), the disengagement theory (Cummings and Henry, 1961), and the continuity theory (Neugarten et al, 1968).

Burbank (1986) supports an individualized phenomenologic approach to explore the meanings of events in older persons' lives using the techniques of life review (discussed further in the Reminiscence Intervention section of this chapter) to study the psychosocial aspects of aging.

These theoretical explorations, although controversial, must continue to provide guidance for the care of our elderly. The intervention and outcome research generated by theoretical advancement provide the practical directions for nursing practice and support the interventions described for the diagnosis Diversional Activity Deficit. To date, no specific empirical testing of this diagnosis has been located, although considerable research base has been located concerning applicable interventions and subsequent outcomes.

ETIOLOGIES/RELATED FACTORS AND DEFINING CHARACTERISTICS

Etiologies/related factors and defining characteristics listed by NANDA (Carroll-Johnson, 1989) are compared with those described by Rantz (1986a) in Table 25.1. There is low consensus among authors for the majority of etiologies and defining characteristics, which could be due to the populations used as a frame of reference for specification of etiologies or defining characteristics (Carpenito, 1983; Gettrust et al, 1985; Gordon, 1982; Rantz 1986a; Rubenfeld, 1986). Etiologies listed by most authors are environmental lack of diversional activity (monotonous environment/lack of stimulation); long-term hospitalization (confinement); frequent lengthy treatments; lack of motivation with signs of depression; immobility or inactivity (impaired mobility/decreased activity tolerance); and lack of skills (knowledge/interest) to perform an activity (hobby).

Defining characteristics listed by most authors include statement of boredom; statement of wishing there were something to do, to read, and so on; (frequent) daytime napping; flat facial expression (affect/depression).

Differential Diagnosis

Other NANDA diagnoses that are closely related to Diversional Activity Deficit are Social Isolation (see Chapter 44) and Impaired Social Interaction.

The defining characteristics of the diagnoses are very similar in content, although the items are worded differently (Table 25.2). The etiologies of Impaired Social Interaction, Social Isolation, and Diversional Activity

Table 25.1

Diversional Activity Deficit

NANDA (CARROLL-JOHNSON, 1989)	RANTZ (1986a)

NANDA (CARROLL-JOHNSON, 1989)

Related Factors/Etiologies

Environmental lack of diversional activity
Long-term hospitalization
Frequent, lengthy treatments

RANTZ (1986a)

Related Factors/Etiologies

High: Immobility or inactivity (impaired mobility, decreased activity tolerance)
        Personal choice or preference
        Prefers to stay in room
Medium: Sensory deficits
        Daytime napping
Low: Lack of motivation with signs of depression
        Lack of skills (knowledge/interest) to perform activity
        Impaired verbal communication
        Pain
        Confusion

Ranked by high, medium, and low frequency in an elderly long-term care population

Defining Characteristics

Patient's statement regarding the following:
    Boredom
    Wish there was something to do, to read, etc
    Usual hobbies cannot be undertaken in hospital

Defining Characteristics

High: Frequent daytime napping
        Refused recreational therapy programs
        Attends selective recreational therapy programs
        Sensory deficits
        Needs encouragement/director to participate in recreation/therapeutic programs
        Isolates self; spends most of day in room by choice
Medium: Statement of boredom
        Confusion
        Weakness and fatigue
        Few leisure skills or independent hobbies
        Dislikes peers/rude to peers
        Limits contacts with peers and staff
        Does not check recreational therapy unit calendar
Low: Flat facial expression (affect/depression)
        Refuses recreational therapy programs off the unit
        Visitors/family restrict participation in recreational therapy
        Watches TV in own room
        Decreased activity tolerance
        Pain
        Impaired verbal communication

Ranked by high, medium, and low frequency of occurrence in an elderly long-term care population

---

Deficit are all highly correlated in content as well as wording of the items. It appears that Social Isolation is a broader phenomenon, of which Impaired Social Interaction is a part. Although the focus of Diversional Activity Deficit is "the decline of environmental stimulation from, and/or decreased interest or engagement in, recreational/leisure activities," it appears that this condition could easily result *from* Social Isolation or Impaired Social Interaction occurring in a client. However, Diversional Activity Deficit may occur without either of the related diagnoses; likewise, either related diagnosis may occur without Diversional Activity Deficit.

ASSESSMENT

Assessment of the elderly for Diversional Activity Deficit begins with collection of data concerning key defining characteristics (Table 25.2). Observation of frequent daytime napping, flat facial expression, and statements

Table 25.2

Defining Characteristics of Related Diagnoses

DEFINING CHARACTERISTICS	DIAGNOSES		
	Social Isolation*	Diversional Activity Deficit[†]	Impaired Social Interaction
Statement of boredom		X	
Statement of wish there were something to do		X	
Frequent daytime napping		X	
Sad, dull affect	X	X	
Absence of supportive significant other(s)— family, friends, group	X		
Inappropriate or immature interests for developmental age or stage	X		
Uncommunicative	X		
Withdrawn	X	X	
No eye contact	X		
Preoccupation with own thoughts	X	X	
Repetitive, meaningless actions	X		
Projects hostility in voice, behavior	X	X	
Seeks to be alone or exists in subculture	X	X	
Evidence of physical and/or mental handicap or altered state of wellness	X	X	
Shows behavior unaccepted by dominant culture, group	X		X
Expresses feelings of aloneness imposed by others	X		
Expresses feelings of rejection	X		X
Experiences feelings of difference from others	X		
Expresses values acceptable to subculture, but unable to accept values of dominant culture	X		
Inadequacy in or absence of significant purpose in life	X		
Inability to meet expectations of others	X		
Verbalized or observed inability to receive or communicate a satisfying sense of belonging, caring, interest or shared history			X
Dysfunctional interaction with peers, family and/or others		X	X
Family report of change of style or pattern of interaction			X
Insecurity in public	X		X
Expresses interests inappropriate to developmental age or stage	X		
Feelings of uselessness	X		
Doubts about ability to survive	X		
Altered thought processes	X	X	
Sleep disturbances	X	X	
Inability to make decisions	X		
Change in nutritional intake (overeating or anorexia)	X	X	
Paranoia	X		
Mistrust	X		
Hallucinations: auditory, visual, kinetic	X		
Feelings of inferiority	X		
Depersonalization	X		
Feeling otherness	X		
Lack of attention	X		
History of limited community/social contacts	X		
Failure to interact with others nearby	X	X	
Time passes slowly	X	X	
Sensory deficits (sight, hearing, etc)	X	X	

* Defining characteristics of Social Isolation compiled from Kim (1984), Gordon (1985), Carpenito (1983), Fischer & Schwartz (1986), Rantz (1986b).
[†] Some defining characteristics of Diversional Activity Deficit or Impaired Social Interaction are worded differently from Social Isolation, but content was judged as similar.

Table 25.3

Instruments Used to Measure Impact of Interventions for Diversional Activity Deficit and Related Diagnoses

MEASUREMENT/AUTHOR	INTERVENTION
Geriatric Depression Scale, Mental Status Questionnaire, Set Tests for Dementia (Brink & Curran, 1985)	Reminiscence
Raven Standard Progressive Matrices (Hughston & Merriam, 1982)	Reminiscence
Evaluation Tool for Reminiscence Group Therapy (Baker, 1985)	Reminiscence
Eye contact, smile, tactile contact, verbal response time, number of words in response, number of questions asked, less verbalizations of violence and delusions (Andrysco, 1982)	Pet therapy
Heart and respiratory rates, blood pressure, ECG rhythm (Atterbury et al, 1983; Baun et al, 1984; Cusack & Smith, 1984; Gordon et al, 1983; Rocke, 1984)	Pet therapy and exercise therapy
Multi-Level Assessment Tool (Hamilton, 1985)	Pet therapy and music therapy
Evaluation of "A Dog in Residence—the JACOPIS Study" (Cusack & Smith, 1984)	Pet therapy
Verbalization, smile, look toward stimulus, eyes open, lean toward stimulus (Robb et al, 1980)	Pet therapy
Lawton's revised Philadelphia Geriatric Center Morale Scale, Rotter's Locus of Control Scale, Duke University's Older Americans Resources and Services Multi-Dimensional Functional Assessment Questionnaire (Robb & Stegman, 1983)	Pet therapy
State-Trait Anxiety Inventory (Frank, 1985)	Music therapy
Rhythm or sound attempt, extremity or body movement, emotional expression and smiles (Olson, 1984)	Music therapy
Modified Hartsock Music Preference Questionnaire, Questionnaire to Evaluate the Effects of Music Therapy (Buckwalter et al, 1985)	Music therapy
Philadelphia Geriatric Center Morale Scale, Rosenberg Self-Esteem Scale (Goldberg & Fitzpatrick, 1980)	Exercise therapy
Functional Life Scale, a constructed activity scale, Beck Depression Inventory (Parent & Whall, 1984)	Exercise therapy
Spielberger State-Trait Anxiety Scale (Yesavage, 1984)	Exercise and relaxation therapy
Engagement (McCormack & Whitehead, 1981)	Arts and crafts
1979 Long-term care minimum data set (Greene & Monahan, 1982)	Visitation
Activity, alertness rating, time spent visiting with peers (Beck, 1982)	Responsibility-inducing activities

of boredom or wishing there were something to do should draw attention to the possibility of this diagnosis.

The literature reviewed did not reveal any comprehensive assessment tool(s) to identify or quantify the diagnosis of Diversional Activity Deficit; however, many instruments have been used to measure the impact of interventions targeted to address this and related diagnoses (Table 25.3). Most tools were also used as premeasurements to establish baselines for measuring effectiveness.

Further Analysis of Diversional Activity Deficit in the Dependent Elderly

The Proceedings of the Fifth National Conference on Nursing Diagnosis (Kim et al, 1984) included research suggestions for the diagnosis Diversional Activity Deficit:

1. How often is this diagnosis used in the clinical setting?
2. Why is this diagnosis perceived as useful?
3. Concurrent or retrospective audit:
   a. Which signs and symptoms do nurses use to identify this diagnosis?
   b. How do nurses decide which activities are appropriate?
4. How is this diagnosis related to the developmental stage of the clients?

To explore these questions in a geriatric setting, medical records of residents in a 328-bed skilled nursing facility from 1983 to 1986 were examined for the nursing diagnosis Diversional Activity Deficit (Rantz, 1986a).

From 1983 to 1986 the diagnosis Diversional Activity Deficit or Potential for Diversional Activity Deficit was recorded for 66 residents. This diagnosis ranked 15th in frequency when compared with other diagnoses identified in the primarily geriatric population. The etiologies and defining characteristics were identified from the 66 care plans and grouped into general frequency categories of occurrence. The approaches most frequently identified on the Diversional Activity Deficit care plans were:

Encourage participation in recreational therapy activities

Praise involvement

Prompt resident to attend activities (if able to attend recreational therapy independently)

Assist resident to activities (if unable to attend recreational therapy independently)

Praise independent leisure activities (eg, reading, talking, crocheting, writing letters, visiting)

Encourage resident to view recreational therapy calendar and choose which groups to attend; schedule nap (or other ADL activities) accordingly

Promote one-to-one staff visits (nursing, recreational therapy, social services)

Encourage and praise resident to continue socializing with residents on the unit

Encourage resident to wear hearing aid and assist with adjustment as necessary

Use kind, firm approach and encourage resident to spend time out of room after meals

The focus of the one-to-one interactions and recreational therapy programming will be developed in greater detail as interventions for the diagnosis Diversional Activity Deficit. Bulechek and McCloskey (1985) suggest music therapy, reminiscence therapy, and support groups. Carpenito (1983) and Gettrust et al (1985) suggest a number of activities as shown in Table 25.4.

The interventions discussed in greater detail in the Nursing Interventions section of this chapter are reminiscence therapy, pet therapy, and music therapy. Other important interventions for this diagnosis include exercise therapy, relaxation exercise, art therapy and crafts, visita-tion, responsibility-inducing activities, residents as volunteers, and intergenerational programs.

CASE STUDY

Diversional Activity Deficit

Harold, an 80-year-old man, was admitted to the nursing home 3 years ago. His admission history included osteoarthritis, depression, and cystostomy secondary to prostatic cancer; additional current diagnoses include hiatal hernia, arteriosclerotic heart disease, congestive heart failure, peripheral vascular disease, and cardiomegaly post-CVA. He has several peripheral open areas. The social history revealed that he was a farmer and a widower for many years.

Harold can propel himself slowly in a wheelchair; he is dependent for most activities of daily living (ADLs). He is disoriented to time and place, and discussions with staff reveal he believes he is still living on his farm and his wife is alive. Preferring to stay in his room, Harold resists activity and involvement with staff or peers.

His nursing care plan includes the diagnosis Diversional Activity Deficit due to confusion. The defining characteristics include being confused and disoriented to time and place; verbalizing boredom; napping in the daytime; being unable to undertake previous leisure/work activities; resisting attendance at recreational therapy activities; frequently expressing negative attitudes; having no current leisure skills or independent hobbies; having minimal interaction with staff, peers, or visitors; spending

Table 25.4

Activities/Interventions Suggested by Previous Authors for Diversional Activity Deficit

CARPENITO (1983)	GETTRUST et al (1985)	RUBENFELD (1986)
Vary daily routine	Assess current and past hobbies/activities	Assess usual pattern of diversional activities
Include the individual in planning schedule for daily routine	Assist in selection and scheduling of an activity seen as imporant/valuable	Assess perception of ability to engage in usual diversional activities
Plan time for visitors	Praise efforts	Encourage to continue menaingful activities
Vary physical environment—light, flowers, pictures, bulletin boards; provide window	Suggested activities:	Encourage to identify personally meaningful activities
Provide reading materials, radio, TV, books, or tapes	Passive—radio, cassettes, reading (large print or talking books), television, pictures	Focus on the capabilities not the deficits
Plan a daily activity	End product—macrame, rug-hooking, knitting, painting	Orient to options such as recreational therapy
Use a volunteer for reading or helping with an activity	Active—modeling clay, exercising, ball toss, playing musical instrument	Support the individual in chosen activity; adapt environment as necessary
Encourage sharing of feelings and experiences	Group activities	Provide positive feedback
Help to work through feelings of anger and grief	Volunteer visiting	Evaluate perception of chosen activity and allow for change of plans if activity unsatisfactory
	Continue previous hobbies	
	Occupational therapy consult	
	Community organizations referral	

most of his time in his room alone; and watching television occasionally in his room.

NURSING INTERVENTIONS

Reminiscence Therapy

Purpose of Reminiscence Therapy The literature suggests that the purpose of reminiscence is to maintain self-esteem, to stimulate thinking, and to enhance and support the natural healing process of life review so that the client can find meaning, worth, and acceptance of what life has been (Ryden, 1981). Many times the terms *life review* and *reminiscence* are used interchangeably. Use of life review as a form of intervention with the elderly was first advocated by Butler (1963). Butler and Lewis (1977) propose that life review provides opportunities to resolve past conflicts, leads to a new understanding of life, and leads to feelings of accomplishment and of having tried to do one's best. However, reminiscence, or the recall of past events, is only a part of the developmental process termed *life review*. Reminiscence initiates and facilitates the internal life review and assists each individual in gaining self-acceptance and other positive outcomes (Molinari and Reichlin, 1984–1985; Sable, 1984).

Reminiscence is common after a loss. Hamner (1984) views reminiscence as an adaptive process representing a natural healing process whose purpose is to achieve a sense of closure. Viewing reminiscence as a healthy process and using it as therapeutic measure may enable the aged person to gain hope and security. Reminiscence may be used as an intervention to assist the aged, in spite of their losses, to maintain ego integrity through eliciting past and/or present successes.

The single greatest advantage of the use of this approach with the aged is its encouragement of active and spontaneous participation, which in turn promotes socialization and personal contact (Cook, 1984). The intervention is used frequently in groups and is often beneficial, as group members are able to share experiences with, empathize with, and offer support to one another (Sable, 1984). Reminiscence may be used as individual therapy to identify areas of past conflict and assist the elderly to achieve resolution, resolve regrets, work through fears of death, and provide substance for emotional and family legacies (King, 1982).

CASE STUDY

Reminiscence Intervention

Original interventions for Harold included one-to-one staff visits focused on reminiscence topics of farming. The music therapist gained Harold's participation in a music discussion group that focused on reminiscing about songs from the early 1920s to the present.

Two months after Harold's admission, his dog, Shelley, joined Harold in his room at the nursing home, and the staff assisted with feeding and walking. Although Harold's confusion was not alleviated, Shelley became an additional reality focus for interactions between Harold and staff and visitors. She provided the needed stimulation for more exercise for Harold, and she promoted a sense of responsibility in Harold because she needed his care, attention, and love.

Reminiscence Group Therapy Reminiscence therapy would be appropriate for use with clients having Diversional Activity Deficit etiologies of environmental lack of diversional activity (monotonous environment/ lack of stimulation); long-term hospitalization (confinement); frequent, lengthy treatments; lack of motivation with signs of depression, immobility, or inactivity (impaired mobility/decreased activity tolerance); lack of skills (knowledge/interest to perform an activity/hobby); impaired sensory functions; or social isolation.

Recent application of reminiscence has been in groups of confused elderly (Baker, 1985; Cook, 1984; Huber and Miller, 1984; Lesser and Lazarus, 1981); in both inpatient and outpatient group psychotherapy (King, 1982; Lesser and Lazarus, 1981); in group therapy for the regressed, fragile, rigidly defended psychotic elderly (Lesser and Lazarus, 1981); and in groups of depressed elderly (Huber and Miller, 1984; Sable, 1984). Most groups were not homogeneous regarding participant problem; most contained participants with various problems ranging from mild to severe depression, psychosis, mild to severe confusion, or memory loss.

Ebersole and Hess (1981) recommend group reminiscing for the cognitively impaired, the psychologically disturbed, and the depressed elderly. They recommend organizing the groups homogeneously based on the client problem. Group reminiscing for the cognitively impaired is recommended because the process of sharing may bring latent memories to the surface and connect missing links in memory chains.

Application of reminiscence group therapy is not limited to institutionalized elderly. It also has been used for groups in independent living arrangements (Hughston and Merriam, 1982; Perrotta and Meacham, 1981–1982) or groups of participants from a mixture of independent and institutional living arrangements (Huber and Miller, 1984; Parsons, 1984; Walker, 1984).

Planning the Group The number of participants, the length of time the group meets, the open or closed nature of the group, the topics of discussion, and the functional abilities of the participants can all vary according to the setting, the personal qualities of group members, and the preferences of group leaders (Cook, 1984). Generally groups are held one or two times per week, last from 45 minutes to over 1 hour, and are run for several weeks/months duration.

Although authors reviewed recommended that baseline assessments be completed for each member, measuring affect, attention span, concentration, orientation, and interpersonal skills prior to group initiation, none recommended specific tools and many pointed to the need for a comprehensive objective measurement tool assessing these areas.

Baker (1985) developed an evaluation tool to measure responses of individual participants in the reminiscence group she conducted.

Advance planning should include meeting time, dates, location, and topics. Baker (1985) assigned participant roles to specific group members, and the responsibility for those roles rotated from member to member each week. The group roles were welcoming chairperson; song leader; poetry leader; hostess; hostess's assistant; chair arranger; secretary; cleanup person.

The location for conducting the groups should be conducive to conversation but may vary depending on facilities and participant needs. Huber and Miller (1984) conducted most meetings in a lounge area; other meetings were held on a patio in the fresh air and warm sunshine or in a patient's room where the patient acted as a gracious hostess.

Topic Selection Sable (1984) suggests selecting group topics based on the life experiences recorded in resident histories in the resident clinical reocrds. Cook (1984) suggests a more flexible approach, with leaders initiating early discussion by seeking memories of childhood days and gradually progressing in chronologic order through adulthood. Both Sable and Cook emphasize the necessity of progressive chronologic discussion.

The group leaders may assume responsibility for topic selection and introduction at each session (Cook, 1984; Sable, 1984) or share that responsibility with participants. Initial group topics may be planned by leaders and expanded by participants (Huber and Miller, 1984). Discussion topics may be suggested at the end of group meetings to select the topic for the next meeting and assign roles for leadership of the next meeting (Baker, 1985). Results of Schafer's (1985) study indicate that it is important for participants to exert control over the nature of the program.

Music is a frequently cited effective cue that sparks spontaneous reminiscing. King (1982) points out that those participants with impaired hearing may be able to hear music better than speech because music is rhythmically patterned and potentially familiar.

Conducting the Group Participants should be reminded of the session approximately 30 minutes before it begins.

Those who require assistance should be escorted to the meeting place. Sable (1984) recommends beginning the group with a few minutes of sensory integrative activity such as balloon volleyball, parachute activities, olfactory stimulation tasks, or tactile stimulation. She cites increased group interaction following these activities.

Both Baker (1985) and King (1982) cite music as a particularly effective warm-up technique for the reminiscing group process. Baker began the group with music related to the discussion for the day, followed by exercises and relaxation techniques to prepare the mood for discussion. After the warm-up techniques, the topic for the discussion is introduced. Open-ended questions that invite participants to share with the group stories or experiences from their past are particularly effective. As discussion progresses it is important to reinforce reminiscing behavior to facilitate continued recall. Group members may experience positive or negative feelings brought about by their reminiscences. The leader should empathize with and acknowledge these feelings (Ryden, 1981).

Depressed individuals in the group may ruminate about past inadequacies or illnesses. The leader may interrupt a long recitation of painful events with other open-ended questions designed to refocus such individuals.

CASE STUDY

Reminiscence Therapy for Confused Elderly

A group of confused elderly nursing home residents were selected to participate in a 45-minute reminiscence group that was conducted weekly for 8 months (Cook, 1984). Changes were observed in the demeanors and in certain behaviors of the regular participants. The energy level, extent of confusion, and willingness or ability to participate varied from member to member and session to session. However, the group leaders noted gradual but steady changes on the part of all participants who attended with regularity. Members appeared more alert, the length of verbal contributions increased, and spontaneous addition of details increased. Humor and laughter were more frequently shared.

Signs of carryover effects into the day-to-day lives of some participants were noted. On two separate occasions, one member, whose attention was typically devoted exclusively to her plate, recognized others seated at adjacent tables in the dining room and identified them as members of the group. On several occasions, she and other members went to the meeting place unaccompanied. She began staying out of her room for longer periods and sometimes voluntarily joined other activities, all of which were new behaviors for her. The length of time the members spent socializing before and after the session dramatically increased. Several persons would continue to sit together—sometimes talking, sometimes not—for as long as half an hour.

The results of the experience with this reminiscence group suggest that this intervention is an effective treatment for Diversional Activity Deficit for institutionalized elderly who are isolated and confused. Participants reviewed some of their heritage, exercised cognitive and memory functions, and grew in self-esteem; they socialized while recalling past accomplishments and pleasant times. These behaviors carried over into day-to-day living, which continued to intervene in their diagnosis.

Music Therapy

Music is an aural stimulant that evokes physical and psychologic responses. Hennessey (1989) has been a leader in developing music therapy combined with reminiscence and exercises. Music provides for self-expression and allows individuals to communicate attitudes, feelings, and moods nonverbally, all of which can lead to an enhanced self-image. Musical activities often occur in groups and necessitate cooperation that fosters social interaction in addition to providing entertainment and recreation. For further information on the effects of music therapy, refer to Buckwalter et al, 1985.

Three principles of music therapy were identified from the early clinician work with music therapy: (1) the establishment or reestablishment of interpersonal relationships; (2) the bringing about of self-esteem through self-actualization; and (3) the use of the unique potential of rhythm to energize and bring order (Gaston, 1968).

The improvement in physical and mental functioning (Michael, 1976) is frequently cited as the purpose of music therapy programs designed for elderly populations in long-term care settings. Programs focusing on the use of music to facilitate exercise, reality orientation, social interaction, and reminiscence have been implemented (Olson, 1984; Palmer, 1983; Schwab et al, 1985).

Application of the Music Therapy Intervention

This intervention would be appropriate for use with clients having Diversional Activity Deficit etiologies of monotonous environment/lack of stimulation, confinement, frequent/lengthy treatments, lack of motivation with signs of depression, impaired mobility/decreased activity tolerance, lack of skills (knowledge/interest) to perform an activity/hobby, impaired sensory functions, or social isolation.

Music therapy is an effective intervention that can be targeted for individual elderly residents or groups of residents. As a single resident activity it may be specifically designed to address Diversional Activity Deficit and also to alleviate a variety of conditions such as pain, anxiety, depression, and nausea/vomiting or to enhance other conditions such as self-expression, self-esteem, and relaxation (Buckwalter et al, 1985; Frank, 1985). Audiocassette players with lightweight headphones make it possible to design specific music tapes to meet individual needs and preferences.

Although most authors commented about music selection that coincided with ethnic, cultural, and religious heritage (Kartman, 1977, 1984; Needler and Baer, 1982; Palmer, 1983), assessment tools were not discussed. The Modified Hartsock Music Preference Questionnaire and the Questionnaire to Evaluate the Effects of Music Therapy by Hartsock are printed in entirety and discussed by Buckwalter et al (1985).

Group Selection

Music therapy can be an effective intervention for a wide range of groups of elderly, varying from severely cognitively impaired elderly (Baker, 1985; Heaman and Moore, 1982; Kartman, 1977, 1984; Needler and Baer, 1982; Palmer, 1983) to functionally and psychologically independent elderly (Ebersole and Hess, 1985; Kartman, 1984; Palmer, 1983). Hamilton (1985), following her comparative study of music and pet therapy interventions, recommends cognitively homogeneous group selection. Kartman (1977) used this same principle when grouping residents for two music therapy groups to facilitate group interaction about the music selections. Reminiscence frequently is used in combination with music therapy. Ebersole and Hess (1985) recommend cognitively homogeneous groups to make reminiscence groups most effective.

Kartman (1977) also used ethnic and cultural similarities to facilitate group effectiveness. The similarities of cognitive impairment, culture, and ethnic background provided direction for music selection, and the group discussion was sparked by the selection. Improved ability to relate to others and increased socialization and social awareness are cited as positive outcomes from these groups.

Using Music Therapy With Other Therapies

Music therapy frequently is combined with other therapeutic approaches such as exercise, remotivation, reality orientation, reminiscence, or pet therapy. Residents who have often resisted exercise to increase tolerance, build strength, and enlarge range of motion may readily join in with maracas as a member of a mariachi band. They accomplish those same exercise goals and *enjoy* the experience (Palmer, 1983). Flag activities, clapping, kicking, and stamping are made enjoyable through music while meeting exercise goals. March music and old folk songs are used in the "Armchair Aerobics" class at one Wisconsin nursing home (Palmer, 1985) to facilitate the exercise effectiveness.

Needler and Baer (1982;503) combined movement, music, and remotivation within a group structure for regressed elderly. Physically, all required total care. Needler and Baer summarized the effectiveness of their group:

The combination of music, movement, and remotivation within a group structure maintains and/or re-establishes physical and mental alertness, expands capabilities, stimulates socializing interactions, and reintroduces awareness of the outside world. Residents relax, laugh, communicate feelings and thoughts, remember, create, develop friendships and celebrate together.

Baker's (1985) reminiscence therapy groups began with a welcome, which was followed by songs related to the day's discussion. The songs were valuable in stimulating memories and facilitating discussion. Palmer (1983) used the same combination of techniques. Residents were encouraged to recall not only the words to songs from their youth, but also when they had learned the songs and other events associated with the songs. This recall stimulated mental function and interaction with their peers as they shared similar experiences. The therapist's role was to promote social interaction and to help residents put responses into perspective with reality.

Reality orientation and remotivation interventions have been combined with music therapy. Discussions of current events and news of the day are facilitated by appropriate choices of related music (Kartman, 1984). The dimension of pet therapy was added to the above combination when a nursing home conducted a pet show (Heaman and Moore, 1982). Songs related to the animals were played as residents gathered and dispersed for the program. Questions prior to and following the program focused on the event and assisted to draw the residents toward reality.

Conducting the Group Music can be used in large recreational groups (Ebersole and Hess, 1985) or in large groups with a therapeutic focus such as Heaman and Moore's (1982) pet show conducted for 65 residents. Small groups of 4 to 12 (Needler and Baer, 1982) or 5 to 8 residents (Kartman, 1977) were used to facilitate discussion, individual remotivation, reality orientation, or reminiscence with individual residents.

The small group session follows a basic format (Needler and Baer, 1982):

1. Residents are greeted and made comfortable.
2. A topic is introduced.
3. The topic is developed through discussion, visual aids, music, movement, or other creative modalities.
4. The meeting concludes with a mutual sense of appreciation.

Music is an excellent tool to facilitate topic introduction and development. For example, "Yankee Doodle" and other patriotic songs lead into national holiday (eg, the Fourth of J4uly) discussions. Needler and Baer (1982) describe the excellent response to patriotic music. Residents readily sing, clap, tap, march in place, and stand, if able.

As the topic is developed, other aspects of the topic are expanded, and their effects on people are explored (Needler and Baer, 1982). The group leader must be flexible as the music triggers related memories, thoughts, and feelings, which are discussed. Discussions from one session may spark topics for the next or subsequent sessions.

Discussion groups that use music, reminiscence, remotivation, and reality orientation are generally 45 to 60 minutes in length. They may be conducted daily, two or three times per week, or weekly, depending on the objectives of the therapy (Ebersole and Hess, 1985; Hamilton, 1985; Kartman, 1977, 1984; Needler and Baer, 1982).

Direction for Future Research Music therapy as a specific single intervention for the geriatric long-term care population needs further attention. Anecdotal case reports of the impact of music group therapy compose the bulk of the geriatric music therapy literature base. A confounding variable is the frequent combination of music with other therapeutic approaches. Evaluation of the effectiveness of music therapy separate from and in combination with other clusters of therapeutic approaches is needed.

CASE STUDY

Music Therapy Intervention

Anna is a 101-year-old tiny Polish woman who was admitted to the nursing home 2 years ago. Medical diagnoses include irreversible dementia (Alzheimer's disease), severe hearing deficit, blindness, and status post right cataract surgery. Nursing diagnoses include Self-Care Deficit: Bathing/Hygiene, Level II, related to uncompensated cognitive perceptual impairment; Potential for Injury related to risk factors of organic brain syndrome, confusion, wandering, blindness; Impaired Physical Mobility, Level II, related to decreased strength and endurance; Altered Thought Process related to cognitive impairment; and Diversional Activity Deficit related to sensory impairment and social isolation. She speaks Polish with some English phrases and understands some English, but a severe hearing deficit makes understanding the communication from the staff very difficult for her.

Although Anna can dress and undress herself, she needs much supervision with hygiene and toileting. She can use a walker with help and can feed herself with orientation to her tray. The nursing staff described Anna as unable to communicate. One of her nurses explained, "Sometimes I can sense that Anna has pain and I will take my hand and touch parts of her body. She will then take my hand and put it on the part that seems to hurt." She does talk with her grandson, who visits several times a week and understands Polish. She prefers to spend most of her time in her room lying on her bed and is frequently resistive when staff intervene or encourage her to spend some time in the dayroom.

Because of Anna's sensory deficit, participation in discussion groups, games, crafts, or even one-to-one attention proved unsuccessful. The music therapist decided to try the medium of music. As she placed her guitar on Anna's knees and began strumming, Anna's hands gently touched the guitar. Anna seemed to sense the vibrations, and her face broke into a large smile.

The one-to-one sessions continued over many months, and gradually Anna became less resistive. Now, when the music therapist approaches Anna, she gently touches Anna's arm and speaks into her right ear, "Musica." Anna takes the music therapist's hand and follows her to her room, where she can touch the guitar while the therapist plays. Anna sings Polish songs that seem to have apparent meaning for her and fit the vibrations of the guitar. At times Anna taps the same rhythm the therapist plays on the guitar. Two years ago Anna refused all therapeutic activities. Now, however, other staff members have successfully included Anna in other music groups.

Pet Therapy

Cusack and Smith (1984) describe the results of pet therapy as extraordinary: Animals provide individuals with distinct physiologic, psychologic, and social benefits that keep them healthy and happy. Pets of all kinds can play an important role in helping maintain emotional stability; a pet may be the only remaining link with reality for some people (Frank, 1984). Pets can be the catalyst for engaging withdrawn residents. Touching animals stimulates conversation and may create a bridge to the real world (Heaman and Moore, 1982). Visiting animals often stirs up fond memories and prompts residents to talk of pets they had in the past (Silverman, 1985). Pets can provide the focal point to stimulate effective reminiscence discussions with nursing home residents.

Pets as companions provide constant, unquestioning sources of comfort and affection, enrich feelings of self-esteem, act as facilitators for interpersonal relations, provide tactile reassurance, relieve feelings of despondency and depression, and stimulate patient responsiveness. More regressed patients seem to incorporate the animals' presence into their own highly personalized reality and are able to use it as a bridge to external reality (Brickel, 1980–1981).

For those nursing home residents who can participate in the care of the pet, having a pet can help satisfy the need to nurture (Erickson, 1985). Caring for a pet fosters a sense of responsibility, strengthens self-esteem, stimulates exercise, and offers the social benefit of stimulating conversation among residents, staff, and visitors. Pet therapy facilitates the alleviation of loneliness, depression, helplessness, and social withdrawal (Andrysco, 1982).

Application of the Pet Therapy Intervention Pet therapy would be appropriate for use with clients having Diversional Activity Deficit etiologies of monotonous environment/lack of stimulation, confinement, lack of motivation with signs of depression, impaired mobility, impaired sensory functions, or social isolation. Pet therapy can be implemented in a variety of ways, depending on the staff's commitment to the value of the intervention.

Visitation Programs Visitation programs may be organized by community organizations such as humane societies, dog clubs, churches, or other volunteer groups or by individuals willing to sponsor the program. Cusack and Smith (1984) offer some practical guidelines for such interested sponsors:

1. Animals should be well-groomed, clean, and healthy.
2. The pet should have some training and socialization prior to participation in a pet visitation program.
3. The pet's temperament should be sociable, friendly, and relaxed.
4. If animals other than cats and dogs are considered for the program, discussions with the facility should be handled in advance to assure that some residents do not have an aversion to these animals.
5. Sponsors should be punctual, follow institution rules and regulations, and introduce themselves to the staff on duty.
6. Elimination functions should be accomplished prior to entrance to the facility. If nursing home grounds are used for this function, the pet owners should have plastic bags to assist with cleanup.
7. When approaching residents, sponsors should always ask if they like the type of animal accompanying them. For example, "Hello, my name is Mary, and this is Topper. Do you like dogs? Would you like to pet the dog?" would be appropriate.

Pet Shows Volunteer organizations may be a resource for organizing pet shows (Heaman and Moore, 1982). The pet show provides subject matter for reality orientation questions such as, "What's going to happen today?" and "Where will the pet show be held?" After the event, asking what happened today, what animals were there, and so forth reinforces the therapeutic process facilitated by the pet show. The animals stimulate conversation and create a bridge to the real world. Residents share experiences from their past and appreciate each other's experiences.

Resident Pets Resident pets provide the opportunity for residents to develop a long-term human–animal bond and reap the benefits of that relationship. Nurses are the critical link in long-term care to facilitate the success of a resident pet therapy program. The resident benefits must be understood and promoted to assist nursing staff to accept some responsibilities in the care and management of the pet.

Suggested resident pets include dogs, cats, birds, rabbits, small caged rodents, or fish (Cusack and Smith, 1984; Erickson, 1985). Caged animals frequently are selected because they require minimal care, and responsibilities for care are easier to define/assign. Companionship benefits of these pets have been described as effective. Dogs, however, are most popular because of their clear and uncritical affection, tactile comfort, perpetual child-like dependence, and burglar alarm function (Erickson, 1985).

If a facility is committed to having a dog in residence, Cusack and Smith (1984) describe some practical factors to be considered:

1. *Size.* If the residents are primarily infirm and immobile, a smaller dog that can sleep comfortably on a lap or in bed is most suitable. If there are residents who are mobile and can participate in the care of the dog, a larger dog might provide more opportunity for play and exercise.
2. *Grooming.* Generally, dogs with short fur require less grooming.
3. *Age.* In most cases, a dog who is housebroken and has completed the rudiments of basic obedience training is recommended. Additionally, after 9 to 10 months, personality traits are defined, so selection for appropriate temperament is easier.
4. *Health.* The animal should be healthy and free from disease. Advance planning for routine veterinarian care is essential. The dog should be neutered, ideally before being brought into the institution.
5. *Temperament.* This is the single most important criterion for selecting an in-residence dog. The dog should be friendly, outgoing, obedient, well-mannered, alert, and calm; it should not be aggressive, high strung, boisterous, unruly, noisy, or fearful. The dog must acclimate to wheelchairs, walkers, and individuals with impaired motor coordination.
6. *Housing.*
   a. If housing the dog outdoors, the area should be fenced with appropriate protection for the animal but located so residents can watch him. Walking the dog two or three times per day is still essential for exercise. Regular cleanup of the yard is required.
   b. A variety of locations can be used to house the pet inside the institution. His "home" may be the activity room, an office, a patient's room, sunroom, and so on. Requirements that the pet not be allowed in areas where residents eat or where food is prepared must be met.

7. *Feeding.* A routine should be established so the dog is not overfed by many residents offering treats. Reponsibilities for feeding and watering should be very clear to residents and staff.

Resident pets in elderly independent housing could provide the same benefits reaped by residents in long-term care who are involved with pet therapy. In his study about pet ownership Lawton et al (1984) expected to find that elderly persons in independent housing were likely to own a pet. He found the contrary, however. Residents cited low income, urban living, and housing prohibitions on pets as reasons for living without pets. Lawton suggests that social pressure be applied to remove these barriers to pet ownership for the elderly in independent living arrangements.

CASE STUDY

Pet Therapy Intervention

After an initial disappointment with a resident pet at a 328-bed nursing home in Elkhorn, Wisconsin, a committed nucleus of staff on one unit decided to try another dog. This time a day-shift employee brought a mixed black labrador puppy to work several times per week. The residents thoroughly enjoyed holding and watching the puppy and looked forward with anticipation to her coming each day. Dorothy, a severely handicapped resident with little upper body movement who was confined to an electric wheelchair, managed to hold the puppy for hours. A highlight of her day was taking the puppy outside to the courtyard area to play.

As the puppy grew, so did the attachment of the residents and staff. A contest was held to select the puppy's name; "Missy" was finally selected. To facilitate Missy's training, the day-shift employee continued to take the dog home each night until housetraining was completed. The recreational therapy staff established a noon hour routine of a long leash walk to promote exercise and leash training. As training was accomplished, planning for Missy to begin staying at the agency 24 hours per day was begun. Adjustments in afternoon and night-shift schedules and routines were made. Along the way, problems were resolved because residents and staff were committed to making this attempt for a resident pet therapy dog successful.

Missy selected a location in one resident's room for sleeping, another favorite resident for walking, and other residents for playing. She became very protective of her residents, their families, and her staff. Missy could readily differentiate between them and residents/staff/visitors from other units. At the appropriate time she was neutered. Missy became an integral part of the unit and a focal point in many residents' lives.

SUMMARY

This chapter discussed the potential incidence of the nursing diagnosis Diversional Activity Deficit in the dependent elderly. The multiple factors that can impede involvement of the elderly in diversional activities and the potential negative effects were identified. The need for empirical testing of this diagnosis was addressed.

The nurse in long-term care settings has a wide variety of interventions to use in achieving positive outcomes for Diversional Activity Deficit. The interventions discussed in detail were reminiscence therapy, music therapy, and pet therapy. A listing of the instruments that can be used to evaluate outcomes is included.

References

Allen J: Exercise Program. Pages 198–219 in: *Nursing Interventions: Treatments for Nursing Diagnoses.* Bulechek G, McCloskey J (editors). Saunders, 1985.

Andrysco R: A study of ethologic and therapeutic factors of pet-facilitated therapy in a retirement nursing community. *Dissertation Abstracts Internat* (July) 1982;43(1B):290.

Atterbury C, Sorg J, Larson M: Aerobic dancing in a long-term care facility. *Physical Occup Ther Geriat* (Spring) 1983; 71–73.

Baker N: Reminiscing in group therapy for self-worth. *J Gerontol Nurs* (July) 1985; 11:21–24.

Baun M et al: Physiological effects of human companion animal bonding. *Nurs Res* (May/June) 1984; 33:126–129.

Beck P: Two successful interventions in nursing homes: The therapeutic effects of cognitive activity. *Gerontologist* 1982; 22:378–383.

Brennan P, Steinberg L: Is reminiscence adaptive? Relations among social activity level, reminiscence, and morale. *Internat J Aging Human Develop* 1983-1984; 18:99–110.

Brickel C: A review of the roles of pet animals in psychotherapy and with the elderly. *Internat J Aging Human Develop* 1980–1981; 12:119–128.

Brink R, Curran M: Geriatric depression scale reliability: Order, examiner and reminiscence effects. *Clin Gerontol* 1985; 3:57–60.

Buckwalter K, Hartsock J, Gaffney J: Pages 58–74 in: *Nursing Interventions: Treatments for Nursing Diagnoses.* Bulechek G, McCloskey J (editors). Saunders, 1985.

Bulechek G, McCloskey J: *Nursing Interventions: Treatments for Nursing Diagnoses.* Saunders, 1985.

Burbank PM: Psychosocial theories of aging: A critical evaluation. *ANS* (Oct) 1986; 9:73–86.

Butler R: The life review: An interpretation of reminiscence in the aged. *Psychiatry* 1963; 26:65–76.

Butler R, Lewis M: *Aging and Mental Health,* 3d ed. Mosby, 1977.

Carpenito L: *Nursing Diagnosis: Application to Clinical Practice.* Lippincott, 1983.

Carroll-Johnson R (editor) : *Classification of Nursing Diagnoses: Proceedings of the Eighth Conference.* Lippincott, 1989.

Cook J: Reminiscing: How it can help confused nursing home residents. *J Contemp Soc Work* 1984; 90–93.

Cummings E, Henry WE: *Growing Old.* Basic Books, 1961.

Cusack D, Smith E: *Pets and the Elderly—The Therapeutic Bond.* Hawthorne Press, 1984.

Ebersole P, Hess P:*Toward Healthy Aging Human Needs and Nursing Response.* Mosby, 1981.

Erickson R: Companion animals and the elderly. *Geriatr Nurs* (Mar/Apr) 1985; 92–96.

Fischer K, Schwartz M: Social isolation. Pages 1935–1941 in: *Clinical Nursing.* Thompson J et al (editors). Mosby, 1986.

Frank J: The effects of music therapy and guided visual imagery on chemotherapy induced nausea and vomiting. *Oncol Nurs Forum* (Sept/Oct) 1985; 12:47–52.

Frank S: The touch of love. *J Gerontol Nurs* (Jan) 1984; 10:29–31,35.

Gaston E (editor): *Music in Therapy.* MacMillan, 1968.

Gettrust K, Ryan S, Engelman D: *Applied Nursing Diagnosis: Guides for Comprehensive Care Planning,* Wiley, 1985.

Goldberg W, Fitzpatrick J: Movement therapy with the aged. *Nurs Res* (Nov/Dec) 1980; 29:339–346.

Gordon M: *Manual of Nursing Diagnosis.* McGraw-Hill, 1985.

Gordon M: *Nursing Diagnosis: Process and Application.* McGraw-Hill, 1982.

Gordon N et al: Assessment of a geriatric exercise programme using ambulatory electrocardiography. *SA Med J* (July) 1983; 64:169–172.

Greene V, Monahan D: The impact of visitation on patient well-being in nursing homes. *Gerontologist* 1982; 22:418–423.

Hamilton G: The roles of pet and music therapy in providing sensory stimulation to institutionalized elderly persons. *Dissertation Abstracts Internat* (Oct) 1985; 46:(4A):1059–1060.

Hamner M: Insight, reminiscence, denial, projections: Coping mechanism of the aged. *J Gerontol Nurs* (Feb) 1984; 10:66–68, 81.

Havighurst FJ, Albrecht R: *Older People.* Longmans Green, 1953.

Heaman D, Moore J: A pet show for remotivation. *Geriatr Nurs* (Mar/Apr) 1982; 108–110.

Hennessey M: Music therapy. Pages 198–210 in: *Working With the Elderly: Group Process and Techniques,* 2d ed. Burnside I (editor). Jones and Bartlett, 1989.

Huber K, Miller P: Reminiscence with the elderly—DO IT! *Geriatr Nurs* (Mar/Apr) 1984; 84–87.

Hughston G, Merriam S: Reminiscence: A nonformal technique for improving cognitive functioning in the aged. *Internat J Aging Human Develop* 1982; 15:139–149.

Johnson-Pawlson J, Koshes R: Exercise is for everyone. *Geriatr Nurs* (Nov/Dec) 1985; 322–325.

Kartman L: The use of music as a program tool with regressed geriatric patients. *J Gerontol Nurs* (July/Aug) 1977; 3:38–42.

Kartman L: Music hath charms . . . *Gerontol Nurs* (June) 1984; 10:20–24.

Kaye V: An innovative treatment modality for elderly residents in a nursing home. *Clin Gerontol* 1985; 3:45–51.

Kim M, McFarland G, McLane A: *Classification of Nursing Diagnoses: Proceedings of the Fifth National Conference.* Mosby, 1984.

King K: Reminiscing psychotherapy with aging people. *JPNMHS* (Feb) 1982; 20:21–25.

Lawton M, Moss M, Moles E: Pet ownership: A research note. *Gerontologist* 1984; 24:208–210.

Lesser J, Lazarus C: Reminiscence group therapy with psychotic geriatric impatients. *Gerontologist* 1981; 21:291–296.

McCormack D, Whitehead A: The effect of providing recreational activities on the engagement level of long-stay geriatric patients. *Age Ageing* 1981; 10:287–291.

Michael D: *Music Therapy: An Introduction to Therapy and Special Education Through Music.* Charles C. Thomas, 1976.

Molinari V, Reichlin R: Life review reminiscence in the elderly: A review of the literature. *Internat J Aging Human Develop* 1984–1985; 20:81–92.

Needler W, Baer M: Movement, music and remotivation with the regressed elderly. *J Gerontol Nurs* (Sept) 1982; 8:497–503.

Neugarten BL, Havighurst RJ, Tobin SS: Personality and patterns of aging. Pages 173–177 in: *Middle Age and Aging.* Neugarten BL (editor). University of Chicago Press, 1968.

North American Nursing Diagnosis Association (NANDA): *Diagnosis Review Committee. Guidelines for General Assembly, "Review and Comment" of Proposed Diagnoses.* NANDA Biennial meeting, March, 1986, St. Louis, Mo.

Olson B: Player piano music as therapy for the elderly. *J Music Ther* 1984; 21:35–45.

Palmer M: Music therapy in a comprehensive program of treatment and rehabilitation for the geriatric resident. *Activities, Adaptation and Aging* 1983; 3:53–59.

Palmer M: Clinical news, gerontological nursing: Sitting Fit. *Am J Nurs* (Mar) 1985; 236, 242.

Parent C, Whall A: Are physical activity, self-esteem, and depression related? *J Gerontol Nurs* (Sept) 1984; 10:8–10.

Parsons W: Reminiscence group therapy with older persons: A field experiment. *Dissertation Abstracts Internat* (Oct) 1984; 45(4A):1040–1041.

Perrotta P, Meacham J: Can a reminiscing intervention alter depression and self-esteem? *Internat J Human Develop* 1981–1982; 14:23–30.

Rantz M: Unpublished data of Diversional Activity Deficit care plans prepared for geriatric patients from 1983 to 1986 in a 328-bed midwestern long-term care facility. Elkhorn, WI, 1986a.

Rantz M: Unpublished data of Social Isolation care plans prepared for geriatric patients from 1983 to 1986 in a 328-bed midwestern long-term care facility. Elkhorn, WI, 1986b.

Robb S, Stegman C: Companion animals and elderly people: A challenge for evaluators of social support. *Gerontologist* 1983; 23:277–282.

Robb S, Boyd M, Pristash C: A wine bottle, plant and puppy: catalysts for social behavior. *J Gerontol Nurs* 1980; 6:721–728.

Rocke L: Adaptive fitness course for nursing homes, institutions, and homes for the aged. *Nurs Homes* (Nov/Dec) 1984: 41–43.

Rubenfeld M: Diversional Activity Deficit. Pages 2095–2099 in: *Clinical Nursing.* Thompson J et al (editors). Mosby, 1986.

Ryden M: Nursing intervention in support of reminiscence. *J Gerontol Nurs* (Aug) 1981; 7:461–463.

Sable L: Life review therapy: An occupational therapy treatment technique with geriatric clients. *Physical Occup Ther Geriatr* 1984; 3:49–54.

Schafer D: Reminiscence groups and the institutionalized elderly: An experiment. *Dissertation Abstracts Internat* (Oct) 1985; 46(4A):1060.

Schuster B: The effect of music listening on blood pressure fluctuations in adult hemodialysis patients. *J Music Ther* 1985; 22:146–153.

Schwab M, Rader J, Doan J: Relieving the anxiety and fear in dementia. *J Gerontol Nurs* (May) 1985; 11:8–15.

Silverman F: Dogs and the elderly: The perfect prescription for companionship. *Nurs Homes* (Jan/Feb) 1985; 1:33–34.

Walker L: The relationships between reminiscing, health state, physical functioning, and depression in older adults. *Dissertation Abstracts Internat* (Nov) 1984; 45(5B):1432.

Yesavage J: Relaxation and memory training in 39 elderly patients. *Am J Psychiatry* (June) 1984; 778–781.

V

Sleep–Rest Pattern

MERIDEAN MAAS, PhD, RN, FAAN
KATHLEEN BUCKWALTER, PhD, RN, FAAN

Overview

SLEEP DISTURBANCES ARE AMONG THE CHIEF complaints of the elderly. In Chapter 27 on Sleep Pattern Disturbance, Hammer explores the dimensions of normal sleep changes associated with the aging process, and the deleterious effects of medications and institutional routines (eg, vital signs every 4 hours) on healthy sleep patterns. The significance of daytime drowsiness is further examined. Numerous factors, including medical conditions, anxiety and depression, territorial affronts, boredom, and fatigue, are discussed as potential etiologies for this diagnosis that are amenable to nursing interventions. Hammer argues that specificity concerning the type of sleep disturbance is essential for the most appropriate nursing intervention to be initiated and evaluated. In Chapter 27 she describes several such interventions, including environmental manipulation, relaxation techniques, and therapeutic touch.

26

Normal Changes With Aging

DONNA BUNTEN, MA, RN

MARY A. HARDY, PhD, RN, C

Definition:

The sleep–rest pattern describes patterns of sleep, rest, and relaxation.

RESEARCH DOCUMENTS THAT CHANGES IN SLEEP OCcur with aging. It is necessary for nurses and other health professionals to have an understanding of normal sleep pattern changes of the elderly before they can identify sleep pattern disturbances.

Normal changes associated with aging that can be identified through electroencephalogram (EEG) tracing include the proportion of rapid eye movement (REM) and non-rapid eye movement (NREM) (stages 1, 2, 3, and 4) sleep time (Colling, 1983; Mendelson, 1984; Miller and Bartus, 1982; Reynolds et al, 1985). (See Chapter 27 for further discussion of the sleep stages.) Researchers have found that total sleep time and the proportion of REM to NREM sleep remain constant from ages 20 to 60. The average length of sleep time decreases to 6 hours by age 70 as compared to the 7.5 hours averaged in earlier adulthood or the 14-hour sleep pattern in infancy (Long, 1987). The sleep time itself changes in character, showing a progressive decrease with aging in stages 3 and 4 sleep throughout adulthood, with the older person experiencing almost no stage 4 or REM sleep (Bahr, 1983; Clapin-French, 1986). That is, REM sleep tends to occur in the same number of episodes, but those episodes are of shorter duration (Miles and Dement, 1980).

Sleep efficiency also declines with advancing age. As early as age 40, nocturnal awakenings become more frequent, and the amount of time spent in bed increases. Therefore, more time is needed in bed to get the restorative sleep that a younger adult can achieve in less time. Older persons may complain that it takes them a longer period of time to fall asleep after getting into bed. This is seen as a normal age-related change in sleeping. These changes markedly increase total waking time; the elderly may nap during the day in an attempt to increase total sleep time (Clapin-French, 1986).

Another change is circadian asynchrony. The sleep of the elderly is often fragmented by awakenings, which in turn are fragmented by periods of drowsiness or sleep. Thus the overall circadian cycle of sleeping and waking loses some of its strength. This may become a problem for some elderly persons because of awakening from pain, nocturia, or institutional regimens and routines. Hayter (1983) found that after the age of 75 there is a marked increase in time spent in bed, including or excluding naptimes, the number of naps taken, the length of time napping, the number of nighttime awakenings, and the amount of variability in sleeping behaviors in the frail elderly. Miller and Bartus (1982:283) concluded that the occurrence of "changes in sleep, cognitive function and response to medications in old age may all be more strongly linked to the asynchrony of biological cycles than we presently suspect."

The combined changes in sleep patterns associated with aging mean that the elderly may require more total time in bed to gain enough restorative sleep or quality sleep. If that time in bed is frequently disturbed, the elderly person will require even more time in bed or will be chronically sleep deprived. Because of their overall health status, the elderly often lack the physical and mental activity/exercise needed to induce quality sleep (Agate, 1986). Other physiologic and psychosocial conditions such as pain and anxiety that may be contributing factors to disturbed sleep patterns in persons of all ages may compound the concern the elderly have over significantly changing sleep patterns.

References

Agate J: Common symptoms and complaints. In: *Clinical Geriatric, III.* Rossman I (editor). Lippincott, 1986.

Bahr R: Sleep-wake patterns in the aged. *J Gerontol Nurs* 1983; 9:534–540.

Clapin-French E: Sleep patterns of aged persons in long-term care facilities. *J Adv Nurs* 1986; 11:57–66.

Colling J: Sleep disturbances in aging: A theoretic and empiric analysis. *ANS* 1983; 6:36–44.

Hayter J: Sleep behaviors of older persons. *Nurs Res* 1983; 32:242–246.

Long ME: What is this thing called sleep? *Nat Geograph* 1987; 172:787–821.

Mendelson W: Sleep after forty. *Am Fam Physician* 1984; 29(1): 135–139.

Miles L, Dement W: Sleep and aging. *Sleep* 1980; 3(2):119–202.

Miller N, Bartus R: Sleep, sleep pathology, and psychopathology in later life: A new research frontier. *Neurobiol Aging* 1982; 3:283–286.

Reynolds C et al: Sleep of healthy seniors: A revisit. *Sleep* 1985; 8(1):20–29.

27

Sleep Pattern Disturbance

Barbara Hammer, MA, RN, C

Sleep is important to well-being and is generally accepted as one of the basic human needs necessary for survival. Sleep serves to rest and restore the body (Ebersole and Hess, 1981; Gambert and Duthie, 1981; Gress et al, 1981; Mitchell, 1973; Nightingale, 1859). When a person receives an inadequate amount and/or quality of sleep, his or her total well-being suffers (Kleitman, 1939; Oswald, 1962; Rutenfranz, 1981; Webb, 1975). This becomes significant to the elderly, as sleep pattern disturbances are among their most frequent complaints (Hayter, 1983).

Nightingale (1859;25), in her *Notes on Nursing*, emphasized the importance of adequate sleep and rest for any individual.

Never to allow a patient to be waked, intentionally or accidentally, is a "sine qua non" of all good nursing. If he is roused out of his first sleep, he is almost certain to have no more sleep. It is a curious but quite intelligible fact that, if a patient is waked after a few hours instead of a few minutes sleep, he is much more likely to sleep again.

NORMAL SLEEP

Despite the fact that sleep is a universal occurrence for all individuals and affects total health and well-being, sleep has yet to be clearly defined. No matter what definition is used, all descriptions of sleep agree that one necessary criterion of sleep is its reversibility; that is, a person who is asleep can be aroused (Kleitman, 1939; Miles and Dement, 1980).

Sleep is controlled by the brain stem and is composed of cycles lasting approximately 85 to 95 minutes, varying from 45 to 60 minutes in the neonate and up to 120 minutes in adults (Kleitman, 1939). The average adult has approximately four to six of these cycles nightly, for a total of about 7 1/2 hours of sleep daily (Kleitman, 1939; Miles and Dement, 1980; Oswald, 1962; Webb, 1968).

The first part of the sleep cycle, which occupies approximately 75% to 80% of the total sleep time, is called slow-wave sleep (SWS) or non-rapid eye movement (NREM) sleep. This NREM sleep is composed of four stages, known as stages 1 through 4. A fifth stage is referred to as rapid eye movement (REM) sleep and occupies the remaining 20% to 25% of total sleep time.

Twenty to 30 minutes elapse between initially falling asleep and progressing to NREM stage 4 sleep. During this time, the physiologic signs, such as blood pressure and pulse, begin to slow or decrease, and muscle tone decreases. The electroencephalogram (EEG) tracing becomes slower and more rounded as the person enters into deeper stages of sleep, until at stage 4, the tracing appears as very large, slow waves. At this point, the process begins to reverse: The sleep goes from stage 4 to stage 3, stage 2, sometimes stage 1, and then enters the fifth stage of sleep, REM sleep, the state of deep sleep that has the most restorative value.

In addition to rapid eye movements, REM sleep is characterized by an increase in brain temperature and activity, irregular respirations, occasional sleep talking, an increase in minute muscle activity, and dreams or nightmares (Brill and Kilts, 1980). The EEG tracing again becomes quite varied and active, not unlike that of waking.

With the end of REM sleep, approximately 10 to 20 minutes, one sleep cycle has been completed. The next cycle begins with entry into NREM stage 2. As the night continues, the character of the sleep cycle changes so that the length of NREM sleep periods decreases while REM periods increase in length. The last one or two sleep cycles may not contain any stage 3 or stage 4 NREM sleep (Berger, 1969).

Changes in sleep patterns occur with aging. See Chapter 26 for a discussion of these changes.

SIGNIFICANCE FOR THE ELDERLY

There are no set requirements of sleep for any one individual, although the elderly may require 6 to 7 hours per day. No one sleep pattern appears to be the most beneficial to the elderly (eg, 6 hours of uninterrupted sleep or 6 hours with 2 hours of daytime naps). The amount of sleep needed varies according to each elderly person's own social and physiologic clocks (Schrimer, 1983). However, at least three sleep cycles (or 4 1/2 hours) of uninterrupted sleep a night should be obtained to avoid suffering from chronic sleep deprivation.

In a study of 180 nursing home residents (Cohen et al, 1983) in which both the residents and the nurses rated quality of sleep, it was found that nurses' ratings did not discriminate sleep problems and correlated poorly with the residents' own ratings. This is a significant finding because nurses may be administering hypnotic medications for sleep deficits in the elderly based on invalid data. Long-acting benzodiazepines, such as flurazepam (Dalmane), may induce confusion, disorientation, or daytime sleepiness, or may affect breathing and its control during sleep (Guillenimault and Silvestri, 1982).

Consequences of Chronic Sleep Deprivation

Because of stereotypes that the elderly sleep a lot of the time, daytime sleepiness is often overlooked as a symptom of sleep disturbance. When an elderly person is chronically deprived of uninterrupted sleep cycles, for whatever reason, the consequences become noticeable but frequently are not identified as a symptom of sleep disturbance.

The elderly person who is awakened every 2 hours throughout the night for turning and incontinency checks frequently will be unable to feed or dress himself or herself or perform other activities of daily living (ADLs) the following morning. This person may be unable to function because of chronic sleep deprivation.

Daytime symptoms thought to be part of the aging process may be signs or symptoms exhibited secondary to sleep deprivation. These symptoms include "loss of ability to perform highly skilled tasks in a rapid fashion, to resist fatigue, to maintain physical stamina, to unlearn or discard old techniques, and to apply the rapid judgment needed in changing and emergency situations" (Bahr, 1983).

Nurses need to be aware of the implications of daytime sleepiness and reassess the elderly individual's routine, such as turning or incontinence checks. Rescheduling of the morning routine to later in the day may allow the elderly person to be more alert and able to participate in activities. These are interventions nursing can and should do independently to help elderly persons obtain an adequate amount of quality sleep and remain maximally functional.

NANDA DEVELOPMENT OF SLEEP PATTERN DISTURBANCE

The North American Nursing Diagnosis Association (NANDA) officially accepted the nursing diagnosis Sleep Pattern Disturbance (SPD) for testing at the 1980 conference (Kim and Moritz, 1982), and no further changes have been made in subsequent NANDA Conferences (Carroll-Johnson, 1989). This author proposes that subdiagnoses, such as latency or difficulty falling asleep, fragmented or interrupted sleep, and early A.M. awakening, should be developed based on specific etiologies to describe more accurately the client behaviors seen and to serve as a better basis for interventions (see Table 27.1).

ETIOLOGIES/RELATED FACTORS

No matter what tool is used, the elderly client with Sleep Pattern Disturbance can be specifically identified and appropriate nursing interventions can be implemented only when the nurse has completed a thorough and systematic assessment. Specificity concerning the type of disturbance is essential for the most appropriate nursing interventions to be initiated and evaluated.

Table 27.1

Sleep Pattern Disturbance

NANDA (CARROLL-JOHNSON, 1989)	HAMMER
Definition	**Definitions**
Disruption in sleep time causes discomfort or interferes with desired lifestyle	LATENCY Onset of sleep being greater than 30 minutes (Cohen et al, 1983:79) INTERRUPTED Three or more nightime awakenings (Cohen et al, 1983) EARLY A.M. AWAKENING Less than 6 hours sleep per night (Cohen et al, 1983)
Related Factors/Etiologies	**Related Factors/Etiologies**
Sensory alterations: 　Internal factors 　　Illness 　　Psychologic stress 　External factors 　　Environmental changes 　　Social cues	LATENCY Internal factors 　Pain/discomfort Environmental changes Institutionalization with resulting staff expectations for change of routine INTERRUPTED External factors 　Nursing procedures Internal factors 　Pain/discomfort, meds 　Anxiety EARLY A.M. AWAKENING Internal factors 　Psychologic stress 　Pain/discomfort Environmental changes 　Depression
Defining Characteristics	**Defining Characteristics**
*Verbal complaints of difficulty falling asleep *Awakening earlier or later than desired *Interrupted sleep *Verbal complaints of not feeling well rested Changes in behavior and performance 　Increased irritability 　Restlessness 　Disorientation 　Lethargy 　ListlessnessPhysical signs 　Mild, fleeting nystagmus 　Slight hand tremor 　Ptosis of eyelid 　Expressionless face 　Thick speech with mispronunciation and incorrect words 　Dark circles under eyes 　Frequent yawning 　Changes in posture 　Not feeling well rested	LATENCY *Verbal complaints of difficulty falling asleep Changes in behavior and performance Increasing irritability INTERRUPTED *Verbal complaints of not feeling well rested EARLY A.M. AWAKENING Subjective statements of fear of dying

*Critical indicators.

Sleep disturbances are most often categorized as sleep latency, fragmented or interrupted sleep, or early A.M. awakening (see Table 27.1).

Medical Conditions

The most frequently identified etiology of Sleep Pattern Disturbance in the elderly is that of discomfort caused by an illness (eg, pain or respiratory distress). This can be the cause of any of the three sleep disturbances.

In patients suffering from duodenal ulcers, the most prevalent sleep disturbance is frequent awakening caused by pain. Karacan and Williams (1983) state that ulcer patients secrete 3 to 20 times more gastric acid during sleep than do normal subjects during REM sleep.

In persons suffering with cardiovascular disease, anginal pain is likely to strike during REM sleep and cause wakefulness, and sometimes even death (Karacan and Williams, 1983; Lerner, 1982). Sometimes the person will awaken without even knowing why.

Medications prescribed for hypertension have an effect on the central nervous system and may cause sleep disturbances (Bengtsson, 1980).

Pain, for whatever reason, will prevent and/or interrupt sleep, depending on its severity. If the person is able to sleep at all, the sleep is disturbed and of poor quality. The person will frequently voice the complaint, "I feel as if I haven't slept at all." It is this type of statement that the nurse needs to assess further.

Nocturia is another frequent complaint of the elderly, occurring in the first third of the night during NREM sleep. If the person is left wet, it has been found that the discomfort of being wet depresses stages 3 and 4 sleep for several hours. If the person is awakened and changed, his or her sleep will return to normal (Williams, 1971).

Anxiety and Depression

Another major etiology of Sleep Pattern Disturbance in the elderly is anxiety, frequently caused by depression (Colling, 1983; Davignon and Bruno, 1982; Karacan and Williams, 1983; Mendelson, 1984; Quan et al, 1984). Anxious elderly persons tend to complain more of insomnia and of multiple awakenings throughout the night. Depression typically is associated with symptoms of unusually early morning awakenings, inability to return to sleep, and changes in REM sleep (Miles and Dement, 1980).

Patients with chronic obstructive pulmonary disease (COPD) frequently suffer from "anxiety" attacks, in which they complain of not getting enough oxygen. Lying in a prone position will cause dyspnea and stasis of mucus (Lerner, 1982). Colling (1983;41) suggests that the frequent arousals of the elderly patient with COPD may be a "physiologically adaptive response to improve ventilation in response to hypoxia."

Territorial or Environmental Affronts

Another major etiology of Sleep Pattern Disturbance is that of conditions producing noise, light, changes in temperature and humidity, or other related environmental affronts to the elderly person as described by Yura and Walsh (1978). Other potential territorial affronts (Quan et al, 1984) occur from hospitalization or institutionalization, such as medical and nursing regimens that interfere with sleep through frequent awakenings (eg, medication administration and vital signs). Sounds unnoticed in the daytime are amplified at night (Gress and Bahr, 1981), which may disturb sleep.

Boredom or Fatigue

The final major etiology of Sleep Pattern Disturbance to be reviewed is boredom or fatigue. Because many elderly persons are retired and normally are not under any rigid schedule of obligations, their daily routines, including sleep–wake times, undergo change. They may start arising later and taking afternoon naps, making it impossible to maintain a pattern of 6 to 8 hours of uninterrupted sleep at night (Davignon and Bruno, 1982).

Carskadon et al (1982) looked at sleep fragmentation in the elderly and its relationship to daytime sleep tendency. In this study significant correlations between sleep fragmentation and the feeling of daytime well-being in the elderly were found. Subjects perceived their sleep as becoming "worse" and complained of fatigue throughout the day. Thus, they spent more time in daytime naps, trying to compensate for their feeling of fatigue.

ASSESSMENT

The literature reveals several assessment criteria to identify sleep patterns or a sleep history. Lerner's Self-Assessment Test (1982) provides the nurse with information about the aged client whose sleep problems might result from inactivity, isolation, or boredom. Schrimer (1983) suggests guidelines for obtaining a sleep history, going from general, open-ended questions to more specific questions about symptoms of sleep deprivation.

Clapin-French (1986), in her study of aged persons in long-term care facilities, developed a nursing sleep history that looked at the client's preadmission and postadmission sleep patterns. She addressed such items as aids to sleep, medication if any, atmosphere, number of pillows used, usual number of hours sleep per night, and naps taken.

Many assessments are simply a matter of nursing personnel marking on a chart every 30 to 60 minutes whether or not a client is asleep, without really knowing if the person is truly asleep or just lying there with eyes closed. In addition, clients' subjective statements of their perception of the quality of their sleep are often used as a basis for nursing and/or medical intervention.

If possible, the client should keep a sleep-wake diary for 14 days. Daily entries should include physical activities, meal times and intake, mental activities with the time of day, time and length of daytime naps, evening and bedtime activities (TV, reading, exercise), presleep state of mind, number of night awakenings, and wake-up time in the morning (Reynolds et al, 1985).

Yura and Walsh (1978) cite that the nurse must also assess such areas as the territorial environment, personal preference of dress for sleep, presleep rituals, presleep activities, and personal sleep patterns to determine specific etiologies and interventions.

Assessment Guides 27.1 and 27.2 show tools the nurse can use to obtain subjective data from the client through the use of a sleep history and a sleep-wake diary and objective data through a sleep-wake diary maintained by nursing staff. Following use for a minimum of 5 days, including a weekend when staffing patterns may be less, more specific questions may be directed to the client if needed. Johns (1971) stated that no one method can give enough information to permit neglect of any other method.

CASE STUDY

Sleep Pattern Disturbance

George, a 62-year-old white man, had lived alone prior to admission to a long-term care facility. He had recently fallen on the street, fracturing some ribs, and the previous week he had had a cataract extraction. Because he had only distant family, the hospital's Social Services Department felt he was unable to care for himself adequately and arranged for his admittance for nursing care. George had worked intermittently the past 10 years as a bartender/short-order cook. His hours of work were from 6 P.M. until 2 A.M. when the bar closed, or until the cleanup work was completed.

After his first 3 days in the facility, nursing staff were complaining that George was a "real grouch" and was swearing at them whenever they tried to help him or get him to do anything. Every night the staff found him sleeping in his clothes and using his winter coat as a blanket.

His primary nurse, who worked 11 A.M. to 7 P.M., had an opportunity to interview him over the first several days following admission, as she usually found him in a lounge watching TV and smoking. Finally one night, George

asked, "Why do I have to be awakened at 6:30 A.M. in order to get to breakfast before 8 when I never eat it? I haven't been going to bed until 4 or 4:30 A.M. I also don't like taking a shower so early." Further questioning revealed that he normally went home from work, drank a couple quarts of beer, and went to bed around 5 or 6 A.M. Around noon he would awaken and fix himself some soup and a sandwich and have some more beer. Sometime during the evening he grilled himself some type of sandwich or steak and french fries. These were the extent of his daily activities, with an occasional trip to the grocery store or laundromat. His primary nurse identified a nursing diagnosis of Sleep Pattern Disturbance: latency related to environmental changes, evidenced by verbal complaints of difficulty falling asleep and changes in behavior and performance.

NURSING INTERVENTIONS

Environmental Structuring

Environmental, or territorial, manipulation is an important intervention, as it can contribute much toward decreasing both sleep latency and sleep interruptions. While we sleep we do not become oblivious to our environment but remain sensitive to relevant sound (Webb, 1975). Cohen (1968) found intermittent sounds to be more annoying than continuous sounds. Dlin et al (1971) also found activity and noise, in addition to nursing procedures, to be the greatest deterrents to sleep.

Although the nurse does not have total control over the medical regimen, she or he should advocate for medication and treatment schedules that interfere least with sleep.

When making routine rounds, nursing staff frequently change the pattern of residents to be checked. Although it may be boring for the staff to maintain a set pattern, it is necessary so that clients are awakened at approximately the same time of the sleep cycle each night, in order to maintain the integrity of the cycle.

In addition, the nurse should use the minimal amount of light required for the task and protect any other clients sharing the room from being awakened unnecessarily.

Instead of automatically prescribing "turn every 2 hours" for an elderly client to prevent pressure sore formation, the nurse should assess the client's ability to make spontaneous body movements and should also assess other potential risk factors such as those Norton (1962) proposed. If the person is not truly at risk for pressure sore formation and is capable of making spontaneous body movements, then an every-4-hour turning schedule, or even no turning at all, may be more appropriate.

Nursing staff can do much to create a restful attitude. The bed linens should be clean, dry, and wrinkle-free. The room should have minimal noise and light and be at a comfortable temperature. Providing the client with a compatible roommate is also helpful to ensure a good night's rest.

If the elderly person prefers to listen to music while going to sleep, it should be of a quiet, relaxing nature. The music should be from a radio as opposed to TV because the flicker from the TV screen can also interfere with sleep.

One of the most important interventions for sleep latency is the establishment of a pre-bedtime routine and a soothing sleep environment for the client. Much of this can and should be done through patient education if the person is capable. This should include a "winding-down" period in which the person doesn't have any extreme physical or mental stimulation within 2 hours of bedtime. Exercise causes an increase in body temperature, which is in conflict with sleep because the body temperature drops during sleep (Demarest, 1986). Mental stimulation or stress prior to sleep tends to prolong its onset (Schrimer, 1983).

The client should be dressed in loose-fitting night-clothes of the style to which they are accustomed (gowns or pajamas). The pre-bedtime routine should include such things as oral and personal hygiene and possibly a bedtime snack if within the elderly person's diet. Clients should be encouraged to empty their bladder; or if clients are incontinent, nursing staff should make sure their bed and/or incontinency undergarment is dry.

A regularly scheduled time for bed should be maintained. However, if unable to fall asleep after 20 to 30 minutes, the elderly person should get up and engage in a quiet activity like reading or listening to quiet music. This will help to maintain the "conditioned" response that a bed is for sleep. If the person is unable to relax, the nurse might try some relaxing techniques, such as a backrub accompanied by soft conversation (Bahr, 1983).

The nurse should instruct the client that caffeine is a stimulant found in coffee, tea, soft drinks, many nonprescription drugs, and many foods. If a cup of coffee or tea is important to the client with his or her evening meal or bedtime snack, suggest a decaffeinated or herbal type (Demarest, 1986). The traditional glass of warm milk at bedtime to help foster sleep actually has a scientific basis. Milk contains L-tryptophan, which has been identified as a sleep inducer (Hoch and Reynolds, 1986). In addition, elderly persons frequently associate milk with the security and nurturing they felt as an infant (Schrimer, 1983). However, the nurse should inform the client that eating or drinking to excess before going to bed increases the workload of the heart and makes it more difficult to fall asleep (Demarest, 1986). Also, if the client awakens after being asleep, do not encourage him or her to eat, as this can be a covert reward for waking up (Demarest, 1986).

CASE STUDY

Nursing Interventions

Because of the cataract extraction, George received ophthalmic drops at midnight and 6 A.M. This necessitated staff awakening him at least once a night and sometimes twice if he decided to go to bed before midnight (which he started to do, saying, "There's nothing to do at this hour if you can't see TV and I can't"). Staff had to turn on a light in order to see to instill the drops and reapply the eyeshield, and they had to talk to him in order to orient him.

George's roommate's care included turning and repositioning every 2 hours with Attends (an adult incontinency undergarment) changes, which required staff to turn on his light and pull hard to shut the dividing door. The roommate would then yell out in his confused state, and 10 minutes or more would elapse before he settled down again. George was unable to sleep through all of this commotion. This was identified as a Sleep Pattern Disturbance: Interrupted Sleep (see Table 27.1).

Four weeks following George's admission, his roommate died, leaving George alone in the room. Thinking George would like this, the staff made no attempt to give him a roommate. However, George again became irritable with staff and demanded he was well enough to go home. Finally, following an altercation with another resident over which TV program to watch, his primary nurse confronted him. He admitted he wasn't sleeping well because he woke up around 3:30 A.M. and lay awake thinking about dying. He confessed he was afraid in the room by himself, that "my heart might give out on me and you wouldn't know all night." The nursing diagnosis Sleep Pattern Disturbance: Early A.M. Awakening was established (see Table 27.1). George was then moved to another room with a roommate who went to the bathroom independently during the night and with whom George was acquainted.

Because the facility believed George should maintain control of his own life as long as feasibly possible, the primary nurse agreed to tell staff to let George wake up whenever he wanted. The nurse also made arrangements for dietary services to fix him a bedtime snack of a meat sandwich, fruit, and a high-protein liquid supplement that George could eat at his chosen time. The 3 to 11 P.M. staff assisted him with his shower early in their shift, since this was the time he was used to taking it, just before going to work.

After 4 months, George was going to bed at 10:30 P.M. following the news, when his roommate went to bed. George now gets up at 7 A.M. and joins his roommate for breakfast. His eyedrops, which have been changed to a twice-daily schedule, are administered during his waking times. Staff report more interaction between George and other residents and increased participation in social activities. When questioned, George stated, "I've never had it so good." George no longer has Sleep Pattern Disturbance and no longer demonstrates any physical signs of SPD such as dark circles under his eyes or frequent yawning. Instead, he has adjusted to institutionalization, while maintaining as much of his individuality as possible.

Relaxation Techniques

Relaxation techniques are independent interventions that a nurse may initiate in an effort to promote sleep. Elderly clients may do slow, deep breathing exercises to induce calm and alleviate tension. Progressive muscle relaxation, in which the muscles are systematically tensed and relaxed, is another way to help alleviate tension. Some elderly clients may even benefit from a relaxation technique such as imagery: visualization, in which persons visualize a relaxing scene from their past, or meditation, in which persons focus attention on a specific image or thought and change their level of awareness.

Therapeutic Touch

Therapeutic touch is a lesser-known technique that could be used to help promote sleep in the elderly. Much skepticism continues about this controversial technique, however (Raucheisen, 1984; Sandroff, 1980).

Krieger (1975) introduced therapeutic touch as an independent nursing intervention. The four phases of therapeutic touch are centering, assessment, balancing, and energy transfer. The entire process takes about 10 minutes. Braun et al (1986) studied the use of therapeutic touch to improve the sleep of elderly nursing home residents and found it effective in enhancing their sleep quality.

Even if the nurse doesn't practice therapeutic touch, the idea of "laying-on of hands" might prompt the nurse to give a backrub, a hug, or a comforting touch rather than just verbal soothing to reduce stress or anxiety in a sleepless elderly person (Sandroff, 1980).

OUTCOMES

The final phase of the nursing process, evaluation of outcome criteria, is one of subjectivity as well as objectiv-

ity. Subjectively, the client must feel rested on awakening from a night's sleep, while objectively looking and acting rested.

An absence of frequent yawning, dark circles under the eyes, thick speech, unusual fatigue, and/or irritability are signs the nurse can easily assess. The client's increased participation in activities of daily living is another objective method the nurse can use to evaluate the effectiveness of nursing interventions. The client's decreased use of sedatives, hypnotics, and tranquilizers to promote sleep is yet another method of evaluation.

The nurse should determine the length of time the client actually sleeps by monitoring the client's sleep-wake status throughout the night; this is easily done in the institutional setting. The client should sleep for at least a 90-minute period, through a complete sleep cycle, and preferably for 4 to 5 hours without awakening.

This won't happen overnight but should occur within several days of the implementation of nursing interventions to eliminate or reduce the amount of sleep disturbance. The length of time required to obtain the outcome criterion of 4 to 5 hours of sleep will depend on the etiology, the severity and chronicity of the sleep disturbance, and the consistency of application of the interventions.

SUMMARY

Nightingale (1859) viewed uninterrupted sleep as essential to well-being. It is just as important today as it was over a century ago and is something nursing should and can help control. Differentiation of the nursing diagnosis through thorough assessment and identification of the etiology is necessary before action can be taken. Many of the actions are ones nurses are capable of initiating independently. Desired outcomes should be defined so that the effectiveness of the interventions can be assessed. Because nurses frequently have 24-hour contact with the elderly, or at least the most frequent contact, they are in the best position to assist the elderly in obtaining quality sleep or rest.

ASSESSMENT GUIDE 27.1

Sleep Pattern Assessment

Subjective:

Initiation:

1. How long do you think you should sleep at night?
2. How long do you actually sleep at night?
3. Does this vary greatly from night to night, or is it relatively constant?
4. What time do you usually like to retire?
5. How long does it take you to fall asleep?

Interruptions:

6. How many times do you awaken during the night?
7. What awakens you?
8. During what part of the night do you awaken?
9. Do you have trouble falling back to sleep?
10. How long does it take for you to fall back to sleep?
11. Do you or your roommate require nursing care during the night?

Quality:

12. Is your sleep quiet or restless?
13. Do you feel rested and refreshed when you awaken?
14. Do you think you receive enough sleep?
15. Do you dream? (describe amount, nature, and emotional character of dream)

Pre-bedtime routine:

16. Do you use any medications to help you sleep?
17. Do you require anything special to help you sleep (eg, pillows, position, drink/food)?
18. Describe your normal pre-bedtime routine.

Habits:

19. What time do you usually awaken in the morning?
20. What time do you actually get out of bed?
21. Do you take naps during the day?
22. If yes, how many and for how long?
23. Describe the amount and type of exercise/activity you do during the day
24. Additional comments:

ASSESSMENT GUIDE 27.2

Daily Patient Sleep History

	Day 1	Day 2	Day 3	Day 4	Day 5	Day 6	Day 7
Time went to bed							
Time went to sleep							
Time of arising							
Number of times awake							
Any difficulty in returning to sleep							
Awoke feeling rested							
Awoke feeling tired							

Additional comments:

SLEEP ASSESSMENT

Date: Time of Assessment	Awake/asleep (A = awake/S = asleep)	Nursing Procedure (P = patient/R = roommate)	Comments: (Physical characteristics, eg, yawning, dozing, decreased attention span)
0030			
0100-etc Done Q. 30 Minutes			

References

Bahr R: Sleep-wake patterns in the aged. *J Gerontol Nurs* 1983; 9:534–539.

Bengtsson CJ: Sleep disturbances, nightmares and other possible central nervous disturbances in a population sample of women, with special reference to those on antihypertensive drugs. *European J Clin Pharmacol* 1980; 17:173–177.

Berger R: The sleep and dream cycle. In: *Sleep: Physiology and Pathology.* Kales A (editor). Lippincott, 1969:17–32.

Braun C, Layton J, Braun J: Therapeutic touch improves residents' sleep. *Am Health Care Assoc J* (Jan) 1986; 48–49.

Brill E, Kilts D: *Foundations for Nursing.* Appleton-Century-Crofts, 1980.

Carroll-Johnson R (editor): *Classification of Nursing Diagnoses: Proceedings of the Eighth Conference.* Lippincott, 1989.

Carskadon M, Brown E, Dement W: Sleep fragmentation in the elderly: Relationship to daytime sleep tendency. *Neurobiol Aging* (Winter) 1982; 3:321–327.

Clapin-French E: Sleep patterns of aged persons in long-term care facilities. *J Adv Nurs* (1986); 11:57–66.

Cohen A: Noise effects on health, productivity, and well-being. *Trans NY Acad Sci* 1968; 30:910–918.

Cohen D et al: Sleep disturbances in the institutionalized aged. *J Am Geriatr Soc* 1983; 31:79–82.

Colling J: Sleep disturbances in aging: A theoretic and empiric analysis. *ANS* (Oct) 1983; 36–44.

Davignon D, Bruno P: Insomina: Causes and treatment, particularly in the elderly. *J Gerontol Nurs* 1982; 8:333–336.

Demarest C: Insomnia, helping your patient get some sleep. *Patient Care* (Feb) 1986; 15:61–71.

Dlin B, Rosen H, Dickstein K: The problems of sleep and rest in the intensive care unit. *Psychosomatics* 1971; 12:155–163.

Ebersole P, Hess P: *Toward Healthy Aging: Human Needs and Nursing Response.* Mosby, 1981.

Gambert S, Duthie E: Sleep disorders: Coping with a waking nightmare. *Geriatrics* (Sept) 1981; 36:61–66.

Gress L, Bahr R, Hassanein R: Nocturnal behavior of selected institutionalized adults. *J Gerontol Nurs* (Feb) 1981; 7:86–92.

Guillenimault C, Silvestri R: Aging, drugs, and sleep. *Neurobiolog Aging* (Winter) 1982; 3:379–386.

Hayter J: Sleep behaviors of older persons. *Nurs Res* 1983; 32:242–246.

Hoch C, Reynolds C: Sleep disturbances and what to do about them. *Geriatr Nurs* 1986; 7:24–27.

Johns M: Methods for assessing human sleep. *Arch Intern Med* 1971; 127:484–492.

Karacan I, Williams R: Sleep disorders in the elderly. *Am Fam Physician* 1983; 27:143–152.

Kim M, Moritz D: *Classification of Nursing Diagnoses: Proceedings of the Third and Fourth National Conferences.* McGraw-Hill, 1982.

Kleitman N: *Sleep and Wakefulness.* University of Chicago Press, 1939.

Krieger D: Therapeutic touch: The imprimatur of nursing. *Am J Nurs* 1975; 75:784–787.

Lerner R: Sleep loss in the aged: Implications for nursing practice. *J Gerontol Nurs* 1982; 8:323–326.

Mendelson W: Sleep after forty. *Am Fam Physician* 1984; 29:135–139.

Miles L, Dement W: Sleep and aging. *Sleep* 1980; 3:119–202.

Mitchell P: *Concepts Basic to Nursing.* McGraw-Hill, 1973.

Nightingale F: *Notes on Nursing.* Harrison and Sons, 1859.

Norton D: An investigation of geriatric nursing problems in hospital. *National Corporation for the Care of Old People,* 1962.

Oswald I: *Sleeping and Awakening: Physiology and Psychology.* Elsevier, 1962.

Quan SF, Bamford CR, Beutler LE: Sleep disturbance in the elderly. *Geriatrics* 1984; 39(9):42–47.

Raucheisen M: Therapeutic touch: Maybe there's something to it after all. *RN* (Dec) 1984; 49–51.

Reynolds C F et al: Sleep of healthy seniors: A revisit. *Sleep* 1985; 8:20–29.

Rutenfranz J: Shift work research issues. In: *Biological Rhythms, Sleep, and Shift Work.* Johnson L (editor). SP Medical and Scientific Books, 1981:165–196.

Sandroff R: A skeptic's guide to therapeutic touch. *RN* (Jan) 1980; 25–31 + .

Schrimer M: When sleep won't come. *J Gerontol Nurs* 1983; 9:16–21.

Webb W: *Sleep: An Experimental Approach.* MacMillan, 1968.

Webb W: *Sleep, The Gentle Tyrant.* Prentice-Hall, 1975.

Williams DH: Sleep and disease. *Am J Nurs* 1971; 71:2321–2324.

Yura H, Walsh M: *Human Needs and the Nursing Process.* Appleton-Century-Crofts, 1978.

VI

Cognitive–Perceptual Pattern

MERIDEAN MAAS, PhD, RN, FAAN
KATHLEEN BUCKWALTER, PhD, RN, FAAN

Overview

ALTERATIONS IN COGNITION AND PERCEPTION affect many elderly and can precipitate institutionalization. In Chapter 29, Hall sets forth her conceptual model, Progressively Lowered Stress Threshold, which guides the practitioner in the four levels of assessment and intervention of clients with Altered Thought Processes: Dementia. This heuristic contribution developed logically from the cluster of losses and behavioral states associated with this nursing diagnosis. In the development of the chapter, Hall organizes her discussion by reversible and irreversible etiologies. She presents detailed care plans and goals and gives special attention to the problems of combative reactions and wandering.

Although the topic of pain in the elderly could consume a book itself, Clinton and Eland (known internationally for her work in children's pain) provide a salient overview of this important and often overlooked topic in Chapter 30 on Pain. The authors identify and discuss biologic, neurologic, ischemic, musculoskeletal, chemical, physical, and psychologic sources of pain with regard to acute, chronic, and malignant pain in the elderly. A number of clinically useful assessment tools are set forth and critiqued for use with the elderly. Clinton

and Eland examine intervening factors, such as the effects of drugs, that influence pain tolerance and treatment. Interventions highlight both pharmacologic and nonpharmacologic approaches, such as relaxation, humor, distraction, teaching, and transcutaneous electrical nerve stimulation.

In Chapter 31 Drury and Akins explicate the diagnosis Sensory/Perceptual Alterations, combining the approaches of the North American Nursing Diagnosis Association (NANDA) and Marjorie Gordon. Four specific diagnoses are set forth. Drury and Akins analyze three of the diagnoses: Sensory/Perceptual Alterations: Uncompensated; Sensory/Perceptual Alterations: Excess; and Sensory/Perceptual Alterations: Deficit. Weitzel discusses the fourth specific diagnosis, Unilateral Neglect, in Chapter 32. The authors describe assessment procedures and tools along with several nursing interventions that are recommended for these diagnoses.

Weitzel emphasizes that Unilateral Neglect is the result of pathology and not normal aging, which largely differentiates the diagnosis from other altered sensory perceptions. Weitzel describes etiologies and related deficits for the diagnosis and specific assessment criteria for the nurse to use with a client with brain injury. Environmental structuring to compensate for the elderly person's neglect of stimuli and specific intervention strategies for inattention and denial are discussed.

In Chapter 33, Rakel addresses Knowledge Deficit, a common problem among the elderly. She develops the concept of alterations in knowledge and distinguishes it from alterations in learning and thought processes. The intervention of patient education is selected as the treatment of choice for this diagnosis, with patient counseling, contracting, support groups, values clarification, reminiscence therapy, remotivation therapy, sensory retraining and relaxation therapy discussed as supplemental approaches. The notion of "readiness to learn" is emphasized, and assessment strategies are set forth. Obstacles to learning are also examined.

28

Normal Changes With Aging

MARY A. HARDY, PhD, RN, C
DONNA BUNTEN, MA, RN
JANICE DRURY, RN
JACKIE AKINS, BSN, RN, C

Definition:

The cognitive–perceptual pattern describes the sensory/perceptual and cognitive pattern.

SENSORY ORGANS RECEIVE AND CARRY MESSAGES FROM the external world; cognitive processes interpret the messages received with the help of information from the memory banks. The possibility of changes in intelligence in the elderly has been studied extensively, but in general it has been found that intelligence remains relatively stable in later adulthood. Some researchers suggest that there may be a decline in "fluid intelligence," which involves tasks not influenced by prior knowledge, whereas "crystallized intelligence," or tasks that require knowledge that is acquired during one's lifetime, shows little or no change (Horn and Donaldson, 1976). Intelligence that relies on accumulated experience sets the elderly apart from other age groups and presents an area for much continued growth. Criticism about findings that reflect decreased fluid intelligence has been based on the speed factor that is frequently required in testing situations. The elderly are at a disadvantage when time limits are imposed, as perception and reaction times are somewhat slowed with normal aging. The elderly also do not practice skills that underlie fluid tasks. However, it has been demonstrated that with training, older persons can compensate for declines in fluid abilities.

With aging, the ability to acquire new information decreases, but once information is learned, subsequent recall is the same or almost the same in the elderly as in younger persons (Botwinick, 1978). This decreasing rate of information processing is more apparent with the higher order processes than with the sensory-motor processes (Cerella, 1985). A variety of other factors such as certain medications (anticholinergics, antidepressants, and antihypertensives), vitamin deficiencies, and metabolic disturbances can also affect a person's rate of learning. Thus, slowing the pace of instruction is important when teaching the elderly.

Age differences may be exhibited in testing conditions. If the elderly are distracted by competing stimuli during testing, their learning and memory are more disrupted than in younger subjects (Craik, 1977). Success might be impaired if the elderly are given too much material to process at once, if the material is not meaningful to them, and if the speed of response required is not paced appropriately (Cunningham, 1980; Light et al, 1982; Lorge, 1936; Poon, 1985).

Deterioration in ability to solve problems, increased difficulty organizing complex material (Knox, 1977), and increased cautiousness with aging may account in part for apparently slowed cognition (Tobin, 1977). Given the factors that impede and expedite learning in the elderly, it is apparent that a stimulus of greater intensity is needed to reduce competing stimuli. Additionally, many elderly proceed more cautiously because they want certainty before being willing to make a response. Studies have shown that if some risk is unavoidable, old and young people do not differ in their degree of cautiousness but, if given the opportunity to avoid risk totally, older people are more likely to take that route (Gribbin, 1976).

As an individual ages, the perceptual processes that determine cognition and manipulation of data and output (behavior) according to life patterns remain unchanged. Mental capacities are generally among the last to decline. Older adults do as well as young adults on all tests of intellectual performance when unlimited time is allowed for completion.

However, sensory system reception changes as a result of aging. An overall slowing is experienced with some decrease in, not total loss of, efficiency. As the senses provide the means by which the elderly interact with and interpret the world, a decrease in functional ability of the senses has a marked impact on behavior.

Overall vision changes begin in the fourth decade of life. These include gradual loss of accommodation (ability to focus vision), increased lens opacity, yellowing of the lens, and senile miosis with decreased peripheral vision (Buseck, 1976; Corso, 1971; Snyder et al, 1976). Ordinarily, vision loss as a result of aging is a gradual process. Most elderly may never become "totally blind" but will experience deficits in vision. Vision changes include the following:

1. With a gradual loss of accommodation, more time is needed for the elder to refocus when looking from one distance to another. Blurring occurs and the ability to discriminate fine visual acuity/detail becomes difficult. Actual loss of rods and cones within the retina of the aging eye (which convert light waves to electrical impulses) also results in a less distinct image being sent to the brain. Corneal scarring from years of environmental exposure may further diminish visual acuity or accuracy. These visual changes affect ability to manipulate objects within the environment. Because a significant amount of meaning/intent of conversation is given through nonverbal cues, this loss diminishes the elder's ability to understand messages being communicated, resulting in a decreased ability to interact socially with persons in that environment.

2. An increased sensitivity to glare occurs because light rays entering the eye tend to scatter as a result of increased lens and corneal opacity. Additionally, portions of the sclera become thinned, allowing unfocused bits of light to enter the inner chamber of the eye.

3. Cataracts (yellowing with increased opacity of the lens) are common among the elderly. Yellowing of the cornea further blurs vision and affects color perception. There is a decreased ability to discriminate between close colors in the spectrum, especially in the blue/green range.

4. Increasing rigidity of the iris with resultant decrease in the diameter of the pupil and a reduction in the blood supply reaching the macula decreases the amount of light reaching the retina and reduces acuity of night vision.

5. Visual fields or peripheral vision is affected by diminished pupil size and may be further compromised by decreased muscle tone, resulting in ptosis, or drooping of the upper eyelids. The ability to gaze in differing directions—horizontally, vertically, or diagonally—is reduced because of decreased muscle tone and/or by changes in innervation by the oculomotor, abducens, and trochlear nerves.

Auditory changes begin to be noticed at approximately age 40. Onset is significantly affected by lifestyle (eg, occupational noise, leisure time choices) and thus may be noticed at a much younger age. For instance, the possibility of reduced conduction time in the acoustic nerve as a result of elevated environmental lead levels has recently been identified (Voke, 1980). In addition, hearing loss or impairment is a common side effect of some medications (eg, anti-inflammatory drugs and antibiotics).

The three most common hearing losses include conductive, sensorineural, and central. Conductive hearing loss generally is a mechanical problem involving the transfer of sound waves through the outer and middle ear to the inner eardrum, where they are converted to electrical impulses. This may be caused by environmental damage to the outer ear (pinna), arthritic stiffening of the stapes, or decreased flexibility of the conductive membranes, eardrum, or oval window. Often cerumen, or wax, which is normally absorbed in the younger person's ear, becomes hard and dark and collects. This buildup is thought to occur when cilia become coarse and stiff and less effective at propelling residue to the external canal opening. Unfortunately, accumulation of cerumen blocks the ear canal, often causing deafness (Bernardini, 1985; Matteson, 1979). The result is a muffling of sounds at all frequency ranges. This makes speech discrimination difficult. Sensorineural loss (presbycusis) in the inner ear affects the ability to identify portions of speech, particularly high-pitched sounds like *s*, *t*, *f*, *g*, and *d*, making conversation nearly unintelligible (Corso, 1971). Central hearing loss occurs because of damage to the acoustic nerve. This impairs transfer of stimuli to the brain, or within the brain itself, and subsequently impairs interpretation of the sound signals.

Auditory and visual perception have been studied extensively, and changes associated with normal aging have been described. Research in the areas of taste and smell is sparse by comparison, perhaps because of the abstract nature of these sensations and the difficulties presented in trying to quantify them. Changes in the character of the olfactory epithelium, a decrease in the number of sensory cells in the nasal mucosa and olfactory bulb, and decreased visual perception are thought to be the main factors contributing to the decreased sense of smell associated with aging. Some of these changes are not normal to aging but are common because of the number of elderly exposed for years to environmental irritants such as dust, pollution, and smoking.

The ability to taste all four flavors (sweet, salt, bitter, sour) begins to decline after age 50. Generally, sour is the last taste lost. Changes are the result of actual loss of taste buds with decreased perception of the taste sensation (Colavita, 1978), so that higher concentration of seasoning in food is necessary to reach a threshold level for perception. Unfortunately, other chronic problems requiring food restrictions, such as low-salt diets and restricted seasoning, may put the elder in a "double bind" with regard to tasting food. Other factors affecting the taste sensation are temperatures of food, oral hygiene, intactness of the sense of smell, and prevalent use of dentures among the elderly. Although at least half of the elderly experience loss of teeth and/or the use of dentures, dentures are less than 35% as effective as natural teeth in the functions of tasting, swallowing, chewing, and sensing temperatures of food and fluids.

Although a uniform dulling of sensation occurs during aging, great variation among individual perception of touch exists at any age. In other words, thresholds for recognition, as a result of aging, change little within the individual over time (Hollinger, 1980). Long-term exposure to the environment causes some decrease in perception of or sensitivity to tactile sensations. Hollinger (1980) suggested that the decrease in touch sensitivity is possibly due to a generalized thinning of epidermal layers, giving the skin a transparent appearance and resulting in a slight decrease in touch sensitivity in many individuals. Loss of cutaneous sensations, which have been found to be impaired or altered in the elderly, include sensitivity to noxious stimuli such as pain, hypothermia or hyperthermia, and a decrease in joint mobility, especially of the lower extremities (Hollinger, 1980).

References

Bernardini L: Effective communication as an intervention for sensory deprivation in the elderly client. *Top Clin Nurs* 1985; 6(4):72–81.

Botwinick J: *Aging and Behavior*, 2d ed. Springer, 1978.

Buseck SA: Visual status of the elderly. *J Gerontol Nurs* 1976; 2(5):34–39.

Cerella J: Information processing rates in the elderly. *Psycholog Bull* 1985; 98(1):67–83.

Colavita FB: *Sensory Changes in the Elderly*. Charles C. Thomas, 1978.

Corso J: Sensory processes and age effects in normal adults. *J Gerontol* 1971; 26(1):90–103.

Craik FIM: Age differences in human memory. In: *Handbook of the Psychology of Aging*. Birren JE, Shaie KW (editors). Van Nos Reinhold, 1977.

Cunningham WR: Speed, age, and qualitative differences in cognitive functioning. In: *Aging in the 1980s*. Poon LW (editor). American Psychological Association, 1980.

Gribbin K: Cognitive processes in aging. In: *Nursing and the Aged*. Burnside I (editor). McGraw-Hill, 1976.

Hollinger LM: Perception of touch in the elderly. *J Gerontol Nurs* 1980; 6:741–746.

Horn JL, Donaldson G: Age differences in fluid and crystallized intelligence. *Am Psychol* 1976; 26:107–129.

Knox AB: *Adult Development and Learning*. Jossey-Bass, 1977.

Light LL, Zelinski EM, Moore M: Adult difference in reasoning from new information. *J Experiment Psychol* 1982; 8:435–447.

Lorge I: The influence of the test upon the nature of mental decline as a function of age. *J Educ Psychol* 1936; 27:100–110.

Matteson MA: A report of sensory assessment at a senior citizens' center. *J Gerontol Nurs* 1979; 5(1):39–41.

Poon LW: Differences in human memory with aging. In: *Handbook of the Psychology of Aging*. Mortimer JA, Schuman LM (editors). Oxford University Press, 1985.

Snyder LH, Pyrek J, Smith KC: Vision and mental function of the elderly. *Gerontologist* 1976; 16:491–495.

Tobin JB: Normal aging: The inevitability syndrome. In: *Readings in Aging and Death: Contemporary Perspectives*. Zarit SH (editor). Harper and Row, 1977.

Voke J: Aspects of hearing one: Physiology of the ear. *Nurs Times* (Aug) 1980; 15:28–30.

29

Altered Thought Processes: Dementia

Geri Richards Hall, MA, RN

Altered Thought Processes: Dementia (ATPD), due to progressive degeneration of the cerebral cortex, is a common nursing diagnosis among older adults, affecting about 5% to 7% of people over age 65 (Office of Technological Assessment, 1987). The number of people with ATPD is expected to increase proportionately as the population ages.

Eighty percent to 90% of people with ATPD will be cared for in their home, during at least the early stages of their illness. Because of the prolonged duration of the disease and the lack of funding for professional nursing services (Office of Technological Assessment, 1987), care will be provided by family members with little or no nursing involvement. Care of persons with ATPD in the hospital setting is limited to short periods of time and to persons who have acute conditions.

In order to focus on the rationale for care and development of a comprehensive care plan, this chapter will focus on the elderly client with Altered Thought Processes: Senile Dementia of the Alzheimer's Type (SDAT), which is the most common dementia among elderly persons. However, the principles of care are applicable to all settings and to most specific types of dementia. Modified care plans based on the conceptual model described are being used in homes, day-care settings, foster homes, and hospitals.

Care of the resident with dementia has been largely a trial-and-error process. Behavior such as wandering or violence is generally thought to occur randomly without cause. Interventions for antisocial outbursts usually consist of the use of physical and chemical restraints while keeping the resident in a highly stimulating environment. This mandates high resident/staff ratios, increasing the cost of care (Cox, 1985; Heaney, 1983; Mace and Rabins, 1981; Schafer, 1985). Most care is based on the notion that confused persons should be reoriented to their surroundings and rehabilitated through maximizing sensory input, providing reality orientation therapy, reeducating for lost skills, and supporting caregivers (Glosser and Wexler, 1985; Heaney, 1983; Holden and Woods, 1982; Mace and Rabins, 1981; Ridder, 1985). Because these approaches are usually unsuccessful, this had led to enormous frustration among caregivers, gerontologic nurses, and the nursing home industry, causing occasional rejection of residents bearing the diagnosis of SDAT.

ETIOLOGIES/RELATED FACTORS AND DEFINING CHARACTERISTICS

The diagnosis Altered Thought Processes is defined by the North American Nursing Diagnosis Association (NANDA) as "a state in which an individual experiences a disruption in cognitive operations and activities" (Carroll-Johnson, 1989;553). The NANDA related factors/etiologies and defining characteristics are listed in Table 29.1 and contrasted with the author's etiologies and behavioral symptom clusters (defining characteristics) for Altered Thought Processes: Dementia. The NANDA behaviors tend to be less specific and provide less direction for the development of a care plan that incorporates the pathophysiology of cortical degeneration. At this time, there are no published research studies validating the defining characteristics of Altered Thought Processes. The most comprehensive reviews of behaviors that occur with degeneration of the cerebral cortex are in the medical literature.

In the 1960s, the symptoms associated with Alzheimer's disease were categorized into three groups of losses: cognitive, affective, and conative (planning) or functional. The presence of several behavioral symptoms in each group or cluster appeared to be indicative of a dementing illness. However, the symptoms still allowed for enormous variety in clinical presentation among individuals (Ballinger, 1982; Gottfries et al, 1982; Venn, 1983). Researchers noted the presence of other symptoms, such as confusion, agitation, night wakening, wandering, and combative behavior, but failed to incorporate these into existing clusters or a new cluster. Hall and Buckwalter (1987) incorporated these symptoms into a separate cluster, entitled "progressively lowered stress threshold." The behavioral symptom clusters (defining characteristics) are listed in Table 29.1.

These behaviors are consistent with the deterioration found on positron emission tomography (PET) scans and on autopsy. Researchers report that scans demonstrate significant deterioration in the posterior parietal and occipital lobes of the brain and in the hippocampus. These areas are responsible for receiving stimuli, assigning meaning, and coordinating responses. This function is called cerebral integration and helps to explain the clusters of symptoms presented by residents with ATPD (Burns and Buckwalter, 1988).

Irreversible Causes

ATPD due to progressive degeneration of the cerebral cortex is a diagnosis that describes behaviors indicating a lack of integration among stimuli, perception, and responses to stimuli.

The pathologies causing degeneration of the cerebral cortex are varied; however, the resulting behaviors are relatively similar for all causes of dementing illnesses. The most common cause is Alzheimer's disease. Thought to cause about 60% of diagnosed dementias, Alzheimer's disease can be broken into two types: senile dementia of the Alzheimer's type (SDAT) and presenile dementia. Both are characterized by generalized cortical atrophy, widening of the cortical sulci, enlargement of the ventricles, and histologic changes including senile plaques, neurofibrillary tangles, and granulovacuolar degeneration of the neurons (Burns and Buckwalter, 1988; Heston and White, 1983; Mace and Rabins, 1981; Mackey, 1982–1983). Both types are also characterized by an insidious onset and inexorable progression.

A second major cause of degenerative decline in the cerebral cortex is multiple infarctions, or strokes. Multi-infarct disease (MID) is thought to account for about 10% of dementing illness. Although the onset of the disease may be slow, MID is characterized by a steplike progression as each new stroke occurs. Combinations of SDAT and MID account for another 17% of dementing illnesses (Heston and White, 1983; Office of Technological Assessment, 1987).

The last 13% of dementing illnesses are rare and occasionally reversible dementias. Pick's disease is a progressive dementia characterized by the formation of Pick's cells, primarily in the frontal and temporal lobes. The patient exhibits amnesia, aphasia, and losses of socially appropriate behavior and inhibitions.

Creutzfeldt-Jakob disease (CJ disease) is an infectious disease thought to be caused by a slow virus. It is characterized by a rapid onset and progression. The patient exhibits myoclonus in addition to the demented behaviors. Life span is usually 12 to 18 months after symptoms appear. Because of the viral nature of the disease, the resident should be placed on blood and secretion/excretion precautions. However, to date there are no documented cases of nursing personnel contracting the disease from an infected patient.

Normal pressure hydrocephalus (NPH) is a reversible dementia characterized by the early onset of aphasia, incontinence, and ataxia. The excess accumulation of fluid in the cranial cavity causes the ventricles to enlarge, compressing the cortex. The disease is treated by implanting a shunt in a ventricle to drain excess fluid.

Toxic substance ingestion, including alcohol, barbiturates, opioids, cocaine, amphetamines, hallucinogenics, caffeine, and tobacco, may cause dementia. Carbon monoxide and some metals, such as lead, may also cause dementia. In some cases the dementia may resolve with the cessation of substance use.

Emotional disorders such as depression and schizophrenia are frequently mistaken for dementia because they tend to mimic the symptoms. Both depression and schizophrenia are treatable disorders.

Table 29.1

Etiologies/Related Factors and Defining Characteristics of Altered Thought Processes and Altered Thought Processes: Dementia

ALTERED THOUGHT PROCESSES	ALTERED THOUGHT PROCESSES: DEMENTIA
NANDA (Carroll-Johnson, 1989)	*Hall*

ALTERED THOUGHT PROCESSES

NANDA *(Carroll-Johnson, 1989)*

Definition: A state in which an individual experiences a disruption in cognitive operations and activities

Etiologies/Related Factors

Physiologic changes
Psychologic changes
Loss of memory
Impaired judgment
Sleep deprivation

ALTERED THOUGHT PROCESSES: DEMENTIA

Hall

Etiologies/Related Factors

Irreversible dementing illness (progressive degeneration
of the cerebral cortex)
    Alzheimer's disease:
    1. Senile dementia of the Alzheimer's type (SDAT)
    2. Presenile dementia
    Multi-infarction disease (MID) or strokes
    Combinations of SDAT and MID

Occasionally reversible dementing illnesses
    Pick's disease
    Creutzfeldt Jakob disease
    Normal pressure hydrocephalus
    Toxic substance ingestion
    Emotional disorders
    Degenerative neurologic diseases
    Conditions affecting the structure or integrity of the brain
    Metabolic disorders
    Infections
    Autoimmune diseases
    (Heston & White, 1983; Mace & Rabins, 1981; Mackey,
    1982–1983; Office of Technological Assessment, 1987;
    Wolanin & Phillips, 1981)

Reversible acute confusional syndrome
    Pathophysiologic changes—delirium
    Stress
    Environmental factors
    Loss of meaning and pattern in routine
    Alterations in self-image

Defining Characteristics

Inaccurate interpretation of environment
Cognitive dissonance
DistractibilityMemory deficit or problems
EgocentricityHyper/hypovigilance
Decreased ability to grasp ideas
Impaired ability to make decisions
Impaired ability to problem solve
Impaired ability to reason
Impaired ability to abstract or conceptualize
Impaired ability to calculate
Altered attention span—distractibility
Commands; obsessions
Inability to follow
Disorientation to time, place, person, circumstances, events
Changes in remote, recent, immediate memory

Defining Characteristics

Irreversible dementing illnesses
1. Cognitive or intellectual losses: loss of memory, initially for
   Progressive degeneration of the cerebral cortex (SDAT) recent events; loss of time sense; inability to abstract, such as
   understanding safety needs; inability to make choices and
   decisions, to problem solve and reason; poor judgment; altered perceptions; loss of language abilities
2. Affective or personality losses: loss of affect; diminished inhibitions, characterized by emotional lability, spontaneous
   conversation and loss of tact, loss of control of temper, inability to delay gratification; decreased attention span; social
   withdrawal; loss of recognition of others, environment, and,
   eventually, self (agnosia); increasing self-preoccupation; antisocial behavior; confabulation, perseveration, psychotic features such as paranoia, delusions, and pseudohallucinations;
   increased fatigue with exertion or cognition, loss of energy
   reserve

Table 29.1

Etiologies/Related Factors and Defining Characteristics of Altered Thought Processes and Altered Thought Processes: Dementia (*Continued*)

ALTERED THOUGHT PROCESSES	ALTERED THOUGHT PROCESSES: DEMENTIA
Delusions Ideas of reference Hallucinations Confabulation Inappropriate social behavior Altered sleep patterns Inappropriate affect *Other Possible Defining Characteristics* Inappropriate/nonreality-based	3. Conative or planning losses: loss of general ability to plan activities, especially those requiring thought to set goal, organize, and carry out; functional loss starting with high-level and transportation and progressing to losses in ADLs in generally the following order: bathing, grooming, choosing clothing, dressing, mobility, toileting, communicating, and eating (Reisberg, 1982); motor apraxia (the inability to plan and coordinate voluntary motor activity) 4. Progressively lowered stress threshold: catastrophic behaviors characterized by cognitive and social inaccessibility; purposeful wandering; violent, agitated, or anxious behavior; purposeless behavior; withdrawal or avoidance behavior such as belligerence; compulsive repetitive behavior; other cognitively or socially inaccessible behaviors

Degenerative neurologic diseases such as Parkinson's disease, Friedreich's ataxia, progressive supranuclear palsey, Wilson's disease, multiple sclerosis, and Huntington's chorea may cause cognitive loss.

Conditions such as tumors, subdural hematoma, trauma, or conditions causing insufficient oxygenation affect the structure or integrity of the brain. Some of these conditions may be amenable to medical treatment.

Disorders affecting the thyroid, liver, kidney, parathyroid, or adrenal glands will produce decreased cognitive function. Vitamin B_{12} deficiency will also produce dementia. Many of these dementias are reversible with treatment.

Infections such as tuberculosis; syphilis; and fungal, bacterial, and viral infections such as meningitis or encephalitis can produce dementia. Persons with acquired immune deficiency syndrome (AIDS) may develop an encephalitis in the later stages of the disease. Autoimmune diseases such as temporal arteritis and lupus erythematosis can also cause dementialike syndromes (Heston and White, 1983; Mace and Rabins, 1981; Mackey, 1982–1983; Office of Technological Assessment, 1987; Wolanin and Phillips, 1981).

Reversible Causes

Thought process alterations may also occur from pathophysiologic changes in biologic compounds; these alterations are reversible if treated. Usually referred to as delirium or acute confusional syndrome, these alterations in behavior have a rapid onset. They are transient and result in an altered state of awareness that is cognitively and socially inaccessible. The resident's normal thought processes are impaired and may present as disoriented,

inattentive, or functionally impaired. Socially inaccessible behavior implies those behaviors that prevent adequate communication between resident and staff, such as withdrawal, belligerence, noisy behavior, or purposeful wandering. Once the underlying medical condition is treated, the condition disappears (Lipowski, 1980; Wolanin and Phillips, 1981; Zarit, 1980). Acute confusional states can also be caused by stress, environmental factors, loss of meaning and pattern in routine, or alterations in self-image. Acute confusional syndrome occurs in both healthy people and those with dementia syndromes. The relationship of the etiologies of Altered Thought Processes is diagrammed in Figure 29.1.

PROGRESSION OF ALTERED THOUGHT PROCESSES: DEMENTIA

The dementing process is inexorably progressive. There are many descriptions of disease stages; however, for planning nursing care, four distinct stages of functional decline with SDAT are noted in Table 29.2.

Behavioral States

Clients with ATPD exhibit three main types of behavior: baseline or normative, anxious, and dysfunctional. Although these three behavioral states are present throughout the disease, normative behavior is replaced increasingly with anxious and dysfunctional behavior as the disease progresses. Baseline or normative behavior is

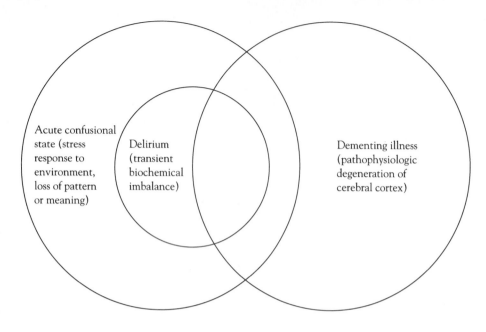

Figure 29.1

The relationship of etiologies of alterations in thought process. (Adapted from Wolanin M, Phillips L: Confusion: Prevention and Care. Mosby, 1981.)

generally a calm state incorporating the cognitive, affective, and conative behavioral losses with the premorbid personality and lifelong cultural and coping patterns. Behavioral symptoms from each cluster will be present in all clients with ATPD; however, clients will exhibit their symptoms differently. Presentation of symptoms is thought to be dependent on size and location of lesions within the cerebral cortex, premorbid personality, cultural and ethnic affiliations, and external demands and resources (Hall and Buckwalter, 1987).

Baseline Behavior Baseline behavior is functional behavior that is characterized by two features. The resident is cognitively accessible, meaning that there is a basic awareness of the environment and the ability to interact calmly and function within the limits of the neurologic deficit. The resident is also socially accessible, meaning he or she is able to communicate needs and respond to the communications of others.

Anxious Behavior Anxious behavior occurs when the resident feels stress. The resident may complain of feeling uneasy. Eye contact is usually lost, and there is a perceptible increase in psychomotor activity as the resident attempts to avoid offending stimuli: For example, the resident may attempt to leave or return to his or her room. Although anxious, the resident is still able to communicate with staff and family.

Dysfunctional Behavior Dysfunctional behavior results if the stress level is allowed to continue or increase. Catastrophic events are sudden changes from baseline behavior characterized by cognitive and social inaccessibility. The patient is unable to communicate effectively with

others and is unable to use the environment in a functionally appropriate manner (Wolanin and Phillips, 1981). Most catastrophic episodes are characterized by fearfulness, panic, and vigorous attempts to avoid offensive stimuli (Hall et al, 1986). Examples of catastrophic behavior are confusion, purposeful wandering, night wakening, "Sundowner's syndrome," agitation, fearfulness, panic, combativeness, or sudden withdrawal. These behaviors usually appear suddenly and last a relatively short period of time. They are rare in the early stages of the disease but increase in frequency and intensity with disease progression (Hall, 1986).

Several basic types of wandering occur in residents with ATP:SDAT. Not all wandering is purposeful and the result of a stress response. The types of wandering will be discussed in the section on interventions.

Caregivers often cite dysfunctional or catastrophic episodes as reasons to institutionalize patients in nursing homes or in acute care facilities. When the institutionalized patient becomes catastrophic, staff usually try to segregate and/or restrain the patient physically or chemically (Greene et al, 1985; Ridder, 1985; Wolanin and Phillips, 1981). These reactions need not occur (Hall et al, 1986; Wolanin and Phillips, 1981).

Catastrophic behaviors were recognized to be stress related in the early 1960s. In a survey of relocated elderly, Aldrich and Mendkoff (1963) discussed the role of stress in producing dysfunctional behavior. Lawton and Nahemow (1973) suggest that functional behavior is likely to occur when the external demands (stressors) on the older individual are adjusted to the level to which the person has adapted. It is logical that persons with ATPD need their environmental demands modified to compensate for their declining ability to adapt.

Table 29.2

Stages of Altered Thought Processes Due to Progressive Degeneration of the Cerebral Cortex

1. Forgetful—The client has begun to forget and lose things, expressing awareness of the problem and compensating for losses. This might compromise job performance, but a problem is not diagnosable at this time. Problems are usually attributed to stress, illness, or fatigue. Depression is not uncommon.

2. Confused—The client has difficulty with maintenance activities such as money management, legal affairs, occupational affairs, transportation and driving, home maintenance, housekeeping, and cooking. Family members are aware of problems and may seek medical attention for the client. Client may deny problem but gives frequent "clues" about "losing my mind." Client may become depressed and withdraw from occupational and social activities. Personality changes become evident. Client has difficulty functioning in strange environments, such as on vacation. Behaviors related to lowered stress threshold occur when under extreme stress, fatigue, change, or illness. Clients living alone may be placed in day care or long-term care because of compromised safety or inability to manage necessary tasks.

3. Ambulatory dementia—Functional losses in activities of daily living occur in approximately the following order: loss of bathing; grooming; choosing clothing; dressing; gait and mobility; toileting, communication, reading, and writing skills. The client begins to withdraw from the family group, becoming increasingly self-absorbed. Depression resolves, and the person appears to be unaware of losses at times. Stress-threshold behaviors are common, and the person may be up at night, wandering, confused, agitated, pacing and/or belligerent. Client may become combative or withdraw. Communication becomes increasingly difficult as the client has increasing difficulty in understanding written and spoken language and in finding words. The client may return to using a primary language, which also may be distorted. Frustration is very common. The client's ability to reason, recognize others, and plan for safety is impaired. Families usually place the client in long-term care during the ambulatory-dementia stage.

4. End stage—The client no longer ambulates and has little purposeful activity. Recognition of family, self in a mirror, or body parts is generally gone; however, the client may experience moments of lucidity. The client is mute or may scream or yell spontaneously. The client forgets how to eat, and loses much of his or her body weight. Problems associated with immobility, such as decubitus ulcers, urinary tract infections, contractures, and aspiration pneumonia are common. As the client becomes more vegetative, death usually results from pneumonia or another complication.

Source: Hall GR: Care of the patient with Alzheimer's disease living at home. *Nurs Clin North Am* 1988; 23(1):31–46.

Verwoerdt (1980) described catastrophic behaviors as primary anxiety resulting from an overwhelming influx of external or internal stimuli. The stimuli create psychologic states of stress to deal with the stressors when mastery is unobtainable, resulting in altered mental mechanisms and behavior patterns. Verwoerdt described the behavior created by primary anxiety as "primitive responses of painful displeasure." Mild cases may include restlessness, tension, or irritability. Severe cases are manifested by rage and defensive attempts to reestablish a stimulus barrier by avoidance behaviors such as repression, denial, magical thinking (ignoring danger), and acting out. Verwoerdt cites Cannon's concept of "fight or flight," suggesting that the situation may be resolved by adjusting and organizing the environment for the patient so that spatiotemporal relations remain constant, minimizing the loss of sense of mastery.

Stress and Coping

Adams and Lindemann (1974) identified four biologic mechanisms required for coping: movement, energy production, sensing, and cerebral integrating. If any of these mechanisms are compromised, individuals become disabled in their ability to cope with the environment. The first three mechanisms are normally somewhat compromised with the aging process; however, most changes occur slowly, and the person develops compensatory mechanisms. ATPD initially compromises the fourth mechanism. As the disease progresses, all mechanisms become deficient and place the individual at progressively higher risk for dysfunctional coping.

The role of stressors in producing dysfunctional behavior in the healthy person is diagrammed in a concep-

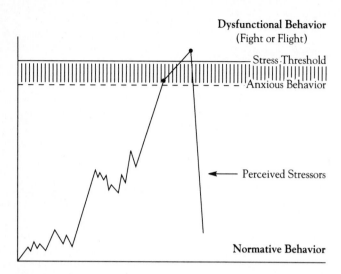

Figure 29.2

Stress threshold in normal individuals.

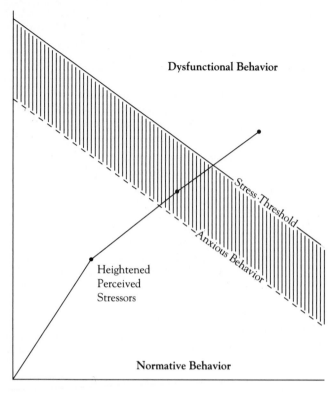

Figure 29.3

Progressively lowered stress threshold.

tual model in Figure 29.2. The model has been adapted for use with persons with ATPD. As the disease progresses and brain cells are lost, the victim becomes less able to receive and process stimuli and information. This, coupled with losses in special senses, mobility, slowed synaptic responses, and diminished energy-producing hormones associated with normal aging, acts to compromise the client's ability to adapt to stress and stimuli. A concomitant progressive decline in the stress threshold, which relies heavily on intact cerebral function, modifies the model as shown in Figure 29.3.

Clients with ATPD report increased levels of stress due to planning deficits, intolerance to multiple stimuli, and increased fatigue from processing information from their environment. This heightens the potential for anxiety, avoidance behavior, and catastrophic behavior (Hall and Buckwalter, 1987).

Woods (1982) cites numerous studies in which psychologists or psychiatrists manipulated the environments of SDAT patients in an attempt to produce increased levels of socialization or other desired responses. Those researchers who decreased environmental stimuli, such as moving the SDAT patients to small groups or decreasing the size of dining groups, noted increases in functional or baseline behavior. Researchers who increased stimuli by moving more chairs into a conversational circle found decreased functional behavior. In fact, the patients repeatedly moved the additional chairs out of the circle, returning them to the wall (Peterson et al, 1977). Lawton (1980) reported similar effects on the SDAT unit at the Philadelphia Geriatric Center. He found that when SDAT patients spent 20% of their time alone in their room, socialization and social contact increased the remaining 80% of the time. He also reported decreased incidence of catastrophic behavior, increased interest in external surroundings, increased meaningful nonsocial behavior, and

decreased need for nursing care. These findings correspond to Lawton and Simon's (1968) "Environmental Docility Hypothesis," which states that as competence decreases, external environmental factors become increasingly important determinants of behavior and affect.

ASSESSMENT

Identification of clients suffering from cognitive loss would assist nurses in determining which clients would benefit from environments and programs that promote safety and maximize function, and in which the patient functions comfortably (Rader and Doan, 1985). Correct assessment of cognitive loss would also facilitate identification of subjects for nursing research in settings where nurses have limited access to comprehensive medical diagnostic services for their clients, for example, rural long-term care settings (Goldenberg and Chiverton, 1984).

Nurses are often expected to provide care to clients experiencing progressive cognitive decline when no medical diagnosis of decline has been established. Studies demonstrate that many nurses have difficulty in recognizing ATPD and in discriminating between acute confusion, depression, or dementia (Lincoln, 1984). Currently, there are no research studies in nursing periodicals that tell how to assess for alterations in thought process. Most nurses rely on the physician's diagnosis of cognitive decline;

however, documentation of mental status may vary in the physician's records. Many clients with ATPD carry no diagnosis of dementing illness. Many are labeled as being senile or as suffering from hardening of the arteries, organic brain syndrome (OBS), probable strokes, or chronic brain syndrome, or their mental status is ignored in the medical record. The nondiagnosis of mental status changes may continue if clients are hospitalized because they may be admitted and treated for an acute problem and discharged without attention to mental status. Nurses are simply expected to plan and provide safe care regardless of the client's behavior.

Nurses have not demonstrated the ability to identify alterations in thought processes consistently. Palmateer and McCarthy (1985), in a study of nurses caring for the elderly, found that although 80% of the nurses felt responsible for evaluating their client's mental status, 36% stated they felt they lacked time to assess mental status of clients on admission. When the mental status examination was completed, the nurses misdiagnosed 72% of the confused clients.

Morgan (1985) reported similar results in a study evaluating the influence of resident and setting characteristics on nurses' perceptions of mental confusion. Subjects were less likely to be assessed as confused when residing in a large institution than when residing in a small one. Nurses were more likely to perceive confusion and communication difficulties if a subject was dependent in activities of daily living (ADLs) or if they were older than the median age for residents in that home. Results of these studies are strengthened by attitudinal surveys that find that nurses stereotype older people, preferring to care for younger clients. These ageist attitudes can affect the care provided and goals set for client recovery (Hatton, 1977; Knowles and Sarver, 1985).

ASSESSMENT TOOLS

Although there are no tools specific to the nursing diagnosis of ATPD, the nursing, medical, and allied health care literature contains numerous assessment instruments and scales for evaluating cognitive loss. Each is designed with a specific purpose. The "Set Test," the "Short Portable Mental Status Questionnaire" (SPMSQ), the "Mental Status Questionnaire" (MSQ), the "Information-Memory-Concentration Test," and the "Mini Mental Status Examination" (MMSE) are brief evaluations of current client mental status. Developed to assist physicians and trained health professionals to determine the need for medical evaluation of altered mental status, health providers occasionally use these tools in making a diagnosis of SDAT. However, this was not their intended purpose. All the instruments involve about 10 items that test recent and past memory and temporal orientation. Quick recall

and ability to abstract and calculate are tested on the SPMSQ and the MMSE. The MMSE also asks the client to carry out simple motor tasks. All are scored to determine the severity of the problem (Blessed et al, 1968; Folstein et al, 1975; Hays, 1984; Isaacs and Akhtar, 1972; Isaacs and Kennie, 1973; Kahn et al, 1963; Pfeiffer, 1975).

Each of the tests has limitations. All studies reviewed using the short assessments for evaluating mental status changes reported false positives with their use (Mattis, 1976; Morgan, 1985; Nagley, 1986; Palmateer and McCarthy, 1985; Winograd, 1984).

A review of instruments assessing for ATPD demonstrates particular problems for nurses assessing residents either on admission or during their stay in the long-term care setting. The first consideration is time and place of the assessment. If a new resident is admitted to the nursing home without a diagnosis of a dementing process, the nurse must establish the diagnosis of ATPD prior to assigning the client a room and roommate. In order to assure a smooth transition, the staff must know of the new resident's mental status prior to providing care. This can be accomplished by requesting a comprehensive medical evaluation for cognitive decline and a descriptive nursing assessment of client behavior and function prior to admission.

Preadmission Assessment

The initial assessment for ATPD should take place prior to admission to the long-term care facility; if possible, the assessment should be done in the client's home. A preadmission assessment in the client's home environment allows the nurse to observe the general stimulus level the client is used to and the family relationships within the environment. Is the home noisy, cluttered, quiet, and/or generally safe? If there are family members living with the client, what are the living arrangements? Does the client spend much time alone? Are family members supportive, or do they challenge the client's losses, finding them embarrassing or annoying? What are the interactions between client and family members?

An initial history of mental status changes should be obtained. Determining the client's premorbid personality, including educational level, occupation, hobbies, relationships with family prior to illness, daily routine, and methods used for relaxation, helps the nurse and staff in identifying the meaning of behavioral patterns and responses after admission. The onset of the mental status changes and any medical conditions that might be contributing to those changes, such as a history of heart disease or hypothyroidism, will help to determine the need for further medical evaluation prior to admission.

It is helpful to discuss the symptom clusters associated with ATP:SDAT with the family, as they will provide additional information when symptoms are mentioned. For example, many families assume memory loss is a normal part of the aging process and attribute other symptoms, such as inability to inhibit behavior, as willfulness. By providing behavioral examples for the family, the nurse will develop a comprehensive understanding of the client's symptom clusters and the global nature of the illness.

The family should be encouraged to describe dysfunctional behaviors, as the demented person will tend to exhibit the same pattern following institutionalization. The nurse will want to determine the onset and duration of stress-related behaviors and any precipitating factors, such as large social gatherings or concern about money. Stress-related events should be described, such as characteristics of wandering or combativeness. Measures to relieve these events should also be discussed. This will assist the nursing staff to determine if the client can be cared for in the nursing home environment and to prevent and/or prepare for such events in the future.

The client's functional level should be assessed both for basic activities of daily living and for maintenance activities such as socialization and daily routine. The nurse will use this information to determine the level of supervision, direction, and assistance required to accomplish bathing, dressing, ambulating, toileting, and eating. The family should be encouraged to share any special techniques or management strategies they use to ensure success.

Assessment of the family and/or caregiver should also take place. The psychosocial history of the family, how they coped with past problems, and perceptions of nursing home placement will all affect client behavior and the care plan. If the family perceives placement as a catastrophe, as failure on their part to care for a family member, or as the breakup of a family, the nurse and social worker must develop special measures to assist with resolving these issues.

Although the preadmission assessment ideally is conducted in the client's home, sometimes this is not feasible, and the assessment may be conducted in a hospital or in the long-term care center. It should not be eliminated because the information gained from the assessment will be used in planning care and providing information to at least the next two shifts of nursing staff following the client's admission to the facility. If the potential resident with ATPD has been in a hospital and/or another long-term care facility, it is helpful to have a policy of gaining a written consent for the director of nursing or a designated nurse to review the nursing notes. The nursing notes will provide clear documentation of the types of behavior observed and potential care or safety problems that might be anticipated.

The preadmission assessment is also a good time to explain the nursing home programs, such as daily routines, specific therapies, and institutional policies, to the client and family. Potential for family involvement with care, programs, and family support mechanisms should be discussed. The preadmission assessment is an especially important event in developing a relationship with the family of a resident with ATPD. Both staff and family need to acknowledge that there is no magic for caring for these difficult residents and a team effort is needed. If family cooperation appears to be a continuing problem, other alternatives for care may need to be discussed (Buckwalter and Hall, 1987).

Ongoing Assessment

Following admission to the facility, assessment continues in several areas. The first level is getting to know the impaired resident. Interviewing the resident with ATPD takes time and special interpersonal skills. Plan to interview the resident early in the day, as fatigue will diminish the resident's ability to attend and communicate. The interview should take place in a quiet area, free from distractions. Make sure that the area does not restrict the resident's movement and that any physical needs are met prior to the assessment. Speak clearly using simple sentences and a low voice pitch. Touch can be used to indicate sincerity and empathy. When phrases are not understood, they should be repeated exactly. The resident with ATPD requires more time to process information and, therefore, to respond. Observe nonverbal behavior while waiting for the resident to respond, and establish the presence of sensory deficits in vision and hearing.

During this assessment, the nurse determines the resident's ability to comprehend the environment and the resident's feelings of safety and worth. Frequently, the interviewer discovers the resident's ability to understand the disease process and how it affects family relationships. These insights help in planning meaningful activities and determining strategies for coping with fearful episodes.

Another aspect of assessment is a continuous evaluation of functional level, including the resident's participation in activities and socialization with other residents and family. This helps to determine disease progression and plan care according to advancement of the disease. For example, during the confused stage of the illness, the resident can rely on self-initiated memory prosthetics such as lists and calendars. During the ambulatory-demented phase, the client must rely on supportive people as reminders.

The third area of ongoing assessment is evaluation of the resident's physical health. Because of the age of most residents with ATPD, it is common to have multiple interacting pathologies with atypical symptom presentation. Quite often, increased confusion may be the only symptom of pain, discomfort, or acute illness. The nurse should physically assess the resident with ATPD on admission to establish a baseline and should assess again every time confusion increases or other symptoms present. Medication use should be evaluated weekly or biweekly depending on the resident's medical condition, since one of the most common causes of acute confusion is medication interactions and reactions (Wolanin and Phillips, 1981).

A fourth area of ongoing assessment is a continuation of evaluation of the family members. By assessing the frequency of family visits and the quality of interactions, the nurse may determine family distress. The family may need additional support or counseling to adjust to the resident's continuing decline and may need assistance in making the nursing home experience and visits easier to deal with.

The fifth area of assessment is the evaluation of stress-related behaviors. When the resident becomes confused or combative, the nurse should determine what caused the behavior in order to prevent reoccurrence. What, if anything, was different about the resident's routine or interactions prior to the event? Identification of causative factors of stress-related behavior will assist the nurse to modify the plan of care to prevent future occurrence (Hall et al, 1986). These factors will be discussed further in the section on interventions. The resident must also be continually assessed for nursing diagnoses that occur concomitantly with the diagnosis of ATPD.

CASE STUDY

Altered Thought Processes: Dementia

Norman was a 72-year-old retired English professor who resided with his wife, Dorothy, in their home of 40 years in a small midwestern college town. Over a period of 3 years, Dorothy noticed Norman becoming increasingly forgetful, disorganized, and distant. Previously methodical, Norman began to make mistakes in the checkbook, miss appointments, and lose possessions. His driving and temper became erratic, problems he blamed on Dorothy. He stopped paying bills, fearful that "they" would take his money. One day, while trying to discuss an article in the newspaper, Dorothy came to the realization that Norman could no longer read. Fearful of the worst, she sought medical attention for Norman.

Norman was diagnosed with senile dementia of the Alzheimer's type by a local physician. Seeking a second opinion, Dorothy took Norman to the medical center in the large university town in which their daughter lived. The diagnosis of SDAT was confirmed. Their daughter, Sue, convinced Norman and Dorothy to move to the university town to be near them. Dorothy sold her home and moved them both to a small apartment near her daughter.

The move caused Norman's symptoms to worsen. In his familiar surroundings he was able to manage on a daily basis without having to plan all activities. Within 6 months he required assistance bathing and dressing. Norman was unable to tolerate the unpacked boxes from the moving, so Dorothy stayed up nights to unpack while he slept. In order to gain rest, Dorothy located a companion to stay with Norman during the day, but, after the first day, he would not allow the companion in the house.

Normal began to think that pictures of people on the wall were real. Television made him think there were children in the room. In fear, he broke two mirrors. One night Norman woke Dorothy repeatedly, fearful that the apartment was on fire. After 3 days of this fearful behavior, he handed her a book in which he had found a picture of children sitting around a campfire, and he screamed "Fire, fire!"

In the next 2 weeks, Norman began to wander away from the apartment. Fearful for his safety and exhausted from lack of sleep, Dorothy contacted a local nursing home. After much anguish and without the support of friends or children, Dorothy decided she had to place Norman in a care facility. The nurse and social worker made the initial assessment at the couple's apartment. A nursing diagnosis of Altered Thought Process: Dementia was established. A thorough assessment and social history were also completed.

NURSING INTERVENTIONS

Interventions for residents with ATPD are based on the provision of a supportive environment that maximizes their level of safe function and comfort within the nursing home community without compromising the needs, rights, and quality of life for lucid residents. This includes enhancing the quality of visits by family and friends through interventions that increase their awareness, understanding, and comfort. Increased visitor comfort will diminish stressors for the resident.

Maximizing functional level is obtained by reducing stress, thus preventing excess disability. Excess disability may be defined as a reversible deficit that is more disabling than the primary condition. Excess disability exists when the disturbance of functioning is greater than might be accounted for by basic physical illness or cerebral pathology (Dawson et al, 1986). The most common sources of excess disability for residents with ATPD are listed in Table 29.3. They may occur alone or in combination.

Although most dementing illnesses that cause Altered Thought Processes are progressive, the rate of behavioral change is not consistent. Most residents exhibit good and bad days rather than a single behavioral pattern. "Bad days" may be attributed to the presence of internal or external stressors that serve to worsen symptoms, most

Table 29.3

Common Causes of Excess Disability

1. Fatigue
2. Change in routine, caregiver, or environment, such as holiday decorations or a visit home
3. Competing or misleading stimuli, or high stimulus activity, such as a band concert, lunch in the crowded dining room, prolonged visit from family, television, mirror images, or potentially frightening pictures of people or animals
4. Stress or frustration from trying to function beyond limits imposed by ATP:SDAT or others, such as trying to participate in reality orientation therapy; trying to bathe, choose clothing, or dress when no longer able to accomplish independently; having other residents, staff, or others constantly telling resident he or she is wrong or to try harder; trying to relearn lost skills; or being physically restrained
5. Physical illness, discomfort, pain, or medication reaction

Source: Hall G, Buckwalter K: Progressively lowered stress threshold: A conceptual model for care of adults with Alzheimer's disease. *Arch Psychiatr Nurs* (Dec)1987; 1(6):399–406.

without worsening the pathophysiology of the disease. These stressors produce excess disability and may be controlled by nursing interventions to prevent or eliminate behavioral complications.

The goals of maximizing resident safety, comfort, and function and preventing complications associated with chronic illness and increasing immobility require attention to all details within the resident's environment. To accomplish this, the staff must assume a prosthetic or helping posture, compensating for the resident's losses rather than increasing the resident's stress levels by encouraging reeducation or rehabilitation for lost abilities. When the staff assumes responsibility for compensating for lost abilities, resident stress is diminished and some spontaneous increase in level of function is observed. This increase may be attributed to the resolution of excess disability by elimination of stress (Dawson et al, 1986; Hall and Buckwalter, 1987).

One method of gaining staff and family understanding of the impact of excess disability is to use an analogy of an amputee. Most adults can imagine a person who has lost a leg. When asked to envision the amputee being instructed to walk without benefit of a prosthesis, crutches, or other device, most will understand the frustration and anger the amputee would experience after repeated falls. Residents with ATPD experience the loss of cerebral cortex, which impairs their ability to integrate sensory input, use intellect, and respond to their environment in the manner anticipated by society. When these losses are challenged rather than supported, residents complain of frustration, anger, fear, and increased awareness of their limitations.

This prosthetic/orthotic approach to care begins in the confused stage of the illness. During this phase residents rely on memory prosthetics such as lists, calendars, and clocks to negotiate in their environment. As the disease progresses, the resident must rely increasingly on people to provide cues that remind them of when, where, and how to function.

Short-range goals are developed to compensate for specific losses and to prevent behavioral complications. During the confused phase of the disease, clients begin to experience frustration, anxiety, and an occasional stress reaction. Therefore, in planning care for the client, the nurse can decide how much stimulus and stress the resident is able to manage by listening to client reactions and observing for anxiety-related behavior. Anxiety-related behavior might include an increase in psychomotor activity, increased or decreased verbalization, a loss of eye contact, complaints of feeling uncomfortable or nervous, and/or an attempt to avoid or retreat from the offensive situation (Nowakowski, 1985).

In planning care for the person with ATPD, the nurse assumes the following:

1. The resident exists in a 24-hour continuum. Care cannot be planned or evaluated on an 8-hour shift basis. If the resident has a problem during the night shift, some changes need to be implemented during the day shift.
2. The confused or agitated client is not comfortable and should be regarded as frightened. All residents have the right to be comfortable.
3. All behavior is rooted and has meaning; therefore, all catastrophic and stress-related behaviors have a cause.
4. All humans require some control over their person and their environment and need some degree of unconditional positive regard.
5. There are certain basic caring functions that, because of the need to consider the good of all residents, the institution cannot always provide. Therefore, the

institution must coordinate care with the societal structure (eg, family unit) that can provide for those unmet needs, for example the provision of special celebrations for a resident on a religious holiday (Buckwalter and Hall, 1987).

The principles of planning care for residents with ATP: SDAT are as follows:

1. The staff should work to maximize the resident's level of safe functioning by supporting cognitive, affective, conative, and stress-threshold losses, using staff and environment as memory prosthetics.
2. The staff should communicate with the resident both verbally and nonverbally in a manner that conveys unconditional positive regard.
3. Behaviors that indicate anxiety should be used in determining limits of levels of activity and stimuli.
4. Staff and family should be taught to listen to the resident to determine reasons for activity and behavior. Some behavior will be rooted in the resident's early life. Staff must, therefore, have insight into the resident's social history.
5. The environment may be the cause of stress and can be modified to support losses and enhance safety.
6. Staff must provide ongoing education, support, care, and problem solving for family and significant others.

The nurse should plan interventions that are appropriate for the resident's level of coping. The use of a consistent routine has been shown to be effective in reducing stress, as the resident does not need to rely on planning skills for most activities (Schwab et al, 1982). Rest periods are provided on a regular basis to compensate for the increased fatigue level and to allow stress levels to decrease. These rests do not potentiate night wakening. Without measures to diminish stress and fatigue, the resident's day might be diagrammed as shown in Figure 29.4.

During a typical day the resident experiences high stress levels when performing the morning activities of daily living. Rather than being afforded the opportunity to rest, compensating for fatigue and high stress, the resident may be sent to activities or a therapy session. At lunchtime, the resident enters the communal dining room, where there may be 50 or more residents. Nurses are passing medications; people are passing trays; assistants are feeding other residents; others are collecting trays; music may be playing and the general noise level is loud. The fatigued resident with ATPD attempts to leave. This is an example of avoidance behavior stemming from anxiety. A nursing assistant returns the resident to the table where there are three or four people talking and a tray with multiple food choices. The resident eats little of the meal and leaves.

The resident may get some opportunity for rest in the afternoon, but may have visitors or another activity. Late in the day or during the night, the resident crosses the lowered stress threshold and becomes dysfunctional. The resident is confused, agitated, combative, or up at night.

Using a care plan that compensates for fatigue and other losses, the resident's stress level may be diagrammed as in Figure 29.5. The resident's stress level is reduced in accordance with his or her ability to tolerate activity without anxiety. Stress-related dysfunctional behavior is prevented if the stress threshold is not surpassed.

Special Problems

Combative Reactions Although a care plan is identified, anticipate that additional problems and needs will arise for the resident with ATPD as the pathophysiologic process progresses. One of the more common problems to arise in the long-term care setting is the combative reaction. Combative episodes create the potential for injury to resident, staff, other residents, and visitors and increase fear of all residents with ATP:SDAT. This may promote the permanent isolation of the combative resident from other residents and visitors; exclusion from normative social activities; increased use of tranquilizing medications, which tend to limit function; the use of soft tie restraints, which limit mobility and worsen resident fear; and staff fear of the resident, which may limit the amount of contact with the combative resident. In some states a combative resident must be discharged from the long-term care center once an episode involving another resident has occurred.

In assessing a combative episode the nurse should recognize that in most residents with ATPD, combative

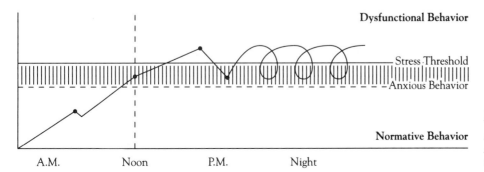

Figure 29.4

A typical day for the resident with ATP:SDAT in an unstructured long-term care program.

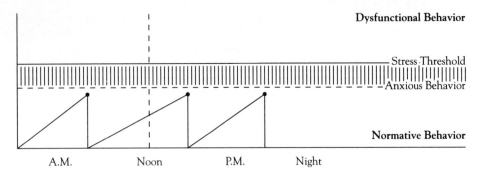

Figure 29.5

Planned activity levels for the resident with ATP:SDAT.

behavior is the last resort for coping with fear and frustration. The cause of the episode should be determined and eliminated, if possible. Common causes of combative episodes, in addition to those listed in Table 29.3, are listed below:

- Negative, restrictive feedback from staff, residents, and visitors
- Restraints
- Misinterpretation of environmental stimuli, especially material on television
- Misinterpretation of boundaries and ownership
- Nonrecognition of familiar persons or mistaking other residents for spouse, family members, or persons who trouble them
- Fear of water or resistance to an activity such as bathing

It is essential to assess the situation and control it quickly to prevent injury and minimize the amount of intervention required, such as medication. The combative resident should be quickly separated from offensive stimuli with as little contact to the agitated resident as possible. For example, if the combative resident is in another resident's room, the other resident might be asked to step outside while the staff works with the combative resident. If the incident involves a staff member, it is best to have another staff member deal with the crisis calmly under the direction of the nurse.

The combative resident should be regarded as frightened, and interventions should focus on removing fear. Allow the combative resident to maintain a sense of personal control through the use of retained social graces. Statements by staff such as "I could use a glass of juice" or "I know this doesn't look familiar, but this is the room I reserved for you this evening" can help the resident to regain a sense of mastery without reinforcing that they are confused or wrong again.

Another successful technique is to focus on the feeling behind the action. "It must be frustrating to have people tell you you're wrong." "Mrs. Jones does resemble your wife. Are you lonely for her now?" This method provides the resident the opportunity to state feelings and needs that may have been buried. It is often surprising how

articulate a resident with a communication deficit can be when agitated.

Residents who repeatedly become combative or agitated, despite reductions in stimuli and increases in rest periods, may require use of a tranquilizer or might benefit from a special care environment designed for persons with ATPD.

Persons who have used violent behavior as a lifelong coping mechanism for stress may present a significant ongoing problem with combative behavior. The resident who has a history of spouse abuse, child abuse, or other regular violent acts may use violence as a method of controlling others and coping with the environment. This is characterized by two features. The resident usually expresses no fear when combative and tends to be combative with people as they become more familiar. Lifelong patterns of violence should be identified prior to the resident's admission to the facility and a determination made concerning the facility's ability to provide care without compromising the rights of other residents.

Wandering Another special care problem is wandering. Wandering is generally considered to be leaving the nursing unit or nursing home without supervision or sanctions from the staff. Wandering differs from pacing in that the resident actually elopes from the specified environment and is generally considered to be at risk for injury. There are several reasons why residents wander (Rader and Doan, 1985). They may be following environmental cues, acting on a reminiscent delusion such as needing to go to work, or feeling frightened and trying to escape. Care must be taken to assess the behavioral characteristics of the resident who wanders in order to determine appropriate interventions that do not impose excessive restraint.

Interventions from the diagnosis Potential for Injury should be reviewed (see Chapter 3); however, the nurse must educate staff and family that the resident will be unable to assess and self-monitor for danger and potential injury. There are increasing numbers of sophisticated alarms, door locks, and resident monitoring systems available to assist with preventing or minimizing injury to residents who wander. The nurse must recognize that the best alarm only alerts staff that injury may have already occurred. Staff must be trained to respond to alarm systems immediately. A response time of a minute or less may not be adequate to prevent a fall down stairs at a fire exit. Wandering drills and regular inservice programs need to be presented on the safety needs of residents who wander.

Additional considerations for residents who wander include having current pictures available to provide searchers for a lost resident, encouraging visitors and staff to remove keys from their cars, and educating family visitors on the problem of wandering. In order to bypass misunderstandings about negligence once wandering has occurred, some facilities are having families sign consents indicating they understand policies not to restrain wanderers unnecessarily.

The Family

Families of residents with ATPD often require special attention. Frequently they are grieving the loss of a family member to a disease they do not understand. The disease process is usually long, leaving the family—especially the spouse—in a period of continuing crisis. Old roles become inadequate as the resident's ability to recognize, communicate, function, and judge safety declines. The family experiences moral dilemmas with placement, advocacy, and decision making about terminal care without helpful input from the client with ATPD, who may refuse in-home services, nursing home placement, or any help from family or professionals (Mace and Rabins, 1981).

Many long-term care facilities have found that support groups for family members help to ease stress. Peer counseling from one trained family member to others is another successful intervention. Be aware of the family burden, and offer empathy and support throughout. Some families may find tips on how to visit helpful, such as preplanning an activity to use during the visit. Others might want to attend care-planning meetings. It may be helpful to have one primary nurse to interact with a resident's family, developing a bond that will help both family and staff provide better care for the resident.

CASE STUDY

Nursing Interventions

Returning to the nursing home after the preadmission assessment, the nurse met with both the day-shift staff and the evening-shift staff on the unit where Norman would be housed. The staff was briefed on Norman's background and behavioral symptoms. A tentative case plan was identified, consisting of having Norman spend the first several days in a consistent routine on the nursing unit until he adapted to the stimulus level within the facility. He was admitted to a unit with several confused residents, as these residents tend to seek each other out, providing positive regard for each other. Norman would have rest periods at 9:30 A.M. and 1:30 P.M. in his own recliner in his room. His room was kept free of misleading pictures and television, and all mirrors were removed.

The morning of admission, Sue brought her father's recliner and personal belongings to the facility. Norman was admitted before lunch in order to take advantage of his better time of day. The staff oriented Norman to his room and hall, serving lunch to him and Dorothy in his room. Dorothy then joined the director of nursing for a family orientation. She was encouraged to visit freely but to choose which time of day was best and incorporate it into Norman's routine. Dorothy was introduced to a family member of another resident with ATPD who would remain her peer counselor throughout Norman's stay. Dorothy was encouraged to attend care-planning sessions and the monthly family support group. She was encouraged to bring care problems to the director of nursing, social worker, and/or administrator when they arose.

On admission, Norman was taking large doses of the neuroleptic medication Mellaril 225 mg per day. After several days, he appeared to be able to handle access to the entire facility, including the dining room. When shown the facility, he had difficulty walking and became incontinent of urine. That night he was awake and confused. The next day he left the facility repeatedly. The nurses placed two strips of yellow tape at either end of the hallway to his nursing unit. Norman stopped the director of nursing in the hall and pointed to the tapes, saying "At last, I know my boundaries. I won't wander off now." Norman did not wander again.

The night wakening continued. The nurses made a decision to feed Norman at a small table in his room with two other residents. Night wakening ceased. Over the months that ensued, Norman's Mellaril was slowly decreased until he became agitated without it when the stimulus level and level of activity could no longer be reduced. He was then maintained on 25 mg at bedtime. As the medication was reduced, Norman's gait and continence improved. This improvement, however, was not permanent.

Two years later Norman ceased to ambulate. After 10 more months of dependent care, he became unable to eat. Dorothy agonized over the decision to pass a nasogastric tube. With support from the staff, she decided on the tube. One year later Norman died. Dorothy was unable to sever her ties with the nursing home staff. Surprised by her grieving at Norman's death, for which she had prayed so long, Dorothy has become a peer counselor, helping other families.

OUTCOMES

The plans of care discussed in this chapter may be evaluated objectively to assess resident comfort and safety using the following measures:

- Hours of sleep at night should increase, and episodes of confused night wakening should decrease.
- Resident weight should stabilize or increase without special supplements. Food intake from the tray will increase and caloric expenditure will decrease as pacing and agitation disappear.
- Episodes of combative behavior will be eliminated. Agitated episodes will diminish or be eliminated
- Resident socialization will increase, including voluntary participation in small-group activities.
- Functional level may improve briefly as excess disability disappears.
- Sedative and tranquilizer needs will decrease.
- Once families understand the care program, satisfaction with care and empathy with staff will increase (Hall et al, 1986).

SUMMARY

Care of the client with Altered Thought Processes: Dementia due to progressive degeneration of the cerebral cortex is one of the largest challenges for geriatric nurses. Wracked with behavioral alterations, the client may be unable to communicate needs and wishes. Clients may refuse all attempts at care or assistance for reasons that are not apparent to the family or nurse.

To decrease the burden, there are few techniques that have been substantiated consistently by nursing or other research. Such research, when undertaken, is compromised because of the difficulty of evaluating results in subjects with communication and reasoning deficits. Subject selection and attrition are also problems because clients are often unable to consent to be studied or regress beyond a point where they can participate in a study.

It is helpful to plan nursing care for these clients using a conceptual model, which focuses interventions and provides outcomes for measurement. Progressively lowered stress threshold is a model that encourages caregivers to individualize care by using client responses to determine activity tolerance. Already in use in client homes, integrated nursing homes, special care units, hospitals, and adult day programs in the Midwest, the model has been shown to be an effective guide to increasing client comfort and minimizing behaviors that might have required medication or physical restraint.

References

Adams J, Lindemann C: Coping with long term disability. In: *Coping and Adaptation.* Coelho G, Hamburg D, Adams J (editors). Basic Books, 1974.

Aldrich C, Mendkoff E: Relocation of the aged and disabled: A mortality study. *J Am Geriatr Soc* 1963; 11:185–194.

Ballinger B: Cluster analysis of symptoms in elderly demented patients. *British J Psychiatry* 1982; 140(3):257–262.

Blessed G, Tomlinson B, Roth M: The associations between quantitative measures of dementia and senile change in the cerebral grey matter of elderly subjects. *British J Psychiatry* 1968; 114(3):797–811.

Buckwalter K, Hall G: Families of the institutionalized older adult: A neglected resource. In: *Aging, Health, and Family: Long Term Care.* Brubaker T (editor). Sage, 1987.

Burns E, Buckwalter K: Pathophysiology and etiology of Alzheimers disease. *Nurs Clin North Am* 1988; 23(1):11–29.

Carnevali D, Patrick M: Health care for elderly: Nursing's area of accountability. In: *Nursing Management for the Elderly.* Carnevali D (editor). Lippincott, 1979.

Carpenito L: *Nursing Diagnosis: Application to Clinical Nursing Practice.* Lippincott, 1983.

Carroll-Johnson R (editor): *Classification of Nursing Diagnoses: Proceedings of the Eighth Conference.* Lippincott, 1989.

Coffman T: Under what conditions is relocation stress fatal to geriatric patients? Paper presented at the meeting of the Eastern Psychological Association, Philadelphia, April 1983.

Cox K: Milieu therapy. *Geriatr Nurs* 1985; 6(3):152–154.

Dawson P et al: Preventing excess disability in patients with Alzheimer's disease. *Geriatr Nurs* 1986; 7(6):298–330.

Edelson J, Lyons W: *Institutionalized Care of the Mentally Impaired Elderly.* Van Nos Reinhold, 1985.

Folstein M, Folstein S, McHugh P: Mini-mental state: A practical method for grading the cognitive state of patients for the clinician. *J Psychiatr Res* 1975; 12:189–198.

Glosser G, Wexler W: Participant's evaluation of educational/support groups for families of patients with Alzheimer's disease and other dementias. *Gerontologist* 1985; 25(3):232–236.

Goldenberg B, Chiverton P: Assessing behavior: The nurse's mental status exam. *Geriatr Nurs* 1984; 5(2):94–98.

Gottfries C et al: A new rating scale for dementia syndromes. *Gerontology* 1982; 28(SZ):20–31.

Greene J et al: Management of Alzheimer's disease. *J Tenn Med Assoc* 1985; 78(1):16–23.

Hall GR: Care of the patient with Alzheimer's disease living at home. *Nurs Clin North Am* 1988; 23(1):31–46.

Hall G, Buckwalter K: Care of the complex client with progressive alterations in thought processes. In: *Home Care Situations of Complex Clients.* Strandell C, Kaza-Matusinic (editors). Aspen, 1989.

Hall G, Buckwalter K: Progressively lowered stress threshold: A conceptual model for care of adults with Alzheimer's disease. *Arch Psychiatr Nurs* (Dec) 1987; 1(6):399–406.

Hall G, Kirschling M, Todd S: Sheltered freedom: The creation of a special care Alzheimer's unit in an intermediate level facility. *Geriatr Nurs* 1986; 7(3):132–136.

Hatton J: Nurses' attitudes towards care of the aged: Relationship to nursing care. *J Gerontol Nurs* 1977; 3(3):21–26.

Hays A: The set test to screen mental status quickly. *Geriatr Nurs* 1984; 5(2):96–97.

Heaney L: Nursing goals in Alzheimer's disease. *Contemp Admin Long-Term Care* 1983; 6(7):26–27.

Heston L, White J: *Dementia: A Practical Guide to Alzheimer's Disease and Related Illnesses.* Freeman, 1983.

Holden U, Woods R: *Reality Orientation: Psychological Approaches to the Confused Elderly.* Churchill Livingstone, 1982.

Isaacs B, Akhtar A: The set test: A rapid test of mental functions in old people. *Age Ageing* 1972; 1(11):222–226.

Isaacs B, Kennie A: The set test as an aid to detection of dementia in old people. *British J Psychiatry* 1973; 123(10):467–470.

Kahn R et al: Brief objective measure for determination of mental status of the aged. *Am J Psychiatry* 1963; 117(2):326–328.

Kim M, McFarland G, McLane A: *Classification of Nursing Diagnoses: Proceedings of the Fifth National Conference.* Mosby, 1984.

Knowles L, Sarver V: Attitudes affect quality of care. *J Gerontol Nurs* 1985; 11(8):35–39.

Lawton M: Psychosocial and environmental approaches to the care of senile dementia patients. In: *Psychopathy in the Aged.* Cole J, Barrett J (editors). Raven Press,1980.

Lawton M, Nahemow L: Ecology and the aging process. In: *Psychology of Adult Development and Aging.* Eisdorfer C, Lawton M (editors). American Psychological Association, 1973.

Lawton M, Simon B: The ecology of social relationships in shared housing for the elderly. *Gerontologist* 1968; 8:108–115.

Lincoln R: What do nurses know about confusion in the aged? *J Gerontol Nurs* 1984; 10(8):26–33.

Lipowski Z: Organic mental disorders: Introduction and review of syndromes. In: *Comprehensive Textbook of Psychiatry.* Kaplan H, Freedman A, Sudock B (editors). Williams and Wilkins, 1980.

Mace N: Facets of dementia. *J Gerontol Nurs* 1984; 10(2):92.

Mace N, Rabins P: *The 36 Hour Day.* Johns Hopkins University Press, 1981.

Mackey M: OBS and nursing care. *J Gerontol Nurs. Alzheimer's Disease: An In-Depth Report 1982–1983;* (Suppl): 3–11.

Mattis S: Mental status examination for organic mental syndrome in the elderly patient. In: *Geriatric Psychiatry.* Bellack R, Karasu B (editors). Grune and Stratton, 1976.

Morgan D: Nurses' perceptions of mental confusion in the elderly: Influence of resident and setting characteristics. *J Health Soc Sci* 1985; 26(2):102–112.

Nagley S: Predicting and preventing confusion in your patients. *J Gerontol Nurs* 1986; 12(3):27–31.

Nowakowski L: Accent capabilities in disorientation. *J Gerontol Nurs* 1985; 11(9):15–20.

Office of Technological Assessment: *Losing a Million Minds: Confronting the Tragedy of Alzheimer's Disease and Other Dementias.* U.S. Congress, 1987.

Palmateer L, McCarthy J: Do nurses know when patients have cognitive deficits? *J Gerontol Nurs* 1985; 11(2):6–17.

Palmer M: Alzheimer's disease and critical care. *J Gerontol Nurs. Alzheimer's Disease: An In-Depth Report 1982–1983;* (Suppl): 13–16.

Peterson R et al: The effects of furniture arrangements on the behavior of geriatric patients. *Behav Ther* 1977; 8:464–467.

Pfeiffer E: A short portable mental status questionnaire for assessment of organic brain deficit in the elderly patients. *J Am Geriatr Soc* 1975; 23(10):433–441.

Rader J, Doan J: How to decrease wandering, a form of agenda behavior. *Geriatr Nurs* 1985; 6(4):196–199.

Rafal R: Clustered losses in Alzheimer's disease. Unpublished paper, 1982.

Reisberg B: The global deterioration scale for assessment of primary degenerative dementia. *Am J Psychiatry* 1982; 139(9):1136–1139.

Reisberg B: An ordinal functional assessment tool for Alzheimer-type dementia. *Hosp Community Psychiatry* 1985; 36(6):593–595.

Ridder M: Nursing update on Alzheimer's disease. *J Neurosurg Nurs* 1985; 17(3):190–200.

Schafer S: Modifying the environment. *Geriatr Nurs* 1985; 6(3):157–159.

Schneider E, Erm M: Alzheimer's disease: Research highlights. *Geriatr Nurs* 1985; 6(3):136–138.

Schwab M, Rader M, Doan J: Relieving the fear and anxiety in dementia. *J Gerontol Nurs* 1985; 11(6):8–15.

VanHoesen G, Damasio A: Neural correlates of cognitive impairment in Alzheimer's disease. In: *The Handbook of Physiology: Higher Functions of the Nervous System.* Plumb F (editor). Washington, D C: Mathers Foundation, 1987.

Venn R: The Sando clinical assessment geriatric (SCAG) scale: A general purpose psychogeriatric rating scale. *Gerontology* 1983; 29(3):185–198.

Verwoerdt A: Anxiety, dissociative and personality disorders in the elderly. In: *Handbook of Geriatric Psychiatry.* Busse E, Blazer D (editors). Van Nos Reinhold, 1980.

Winograd C: Mental status tests and the capacity for self care. *J Am Geriatr Soc* 1984; 32(1):49–55.

Wolanin M, Phillips L: *Confusion: Prevention and Care.* Mosby, 1981.

Woods R: The psychology of aging: Assessment of defects and their management. Pages 68–113 in: *The Psychology of Later Life.* Levy R, Post F (editors). Blackwell, 1982.

Zarit S: *Aging and Mental Disorders: Psychological Approaches to Assessment and Treatment.* Free Press, 1980.

30

Pain

PATRICIA CLINTON, MA, RN
JO ANN ELAND, PhD, RN

BROWNING (1864) WROTE "GROW OLD ALONG WITH me—the best is yet to be." However, for many elderly persons at home or confined to institutional facilities, the "best" will never arrive because of the specter of pain that is their constant companion. However, pain and discomfort do not have to be part of the aging process. Through the use of the nursing process, nurses can make a difference in the quality of life for the elderly client.

It is important to recognize that the discussion of the elderly person's pain experience is not limited to the dependent elderly. The majority of the elderly population (approximately 65%) live in some type of private or semiprivate residence (Blazer and Siegler, 1984). Despite the common misconception that many elderly are cognitively impaired, organic mental disorders affect only between 5% and 10% of persons over age 65 (Blazer and Siegler, 1984:112), although many elderly may be depressed.

The purpose of this chapter is to provide nurses with the information by which to understand, assess, and intervene in the elderly person's pain experience. When appropriate, specific suggestions for the dependent elderly or those with cognitive impairment will be made. The reader is also referred to Chapter 29 on Altered Thought Processes for further clarification.

CONCEPTUAL DEFINITION

There are many definitions of pain, conceptual and operational, that attempt to describe the unique and subjective phenomenon of pain. The complexity of the pain experience is attributable to the interrelationship of the physiologic and psychologic (including the cognitive and motivational aspects) components of pain.

Sternbach (1968) defines pain as a personal, private sensation of hurt that protects the body by signaling the presence of current or impending tissue damage. Although this definition is useful, it does not explain how the pain experience can vary so greatly among individuals.

Melzack and Wall (1965) proposed the gate control theory of pain that recognizes how cognitive, motivational, and physiologic factors combine to create a unique individual pain response. The theory recognizes the importance of an individual's past pain experience, culture, and attitudes in the overall perception and response to pain.

It is important that nurses who work with the elderly incorporate an operational definition of pain in their standard of care. McCaffery's (1979;11) definition of pain focuses on the individual experience of pain: "Pain is whatever the experiencing person says it is, existing whenever he says it does." When pain is operationalized in this way, the nurse has the freedom to employ many forms of therapy to relieve the patient's discomfort.

The nursing diagnosis Altered Comfort: Pain was accepted at the Fourth National Conference of the North American Nursing Diagnosis Association (NANDA) in 1980 (Kim and Moritz, 1982). At the Seventh Conference the related diagnosis Altered Comfort: Chronic Pain was accepted (McLane, 1987). At the Eighth Conference the labels Altered Comfort: Pain and Altered Comfort: Chronic Pain were changed to Pain and Chronic Pain, respectively (Carroll-Johnson, 1989). Table 30.1 presents these diagnoses, contrasting NANDA related factors and defining characteristics with those emphasized in this chapter.

SIGNIFICANCE OF PAIN FOR THE ELDERLY

To assess or plan appropriate interventions for the elderly person in pain, the nurse must understand the significance of pain for the individual. For an elder with a long history of chronic pain, episodes of acute pain may be underreported. Coping mechanisms appropriate for chronic pain are not usually beneficial in episodes of acute

Table 30.1

Etiologies/Related Factors and Defining Characteristics of Pain and Chronic Pain

DIAGNOSIS: PAIN (CARROLL-JOHNSON, 1989)

Definition:	A state in which an individual experiences and reports the presence of severe discomfort or an uncomfortable sensation
Defining Characteristics:	*Major:* Subjective: Communication (verbal or coded) of pain descriptors. Objective: Guarding behavior, protective; self-focusing; narrowed focus (altered time perception, withdrawal from social contact, impaired thought processes); distraction behavior (moaning, crying, pacing, seeking out other people or activities, restlessness); facial mask of pain (eyes lack luster, "beaten look," fixed or scattered movement, grimace); alteration in muscle tone (may span from listless to rigid); automatic responses not seen in chronic stable pain (diaphoresis, blood pressure and pulse change, pupillary dilatation, increased or decreased respiratory rate)
Related Factors:	Injuring agents: biologic, chemical, physical, psychologic

DIAGNOSIS: CHRONIC PAIN

Definition:	A state in which the individual experiences pain that continues for more than 6 months in duration
Defining Characteristics:	*Major:* Verbal report or observed evidence of pain experienced for more than 6 months. *Minor:* Fear of reinjury; physical and social withdrawal; altered ability to continue previous activities; anorexia; weight changes; changes in sleep patterns; facial mask; guarded movements
Related Factors:	Chronic physical/psychosocial disability

DIAGNOSIS: PAIN (CLINTON/ELAND)

Defining Characteristics:	Same as Carroll-Johnson, 1989
Etiologies/Related Factors:	Biologic: Inflammation, eg, rheumatic arthritis, temporal arteritis. Neurologic, eg, herpes zoster, headaches. Ischemic, eg, intermittent claudication. Musculoskeletal, eg, osteoporosis, pathologic fractures. Chemical, eg, cell damage and inflammation. Physical, eg, trauma, fractures. Psychologic, eg, depression

DIAGNOSIS: CHRONIC PAIN

In addition to Carroll-Johnson:

Defining Characteristics:	Self-focusing, social withdrawal, altered time perception, impaired thought processes, depression
Etiologies/Related Factors:	Arthritis, peripheral vascular disease, neuropathy, 2° diabetes, systemic lupus erythematosus, scleroderma, lower back pain, malignancies

pain. The tolerance for chronic pain that individuals develop does not prepare them for acute pain (Wachter-Shikora and Perez, 1982).

This may not be understood by the elderly person who is unable to distinguish between chronic and acute episodes of pain. For many dependent elderly, waiting is a way of life. Many elderly fiercely cling to their independence and are therefore reluctant to admit to pain for fear of losing their autonomy.

Living with chronic pain may condition the elderly to believe that one must "put up with" a certain amount of pain. For example, Oliver (1984) reports that abdominal pain in the elderly is frequently underreported and misdiagnosed with serious consequences. Perforations of the appendix or duodenal ulcers may produce only mild discomfort but can contribute significantly to an increase in mortality.

For some elderly, pain and death may be synonymous. It is not uncommon to encounter an elderly person who has had little or no previous experience with pain (Wachter-Shikora, 1983). The sudden onset of pain may be interpreted as the forerunner of a serious or perhaps terminal illness. The anxiety and fear associated with this interpretation frequently leads to increased pain perception. In contrast, elders whose pain has become insufferable may view death as a release from suffering. The nurse should explore the meaning of pain as it relates to the individual person.

A recurrent theme in the literature notes the myth that pain and discomfort are a natural part of the aging process. Elderly persons who complain of pain frequently are characterized as malingerers or manipulators (Wachter-Shikora, 1983). Dependent elders may have difficulty in adapting to changes, and this may intensify the pain experience. Changes in routine and medication, and unfamiliar settings can lead to confusion and fear of losing control of their lives.

ETIOLOGIES/RELATED FACTORS

Etiology is an integral part of the nursing diagnosis. Not only does it more accurately describe the problem, but it also may suggest specific interventions. This is most evident in the nursing diagnosis for pain. The etiology of the pain episode can be attributed to four injuring agents: (1) biologic, (2) chemical, (3) physical, and (4) psychologic.

Biologic Agents

Etiologies attributable to biologic injuring agents include inflammation, neurologic conditions, ischemic conditions, and/or musculoskeletal conditions. Inflammatory pain is due to a combination of factors including sensitization, pressure, temperature changes, and chemicals released from injured cells. For example, the pain associated with rheumatoid arthritis, estimated to affect 80% of persons of retirement age (Kolodney and Klipper, 1976), results from the inflammatory process within the involved joints. Although researchers do not believe the joint surface itself is particularly sensitive, the tissue destruction associated with the disease process results in inflammation that denudes nerve fibers, a process known as sensitization (lowered pain threshold of the innervating fibers). This causes increased pressure on the nerve endings that in turn gives rise to increased release of chemicals from damaged cells. This chemical release is further enhanced by vasodilation and increases in temperature (Eland, 1981a; Melzack and Wall, 1983).

Neurologic Conditions Pain that is neurologic in etiology is seen in herpes zoster and is thought to be related to destruction of the large fibers by the virus. The incidence of herpes zoster is particularly high in the elderly population, and the severity of the illness and resulting complications are also correspondingly higher than for other age categories (Harnish, 1984). The overall rate of herpes zoster is three to five cases per 1000 persons each year. This rate triples (15 per 1000) in persons over age 70 (Hallal, 1985). The pain is most often described as tingling, burning, or itching, but may also be deep and/or dull in nature.

Headaches in the elderly should be evaluated in the same manner as in younger patients. The specific etiology of headaches can be neurologic but may also be related to inflammatory processes (temporal arteritis), ischemic conditions (cerebrovascular disease with transient focal ischemia), or muscle tension.

Ischemic Conditions Ischemic pain may be caused by a buildup of lactic acid in the affected tissues or by the release of chemicals such as bradykinins and histamine from the damaged cells. Ischemic pain can be seen in several forms. Intermittent claudication presents with aching, persistent, cramping pain following exercise of the affected extremity and is relieved by rest. Pain at rest is caused by severe ischemia of the tissues and sensory nerve terminals usually localized in the digits, and is described as a severe ache or gnawing pain. Pain of ischemic neuropathy is usually seen late in the course of obstructed circulatory flow to the lower extremities and may also be associated with paresthesias. The pain may be quite severe and generally follows the distribution of the peripheral sensory nerves (Bullock and Rosendahl, 1984).

Musculoskeletal Conditions Pain originating in the musculoskeletal structures can be described as a deep, aching, poorly localized pain when bone is involved, or as sharp or dull pain that is aggravated by movement when muscles, tendons, and/or ligaments are involved. Low back pain is a significant problem among the elderly. In a recent study in Iowa, 20% of persons over the age of 65 living in two rural counties reported low back pain (Lavasky-Shulan et al, 1985). Musculoskeletal problems can be the source of headaches, as previously discussed, or indicators of more serious pathology such as osteoporosis or malignancies resulting in pathologic fractures.

Chemical Agents

When cells are damaged they release various chemical substances, such as potassium ions and adenosine triphosphate (ATP), which cause pain. Additionally, bradykinins are released from injured cells and produce pain by excitation of the nerve fibers as well as vascular changes. As tissues become inflamed, the compound prostaglandin is released. Prostaglandins sensitize nerve endings, which makes them more vulnerable to being fired by other agents (Melzack and Wall, 1983).

Physical Agents

The diminished sensory perceptions of some elderly persons may make them more susceptible to injury, with a resultant increase in the incidence of injuries due to trauma. For example, poor vision may lead to falls that can result in fractures. Hip fractures are the primary cause of more than 200,000 hospital admissions each year with persons over age 65 sustaining 84% of all such fractures (Baker et al, 1984) (see also Chapter 3).

The pain that accompanies the injury may be due to the release of irritating chemicals at the site of the tissue damage, to nerve compression, or to stretching and tearing of tissue. In an attempt to protect the injured site the elder may demonstrate splinting movements, which can cause muscle contraction. If the splinting continues, anaerobic metabolism within the muscle tissue causes an accumulation of lactic acid that irritates small fibers and results in further pain.

Psychologic Agents

Depression is a common and significant problem in the elderly population. One study suggests that 25% of the elderly surveyed reported moderate to severe depression (Freedman, 1982). Furthermore, Lindsay and Wyckoff (1981) report that 59% of elders requesting treatment for depression also complain of recurring pain, and conversely, 87% of elderly persons in pain clinics have depression. Thus, an important consideration in assessing depressed elderly persons is to evaluate their pain status (see Chapter 35).

TYPES OF PAIN

Pain is also classified by the duration of time that the response is experienced. Acute pain in the elderly is defined as pain lasting less than 6 months. Pain that lasts more than 6 months and is not caused by a malignancy is defined as chronic benign pain. Malignant pain is a complex phenomenon associated with cancer that can have characteristics of both acute and chronic pain for the elderly.

Acute Pain

Common medical diagnoses that are ordinarily manifested as acute pain include fractures or joint replacements, bowel obstruction requiring surgical intervention, and muscle sprains and strains. In each of these situations pain may be the presenting symptom that leads the elderly person to seek medical care. The pain associated with these conditions is generally short lived and is handled pharmacologically.

Chronic Pain

Medical diagnoses associated with chronic pain ordinarily involve underlying pathology. Arthritis, peripheral vascular disease, neuropathy secondary to diabetes, systemic lupus erythematosus, scleroderma, and lower back musculoskeletal disease are among the most frequent pathologies. Chronic pain presents health care professionals with complex ethical dilemmas interwoven with other issues such as independence, compliance, immobility, depression, and quality of life issues. The pain producing pathology is not going to disappear or cause death, but it will seriously affect the quality of life. The reader is referred to the chapters in this text on immobility (Chapter 23) and reactive depression (Chapter 35).

Pain relief alternatives include surgery, neurosurgical pain relief procedures, nerve blocks, nonnarcotic analgesia, physical therapy, biofeedback, relaxation, and imagery. The elderly often spend thousands of dollars every year, if they can afford it, in their continual search for pain relief. For some older individuals, one, or a combination, of these approaches will provide adequate relief. For an unfortunate few, none of these alternatives will provide pain relief or allow them to be functional, even in a limited sense.

Malignant Pain

Matthews et al (1973) have identified the five leading causes of cancer-induced pain as (1) bone destruction with infraction; (2) infiltration or compression of nerves; (3) obstruction of a viscus or vessel; (4) infiltration or distention of integument or tissues; and (5) inflammation, infection, or necrosis of tissue. Acute pain symptoms, including the stress response, will be present as the disease process advances and creates a new problem. Acute pain associated with malignancy is present in the elderly person with cancer who develops a bowel obstruction from tumor growth. The elderly person may also have an underlying chronic pain such as arthritic bone pain, in which there is almost no pain in remission, but during exacerbation the pain may prohibit most activities of daily living.

DEFINING CHARACTERISTICS

To assess the elderly person for pain the nurse looks for subjective and/or objective evidence that will specifically define the problem. The official classification of nursing diagnoses provides a list of defining characteristics that identifies data supporting a diagnosis of pain (see Table 30.1). Although this list is quite inclusive it is not exhaustive. Because of the uniquely individual pattern of pain responses, each elderly person may present with subtle, yet nevertheless definitive, signs of pain. Therefore, when seeking supporting data for this diagnosis, the nurse should also consider the individual's daily routines for changes in patterns.

Subjective Defining Characteristics

Melzack and Torgerson (1971) have generated an extensive list of verbal descriptors, common to the adult vocabulary, that characterize the sensory, affective, evaluative, and temporal components of pain. The nurse needs to be aware of the elderly person's pain vocabulary as well as his or her sociocultural and personal value system in order to assess pain status accurately. In the elderly, as is common with the young child, language or vocabulary can be a problem because of aphasia or dementia. Not being able to find the right word to describe pain can be extremely frustrating. Perceptual deficits are common in several neurologic problems (eg, stroke, dementia) and may severely limit the elderly client's ability to describe the pain verbally. For example, an elder may deny "pain" but admit to a "soreness" in the leg or may be unable to identify the part of the body where the pain is located.

Coded descriptors of pain can minimize confusion in terminology. Visual analog scales (VAS), as illustrated in Figure 30.1, provide the elderly person with a convenient method for rating pain. Based on a number scale, for example 1 to 10, the individual can describe the intensity of the painful episode. The ability to describe the intensity or quality of the pain is important for a number of reasons. First, it provides the nurse with baseline information by using a quantified intensity scale that is less likely to be misinterpreted than verbal descriptors. Similarly an objective rating of the pain is established for the elder's own use. Finally, both the nurse and the elderly

A. Visual Analog Scale

No pain   Extreme pain

B. Graphic Rating Scale

No pain   Mild   Moderate   Severe   Extreme pain

C. Melzack and Torgeson Scale

Mild   Discomforting   Distressing   Horrible   Excruciating

D. 0–100 Numeric Scale

0   10   20   30   40   50   60   70   80   90   100

No pain   Moderate pain   Unbearable pain

Figure 30.1

Types of pain scales (Source: Stewart ML: Measurement of clinical pain. Chapter 5 in: Pain: A Source Book for Nurses and other Health Professionals. Jacox A, editor: Little, Brown, 1977).

person have an objective scale to evaluate progress toward pain relief.

Vocalizations are sounds other than language. These include crying, sobbing, moaning, whimpering, and many others. If the pain is very sudden or unexpected, these responses are often involuntary (Johnson, 1977).

Verbal and coded descriptors are useful in both the assessment stage and the evaluative stage of the nursing diagnosis. Because these descriptors are subjective, the nurse must also be cognizant of the intervening variables that might influence the elderly person's pain experience. Intervening variables that are important to assess for the diagnosis and management of pain are discussed later in this chapter.

Objective Defining Characteristics

Individuals in pain will often exhibit guarding or protective behavior. Favoring a limb or attempting to immobilize an injured body part can indicate pain. The nurse needs to evaluate the client's body movement and positioning. With the high incidence of arthritis and back pain in the elderly, a statement by the nurse such as "You seem to be limping. Is your leg bothering you?" invites the elder to respond and demonstrates that the nurse has observed that the individual is having some difficulty.

Elderly people in pain may exhibit self-focusing behavior and may become oblivious to others around them. This can be misinterpreted as being reclusive or uncaring of others. Self-focusing is particularly true of elders with chronic pain. Either through their own withdrawal from relationships or because of avoidance by significant others, their social interactions can become more and more limited. It is useful to ask such questions as "Do you get the opportunity to see many of your friends?" or "How often do you go out socially in a week? in a month?" The answers may illuminate a problem that the elderly person has not been willing to discuss for fear of "burdening the nurse with my problems."

A narrowed focus is also indicative of pain. Although similar to self-focusing, it would also include such phenomena as altered time perception and impaired thought processes, both of which occur in dementing processes in the elderly. Careful assessment is necessary to evaluate whether these alterations are due to drug interactions or to a preexisting pathophysiologic condition. For some elderly, all of these variants may be operating, and pain as a precipitator may be overlooked.

Distraction is a common characteristic of pain. The elder may appear restless or fidgety, often pacing up and down the room. Rather than withdrawing into isolation, the person may seek out new people and/or activities.

Distraction is a coping mechanism that can be very effective in relieving pain. It is important to recognize it as a defining characteristic as well.

For some elderly persons, the only clue the nurse may observe that would indicate they are experiencing pain might be what is known as the "facial mask of pain." Facial contortions such as grimacing, wrinkling, or clenched teeth are readily apparent. The elder, however, may project only a rather somber expression (Johnson, 1977). This should indicate the importance of careful observation on the part of the nurse to determine if the elderly person is exhibiting any change in facial characteristics.

Nurses have been instructed that an individual who is in pain will exhibit muscle tension such as a clenched fist. However, through trial and error, the elderly person may have learned the value of muscle relaxation to relieve pain. Direct statements such as "You seem quite relaxed. Does this help you relieve some pain you are having?" offer the elder the opportunity to describe the pain experience.

Unlike elderly individuals who have chronic pain and have adapted to it, those suffering from acute pain will exhibit certain autonomic responses that are readily observable to the nurse. For those elders in chronic pain, the responses of the autonomic nervous system are altered or diminished and are therefore less conspicuous. Table 30.2 summarizes these responses (defining characteristics).

Another defining characteristic that the nurse should be aware of is a change in sleeping pattern. Is the elderly person sleeping more or less? Pain often robs the individual of desperately needed sleep. When pain control is attained, the initial response may be many hours of uninterrupted sleep, the body's way of compensating for the deficit. In the absence of pain control, the elder may use sleep as an escape from pain and spend an increasing amount of time sleeping or dozing. To evaluate any changes in the elderly person's sleep patterns properly, the nurse should also be aware of the changes in the sleep cycle associated with aging (Bullock and Rosendahl, 1984) (see Chapter 27).

Changes in eating habits can also signal pain. Anorexia is common with acute pain and chronic pain due to malignant pathology. The elderly are at particular risk for protein deficiencies. If protein malnutrition occurs, the distribution of drugs can be altered because of a decreased availability of protein binding sites with which they can bind. Weight loss further debilitates the elder and contributes to additional health problems. Weight gain can also be a problem for the chronic pain sufferer whose only pleasure in life is eating (Meinhart and McCaffery, 1983;254). Altered eating patterns, weight gain, and weight loss are all signs that warrant investigation as possible indicators of pain (see Chapter 9).

Table 30.2

Autonomic Responses to Pain

RESPONSE	SYMPATHETIC STIMULATION	PARASYMPATHETIC STIMULATION
Pupil size	Dilated	Constricted
Perspiration	Increased	No effect
Rate and force of heart rate	Increased	Decreased
Blood pressure	Increased	Decreased
Depth and rate of respiration	Increased	No effect
Urinary output	Decreased	No effect
Peristalsis of GI tract	Decreased	Increased
Basal metabolic rate	Increased	No effect

Source: Johnson M: Assessment of clinical pain. Chapter 6 in: *Pain: A Source Book for Nurses and Other Health Professionals.* Jacox AK (editor). Little, Brown, 1977.

INTERVENING VARIABLES

Intervening variables are modifiers such as psychologic and physiologic factors, drug effects, or cultural gender variables that either inhibit or promote the elderly's response to proposed interventions. When obtaining a history of the elderly person, it is important to identify the constraints, capabilities, and/or resources available to the elder.

Psychologic Changes

For some elderly persons pain will be a new experience, whereas for others it will be a well-known phenomenon. Past pain experiences are important considerations in planning appropriate interventions for pain relief. The nurse needs to determine what type of pain the elderly person has experienced in the past and how the elder has coped with that pain.

Coping mechanisms are developed over a lifetime of experiences. Depending on a host of variables, children learn how to cope with pain, and many of these coping strategies are carried over into late adulthood. Wachter-Shikora and Perez (1982) report that many of the elderly persons they interviewed had not had experience with painful episodes. Complaining of pain may be a socially acceptable way of indicating unmet needs or concerns. For the elderly person faced with declining health and multiple losses, complaints of pain may bring attention and result in concern and some degree of caretaking by friends or relatives (Kwentus et al, 1985).

In institutions, the elderly person's pain behavior may cause conflict between the elder and the staff. McCaffery's (1979) definition of pain states that pain exists whenever the client says it does. Yet frequently the elderly person is dismissed as a chronic complainer or malingerer who is exaggerating his or her pain. The nurse can evaluate an individual's pain behavior by observing that person both when he or she is alone and when he or she interacts with others. The family can often provide useful information concerning the elderly person's pain behavior.

Physiologic Changes

A number of physiologic changes accompany old age. The inflammatory response is diminished as the result of a decline in the body's humoral and cell-mediated responses. For example, complaints of abdominal pain due to infection may be misdiagnosed because fever and leukocytosis are absent or diminished. Instead, the elderly person might present with signs of confusion, anorexia, and/or tachycardia (Oliver, 1984).

Evidence exists, although some of it is contradictory, that the elderly experience changes in pain threshold and pain tolerance. Pain threshold is the point at which pain is first perceived, and pain tolerance is the amount of pain sensation the person is willing to endure. These changes may in part explain reports in the literature that suggest that the elderly frequently do not report pain as a major presenting symptom in myocardial infarction (McDonald, 1983; Rodstein, 1956). Sherman and Robillar (1980) report that cutaneous pain sensitivity decreases with age, but it is unclear if the association between age and pain threshold is due to central nervous system (CNS) changes (information processing) or peripheral changes (changes in the skin) or both.

Several authors report that the elderly appear to tolerate more pain. The authors use words such as *stoic, resigned,* and *tolerance* to describe their patients (Kwentus et al, 1985; Oliver, 1984; Wachter-Shikora and Perez,

1982). Much of this evidence is based on observations of the elderly rather than on empirical data and therefore should be viewed with caution. Clinicians should evaluate their elderly clients who minimize pain as to whether their pain behavior is consistent with pathologic evidence that would suggest pain.

Metabolic changes within the brains of elderly persons, due to a decreased number of neurons, result in a weakening of the transmission of signals from the brain to body parts, which may alter the threshold for arousal in the various organ systems. Of particular significance is a reduced level of norepinephrine, which is associated with depression (Bullock and Rosendahl, 1984), and a functioning antinoceptive system (responsible for reducing painful stimuli) (Meinhart and McCaffery, 1983).

Drug Effects The elderly experience metabolic changes that are responsible for significant drug effects. Alterations in liver function, secondary to chronic disease or decreased perfusion, can lead to a prolonged duration of action of drugs so that the danger of accumulation is a significant threat (Malseed, 1985). In some cases, prolonged duration of a drug can be advantageous. Kaiko (1980) reports that morphine has a higher duration of pain relief in the elderly, which is thought to be due to the positive correlation between age and increased plasma elimination half-life (see Chapter 4).

Alterations in renal and hepatic functions can result in toxicity (Pfeiffer, 1982). The renal system undergoes significant changes with advancing age, and the amount of drug that can be filtered and excreted at any given time is substantially reduced (Bullock and Rosendahl, 1984; Kwentus et al, 1985; Malseed, 1985). Changes in the gastrointestinal (GI) tract of the elderly can also result in a slower rate and a less consistent absorption of drugs (Malseed, 1985).

Distribution of drugs can be affected in the elderly because of decreased cardiac output, decreased hepatic enzyme activity, lower plasma albumin levels, smaller body size, and increased deposition of fat that replaces muscle (Kwentus et al, 1985; Malseed, 1985). Clinicians should keep these effects in mind when calculating drug dosages.

The increased number of drugs taken by the elderly can lead to drug interactions. For example, nonsteroidal anti-inflammatory drugs (NSAIDs) can displace other drugs from protein-binding sites (Kwentus et al, 1985). Aside from drug interactions, the elderly frequently take multiple drugs, which can lead to confusion in dosage, either skipping doses or repeating doses.

Changes in receptor site sensitivity due to aging may account for the increased effect of certain drugs such as barbiturates. The decrease in hormonal activity that accompanies the aging process may alter a drug's effect or increase the drug's toxicity. Steroids, for example, should be used cautiously in the elderly because of the increased likelihood of glucose intolerance, osteoporosis, and susceptibility to infection (Kwentus et al, 1985; Malseed, 1985).

Culture

The nurse must consider an individual's cultural background when investigating pain. One's ethnic background may dictate certain acceptable pain behaviors and expressions. However it is essential that the nurse avoid stereotyping the elderly individual. The myth of the stoic Asian is as damaging as the myth of the loudly complaining Jew or Italian. The elder's cultural background should be used as a framework for understanding the individual's pain response and for developing appropriate interventions. Several researchers have identified various traits that seem to be associated with certain ethnic and religious groups. Zbrowski's (1952) classic study found Jews and Italians to be more vocal in their pain response, whereas Old Americans (Zbrowski's term) and Irish avoided vocal manifestations of pain. Table 30.3 summarizes Zbrowski's conclusions on various ethnic interpretations and responses to pain. It may serve to sensitive the nurse to the possibility of ethnically-conditioned responses by elderly patients.

Gender

Reports in the literature differ considerably regarding gender differences with respect to pain. However, the consensus seems to be that the pain threshold is similar for men and women, whereas pain tolerance is greater in men. One study suggests that older women do not have the discriminatory sensitivity to mild sensations that older men do (Clark and Mehl, 1971). Although this difference in pain tolerance is not completely explained, cultural and social variables must be taken into account.

In addition, gender differences have been noted among health practitioners and their perceptions of pain in their clients. Armitage et al (1979) report that male physicians tend to take a man's illness more seriously and conclude that this may be in response to the stereotype of the stoic man and hypochondriachal woman. Pilowsky and Bond (1969) note that overall, older patients receive less powerful analgesics. They also report that female nurses respond with more concern for female patients and are more likely to give the female patients more powerful analgesics. In contrast, Cohen's (1977) study of postoperative pain relief suggests that women receive less powerful postoperative analgesics than do men.

Awareness of gender stereotypes should alert nurses to consider each elderly person as an individual. As an intervening variable, the gender of the clinician may have more implications for medical and nursing actions than do gender differences among clients.

Table 30.3

Influence of Culture on Pain

CULTURAL GROUP	INTERPRETATION/RESPONSE
Old American	Future oriented; concerned with implications of pain; certain types of pain are expected or considered normal; avoids vocal expressions of pain; attempts to minimize reflexive responses
Jewish	Future oriented; concerned with significance of pain; frequently expresses pain to other in order to gain sympathy and assistance; readily seeks out medical assistance
Italian	Present oriented; concerned more with pain sensation than its implications; rarely complains of pain to family but likes to have them around for distraction; readily seeks medical aid and treatment
Irish	Future oriented; reluctant to discuss pain; prefers to suffer alone; appears proud of ability to handle pain; uses relaxation or fighting to deal with pain
Chinese	Yin-Yang philosophy of dynamic equilibrium; body viewed as gift from parents with self-imposed responsibility to care for self; may ignore symptoms to avoid becoming burden; alternative health practices (eg, acupressure/acupuncture) frequently used
Japanese	Self-control, resignation, gratitude, and forebearance highly valued; when ill willing to submit to care by others; feelings most often communicated nonverbally; first generation most stoic; in general refrains from any expression of pain; will not ask for or expect pain medication
Black	Frequently denies existence of pain; reluctant to ask for pain relief or seek medical assistance; may subscribe to uncommon ideologies
Hispanic	Present oriented; stoicism valued; suffering viewed as positive experience in which to do penance; modesty highly valued by both sexes; folk medicine commonly practiced

ASSESSMENT

Two assessment activities are required on an ongoing basis for elderly persons with cancer: These activities will be discussed separately. First, find out where each pain is located, how severe it is, what the client thinks is causing the pain, whether the pain has been experienced previously, and, if so, what did/did not work to relieve the pain. It is also important for the nurse to find out which pain the client wants relieved first. Unfortunately, professionals often categorize a client's pain by virtue of the primary pathology (eg, cancer clients have pain due to cancer). This assumption can result in the misdiagnosis of the cancer client's pain, which might be caused by an unrelated antecedent (eg, heart attacks, gout, constipation, or myofascial pain).

The following situations illustrate the importance of adequate assessment of malignant pain.

CASE STUDY

Pain, Mrs. R.L.

Mrs. R.L., a 70-year-old woman with terminal leukemia, was assumed to be in total body pain, was bedfast because of the pain, had refused food for the previous week, and was receiving 270 mg of subcutaneous morphine per hour. Closer evaluation revealed the pain she most wanted relieved was from her trapezious muscle, which was in spasm. Application of a transcutaneous electrical nerve stimulator (TENS) to the motor loci of the muscle resulted in complete relief of pain in the trapezious except for an ache (the result of the buildup of lactic acid and cellular by-products), which disappeared in 2 days. Twelve hours after application of the TENS unit she left her house and went out to a congregate meal site for lunch. Approximately a week later she attended her pinochle club and returned to her volunteer activities three mornings a week at her local hospital.

CASE STUDY

Pain

A 70-year-old man was hospitalized with recurrent cancer of the prostate with extensive bony metastasis. Because of the extent of his disease process, the client decided he wanted no further treatment and wanted to return home as soon as his pain was under control. One afternoon he became diaphoretic and tachycardic, his blood pressure became elevated, and he told the nurse he was in pain. The nurse notified the staff physician, who came to the patient's bedside and decided that the client's disease process was probably more extensive than had previously been thought and that death would probably occur in a few hours. A short time later a junior medical student walked by the client's room and observed the client's distress. He entered the room and almost immediately went to the nurses' station and announced that the client was having a heart attack. No one had asked the client any specifics about the pain he was experiencing and assumed the pain he was reporting was due to malignant disease. When the medical student asked the client where his pain was, he gave the characteristic description of crushing chest pain that was radiating down his left arm. The client was sent to the cardiac care unit, where he recovered from his myocardial infarction, was later released, and lived several more months.

The second important assessment activity is to distinguish whether the elderly patient is in severe or overwhelming pain. An elderly person in overwhelming pain has the following characteristics: sleeplessness, loss of morale, fatigue, irritability, restlessness, inability to be distracted, and complaints of severe pain (Twycross and Lack, 1983). Often the elder or family tells the professional that the client has not slept for a number of days or weeks. The dark circles under the eyes of both the elderly person and their family members validate the loss of sleep. Elders are prevented from falling asleep by the pain, or, if they fall asleep, it is not a sound sleep, and they often are awakened by the pain. Before any other pain relief modality can receive an appropriate evaluation, the elderly person must be allowed to rest, sleep, and restore the body's energy.

Sleep will occur naturally when the elderly person is pain free. Pain relief is often achieved by administering morphine until the person reports no pain. This action breaks the cycle of pain: insomnia—fatigue—pain. Institutional policy may dictate where morphine may be given. Some home health care providers insist on hospitalization for morphine titration, whereas others permit administration in the home setting if the nurse stays for 3 to 4 hours after repeated administration. If a terminally ill person is hospitalized for titration, it is important to indicate to them that they will go home in 48 to 72 hours with their pain under control. Once the pain cycle is broken, morphine needs to be given around the clock to allow the person to sleep, rest, restore his or her energy, and remain pain free.

When the elderly individual is finally pain free, sleep may last 24 hours a day for 2 to 3 days. This can be disquieting to nurses and families, who fear they may have harmed the elder and that sleep is an undesirable side effect of the drug. When aroused from this sleep an elderly person behaves like any person who has been sleeping soundly. The speech pattern is appropriate for a sleepy person, and the respiratory rate remains slightly lower than what it is was prior to the administration of morphine. Pain is a potent stimulator of epinephrine release, and when the stimulus (pain) is removed, the pulse, respiratory rate, and blood pressure will drop predictably in response to the

decreased levels of epinephrine. After 2 or 3 days of sleep and rest, elderly persons will wake up, and often families report that they are their "former selves."

When the cycle of pain has been broken for 2 to 3 days, a complete pain assessment is imperative. Elderly persons in overwhelming pain initially report that they hurt "everywhere" and cannot be specific when asked to identify individual pains that are causing them the most hurt. When the elder and family are rested, other pain relief options can be explored, including decreasing the dose of morphine or trying nonsteroidal anti-inflammatory drugs, using relaxation modes such as imagery, distraction, or taking trips out of the home.

ASSESSMENT TOOLS

The importance of obtaining accurate data in an organized manner that will provide a complete picture of the elderly person's pain cannot be overstated. This information is necessary for identifying the type and quality of pain the elder is experiencing. It guides the nurse in identifying the etiology, which is needed to develop appropriate interventions, and it provides a means by which to monitor the effectiveness of the interventions. A number of tools for assessing pain are available, and the nurse should choose those that are most suitable to a particular elderly person. Criteria for choosing an assessment tool include the elderly individual's verbal, physical, and cognitive capabilities. To assess the elder adequately and to accommodate any limitations that are present, it may be necessary to adapt a particular tool or combine parts of several tools. The goal is to find the tool(s) that will provide the most complete picture of the elderly person's pain.

The quickest and most simple of the standardized assessment tools is the visual analog scale. This type of scale should be standardized to 10 centimeters in length, with the numbers 0 and 10 at either end (Melzack and Wall, 1983). When descriptors such as mild, moderate, and severe are used in conjunction with the visual analog scale, it is known as a graphic rating scale (Stewart, 1977).

There are advantages and disadvantages to using these types of scales. Whenever words are used, there is the possibility of different interpretations by the elderly and staff concerning their meaning. The scale should use as few descriptors as possible to reduce misinterpretation, yet it should be sensitive enough to capture the elderly person's perception of the quality of the pain experienced. Number scales are effective in quantifying pain but do not yield information on the quality of pain being experienced.

Melzack and Torgeson (1971) developed a scale (values 1–5) that used words as pain descriptors and that demonstrated a linear relationship. This scale provides the clinician with a qualitative assessment based on the sensory qualities, the affective qualities, and the evaluative words. It also measures the overall intensity of the pain experienced. The difficulty with this scale is once again that the words used may not be part of the elderly person's vocabulary and therefore not meaningful to the patient.

The 0 to 100 numeric scale is a continuum that provides more sensitivity in rating pain by the individual. It can be used with or without words, depending on the cognitive ability of the elderly individual. The usefulness of numeric scales needs to be balanced with the cognitive capabilities of the elderly person. Depending on the characteristic of pain, qualitative or quantitative, that is being evaluated, one scale may be more appropriate than another. Several studies have demonstrated the reliability and validity of these scales (Berry and Huskisson, 1972; Clark and Spear, 1964; Melzack and Torgeson, 1971; Pilowsky and Bond, 1969; Pilowsky and Kaufman, 1965). The nurse must use his or her clinical judgment to determine which scale would best suit the needs of the elderly person. Interested readers are directed to Stewart (1977) for a more elaborate discussion of these scales. Figure 30.1 demonstrates the various types of scales.

The McGill Pain Assessment Questionnaire is a comprehensive tool useful for an initial intake history (Melzack, 1975). It provides the nurse with a detailed history of past pain experiences, medications used, and other types of treatments sought for pain relief. Information is also elicited on the current pain episode and how it has affected the elderly person in terms of his or her daily activities, including sleeping patterns, eating habits, sexual activities, and work requirements. Information about the quality and location of pain may be obtained.

A serious drawback to this tool is the length of time it takes to complete and the reliance on the vocabulary and cognitive ability of the elderly. For some elderly it may be impractical. For more information on the McGill tool the reader is referred to studies by Dubuisson and Melzack (1976), McCaffery (1979;288–293), and Melzack (1975).

Color has been used successfully to describe pain. Stewart (1977) developed a Pain-Color Scale that uses a yellow–orange to red–black chromatic display to represent pain. Verbal descriptors (no pain and worst possible pain) are used in conjunction with the color scale to serve as reference points for clients.

Eland (1981b) has developed a tool that uses a body outline, which the client colors using crayons or markers chosen to represent a personal pain scale. The client chooses four colors to represent no pain, mild pain, moderate pain, and worst pain and then uses these colors to pinpoint pain on the body outline. This tool has been used primarily with children because of their limited vocabulary to describe and locate pain. It therefore may be useful for some elderly persons who are experiencing language difficulties.

The use of a pain flow sheet can be invaluable in assessing and monitoring the elderly person's pain status. Meinhart and McCaffery (1983) have developed a pain flow sheet that is quick and easy to use and that could be incorporated easily into the elderlys' records. Aside from its obvious merit in evaluating responses to treatment, it can also be used as a means of limiting dicussions to avoid prolonged focusing on pain. When shared with the elder, the flow sheet can be a positive reinforcer of progress in pain relief. It can also identify peculiar patterns or situations that exacerbate pain, which the elderly person and nurse can then plan for accordingly.

NURSING INTERVENTIONS

The task of choosing an appropriate intervention is made significantly easier when a thorough assessment has been made of the elder's pain. As discussed previously, this must include knowledge related to the etiology of the pain. These antecedent conditions (biologic, chemical, physical, and psychologic) must be understood in relationship to the three components of the pain experience: sensory, motivational, and cognitive.

Because of these unique aspects of pain, it is impossible to match a single intervention with any particular etiology. Knowledge of the pain components and the possible etiologies of pain indicates that the best intervention for pain relief combines methods to alter the pain experience at the sensory, motivational, and/or cognitive level. The importance of establishing mutual goals between the nurse and the elderly person for pain relief should be a primary consideration. When both elder and nurse have shared goals and realistic expectations, the odds for successful pain relief improve.

Use of Analgesics

It has been suggested that as many as half of the elderly do not take their medications as prescribed, and 35% of the elderly misuse drugs to the degree that they experience adverse effects (Smith, 1976; Wandless and Davie, 1977). Any analgesic regimen should be simple, include the fewest number of drugs with the fewest side effects, be easily administered, and cost the least amount possible. The nurse, pharmacist, or physician should give the elderly individual and the family both verbal and written instructions concerning medications (see Chapter 4).

A calendar or some type of recording system for each dose of drug taken can be placed where the elderly person will see it at the appropriate time, such as on the bathroom mirror, on the refrigerator, or by a favorite chair. If at all possible, medication administration should be incorporated into the elder's schedule *before* another of the elderly person's routine activities. An elderly person who goes to congregate meals at noon might put his or her apartment keys beside the medicine as a reminder to take it prior to going to the meal. Obviously, some medications must be taken an hour prior to or after meals, which is more difficult to remember.

Elderly who require an analgesic in the middle of the night should set their alarm and place only *one* dose of analgesic at the bedside (not the entire bottle) along with a glass of water. This prevents taking more than one dose when the person may be drowsy and easily confused.

The least potent analgesics should first be given a trial with appropriate patient education and around-the-clock administration. To achieve maximum pain relief, analgesics must be given around the clock, including the dose in the middle of the night. The initials "p.r.n." when translated for pain relief mean "pain relief nil." Inadequate and fluctuating blood levels of analgesics are the predictable and undesirable results of p.r.n. administration. With p.r.n. administration the individual's level of pain peaks to the point where a usual dose that would be expected to relieve pain does not. Doses of analgesics given p.r.n. that are thought to be relieving pain often do not do so; they just *sedate*. The pain itself remains, but the sedative effect allows the individual to sleep. When individuals are not sleeping their pain is uncontrolled. The physician who is made aware of the uncontrolled pain is likely to order a larger dose of the analgesic or change to a stronger analgesic when all that was needed was for the nurse to administer the analgesic around the clock. If a person begins to develop side effects such as tinnitus, the *dose* should be altered, *not* the frequency of administration.

Administering analgesics on a regular basis is an appropriate intervention to "keep ahead of pain." For example, an elderly person who is 24 hours postoperative from having a fractured hip repaired will experience some degree of pain. Anticipating and preventing pain are desirable outcomes. Pain control decreases the effects of immobility, encourages adequate pulmonary oxygenation, and allows adequate rest. The fracture and associated surgery have activated the stress response. Pain in the postoperative period ensures a continual release of epinephrine, which increases myocardial oxygen demands, increases cardiac output, and intensifies preexisting cardiovascular pathology.

Drug interactions can be a significant problem for any elderly individual with multiple health problems who may be taking a variety of pharmacologic agents. Before initiating a pharmacologic approach to pain control, it is imperative that the nurse discuss all of the elderly person's medications with a competent clinical pharmacist or with the primary physician, who is aware of all the elder's medical problems. Often "parts" or systems of elders are parcelled out to various specialty physicians with no one knowing about the whole person.

As discussed previously, elderly individuals' renal, hepatic, and gastrointestinal metabolism may be significantly different in the latter stages of life. Narcotic analgesics will have a longer half-life, and the by-products of metabolism will be circulating longer because of metabolic changes within the liver and kidney. The gastrointestinal system has a decreased ability to absorb drugs and may be more sensitive to drugs that can cause gastric upset.

The following sections are not meant to be inclusive but consider some of the most frequently prescribed analgesics for the elderly in the United States.

Narcotic Analgesics

After numerous interventions and nonnarcotic analgesics have proved unsuccessful in providing pain relief for chronic benign pain, the question of whether to prescribe narcotic analgesics is raised. Unfortunately the consistent use of a narcotic analgesic for nonmalignant chronic pain is not viewed in the same context as the consistent use of insulin, diuretics, antihypertensives, or cardiotonics prescribed for other chronic conditions.

The authors advocate long-term use of narcotic analgesia for chronic benign and malignant pain when nonnarcotic drugs have been unsuccessful in achieving pain relief, despite around-the-clock administration that includes appropriate dosages and an adequate trial period for evaluation. Second, narcotic analgesia is recommended when nerve blocks, TENS, surgery, and other nonpharmacologic interventions have been evaluated for the specific elderly person and found to be either inappropriate or ineffective. Finally, narcotics should be prescribed when pain has reduced an elderly person's quality of life to social isolation, depression, immobility, and withdrawal.

Some health care providers will never be comfortable in prescribing or administering a narcotic analgesic for long-term use when the preceding criteria have been met. The clients of these health care providers will lead a predictable life of social isolation, intense anger, dependency, depression, and immobility, and a significant number of them will commit suicide. If asked, many will tell you that they envy cancer patients because "cancer patients get to die and I have to live with my pain."

Professionals who prescribe or administer narcotics on a long-term basis face an ongoing educational process directed toward their peers, clients, and clients' families, which includes the following information:

1. Long-term narcotic use in the elderly person's particular situation does not put him or her in the same category as a person who abuses drugs and is psychologically addicted.
2. Gradually increasing a dose of a narcotic will not result in the client's death by respiratory depression.

3. Treating chronic or malignant pain with narcotics does not mean that death is imminent; it may actually result in the elderly individual wanting to live longer because pain is no longer a problem.

4. Initially individuals who have suffered for months or years may sleep for a few days when pain is brought under control because they are exhausted from fighting pain. This will not be a long-term consequence of pain relief if the drug is appropriately titrated.

5. Narcotics can be titrated, enabling the person to be "awake," but the pain itself will be "asleep." Titrating a narcotic to achieve optimal pain relief may take 2 weeks and will require ongoing evaluation.

6. The individual needs the narcotic just as much as he or she might need insulin, diuretics, antihypertensives, or cardiac drugs, and just as the need for those drugs will increase with time, so will the need to increase the narcotic (Twycross and Lack, 1983).

A daily balancing act for health professionals is the titration of a dose of narcotic analgesic that will provide pain relief without sedation and have the least number of undesirable side effects. Constipation is the most common undesirable side effect in clients who receive narcotic analgesia. Constipation can be as problematic as the pain itself, especially for the elderly person. When an elderly person is placed on a narcotic, an aggressive bowel program should also be initiated. The reader is referred to Chapters 14 and 16 for more specific information on constipation and incontinence. For some elderly who have urinary retention problems, such as those with prostatic problems, the cholinergic action of many of the narcotic drugs will accentuate the problem. Although urinary retention and/or constipation should not prevent prescribing or administering narcotics, nurses should anticipate the need for further intervention and have a working plan if either problem presents itself. The following paragraphs briefly discuss some of the most frequently prescribed narcotics and their advantages and disadvantages in the elderly population.

Meperidine (Demerol) Meperidine is a poor choice of analgesic for the elderly population for two reasons. It has a by-product of metabolism called normeperidine that has a long half-life and causes CNS excitation ranging from restlessness and confusion to seizures (Kaiko et al, 1983). The peak blood levels of meperidine occur 90 minutes after administration, and all traces of the drug are gone within 2 to 2 1/2 hours (Halpern, 1984). Between 40% and 60% of the drug is taken to the liver by the portal vein and metabolized soon after oral administration. In the elderly with impaired liver function, as much as 80% of the drug is detoxified in this manner. An oral dose of 200 to 300 mg of meperidine is required to obtain the equivalent effect of 75 to 100 mg of intramuscular meperidine (Mather, 1986). Intramuscular meperidine is painful on injection and leaves large painful lumps in tissue.

Methadone Methadone can be a useful drug for the elderly because it does not have to be administered often. However, it has an 18-hour half-life in adults. If methadone is used, it must be closely monitored because of the preexisting metabolic changes in the elderly. Titration of the dose can be difficult, and if overdose results, the accompanying respiratory depression can last 3 or more days.

Oxycodone (Percodan, Percocet) Percodan or Percocet contains a small amount of narcotic (5 mg) and, if care is taken, can be used for the elderly. The use of either drug for severe pain is questioned because clients often take two or three tablets at a time to relieve pain. The effect of this many tablets over a short period of time is toxicity of salicylate (Percodan contains 225 mg of aspirin) or acetaminophen (Percocet contains 325 mg of acetaminophen). Many physicians who treat chronic pain clients believe that Percodan and Percocet have a higher incidence of unpleasant cognitive side effects, including nightmares, hallucinations, and an inability to process information (Doughtery, 1986).

Codeine Codeine is a useful drug for the elderly, and when combined with aspirin or acetaminophen, the results can be very beneficial. However nausea, vomiting, and severe constipation often accompany its use. Codeine is less expensive if ordered by itself instead of in combined form with aspirin or acetaminophen (eg, Percodan, Percocet, Tylenol #3). When combination drugs are prescribed, such as Tylenol #3 or Empirin #3, clients pay extra money for the convenience of two drugs in one tablet.

Heroin Heroin has become more a political issue in the United States than a medical one. The hospice system in England, using double blind research designs, found heroin to be no more beneficial than morphine. When sophisticated assays became available, it was determined that heroin, after deacetylization by the liver, is converted to a substance that is chemically almost identical to morphine (Twycross and Lack, 1983).

Morphine Morphine is probably the drug of choice for severe pain in the elderly. The half-life is sufficiently short to make titration relatively easy, it has no undesirable by-product buildup, and it causes no more constipation than other narcotics. There is increasing evidence that morphine, when combined with aspirin or another NSAID, effectively alleviates the pain of bone metastasis

(Foley, 1985). Additionally, it is available in several different oral preparations of varying strengths. The oral forms include liquid, quick release tablets, and slow release enteric-coated tablets. The enteric-coated tablets are very small and are in a wax base that allows the tablet(s) to bypass the first pass metabolism because they are absorbed in the small bowel. Manufacturers are also developing sublingual and skin patches containing morphine that will also bypass the first pass metabolism and should be available in the near future.

Morphine can be given subcutaneously either by single injection or by constant infusion using a small portable pump. The small portable pumps (approximately 3 × 3 × 1 inch) allow the elderly person to ambulate and not be dependent on a large cumbersome intravenous pump (Twycross and Lack, 1983).

Recently morphine has been administered via an implanted catheter in the epidural or intrathecal space. The advantages of this delivery system are thought to include better pain relief with smaller amounts of the drug. The disadvantages include the cost, the necessity of undergoing the procedure for catheter placement, and the potential for dislodging the catheter (Coombs et al, 1983; Malone et al, 1985).

Nonnarcotic Analgesics

Elderly persons with sprains and strains should receive aspirin, acetaminophen, or another NSAID around the clock to relieve pain. Application of ice packs followed by heat will help reduce the pain and swelling of tissue. For elders who have undergone surgical procedures, it is advisable to give around-the-clock narcotic analgesia for the first 48 to 72 hours postoperative and then switch to a NSAID. Pain caused by surgical intervention must be alleviated to prevent postoperative pneumonia, which can be particularly devastating in the elderly. Nurses who are concerned about respiratory depression in the elderly should be reminded that pain itself is a potent respiratory stimulant. For further discussion the reader is referred to the section of this chapter that deals with the use of analgesics in the elderly.

Aspirin The most frequent problem with aspirin administration in the elderly population is gastrointestinal irritation, which is sometimes alleviated with an antacid or by giving the drug in an enteric-coated tablet. Aspirin can be purchased in a tablet form that contains an antacid (Ascriptin), which is another convenience product that is more costly than taking aspirin plus liquid antacid. It has been recently discovered that 900 to 1000 mg may be an appropriate dose of aspirin. Previously, 600 mg was thought to be the maximum dose (Flower et al, 1985; Twycross and Lack, 1983). Timed release aspirin preparations that have to be taken less frequently are often

beneficial, but are costly and beyond the financial resources of many elderly.

Acetaminophen (Tylenol, Datril) Acetaminophen causes less irritation to the gastrointestinal tract than aspirin. Its action at the cellular level is different than aspirin, and acetaminophen has no anti-inflammatory action. As with aspirin, acetaminophen can be used with various amounts of codeine to provide greater pain relief than either drug used separately.

Nonsteroidal Anti-Inflammatory Agents Nonsteroidal anti-inflammatory agents represent a classification of drugs that provide pain relief by (1) reducing prostaglandin production; (2) blocking other mediators derived from prostaglandin; and (3) blocking the generation of impulses by pain fibers when given prophylactically. The drugs phenylbutazone (Butazolidin) and indomethacin (Indocin) are probably the oldest drugs in this category but were not effective in the elderly because of severe gastrointestinal irritation. There are approximately 20 "new" drugs in this classification, including ibuprophen (Motrin, Advil), naproxen (Naprosyn), sulindac (Clinoril), tolmetin (Tolectin), and piroxicam (Feldene). The introduction of these drugs has greatly aided pain control, but clinical knowledge about their actions and side effects is not yet specific enough to enable physicians to prescribe a specific NSAID for a specific diagnosis. Clients may try several different NSAIDs before finding the drug that provides the greatest relief with the least number of side effects. The majority of these drugs are also metabolized by the liver and excreted by the kidney, and some cause more gastric distress than others.

Corticosteroids Corticosteroids have a place in pain control, although their side effects should never be minimized. When all other drugs have been tried, steroids are used in degenerative conditions such as systemic lupus erythematosus or arthritis. Steroids are often used in combination with other analgesics to reduce the pain within both the peripheral system and the central nervous system of terminal cancer patients. Dexamethasone (Decadron) can be used to reduce intracranial pressure and stop the headache associated with central nervous system lesions. Peripherally, corticosteroids can act as a "cushion" between the malignant tumor and the nerve fiber itself, providing significant pain relief. Steroids also improve appetite and often promote a sense of well-being, which may be a beneficial effect for cancer clients (Twycross and Lack, 1983).

Tricyclic Antidepressants There is research and clinical evidence to suggest that tricyclic antidepressants have an analgesic effect (Butler, 1984). Administration of tricyclic antidepressants to geriatric clients with preexisting cardiovascular disease can cause significant orthostatic hypotension. The drugs amitriptyline and imipramine are most likely to cause orthostatic changes. For this reason, secondary amines such as nortriptyline and desipramine should be used with the elderly (Balderssarini, 1980). Whether or not the drugs have a specific analgesic effect of their own is probably of no consequence to the patient or family because relief from depression that often accompanies chronic or cancer pain results in many changes that make living easier for all. Elderly individuals have a right to be free of their pain, and an antidepressant may well provide quality to the remainder of their life.

Gate Control Theory

The most widely accepted theory of pain is the gate control theory proposed by Melzack and Wall (1983). The gate control theory, based on a conceptual framework that addresses all three components of the pain phenomenon, provides the clinician with the theoretical foundation for employing any number of pain relief measures.

According to this theory, pain impulses can be modulated by the opening and closing of a gate. When the gate is open the pain impulses are readily transmitted; when the gate is closed the impulses are not transmitted. If the gate is partially open, only some of the impulses can be transmitted. This gating mechanism is controlled by the interaction of three systems. The substantia gelatinosa, located in the dorsal horn of the spinal column, acts as a gate control system that modulates the afferent patterns before they activate the transmission (T) cells. The central control trigger, located in the cerebrum and thalamus, activates certain brain processes that exert control over sensory input. Stimulation of these processes activates descending efferent fibers, which in turn influence afferent conduction at the earliest synaptic levels of the sensory structures of the body. Finally, spinal cord T cells, which are responsible for projecting information to the brain, can be modulated concerning the amount of information projected to the brain. The T cells activate neural mechanisms that make up the action system responsible for perception and response. These neural mechanisms have the ability to open or close the gate that controls the flow of nerve impulses from the peripheral fibers to the central nervous system.

Nursing interventions should be based on empirical research and a sound theoretical foundation. The gate control theory provides the nurse with the knowledge necessary to make informed choices concerning appropriate interventions tailored to meet the client's needs.

Alteration of Central Control   Interventions to alter central control involve techniques that affect either the cognitive component of pain or the motivational-affective component of pain by activating the central control trigger. The central control processes are more open to suggestion when fear and anxiety are decreased (see Chapters 38 and 39).

Cognitive Control   Clients who are extremely anxious and fearful often benefit from being given information. Johnson (1972) demonstrated that clients experienced less distress and tension when procedures were described and sensations likely to be experienced were explained. With the reduction of anxiety there is usually a reduction in pain perception.

It is important to prepare elderly clients for various procedures or nursing interventions. For example, dependent elders with total hip replacement may resist beginning ambulation by the second or third postoperative day because they fear pain and injury to the operative site. Careful explanations by the nurse, prior to surgery and again immediately postoperatively, about the importance of early ambulation, how to move properly, and what sensations are likely to be experienced will both increase cooperation and lessen discomfort.

Another example of cognitive control is the placebo response. If the individual believes that a medication will relieve pain, the effects of the medication can be enhanced. The use of positive suggestion demonstrates to clients that the nurse cares that they are experiencing pain and that together they will find relief of pain. When a trusting relationship has been established with the elderly person, the nurse can use positive suggestion as a pain relief measure.

It is important to remember that placebo responders are not feigning pain. In the past, individuals were often given placebos to discriminate physiologic versus imagined pain. Research has demonstrated that a true and positive placebo response cannot be used to make that discrimination (McCaffery, 1979). It has been suggested that endorphins are responsible for the placebo response (Levine et al, 1978). Placebo responders are able to synthesize or better use the body's production of endorphin, which acts to alleviate pain chemically. If, however, the person discovers that a placebo has been given, and in essence realizes that she or he has been tricked, the ability to stimulate endorphin production to relieve pain will be lost.

Motivational-Affective Control

Relaxation   Interventions appropriate for their effect on the motivational-affective component of pain include relaxation, distraction, and comfort measures. Several different methods of relaxation are available to clients. Some are quite simple, whereas others require considerable training and practice to be effective. Deep breathing and selective tightening and relaxation of specific muscle groups are fairly simple techniques to learn, whereas techniques such as meditation, zen, and yoga require the assistance of someone trained in these arts (McCaffery, 1979).

The simple forms of relaxation may be adequate for episodes of acute pain. The nurse instructs the elderly person to take several deep, slow breaths and think about a particularly pleasant experience, for example a warm spring day; this refocuses the elder's attention and reduces anxiety. This is often enough to relieve considerable muscle tension. In an experimental study, Bobey and Davidson (1970) reported that relaxation techniques are the most effective methods for controlling painful stressors. The use of pictures to recall pleasant times can facilitate relaxation techniques. By encouraging the client to give detailed descriptions of the picture, attention is focused on something other than pain. For the elderly person, pictures from the past are often recalled better than more recent pictures (McCaffery, 1979). Environmental modifications and comfort measures such as soft lighting, comfortable room temperature, quiet music, or a back massage can help create the appropriate mood for relaxation techniques.

Distraction Distraction as an intervention for pain is based on the research of Melzack et al (1977). According to McCaffery (1979;27):

> *Normal or excessive sensory input may relieve pain. It appears that the reticular system in the brain stem can inhibit incoming stimuli, including pain, if the person is receiving sufficient or excessive sensory input. The brain stem may then project inhibitory impulses that help close the gate to the transmission of pain impulses.*

Distraction as a technique that can be readily used by the elderly requires that the nurse explore with elders their interests and previous use of distraction. With this information several alternatives can be suggested, and the elder can choose what is especially appealing.

Distraction in the form of music, particularly helpful when earphones are employed, can be useful, as can television or visitors. The release of endorphins during auditory stimulation is thought to be responsible for the placebo effect (McCaffery, 1979). Endorphins are opiate-like substances produced by the body that act as neuro-modulators. Endorphins inhibit neurotransmitter substances, thus closing the gate and modifying the noxious stimuli. Endorphin release can be stimulated by the use of TENS, acupuncture, and auditory stimulation, and appears to be the mechanism behind the placebo response and biofeedback techniques.

Humor is another effective distraction technique. Cousins (1979) attributes his remarkable recovery from a severely debilitating and painful collagen disease to daily sessions of belly laughing. A wide variety of humorous video and audio tapes are available to provide hours of joyous entertainment.

By refocusing attention to a stimulus other than pain, the individual begins to feel some control over the pain episode. This in turn can reduce anxiety and tension and break the cycle of pain. When used in conjunction with other pain relief measures, distraction can increase pain relief. However, the elderly person should also realize that when the distraction is discontinued awareness of the pain usually returns. Distraction should not be used indiscriminately, and it is important that the elder be informed of its effects and limitations (McCaffery, 1979).

Comfort Measures Much can be done in extended care facilities, and to a somewhat more limited extent in acute care settings, to make the environment as homelike and comfortable as possible and provide a normal sensory environment. Encourage family to bring in pictures and familiar objects from home when they visit. Some facilities allow small animals, dogs or cats, to visit occasionally and in some cases become permanent residents. (See Chapter 25 for more on pet therapy.)

Planning social activities, such as bingo or card parties, can help relieve boredom and monotony. Interaction with other residents and staff decreases social isolation and draws attention away from self. Another innovative practice is to integrate nursing home facilities into the community. It is not unusual to see child day-care centers next to a senior citizens home. Both age groups benefit from this interaction. In one Ohio nursing home–child care center, an elderly woman was observed rocking her small great granddaughter, who was hydrocephalic, for long periods of time. As a result, staff at the center reported a significant decrease in physical complaints by the woman (Sommers, 1985).

The importance of comfort measures such as room temperature, backrubs, and lighting cannot be stressed enough. Providing cool, crisp bed linens or a cup of tea and listening to the dependent elder's concerns can provide immeasurable comfort. Another way to provide comfort and indicate a sense of concern is to learn as much as possible about the elderly person's lifestyle, routines, likes, and dislikes. Change is difficult for everyone, and when possible, the individual's daily routines should be preserved. A refreshing night's sleep can increase pain tolerance during the day. To ensure a good night's rest, explore with the elderly person what she or he did at home. Was there a bedtime snack? A soak in a hot tub? These rituals can be accommodated in almost any setting.

Caring Although it is given little attention in the literature, the attitude of caring that the nurse projects is a critical ingredient in pain relief. Dependent elderly who perceive their caregivers as cold and uncaring will not receive the maximum benefit from any pain relief intervention. Often the elderly person has few peers or family and is lost in the overwhelming maze of a complex health care system. The nurse is often the only consistent and knowledgeable caregiver who genuinely cares about what happens to the elderly person and can act in the person's behalf. It is possible that the individual's perception of caring is capable of eliciting exogenous endorphin release. Regardless of the mechanism, it is a powerful intervention and conveys a message of deep concern to the elderly person, restores his or her sense of dignity, and maintains the bond of human compassion.

Patient Teaching   Clients are often more willing to express concerns and ask questions of nurses that they will not ask their physicians or other caregivers. The experienced nurse who is faced with an inability to answer a question should respond by saying, "I don't know the answer to that question but I will find out and get back to you." The nurse then consults the appropriate resource to obtain the answer to an elderly person's question.

An appropriate intervention for pain relief may not benefit a client because of the elderly person's failure to understand the instructions for its use. TENS units can provide pain relief for many individuals, but the devices themselves may seem complex to the elderly person. The elder's ability to learn information about a TENS unit during a teaching session at the physician's office may be confounded by any combination of the following:

1. Having visual and auditory difficulties
2. Having some degree of cognitive clouding that prevents them from understanding
3. Experiencing cognitive side effects of medication
4. Fearing that their transportation home may be waiting for them
5. Fearing electricity
6. Fearing that they will be damaged by the device
7. Having to go to the bathroom and not knowing where one is
8. Worrying about the cost of the device
9. Fearing that the device will cause more pain when applied to the painful area
10. Worrying that they will not be capable of operating the device or securing the electrodes
11. Fearing that they are not going to get well

Such an extensive list of factors should not prevent the elderly from receiving pain relief intervention but should dictate a consistent, individualized nursing approach. Learning sessions may have to be brief, with information broken down into several units presented (and perhaps repeated) over several days or weeks. If the elderly person has an ability to read, written instructions at the elder's level of understanding can be helpful because the client can pursue them at his or her own pace and read them more than once. For a detailed discussion of the diagnosis Knowledge Deficit, the reader is referred to Chapter 33.

Beyond health problems the elderly are faced with an additional set of stressors, which may include bereave- ment, retirement, and relocation. In the context of pain, these stressors become intervening variables that can intensify the elderly individual's pain experience. It has been suggested that social support and the maintenance of one's social networks can alleviate some of the isolation that accompanies bereavement, retirement, and/or reloca- tion (Kulys and Tobin, 1980; Treas and Simons, 1977). Social support appears to act as a buffer against negative health outcomes (Minkler, 1985), and, although much research is still needed in this area, the implications of its impact in achieving a better quality of life for the elderly should not be overlooked. Health care professionals should assist elderly persons in maintaining contact with support networks and encourage the development of new members in their support network.

Dependent elderly who are restricted in activities of daily living, who are confined to bed, or who use accessory muscles to splint pain develop myofascial pain that is technically unrelated to their primary pathology. Myofas- cial pain often becomes a problem of equal magnitude to the pain produced by the primary pathology, and clients often request it have first priority in pain relief. Nonspe- cific massage, vibration, rubbing, acupressure, or applica- tion of heat or cold often makes myofascial pain diminish for a brief period of time. If more specific attention to the motor loci (trigger point, acupuncture point) of the painful muscle(s) is applied, dramatic pain relief is obtained (Melzack, 1981; Melzack et al, 1977; Travel and Rinzler, 1952). The most comprehensive resource on myofascial and referred pain, which has excellent drawings of the trigger points, is Travel and Simons's *Myofascial Pain and Dysfunction: The Trigger Point Manual* (1983).

Muscle Spasms   Muscle spasms such as those experienced by Mrs. R.L. in the case study noted earlier can be effectively treated with muscle stimulation techniques. Massage, rubbing, pressure, vibrators, and/or heat or cold applied to these areas can result in greater relief than nonspecific activity directed over a larger area. The worst pain of the muscle spasm can be alleviated, but an ache or dullness will remain for 2 to 3 days after the spasm has been stopped. A NSAID administered on an around-the- clock basis will help to alleviate the dull ache that remains, and heat will cause vasodilation, which will allow the lactic acid and other painful by-products of muscle spasm to leave the area more quickly. A muscle that has been in spasm for a prolonged period may require intervention to the motor loci every 3 hours to stop the worst pain. The trigger points can be marked with an indelible marker to identify specific points to be stimulated by family members or other caregivers.

Heat and cold must be carefully monitored by frequent visualization and inspection of the body part because sensation to the area may be altered as a result of decreased blood supply or peripheral neuropathy, and/or cognitively the elderly person may not have an accurate perception of what is "hot" or "cold." Specifically, an elderly person may be burned or develop frostbite because he or she does not perceive the hot pack or ice pack as "too hot" or " too cold."

Transcutaneous Electrical Nerve Stimulators (TENS) TENS deliver a small amount of electrical energy to the painful muscle and will often relieve pain more efficiently than massage, ice, or heat. The concept of electrical stimulation dates back to the ancient Egyptians, who used the Egyptian lung fish in buckets of water to provide relief of pain from gout. The devices used today represent a technology that has undergone many important changes both technically and in clinical application. If a client has not received pain relief in the past from a TENS unit, pain relief may be possible now because of the changes in both domains. The margin of safety is wide and the risks few. TENS units should not be used in pregnant women or in patients with demand pacemakers.

TENS units deliver small amounts of energy to the skin through surface applied electrodes. Early models of TENS were large and cumbersome and made buzzing noises. Now most units are the size of paging devices and make no noise. Some have rechargeable batteries. Prior to the development of new electrode gels, skin breakdown was a significant problem. Additionally, electrodes have been developed that are of varying sizes and shapes and can be used for more than one application. Some can be left on the skin for 3 to 4 days.

TENS technology has primarily been in the hands of physical therapists, and they remain an excellent source of information for nurses who can continue to work with the client on a day-to-day basis. In outpatient and inpatient settings, the nurse spends more time with clients than does any other professional. The nurse can identify the client who might benefit from a TENS and request a prescription from a physician for the device. If the physician is unfamiliar with TENS, sharing current printed information with the client is advisable, as is a discussion of why the nurse feels a particular client will benefit from TENS. If the nurse is unfamiliar with TENS, a referral to an experienced physical therapist is indicated. To maximize the effect of the TENS, the nurse should understand what stimulation parameters have been recommended by the therapist, how frequently to stimulate, and how often. Many medical supply dealers allow rental of a TENS unit and, if successful, the rental cost applies to the purchase price. Many third-party payers will cover up to 80% of the cost of rental or purchase price. There are many devices on the market. TENS can also be used in surgical incision pain and a variety of soft-tissue injuries. The reader is referred to Mannheimer and Lampe (1984) for a comprehensive source on TENS use.

OUTCOMES

Evaluation is an important aspect of the nursing process. By objectively evaluating the success or failure of specific interventions, determined by the defining characteristics, the nurse is able to make informed decisions regarding the individual's care plan. Evaluation is also necessary because client needs change. An awareness of changing pathology should indicate a change in treatment. As the client's condition improves or declines, previously effective interventions may need to be abandoned and new ones tried.

The nurse should not overlook the client's involvement in evaluating pain relief measures. Once again this underscores the advantages of mutual goal setting. By exploring expectations and defining goals and limitations, both the nurse and the client are active participants and continue to work as a team.

The nurse can use several evaluation criteria to judge the success or failure of a care plan for pain. Ideally the care plan will incorporate several methods of pain control. For example, aside from the use of analgesics, the nurse might also employ the use of relaxation and the stimulation of large diameter fibers to reduce transmission of painful impulses. By understanding why a particular intervention is used and what component of the pain episode it affects, alterations can be made in the care plan to maximize its effectiveness and tailor it to the client's current needs.

Physical Indicators

The nurse should look and feel for a relaxation of the skeletal muscles. This is an indication of decreased muscle tension and a reduction of fear and anxiety. Confirming this observation reinforces the elderly person's belief in the effectiveness of the intervention and promotes a sense of well-being.

Elimination of pain postures is also indicative of pain relief in that the elder no longer needs to protect a joint or a limb with a rigid posture. As muscles relax, rigid posturing should continue to decrease with an accompanying increase in activity level and mobility.

Behavioral Indicators

The individual who is relatively pain free often demonstrates an increase in activity level. This also promotes further pain control by increasing circulation and promoting a sense of self-worth. Whenever possible, the nurse should reinforce and encourage the client to "keep up the good work."

When pain no longer rules the body, the individual's attention span is increased, and the client can once again participate in activities or hobbies that formerly brought pleasure. This sense of accomplishment further enhances the individual's sense of well-being and continues to weaken the cycle of pain. There should also be a noticeable focus of attention away from pain. Social interactions should increase and the client should become less isolated. When pain is no longer the central focus of one's day, the body has more energy to devote to pleasurable activities and pleasant conversation.

Once the fearful grip of pain is broken there should be an almost immediate increase in the ability to rest, relax, or sleep. It is not uncommon for a person who has been experiencing excruciating pain of long duration to sleep for quite extended periods of time. Such severe pain leaves the body exhausted, and once relief is obtained, the body acts to replenish its resources.

Verbal Indicators

Successful interventions should result in a decreased use of pain references during conversations and in an overall decrease in specific complaints of pain. Although pain may not be entirely eliminated, the nurse should listen carefully for qualitative descriptions that indicate a lessening of intensity of the pain. For example, in reference to the McGill Pain Questionnaire, words that describe extremely severe pain might include *unbearable, torturing,* or *pounding.* If these descriptors are replaced by words such as *annoying, nagging,* or *flickering,* the intervention has been successful.

Finally, the client should describe fewer or absent pain sensations. The nurse might say to the patient, "Yesterday you rated your pain as an eight. How would you rate it today?" It is also important to ascertain whether the location and quality of the pain are the same or different.

Evaluation Tools

The visual analog scales or verbal descriptor scales can be used to evaluate an intervention as well as to assess a painful episode. Likewise the use of body outlines, with or without color, can aid the nurse in providing data for measures of pain relief.

Meinhart and McCaffery (1983;361) also suggest the use of a pain flow sheet to mark a client's progress. Not only is this useful to the medical staff, but it can also reassure the client that progress is being made. Many times the client can be actively involved in recording data on the flow sheet. For example, it may be useful to have the client record pain ratings at various times. Often this can demonstrate a pattern to the client that will enhance the prescribed plan of care.

SUMMARY

Caring for the elderly person must include an assessment and evaluation for pain with appropriate interventions based on clinical judgments. The myth that pain and old age go hand in hand must be dispelled.

Assessment begins with a thorough health history and an evaluation of the elderly person's pain status. Consideration must be given to the intervening variables that can affect the proposed interventions.

Interventions should be prescribed so as to affect the cognitive, motivational, and/or physiologic components of pain. This may include a variety of measures ranging from simple comfort measures to pharmacologic therapy or transcutaneous nerve stimulation.

Finally, the elderly patient must be continually evaluated to determine the success of the prescribed interventions. This is an ongoing process that changes as the elderly person's needs and condition change.

By the effective use of the nursing process in the intervention for pain in the elderly the nurse can assure the patient a better quality of life. If we cannot promise our elderly that the best is yet to be, we can strive to make their lives as pain free as possible.

References

Armitage KJ, Schneiderman LJ, Bass RA: Responses of physicians to medical complaints in men and women. *JAMA* 1979; 241(20):2186–2187.

Baker SP, O'Neill B, Karpf RS: *The Injury Fact Book.* Lexington Books, 1984.

Balderssarini RJ: Drugs and the treatment of psychiatric disorders. In: *The Pharmocological Basis of Therapeutics.* Gillman AG, Goodman LS, Gilman A (editors). Macmillan, 1980.

Berry H, Huskisson EC: A report on pain measurement. *Clin Trials* 1972; 9:13.

Blazer D, Siegler IC: *A Family Approach to Health Care of the Elderly.* Addison-Wesley, 1984.

Bobey MJ, Davidson PO: Psychological factors affecting pain tolerance. *J Psychosom Res* 1970; 14:371–376.

Browning R: "Rabbi Ben Ezra." In: *The Complete Poetical Works of Browning.* Scudder HE (editor). Houghton Mifflin, 1895.

Bullock B, Rosendahl D: *Pathophysiology.* Little, Brown, 1984; 808–821.

Butler S: Present status of tricyclic antidepressants in chronic pain. In: *Advances in Pain Research and Therapy.* Benedetti C (editor). Raven Press, 1984.

Carroll-Johnson, R (editor): *Classification of Nursing Diagnoses: Proceedings of the Eighth Conference.* Lippincott, 1989.

Clark PRF, Spear FG: Reliability and sensitivity in the self-assessment of well being. *Bull British Psychol Soc* 1964; 17 (55):18A.

Clark WC, Mehl L: A sensory decision theory analysis of the effect of age and sex on d', various response criteria, and 50% pain threshold. *J Abnormal Psychol* 1971; 78:202–212.

Cohen FL: Postsurgical pain relief: Patients' status and nurses' medication choices. *Pain* 1977; 9:265–274.

Coombs DW et al: Relief of continuous chronic pain by intraspinal narcotics infusion via an implanted reservoir. *JAMA* 1983; 250(17):2336–2339.

Cousins N: *Anatomy of an Illness as Perceived by the Patient: Reflections on Healing and Regeneration.* Norton, 1979.

Doughtery R: Personal communication, May 11, 1986.

Dubuisson D, Melzack R: Classification of clinical pain descriptors by multiple group discriminant analysis. *Experiment Neurol* 1976; 51:480–487.

Eland JM: Pain. Chapter 9 in: *Concepts Common in Acute Illness.* Hart LK, Reese JL, Fearing MO (editors). Mosby, 1981a.

Eland JM: Minimizing pain associated with prekindergarten intramuscular injections. *Issues Compr Pediatr Nurs* 1981b; 5:361.

Flower RJ, Monceda S, Vane JR: Analgesics, antipyretics, and anti-inflammatory agents: Drugs employed in the treatment of gout. In: *Goodman and Gilman's The Pharmacological Basis of Therapeutics,* 7th ed. Gilman A (editor). Macmillan, 1985.

Foley KM: The treatment of cancer pain. *N Engl J Med* 1985; 313:84–95.

Freedman N: Depression in a family practice elderly population. *J Am Geriatr Soc* 1982; 30:372–377.

Hallal JC: Understanding zoster and relieving its discomfort. *Geriatr Nurs* 1985; 6(2):74–78.

Halpern L: Drugs in the management of pain: Pharmacologic and applied strategies for clinical utilization. In: *Advances in Pain Research and Theory,* Vol 7. Raven Press, 1984.

Harnish JP: Zoster in the elderly: Clinical, immunological, and therapeutic considerations. *J Am Geriatr Soc* 1984; 32(11):789–793.

Johnson JE: Effects of structuring patients' expectations on their reactions to threatening events. *Nurs Res* 1972; 21:489.

Johnson M: Assessment of clinical pain. Chapter 6 in: *Pain: A Source Book for Nurses and Other Health Professionals.* Jacox AK (editor). Little, Brown, 1977.

Kaiko RF: Age and morphine analgesia in cancer patients with post-operative pain. *Clin Pharmacol* 1980; 28:823–826.

Kaiko RF et al: Central nervous system excitatory effects of meperidine in cancer patients. *Ann Neurol* 1983; 13(2):180–185.

Kim MI, Moritz DA (editors): *Classification of Nursing Diagnoses: Proceedings of the Third and Fourth National Conferences.* McGraw-Hill, 1982.

Kolodney AL, Klipper AR: Bone and joint disease in the elderly. *Hosp Pract* 1976; 11:91–101.

Kulys R, Tobin SS: Older people and their responsible others. *Soc Work* 1980; 138–148.

Kwentus JA et al: Current concepts of geriatric pain and its treatment. *Geriatrics* 1985; 40(4):48–57.

Lavasky-Shulan M et al: Prevalence and functional correlates of low back pain in the elderly: The Iowa 65 + rural health study. *J Am Geriatr Soc* 1985; 33:23–28.

Levine JD, Gordon NC, Fields HL: Evidence that the analgesic effect of placebo is mediated by endorphins. Page 18 in: *Pain Abstracts 1;* Seattle: International Association for the Study of Pain, 1978.

Lindsay PG, Wyckoff M: The depression pain syndrome and its response to antidepressants. *Psychosomatics* 1981; 22:571–577.

Malone BT, Beyer R, Walker J: Management of pain in the terminally ill by administration of epidural narcotics. *Cancer* 1985; 55(2):438–440.

Malseed RT: *Pharmacology: Drug Therapy and Nursing Considerations,* 2d ed. Lippincott, 1985.

Mannheimer JS, Lampe G: *Clinical Transcutaneous Electrical Nerve Stimulation.* Davis, 1984.

Mather LE: Pharmokinetic studies of meperidine. In: *Advances in Pain Research and Theory.* Foley KM, Inturrisi CE (editors). Raven Press, 1986.

Matthews G, Zarrow V, Osterholm J: Cancer pain and its treatment. *Sem Drug Treat* 1973; 3(1):45–72.

McCaffery M: *Nursing Management of the Patient with Pain,* 2d ed. Lippincott, 1979.

McDonald JB: Coronary care in the elderly. *Age Ageing* 1983; 12:17–20.

McLane AM (editor): *Classification of Nursing Diagnoses: Proceedings of the Seventh Conference.* Mosby, 1987.

Meinhart NT, McCaffery M: *Pain: A Nursing Approach to Assessment and Analysis.* Appleton-Century-Crofts, 1983.

Melzack R: The McGill Pain Questionnaire: Major properties and scoring methods. *Pain* 1975; 1:277–299.

Melzack R: Myofascial trigger points: Relation to acupuncture and mechanisms of pain. *Arch Phys Med Rehab* 1981; 62:114–117.

Melzack R, Stillwell DM, Fox EJ: Trigger points and acupuncture points for pain: Correlations and implications. *Pain* 1977; 3:3–27.

Melzack R, Torgerson WS: On the language of pain. *Anesthesiology* 1971; 34:50–59.

Melzack R, Wall PD: Pain mechanisms: A new theory. *Science* 1965; 150:971–975.

Melzack R, Wall PD: *The Challenge of Pain.* Basic Books, 1983.

Minkler M: Social support and health of the elderly. Chapter 10 in: *Social Support and Health.* Cohen S, Syme SL (editors). Academic Press, 1985.

Oliver N: Abdominal pain in the elderly. *Australian Fam Physician* 1984; 13(6):402–404.

Pfeiffer RF: Drugs for pain in the elderly. *Geriatrics* 1982; 37(2):67–76.

Pilowsky I, Bond MR: Pain and its management in malignant disease. *Psychosom Med* 1969; 31:400–404.

Pilowsky I, Kaufman A: An experimental study of atypical phantom pain. *British J Psychiatry* 1965; 111:1185.

Rodstein M: The characteristics of non-fatal myocardial infarction in the aged. *Arch Intern Med* 1956; 98:684–690.

Sherman ED, Robillar E: Sensitivity to pain in the aged. *Can Med Assoc J* 1980; 83:944.

Smith DL: Patient compliance with medical regimens. *Drug Intel Clin Pharm* 1976; 10:386–393.

Sommers K: The geriatric mix: Child care in the nursing home. *Nurs Homes* 1985; 34(4):27–30.

Sternbach RA: *Pain: A Psychological Analysis.* Academic Press, 1968.

Stewart ML: Measurement of clinical pain. Chapter 5 in: *Pain: A Source Book for Nurses and Other Health Professionals.* Jacox A (editor). Little, Brown, 1977.

Travel J, Rinzler SH: The myofascial genesis of pain. *Postgrad Med* 1952; 11:425–434.

Travel J, Simons R: *Myofascial Pain and Dysfunction: The Trigger Point Manual.* Williams & Wilkins, 1983.

Treas J: Family support systems for the aged: Some social and demographic considerations. *Gerontologist* 1977; 17:486–491.

Twycross RG, Lack SA: *Symptom Control in Far Advanced Cancer: Pain Control.* Pitman, 1983.

Wachter-Shikora N: The elderly patient in pain and the acute care setting. *Nurs Clin North Am* 1983; 18:395–401.

Wachter-Shikora N, Perez S: Unmasking pain. *Geriatr Nurs* 1982; 3(6):392–393.

Wandless I, Davie JW: Can drug compliance be improved? *British Med J* (Feb) 1977; 1:359–361.

Zbrowski M: Cultural components in response to pain. *J Soc Iss* 1952; 8:16–30.

31

Sensory/ Perceptual Alterations

JANICE DRURY, RN
JACKIE AKINS, BSN, RN, C

PERCEPTION IS THE PROCESS OF INTEGRATING, CLASSI-fying, discriminating, and assigning meaning to stimuli. The human individual is oriented to surroundings through the ability to receive and organize information. Stimuli are gathered through sensory receptors. The senses, then, may be thought of as the gateways to the central nervous system. They "furnish the primary data of our knowledge of the external world, and serve as a feedback mechanism to tell us how well we are adjusting to the physical, geographical, and social aspects of the world in which we live" (Avant and Helson, 1973;337).

This chapter discusses what happens when elderly persons experience loss in these integrative or adjustment mechanisms of sensory perception, the resulting behavior, and the nursing assessment and interventions for these losses.

DETERMINATION OF THE DIAGNOSIS

At the Seventh Conference, the North American Nursing Diagnosis Association (NANDA) identified two diagnostic labels in the area of sensory/ perceptual dysfunction: Unilateral Neglect and Sensory/Perceptual Alterations (S/PA): visual, auditory, kinesthetic, gustatory, tactile, olfactory. Unilateral Neglect is defined as perceptual unawareness of or inattention to one side of the body. S/PA is defined as a state in which an individual experiences a change in the amount or patterning of incoming stimuli accompanied by a diminished, exaggerated, distorted, or impaired response to such stimuli (Carroll-Johnson, 1989;551). The concept of Sensory/Perceptual Alterations is complex. Alterations affect one's ability to maneuver physically within the environment, respond to the demands of the environment, and react to the cognitive and affective implications of that environment.

Gordon (1987;178–184) differentiates Sensory/ Perceptual Alterations into three more specific diagnoses. The first is Sensory/Perceptual Alterations: Uncompensated Deficit, a state in which the individual experiences or is at risk of experiencing uncompensated loss of acuity in (or absence of) vision, hearing, touch, smell, taste, or kinesthesia. Assessment and intervention are directed toward the etiologies to alleviate or compensate for losses in the sensory systems and facilitate optimal functioning in the environment. The second specific diagnosis is Sensory/Perceptual Alterations: Input Excess (or sensory overload), defined as environmental stimuli greater than habitual level of input and/or monotonous environmental stimuli. Assessment and treatment strategies focus on the individual's ability to cope with environmental demands and on adjustment of the environment to reduce stimuli. The third diagnosis, Sensory/Perceptual Alterations: Input Deficit (sensory deprivation) is defined as reduced environmental and social stimuli relative to habitual (or basic orienting) level. It is important that the elder's cognitive abilities are assessed for optimal functioning. The last two diagnoses address the elder's response to a change or disruption in the quality or quantity of incoming stimuli that affects physiologic, emotional, cognitive, and affective domains. Although these diagnoses have similar and overlapping etiologies (see Table 31.1), the defining characteristics and implications for nursing assessment and intervention differ.

The NANDA diagnosis Unilateral Neglect addresses an alteration in perceptions but differs from the other S/PA diagnoses in defining characteristics as a result of defect or damage within the individual and the internal response to these losses. Thus, etiology and focus of intervention are different and are addressed in Chapter 32. The three previously defined diagnoses, S/PA: Uncompensated; S/PA: Excess; and S/PA: Deficit, are closely connected with the interaction with the environment (physical and social) and the quantity or quality of that interaction with each other. The four diagnoses are needed for the accurate assessment and planning of care for S/PA of the elderly.

SIGNIFICANCE FOR THE ELDERLY

Changes within the sensory systems have great impact on how the elder functions in the environment. Overall blurring and other vision changes put the elder at risk for injury such as falls or incorrect choices in medications or containers of substances. Cues helpful in determining appropriate behavior or choices can be misinterpreted or lost. Participation in hobbies or other leisure time activities becomes more difficult. The person may stop reading the daily newspaper or may not be able to drive. Aside from loss of intrinsic enjoyment derived from leisure time activities, the individual begins to experience some social isolation through lack of contact.

The muffling of sounds with decreased discrimination of conversational speech also has implications for safety. Warnings, such as verbal messages or alarms, may be misunderstood or missed entirely. Orientation cues, such as the ticking or chiming of a clock, or background environmental sounds become muffled or lost. Partial or no reception of messages interferes with cognitive interpretation and response (eg, perception of the word *sing*

instead of *thing*, or *fine* rather than *sign*). The resultant error in response (and the elder who made it) may then be labeled as confused, irrational, or inappropriate. Affective changes ranging from acceptance or resignation to shyness to defensiveness to bitterness and hate have been associated with hearing loss (Iveson, 1979). Sound not only makes us constantly aware of our environment but also assures us of our separate existence within a physical and social context (Conover and Cober, 1970).

A safety concern associated with losses in taste and smell is the inability to perceive warnings of danger, such as smoke, spoiled foods, ingestion of poisonous substances, or gas. Losses of acuity in individual senses of smell, taste, and vision interact so that the total loss is greater than the sum of the individual losses. Implications for the decrease in smell, taste, and vision in the elder must also include the psychosocial importance of food in American culture and social interaction during the dining experience. Adequacy of nutritional intake may be affected.

Tactile sensations provide the individual with warnings of heat, cold, and pain. Susceptibility to conditions of hypo- or hyperthermia or physical injury is increased. Touch provides information about the relationship between the environment and self. Incomplete information alters the appropriate response to the environment. Barnett (1972;102) identifies that the "first and most fundamental means of communicating is through some form of touch." For many persons, touching and being touched become associated with acceptance (Montagu, 1971;4–5).

Nurses' own attitudes regarding the elderly are important determinants of the behavior of caregivers and the elderly. Because the nurse may reflect a negative perception of the elderly, assessment, diagnosis, and accurate prescription of therapy(s) may be affected. Although nurses recognize the social and psychologic aspects of nursing care, treatment for the elder is often viewed in terms of palliative or custodial care. Prescriptions for care frequently focus on physical and medical needs rather than on psychosocial or emotional needs and compensatory interventions (Hefferin and Hunter, 1975; Wolk and Wolk, 1971). Conventional supportive therapy— supporting, nurturing, listening, counseling, and manipulating the environment—is sometimes regarded as second rate. It is not "real therapy" with respect to the challenge and professional skill required (Kastenbaum, 1963). Attitudes not only influence the kind or amount of intervention prescribed for the elderly but may influence whether they receive any treatment at all. Opportunities may not be provided to assess or draw out functions assumed to be lost. Snyder et al (1976;494) indicate that less than one fifth of all older persons receive vision care of any kind, and older persons in institutions may receive less frequent visual care than elderly persons in communities at large.

Table 31.1

Definitions, Etiologies, and Defining Characteristics of Sensory/Perceptual Alterations

CARROLL-JOHNSON (1989)	GORDON (1987)	DRURY/AKINS
S/PA: Visual, Auditory, Kinesthetic, Gustatory, Tactile, Olfactory		

S/PA: Visual, Auditory, Kinesthetic, Gustatory, Tactile, Olfactory

CARROLL-JOHNSON (1989)	GORDON (1987)	DRURY/AKINS
Definition A state in which an individual experiences a change in the amount or patterning of incoming stimuli accompanied by a diminished, exaggerated, distorted, or impaired response to such stimuli	*Definition* Uncompensated loss of acuity or absence of vision, hearing, touch, smell, or kinesthesia and/or integration	
Etiologies Environmental factors therapeutically or socially restricted Altered sensory reception, transmission, integration Chemical alteration endogenous/exogenous Psychologic stress	*Etiologies* None listed, but may be etiology for other	*Etiologies* Altered sensory reception including normal age-related changes and diseases (Authors add these etiologies to those listed by McLane and Gordon)
Defining Characteristics Disoriented in time, in place, or with persons Altered abstraction Altered conceptualization Change in problem-solving abilities Reported or measured change in sensory acuity Acuity Apathy Change in usual response to stimuli Indication of body-image alteration Restlessness Irritability Altered communication patterns Disorientation Lack of concentration Daydreaming Hallucinations Noncompliance Fear Depression Rapid mood swings Anger Exaggerated emotional responses Poor concentration Disordered thought sequencing Bizarre thinking Visual and auditory distortions Motor incoordination Complaints of fatigue Alterations in posture Change in muscular tension Inappropriate responses	*Defining Characteristics* *Vision*—inability to read newsprint or identify objects or persons *Hearing*—inability to identify whispered sounds or normally voiced words *Smell*—inability to identify odors *Touch*—inability to discriminate various qualities or tactile sensations or absence of tactile sensations *Kinesthesia*—inability to identify extent, direction, or weight of movement of body or part	*Defining Characteristics* Taste—inability to identify tastes (Added to those listed by Gordon)

(Continues)

Table 31.1

Definitions, Etiologies, and Defining Characteristics of Sensory/Perceptual Alterations (*Continued*)

CARROLL-JOHNSON (1989)	GORDON (1987)	DRURY/AKINS
S/PA: Input Excess		
Definition NANDA does not list this diagnosis separately	*Definition* Environmental stimuli greater than habitual level of input and/or monotonous environmental stimuli	
	Etiologies Environmental complexity/monotony	*Etiologies* Environmental complexity internal/external Diminished discriminatory cognitive functioning Decreased coping
	Defining Characteristics Irritability, anxiety Restlessness Disorientation (periodic or general) Sleeplessness Reduction in problem-solving ability, work performance Complaints of fatigue Increased muscle tension Uninterrupted and/or unchanging stimuli (motor, monitor, light, voices) Complex environment relative to cognitive capabilities to handle sensory input	*Defining Characteristics* Irritability Restlessness Confusion General anxiety Sleeplessness Fatigue Muscle tension Reduced problem-solving ability Reduced work performance Environmental monotony Environmental complexity
S/PA: Input Deficit		
Definition NANDA does not list this diagnosis separately	*Definition* Reduced environmental and social stimuli relative to habitual (or basic orienting) level	
	Etiologies Isolation (restricted environment)	*Etiologies* Uncompensated visual/hearing deficit Therapeutic environmental restriction (isolation, bed rest, traction) Socially restricted environment (homebound, institutionalization, age debilitation) Impaired communication Immobility Decreased sensory stimuli (quality/quantity)
	Defining Characteristics Alert with periodic disorientation, general confusion, or nocturnal confusion Hallucinations Apathy Auditory, visual, reality-orienting, or time-orienting input reduced or absent Limited proprioceptive input Presence of uncompensated visual or hearing deficits	*Defining Characteristics* Same as Gordon, 1987

SENSORY/PERCEPTUAL ALTERATIONS: UNCOMPENSATED DEFICIT

Sensory/Perceptual Alterations: Uncompensated (S/PA: Uncompensated) identifies changes within the sensory systems that result in altered ability to interact with the environment. Commonly the cause for this change or loss in the elder is related to the normal process of aging. Aging occurs at different rates for different individuals and even within the organ systems of an individual. Changes in the senses, as in the whole body, occur at different times for different individuals. These changes affect and are affected by one another. They occur as the individual ages but are also a result of living in the world. Multiple theories have been advanced to explain the aging process. No one theory seems comprehensive enough at this time; however, the "wear and tear" theory of the deterioration associated with aging in conjunction with other theories does seem to help explain some of the loss exhibited in the sensory systems (Ebersole and Hess, 1981). Aging in other systems also affects the efficiency of the senses (eg, loss of muscle strength, endurance, and agility; slowing of conduction velocity or speed of impulse transmission in the nerves; and synaptic delay caused by decrease in the amount of neurotransmitters) (Bloom et al, 1985;275).

Etiologies of S/PA: Uncompensated are summarized in Table 31.1. Nursing assessment and intervention are discussed separately for each sense.

Assessment of Sensory/Perceptual Alterations: Uncompensated Deficit

Assessment of sensory function, specifically for S/PA: Uncompensated, can be inexpensive and fairly simple. It is important to include assessment of how the elder manipulates and functions within the surroundings. For optimal results, tests of functional abilities need to be conducted in quiet, uncluttered surroundings with balanced lighting. Because these may be new experiences for elders, expectations or goals of testing related to possible practical application of the results should be clearly explained with ample time allowed for processing of the information and for feedback. Signs and symptoms of S/PA: Uncompensated are summarized in Table 31.1.

Vision A standard Snellen vision chart is used to determine visual acuity. For persons not able to read letters, directional arrows or pictures may be used. Various print sizes for signs, magazines, or newspapers can be used to measure what the literate individual can interpret. Pictures can be used for individuals who are not able to read. Visual fields should be checked to assess the scope of peripheral gaze. Examination of the inner eye is often very difficult because of corneal scarring or presence of cataracts. The nurse must remember that the focus of assessment is on the individual's ability to maneuver and function in the environment.

Hearing The first step in the assessment of hearing is to check the ear canals for mechanical obstruction. If cerumen is present, a softening product is recommended to clear the canal. After this is accomplished, visualization of the canal with an ophthalmoscope should reveal a healthy pink membranous lining without open or irritated areas or drainage. The eardrum is normally a pearly silver–gray flat-looking disc. Bulging of the membrane may indicate a buildup of pressure or infection. Hearing then may be assessed using a tuning fork, loud ticking clock, or verbal cues to determine auditory accuracy at measured distances.

Smell and Taste Smell and taste are best assessed by offering various common scents, such as coffee, garlic, vinegar, nutmeg, and cinnamon, and common tastes, such as popcorn (with and without salt) and lemonade (with varying amounts of sweetness), for identification. Time between samples must be allowed so that overlapping sensations don't occur.

Touch The sensation of touch may be determined first by touching the individual with wisps of cotton and having the individual identify when he or she is being touched. After some notion is gained about intactness of touch sensation, discrimination of touch can be determined by using a safety pin and having the individual identify if the sensation is sharp (using the point end) or dull (using the hinge end). Using two pins at the same time at varying distances apart helps measure the accuracy of discrimination. Further testing should include identification of various textures of fabrics or common objects by touch.

The reader is referred to Bates (1979) or a general physical assessment text for more detailed assessment information. Additionally, the elder may need to be referred to appropriate specialists for more definitive examination.

CASE STUDY

Sensory/Perceptual Alterations: Uncompensated Deficit

J.C. is a 70-year-old white man who lives in a long-term care facility, where he has resided since 1961. He has no history of drug or alcohol abuse. Current medical diagnoses include (1) bilateral blindness with ocular opacity secondary to detergent burns several years ago; (2) obesity;

(3) kyphoscoliosis; and (4) history of iron deficiency anemia. Medications include aspirin (ASA), Theragran-M, Metamucil, Trilisate, vitamin C, and Senokot. Generally, J.C. agrees to and is cooperative with measures implemented to promote good health. He was married once and divorced after 2 years, but has no children. He has had no contact with his ex-wife since their divorce. J.C.'s family consists of a sister who lives 60 miles away and visits approximately once every 2 months. He has one niece in Colorado who writes. He does not seem bothered by a group living situation and has formed a close relationship with another resident who was temporarily housed on the same unit, but after 2 months moved to a different unit. Since the friend's transfer to another unit, the friend has maintained contact, and J.C. looks forward to and enjoys these visits.

J.C. is oriented to his unit's environment and current events occurring within this environment. He has an eighth grade education and worked as a laborer most of his life. Language and conversation are consistent with education and occupation. Generally, J.C. is able to remember, tell, and respond to jokes or broad nuances of conversation. His facial and nonverbal gestures are expressive and consistent with verbal content. He doesn't appear to be anxious, defensive, or fearful and seems to trust that he won't be harmed and that his needs will be met. J.C. smiles frequently and often thanks staff for their care. At this time, he is considered competent, able to handle his own financial affairs, and able to make decisions requiring informed consent. Generally, he is able to understand requests and expectations.

He is blind in both eyes, and hearing is slightly diminished bilaterally. He can hear speech when the volume is increased. He was referred to an audiologist, who recommended amplification with a hearing aid to be used in the right ear. With the hearing aid J.C. hears voices at normal speaking tones up to 10 to 15 feet away. His tympanic membranes appear normal. Although J.C. wears dentures, he likes all foods and truly enjoys meals. When asked to identify various tastes and smells on his meal tray, he is almost always accurate. He responds to light touch and is able to discriminate between various textures. His gait is somewhat ataxic, and he prefers that staff walk backward in front of him and hold his hands. J.C. walks approximately 100 to 150 yards, then begins to complain of pain in his knees. Joints are slightly stiffened, but he is able to go through 100% active range of motion if initially supported in the movement. X-rays show moderate degenerative changes in both knees with some calcification in joint spaces, particularly in the right knee. J.C. is able to assist with activities of daily living (ADLs).

Interventions for Sensory/Perceptual Alterations: Uncompensated Deficit

Creativity and common sense are vital in developing alternative techniques appropriate for the elderly individual with S/PA: Uncompensated. Four nursing intervention strategies are appropriate for the diagnosis of S/PA: Uncompensated. These are environmental structuring for enhanced sensory function/interpretation; provision, care, and use of assistive appliances; referral to appropriate specialized clinicians, and teaching/counseling of the elder, significant others, or nursing staff.

Environmental Structuring Careful assessment and manipulation of the environment to compensate for the elder's sensory losses is essential. The aim for compensating visual deficits is to add additional color and contrast, making the environment easier to see and interpret. Use of bright (not glaring) contrasting colors helps elders identify living spaces, corners, and staircases. "Warm" colors in the red/yellow range are more easily distinguished than blue/green colors, which are more frequently perceived as grays (Sullivan, 1983;230). The use of red/yellow colors in the environment enhances depth perception. Contrasting strips along the edges of stairs or at the bottom of walls also facilitate depth perception. Lighting without glare within living areas is recommended. "Close work is done best when the light on the task at hand is three times brighter than the background light" (Sullivan, 1983;232). Multiple sources of light are best. Glare can be minimized by reducing the number of reflective surfaces (eg, large areas of glass, high-gloss wall/floor finishes). Sudden contrasts between bright sunlight and shade or between indoors and outdoors can compromise vision until adaptation takes place (Yurick, 1980). Sunglasses, hats with broad brims, and umbrellas are recommended for use during outdoor excursions. Night-lights to facilitate transition from light areas to dark areas are invaluable. Handrails and large print or pictorial directional signs, calendars, and clocks to assist with locating places or orientation are recommended. Consistent placement of objects within the environment is also important (Sullivan, 1983). Traffic patterns through rooms should be kept clear of clutter, with wide spaces left between furniture to facilitate movement and prevent injury.

For enhancing hearing, auditory cues and directions given in quiet surroundings are heard best. Reducing background noise, speaking clearly face to face with the elderly person, adjusting voice volume and pitch, and limiting the number of persons in groups to four or five are also ways to enhance audition.

The addition of spices allowed within the therapeutic diet to foods will enhance flavors and increase perception of taste. Because food must be in solution for the taste buds to sense flavor, taking fluids with solid foods may improve taste, especially if the elder's mouth is dry as a result of disease, medications, or reduced salivation. An unhurried meal that looks, smells, and tastes good and that is served in pleasant, sociable surroundings increases the pleasure of dining as well as the appetite.

A variety of textures in the environment increase object recognition. Consistency in furniture placement assists elders to orient themselves in the environment. Multiple tactile sensations enhance the elderly's ability to experience their surroundings to the fullest. This promotes orientation and independence.

Provision, Care, and Use of Assistive Devices

Optimal care of assistive devices (eg, eyeglasses, hearing aids) includes maintenance of proper fit and cleansing. Clearing of cerumen from hearing aids, checking correct placement and fit, and checking batteries are important nursing interventions. Other devices that can assist the elder include hand-held or tablestand magnifying glasses or large print items; telephones with extra loud bells or lights for the hearing impaired; telephone dial covers with enlarged numbers; telephones with programmed dialing of often-used or emergency numbers; amplifiers for telephone receivers; and clocks that chime or recite the time. Properly fitting dentures are essential and must be kept clean to enhance flavors of food.

Referral to Appropriate Specialized Clinicians

Referrals to an appropriate specialist—ophthalmologist/optometrist, audiologist, occupational therapist, or physical therapist—for detailed examination should be considered. Various specialized resources (eg, Commission for the Blind) can provide further information and suggestions for care. When no other solution is readily apparent, brainstorming with resource people can help to identify new approaches.

Teaching/Counseling

The priority for assessment needs to be conveyed to the elder and others. Societal role expectations of mental impairment and behavioral frailty can affect the self-image of the elder and become a self-fulfilling prophecy (Lawton, 1970). When sight or hearing are no longer primary ways of gaining information to function efficiently, alternative techniques must be developed, and time for ventilating feelings or grieving about sensory losses must be allowed. Identification of coping strategies then follows. A "functional" perspective is positive, focusing on the elder's capabilities rather than on his or her disabilities.

It is important to check glasses or hearing aids to maintain their function and to enhance reception of messages. The nurse should gain the elder's attention before starting the message, speak slowly with careful enunciation of words, and generally lower the pitch of the voice while not increasing the volume. Because some elderly require a higher pitch, testing the hearing of each elderly person is recommended. Increased volume forces the pitch of the voice into higher frequencies and further decreases comprehension. The nurse should also stand facing the elder to facilitate lipreading and use of nonverbal gestures to reinforce meaning. The nurse should provide information about any examination and allow the client time to practice expectations of examination situations prior to appointments with consultants. The nurse also should provide instructions in proper care and use of adaptive devices. Again, this includes allowing time for hands-on practice, giving step-by-step instructions and written cues for use, and sharing mutual goals for use of the aid.

The nurse and client may use a variety of techniques to compensate for the client's sensory losses. Discussing environmental strategies with the elder, encouraging the elder to use multiple or alternate senses, and assisting the elder to focus on other environmental cues help to compensate for areas of deficit. Clients with compromised vision may skim the walls and articles of furniture with a hand (touch) to orient themselves to position. The nurse may call attention to the draft coming from the window to help orient the client spatially to the room. Or the nurse may identify the smell and sounds of food preparation to orient the elder to time of day. The elder may learn lipreading skills to augment hearing.

CASE STUDY

Nursing Interventions

J.C. has Sensory/Perceptual Alterations: Uncompensated Visual Loss. Goals for nursing interventions are directed toward optimizing J.C.'s functioning within his environment. Because he is blind, the stimulation of other senses is important. Auditory cues are enhanced through use of his hearing aid, a talking clock, and a radio. J.C.'s ears are checked monthly for cerumen, and softening drops are used to clear wax if needed. When on the unit, J.C. sits near the nursing station where folks are talking, which helps him keep oriented to time, activities, and "current events." To increase the variety of his interactions, staff bring in children and/or pets when attending off-shift meetings or getting paychecks. J.C. remembers and enjoys the interaction he has with them.

J.C. is encouraged to perform as much of his own ADLs as possible. He washes himself when assisted to the bathroom and his care articles are laid out. He is able to put on his shirt and trousers, button his shirt, and zip his trousers once the clothing is handed to him. Staff help with the TED hose and shoes. J.C. combs his hair and shaves himself with an electric razor. Hygiene articles are routinely kept in the same place so that J.C. is able to locate them. As identified in the assessment, J.C. has full dentures, which fit well. He is able to accomplish his own oral care, rinsing his mouth with Cepacol, then brushing his dentures after toothpaste is applied to the toothbrush (sometimes requiring staff assistance). J.C. is able to feed himself after the meal tray is "set up" by staff (milk carton opened, condiments added, placement of food identified). He uses adaptive feeding aids, a large tablespoon and plate guard, to assist him.

Summary

Deficits in the sensory systems affect the elder's ability to function within his or her environment. Accurate assessment by the nurse to identify the elder's actual disabilities is needed. Validity of this assessment depends on the nurse's awareness of attitudes and stereotypes about aging and the aged person. Without diagnosis and appropriate intervention based on actual status, the elder is unnecessarily limited. As will be discussed in the following sections, the elder's sensory perceptions can then become further compromised. Compensation for losses in the sensory organs is usually accomplished by minimizing loss and focusing on remaining abilities. The creativity needed on the part of the nurse to accomplish this is rewarded by the increased dignity and quality of life for the elder.

SENSORY/PERCEPTUAL ALTERATIONS: INPUT EXCESS

The nursing diagnosis Sensory/Perceptual Alterations: Input Excess (S/PA: Input Excess), sensory overload, deals with the loss of ability to sort or respond appropriately to incoming stimuli. The complexity of the elder's environment has a great deal to do with his or her responses to it. Exposed to a variety of stimuli, some of which have meaning and some of which do not, we learn selective perception to screen the stimuli received and direct appropriate responses in order to avoid sensory overload and loss of "normal" functioning. If excess sensory input is not screened, identified, or compensated for, loss of function may result, be inadvertently reinforced, and become a chronic condition. S/PA: Input Excess is

a multi-sensory experience wherein two or more senses receive stimuli of greater than normal intensity, either suddenly or in rapid succession. This rapid, multi-focused assault of the receptive activities in the brain can lead to behavior immobility (confusion). Each stimulus is not fully interpreted in terms of reality, so that the client's behavior

is related to their own interpretation of reality (Gioiella and Bevil, 1985;535-536).

In recognizing the vulnerability of the elderly to S/PA diagnoses, Carnevali and Patrick (1979;7) state that:

Older persons, particularly those over 70, have a balance to maintain between activities of daily living, demands of daily living, and the increasingly fragile coping resources and support systems that tend to become more precarious with the years.

The tendency to believe that demands lessen with age can be true about certain factors, but many demands continue, such as basic living requirements. New demands may be added as a result of role and status changes, possible shifts in financial priorities and resources, and increased risks for health problems. At the same time that new demands are added, support systems and available resources often diminish. Bloom et al (1985;275) describe senescence, or the process of aging, as the "progressive loss of restorative and adaptive responses that serve to maintain normal functional capacity." They also address the issue that "measurements made on the old and the very old may simply reveal the factors that are conducive to survival rather than the changes that lead to decline."

Etiologies/Related Factors of Sensory/Perceptual Alterations: Input Excess

Gordon (1987) identifies only one etiology, environmental complexity/monotony, for the diagnosis S/PA: Input Excess. The authors identify an additional etiology, diminished discriminatory cognitive functioning. Both etiologies may be compounded by decreased coping abilities in the elderly, with the possibility of overload of the individual senses (eg, chronic pain).

Environmental complexity is described as the surroundings of an individual, which include the noise and activity level, numbers of persons, familiarity, intensity of colors and light, furnishings, odors, demands, stability, or frequency of changes. Another important factor to be considered in the environment, but less easily measured, is the milieu or feeling tone of interactions of persons within the environment. One example of environmental complexity is the changing of shifts in a nursing care setting. Synder et al (1976) report that wandering and confusion increase during these busy and noisy times. These behaviors are two defining characteristics of S/PA: Input Excess.

Environmental monotony can best be described as frequent, repetitive, meaningless stimuli in the environment. The person is subject to monotony either because of distorted perceptions or because of the actual inability to act to change the environment. This inability can be physiologic or psychologic, perceived or real.

A good example of a monotonous sound is the ticking of a clock. To some people this continuous sound is reassuring or even calming. For others, it is a constant unrecognizable noise that irritates or contributes to a situation of input excess with its continuous assault on the receptive system.

Environmental monotony is not limited only to noise. Scott and Crowhurst (1975;22) explain, "Many have grown old in our institutions, and face a future of 3 meals a day, a roof, a bed, the best of intentions from all disciplines, but above all, the crushing boredom of their daily routine." Both environmental complexity and monotony are dependent on internal perception as well as external stimuli. That is, the way the stimuli are interpreted by the individual determines the level of complexity or montony. This is directly related to the etiology of diminished discriminatory cognitive functioning.

Experiments have shown that the synthesis of change and stability in the environment is necessary for the maintenance of a healthy ego (Burnside, 1988;131). However, the exact mechanisms involved in perception of this environment are poorly understood. Schultz (1965) and Gioiella and Bevil (1985) discuss the role of the reticular activating system (RAS) on the input of sensory information to the brain.

The RAS monitors incoming and outgoing stimuli and becomes attuned to a certain level of activity which is projected to the cortex. The RAS functions optimally only within this specific range of stimulation, that is, it can only adapt within certain limits. This level is required for normal perception, learning, and emotion. When this regulatory system is upset by disturbances in sensory input, including increases, decreases, and distortions of stimuli, the organism is no longer able to project a normal level of activation to the cortex. It makes compensatory adjustments to regain equilibrium. If these adjustments fail, behavior becomes disorganized (Gioiella and Bevil, 1985;508).

Others have discussed the "optimal level of stimulation and sensoriatases, or the drive for sensory variation" (Wolanin and Phillips, 1981;173). All individuals have the need to attempt to control the degree and variety of stimuli that is comfortable for them. The individual constantly tries to maintain an optimal level of stimuli, which would define a sense of equilibrium. Thus, sometimes the individual needs to limit incoming messages, as in sensory overload, and sometimes the individual needs to increase the stimuli, as in sensory deficit. When an individual is functioning at an optimal cognitive level, this is usually successful. However, if there are any limitations in this system, stress may occur as the individual tries to adapt. This stress can cause two major reactions in the body: the disruption of a particular neurophysiologic or

organ system in and of itself and the suppression of normal immunologic functions, leading to increased susceptibility to disease (Bloom et al, 1985;293; Sutterley and Donnelly, 1979).

Because of the loss of discrimination abilities and the need to conserve resources to achieve stability in the environment, the elderly person may use perceptual and cognitive mechanisms to reduce the complexity of the environment (Hall, 1983). This may result in some maladaptive behavior, the use of more primitive cognitive styles, and more dependence on others.

Normal age-related changes and/or disease processes that alter cognitive functioning influence the elder's ability to cope and may increase stress for the individual. The stress may be aggravated by other factors (medication, sleep deprivation, chronic pain), producing anxiety. The stress stems from the inability to respond to stimuli appropriately and from negative feedback received from others. Sensing that the response is somehow incorrect, the elder can feel pressure to produce a more "normal" response.

In an effort to deal with situations and perceived changes, many elders feel overwhelmed. Initially, the response to S/PA: Input Excess is similar to any stress. If it is interpreted as "too much to handle," the person will withdraw, limiting stimulation, and S/PA: Input Deficit can occur (Akins, 1986). Many factors affect one's ability to handle stress. Past life experiences of coping with stress and the success of the mechanisms employed can reduce fear and lessen anxiety when facing a new situation. The perception of the stressor and its intensity, along with the timeliness or "pyramiding effect" of stressors, needs to be considered. One's value system, family and peer relationships, support systems, and internal feelings can all be a part of the interpretation of stress and its effect on the individual.

Response to stress is dependent on the interaction of three important factors: the elder's perception and interpretation of life events, the timing of the stressor in relation to other demands, and the resources available to the individual. The nurse needs to be aware of all of these factors of stress and how they potentiate and compound each other. Some stress is needed to complete tasks. If there were no consequences for not completing a job, an assignment, or a behavior, it is doubtful that people would be as motivated to perform. However, when stress reaches the point of demanding more than a person can successfully cope with, it can become distress, displayed as anxiety.

Assessment of Sensory/Perceptual Alterations: Input Excess

Assessment of the elder experiencing S/PA: Input Excess is similar to all Sensory/Perceptual Alterations diagnoses. A baseline of cognitive functioning needs to be established for each individual. The mental status test is aimed at discerning cognitive processing abilities in relation to the person's functional level within the environment. Demanding absolute reality and "correct answers" from an already overloaded sensory system places additional stress on the individual. In addition to identification of functional behaviors, the nurse assesses for behaviors that depart from the elder's baseline behavior that may indicate anxiety and stress reaction.

Defining Characteristics of Sensory/Perceptual Alterations: Input Excess

Anxiety is a vague feeling of dread, a foreboding of an unknown danger, and is one of the key symptoms of S/PA: Input Excess. Reaction is "accompanied by unconscious alterations in behavior that transfer the anxious feeling to more specific and observable symptoms" (Ebersole and Hess, 1981). Examples of such symptoms include regression, disorganization, perseveration, frantic overactivity, exaggerated emotional reactions, disturbed memory, inability to concentrate, decreased problem-solving ability, suspiciousness, illusions, hallucinations, delusions, phobias, and an inability to carry out usual appropriate social behaviors. Also to be considered are the coping mechanisms of denial, displacement, and fantasy (Ebersole and Hess, 1981).

Research in the identification of the specific responses and behavioral changes of S/PA: Input Excess in humans has been limited. However, a study of steel workers revealed that men who worked in noisy conditions were more aggressive, distrustful, and paranoid than those working in quieter conditions (Berland, 1972). This may have implications for the elderly. Increased congestion, crowded conditions, and noise provide more stimuli than can be successfully processed for an appropriate response. Burnside (1988;1018) notes that coping mechanisms that were operational in earlier years may not function successfully for the elderly. The state of exhaustion may occur sooner for the older adult.

When the individual employs coping mechanisms and is unsuccessful in reaching the optimal level of stimulation, the resulting behaviors include an accentuated use of one mode of behavior; less organized (from normal) behavior; demonstration of greater sensitivity to the environment with decreased tolerance level; presence of behaviors reflective of alteration of usual physiologic activity, such as the speed at which a person would talk; and distortion of "reality" if problem solving is decreased (Thierer, workshop presentation, 1978). Stimuli that require maximum endurance can be recognized by racing thoughts, scattered attention, restlessness, and aberrant thoughts or actions (Ebersole and Hess, 1981). Other

observable symptoms include disorganized thinking, erratic or restless movement, or emotions ranging from anger to apathy.

CASE STUDY

Sensory/Perceptual Alterations: Input Excess

W.L. is a 91-year-old man. He has been institutionalized for 2 years at three different long-term care facilities. His wife lives with their daughter within a few miles of the facility. Prior to being institutionalized W.L. lived on a farm that he and his wife had owned for 60 years. They had six children, one of whom visits daily. The others live farther away and do not visit frequently. W.L. made his wife promise in their younger years that he would never have to leave the farm.

When admitted, he was assessed by his primary nurse. His wife, R.L., was present during the assessment. He was disoriented to time and place and often yelled out his responses. He often responded inappropriately to questions and did not open his eyes during the interview. R.L. often interjected appropriate answers for W.L. when he answered inappropriately, and she tried to encourage him to cooperate. W.L. would often cup his hand to his right ear when listening. W.L. did not help to turn or cooperate with the nurse during the physical assessment. In fact, he strongly resisted being touched by the nurse or by instruments used for assessment (eg, stethoscope, otoscope). W.L. was bedfast except for the few times he would get out of bed with the staff's assistance. His wife related that he hadn't walked for several months and had nearly died with a urinary tract infection.

R.L. also related that it was extremely dangerous to get W.L. up because he had "fainting spells." She wondered if it was related to his diabetes or some other etiology. In the last years on the farm she did the majority of the yard and garden work. They lived mainly on foodstuffs from their garden. R.L. regulated the meals and W.L.'s medication. He took pain medication at least three times daily for arthritic discomfort. At times he was on prescribed codeine; if not, he used ASA. W.L. states he does not like to take medications because they are "harmful additives to the body." However, the physician has prescribed several medications. Major medical diagnoses are hard of hearing, adult onset non-insulin-dependent diabetes mellitus, chronic urinary tract infections from neurogenic bladder and urinary retention, past history of hydrocele, congestive heart failure, and chronic obstructive pulmonary disease.

Nursing staff from the previous care facility reported that W.L. was demanding, demented, confused, and occasionally combative. At the very least he was noncompliant with their routines. R.L. is adamant that staff did not understand W.L.'s needs. R.L. relates that sometimes W.L. "yells out about being on the rifle range or being back in the war" when staff initiate personal cares or treatments. Staff viewed this as further validation that W.L. was confused and demented. No mental status assessment was documented in his referring records.

W.L. does not wear glasses now, although he has in the past. According to his wife, he has never had his hearing tested. W.L. tries to feed himself and hates pureed food. He is edentulous, but R.L. states he has been so for 30 years and can eat steak with no problem.

Interventions for Sensory/Perceptual Alterations: Input Excess

Interventions for S/PA: Input Excess are directed toward the reduction of stress either perceived or real. These include calming strategies: environmental structuring to modify or decrease the amount of stimuli; and teaching/counseling.

Calming Strategies   When stress reactions in elders cause bizarre or aggressive behavior, this has to be dealt with in a positive fashion while taking care to ensure safety of the elder, the caregiver, and any other persons that may be affected and initiating environmental structuring to reduce excess sensory input. There may be beneficial effect from a quiet "time-out" period or from one-to-one contact with staff. Gentle touch and an unconditional acceptance portrayed by caregivers leads to a feeling of being secure and safe. Even if the nurse is not sure what the elder is experiencing, chances are the gentle, calm, caring approach will help to reduce the elder's stress. In addition, it is essential to assess what the elder perceives as reality and intervene according to that reality.

Group therapies are sometimes helpful in promoting feelings of productiveness or worthiness if extraneous stimuli are controlled. Therapies that enhance self-esteem and familiarity with the environment include music, exercise, reminiscence, and art. Large-group activities will likely not be the first step in intervening with an extremely agitated individual. To prevent severe distress, or in cases of low to moderate anxiety, small-group techniques may refocus energy into appropriate behavior responses. When intervening in the acute situation group leaders may use relaxation techniques to prevent the stress response.

Environmental Structuring   Modifying environmental complexity is an important factor in helping to alleviate excess stimulation. Simplifying the environment includes considering color combinations and intensity or brightness of colors and light; eliminating clutter; decreasing quantity while increasing meaningfulness of sound; and identifying traffic patterns and the placement of the elder in relation to these areas. Caregivers should be aware that their actions and activity patterns may add to the environmental chaos or become a positive contribution to the therapeutic milieu. A private space for the elder and his or her personal possessions should be provided for a "time-out." When stressed, a "time-out" in this familiar and secure space is beneficial. However, any quiet or calm area will serve this purpose. Designating this area in advance alerts all caregivers to avoid and/or monitor traffic flow or noise levels when this area is in use.

Although it is important for the caregiver to maintain a reliable and consistent care routine, it must be done with concern for the individual as such and not just as "part of the routine." The caregiver should explain concisely with the intent of gaining consent and allowing the elder choice and control. It is of great value for caregivers to wear large print nametags and to identify themselves verbally to the elder.

Documentation of expected behavioral responses in the care plan and of effects of interventions is essential. It is equally important to note conditions that precipitate anxious behavior so that appropriate reinforcement, either positive or extinguishing, can be initiated. Reinforcement may include redirecting the elder's activities or attention, channeling thought processes, or focusing on the most workable interventions. The elder should be referred to appropriate clinicians to correct sensory losses. The client should also have a medical evaluation to determine if there are physiologic reasons for observed behaviors. Evaluation by a psychologist or psychiatrist to further define parameters of cognitive functioning, intelligence, or other patterns of behavioral significance may be beneficial. The nurse may collaborate with clinicians working with Alzheimer's disease and those having specialized knowledge in the areas of stress reduction measures, low input environments, and other therapeutic approaches for relaxation.

Teaching/Counseling   Teaching/counseling in S/PA: Input Excess is important to both the elder and the involved caregiver. Education is directed toward an understanding of the variables that affect the central processing system in the brain and result in the symptoms of S/PA: Input Excess. "Venting" sessions for caregivers help to alleviate or prevent buildup of stress. These sessions also help caregivers to recognize the impact of their attitudes, stereotypes, and value systems on the environmental milieu.

Education concerning holistic health practices such as nutrition and physical activity can facilitate the elderly individual's strengthening defenses against disease and thus can decrease the negative effects of stress. Planned daily exercise in groups or individually promotes feelings of wellness and accomplishment. Providing planned times for the release of stress may enhance calmer, more appropriate interactions for the remainder of the day.

CASE STUDY

Nursing Interventions

Interventions are determined by the goals that W.L. and R.L. set, which include (1) to feel safe and secure; (2) to control the environment optimally; (3) to use a mode of communication to make needs known; and (4) to correct or compensate sensory losses.

At the preadmission assessment, staff gave R.L. information concerning the resources available at the facility. W.L.'s current activities of daily living were identified with R.L. as well as her preferences for W.L's care. Documentation from the nursing staff at the previous care facility was reviewed. Obtaining the history at this time aided in building rapport between R.L. and W.L. and the primary nurse. W.L. was included as much as possible. A temporary plan was made with R.L.'s input before admission.

W.L. was referred for speech and hearing evaluations as well as for an eye examination. A medical referral was made to review medications and concerns R.L. had regarding medical diagnoses. An assigned primary caregiver was initiated to orient W.L. to his room arrangements and call system. A care conference was held to share the plan regarding W.L.'s needs. Specific approaches were outlined to minimize the possibility of aggression when W.L. interacted with staff. To facilitate the interaction, caregivers were encouraged to touch W.L. on the upper shoulder to let him know that they were near. Caregivers were also encouraged to use a calm, low voice and to speak into W.L.'s right ear. A hearing aid was attempted but was unacceptable to W.L. for comfort and effectiveness reasons. A phonic ear was placed, and R.L. and staff worked diligently to help W.L. adjust to this prosthesis. Use of the adaptive device was rewarded by W.L. being able to hear taped church services from his hometown and letters from relatives read by R.L. Eventually, W.L. was able to participate in normal conversational levels of speech and direct his care routine. After communication was established, a TENS unit for p.r.n. pain control was initiated. Staff manipulated the settings of the unit with W.L. giving feedback regarding effectiveness of interventions.

All medication was evaluated, and a pain medication was added. W.L.'s diabetes was found to be controlled most effectively by diet. Timoptic drops (gtts) were prescribed for glaucoma after ophthalmologic evaluation; however, there was no way to increase vision. An observant caregiver discovered W.L.'s light sensitivity one sunny afternoon. It was noted that W.L. became more restless and experienced pain in his eyes when he was in direct sunlight. Sunglasses relieved the pain and the resultant restlessness.

To help W.L. have some control, referrals were made to Occupational Therapy and Physical Therapy. The therapists prescribed a plate guard and a big tablespoon, which greatly enhanced W.L.'s self-feeding ability. He also learned to hold his eyelid open so that the timoptic gtts could be put into his eye, and he became much less resistive to the treatment.

The primary nurse spent much time with W.L. to assess various care approaches and times to minimize the continued combativeness. She asked R.L. to provide reassurance by holding W.L.'s hand or arm during cares. W.L. learned to direct how and when he wanted to be turned. He even helped to lift himself with an over-bed trapeze.

W.L.'s condition could easily have been mistaken for sensory deprivation when in reality it was S/PA: Input Excess. W.L. experienced both complexity of a new environment with little cognition of what was happening or why and a constant input of monotonous sounds and sights to the brain that conveyed little meaning. He experienced much distortion in sensory input as a result of actual loss in the sensory organs. Even with some compensation, deficits remained that made interpretation and screening of stimuli stressful. However, with much trial and error and one-to-one time by clinicians, most of the couple's goals were met. This was accomplished after approximately 1 full year of working with this elderly couple.

Summary

The diagnosis of S/PA: Input Excess requires an astute nurse to assess the reality of the personal and environmental situation within the context of the elder's perception of that reality and his or her ability to cope. Unfortunately, the most effective interventions are often found by trial and error because of the lack of specific research. S/PA: Input Excess cannot always be avoided, but the symptoms can be minimized.

SENSORY/PERCEPTUAL ALTERATIONS: INPUT DEFICIT

Sensory/Perceptual Alterations: Input Deficit (S/PA: Input Deficit) has been variously described as sensory deprivation, sensory isolation, perceptual deprivation, reduced sensory stimulation, confinement, isolation, and sensory isolation. This portion of the chapter will refer to S/PA: Input Deficit as reduced physical or social environmental stimuli relative to a habitual (or basic orienting) level. Initial interest and work in this area began in the mid- to late 1950s following the Korean Conflict prisoners' of war experiences with sensory deprivation and "brainwashing." Research that followed was done in controlled settings with observation of volunteers' re-

responses to deprived conditions (ie, placement under water, isolation from any human contact). Although these studies are old, they have proved to be classic references for later studies. Research done since 1958 to 1965 has concentrated on surgical manipulation of animals and patient response in health care settings (patients in iron lungs, patients undergoing cataract surgery, patients in intensive care units [ICU]). Some research has continued on the effects of ICU settings on the individual. However, nothing has been done in the incidence of S/PA: Input Deficit in the elderly population, particularly those who are institutionalized.

Several theories have been advanced to describe the condition of S/PA: Input Deficit. These can be broadly grouped into five categories. First, the *physiologic* category addresses the need for the human brain to experience change, complexity, and surprise to maintain the functions of attention (and concentration), arousal, wakefulness, and consciousness (Ernst et al, 1978; Heron, 1961; Oster, 1979; Schultz, 1965; Selye, 1956; Ziskind, 1958). As a result of aging of brain cells, the elderly experience a decreased capacity to respond adequately to environmental stimuli. Remaining cells require stimulation for continued growth and activity and to enhance mental functioning (Hirschfeld, 1985). Lack of this stimulation further reduces the adaptive function of the individual. Thus S/PA: Input Deficit speeds up the degenerative changes normally associated with aging and enhances the loss of functional cells in the central nervous system (CNS).

The second category, *personality*, involves ego, body-field orientation, and the "need for stimulation to find ordered relationships" (Freedman et al, 1961;20). With the breakdown of internalized order, it becomes increasingly difficult for the individual to test reality and modify old schema, and for adaptation and accommodation to occur. The ego then turns inward in the absence of meaningful external stimuli (Freedman et al, 1961). Decreased reception of information from the external world as a result of age-related changes in the senses "makes that world a lonely and frightening place. And, in depression or anxiety the person tends to withdraw into the internal world, projecting apathy to the surroundings" (Ernst et al, 1978;472).

The third category, *drive/need* or "stimulus hunger," is generated when variation, intensity, and meaningfulness of external and kinesthetic stimuli are reduced to a minimum for arousal (Maddi, 1961), as described in the previously discussed physiologic theories. Associated behaviors are an effort to increase sensory impact. Negative or positive affect results—negative when activation level differs markedly from normal levels, positive when associated with shifts toward a more normal level (Davis et al, 1960; Freedman et al, 1961; Lambert and Levy, 1972; Oster, 1979; Zuckerman et al, 1970).

Institutionalization for the elderly may involve prolonged and monotonous immobilization. Freedman et al (1961) state that active movement and visual input (feedback) are necessary for adaptation in a disarranging experience. Arie (1973) linked dementia of the elderly to restricted mobility.

In the fourth category, *social influence*, the significance of others is a part of the individual's environment. Communication with others promotes cognitive activity such as logical reasoning.

The elderly experience many social losses, for example, positions or roles, familiar homes, and significant others. Carter and Galliano (1981;342) observed that "lifestyle and general environment didn't appear to add to social isolation, rather, interpersonal withdrawal and isolation became a defense." As a result of the aging process, which was discussed in the section on S/PA: Uncompensated Deficit, individuals experience barriers to communication because of hearing and visual losses. Thus, older persons may purposefully limit interaction with others, fearing that their slow or inaccurate information processing may be interpreted as a sign of deterioration (senility) (Kogan and Shelton, 1962). This fear appears to have merit and is true of staff–client interactions in institutions. Gilbert (1984) found that nurses interacted 15% of the time with more oriented clients and only 5.6% of the time with confused clients.

The fifth category includes *cognitive* or *perceptual* theories. The basis for these theories have been touched on in the preceding discussion. Heron (1961) supports the necessity of varied sensory input for normal mentation. Under deprivation conditions, realistic interpretation of perception cannot be made. The goal of perception of environmental stimuli is to arrive at an appropriate response (Bower, 1967; Freedman, 1961). Freedman et al (1961;70) found "that it is the absence of meaning or order, rather than the specific nature of the stimulus field, which degrades perceptual organization."

The institutional environment, although bright and cheerful, tends to be unchanging. Schedules and staff routines become priority goals. Gilbert (1984;47), in a study of nurses' communication with the institutionalized elderly, found that unless the patients were sufficiently active or motivated to go for a walk themselves or ask for assistance, they remained in their armchairs uninterrupted by nursing staff. Patients spent very little time in purposeful activity, and some of the more confused patients showed destructive and attention-seeking behaviors.

Pain-killers, sedatives, and minor tranquilizers further reduce awareness of stimulation and impair sensory discrimination. If the individual is institutionalized, the nature of the presenting illness, or more likely the treatment of that illness, may result in a drastic reduction in the amount of everyday stimulation. Although it has been over 30 years since the first experiments in S/PA: Input Deficit were conducted, unification or standardization of the diagnosis has not been accomplished. However, five broad etiologies of S/PA: Input Deficit are generally agreed on. These etiologies are listed in the following section.

Etiologies/Related Factors of Sensory/Perceptual Alterations: Input Deficit

1. *Decreased quantity of stimuli.* The individual literally receives fewer stimuli through one or more sensory modalities or from environmental restrictions.
2. *Decreased quality of stimuli.* This refers to a decrease in intensity, patterning, or meaningfulness of stimuli. That is, there is a qualitative change in sensory input.
3. *Decreased mobility/movement.* This refers not only to an inability to change location but also to restriction of the kinesthetic experience.
4. *Isolation or loss of socialization.* This refers to feelings of "aloneness," which Bentz (1978;1300) identified as an "awareness of and absence of meaningful integration with other individuals or groups of individuals."
5. *S/PA: Input Excess.* As discussed previously, this can lead to social withdrawal in order to decrease sensory input.

Assessment of Sensory/Perceptual Alterations: Input Deficit

The nurse must make a careful, thorough assessment to determine the diagnosis S/PA: Input Deficit. The condition is easily misdiagnosed as altered thought processes: confusion or disorientation; a result of normal aging; grieving; diversional activity deficit; translocation syndrome or ineffective coping: manipulation or noncompliance. Symptoms of S/PA: Input Deficit may be vague and highly variable. Characteristically, these behaviors do respond promptly to appropriate manipulation of the sensory and social environment. Therefore, diagnosis is made on a "rule-out" basis, eliminating such causes as physiologic conditions, reversible and irreversible dementias, or recent change in lifestyle.

Defining Characteristics of Sensory/Perceptual Alterations: Input Deficit

A variety of behaviors occur as a result of S/PA: Input Deficit. Signs and symptoms cluster into the general areas of physiologic, cognitive, perceptual, emotional, and behavioral (Table 31.1). These range from mild to very severe expression. In general, symptoms may occur as early as 2 to 3 hours after the person is placed in a

deprived situation, and this condition of input deficit may become chronic.

Cognitive–perceptual changes include feelings of boredom, reduced awareness, difficulty concentrating, loss of contact with surroundings (disorientation), delusional thoughts, and hallucinations, used here in the sense of perception without object (Heron, 1961).

Initial emotional reactions to S/PA: Input Deficit may be positive: The individual may enjoy the experience of "peace and quiet" or "no interruptions." As length of time increases, however, the person becomes noticeably irritable. The client with S/PA: Input Deficit experiences tedium stress, including worry, anxiety, and feelings of inner tensions, and is often concerned with the passage of time. The individual may also show signs of depression, fear, and paranoid symptoms varying from mild to outright panic.

Motor behaviors exhibited seem tied to the progressive deterioration of perceptual–cognitive and emotional functioning. Initially, there is restless "settling-in" activity followed by a relatively inactive period. Later behaviors (whistling, tapping) indicate a need for movement and stimulation. These movements may progress to very restless, random movement to the point where the person attempts to escape. Alternatively, the person may become totally passive and withdraw from the surroundings.

CASE STUDY

Sensory/Perceptual Alterations: Input Deficit

H.B. is an 89-year-old woman. She lives with her 53-year-old daughter. H.B. was born and spent most of her adult life in a small town of 900 people, 15 miles away from where she is currently living. She was married and raised four children. Her socioeconomic status was lower middle class. H.B. was involved in Eastern Star, a card club, the Christian Church, and Bible study. She received an eighth grade education.

As H.B. became less mobile as a result of degenerative arthritis and as her friends began to die, she sold her home and moved in with her daughter. Both viewed this as positive, as they had always had a close relationship and compatible personalities. H.B. helped with light housework—dusting, doing dishes, and preparing meals. Her daughter was divorced and worked as a bank clerk at the local bank. Besides her activities in the community, church, and Senior Citizen group, H.B. kept in touch with her brother, sister, and friends through letters. She also subscribed to her old hometown paper. Reading and working crossword puzzles were life-long leisure activities, and she followed her favorite "soap" on TV. H.B. had no significant medical conditions other than the degenerative arthritis of the hips, for which she took buffered aspirin

(600 mg) four times each day. This resulted in some dull pain all of the time, which intensified with movement of the joints. Two years after moving in with her daughter, H.B. admitted that her vision was "pretty blurry" and was seen by an ophthalmologist. He found bilateral cataracts. H.B. denied that her vision interfered with her lifestyle at that time and stated that it was just something to be expected at her age. She refused treatment because "it wasn't worth the money."

The following year, it was noted that H.B. was beginning to stay home rather than go to Fellowship and Senior Citizen meetings, and she missed an occasional Bible study. She was not seen reading or working puzzles. Usually very prompt about mailing out Christmas cards, she put off working on them, even requesting her daughter to "pick some out for me—I don't care." During this time she becamse slightly irritable, making comments that she "used to have (an object) but I sure wouldn't know where it is now. I suppose it was just sold with the house." This statement was repeated at various times, becoming an underlying theme. H.B. developed a snappish quality to her voice: "Well, I don't know what you're talking about" or "I guess I'll just have to do what I'm told."

As severe winter weather set in, H.B. only left the house on Sunday mornings for church. Social visiting and special events were cancelled because of the bad weather. The usual daily routine became more routinized with fewer interruptions. H.B. got up with her daughter, and they fixed breakfast and ate together. After H.B.'s daughter left for work, H.B. turned off the radio to "save electricity." She then dusted, if necessary, changed clothes, made her bed, and then sat in her easy chair dozing until it was time to begin the noon meal. The TV was not turned on during the morning. Her daughter began to notice some discrepancies between what was prepared and the planned menu, sometimes noting a substitution of food or an omission. H.B. also began requesting specific instructions for the actual food preparation. At lunch, the TV was turned to H.B.'s "soap." H.B. and her daughter had always discussed the plot, but during this time H.B. would remark she "really didn't follow the meaning anymore." After lunch and completion of the show, the TV was again turned off. H.B. spent the remainder of the afternoon sitting in the easy chair. She rarely turned any lights on in the late afternoon, again so as not to "waste electricity."

Interventions for Sensory/Perceptual Alterations: Input Deficit

General nursing interventions appropriate for S/PA: Input Deficit include environmental structuring; mobilization of the individual; increasing opportunities for socialization; individual teaching/counseling; and referral to appropriate specialized clinicians for consultation. Goals of specific nursing interventions are directed toward minimizing or eliminating etiologies of S/PA: Input Deficit and reversing the signs and symptoms.

Environmental Structuring Increasing the quantity and/or quality of sensory input through environmental structuring or manipulation as described under S/PA: Uncompensated Deficit is often effective. The physical environment should be enriched through appropriate use of colors, sounds, and tactile sensations. If the elderly person is in a long-term care institution, the nurse should give careful consideration to the elder's placement on the unit, for example where "people-watching" can take place and involvement with unit activities occurs or near a window to observe the weather and outdoor activities. The nurse may plan supervised outdoor activities to allow the elder to experience the sun, breezes, soil, and smells. The only limitation in promoting variety within the environment is the nurse's creativity. Stimulation of multiple senses at one time increases the impact of the sensory experience. Meaningful stimulation can be provided to reinforce or accommodate the individual's history, preferences, and responses to previous stimuli.

Mobilization of the Individual It is essential that movement in all directions be encouraged. This may be accomplished through formal or informal group or individual exercise programs, or the caregiver may assist the individual to maintain the ability to seek variety in the environment by moving to different locations. Movement can also be provided in individual self-care activities. Family and staff caregivers need to provide opportunities and assistance if the individual is unable to move. Passive range-of-motion exercises stimulate kinesthetic sensations within joints and muscles of dependent elders.

Increasing Opportunities for Socialization Promotion of social interactions can be facilitated either on a one-to-one basis or in group settings. Nurses can work with friends, relatives, and significant others to enhance interpersonal contact for the elder. Group work with the elderly on various topics has been found to be beneficial; therapies may include socialization, reminiscence, sensory stimulation, and reality orientation (Burnside, 1988). The elder may need assistance in making arrangements for transportation to attend social activities. To assist the elder in maintaining social contact, the nurse may use written or telephone reminders to attend meetings or arrange transportation. Maintenance of communication provides a sense of security, self-esteem, and dignity. The family may use video- or cassette-tape recordings to send personalized messages to the elder; this enhances social contact and reinforces the elder's sense of identity and esteem.

When the individual is confused, communication must be modified to be effective. Nowakowski (1985) recommends that the caregiver talk to the person "behind" the dysfunction, focusing on client strengths. Communication strategies include using short words and simple sentences; communicating without making demands; using purposeful and slow speech; enunciating words; allowing time to respond; asking one question at a time and repeating exactly if necessary; asking questions that can be answered with yes or no; maintaining eye contact; moving slowly; listening carefully; treating the person as an adult; being honest if you don't understand; using nonverbal techniques such as visual cues and gestures; interpreting gestures; and using touch. The nurse should document those interventions that are effective.

Individual Teaching/Counseling   Teaching the elderly person to identify a sensory-deprived environment and its implications gives the person the opportunity to control and minimize its impact. Teaching strategies are discussed earlier in this chapter. Referral to appropriate specialized clinicians for consultation and correction of sensory losses to optimize sensory input (quantity of stimuli) is an important intervention that nurses are in a key position to initiate.

CASE STUDY

Nursing Interventions

H.B.'s daughter contacted the local Visiting Nursing Service, and the nurse came to the home and assessed H.B. The nurse determined that a second visit to the ophthalmologist was warranted, and an appointment was scheduled. The nurse reviewed the examination routine with H.B. and helped her practice the routine. Evaluation showed H.B's vision to be severely impaired, and with her permission, cataract surgery was scheduled. An intraocular lens replacement was performed on the right eye, which was the more advanced cataract. During hospitalization, H.B.'s roommate was a 76-year-old woman from her old hometown. She too was awaiting cataract surgery, and the women spent many hours discussing fears of surgery and reminiscing. The nurse noted a possible hearing loss and examined H.B.'s ears, discovering that H.B. had a moderate buildup of cerumen, which was corrected. On the second day after return to her daughter's house, H.B. commented,"Why there's a shovel on the steps of the empty house across the street." Much laughter followed the comment, since the shovel had been there all winter. H.B.'s vision improved rapidly, evidenced by subjective comments, renewed reading of the hometown paper, more active observing of the cardinal outside in the bird feeder, renewed correspondence with family and friends, and her return to the weekly Bible studies and Senior Citizen

meetings. The negative comments and apparent forgetfulness disappeared.

H.B. experienced S/PA: Input Deficit as a result of cataracts impinging on her visual acuity. The normal diminishment in hearing due to aging was increased by a moderate cerumen buildup. Her concern about energy consumption when turning on the TV, radio, or lights also added to the input deficit condition. The quality of sensory stimulation decreased as H.B.'s routine became monotonous, partly because of her withdrawal from social activities (not getting out as a result of bad weather), but also because of isolation due to the inability to read the hometown paper and difficulty in writing letters. The bad weather and the physical pain caused by arthritis also decreased mobility. Thus, H.B. spent a lot of time sleeping in her chair, exhibited mental cloudiness and forgetfulness, and had difficulty in performing her usual tasks (eg, preparing meals). Her emotions ranged from apathetic to slight irritability. She quit attending many activities and reading.

H.B.'s sensory perceptual function (vision) was improved as a result of the cataract surgery. If this had not been an option, nursing interventions directed toward increasing variation in the physical and social environments would have been beneficial. Some alternative suggestions might have been use of large-print instructions about meal preparation, with telephone follow-up mid-morning for possible questions/comments; use of large-print books/ magazines and magnifying devices to enlarge print further; use of remote control to facilitate use of TV by decreasing painful movement; discussion and demonstration with H.B.'s daughter about actual costs of electrical use; routine ear checks to prevent cerumen buildup; use of an elevated chair seat to ease effort needed to arise from the chair; and use of warm packs and active range-of-motion exercises to maintain mobility. The nurse might also facilitate attendance of activities by arranging for transportation or might encourage phone contacts with local friends and/or visitation by these friends.

SUMMARY

As described in the preceding sections, the elderly are at risk for three specific diagnoses of Sensory/ Perceptual Alterations. Goals identified are based on the focus of the specific diagnosis. In general, the goal of intervention for S/PA: Uncompensated Deficit is that the individual functions maximally within the environment given the sensory deficits. For S/PA: Input Excess, the desired outcomes are that the individual is without signs and symptoms of anxiety or stress and that the individual doesn't withdraw into a situation of sensory deprivation. The goal for S/PA: Input Deficit is for the individual to maintain or return to optimum cognitive functioning.

The three diagnoses described are often not clearcut. After data have been gathered and a baseline established, the nurse must continue careful monitoring in order to distinguish the appropriate diagnosis and intervention strategies.

A review of current literature reveals that little research has been published using the NANDA nomenclatures (Maas and Hardy, 1988), although there has been a great deal of research in the areas of stress and sensory overload. Studies of the effects of deprivation on hospitalized humans were generally in intensive care units or of individuals (not necessarily the elderly) having eye surgery. Aging of the sensory systems and its impact on the individual has not been systematically studied. Research specific to this population is needed. Certainly, the need for assessment tools and effective interventions in dealing with Sensory/Perceptual Alterations should be a priority. These diagnoses are clearly in the realm of nursing practice to identify and treat. However, to validate the nurse's assessment, diagnoses, and interventions, a research base is needed.

References

Akins J: Sensory perceptual alteration-deprivation: The institutionalized elderly a population at risk. Unpublished paper, 1986.

Arie T: Dementia in the elderly: Management. *British Med J* 1973; 4(5892):602–607.

Avant LL, Helson H: Theories of perception. Pages 419–450 in: *Handbook of General Psychology*. Wolman B (editor). Prentice-Hall, 1973.

Barnett K: A theoretical construct of the concepts of touch as they relate to nursing. *Nurs Res* 1972; 21(2):102–110.

Bates B: *A Guide to Physical Examination*, 2d ed. Lippincott, 1979.

Bentz JE: Short-term sensory reduction used as a therapeutic aid in enhancement of self-concept. *Psycholog Rep* 1978; 42(3):1299–1304.

Berland T: Noise: Our quiet pollution. *Sci Activities* (Jan) 1972: 10–14.

Bloom FE, Lazerson A, Hofstader: *Brain, Mind and Behavior*. Freeman, 1985.

Bower HM: Sensory stimulation and the treatment of senile dementia. *Med J Australia* 1967; 1(22):1133–1118.

Burnside IM: *Nursing and the Aged*, 3d ed. McGraw-Hill, 1988.

Carnevali D, Patrick M: *Nuring Management for the Elderly*. Lippincott, 1979.

Carroll-Johnson R: *Classification of Nursing Diagnoses: Proceedings of the Eighth Conference*. Lippincott, 1989.

Carter C, Galliano D: Fear of loss and attachment. *J Gerontol Nurs* 1981; 7(6):342–349.

Conover M, Cober J: Understanding and caring for the hearing-impaired. *Nurs Clin North Am* 1970; 5(3):497–498.

Davis JM, McCourt WF, Soloman P: The effect of visual stimulation on hallucinations and other mental experiences during sensory deprivation. *Am J Psychiatry* 1960; 5:106.

Ebersole P, Hess P: *Toward Healthy Aging: Human Needs and Nursing Response*. Mobsy, 1981.

Ernst P et al: Isolation and the symptoms of chronic brain syndrome. *Gerontologist* 1978; 18(5):468–474.

Freedman S: Sensory deprivation: Facts in search of deprivation theory. *J Nervous Mental Disorders* 1961; 132:17–21.

Freedman SJ, Grunebaum HU, Greenblatt M: Perceptual and cognitive changes in sensory deprivation. In: *Sensory Deprivation*. Solomon P, Kubzansky P, Leiderman P, et al (editors). Harvard University Press, 1961:58–71.

Gilbert M: Challenging steoreotypes. *Nurs Mirror* 1984; 158(16):42–43.

Gioiella EC, Bevil CW: *Nursing Care of the Aging Client*. Appleton-Century-Crofts, 1985.

Gordon M: *Manual of Nursing Diagnosis*. McGraw-Hill, 1987.

Hall B: Toward an understanding of stability in nursing phenomena. *ANS* 1983; 5(3):15–20.

Hefferin EA, Hunter ARE: Nursing observation and care planning for the hospitalized aged. *Gerontologist* 1975; 15:57–60.

Heron W: Cognitive and physiological effects of perceptual isolation. Pages 6–33 in: *Sensory Deprivation*. Solomon P et al (editors). Harvard University Press, 1961.

Hirschfeld M: Self-care potential: Is it present? *J Gerontol Nurs* 1985; 11(8):29–34.

Iveson L: To be deaf . . . Views from the people who are. *Nurs Care* 1979; 11:17–18.

Kastenbaum R: The reluctant therapist. *Geriatrics* 1963; 18:296–301.

Kogan N, Shelton FC: Beliefs about old people: A comparative study of older and younger samples. *J Genetic Psychol* 1962; 100:93–111.

Lambert W, Levy LH: Sensation seeking and short-term sensory isolation. *J Personality Soc Psychol* 1972; 24(1):46–52.

Lawton MP: Assessment, integration, and environments for older people. *Gerontologist* 1970; 10:38–46.

Maas M, Hardy MA: A challenge for the future. *J Gerontol Nurs* 1988; 14(3):8–13.

Maddi SR: Exploratory behavior and variation-seeking in man. Pages 253–277 in: *Functions of Varied Experience*. Fiske DW, Maddi SR (editors). Dorsey Press, 1961.

Montagu AM: *Touching: The Human Significance of the Skin*. Columbia University Press, 1971.

Nowakowski N: Accent capabilities in disorientation. *J Gerontolog Nurs* 1985; 11(9):15–20.

Oster C: Sensory deprivation and homeostasis. *J Am Geriatr Soc* 1979; 27(8):389–396.

Scott D, Crowhurt J: Reawakening senses in the elderly. *Canad Nurse* (Oct) 1975; 21–22.

Schultz D: *Sensory Restriction: Effects on Behavior*. Academic Press, 1965.

Selye H: *The Stress of Life*. McGraw-Hill, 1956.

Snyder LH, Pyrek J, Smith KC: Vision and mental function of the elderly. *Gerontologist* 1976; 16(6):491–495.

Sullivan N: Vision in the elderly. *J Gerontol Nurs* 1983; 9(4):228–235.

Sutterly DC, Donnelly FG: Stress and health: A survey of self-regulation modalities. *Top Clin Nurs* 1979; 1:1.

Thierer J: Physiological and psychological manifestations of stress. Unpublished workshop presentation, 1978.

Wolanin MO, Phillips L: *Confusion: Prevention and Cure.* Mosby, 1981.

Wolk RL, Wolk RB: Professional workers' attitudes toward the aged. *J Am Geriatr Soc* 1971; 19(7):624–639.

Yurick AG: Vision in the elderly person and the nursing process. In: *The Aged Person and the Nursing Process.* Yurick AG, Robb SS, Spier BE (editors). Appleton-Century-Crofts, 1980.

Ziskind E: Isolation stress in medical and mental illness. *J Am Med Assoc* 1958; 168:1427–1431.

Zuckerman M et al: Sensory deprivation versus sensory variation. *J Abnormal Psychol* 1970; 76(1):76–82.

32

Unilateral
Neglect

ELIZABETH A. WEITZEL, MA, RN

UNILATERAL NEGLECT IS THE STATE IN WHICH AN individual is perceptually unaware of and inattentive to one side of the body (Carroll-Johnson, 1989). This condition is the result of brain damage that alters perception, and it may be related to other perceptual problems following brain injury, such as trauma, tumor, or cerebrovascular problems. The lesion is most likely to be in the right parietal lobe, the rate being estimated as low as 3:1 and as high as 16:1 for the right lobe being affected versus the left (Riddoch and Humphreys, 1983; Weinstein and Friedland, 1977). Therefore, Unilateral Neglect is most frequently associated with left hemiplegia, a condition that often afflicts the elderly who have had a cerebrovascular accident (CVA) of the right brain hemisphere. Sometimes the symptoms are most noticeable immediately after the lesion occurs, subsiding with recovery of other functions. However, some or all of the symptoms may persist and influence rehabilitation (Dudas, 1986). There is also some evidence that men are more likely to have overt symptoms, perhaps related to functions being more rigidly segregated by hemisphere in the male, with verbal functions on the left and spatial functions on the right (Geshwind and Behan, 1982; McGlone, 1978).

Theories of the underlying deficit that results in Unilateral Neglect include disorders of (1) sensory input; (2) internal representation of space; and/or (3) attention to stimuli contralateral to the lesion. Studies by Riddoch and Humphreys (1983) support disordered attention as a primary part of the deficit. This knowledge is important when choosing interventions.

SIGNIFICANCE FOR THE ELDERLY

If Unilateral Neglect is not diagnosed and treated in the elderly, there is potential for injury to the affected side through neglect of hygiene or trauma. The older person may not recognize the affected side as part of his or her body. This means the person may be unaware of the potential for danger, the need for hygiene, and the effects of trauma to the affected side. Thus, older persons may accidentally burn, bruise, or cut their affected side and be completely unaware of pain or bleeding (Siev and Freishat, 1976).

When caring for the elderly client, behaviors related to Unilateral Neglect may be misdiagnosed as other psychologic problems or mental deterioration, leading to inappropriate or ineffective interventions (Gorelick, 1986). It is important that the nurse, who is aware of hygiene and other behaviors, assess for Unilateral Neglect when brain damage has occurred. Other sensory losses with aging will exaggerate Unilateral Neglect and compound its effects on functioning. Compensating for these losses is important and should take place before making a final determination about the extent of neglect present.

The elderly are at risk for developing Unilateral Neglect because both CVA and subdural hematoma occur more frequently with advanced age.

CURRENT STATUS OF THE DIAGNOSIS

Unilateral Neglect was added as a subdiagnosis under Altered Sensory Perceptions in 1987 by the Seventh Conference of the North American Nursing Diagnosis Association (NANDA). Unilateral Neglect is differentiated from Sensory/Perceptual Alterations in the elderly (see Chapter 31) in that it is the result of pathology, not of normal aging. Unilateral Neglect results from damage to brain tissue and not from alterations in the environment. It may result in some of the same behaviors as other altered sensory perceptions, but only as related to perception of one limb or half of the body, and is usually associated with hemiplegia, hemianopsia, or other sensory deficits (Heilman and Valenstein, 1977).

ETIOLOGIES/RELATED FACTORS

CVA is probably the most common cause of Unilateral Neglect in the elderly, but any lesion to the parietal lobe, especially in the right hemisphere, can cause Unilateral Neglect to occur. Occasionally damage to other parts of the brain will result in Unilateral Neglect, but not as consistently as damage to the parietal lobe (Heilman and Valenstein, 1977). Unilateral Neglect is complicated by a variety of deficits that may accompany or account for some of its effects.

Related Deficits

Anosognosia *Anosognosia* has come to mean the unawareness or denial of hemiplegia. (Technically it means unawareness of the disease.) Elderly persons with this deficit will confabulate reasons why they are not walking or using their arm. Sometimes they will deny that the limbs belong to them. For example, an elderly man claimed that his undertaker friend had replaced his arm with one from a cadaver. It is not uncommon for elderly

persons with anosognosia to try to get out of a bed or chair without assistance or proper safety precautions, since they are unaware of functional limitations.

Hemiakinesia *Hemiakinesia* refers to limited or no movement of the affected extremity in the absence of, or out of proportion to, motor dysfunction. For example, if an elderly person is given a pair of gloves, he will typically use the affected hand to put the glove on the unaffected hand, but will not put a glove on the affected hand (Friedland and Weinstein, 1977).

Hemianopsia *Hemianopsia* (also referred to as homonymous hemianopsia) is the loss of one half of the visual field, usually to the affected side. This condition usually occurs in lesions posterior to the optic chiasm and leaves a deficit on the side of hemiplegia if it is also present (Johnson and Cyran, 1979; Nooney, 1986). The elderly person with hemianopsia is not blind in one eye but has lost vision to one side in each eye. Hemianopsia further complicates other deficits because the person is not receiving visual input. Johnson and Cyran (1979) describe assessment and nursing interventions for hemianopsia in more detail.

Hemispatial Neglect *Hemispatial neglect* is inattention to the space located to one side of the midline of a person as well as inattention to this half of the body. Elderly persons with this deficit will ignore voices or objects on the affected side. They may also neglect half of a book or half the meal tray on the affected side. Persons with hemispatial neglect will draw half a flower or the unaffected side of their body normally, whereas the affected side may be omitted or drawn fainter and less distinct. If the older person also has hemianopsia, she will not be aware of the loss of vision to the affected side.

Visual Inattention *Visual inattention*, which can be a part of hemispatial neglect, will cause the elderly person to fail to read words on the affected side. However, when attention is called to the omitted words, they can be read without changing the direction of gaze or moving the head. This characteristic distinguishes visual inattention from hemianopsia, in which the word is not seen unless the older person's head is turned or the gaze is changed to use the functioning half of the eye.

Proprioception *Proprioception* is the ability to know the position of a limb through its sensory input, without looking at it or feeling it with another extremity. Loss of proprioception compounds other deficits for the elderly. When proprioception is lost, safety of the affected limb becomes a problem for older persons.

Other tactile deficits include *allesthesia*, the perception of stimuli to the affected side as being to the opposite limb, and the *extinction phenomenon*. With these deficits, elderly persons can distinguish a single stimulus to their affected side, but if a stimulus is given to both extremities simultaneously, only the stimulus to the unaffected side is perceived. This test is referred to as Double Simultaneous Stimulation (DSS).

Related deficits that need to be differentiated from Unilateral Neglect and that may complicate neglect behaviors include agnosia and apraxia. *Agnosia* is failure of the brain to recognize input from a single sense, such as vision, hearing, proprioception, or touch. The body receives the input, but the brain does not recognize the input as familiar. For example, if you put a key in the hand of an older person with tactile agnosia, while not allowing the key to be seen, and ask them to identify the object, the older person may tell you the hand holds something cold and hard. If the person is allowed to look at the object, he can correctly identify the key. Agnosias may accompany Unilateral Neglect or be present in the absence of Unilateral Neglect. Obviously, having both agnosias and Unilateral Neglect compounds the effect of the deficits for elderly individuals.

Apraxia *Apraxia* is the inability to carry out a learned movement voluntarily, or to plan and execute movement when comprehension and motor abilities are intact. A dependent elderly person with this deficit may scratch with the affected limb unconsciously but be unable to move the limb with precision voluntarily (eg, pick up eating utensils, appropriately fill a spoon and bring it to her mouth). This deficit may appear either with Unilateral Neglect or separate from it. There may also be apraxia of the unaffected side, further compounding the deficit and confusing the assessment. For example, an elderly person with a lesion in the right hemisphere who also has apraxia may have weakness on the left and have difficulty handling a spoon correctly with the right hand for a period of time following the injury (see Assessment Guide 32.1 for an example of differential diagnosis).

Several other deficits common with right hemisphere damage exist, including problems related to monitoring behavior, resulting in lack of inhibition, social inappropriateness, and verbal outbursts. Conceptual deficits such as loss of abstract thinking, loss of appreciation of subtleties, and loss of attention span may also accompany right brain damage. The elderly person's retention of normal speech may mask initial identification of many of these deficits. It is beyond the scope of this chapter to discuss all of these cognitive and psychologic deficits in detail. The classic articles written by Fowler and Fordyce (1972) and the articles by Dudas (1986), Gorelick (1986), and Tellis-Nazak (1986) are resources for more detailed information.

DEFINING CHARACTERISTICS

The major indicator of Unilateral Neglect is consistent inattention to stimuli on the affected side. This is often accompanied by inadequate self-care of the affected side, lack of positioning and/or safety precautions with regard to the affected side, failure to look toward the affected side, and neglect of food or reading material on the affected side (Table 32.1).

ASSESSMENT

Given the above deficits, it is important for the nurse not only to identify the dependent older person who has Unilateral Neglect but to determine the extent of all the deficits before selecting interventions. The first step is to look for signs of Unilateral Neglect following brain injury, especially injury to the right hemisphere. However, this phenomenon should not be ruled out with left hemisphere damage.

The nurse should look for the signs and symptoms of neglect (ie, consistent inattention to stimuli on the affected side of the body, inadequate self-care to the affected side, failure to look toward the affected side, and neglect of food or reading material on the affected side). Assessment Guide 32.2 is an example of a tool that is useful for assessing Unilateral Neglect.

When the nursing diagnosis Unilateral Neglect is identified, the extent of deficits must be assessed. Other health professionals can be helpful in determining the extent of deficits. However, many nurses working with the elderly have limited access to these professionals and must rely on their own assessment. Even when other professionals are available, it is wise for the nurse to compare a client's behavior in a "test" environment with the behavior present in daily self-care and interactions, since abilities may not appear to be the same in both contexts.

Fatigue is another factor that must be taken into account when assessing persons with brain damage, since most deficits will be pronounced and frustration more evident when the person is fatigued (Lezak, 1976). The older person needs to be given the best circumstances to display existing abilities. Assessing the person when rested and away from distractions will result in more accurate data on which to base diagnoses and interventions (see the section on interventions for ways to decrease distractions).

Assessing the elderly person without prejudice is also important. Tellis-Nazak (1986) discusses the effects of attitudes toward aging and stroke on the rehabilitation of older clients. Before assessment is conducted, health professionals, as well as society at large, often share attitudes that assume the older person will not benefit from rehabilitation. This can become a self-fulfilling prophecy if health professionals are unaware of this bias.

Table 32.1

Unilateral Neglect

Definition: The state in which an individual is perceptually unaware of and inattentive to one side of the body (McLane, 1987)

NANDA (CARROLL-JOHNSON, 1989)	WEITZEL
Related Factors/Etiologies	*Related Factors/Etiologies*
Effects of disturbed perceptual abilities, eg, hemianopsia One-sided blindness Neurologic illness or trauma	Brain injury: trauma, tumor, or cerebrovascular problems Disorders of sensory input, internal representation of space, attention to stimuli contralateral to the lesion Limited or no movement of the affected extremity Loss of one half of visual field, usually to the affected side Loss of ability to know the position of a limb through its sensory input, without looking at it or feeling it Perception of stimuli to the affected side as being to the opposite limb. Perception of only stimulus to the affected side when stimulus is given to both extremities simultaneously
Defining Characteristics	*Defining Characteristics*
Consistent inattention to stimuli on an affected side Inadequate self-care Lack of positioning and/or safety precautions in regard to the affected side Does not look toward affected side Leaves food on plate on the affected side	Nonrecognition of affected side as part of the body Unawareness of functional limitations Inattention to the space located to one side of the elder's midline and inattention to that half of the body **Denial:** Function not improved by calling attention to neglected side **Inattention:** Failure to read words on the affected side. When attention is called to the omitted words, they can be read without changing the direction of gaze or moving the head **Major indicators:** Consistent inattention to stimuli on the affected side Inadequate self-care of the affected side Lack of positioning and/or safety precautions with regard to the affected side Not looking toward the affected side Neglect of food or reading material on the affected side

Categories of Extent of Deficit

O'Brien and Pallett (1978) categorize the extent of the deficits resulting in Unilateral Neglect as follows:

Inattention Inattention is the mildest form. These persons can use the affected side and care for it if someone else draws their attention to it.

Unconcern Unconcern describes persons who admit the presence of a disability but may display affect that is inappropriate in proportion to the amount of deficit.

Unawareness Unawareness is described as a transitory state soon after the injury, which clears as sensorium clears. These persons may try activities beyond their ability because they do not recognize the extent of their disability.

Denial Denial is the most severe form of Unilateral Neglect. It includes persons described previously as having anosognosia and is often complicated with hemianopsia, apraxias, and/or agnosias. Persons in denial are not accepting of their disability. It is important to understand that this condition is not part of the normal psychologic reaction to loss in which denial is protective until the psyche is ready to accept the loss. In persons with Unilateral Neglect, the brain has been damaged so that it no longer acknowledges the affected side as being part of the person. It is possible, however, that the extent of this deficit may diminish as the brain heals, so the older person should be reassessed at regular intervals for several months following brain damage.

When analyzing assessment data to develop interventions, it is probably most useful to place older persons in the first three categories (inattention, unconcern, and unawareness) into one general area and those with denial into another. Thus, two distinct diagnoses emerge: Unilateral Neglect: Inattention and Unilateral Neglect: Denial. Each individual will need interventions specific to existing deficits, but there are some definite differences between interventions for these two areas. Table 32.1 summarizes the assessment data that need to be collected that lead to a determination of inattention or denial. In addition, specific deficits such as hemianopsia, apraxia, agnosia, or visual-spatial relationship problems require interventions specifically addressed to these deficits. See Assessment Guide 32.1 for differential diagnosis of these deficits. Table 32.1 compares Weitzel's related factor/etiologies and defining characteristics with NANDA's related factors/etiologies and defining characteristics (Carroll-Johnson, 1989).

CASE STUDY

Unilateral Neglect, T.S.

T.S. is a 70-year-old man whose condition has just stabilized following a thrombolitic stroke affecting the right hemisphere of the brain. When approached from the left, he often does not respond until the nurse is standing in front of him. If the nurse has gained his attention and then moves to his left, he responds and can see objects to which the nurse points. He scratches his head with his left hand but does not wash his left side when bathing. In regard to his visual field, he can see a finger held to the left side of his head after being told it is there, as long as there is not visual stimulation to the right side. Based on these assessment data, the nurse diagnoses Unilateral Neglect: Inattention related to right hemisphere damage as evidenced by lack of response to stimuli from the left side, unless cued.

CASE STUDY

Unilateral Neglect, R.B.

R.B. is a 68-year-old man who had a stroke of undetermined type a year ago, which has left him with hemiparesis of the left leg and hemiplegia of the left arm. He tells the nurse he could walk if he just had new shoes. He will attempt to stand unattended but does not place his left foot flat on the floor or use his quad cane, even though he has been instructed several times to do both. Often he will fall if staff do not intervene. R.B. has no sensation of touch to his left arm, fails to bathe it, and leaves it dangling in the wheel of his wheelchair. When his gaze is directed to the left, he can see his left arm only after turning his head and using the right side of his eyes. He tells the nurse that this is not really his arm, that it belongs to his roommate. Based on these assessment data, the nursing diagnosis is Unilateral Neglect: Denial related

to right hemisphere brain damage as evidenced by failure to respond to stimuli to the left side, even when cued, and by hemianopsia.

NURSING INTERVENTIONS

Interventions will be discussed in three categories: those that are appropriate with both inattention and denial; those specific for inattention; and those specific for denial. Distinguishing these diagnoses on the basis of etiologies is not precise at this time, so the determination will be made based on assessed signs and symptoms. All of the interventions are compensatory, since the etiology of brain damage cannot be reversed by the nurse.

When the diagnosis of Unilateral Neglect is established, certain interventions are appropriate, whether the neglect is inattention or denial. These interventions generally fall into two broad categories: control of sensory input and psychosocial aspects. Nursing literature has little about Unilateral Neglect. Much of the research related to interventions for Unilateral Neglect was conducted several years ago. This is an area that could benefit from clinical nursing research.

Environmental Structuring

Decreasing Environmental and Unaffected Side Stimuli To increase the elder's awareness of stimuli from the affected side, it is important to control the stimuli that may interfere with the individual's ability to concentrate following brain injury. Although there is limited research support for this approach, it is validated through anecdotal observations (Fowler and Fordyce, 1972; Tilton and Maloof, 1982; Wallhagen, 1979). A quiet room without excessive visual stimuli (eg, bright patterns, movement of objects or persons) is important. The presence of hemianopsia or visual inattention may be used to advantage by putting the elderly person's unaffected side toward a wall or partition, thus decreasing input from the remainder of the room. The nurse should move slowly around the patient and speak in concrete terms, giving one instruction at a time and breaking each task into small steps. Verbal instruction may be more effective than visual demonstration, especially if the person has any visual-spatial perception disorder. Some persons have been found to concentrate better when talking on the phone than when looking at the other person. If this ability is evident, encourage phone conversations. Written cue cards of the sequence of steps are sometimes helpful in complex tasks, such as dressing. Encourage the older person to slow down, and discourage impulsive movements. Consistency of care is crucial.

Increasing Stimuli to the Affected Side There is nonsystematic empirical evidence, as well as some research, to support selective increase of stimuli to the affected side to decrease the effects of Unilateral Neglect. Marmo (1974) found that activities such as whole-body rubdown, especially with verbal input about the affected parts being stimulated, helped to increase awareness of the affected side. Marmo also suggests positioning the person prone with the head turned to the affected side to carry out activities of daily living (ADLs) or recreation, and rolling the person over the affected side. This study did not indicate if these activities are effective if the person has Unilateral Neglect: Denial. The nurse should be cautious when using these approaches with elderly persons if they are frail, have limited joint movement, or have respiratory or cardiac problems.

Booth (1982) questions the practice of encouraging the person to perform ADLs in front of a mirror, unless the nurse stays with the person to cue attention to the affected side. However, the older person might be taught to rotate the plate occasionally while eating to counteract the problem of seeing only half the plate. Additional interventions are included in the discussion of inattention.

Psychosocial Aspects The nurse must be accepting of the older person's attempts to perceive, gently correcting inappropriate responses and immediately praising correct responses. It is important that the nurse not overestimate the person's ability simply because the person has intact speech and social skills. As the older person masters one set of tasks, the nurse may gradually increase the amount and complexity of tasks. It is important for the nurse to be alert to mental as well as physical fatigue. When the person who was responding appropriately begins to be inappropriate and/or becomes frustrated, it is time to take a break.

If the elder shows emotional lability or other forms of perseveration (repeating an action or word after its usefulness is past) the nurse should interrupt with a gentle touch to the arm, ensuring the older person's attention, and then move on to the next activity. Sometimes it will be necessary for the nurse to complete a task (eg, feeding, dressing) for the older person if fatigue is a problem and the task needs to be finished. In this case, the nurse should expect successively more of the task to be completed by the older person in future attempts. The nurse should see that the patient's needs are met, while at the same time stimulating the older person to be more independent.

It is important that elderly persons with Unilateral Neglect have a minimum of relocation and as much consistency of staff as possible. Abilities to cope with change will be compromised both by the effects of age and by the effects of the perceptual deficit.

Safety Factors Providing for the safety of the older person with Unilateral Neglect is another important part of the nurse's interventions. This includes ensuring that proper hygiene measures are carried out for the affected part of the body, protecting the affected part, and dealing with inadequate caution on the part of the person who does not realize the extent of the disabilities present. Providing a wide armboard on a wheelchair for support of the affected arm may keep the arm out of the wheels of the chair. Using a sling is usually not advised because it limits any use that remains in the arm and fosters formation of flexion contractures at the elbow, wrist, and fingers. A seatbelt fastened to the wheelchair may be necessary if the older person cannot remember to carry out safety precautions (eg, lock brakes, plant affected foot firmly on floor, or await assistance from staff). The nurse should balance the need for safety with the need for dignity and quality of life.

Family Involvement It is also important for the family to remain involved and be aware of the deficits and interventions appropriate for the older person. Family can assist the staff in frequently reorienting the older person to the affected side and safety precautions, as well as sharing valuable information with the nurse about the older person's usual lifestyle.

Interventions Specific to Inattention

Cuing When a dependent older person has Unilateral Neglect: Inattention, cuing will often increase the ability to function using the affected side of the body. Weinberg et al (1979) improved visual scanning by putting a vertical line along the left edge of the page and numbering the lines of print. The person with inattention learned to look for these cues to increase ability to read the whole page and not lose the place on the page. These same researchers also found that having the person identify where a touch was located on the back and estimating the size of an object could improve awareness, especially when the person was made aware of deficits and a means was provided to correct the deficit with simple cues (Weinberg et al, 1977).

Some nurse clinicians have found that placement of flashing lights or moving objects next to the affected side increases awareness of that side (Olson and Hening, 1973). Others found that wearing a watch, a favorite ring, a bell, or a charm bracelet on the affected arm helped to draw attention to it (Flower and Fordyce, 1972; Olson and Hening, 1973). Placing the bedside table to the affected side may also increase awareness. It is important to approach the older person with Unilateral Neglect: Inattention from the *affected* side to increase awareness. It is also important to minimize stimulation to the unaffected side when trying to increase awareness.

CASE STUDY

Nursing Interventions, T.S.

T.S., previously given the diagnosis Unilateral Neglect: Inattention, will probably benefit from a variety of cuing activities to improve input from the affected side. He should have his room arranged so people approach him from the affected side. Also, his bedside table should be placed to that side. With morning and evening care, he should be asked to identify where he is being touched on his back in a variety of spots. A mobile of favorite objects could be hung within eyesight on his affected side, perhaps having a chime or other noise associated with it. A radio or TV could also be placed next to his affected side to increase auditory input. It is anticipated that these activities would increase independence and awareness of the affected side. After a few weeks T.S. should be reassessed to determine the amount of stimuli he perceives to the affected side without cuing.

Interventions Appropriate for Denial

While the older person's Unilateral Neglect: Denial persists, there is little that can be done to increase awareness of the affected side. Thus, interventions become focused on allowing persons to function as fully as possible within their limitations and to maintain safety. If the denial is so great that the older person fails to recognize any limitations, the nurse may need to become creative in developing ways to protect the person without undue constraint. The interventions for decreasing and increasing selected stimulation are appropriate, since the extent of denial may lessen with time.

The elderly person with denial should have objects arranged on the *unaffected* side to allow the objects to be seen and used. This includes the bedside table, call light, and any other essential objects. Persons with denial should be approached from the unaffected side to avoid startling them or having them reject voices on the affected side. These persons will need a great deal of simplification of tasks and verbal input throughout. The meal tray should be placed on the unaffected side or turned during the meal. Sometimes the visual loss can be used to advantage by placing part of the food out of the field of vision. This decreases the amount of food seen, which may simplify the task of eating.

Interventions for Associated Deficits

Apraxia The older person with apraxia should be helped to guide his or her hand through the correct movement. If the individual has problems with eating, put food in the spoon, place the spoon in his or her hand, and guide movement to the mouth. This may need to be repeated several times before it can be carried out independently. Practicing putting an object in a desired place may help decrease the older person's apraxia (Lord and Hall, 1986). The nurse may empty a bag of soft wrapped candy on the overbed table and have the older person with apraxia pick up the candy, one piece at a time, and place each piece in a wide-mouth cup. When all the candy is in the cup, one piece can be eaten as a reward, if the diet allows. Repeating this activity two to three times a day may increase the older person's ability to use the hand purposefully. The author has used this technique with success. If apraxia causes the older person to confuse the top and bottom of clothing, sewing colored labels in the top may increase independence in dressing.

Agnosia The older person can be helped to learn to use the other senses to compensate for the agnosia. For example, if the older person has tactile agnosia, help this person to learn to look at objects rather than depend on feel for recognition.

Visual-Spatial Relationships Having an uncluttered environment and keeping essential items in easy view will help the older person locate needed items. Teach the older person to stay toward the unaffected side in hallways and doorways to avoid hitting the affected side. Sometimes exercising to increase sitting and standing balance and keeping the head in midline will improve these problems.

Hemianopsia Teach older persons to scan with their eyes and turn their head. If the person has denial, hemianopsia may not be an area that can be corrected, so approach the older person from the unaffected side and move toward the affected side, asking the person to turn her head. When taking older persons with hemianopsia out of their rooms, point out landmarks or color cues in the hallway. Loss of vision to the affected side will mean that the side visualized going down the hall will not be visible to the older person on the way back to the room.

CASE STUDY

Nursing Interventions, R.B.

R.B., previously given the diagnosis Unilateral Neglect: Denial and hemianopsia, will probably be frustrated by any attempts at cuing. Selected stimuli can be given to the affected side but may not change his ability to function. He will need to have his room arranged with articles to his unaffected side, and persons should approach him from the unaffected side. A wide armrest on his wheelchair could increase safety for his affected arm. If R.B. continues to attempt to stand and walk unaided, a seatbelt may be necessary. Because of the denial, R.B. will require closer monitoring by staff than will T.S. However, with time, R.B. may begin to respond to more stimuli on the affected side. If reassessment should confirm this improvement in status, the diagnosis should be changed to Unilateral Neglect: Inattention and interventions altered appropriately.

OUTCOMES

Expected outcomes with the nursing diagnosis Unilateral Neglect are that the neglect behavior will decrease or be compensated and cause fewer problems for the older person in daily activities. Evaluation will necessitate reassessment and comparison of current behaviors against previous data and defined goals.

SUMMARY

The nursing diagnosis Unilateral Neglect is a deficit that may affect older persons following brain injury. It can be displayed as either inattention or denial. Nurses can treat both diagnoses best by structuring the environment. Inattention is most amenable to the intervention environmental cuing. Denial as a result of brain damage is not the same as denial following loss. Denial that results from brain damage is an inability of the brain to function correctly. This denial requires the nurse to compensate for the deficit as long as the denial persists; the person having denial usually is not aware of any deficit or of the extent of the deficit. Ensuring safety and maintaining the elderly person's dignity are major concerns of the nurse.

ASSESSMENT GUIDE 32.1

Differential Diagnosis—Unilateral Neglect

The following items will assist the nurse in differentiating the extent of deficits:
1. Does the person fail to use the affected limb, even though motor ability is present?
   a. Does the person use the limb when cued? Yes = inattention. No = probable apraxia.
   b. Does the person have difficulty using hygiene articles or putting on clothes correctly? Yes = apraxia.
2. Does the person run into walls or door frames, even when there is ample room, or have difficulty walking or steering a wheelchair in a straight line? Yes = visual-spatial problems.
3. Is reading material neglected on the affected side?
   a. When attention is drawn to the missing words, can they be read without moving the gaze? Yes = inattention. No

= hemianopsia and/or denial.
4. When the person is looking at a fixed point in midline, can fingers brought simultaneously from behind the head be detected at the same time? No = visual deficit.
   a. Can a finger be seen on the affected side when moved from midline outward and gaze remains fixed on midline? Yes = visual inattention. No = hemianopsia.
5. If a number of familiar objects are placed close to the midline of an overbed table, can all objects be named or pointed to without turning the head or gaze? No = hemianopsia.
6. When touched on the affected side, is touch perceived? Yes:
   a. Is it perceived accurately where touched? If perceived on the opposite side, this indicates allesthesia.
   b. Is it still perceived if the opposite side is touched at the same time (DSS)? No = extinction.
   No:
      a. Is perception increased if person looks at being touched and receives verbal input about touch? Yes = inattention. No = hemiplegia and/or denial.
7. Does the person have trouble finding an object in a cluttered drawer, miss the cup when pouring liquids into it, or knock things over, even with the unaffected hand? Yes = apraxia and/or visual-spatial relationship problems.
8. Does the person use incorrect terms when referring to familiar objects, not respond correctly to familiar sounds, or fail to recognize familiar objects placed in the hand with eyes closed?
   Yes = agnosia (type dependent on sense not functioning).
9. Does the person have difficulty estimating time passage when though a clock is available?
   a. Can the person read the clock correctly? If no and hemianopsia is not present, may indicate a form of agraphia.
   b. If yes, may indicate time orientation problems.

ASSESSMENT GUIDE 32.2

Assessment Tool for Unilateral Neglect

The following questions will assist the nurse in establishing the presence of neglect:
1. Is there consistent inattention to the affected side?
2. Is there inadequate self-care to the affected side?
   a. Dressing
   b. Bathing
   c. Application of deodorant/cologne
   d. Shaving
   e. Application of cosmetics
3. Is there lack of positioning and/or safety precautions with regard to the affected side?
4. Is food left on the plate on the affected side?
5. Does food remain in the cheek on the affected side?
6. When asked to draw a daisy, is the drawing complete or are petals missing on the affected side?
7. When asked to draw self, is the drawing complete (stick drawing) or are limbs on the affected side missing, distorted, or lighter?
8. When asked to draw the face of a clock, are numbers omitted to the affected side?

References

Booth K: The neglect syndrome. *J Neurosurg Nurs* (Feb) 1982; 14(1):38–43.

Carroll-Johnson R (editor): *Classification of Nursing Diagnoses: Proceedings of the Eighth Conference.* Lippincott, 1989.

Dudas S: Nursing diagnosis and intervention for rehabilitation of the stroke patient. *Nurs Clin North Am* (June) 1986; 21(2):345–357.

Fowler R, Fordyce W: Adapting care for the brain damaged patient. *Am J Nurs* 1972; 72(10):1832–1835.

Friedland RP, Weinstein EA: Hemi-inattention and hemisphere specialization: Introduction and historical review. Pages 1–31 in: *Advances in Neurology*, Vol 18. Weinstein EA, Friedland RP (editors). Raven Press, 1977.

Geshwind N, Behan N: Left-handedness: Association with immune disease, migraine and development of learning disorders. *Proceed National Acad Sci* 1982; 79:5097–5100.

Gorelick PB: Cerebrovascular disease: Pathology, physiology and diagnosis. *Nurs Clin North Am* (June) 1986; 21(2):275–288.

Heilman KM, Valenstein E: Mechanisms underlying hemispatial neglect. Pages 166–170 in: *Advances in Neurology*, Vol 18. Weinstein EA, Friedland RP (editors). Raven Press, 1977.

Johnson JH, Cyran M: Homonymous hemianopsia: Assessment and management. *Am J Nurs* 1979; 79(12):2131–2134.

Kim MJ, McFarland GK, McLane AM: *Pocket Guide to Nursing Diagnoses.* Mosby, 1987.

Lezak MD: *Neuropsychological Assessment.* Oxford University Press, 1976.

Lord JP, Hall K: Neuromuscular reeducation vs. traditional programs for stroke rehabilitation. *Arch Phys Med Rehab* 1986; 67(2):88–91.

Marmo NA: A new look at the brain damaged adult. *Am J Occup Ther* 1974; 28(4):199–200.

McGlone J: Sex differences in functional brain asymmetry. *Cortex* 1978; 14:122–128.

McLane A (editor): *Classification of Nursing Diagnoses: Proceedings of the Seventh Conference.* Mosby, 1987.

Nooney TW: Partial visual rehabilitation of hemianopia patients. *Am J Optometry Physiolog Optics* 1986; 63(5):382–386.'

O'Brien MT, Pallett PJ: *Total Care of the Stroke Patient.* Little, Brown, 1978.

Olson DO, Hening E: *A Manual of Behavior Management Strategies for Traumatically Brain-Injured Adults.* Rehabilitation Institute of Chicago, 1973.

Riddoch MJ, Humphreys G: The effect of cuing on unilateral neglect. *Neuropsychologica* 1983; 21(6):589–599.

Siev E, Freishat B: *Perceptual Dysfunction in Adult Stroke Patients.* Slack, 1976.

Tellis-Nazak M: The challenge of the nursing role in rehabilitation of the elderly stroke patient. *Nurs Clin North Am* (June) 1986; 21(2):339–343.

Tilton CN, Maloof M: Diagnosing the problem in stroke. *Am J Nurs* 1982; 82(4):596–601.

Wallhagen M: The split brain: Implications for care and rehabilitation. *Am J Nurs* 1979; 79(12):2118–2125.

Weinberg J, Diller L, Gordon WA: Visual scanning training effect on reading-related tasks in acquired right brain damage. *Arch Phys Med Rehab* 1977; 58:479–486.

Weinberg J, Diller L, Gordon WA: Training sensory awareness and spatial organization in people with right brain damage. *Arch Phys Med Rehab* 1979; 60:491–496.

Weinstein EA, Friedland RP: *Advances in Neurology*, Vol 18. Raven Press, 1977.

33

Knowledge Deficit

BARBARA RAKEL, MA, RN

KNOWLEDGE DEFICIT HAS BEEN DEFINED AS THE inability to state or explain information or demonstrate a required skill related to disease management procedures, practices, and/or self-care health management (Gordon, 1982). Knowledge deficits are common and affect people of all ages at various times of their lives. If an individual has never experienced a new health condition, such as diabetes; undergone newly prescribed treatments or diagnostic tests; or performed new self-care or health maintenance behaviors, knowledge deficit is possible. With increasingly complex medical technology and patients performing more health care activities at home or in the community setting, knowledge deficits are becoming even more prevalent. Health care practitioners must consider teaching as a more prominent part of their practice.

SIGNIFICANCE FOR THE ELDERLY

The elderly are at risk for Knowledge Deficit. As individuals age, many experience limitations in their capacity for self-care. They may also suffer the loss of role identity and begin to lose control over their environment. They may no longer see themselves as the vital, virile people they once were. Entering a long-term care facility enhances these feelings and intensifies the stigmatization and loss of control over their environment (Taft, 1985). All these forces are negatively correlated with self-esteem, which in turn affects a person's quality of life. Self-control and independence are the cornerstones of feeling good about oneself. Too often older persons are robbed of their self-care capacities in the name of efficiency, protection, or compliance with facility or government regulations (Eliopoulos, 1984). Looking at ways to maximize a person's quality of life is an important aspect of geriatric nursing care.

Increasing geriatric patients' self-care capacity through education can be an effective way of meeting their self-esteem needs. Orem's (1985) self-care model can be used to facilitate this type of nursing. Eliopoulos (1984) uses Orem's model to develop a theoretical framework for gerontologic nursing. She makes the distinction between the nurse helping individuals meet their needs versus performing activities that individuals cannot do for themselves.

Other nursing theorists agree with this approach. Henderson's (1955) classic definition of nursing is, "primarily assisting the individual (sick or well) in the performance of those activities contributing to health or its recovery . . . that he would perform unaided if he had the necessary strength, will, or knowledge." She recognizes lack of knowledge as characteristic of the patient and specifies patient education as an appropriate task of the nurse. Peplau (1952) was equally explicit when defining nursing as, "an educative instrument, a maturing force, that aims to promote forward movement of personality in the direction of creative, constructive, productive, personal, and community living."

Smith (1982) reports a study that also supports this approach. A group of self-care elderly nursing home residents were asked to rate the importance of various care activities. They rated the importance of patient teaching activities and psychosocial activities far above medical and physical care activities. Further, patients rated teaching activities higher than did the nursing staff.

Assisting the elderly to maintain their dignity by teaching them to perform tasks that increase their independence and self-care capacity can have a large impact on their self-esteem and, consequently, their quality of life. However, to accomplish this, nurses must be able to recognize when there is a need for such education. This recognition is benefited from the use of the nursing diagnosis Knowledge Deficit.

CURRENT STATUS OF THE DIAGNOSIS

Knowledge Deficit as a Concept

The diagnosis Knowledge Deficit has been recognized by the North American Nursing Diagnosis Association (NANDA) and has been on their list of accepted diagnoses since the delineation began. Nurses have dealt with this diagnosis in the clinical setting for many years. The literature contains a vast array of articles dealing with the importance of patient knowledge in preparation for various tests or procedures and in relation to newly acquired disease states or self-care limitations. Texts that list potential nursing diagnoses for various medical conditions include Knowledge Deficit as a potential nursing problem for most conditions.

Martin and York (cited in Kim et al, 1984) conducted a study to determine which of the nursing diagnoses accepted by the Fourth National Conference in 1980 were most frequently used by staff nurses. They found that Knowledge Deficit was the third most prevalent nursing diagnosis used in the settings they tested (medical-surgical, obstetric, and rehabilitation patients). The first two were Altered Comfort and Ineffective Breathing Pattern.

The prevalence of this diagnosis can be attributed to many things. One of these is the attention given to legal responsibilities, such as those stated in "A Patient's Bill of Rights" (American Hospital Association, 1975), confirming the patient's right to receive complete information about his or her diagnosis, treatment, and prognosis. Another is reflected in the American Nurses' Association's (1975) statement entitled "The Professional Nurse and Health Education," which professes that the responsibility and accountability of every professional nurse includes teaching the patient and family relevant facts about specific health care needs. In addition, patients themselves are demanding more information about their treatment and care (Corkadel and McGlashan, 1983).

Another reason Knowledge Deficit is so common is its broad scope. It is the only diagnosis, aside from Altered Thought Processes, that deals with the human response pattern "knowing." NANDA's taxonomy places "knowing" (see Figure 33.1) as one of the nine level I concepts. This concept is broken down into three level II concepts: alterations in knowledge; alterations in learning; and alterations in thought processes. It is obvious from the number of blank boxes that this pattern remains incomplete and underdeveloped. Knowledge Deficit is the only diagnosis currently being used that deals with both alterations in knowledge *and* alterations in learning. Further delineation is needed. As Figure 33.1 suggests, knowledge is a separate concept from learning, and confusion occurs with attempts to include aspects of learning under the realm of knowledge.

A study was performed that attempted to develop the diagnosis alterations in learning ability and describe the defining characteristics that distinguish this diagnosis from the diagnosis Knowledge Deficit (Rakel, 1988). It was found that not only are there multiple diagnoses under the area of alterations in learning ability that are relevant to nursing, but the defining characteristics are easily distinguishable from those of Knowledge Deficit. In addition, the results suggested a need to change the NANDA taxonomy by moving Knowledge Deficit to a level above alterations in learning ability.

ETIOLOGIES/RELATED FACTORS

The etiologies proposed by NANDA (Carroll-Johnson, 1989) (Table 33.1) and those published by Gordon (1982), Hurley (1986), Kim et al (1984), and McLane (1987) were inductively generated and not drawn from a research base. Rather, they were offered in the hope of stimulating research in this area. Because Carpenito (1983) does not cite any research base for her list, it is likely that hers also was compiled through induction. Review of the literature, however, revealed no studies designed to identify the causes of Knowledge Deficit. Other studies, though, along with anecdotal literature, offer support for some causes, especially medical

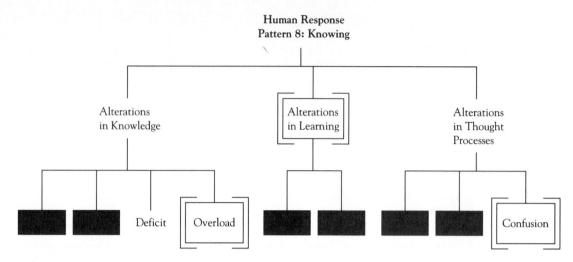

Figure 33.1

Human response pattern 8: Knowing.

conditions (eg, hypertension) and chronic diseases (eg, arthritis). This supports the etiology of "a new orexisting medical condition" stated by Carpenito (1983) (Table 33.1).

Another cause, especially relevant to the elderly, is the need to follow "prescribed treatments (new, complex)" (Carpenito, 1983). Diet treatments, such as low-salt diets for patients with hypertension, and medication prescriptions, especially for the elderly who consume approximately 25% of all drugs used in this country, necessitate the need for knowledge to facilitate adherence to the diet and prevent drug-related complications (Carpenito, 1983; Dall and Gresham, 1982; Donahue et al, 1981; Kern and Gawlinski, 1983).

Another etiology supported by Dall and Gresham (1982) is "information misinterpretation" (Hurley, 1986; Kim et al, 1984). They discuss how research has confirmed that elderly living at home tend to make errors in self-administration of their medications, thereby indicating the need for proper knowledge.

Other articles suggest that the goal of increased self-care and health maintenance (Carpenito, 1983) necessitates a need for knowledge of self-care and health maintenance skills. Resler (1983) and Speers and Turk (1982) discuss the need of patients with diabetes to perform certain skills such as insulin administration, skin and foot care, and food planning for the purpose of achieving self-care and maintaining health. Nelson et al (1984) further discuss the importance of self-care for the elderly and how it necessitates a need for education in medications, emergencies, resources in the community, and coordination of one's own health and welfare needs.

New therapies such as diagnostic tests or surgical procedures, both etiologies listed by Carpenito (1983), are indications that added knowledge is needed. In fact, Pokorny (1985) found that patients undergoing these

therapies were given education without being assessed for defining characteristics of a knowledge deficit. It was simply assumed that new knowledge was needed.

Numerous studies discuss the importance of preoperative instruction and its effects on state anxiety (Shimko, 1981), ability to cough and deep breathe (King and Tarsitano, 1982; Lindeman, 1973; Lindeman and Van Aernam, 1971), postoperative vomiting (Dumas and Leonard, 1963), and length of hospital stay (Healy, 1968; Lindeman, 1973; Lindeman and Van Aernam, 1971) after surgical procedures. Rossi and Haines (1979) also discuss the importance of information prior to diagnostic tests for patients after a myocardial infarction. These findings lend support to these therapies as etiologies for Knowledge Deficit.

It is interesting to note that most of the etiologies supported by the literature were ones stated by Carpenito (1983). None of those listed by Gordon (1982) were referred to in these articles, and "information misinterpretation" is the only one stated by both Kim et al (1984) and Hurley (1986) that was acknowledged by authors. It is possible that learning etiologies are being identified more than causes of knowledge deficits, or that they are viewed the same. Many of the etiologies in the literature refer to learning or a condition of learning (ie, lack of interest or motivation to learn, low readiness for reception of information, cognitive limitations, and so on). The fact that the literature does not support these as etiologies of Knowledge Deficit further suggests that knowledge and learning are separate concepts. A diagnosis (or diagnoses) for learning deficits is needed to incorporate these conditions. These situations exist and are possibly as common as, or more common than, knowledge deficits. It is important to remember, however, that this contention is not based on research, which is desperately needed in this area.

Table 33.1

Etiologies/Risk Factors and Defining Characteristics of Knowledge Deficit

ETIOLOGIES	DEFINING CHARACTERISTICS
NANDA *(Carroll-Johnson, 1989)*	
Lack of exposure	Verbalization of the problem
Lack of recall	Inaccurate follow-through of instruction
Information misinterpretation	Inadequate performance of test
Cognitive limitation	Inappropriate or exaggerated behaviors (eg, hysterical,
Lack of interest in learning	hostile, agitated, apathetic)
Unfamiliarity with information resources	
CARPENITO *(1984)*	
Pathophysiologic:	Verbalizes a deficiency in knowledge or skill
Any existing or new medical condition	Expresses "inaccurate" perception of health status
Situational:	Does not correctly perform a desired or prescribed health
Language differences	behavior because of inadequate knowledge
Prescribed treatments (new, complex)	Does not comply (noncompliance) with prescribed health
Diagnostic tests	behavior
Surgical procedures	Exhibits or expresses psychologic alteration (eg, anxiety,
Medications	depression) resulting from misinformation or lack of
Pregnancy	information
Personal characteristics—lack of motivation, denial of situation, ineffective coping patterns (eg, anxiety, depression)	
Maturational:	
(Children)	
Sexuality and sexual development	
Safety hazards	
Substance abuse	
Nutrition	
(Adolescents)	
Same as children	
Automotive safety practices	
Substance abuse (alcohol, drugs, tobacco)	
Health maintenance practices	
(Adults)	
Parenthood	
Sexual function	
Health maintenance practices	
(Elderly)	
Effects of aging	
Sensory deficits	

DEFINING CHARACTERISTICS

As with the etiologies, the defining characteristics listed by most authors were also inductively generated and not drawn from a research base. However, the literature again supports the validity of some defining characteristics. Baldini (1981), Kim and Grier (1981), Linde and Janz (1979), and Milazzo (1980) tested the effectiveness of various teaching strategies with the use of pretest scores as a baseline to define the need for education, thereby offering support for the defining characteristic "inadequate performance on a test."

Others (Speers and Turk, 1982) described inaccurate follow-through of instructions, inadequate performance on a test, and inaccurate demonstration of a skill as indications of lack of knowledge.

Dall and Gresham (1982) identify questions such as "What's this little pill for?" or "Why do I get dizzy with this pill?" and observations of inaccurate drug-taking behavior as indications that a knowledge deficit exists in elderly patients on medication-taking regimens. These questions lend support to the characteristics verbalization of the problem, verbalization of a deficiency in knowledge or skill, and inaccurate follow-through of instruction.

When discussing the case study of a patient with coronary artery disease, Kern and Gawlinski (1983) reveal how the patient's inadequate understanding of information, information misinterpretation (Gordon, 1982), or statement of misconception (Kim et al, 1984) indicated a knowledge deficit. This patient made statements implying his assumption that sticking to a low-sodium diet simply meant "no salt," not foods containing sodium. This was interpreted as evidence that a knowledge deficit existed and further education was needed.

Three of the proposed characteristics relate to a verbalization by the patient that he or she needs more information, does not remember information previously given, or does not understand it. The literature suggests that not only are patients aware of their own gaps in knowledge (Weiler, 1968), but they are often able to identify accurately areas in which knowledge is needed (Casey et al, 1984).

Pokorny (1985) performed a study designed specifically to identify the presence of the proposed defining characteristics of Knowledge Deficit in a clinical setting. She sought to answer the questions, What defining characteristics are documented when the nursing diagnosis Knowledge Deficit is made? With what frequency does each occur? And, do any of the defining characteristics constitute a critical defining characteristic, that is, one that is present in 95% or more of the cases?

The defining characteristics Pokorny (1985) used were drawn from those proposed by participants in the Fourth National NANDA Conference (Kim and Moritz, 1982) and by Gordon (1982). She found that inadequate knowledge was the defining characteristic most frequently used, followed by verbalized inadequate recall of information and verbalized inadequate understanding of information.

The most commonly encountered behavioral defining characteristic was evidence of inaccurate follow-through of instructions, which was associated with length of hospital stay. No instances of inappropriate or exaggerated behavior as an indicator of Knowledge Deficit were found, nor were defining characteristics found other than those listed on the tool. Also, no critical defining characteristics were identified.

An interesting finding in this study was that defining characteristics were documented in only 51 of the 120 cases studied. There was also a significant association between the absence of documented defining characteristics and the presence of a medical diagnosis involving invasive diagnostic procedures. As Pokorny (1985;650) states, "It may be that nurses considered all patients about to undergo a cardiac catheterization or other invasive procedure to lack the knowledge needed to participate in the procedure and recovery and applied the

diagnosis of Knowledge Deficit without documenting the data to support it." This is consistent with other studies in which education was provided without evidence of prior assessment to support its need (Donahue et al, 1981; Dumas and Leonard, 1963; Healy, 1968; King and Tarsitano, 1982; Lindeman, 1972; Lindeman and Van Aernam, 1971; Mezzanote, 1970; Morisky et al, 1982; Shimko, 1981).

There is also danger in assuming that patient education is the only or most effective intervention for solving a knowledge deficit problem. Other interventions, such as behavior modification, attitude therapy, and remotivation, may more effectively deal with the etiology. However, unless the etiology and defining characteristics are assessed and known, appropriate planning and interventions cannot be instituted. Defining characteristics listed by NANDA (Carroll-Johnson, 1989) are in Table 33.1.

CASE STUDY

Knowledge Deficit

H.K. is an 86-year-old white woman who suffered a right intertrochanteric hip fracture and underwent open reduction and internal fixation of the right hip 5 months ago. Prior to the accident, she had been living alone at home and took pride in her independence. However, after discharge from the hospital, she had to be admitted to a long-term health care facility because she could no longer walk or get around on her own. This upset her, and on admission she stated that her main goal was to learn to walk again so that she could do things for herself and return home.

H.K. is alert; is oriented to time, place, and person; has good communication skills; and is a good historian. Her speech and hearing are within normal limits, and she wears corrective lenses that allow her to do needlepoint. She is pleasant and cooperative and takes part in most of the center's activities. However, H.K. frequently tries to do too many things for herself and avoids calling the nurse until it is absolutely necessary. Occasionally she wets the bed or floor because she is too embarrassed to call for help.

When tested on admission, H.K. displayed good upper extremity strength bilaterally and had adequate range of motion of all extremities. Partial weight-bearing ambulation, with progression to full weight-bearing ambulation, was ordered to facilitate her rehabilitation and increase her independence. However, an assistive device was needed for partial weight-bearing and balance. H.K. had used a cane for assistance in the past, but this did not give her the support she needed now. A walker was indicated, but H.K. stated that she did not know how to use one.

TENTATIVE DIAGNOSIS

Knowledge Deficit related to prescribed treatment of partial weight-bearing ambulation, indicating use of a walker, as evidenced by patient's statement that she does not know how to use one. (See Table 33.2 for other diagnoses ruled out.)

NURSING INTERVENTIONS

Patient Education

Patient education is often the most effective way to resolve a knowledge deficit. Redman and Thomas (1985) state that even though patient education can be used to treat many nursing diagnoses, Knowledge Deficit is one of the most directly relevant diagnoses for this intervention. Most authors who list Knowledge Deficit as a nursing problem include patient teaching or the teaching/learning process as the treatment, implying that they go hand in hand (Carpenito, 1983; Dall and Gresham, 1982; Linde and Janz, 1979; Lorig et al, 1984; Powers and Wooldridge, 1982; Resler, 1983; Rossi and Haines, 1979; Speers and Turk, 1982). If patient education is defined as a teaching/learning process directed toward influencing patient and family behavior through changes in knowledge, attitudes, and beliefs and through the acquisition of psychomotor skills (Carpenito, 1983), the direct correlation between Knowledge Deficit and the teaching/learning process is obvious. It is this close correlation, in fact, that may

account for the confusion that exists between learning problems and Knowledge Deficit.

Other Possible Interventions

Other interventions can be used to correct a knowledge deficit problem if, for example, the knowledge deficit is related to prescribed treatments or medical conditions necessitating lifestyle changes. In these cases, patient contracting, counseling, support groups, self-modification, or values clarification may be more effective than education. At other times enhancement of a patient's learning ability may be needed to deal with a knowledge deficit problem, especially when treating the elderly. (Note: Because learning problems are currently being addressed under Knowledge Deficit, interventions for them will also be discussed here.) Also, elderly patients may have cognitive limitations that affect their learning ability.

Reminiscence Therapy Reminiscence therapy may be used to improve the teaching/learning process. Hughston and Merriam (1982) investigated the effect of a structured reminiscent intervention program on cognitive functioning of the elderly and found that women given learning tasks using material from their past personal lives, rather than new material, had significantly improved cognitive functioning. This suggests that reminiscence therapy may provide an effective educational and counseling strategy with the aged.

Table 33.2

Differential Diagnoses, Case Study, H.K.

SIGNS AND SYMPTOMS	DIAGNOSES RULED OUT	ADDITIONAL DATA NEEDED
Alert/oriented x 3 Good historian	Altered Thought Processes	Distractibility? Ability to think abstractly?
Good communication skills	Impaired Verbal Communication	Degree of auditory comprehension?
Speech and hearing within normal limits		Ability to name objects? Ability to find correct word?
Cooperative Motivated to learn Made consistent progress	Noncompliance	Number of appointments kept? Number of complications?
Pleasant Participates in most of center's activities	Social Isolation	Feelings regarding usefulness, difference from others, aloneness? Support from significant others? Interests appropriate to age?
Speech and hearing within normal limits Wears corrective lenses Alert/oriented x 3	Sensory-Perceptual Alteration	Report of sensory acuity? Change in usual response to stimuli?

Sensory Retraining Sensory retraining can facilitate the teaching/learning process by increasing the amount and variety of sensory information coming into the elderly individual's central nervous sytem. In addition to the sensory changes that occur normally with age, many dependent older individuals further reduce their sensory input by physical and psychologic withdrawal. Sensory retraining is an organized, therapeutic attempt to reactivate all sensory channels and assist the older person in reestablishing and/or maintaining discriminating contact with the environment (Saxon and Etten, 1984).

Remotivation Therapy Lack of motivation to learn due to depression or apathy about their situation may also be a problem with persons who have a knowledge deficit. Remotivation therapy may be indicated with these patients. This intervention actively solicits interest in objective, real-world subjects in an effort to help individuals put their personal problems in perspective and to keep individuals in touch with life outside the institution (Kohut et al, 1983).

Relaxation Therapy Anxiety about a learning situation can affect a person's attention and memory. The effects of relaxation therapy have been shown to increase performance on memory tasks. Yesavage (1984) found that elderly subjects who received relaxation training before learning showed a significant improvement in recalling names and faces than older adults who did not receive this training. This improvement was significantly related to a decrease in anxiety (Yesavage and Jacob, 1984). Subjects with a relatively high level of anxiety before the training showed more improvement after relaxation than those with a previously low level of anxiety (Yesavage et al, 1982).

Research Base for Patient Education

Literature in the area of patient education is unsystematic and inconsistent. There are no comprehensive models into which patient education fits. Therefore, the bulk of the literature is segregated into groupings for specific patient populations, each defining a teaching model around a particular disease entity, with no cross-referencing among them. Such groupings suffer from biases and narrow horizons and are not sufficient by themselves (Redman and Thomas, 1985).

Meta-Analysis

A form of synthesis called meta-analysis has been used to draw some conclusions from the confusing literature in the area of patient education. This approach uses an empirical form of integrating research findings and offers a method by which to draw conclusions about various aspects of patient education that have been tested in a group of selected studies.

These reviews, on the average, find patient education to be positive and clearly better than no teaching at all. However, they also suggest that strictly informational approaches are not the most effective option. Mumford et al (1982) found that psychologic approaches offering emotional support and relief of anxiety were more effective than purely educational methods, and that a combination of both was superior to either alone. A study by Mazzuca (1982) summarized 30 controlled experiments of persons with chronic disease in which the dependent variables included compliance with a therapeutic regimen, physiologic progress of patients, and long-range health outcomes. Efforts to improve health by increasing patient knowledge alone were rarely successful. Instead, behaviorally oriented programs that gave special attention to changing the environment in which patients cared for themselves and that used the patient's own regimen or daily routine to focus the instruction were consistently more successful in improving the clinical course of chronic disease.

Reading (1979) also supported the significance of individual differences influencing the impact of information. He examined the short-term effects of psychologic preparation of patients having surgery and found that, in the studies he reviewed, some patients benefited from an absence of information, whereas others needed extensive teaching. This difference depended on the patient's personality and the nature of the procedure to be undergone.

We can conclude from these reviews that assessing the psychologic status of patients, their perception of the situation, and their learning needs is an important aspect of any patient education intervention. Also, involving patients in the instruction and making the information specific to their home environment and daily regimen will provide patients with a better ability to follow through with and retain the information.

The Teaching/Learning Process

In spite of the popularity of patient education, there is evidence that effective, consistent teaching is not being accomplished. Corkadel and McGlashan (1983;9) state that "while nurses are expected to teach patients, at least in theory, the teaching has generally been unstructured, inconsistent, and often left up to chance." At times, patient education is thought of as simply information availability, regardless of the learning needs of the patient (Swain and Steckel, 1981). This does not adequately represent an educational intervention. If nurses are to be effective teachers they cannot simply concern themselves with the transmission of facts. They must perform the critical function of engaging the patient in the learning process.

The "process" of teaching is the critical key to the success or failure of educational efforts (see Figure 33.2 for an algorithm of one type of process). At least two process approaches are cited in the literature. The most common approach follows the traditional nursing process steps of assessment, diagnosis, planning, implementation, and evaluation (Figure 33.2). Another, used by Green et al (1980), starts with the desired health status and works backward to identify the necessary behaviors; to categorize factors that have direct impact on the behaviors into predisposing, enabling, and reinforcing factors; and to intervene to remove blocks or increase positive forces.

The first approach is most familiar to nurses and relates closely with activities of teaching identified as important in the instructional design literature (Andrews and Ludwika, 1980; Briggs, 1977; Kemp, 1985; Reigeluth, 1983). Experts in patient education (Huckabay, 1980; Redman, 1984; Resler, 1983; Stanton, 1985) use this format when describing the teaching/learning process and when incorporating the various activities of teaching into patient education and health care settings.

Certain elements of the teaching/learning process have been consistently identified as important in the literature and should be considered whenever educating elderly patients. One element is proper assessment of learner needs (discussed under defining characteristics of Knowledge Deficit) and the individual's readiness to learn. This can prevent ineffective teaching and wasted efforts. Many individuals who are normally good learners are affected by their situation in ways that alter their ability to learn and retain information. If learning is to occur, patients must be both willing and able to make use of the instruction. Factors affecting their motivation and ability to perceive information must be assessed before instruction begins. An instrument was developed by the author to assist in evaluating a patient's readiness to learn (see Assessment Guide 33.1). Content validity for this instrument is supported by the feedback of experts.

A second important element in the teaching/learning process is setting specific, measurable learning objectives that indicate what skills and/or knowledge the patient should possess after the instruction. This is a very important step and one that is often ignored. Clear, concise objectives facilitate learning because they (1) let patients know exactly what is expected of them; (2) help the nurse select appropriate content, teaching activities, and media to get the information across; and (3) provide a framework with which to evaluate the patient's learning accurately. For specifics on how to formulate objectives see Grunlund (1978), Kemp (1985), and Redman (1984). Objectives that deal with higher-level learning skills, such as application, synthesis, or problem solving, should be aimed for because patients often need to apply

information/skills and solve problems in their home environment. An objective should state what the learner is expected to accomplish, using verbs that describe observable activities, such as *list*, *describe*, or *choose*.

A third important element in the teaching/learning process is matching content, learning activities, and media to the behavioral objectives. Learning activities are the means by which the patient receives the information needed. It is the responsibility of the nurse/teacher to become familiar with the advantages and disadvantages of learning activity so that the appropriate one can be selected. This also applies to media selection. A variety of materials are available, but the nurse must know how and when to use each one to satisfy the behavioral objectives that have been identified. This requires thorough familiarity with the media (as well as accurate assessment of the patient). Too often the nurse will choose a film or pamphlet without actually reading or viewing it to see if the level of information is appropriate or the points it stresses coincide with the learning objectives.

Evaluate Patient Learning

This step is vital for determining success of the intervention. Unless one evaluates whether or not learning actually occurred, there is no way to know whether the instruction was effective. This is where the careful listing of objectives pays off. If the objectives are stated in behavioral terms, evaluation can specifically measure these outcomes. The accomplishment of the objectives not only provides satisfaction for both the learner and the teacher, but it verifies the effectiveness of the nursing intervention and provides documentation of the nurse's influence. Evaluation can be done throughout the teaching process to provide feedback to learners on how well they are doing and to let the nurse know how the instruction is going, and/or evaluation can be done at the end to measure the degree to which the outcomes were attained.

These steps provide nurses with the skills necessary to become effective teachers. Knowing what methods are most effective for the elderly and developing these to their fullest can provide nurses with the necessary tools to perform this intervention effectively and efficiently.

Patient Education in the Elderly

It is a myth that older adults have little capacity for learning new concepts and skills. Most studies that evaluated the effects of educational programs on the elderly individual were found to be effective. Morisky et al (1982) tested the effects of a health education program designed to address specific needs of patients with hypertension. They found that despite the fact that older patients (>65) had more chronic disease, had more

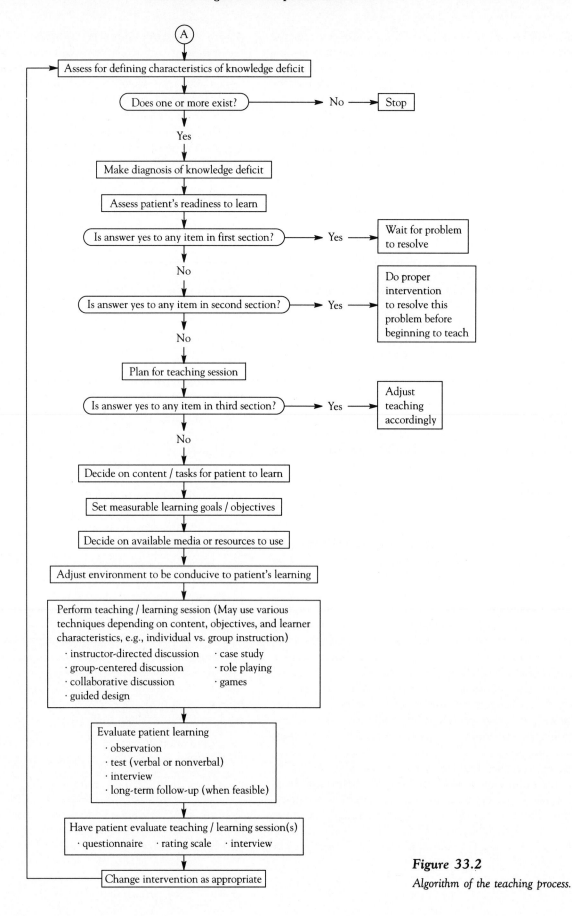

Figure 33.2

Algorithm of the teaching process.

complications from hypertension, and were receiving more complex drug therapies than younger patients (<65) exposed to the same experimental interventions, they demonstrated significantly higher levels of compliance with drug therapy, significantly higher levels of appointment keeping, and no difference in having weight and blood pressure under control at 2-year and 5-year follow-ups.

Lorig et al (1984) studied the effectiveness of a 12-hour, community-based, lay-led arthritis self-management course on 200 elderly people, aged 55 to 94, with arthritis. Those in the 55 to 74 age group showed significant gains in knowledge and decreases in pain for 20 months. In addition, they shared a decrease in disability for 8 months. Those in the 75 to 94 age group showed an increase in knowledge for 20 months and decreased their pain and number of visits to the physician for 8 months.

Check and Wurzbach (1984) conducted a survey to determine how men and women over age 65 perceived learning and whether they thought age was a deterrent. Overall, this group did not associate advanced age with an inability to learn. Although they claimed some difficulty memorizing, they felt that it was possible to learn with proper pacing. There were some differences between the following two groups, however. Intermediate care facility residents expressed an overall sense of tiring more easily and complained more of having difficulty with memory than those in independent living.

Obstacles to Learning As a person ages, changes occur that may become obstacles to learning if they are not properly dealt with.

Vision More than 90% of people 60 years of age or older require some correction of vision. Consequently, when using visual aids with an elderly learner, remember to use the largest, boldface print available; avoid materials combining greens, blues, purples, or violets (reds, yellows, and oranges are preferred); use matte rather than glossy letters to reduce the effects of glare; use a neutral background (eg, light tan) rather than a highly contrasting one to display information; provide adequate lighting with localized "task" lighting whenever possible; allow the elder to control the lighting of the learning environment when possible (eg, controlling the blinds over outside windows, selecting level of overhead illumination) to help minimize glare and facilitate the learner's visibility of important materials; and, finally, allow extra time for dark–light adaptation, turning the light on in increments whenever possible.

Hearing The incidence of some degree of hearing loss is 11.4% among persons 45 to 65 years old, about 40% among persons in their 70s, and 65% in persons over 80. Older adults may attempt to compensate for this loss in hearing by lipreading. Therefore, it is important for the nurse/teacher to face the older learner and speak slowly.

It may also be helpful for the nurse to lower the pitch of his or her voice, since seniors often have difficulty hearing high-pitched tones. Also, eliminating extraneous sounds by keeping the environmental background noise to a minimum will facilitate hearing. The older learner who has to listen with extra concentration to understand what is being said may become easily fatigued. Therefore, keeping sessions short and simple will also facilitate learning and decrease frustration in the hearing impaired.

Slowness Kim and Grier (1981) conducted a study to examine the pacing effects of medication instruction on the learning of elderly patients. They randomly assigned 45 patients to one of three groups: an experimental group receiving medication instruction at a normal pace (159 words per minute), an experimental group receiving instruction at a slower pace (106 words per minute), and a control group not receiving any instruction. They found that patients in the slow-paced group not only had significantly greater gains in scores from the pretest to the posttest than patients in the normal-paced group, but also made significantly fewer response errors during the instruction than did the normal-paced group. Furthermore, the gain in scores of the group receiving instruction at a normal pace did not differ significantly from that of the group who did not receive any instruction.

In addition to the benefits from slower rates of instruction, research suggests that there may be a limited range of rates within which the slowing of speech results in improved comprehension. Schmitt and McCroskey (1981) studied elderly listeners and found that the subjects they tested had significantly better comprehension performance under a time expansion of 140% the normal rate (normal rate being 175 words per minute) but did not show significantly better performance with further slowing to 180% time expansion. This finding was also supported by Schmitt (1983).

Therefore, finding the appropriate pacing of teaching material not only is essential for optimal learning but may require frequent feedback from learners to determine their rate of comprehension. Pausing after each major point to allow time for questions and discussion may aid older adults' ability to process information. Also, using simple, familiar language; opting for less content; and providing more specificity, definition, and application of the information included will help the older person learn. Ascoine and Shimp (1984) found that drug knowledge in 158 elderly cardiovascular patients was improved by a strategy that provided small amounts of specific information, thereby decreasing the possibility of overwhelming the patient.

In addition to a slowing of information processing in the older adult, there is a decline in reaction time. When given more time to respond to a test question or assigned task, older adults are able to improve their performance (McKenzie, 1980). Therefore, allowing adequate time for responding is another factor to remember when teaching the older adult. In general, however, older people learn best when working at their own pace rather than at a pace that is determined by someone else. Fleming and Lopez (1981) found that elderly subjects given control over the learning situation, in the form of self-pacing, performed better on learning tasks than those who were not given control. These effects were seen even when the group not given control learned under the same response time as the self-paced group. Use of self-paced learning techniques such as self-instructional booklets or self-paced modules that permit the older learner to control the presentation pace may, therefore, be the most effective teaching strategy to use with the older adult learner.

Attention There is a decrease in attention span and an increase in distractibility as a person ages. In other words, the ability to fix and maintain attention on a subject is reduced in elders, and they are easily distracted from a task. In addition, the ability to attend to competing tasks simultaneously or in alteration is impaired. Therefore, blocking out distracting noises and/or activities in the surrounding area by moving to a private room or turning off the radio or television may help (Swift, 1984). Also, concentrating on one subject or task at a time and avoiding irrelevant information may facilitate learning. It has been shown that as the amount of irrelevant information increases, the performance of the older person disproportionately declines compared to that of the younger person (Kausler and Hakami, 1982; Rabbitt, 1965).

Task meaningfulness also affects an older person's attention. Adults perform better on meaningful tasks than they do on tasks that they find less meaningful (Gribbin, 1976). Therefore, instruction that is of value to elders and provides solution to their immediate problems will be better learned than instruction that is of no value or does not promise usefulness in the future.

Rigidity It is a common belief that older people are resistant to change. It is not that the elderly have a lowered aptitude for learning; rather the problem is that they have more difficulty "unlearning" their already well-established ways of doing things. Botwinick (1978) found that elderly subjects rigidly stuck with behavioral patterns even when it was apparent that they were no longer effective. Likewise, Ceci and Tabor (1981) found that age was associated with a less flexible style of retrieval on two types of semantic encoding tasks. Young and middle-aged adults were more flexible in retrieving items, switching modes during retrieval, and thereby having greater recall than older adults.

Just because a person is rigid in one respect, however, does not mean he or she is rigid in another. Rigidity has been shown to be more a function of intelligence than of age in some studies (Gribbin, 1976). In addition, it appears that rigidity may be determined by cultural and experiential factors rather than by age.

Cautiousness Cautiousness increases with age and can be viewed as a defense mechanism resulting from the older person's discomfort with uncertainty and/or fear of failure. Calhoun and Hutchison (1981) found that when given the opportunity to avoid making decisions on the Choice Dilemmas Questionnaire, the elderly did so, even under no risk at all concerning the outcome of the decision. This behavior may also affect the elderly person's readiness to learn. If cautiousness is due to an expectation or fear of failure, careful attention to content sequencing—starting with easier topics and working toward the harder areas—may help build confidence and increase readiness to learn in the elderly.

Intelligence Intelligence can be divided into fluid intelligence and crystallized intelligence. Fluid intelligence is characterized by the ability to adapt to new areas, develop new ideas, and perform abstract thinking (conceptualization). It is relatively uninfluenced by formal education. Crystallized intelligence, on the other hand, involves learned or information-based concepts and has a high content of memorized components. Fluid intelligence declines with age, whereas crystallized intelligence tends to maintain itself or grow (Alford, 1982; Gribbin, 1976; Moore, 1983). To compensate for the elderly's decline in fluid intelligence, the nurse can try to tie new material to an old, familiar concept by asking learners for examples from their own lives or asking them what they know about the subject before beginning the teaching. When this is not possible, the use of concrete examples may help.

Problem Solving Along with the ability to conceptualize, the ability to solve problems also decreases with age, which may explain the elderly's rigidity or reluctance to change (Knox, 1977; Lancaster, 1981; Moore, 1983). The nurse can facilitate problem solving by dividing tasks into smaller, more manageable parts; keeping the information simple and concrete; avoiding irrelevant information; and providing frequent examples.

Memory Memory can be categorized into primary memory, which provides short-term or temporary storage, and secondary memory, which provides long-term storage. Memory tasks are impaired as people age and are most severe in tasks that involve abstract, logically disconnected material. Memory impairment is minimal when the information to be remembered is meaningful and logically coherent (Alpert, 1984).

Charness (1985) explains how memory is involved with learning and how old age affects one's memory. He describes a five-stage process. First, the material must be perceived and comprehended. Next, it must be held in some form of dynamic, short-term memory system for at least a few seconds until the third stage of long-term registration has taken place. Fourth, it is held in this long-term storage until it is required for use. Finally, it must be recovered from storage when needed. Registering material in the long-term memory appears to be especially difficult for older people. As discussed previously, they need more trials and longer time free of distractions. Once registered, however, material tends to be well retained. The elderly have difficulty in the fifth stage—that of recovering material from storage. Age differences in retrieving information are frequently found with tasks that require free recall of information. These differences are greatly reduced and even disappear, however, with recognition tasks (White and Cummingham, 1982). Therefore, testing the elderly's knowledge with recognition tasks, such as multiple-choice, true/false, or matching questions, rather than recall tasks, such as fill-in-the-blanks or short answers, will facilitate retrieval.

To aid memory performance, the use of "cues" can also be helpful. Carroll and Gray (1981) discuss a memory development program involving the use of cues, practice, and motivation to improve memory function among nursing home residents. Cues included were clocks, photographs, calendars, seasonal decorations, and the like that provided reinforcement for remembering important information. Practicing activities or rehearsing information was also used to facilitate memory. As mentioned before, relaxation training has been shown to improve name/face recall by decreasing anxiety and increasing attention in the older person Yesavage, 1984; Yesavage and Jacob, 1984; and Yesavage et al, 1982). Likewise, use of imagery techniques has been shown to increase name/face recall in the elderly (Yesavage, 1983; Yesavage et al, 1983).

The most widely used clinical instrument for assessing memory is the Wechsler Memory Scale (Wechsler, 1945), which consists of a series of seven short subtests that provide a rapid, simple examination of memory function. A broad range of applications for this scale have been supported in various studies. However, Bak and Greene (1981) found that levels of education and intelligence seemed to exert a substantial influence on performance of the various subtests in normal elderly adults. Alpert (1984) suggests that memory assessment can be done with tasks that use lists, paired associates, information in a paragraph format, figure drawing, and facial identification.

Factors that should not be forgotten when assessing memory function are the elderly individual's nutritional intake and metabolic status and the medications the individual is taking. A variety of studies have shown the effects of nutritional status, anticholinergic and antidepressant medications, and metabolic disturbances on memory (Branconner et al, 1982; Goodwin et al, 1983; Potamianos and Kellett, 1982).

OUTCOMES

The goal of any teaching intervention is the accomplishment of the stated objectives. These objectives may be in the cognitive, psychomotor, or affective domain and pertain to various levels within each domain. The methods used to evaluate accomplishment of these objectives depend on the verbs used to describe them. For example, if the objective states that the learner will be able to list three benefits of patient education, then an effective method for measuring this would be to have the elderly learner list the benefits verbally or in written form. At other times, however, this relationship may not be as clear. For example, if the objective states that the elderly patient will be able to apply various diet limitations in the home environment, the most appropriate method of evaluation would be to observe the elder making diet choices in the home. Because this is usually not feasible, a less ideal but satisfactory alternative may be to observe the elder simulating a weekly home diet plan.

There are many options available for evaluating patient outcomes. For objectives in the psychomotor domain, measures such as rating scales, checklists, and anecdotal records can be used. Affective domain objectives may require questionnaires, observations, interviews, or rating scales. Finally, objectives in the cognitive domain can be evaluated with a variety of verbal or written tests, such as multiple-choice, true/false, matching, short-answer, or essay tests (Kemp, 1985). There are advantages and disadvantages to each type of measurement, some of which are listed in Table 33.3.

Emphasis has been placed on developing specific evaluation measures for each teaching session. This is not always possible and, for establishment of measurement reliability and validity, may not always be the best technique. For content that is frequently taught with a particular patient population, the development of standard tests of measurement may be beneficial. However, it is necessary for the objectives to coincide with these measures, which may precipitate restrictiveness of teaching and, therefore, be seen as a disadvantage. It is up to each nurse to evaluate the situation and decide what technique and measures are best for each learner.

CASE STUDY

Nursing Interventions

Knowledge Deficit was diagnosed for H.K. based on her verbalization of the problem (ie, statement that she does not know how to use a walker). Assessment of her readiness to learn includes the fact that she expressed a desire to learn to walk again so that she can do things for herself and return home. Because she needs to learn to use a walker in order to achieve this goal, it appears that the teaching goal is congruent with hers. She does not appear to have any of the problems listed in the first section of the readiness to learn tool (Assessment Guide 33.1). Therefore, further assessment of her readiness to

Table 33.3

Types of Evaluation Measurement

TECHNIQUE	ADVANTAGES	DISADVANTAGES
Direct Observation	Performance under real or simulated conditions can be assessed. Task is credible to patient. Measure has good content validity.	Awareness of the observer may affect performance. Training, supervising, using observers costly. Number of patients who may be studied and their locale may be restricted because of the high per-patient cost of observing.
Observational checklist	Simple, objective task to record observations. Observer error low.	Checklist may be long if a multifaceted behavior is measured.
Anchored rating scale	Simple, objective task to record observations. Observer error low. More gradations of judgment allowed than typical of an observational checklist.	Difficult to write behavioral descriptions that differ by equal amounts over an ordered scale. Descriptions may introduce several dimensions into a single rating.
Observational record	Permits routine recording of simple, repetitive behaviors.	Inferences depend on sample of time and fineness of recording unit.
Anecdotal notes	May provide unique insights, illustrations.	May be irrelevant to outcomes of interest.
Critical incidents	Characterize adaptive and maladaptive behavior. May serve as the basis for more structured measurement.	Time consuming to collect and analyze. Focus on behavioral extremes; ignore typical behavior that is not outstandingly adaptive or maladaptive.
Physiological Measures	Measure is accurate. Measure is a good indicator of health status. Measure is responsive to compliance with health care regimen.	Measure may be multiply determined; not affected by teaching outcomes alone. Measure may depend on patient's willingness and ability to perform routine self-testing and recording. Measurement may be costly to obtain and analyze. Measurement may be invasive.
Self-Report	Provides data and insights not available from other sources. Measures cognitive, affective, and performance outcomes directly.	Subject to faking, socially desirable response set. Requires skill in construction of instrument.
Oral self-report	Little reading and no writing required of patient. Contingent questions, probing, and question clarification possible.	Recording burden for interviewer. Responses may be biased by interviewer. Data collection individualized and costly.
Written self-report	Cheap; group administration of instruments is possible.	Reading and recording burdens are placed on patient. Questions are fixed; probes and clarifications cannot be introduced. Possible reduction in response rate or quality resulting from respondent burden.
Open-ended questions	Respondent free to shape reply.	Extent of reply depends on verbal fluency of respondent. Heavy recording burden for respondent or interviewer. Inconsistent dimensions of response across patients. Responses difficult to code and analyze.

Table 33.3

Types of Evaluation Measurement (*Continued*)

TECHNIQUE	ADVANTAGES	DISADVANTAGES
Closed, fixed-alternative questions	Easy recording, coding, processing of data. Limited dimensions for replies. Relative insensitivity to verbal fluency.	Construction of instrument is time consuming. Dimensions on which choices will vary must be anticipated. Choices may be forced among nonsalient options.
Single questions per topic Scales of questions per topic *Self-Monitoring*	Speed, ease of response. Stability of response Recording occurs concurrently with behavior. Access to all behaviors, covert and overt, is possible.	Instability of response. Increased length of instrument. Recording process may be reactive. Quality of record is dependent on patient's cooperation. Self-monitored data may differ from externally observed data.
Records	Noninvasive—supply data without added demands on patients. Nonreactive—relatively insensitive to external manipulation to claim desired outcomes. Relatively low cost of collection.	May not be organized to permit easy access and retrieval. Incomplete and/or inconsistent records. Indirect measures; may not be directly relevant to teaching outcomes.
Patient charts, physician records		May require health care professional to record and interpret relevant data. Privacy considerations may restrict access to records or require hierarchy of obtained consents.
Agency service records, public records and reports	Data may be collected by relatively unskilled workers	Data come from a variety of sources with varying degrees of accessibility, reporting standards, and variable conceptualization.

Source: McSweeney M: Measuring the effect of patient teaching. *Diabetes Educat* 1981; 7(3):9-15.

learn would include whether or not she was in pain, fatigued, or having any other problem described in the second section that would be a barrier to her ability to learn at the time decided on.

Because H.K. is 86 years old, it is likely that she has some of the problems listed in the third section of the readiness tool. Assessment of these will be necessary prior to planning the teaching session, and appropriate adjustments must be incorporated into the teaching/learning sessions. Assessing the rate at which H.K. processes information and responds, and using an adequate pace of instruction will be important. Her attention span may be short and her distractibility high. Therefore, teaching the task when the hallway is quiet, or using a quiet, private room, such as the cafeteria, may be required. Memory impairment and ability to grasp abstract ideas may also be involved, so keeping the instruction simple and concrete, avoiding irrelevant information, and repeatedly stressing important points are also good rules to follow when teaching H.K. Because of the risks involved in learning this task, H.K. may display a great deal of cautiousness. Sequencing the instruction in an organized manner, starting with the easier areas and slowly working toward the more complex ones, may decrease H.K.'s fears and increase her confidence to learn the needed skill.

The next step in the planning process includes the setting of learning objectives. (Deciding on the task for H.K. to learn has already been done—that is, learning to walk with a walker.) This should be done *with* H.K. Learning to use a walker falls under the psychomotor domain and includes perceptual abilities, physical abilities, and skilled movements (Harrow, 1972). Perceptual abilities involve kinesthetic awareness such as a change in body balance, tactile discrimination, and coordination of eye-hand and eye-foot movements. Physical abilities include endurance, strength, and flexibility, and skilled movements are the ability to perform complex actions efficiently. Therefore, possible objectives for H.K. may be that, at the end of the teaching/learning process, she will be able to:

1. Balance with use of the walker
2. Demonstrate appropriate use of the walker
3. Use the walker to perform certain tasks independently, such as going to the bathroom

Resources for teaching H.K. will include a properly fitting walker and any available visual aids, such as demonstrations, pictures, and audiovisual materials, that show correct use of a walker. Written aids may also be used. However, because these would probably describe the process involved, they may be less effective for someone who has difficulty grasping abstract ideas.

Once adjustments have been made to provide a conducive environment and include the factors discussed in section three of the readiness tool, implementation of the teaching/learning session can begin. Individualized, instructor-directed teaching is most appropriate for teaching this type of task to H.K., and multiple sessions may be necessary to achieve the stated objectives. However, at the beginning of each teaching session, it is important to determine H.K.'s readiness to learn (the first and second sections of the tool) before proceeding. In addition, consistently adhering to the adjustments necessary for facilitation of H.K.'s learning ability during each session is important.

Finally, evaluating H.K.'s learning is critical to ensure that she can be left alone to perform certain tasks with the walker. This can easily be done by observing H.K. perform the actions stated in the objectives. Using a rating scale or checklist may be helpful, and this evaluation can be done throughout the teaching/learning process rather than solely at the end. Also, having H.K. evaluate the teaching/learning intervention through verbal questions or interviews along the way can be helpful for changing the sessions to be more effective and beneficial to her. This information will also provide feedback for future patient education interventions.

SUMMARY

This chapter has focused on assessment and diagnosis of Knowledge Deficit and on the process involved in planning, implementing, and evaluating the nursing intervention of patient education. Emphasis has been placed on the importance of increasing the elderly person's quality of life through identification of self-care knowledge needs and on individualization of instruction so that it is meaningful and specific to the older person's lifestyle. Teaching the elderly requires that the nurse recognize special learning needs and take appropriate actions to facilitate learning ability. Involving them in identification of their learning needs, objectives of instruction, and learning formats, as well as obtaining frequent feedback to evaluate their comprehension and make appropriate adjustments, can have a substantial impact on the elderly's learning capacity. Keeping the message simple and the format uncomplicated, allowing time for assimilation, relating material to what is already known, and increasing their sensory capacities can go a long way in aiding elderly learners. Finally, proper evaluation of patient outcomes is necessary to determine whether or not the patient actually learned the information given.

Knowledge deficits are common problems in the clinical setting. They can be effectively treated if proper interventions are performed. Patient education is a commonly used therapy and, with proper planning, implementation, and evaluation, can be a powerful treatment in resolving knowledge deficit problems.

ASSESSMENT GUIDE 33.1

Assessment of Readiness to Learn

If the answer to any to these is "yes," the patient is not ready to learn until it is resolved:

age < 3 years? _____

+ present knowledge adequate? _____

+ critical illness? _____

+ disorientation/confusion? _____

+ altered perception (due to medications, anesthesia, physical condition, etc)? _____

+ intense emotion (anxiety/fear, depression, anger, grief, etc)? _____
+ first stages of adaptation to crisis:

        shock/disbelief? _____

        defensive retreat/denial? _____

If the answer to any of these is "yes," it will have to be dealt with before the patient will be ready to learn and effective teaching can take place:

+ pain? _____

+ fatigue/lethargy? _____

+ physiologic needs (hunger, thirst, warmth, oxygen, etc)? _____

+ safety needs (survival, control, familiarity, etc)? _____

+ love/belongingness needs (loss or absence of loved ones)? _____

+ sensory overload/underload? _____

low or threatened self-concept? _____

bad past experience with health care? _____
inadequate:

        perception of severity of illness? _____

        perception of susceptibility to complications? _____

        perception of ability to control progression or cure condition? _____

perception of actions as too risky to lifestyle? _____

incompatible lifestyle? _____

conflicting goals? _____

lack of nurse–patient rapport? _____

lack of nurse credibility? _____

If the answer to any of these is "yes," the teaching will have to be adjusted accordingly to be effective:

age 3–14? _____

sensory impairment? _____

longer time to process information and respond? _____

short attention span/distractibility? _____

rigidity? _____

cautiousness? _____

(Continues)

ASSESSMENT GUIDE 33.1

Assessment of Readiness to Learn (Continued)

inability to grasp abstract ideas/conceptualize? _____

inability to solve problems? _____

memory impairment? _____

incongruent biorhythms? _____

unfamiliar language? _____

lack of past experience/education? _____

external locus of control? _____

poor financial status? _____

conflicting values/beliefs? _____

References

Alford DM: Tips for teaching older adults. *Nurs Life* (Sept/Oct) 1982; 60–64.

Alpert M: Assessment of cognitive function in the elderly. *Psychosomatics* 1984; 25(4):310–317.

American Hospital Association: *A Patient's Bill of Rights.* The Association, 1975.

American Nurses' Association: *The Professional Nurse and Health Education.* The Association, 1975.

Andrews DH, Ludwika AG: A comparative analysis of models of instructional design. *J Instruct Devel* 1980; 3:2–16.

Ascoine FJ, Shimp LA: The effectiveness of four education strategies in the elderly. *Drug Intell Clin Pharm* 1984; 18:926–931.

Bak JS, Greene RL: A review of the performance of aged adults on various Weschler Memory Scale subtests. *J Clin Psychol* 1981; 37(1):186–188.

Baldini J: Knowledge about hypertension in affected elderly persons. *J Gerontol Nurs* 1981; 7(9):542–551.

Botwinick J: *Aging and Behavior: A Comprehensive Integration of Research Findings,* 2d ed. Springer, 1978.

Branconner RJ et al: Amitriptyline selectively disrupts verbal recall from secondary memory of the normal aged. *Neurobiol Aging* 1982; 3:55–59.

Briggs L: *Instructional Design: Principles and Applications.* Educational Technology Publications, 1977.

Calhoun RE, Hutchison SL: Decision-making in old age: Cautiousness and rigidity. *Intnat J Aging Human Devel* 1981; 13(1):89–97.

Carpenito LJ: *Nursing Diagnosis: Application to Clinical Practice.* Lippincott, 1983.

Carpenito LJ: *Handbook of Nursing Diagnosis.* Lippincott, 1984.

Carroll K, Gray K: Memory development: An approach to the mentally impaired elderly in the long-term care setting. *Intnat J Aging Human Devel* 1981; 13(1):15–35.

Carroll-Johnson R (editor): *Classification of Nursing Diagnoses: Proceedings of the Eighth Conference.* Lippincott, 1989.

Casey E, O'Connell JK, Price JH: Perceptions of educational needs for patients after myocardial infarction. *Patient Educ Counsel* 1984; 6(2):77–82.

Ceci SJ, Tabor L: Flexibility and memory: Are the elderly really less flexible? *Experiment Aging Res* 1981; 7(2):147–158.

Charness N (editor): *Aging and Human Performance.* Wiley, 1985.

Check JF, Wurzbach ME: How elders view learning. *Geriatr Nurs* (Jan/Feb) 1984; 37–39.

Corkadel L, McGlashan R: A practical approach to patient teaching. *J Contin Educ Nurs* 1983; 14(1):9–15.

Dall CE, Gresham L: Promoting effective drug-taking behavior in the elderly. *Nurs Clin North Am* 1982; 17(2):283–291.

Donahue E et al: A drug education program for the well elderly. *Geriatr Nurs* (Mar/Apr) 1981; 140–142.

Dumas RG, Leonard RC: The effect of nursing on the incidence of postoperative vomiting. *Nurs Res* 1963; 12(1):12–15.

Eliopoulos C: A self care model for gerontological nursing. *Geriatr Nurs* (Nov/Dec) 1984; 366–369.

Fleming CC, Lopez MA: The effects of perceived control on the paired-associate learning of elderly persons. *Experiment Aging Res* 1981; 7(1):71–77.

Goodwin JS, Goodwin JM, Garry PJ: Association between nutritional status and cognitive functioning in a healthy elderly population. *JAMA* 1983; 249(21):2917–2921.

Gordon M: *Manual of Nursing Diagnosis.* McGraw-Hill, 1982.

Green LW, Lewis FM, Levine DM: Balancing statistical data and clinician judgments in the diagnosis of patient educational needs. *J Commun Health* 1980; 6(2):79–91.

Gribbin K: Cognitive processes in aging. In: *Nursing and the Aged.* Burnside IM (editor). McGraw-Hill, 1976.

Grunlund NE: *Stating Objectives for Classroom Instruction,* 2d ed. Macmillan, 1978.

Harrow AJ: *A Taxonomy of the Psychomotor Domain.* David McKay, 1972.

Healy KM: Does preopertive instruction make a difference? *Am J Nurs* 1968; 68(1):62–67.

Henderson V: *Harmer and Henderson's Textbook of the Principles and Practices of Nursing*, 5th ed. Macmillan, 1955.

Huckabay LMD: A strategy for patient teaching. *Nurs Admin Q* 1980; 4(2):47–54.

Hughston GA, Merriam SB: Reminiscence: A nonformal technique for improving cognitive functioning in the aged. *Intnat J Aging Human Devel* 1982; 15(2):139–149.

Hurley ME (editor): *Classification of Nursing Diagnoses: Proceedings of the Sixth Conference*. Mosby, 1986.

Kausler DH, Hakami MK: Frequency judgements by young and elderly adults for relevant stimuli with simultaneously present irrelevant stimuli. *J Gerontol* 1982; 37(4):438–442.

Kemp JE: *The Instructional Design Process*. Harper and Row, 1985.

Kern LS, Gawlinski A: Stage-managing coronary artery disease. *Nurs 83* (Apr) 1983; 13(4):34–40.

Kim KK, Grier MR: Pacing effects of medication instruction for the elderly. *J Gerontol Nurs* 1981; 7(8):464–468.

Kim MJ, Moritz DA (editors): *Classification of Nursing Diagnoses: Proceedings of the Third and Fourth National Conferences*. McGraw-Hill, 1982.

Kim MJ, McFarland GK, McLane AM (editors): *Pocket Guide to Nursing Diagnoses*. Mosby, 1984.

King I, Tarsitano B: The effect of structured and unstructured pre-operative teaching: A replication. *Nurs Res* 1982; 31(6):324–329.

Knox AB: *Adult Development and Learning*. Jossey-Bass, 1977.

Kohut S, Kohut JJ, Fleishman JJ: *Reality Orientation for the Elderly*, 2d ed. Medical Economics Books, 1983.

Lancaster J: Maximizing psychological adaptation in an aging population. *Aging* 1981; 31–43.

Linde BJ, Janz NM: Effect of a teaching program on knowledge and compliance of cardiac patients. *Nurs Res* 1979; 28(5):282–286.

Lindeman CA: Nursing intervention with the presurgical patient. *Nurs Res* 1972; 21(3):196–208.

Lindeman CA: Influencing recovery through preoperative teaching. *Heart Lung* 1973; 2(4):515–521.

Lindeman CA, Van Aernam B: Nursing intervention with the presurgical patient—the effects of structured and unstructured preoperative teaching. *Nurs Res* 1971; 20(4):319–332.

Lorig KL, Laurin J, Holman HR: Arthritis self-management: A study of the effectiveness of patient education for the elderly. *Gerontologist* 1984; 24(5):455–457.

Mazzuca SA: Does patient education in chronic disease have therapeutic value? *J Chron Dis* 1982; 35:521–529.

McKenzie SC: *Aging and Old Age*. Scott, Foresman, 1980.

McLane A (editor): *Classification of Nursing Diagnosis: Proceedings of the Seventh Conference*. Mosby, 1987.

McSweeney M: Measuring the effect of patient teaching. *Diabetes Educator* 1981; 7(3):9–15.

Mezzanote EJ: Group instruction in preparation for surgery. *Am J Nurs* 1970; 70:89–91.

Milazzo V: A study of the difference in health knowledge gained through formal and informal teaching. *Heart Lung* 1980; 9(6):1079–1082.

Moore SR: Cognitive variants in the elderly: An integral part of medication counseling. *Drug Intell Clin Pharm* 1983; 17:840–842.

Morisky DE et al: Health education program effects on the management of hypertension in the elderly. *Arch Intern Med* 1982; 142:1835–1838.

Mumford E, Schlesinger HJ, Glass GV: The effects of psychological intervention on recovery from surgery and heart attacks: An analysis of the literature. *Am J Public Health* 1982; 72(2):141–151.

Nelson EC et al: Medical self-care education for elders: A controlled trial to evaluate impact. *Am J Public Health* 1984; 74(12):1357–1362.

Orem DE: *Nursing: Concepts of Practice*, 3d ed. McGraw-Hill, 1985.

Peplau HE: *Interpersonal Relations in Nursing*. Putnam, 1952.

Pokorny BE: Validating a diagnostic label: Knowledge deficits. *Nurs Clin North Am* 1985; 20(4): 641–655.

Potamianos G, Kellett JM: Anti-cholinergic drugs and memory: The effects of Benzhexol on memory in a group of geriatric patients. *British J Psychiatry* 1982; 140:470–472.

Powers MJ, Wooldridge PJ: Factors influencing knowledge, attitudes, and compliance of hypertensive patients. *Res Nurs Health* 1982; 5:171–182.

Rabbitt PMA: An age decrement in the ability to ignore irrelevant information. *J Gerontol* 1965; 20:233–238.

Rakel BA: *Development of a New Nursing Diagnosis: Alteration in Learning Ability*. (Unpublished thesis.) University of Iowa, Iowa City, IA, 1988.

Reading AE: The short term effects of psychological preparation for surgery. *Soc Sci Med* 1979; 13A:641–654.

Redman BK: *The Process of Patient Education*, 5th ed. Mosby, 1984.

Redman BK, Thomas SA: Patient teaching. In: *Nursing Interventions: Treatments for Nursing Diagnoses*. Bulechek GM, McCloskey JC (editors). Saunders, 1985.

Reigeluth CM: *Instructional-Design Theories and Models: An Overview of Their Current Status*. Lawrence Erlbaum Associates, 1983.

Resler MM: Teaching strategies that promote adherence. *Nurs Clin North Am* 1983; 18(4):799–811.

Rossi LP, Haines VM: Nursing diagnoses related to acute myocardial infarction. *Cardiovasc Nurs* 1979; 15(3):11–15.

Saxon SV, Etten MJ: *Psychosocial Rehabilitative Programs for Older Adults*. Charles C. Thomas, 1984.

Schmitt JF: The effects of time compression and time expansion on passage comprehension by elderly listeners. *J Speech Hear Res* 1983; 26:373–377.

Schmitt JF, McCroskey RL: Sentence comprehension in elderly listeners: The factor of rate. *J Gerontol* 1981; 36(4):441–445.

Shimko C: The effect of preoperative instruction on state anxiety. *J Neurosurg Nurs* 1981; 13(6):318–322.

Smith CE: Teaching models: A conceptual analysis for nursing. *J Contin Educ Nurs* 1982; 13(4):5–9.

Speers MA, Turk DC: Diabetes self-care: Knowledge, beliefs, motivation, and action. *Patient Counsel Health Educ* 1982; 3(4):144–149.

Stanton MP: Teaching patients: Some basic lessons for nurse educators. *Nurs Manage* 1985; 16(10):59–62.

Swain MA, Steckel SB: Influencing adherence among hypertensives. *Res Nurs Health* 1981; 4:213–222.

Swift AE: Enhancing intellectual performance in older people. *Home Healthcare Nurse* (May/June) 1984; 23–26.

Taft LB: Self-esteem in later life: A nursing perspective. *ANS* 1985; 8(1):77–84.

Wechsler D: A standardized memory scale for clinical use. *J Psychol* 1945; 19:87–95.

Weiler MC: Postoperative patients evaluate preoperative instruction. *Am J Nurs* 1968; 68(7):1465–1467.

White N, Cummingham WR: What is the evidence for retrieval problems in the elderly? *Experiment Aging Res* 1982; 8(3):169–171.

Yesavage JA: Imagery pretraining and memory training in the elderly. *Gerontology* 1983; 29:271–275.

Yesavage JA: Relaxation and memory training in 39 elderly patients. *Am J Psychiatry* 1984; 141(6):778–781.

Yesavage JA, Jacob R: Effects of relaxation and mnemonics on memory, attention, and anxiety in the elderly. *Experiment Aging Res* 1984; 10(4):211–214.

Yesavage JA, Rose TL, Bower GH: Interactive imagery and affective judgements improve face-name learning in the elderly. *J Gerontol* 1983; 38(2):197–203.

Yesavage JA, Rose TL, Spiegel D: Relaxation training and memory improvement in elderly normals: Correlation of anxiety ratings and recall improvement. *Experiment Aging Res* 1982; 8(4):195–198.

VII

Self-Perception–
Self-Concept Pattern

KATHLEEN BUCKWALTER, PhD, RN, FAAN
MERIDEAN MAAS, PhD, RN, FAAN

Overview

DEPRESSION IS THE LEADING PSYCHIATRIC DISORder among the elderly. In Chapter 35, Reactive Depression, Love and Buckwalter provide a theoretical overview of depression in later life and integrate these psychiatric perspectives with theories of aging. They advocate a multifaceted assessment approach, using physiologic, cognitive, psychologic, social, and economic data. Behavioral, cognitive, social support, and group interventions are highlighted, as well as discussions of somatic therapies (eg, psychopharmacologic and electroconvulsant), with which the nurse must be knowledgeable.

In Chapter 36, Body Image Disturbance, Glick and Eastman discuss disruptions in the way elderly persons perceive or experience their body. These authors view body image as a developmental process, and the chapter differentiates various aspects of that process, including body schema, body self, body fantasy, and body concept. Assessment is presented in terms of history-taking approaches useful with the elderly, and several standardized body image assessment tools are discussed. The authors also discuss four interventions for disturbances in body image with the elderly that have been tested in the literature: psychotherapy, sensory stimula-

tion, exercise and movement therapy, and patient education.

Because of the accoutrements of aging, elderly persons are vulnerable to losses of resources and thus loss of power and control. In Chapter 37, O'Heath examines the problem of Powerlessness in the elderly, particularly emphasizing the effects of institutionalization. The relationship of powerlessness, social learning theory, and locus of control is used as a framework for understanding health behaviors of the elderly as well as behaviors associated with lowered self-esteem, hopelessness, and social isolation. Nurse advocacy to maintain the elderly persons' involvement in decisions and to keep them informed so that they remain in control of their own lives is the principal nursing intervention strategy that is urged.

Chapter 38, Fear, by Cesarone and Chapter 39, Anxiety, by Vogel complement and yet are distinguished from each other. Many fears can assault the dependent elder, and the most common ones, such as fear of pain and suffering, abandonment, loneliness, and meaninglessness, are explicated in Chapter 38. The goals of nursing interventions are to reduce or extinguish the fear and to increase coping abilities. Strategies nurses can use to meet these goals, such as patient education, are set forth.

As discussed by Vogel, signs of anxiety are prevalent among elderly persons and may be manifested in somatic and cognitive symptoms. In Chapter 39, Vogel identifies different types of anxiety (eg, depletion, trait, state, death) and recommends networking for the community-based elderly and providing a supportive atmosphere to counteract anxiety in the institutionalized elder. She argues that nursing interventions must be broad based and multifaceted to deal most effectively with this complex diagnosis.

In Chapter 40, Whall and Parent focus on Self-Esteem Disturbance. Coming from the theoretical perspective of Roy, the authors analyze the concept of self-esteem, discuss it in terms of aging and institutionalization of the elderly, develop the diagnosis Self-Esteem Disturbance, and review assessment of the critical data from which the diagnoses and probable etiologies can be inferred. Nursing interventions that restore, maintain, or promote self-esteem are described along with evaluation of desired outcomes.

34

Normal Changes With Aging

Donna Bunten, MA, RN
Mary A. Hardy, PhD, RN, C

Definition:

This unit describes the self-concept pattern and perceptions of self (eg, body comfort, body image, feeling state).

As Americans age, their quality of life is often affected by decreased vitality, increased vulnerability for physiologic losses, and multiple psychosocial losses. Rapidly advancing technology has enabled us to expect to continue our quality of life while aging. Holistic health care can maintain quality of life, manage the challenges of aging, and as a result, preserve self-esteem (Taft, 1985).

Self-esteem is a part of the much larger concept of self. The self, or individuals' thoughts and emotions about themselves, results from experiences with other people, the ways others act toward them, and their impression of how others view them. One's perception of self normally maintains a certain degree of stability and consistency. But as people grow older their interpersonal networks change, the lifelong series of entrances and exits in social groups continues, and the importance of associations may change. Researchers have suggested that positive feelings about self increase until middle age, when they stabilize or gradually begin to become negative (Kogan and Wallach, 1961; Lowenthal and Chiriboga, 1972).

When considering what factors associated with advancing age may present a potential for lowered self-esteem, the central theme is the cumulative losses associated with growing old. Among these losses are physical health, mental health, functional abilities, meaningful personal relationships, and lifelong roles. Our society remains heavily youth oriented and still embraces ageism, a form of prejudice based on chronologic age (Butler, 1975). The elderly are frequently stereotyped as being mentally, physically, and socially inept as well as being dependent and nonproductive members of society. The obvious impact of society's devaluing of older adults is the potential for negative perceptions of self and self-concept on the part of those elderly who internalize stereotypes.

Social gerontologists have analyzed the relationship of life satisfaction and feelings of self-esteem associated with social activity and inactivity. Currently, the continuity or developmental theories are supported by many who work with and know the elderly. According to the continuity theory (see Table 2, Introductory Chapter) the continuation of a previously established pattern of behavior is perhaps one of the most critical factors in the social and emotional well-being of the aging adult. As people age they try to maintain continuity of preferences, habits, and commitments. If they have been happiest when involved in many social interactions or happiest when retiring and inactive, these patterns will direct their expectations, sense of satisfaction, and self-esteem as they age (Steffl, 1984). Within this theoretical perspective, it is more appropriate to compare interaction levels of the elderly to levels at other stages of their lives. There is no identified optimum level of interaction for any specific age group.

Loss of support, diminished social interaction, and a sense of helplessness and hopelessness are only some of the manifestations of the losses in the aging population. As the elderly become more dependent on others because of emotional and physical losses, many times their usual decision-making roles are either abandoned or taken away by those on whom the elderly person has become dependent. This loss of control over many aspects of one's environment has negative effects on self-esteem, which is particularly evident in the lives of institutionalized elderly. Collaborative decision making between clients and professionals may diminish this loss of control and increase self-esteem. The importance of control in the lives of the elderly is evident in the findings of Langer and Rodin (1976) and Stanwyck (1983). They found that elderly persons provided with opportunities to make decisions were more self-directed, more alert, and more involved with their environment, and had a higher sense of well-being.

References

Butler RM: *Why Survive? Being Old in America.* Harper and Row, 1975.

Kogan N, Wallach M: Age changes in values and attitudes. *J Gerontol* 1961; 16:272–280.

Langer E, Rodin J: The effects of choice and enhanced personal responsibility for the aged: A field experiment in an institutional setting. *J Personal Soc Psychol* 1976; 34:191–198.

Lowenthal M, Chiriboga D: Transitions to the empty nest: Crisis, challenge or relief. *Arch Gen Psychiatry* 1972; 26(1):8–14.

Stanwyck D: Self-esteem through the lifespan. *Fam Community Health* 1983; 6:11.

Steffl BM: Theories of aging: Biological, psychological, and sociological. In: *Handbook of Gerontological Nursing.* Steffl BM (editor). Van Nos Reinhold, 1984.

Taft LB: Self-esteem in later life: A nursing perspective. *ANS* 1985; 8(1):77–84.

35

Reactive Depression

Colleen C. Love, MA, RN, C
Kathleen C. Buckwalter,
PhD, RN, FAAN

Here I am, an old man in a dry month,
Being read to by a boy, waiting for rain.

T.S. Eliot (Harcourt Press, 1971)

This chapter provides the reader with an overview of the theory and research base for the diagnostic concept Reactive Depression. It includes a guide to assessment describing the constellation of behaviors and feelings (signs and symptoms) that are manifested in a depressed elder. A description of a treatment plan with specific interventions and evaluation strategies is included and illustrated with a case study.

SIGNIFICANCE FOR THE ELDERLY

It is important to note that depression is the mot prevalent and most treatable mental disorder of later life. Unfortunately, depression in the elderly is often misdiagnosed or left untreated because of ageist attitudes, social isolation, denial, and ignorance of the normal aging process. Depression robs the elderly of late-life satisfaction, inhibits fulfillment of the developmental tasks of senescence, and financially and emotionally drains the individual, the family, and the larger social system. The life expectancy of a depressed elder may be substantially decreased because symptoms may precipitate or aggravate physical deterioration. Suicide rates among the elderly are more than three times the rates seen in the general population. It has been estimated that between 50% and 80% of elders in long-term care facilities have diagnosable psychiatric disorders with depression chief among them (Stotsky, 1967; Whanger and Lewis, 1975). Traditional institutional care adds additional risk factors, in that patients are often expected to adopt the sick role and remain passive. Institutionalization exposes the elderly to life stressors that are conducive to development of depressive illness.

Health care professionals, lay persons, and elders themselves often equate growing old with growing sad, disengaged, and apathetic. It is *not* normal to be old and sad! Symptoms of depression are often indistinguishable from the "expected" behaviors of growing old and therefore require persistent, sensitive, and skilled observation and assessment to uncover masked depressive states that may mimic, precede, or exist concomitantly with other organic pathologies. Depression in the elderly poses a significant personal and public health problem that requires skilled attention and aggressive intervention. Nurses in a variety of settings (eg, long-term care, community health, psychiatric facilities) are in a critical position to identify and treat depressive conditions among the elderly. The nurse who understands the complex interrelationships among mental health, physical health, and the consequences of drugs commonly used to treat illness in the elderly is in a unique position to make a differential diagnosis of reactive depression and assist elderly clients in improving their affective state (mood). Nurses can employ a variety of interpersonal, as well as group, strategies to help alleviate depression. They also assume an important function in monitoring psychotropic and other medications that may precipitate adverse side effects or cause secondary depression.

DEPRESSION—THEORETICAL OVERVIEW

The diagnosis Depression has not yet been accepted by the North American Nursing Diagnosis Association (NANDA) (Carroll-Johnson, 1989). Gordon's (1982;166) definition of the concept Reactive Depression is provided in Table 35.1.

The definition and indicators for the concept of Reactive Depression suggest that there is an isolated subsyndrome of depression that is primarily a reaction to a real or perceived threat. In accordance with the title and purpose of this chapter, the interventions discussed focus mainly on the treatment of a psychologic response to a stressor of external origin. However, the authors wish to convey that depression, particularly in the elderly, is often characterized by a combination of etiologic factors including biologic, psychosocial, interactional, and developmental concomitants. All of these related factors must be considered when a clinician observes the signs and symptoms of a depressive state. The fact that there is an

observable or articulated stressor (eg, death of a loved one, relocation, loss of physical capacity) preceding behavioral and affective changes consistent with a depressive illness does not preclude the possibility that there are other endogenous or internal contributing factors (eg, biochemical imbalances, drug toxicities, nutritional deficiencies, carcinoma).

Many theories of the etiology of depression exist; however, because of space limitations this chapter will focus only on the integrated theory set forth by Chaisson-Stewart (1985).

Integrated Theory of Depression

The integrated theory of depression posited by Chaisson-Stewart (1985) expands the concept of Reactive Depression and combines the best of four previous psychiatric models: binary view (Kraeplin, 1921); psychotic/neurotic severity model; psychoanalytic interpretations (Freud, 1904; Muslin, 1984); and stress-related models. This theory incorporates the unitary model set forth by Meyer (1905) and others with Selye's (1978) stress theory to arrive at a severity continuum of stress-induced depressive illness that interrelates psychologic and biologic factors throughout. This integrated theory fits well with the clinical presentations observed in practice and allows for a more holistic, multidimensional treatment approach, which is essential when working with the elderly.

Unitary Model The unitary model, elaborated by Meyer (1905), Mapother (1926), Lewis (1934), Hill (1968), and Kendel (1968), described depression on a continuum of maladaptive psychobiologic responses to the stressors of

---

Table 35.1

Depression, Reactive (Situational)

Definition: Acute decrease in self-esteem or worth related to a threat to self-competency

Defining Characteristics

    Expression of hopelessness, despair
    Inability to concentrate, making reading, writing, conversation difficult
    Change, usually decrease in physical activities, eating, sleeping (early morning awakening), sexual activity
    Continual questioning of self-worth (self-esteem)
    Feeling of failure (real or imagined)
    Withdrawal from others to avoid possible rejection, real or imagined. Threats or attempts to commit suicide
    Suspicion or sensitivity to words and actions of others related to general lack of trust in others
    Misdirected anger (toward self)
    General irritability
    Guilt feelings
    Extreme dependency on others with related feelings of helplessness and anger

Etiology: Perceived powerlessness

Source: Gordon M: *Manual of Nursing Diagnosis.* McGraw-Hill, 1982.

life change. This model incorporates the notion that biologic responses come into play, *along with* a psychologic response in varying intensities. Applying Selye's (1978) general adaptation model to the unitary view accentuates the importance of perception in the genesis of depression (Table 35.2). Thus, the physiologic response to stress (automatic and basically the same for all persons) is mediated by the psychologic perception of the stress (which may differ dramatically from person to person). For example, relocation to a nursing facility for one individual may be viewed as a positive life change, providing regular nutritious meals, companionship, and nursing care. For another person, moving to an institutional setting may be perceived as a significant threat to his or her independence, sense of control and self-concept, and this move may trigger a depressive illness. Chaisson-Stewart (1985;57) has used the word *endogenous* as the descriptor for the more severe form of depression and the word *reactive* to describe the milder form of the syndrome. Thus, the diagnostic concept of Reactive Depression, for purposes of this chapter, acknowledges the influence of both somatic and psychosocial factors (particularly those unique to aging), which must be considered when treating depression following a psychologic insult to an elderly person.

THEORIES OF AGING RELATED TO DEPRESSION

There are many variables that have an impact on mental health in late life: cultural and ethnic factors, genetic makeup and heritage, physiologic history, the environment, the family system, relationships, losses, personality composition, and economics. Late-life research efforts and theory development have focused primarily on biologic aging, personality and developmental aspects, and social and interactional factors. Many of these theories contribute to the distinction between normality and pathology regarding depression in the elderly, and some can be translated into therapeutic interventions. For example, interventions such as life review and reminiscence flow logically from Erikson's developmental model (1950), which suggests that life's eighth stage of ego integrity requires meaningful integration of past experiences.

ASSESSMENT

The variety of theories on depression and aging illustrate the need for an individualized, multifactorial, comprehensive assessment. The interview is the initial step in the assessment of an elderly client and the most important procedure in differentiating depression from other psychiatric disorders (Lazarus et al, 1985). Interviewing the elderly requires skill and heightened sensitivity and typically takes more time than with other age groups. The assessment tools included in this chapter may be used in conjunction with the face-to-face interview.

Burnside (1980) suggests that the interviewer attempt to make the interview pleasant for the elderly patient, conveying a sense of empathy, respect, and caring. The interviewer should position herself or himself close to the patient, use touch when appropriate to diminish the patient's anxiety, and be clear in stating the purpose of the interview and the length of time it will take. A skilled diagnostician attends to verbal, nonverbal, and environmental cues, as well as cognitive and behavioral aspects of the client (Kneisl and Wilson, 1984). During the course of the interview, it may become necessary to reiterate the purpose and time frame, as the elderly person may forget or tend to wander mentally and reminisce.

Sensory loss, confusion, communication disorders, cultural influences, shame, and fear of stigmatization may inhibit expression of feelings by elderly persons. Frequently, depressed elders are unaware of their apathetic

Table 35.2

Integrated Model of Depression

EXTERNAL	STRESSOR	INTERNAL
Psychosocial		Physiologic
Death of loved one		Surgery
Relocation		Drug toxicity
Loss of status	BIOLOGIC STRUCTURES	OBS, cancer,
Loss of independence		Organic and neurologic factors
	PERCEPTION	
Psychologic response		Biologic response
	DEPRESSION	
Reactive		Endogenous
	(Severity)	

and withdrawn behavior or assume it is part of getting old. Enlisting interpretations from family and staff members may fill in aspects of the clinical picture. When the client's history is lacking or withheld, the clinician must be persistent and perceptive in uncovering clues to validate a masked depressive state. The interview should take into account:

- Physiologic status, including health, nutritional status, medication, psychiatric, family health history; thorough physical and neurologic exam
- Cognitive functioning mental status exam, including changes in cognition over time, educational level
- Psychologic strengths and symptomatology, coping skills, spirituality, sexuality, suicidal ideation, past attempts at suicide
- Quality and quantity of social support, financial status, and potential for elder abuse

DEFINING CHARACTERISTICS OF DEPRESSION

Despite variations in terminology and etiology, overall the signs and symptoms of depressive disorders remain fairly consistent throughout the life span. Individuals who are depressed will ordinarily look sad, tired, and forlorn. They will usually move very slowly (psychomotor retardation), although in some cases they will appear very anxious and restless (agitation). Often, attention to grooming, hygiene, and self-presentation has been neglected because of a lack of motivation. Depressed individuals are frequently tearful and sometimes are hostile, irritable, and aggressive. The feelings most often reported by depressed individuals include guilt; hopelessness; disinterest in life; isolation; loneliness; lack of pleasure; decreased energy, libido, and appetite; anxiety; emptiness, feelings of failure; inability to concentrate; self-devaluation and reproach; recurrent thoughts of death; and suicidal rumination. Signs and symptoms can include anorexia and weight loss or overeating and weight gain, sleep pattern disturbances (insomnia or hypersomnia), brooding about the past, pessimism, social withdrawal, suicidal ideation or attempt, constipation, tachycardia, somatization, confusion, disorientation, delusions, hallucinations, and paranoia. A markedly depressed elder may be mute and unresponsive to the assessment interview.

DSM IIIR Criteria

The *Diagnostic and Statistical Manual III*, Revised (DSM IIIR), published by the American Psychiatric Association (1987), provides a revised version of the standardized, operationalized criteria for psychiatric illnesses found in the DSM III, 1980. This revised edition is used by most psychiatrists and mental health professionals. Despite the wide application and promising results from extensive validity and reliability measures, clinicians have criticized the third edition's precision in identifying psychiatric phenomena, particularly in the elderly. This criticism stems partly from the necessary limits imposed on a statistical manual (which must group together a wide range of disorders into a limited number of categories) as opposed to a nosologic system, which is expansive and includes all approved terms describing a wide range of identified pathologic conditions. Zung (1980) and Freeman et al (1982) contain more complete discussions of the limitations and advantages of the DSM IIIR.

Depression is included in three main sections in the DSM IIIR (1987) under (1) Affective Disorders; (2) Organic Mental Syndromes and Disorders; and (3) Adjustment Disorders. The diagnostic criteria for Major Depressive Episode as listed in the DSM IIIR is provided in Table 35.3.

With regard to developmentally linked disorders, the DSM IIIR includes only a brief entry, "Phase of Life Problem or Other Life Circumstance Problem," which acknowledges that there are life changes *apparently not due to a mental disorder* that may become a focus for treatment. The DSM IIIR authors have also provided a definition of grief termed "Uncomplicated Bereavement," which may become dysfunctional if it increases in severity or continues for excessive periods after the loss. The DSM IIIR criteria are used to diagnose depression throughout the life span, and the criteria listed in Table 35.3 are applied to the elderly as well.

Unique Characteristics of Depression in the Elderly

There are characteristics of depression specific to the elderly that are not explicitly identified in the DSM IIIR. It is crucial for clinicians to be aware that depressive illness in the elderly, which is amenable to treatment, may mimic other organically based irreversible disorders. Many elderly patients who are thought to be demented may actually have a depressive disorder with misleading cognitive symptoms.

The term *pseudodementia* refers to the depression associated with and often misinterpreted as dementia. Generally, depressive illness manifests itself suddenly, whereas the organic brain syndromes appear more slowly, or in the case of multi-infarct dementia, in a graduated stepwise fashion (Lazarus et al, 1985). Signs of confabulation suggest there may be organicity such as that seen in Alzheimer's disease. Demented patients often become angry and attempt to cover up the cognitive impairment when their memory is tested, whereas depressed elders may not answer questions or simply acknowledge that they don't remember (see Table 35.4).

Table 35.3

Major Depressive Episode

Note: A "major depressive syndrome" is defined as criterion A below.

A. At least five of the following symptoms have been present during the same two week period; at least one of the symptoms was either (1) depressed mood, or (2) loss of interest or pleasure. (Do not include symptoms that are clearly due to a physical condition, mood-incongruent delusions or hallucinations, incoherence, or marked loosening of associations.)
   (1) depressed mood most of the day, nearly every day (either by subjective account, eg, feels "down" or "low," or is observed by others to look sad or depressed)
   (2) loss of interest or pleasure in all or almost all activities nearly every day (either by subjective account or is observed by others to be apathetic)
   (3) significant weight loss or weight gain when not dieting or binge-eating (eg, more than 5% of body weight in a month), or decrease or increase in appetite nearly every day (in children, consider failure to make expected weight gains)
   (4) insomnia or hypersomnia nearly every day
   (5) psychomotor agitation or retardation nearly every day (observable by others, not merely subjective feelings of restlessness or being slowed down) (in children under six, hypoactivity)
   (6) fatigue or loss of energy nearly every day
   (7) feelings of worthlessness or excessive or inappropriate guilt (which may be delusional) nearly every day (not merely self-reproach or guilt about being sick)
   (8) diminished ability to think or concentrate, or indecisiveness, nearly every day (either by subjective account or observed by others)
   (9) thoughts that he or she would be better off dead, or suicidal ideation, nearly every day; a suicide attempt

B. (1) An organic etiology has been ruled out (ie, either there was no new organic factor or change in a preexisting organic factor that precipitated the disturbance), or the disturbance has persisted for at least one month beyond the cessation of the precipitating organic factor
   (2) Not a normal reaction to the loss of a loved one (Uncomplicated Bereavement)

   Note: Morbid preoccupation with worthlessness, suicidal ideation, marked functional impairment or psychomotor retardation, or prolonged duration suggest bereavement complicated by Major Depression.

C. At no time during the disturbance have there been delusions or hallucinations for as long as two weeks in the absence of prominent mood symptoms (ie, before the mood symptoms developed or after they have remitted).

D. Not superimposed on Schizophrenia, Schizophreniform Disorder, or a Delusional Disorder.

Source: American Psychiatric Association. *Diagnostic and Statistical Manual of Mental Disorders,* 3d ed. (Revised.) Washington, DC, 1987.

Organic disorders can also exist concomitantly with depression, and the cognitive impairment may be worsened by the depressive overlay, a situation described as "excessive disability." That is, the elderly patient's condition is compromised beyond what would be expected by the dementing process alone. Judicious use of antidepressant medications, together with brief psychotherapy in the early stages of dementia, has been shown to alleviate excess disability. Although depressive symptoms can be successfully treated in this manner, the course of the irreversible dementia remains inexorably progressive despite treatment.

Another sign of depression, especially in older persons, is excessive preoccupation with physical symptoms (somatization). Indeed, hypochondriacal symptoms seem to increase among depressed elderly, whereas phobic and obsessional symptoms are diminished. Expressing bodily discomfort is often more familiar to older persons than is bringing forth symptoms of psychic pain. Clinicians have noted that because of the stigma associated with mental illness, depressed elderly patients will sometimes "cover up" depression when interacting with others by maintaining meticulous grooming and feigning a cheerful attitude.

Further, elderly depressed persons most often approach their family physician with somatic complaints related to depression rather than going to a psychiatrist or other mental health professional. Be alert for other signs of depressive illness in an elderly patient who consistently focuses on physical problems. Chronic complaints of constipation, headaches, musculoskeletal pain, chest tightness and dyspnea with no physical basis, and chronic gastrointestinal upset may be the result of the depressed elder unconsciously shifting attention away from distressing emotions to physical symptoms, which he or she may feel are more acceptable and less stigmatizing.

ASSESSMENT TOOLS

There are a variety of tools available that can facilitate the assessment of an elderly patient and allow systematic data collection. Any tool used to assess the elderly must have established reliability and validity for use with elderly populations. Tools designed for and tested on other age groups are not likely to provide accurate findings when applied to the elderly. Caution

Table 35.4

Differentiating Dementia and Depression

AFFECT

Labile, fluctuating from tears to laughter, not consistent or sustained; may show apathy, depression, irritability, euphoria, or inappropriate affect. Normal control impaired, suggestible.

Depressed, feelings of despair that are pervasive, persistent. Anxious hypomanic. Not influenced by suggestions. May be flat, withdrawn, sad, tearful.

MEMORY

Decreased attention for recent events; confabulation; perseveration. Irritability when memory tested.

Difficulty in concentration. Impaired learning of new knowledge. Decreased attention with secondary decrease in recent memory. May not respond when tested or will admit can't remember.

INTELLECT

Impaired, decreased as tested by serial 7s, similarities, recent events.

Impaired but can perform serial 7s and can usually remember recent events.

ORIENTATION

Fluctuating with varying levels of awareness. Disoriented for time, place.

May have some confusion, not as profound as in dementia.

JUDGMENT

Poor judgment with inappropriate behavior, dress. Deterioration of personal habits and hygiene. Loss of bowel and bladder control.

May be poor, especially if suicidal, eg, poor grooming. May be careless with medication. May risk personal safety.

SOMATIC COMPLAINTS

Fatigue, failing health complaints with vague complaints of pain in head, neck, back.

Typical complaints as: decreases in sleep, appetite, weight, libido, energy and c/o constipation.

NEUROLOGIC SYMPTOMS

Dysphasia, apraxia, agnosia.

Not present.

Source: Adapted from Zung WWK: Affective disorders. In: *Handbook of Geriatric Psychiatry*, Busse EW, Blazer DG (editors). Van Nos Reinhold, 1980; 357.

must be used even with tools designed for the elderly because multiple extraneous variables may influence the results. For example, sensory loss, time of day, lack of patient cooperation, environmental stimuli, cultural influences, medication, and other factors may affect the scores obtained. Therefore, the use of a combination of tools and multiple trials is recommended to assess cognitive function and mood disorders with the elderly before establishing a definitive diagnosis.

Geriatric Depression Rating Scale (GDRS)

The GDRS was developed as a screening tool to measure depression in the elderly (Brink et al, 1982). The GDRS is a 30-item tool with a simple yes/no response self-report format. It can also be read to an elderly person

who may have visual difficulty. Reliability and validity of the GDRS have been documented for use with the elderly. Concurrent validity has been established for the GDRS against the other most commonly used measures of depression: Zung's Self-Rating Scale for Depression (SDS), the Hamilton Rating Scale for Depression (Ham-D), and Research Diagnostic Criteria (RDC). The GDRS purposely excludes somatic symptoms, which have not been found to correlate well with other measures of well-being and mood disorder items.

Beck Depression Inventory (BDI)

The BDI is an easily administered patient self-report questionnaire that has also been validated for interview administration (Beck, 1967). Items on the BDI were derived clinically on the basis of experience with depressed patients, and each item consists of a graded series (0–3) of self-evaluative statements reflecting severity of the particular symptom.

The BDI has been used in many research studies as a means of identifying the presence of depression and measuring the degree of severity. BDI has been shown to reflect even minor changes in the intensity of depression over time (Beck, 1967) and to discriminate depression from other emotional states such as anxiety. The BDI was designed to include all symptoms integral to the depressive constellation, and its 21 items test the following areas: sadness, pessimism, sense of failure, dissatisfaction, guilt, sense of punishment, self-dislike, self-accusations, self-harm, crying spells, irritability, social withdrawal, indecisiveness, self-image change, work difficulty, sleep disturbance, fatigability, anorexia, weight loss, somatic preoccupation, and loss of libido.

The BDI is easily scored, is quantitatively interpreted, and has well-established reliability and validity. It has not, however, been specifically validated for the elderly. The BDI is copyrighted and should be used with written permission of the author, Dr. Aaron T. Beck. Elderly subjects must be cognitively and physically able to respond to the self-report format.

Observation-Based Rating Scales

Interview and self-report instruments require the patient's cooperation to complete. Severely depressed cognitively impaired elders and those patients with chronic physical or neurologic illnesses are often unable to participate in a structured interview. The need for reliable and valid assessment procedures that do not require the patient's cooperation has led to the development of various observation-based scales.

Sandoz Clinical Assessment-Geriatrics (SCAG)
The SCAG, originally designed for psychopharmacologic research purposes, is an observation-based scale with ratings in 18 dimensions, including an overall impression score (Shader et al, 1974). The SCAG was designed to facilitate the differentiation of dementia from depressive disorders. Interpretations are made from the patient's presenting behavior and response to stimuli. Advanced clinical skill is needed for proper use of this tool.

Nurse's Observation Scale for Inpatient Education (NOSIE)
This tool was developed for evaluation of institutionalized schizophrenic patients over a 3-day period (Honigfeld et al, 1966). Observable responses and behavior of the patient, measuring social competence, social interaction, cooperation and psychotic depression, are rated on a Likert-type scale. The NOSIE has been tested on geriatric populations and demonstrates sound psychometric properties.

This section on assessment has highlighted the diverse and multidimensional nature of depression in the elderly, stressing the need for use of a combination of assessment methods over time. Difficulty in making an accurate differential diagnosis is compounded by increased somatization among the elderly and by coexisting symptoms of depression and dementia.

In the following case study particular attention has been given to aspects of assessment, patient strengths, and adaptive behaviors. To ensure that these often overlooked aspects of the elderly are included, the authors recommend that a specific, regularly updated section of the care plan be devoted to "signs of growth/strengths" (see case study) and that these crucial aspects of the patient (no matter how minimal they may seem) be stressed in *every* form of communication related to the geriatric patient's status (eg, shift report, progress notes, physician rounds, reports given to family members, interactions with the patient). Shifting the focus away from the problems will ensure that the strengths of the patient are fortified and encouraged to progress by all who have contact with the dependent elder.

CASE STUDY

Reactive Depression

Mr. R is an 85-year-old Italian immigrant who is currently residing on the health-related floor in a long-term care facility. His wife is also in the same facility, on the skilled nursing care unit. Mr. and Mrs. R lived independently up until about a year ago when Mrs. R suffered a massive stroke, leaving her comatose. She was described as a doting wife and a meticulous housekeeper. Despite living in this country since they were both 18, she spoke little English, relying on her husband for all interactions outside the immediate household. Mr. R was a mason for 40 years, with an eighth grade education. They had two children: One son died in infancy, and another son died at age 28 from cancer. Since his admission, Mr. R has refused to visit his wife and has demonstrated a variety of behavior changes, becoming progressively agitated and unmanageable. His attending physician ordered Valium 5 mg t.i.d. to control his anxious and combative tendency and Restoril for sleep. The medication seemed to decrease his agitation, although he became more withdrawn during the day, refusing to participate in any ward activities. His disturbed sleep pattern remained unchanged. The staff obtained permission to consult with a geropsychiatric nurse clinician, who then came to the facility to assess the patient.

The nurse introduced herself to Mr. R and stated that she had come to see him because the staff was concerned about the way he had been feeling recently. She asked him if he would be willing to spend some time talking with her to see if together they could figure out why he had not been eating and sleeping well. She explained that she wanted to ask him some questions, and it would take about an hour.

HEALTH HISTORY

Medical records revealed that Mr. R had been essentially healthy during his adult years. Family history was not available. He was on no medication at home and reported no history of alcohol abuse and no history of depression. His appetite had been poor since admission, and he had lost 15 pounds in the past 8 months. He was treated for frequent fecal impactions, for which he received Colace, b.i.d. He had no physical limitations and had been physically active gardening and taking daily walks with the family dog prior to admission.

BIOPSYCHOSOCIAL ASSESSMENT

Mr. R appeared gaunt, disheveled, and tired: His hair was uncombed, and he had several days' worth of stubble on his face. When addressed, he emitted a pervasive feeling of despair with an undercurrent of anger and despondency. The nurse used a Mini Mental Status Exam as a guide to assess his cognitive status. He was reluctant to converse but became less anxious when the nurse touched his arm and asked him to share a cup of coffee with her. Mr. R was oriented in all spheres, with judgment, remote memory, and recent memory intact. His thoughts flowed logically, and he did not demonstrate any perceptual difficulty. His gait was obviously slow though steady. He spoke hesitantly of the many losses he had encountered in his life, both past and recent. When asked what things he did to get through difficult times in the past he looked puzzled, then explained he never considered his needs since his wife's were more important. He indicated that his wife grieved quite openly and demonstratively, and he often felt the need to console her rather than himself. When the nurse broached the subject of his wife's condition it became apparent that he felt irrationally guilty, blaming himself for not having insisted that she see a doctor when she complained of feeling dizzy. "I was always complaining about money, so she didn't want to spend the money on a doctor." Highlights of the nurse's assessment of Mr. R are presented below, illustrating principles of therapeutic communication.

NURSE: Mr. R, do you ever think about killing yourself?

Assessment of suicidal ideation

PATIENT: (withdrawing, angrily) You think I'm crazy, don't you?

Fear of stigmatization

NURSE: (touching his arm, emphasizing her response with direct eye contact) Mr. R, you are *not* crazy. Everything you have said makes perfect sense to me. You are thinking very clearly and logically. (pause) The

Validation, support
Emphasis on strengths

staff and I are concerned about you because you seem blue and down in the dumps most of the time. You aren't eating or sleeping well. You've lost weight, and these things suggest to me that you are feeling depressed. I can understand fully why you are feeling blue. It seems very *normal* to me that you feel sad. (pause) I would like to help you to feel better and maybe even be happy again. (pause, nurse takes his hand) Sometimes when people have suffered great losses they are able to feel better if they can share their feelings with another person. You have been holding your sadness inside for a long time now and it's affecting your health. (pause) I would like to help you. You don't have to suffer alone. I think together we can work this out. Would you be willing to share your feelings with me? (long silence) Only you can tell us how you feel.

Provides concrete evidence

Validation

Expression of caring touch, contact

Validation Education Empathy

Reassurance Seeking patient input, collaboration Reinforcing patient's control

PATIENT: (withdraws his hand and wipes away a tear) If I could sleep better I'd feel better.

Shifting focus from feelings to somatic complaints

NURSE: That's probably very true. Maybe a goal we could work on would be to help you sleep longer at night. (pause) Do you think if you shared your upsetting feelings with me during the day you might feel more restful at night? (long silence, no answer)

Validation Collaboration, mutual goal setting Redirecting

Reluctance

NURSE: I imagine it feels uncomfortable to you to think about sharing your sadness with me. You don't know me very well. (pause) Maybe we could start by talking about some of the good times you've had in your life? Would that feel more comfortable to you?

Validation, empathy Establishing trust by refocusing temporarily on less painful issues, being direct, refocusing on feelings

PATIENT: (pause) Will you come every day?

Seeking clarification suggests acceptance

Based on the assessment interview and historical data, it was agreed that Mr. R was depressed and was given the DSM IIIR diagnosis "Adjustment Disorder with Depressed

Mood." The nursing diagnosis Reactive Depression secondary to loss of companionship and the implications of relocation was also made. Other relevant nursing diagnoses were also identified. These nursing diagnoses are frequently associated with reactive depression in the elderly:

Anxiety
Impaired Verbal Communication
Ineffective Individual Coping
Diversional Activity Deficit
Dysfunctional Grieving
Altered Nutrition: Less Than Body Requirements
Powerlessness
Self-Care Deficit
Self-Esteem Disturbance
Social Isolation
Constipation

> The reader is referred to chapters in this book that describe these diagnoses.

A care plan is discussed following the section on interventions. An important part of the care plan is the list of patient strengths identified through the assessment process:

PATIENT STRENGTHS/ SIGNS OF GROWTH

Is in excellent physical condition; has absence of chronic illness; is completely mobile; is agile and fully ambulatory

Scored 1 on SPMSQ, indicative of intact intellectual functioning

Is nonsuicidal

Resides on the health-related unit, among many other highly functional peers

Is financially secure

Has been assisting his roommate to the dining room recently

Is bilingual; had enjoyed translating magazines and newspapers to his wife

Is knowledgeable about gardening

Possesses adaptive strengths. He has endured significant losses in his life

Had a solid marriage and good relationships with his neighbors in the community and belonged to a paternal organization much of his life, indicating the ability to maintain meaningful relationships

Derived much satisfaction from caring for the family dog

Has strong religious beliefs

Is physically attractive

Has a rich life history, having immigrated from Italy to the United States

Used to make his own wine

Agreed to meet with the geropsychiatric clinician

The list of strengths was made a permanent part of Mr. R's record; it was reviewed and updated at biweekly multidisciplinary care conferences.

NURSING INTERVENTIONS

There is a notable lack of outcome studies that compare the effects of different psychotherapeutic interventions in the over-65 population. Those few studies that are available concur that the elderly are more amenable to therapy than was previously thought. Additionally, a few studies have demonstrated that the combination of psychotherapy and medication has been more efficacious in relieving depression than either intervention alone (Rush and Beck, 1978; Thompson and Gallagher, 1986). This section provides an overview of interventions commonly used with the depressed elderly. Social support and group interventions are particularly useful for treatment of depression among the elderly in long-term care settings where the milieu itself can have therapeutic or destructive effects.

Behavioral Interventions

The behavioral model of depression contrasts directly with the psychoanalytic model, in that unconscious or theoretical *causes* of the depression are not the focus of therapy. Rather, the demonstrated behavior and the observed *results* become the treatment focus, with explicit goals being behavioral change rather than personality change.

The behavioral principles inherent in this model stem from the work of Seligman (1975), who proposed a "learned helplessness" etiology of depression secondary to aversive stimuli and perceived rewards from the depressed or sick role. The depressive behaviors are thought to be reinforced with attention (positive or negative) from the environment. The goal of treatment in this model is to remove the reinforcers, which are believed to perpetuate the sick-role behavior, and shift attention to the healthy aspects of the patient's behavior.

An institutional environment that is limited to "containment" tends to foster or reinforce the negative behaviors of illness and depression (eg, dependency, incontinence, agitation, disorientation, anorexia). In understaffed, overcrowded facilities, the elderly patient who does not exhibit sick-role behaviors risks being left alone because the staff's priority necessarily becomes attending to those patients who are the most ill or the most disruptive. At the same time, if positive signs of growth in each elderly individual are not explicitly recognized and encouraged to progress through reinforcement (attention), they are likely to diminish.

Cognitive Interventions

Beck (1967) focused on the cognitive processes of depression. His contribution is based primarily on the theory that depressive signs stem from the negative "self-talk" characteristic of depressed individuals. This negative triad or cognitive set consists of attitudes and beliefs regarding the self, the world, and the future. Beck characterized depressed individuals as creating their own depression by distorting interpretations of reality, focusing on and reinforcing the negative. Thus, as noted in the integrated model (Chaisson-Stewart, 1985), the individual's perceptions have a profound impact on his or her interpretation and response to situations and stressors. Consistently exaggerating and focusing on the negative is likely to lead to a depressive disorder.

The therapeutic approach consistent with Beck's theory (cognitive therapy) involves the conscious restructuring of the negative thought processes of depressed individuals, using a time-limited (thus efficient) approach. The treatment goal in cognitive therapy is concrete learning to modify conscious thoughts, feelings, and behaviors identified as promoting the depressive state. The therapist and patient collaborate, through mutual goal setting, to achieve the desired cognitive and affective changes.

Vague and "mysterious" approaches to therapy, in which the objectives are not clear and the therapist remains disengaged, are poorly tolerated by most elderly persons. A combination of cognitive and behavioral interventions is promoted by therapists who work with the elderly because of the time efficiency, the reinforcement of self-control and the relative ease with which the technique can be learned by caregivers (Chaisson et al, 1984). The elderly have been found to be more accepting and responsive to cognitive/behavioral approaches because of the collaborative stance of the therapist and the explicitness and practicality of stating specific cognitive and behavioral outcomes, which are easily recognized (reinforced) in the course of therapy. Nurses with psychiatric background can easily introduce the principles of cognitive/behavioral therapy in the long-term care setting, and these principles should be reinforced by all staff members.

Social Support and Group Interventions

Hear that lonesome whippoorwill?
He sounds too blue to fly.
The midnight train is whining low,
I'm so lonesome, I could cry.

Hank Williams (Chappell, 1982)

Humans are social beings. A major component of an individual's identity is derived from membership in social groups. Loss of affiliation with significant groups (family, professional and work group, bridge club, and so on) and loss of social support can lead to identity dissolution, isolation, loneliness, and depression.

Group therapy is considered by many to be a treatment of choice for the elderly. Group work with the elderly is efficient because eight to ten persons can benefit from this intervention at one time. Long-term care facilities are ideally suited for group work because the members are easily accessible, and transportation is not a problem.

Yalom (1975) has identified what he terms "curative factors" in group psychotherapy. Five of these factors have been noted to be particularly beneficial to elderly persons (Table 35.5) (Yost and Corbishley, 1985).

Table 35.5

Curative Factors in Group Work With the Elderly

Socialization	Provides replacement of meaningful relationships and stimulation of social skills. Allows for celebration of holidays and social events and reminiscing among cohorts. Provides opportunities to resume former roles (chairman, secretary, president, etc)
Group cohesiveness	Refers to the "stick togetherness" characterized by group membership. Provides for a sense of belonging (eg, an old cohort group may begin to view themselves as the "biological elite" within a facility). Reaffirms ability to be liked and make friends. Provides for expression of affection and physical contact, esteem, and validation
Universality	Provides a sense of "We're all in this together." Enables members to see themselves in others and to share experiences, successes, and losses
Instillation of hope	Complements universality. Enables members to see that others have suffered and survived similar situations. Members can share adaptive strengths and coping skills.
Altruism	Very important. Members are provided opportunities to feel needed and to help others. Reinforces self-esteem. Often the support and advice received from peers is integrated more readily than "professional advice"

Source: Adapted from: Yost EB, Corbishley MA: In: *Depression in the Elderly.* Chaisson-Stewart GM (editor). Wiley, 1985.

Special Focus of Group Work With Elders

A geriatric group may be designed for a variety of purposes. Severely depressed and cognitively impaired elderly will benefit from sensory stimulation, reality orientation, and remotivation activities. Including persons with a variety of affects may be beneficial in stimulating withdrawn patients and calming anxious members. A cohort group that focuses on reminiscing and life review may facilitate these processes for those members reluctant to engage in reminiscing on a one-to-one basis. Movement, music, art, and psychodrama tend to bring forth creativity and expression of feelings (catharsis) that may not surface without stimulation. The curative factors of "universality" and "instillation of hope" can be especially beneficial for members of a "grievers" or widow's group, since the members can share their loss experiences.

Group work, when applied with sensitivity, caring, planning, organization, skill, and self-investment, can be fun and rewarding. Anecdoctal evidence supports the effectiveness of this intervention with the elderly; however, there are few outcome studies comparing the effectiveness of different types of geriatric group work. Nurses in long-term care settings are in prime positions to explore this cost-effective, therapeutic intervention through ongoing research efforts. For a complete guide to group work with the elderly the reader is referred to *Working with the Elderly: Group Process and Techniques* by Irene Burnside (1984).

Milieu Therapy

We are the children of our landscape; it dictates behavior and even thought in the measure to which we are responsive to it.

Lawrence Durrell (*Justine*, 1957)

Behavioral principles and group process theory form the major theoretical foundations for constructing a therapeutic milieu. Perhaps no other psychotherapeutic intervention has such strong implications for nursing in long-term care settings. The scientific structuring of the environment to promote health, foster individual strengths, and affect personal growth in patients is clearly the nurse's domain. Milieu therapy has preventive as well as therapeutic value and must be a major consideration in all long-term settings providing services to the elderly.

To best meet the needs of each unique elder within a diverse and changeable patient–staff community, the geriatric milieu must be dynamic and evolving. Staff-related factors (nurse/patient ratio, interpersonal variables, attitudes and interactions, staffing patterns and composition, level of skill) have a profound influence on the prevailing atmosphere and therefore must be included in the milieu assessment and structuring. Table 35.6 provides a useful framework for organizing the complex concept of milieu into a workable format. Examples illustrate how to categorize elements in the environment. Once the elements in each long-term care facility have been categorized, the staff, and residents if at all possible (we recommend an ongoing "milieu committee"), can determine, based on individual strengths and needs, which

Table 35.6

Milieu Components

STRUCTURE	CONTAINMENT	SUPPORT	VALIDATION
Regular meal times	Physical aspects of the facility: interior design, safety features, atmosphere, space, privacy, lighting, location, temperature, noise, odors, colors, infection control, restraints, confinement, isolation, "homey"	Nourishment	Reality orientation, feedback, acceptance
Scheduled activities		Medication	Interaction, contact with world
Predictability and routine consistency		Social support	Music, touch, warmth, creative expression, sensory stimulation
Bowel/bladder program		Reassurance	
Shift change		Visitors	
Medication time		P.T., O.T.	Focus on positive aspects of behavior, "downplay" negative
Vital signs		Spiritual expression, consistent, positive	
Regular MD visits	Atmosphere of rooms, roommates	Staff attitudes	Newspaper, TV, 1:1 relationships
Bedtime		Handrails	
Primary nursing	Access to public transportation	Mutual goal setting	Patient autonomy and decision making
Care planning	"Knock before entering"	Exercise	
Evaluation			Excursions outside

Source: Adapted from: Gunderson JG, Will OA, Mosher LR: *Principles and Practice of Milieu Therapy*. Aronson, 1983.

elements should be manipulated or altered to promote health, foster growth, and prevent deterioration.

Pharmacologic Interventions

When concomitant physical illnesses have been ruled out or treated and psychotherapeutic interventions have been ineffective in improving the mood disturbance in a depressed elder, antidepressant medication should be tried, *along with* psychotherapy. Antidepressant medication has been effective in alleviating depression in the elderly; however, caution must be used in the selection of medication and the regulation of dosage. Biologic changes that accompany aging influence the metabolism and excretion of most medications. Additionally, the anticholinergic, cardiovascular, and neurologic side effects of many of the commonly used antidepressants may be pronounced in the elderly. Patients with significant cardiac disease will require particularly judicious use of medication and careful monitoring. Selection of medication will depend on the following (Lazarus et al, 1985;46):

The previous response of a patient or family member (a previous good response, even in a family member, indicates that the same medication should be considered)

The presence of agitation or psychomotor retardation
Susceptibility to hypotension or sedation
Concomitant drug use

Generally, the drugs in the antidepressant class, known as the secondary amines, are as efficacious as the tertiary amines in relieving depression and have the advantage of fewer anticholinergic and sedative side effects. For agitated, depressed elders, more sedating antidepressants may be warranted. The recommended geriatric dosage is always lower than the recommended dosages found in drug handbooks for the general population (usually one-third to one-half lower). It is generally recommended that the daily dosage be divided into two or three doses to avoid the sudden rise in blood levels that may accentuate side effects. Table 35.7 lists the daily dosages and select characteristics of the most commonly used antidepressants (see also Chapter 4 on drug toxicity).

Clinical trials of antidepressant therapy must be accompanied by careful monitoring of vital signs to detect postural changes and cardiac irregularities. The authors recommend that postural (lying and standing) vital signs be monitored t.i.d. initially, and daily thereafter. To prevent falls, patients must be cautioned not to change position too quickly. Output should be monitored to detect urinary retention. Elderly patients may take as long as 2 to

Table 35.7

Characteristics of Selected Antidepressant Drugs

DRUG	LEVEL OF SEDATION	ANTICHOLIN-ERGIC ACTIVITY	DEGREE OF ORTHOSTATIC HYPOTENSION	RECOMMENDED GERIATRIC DOSAGE (MG/DAY)
Tricyclic Tertiary Amines				
Amitryptyline	Very High	Very High	High	25 to 150
Doxepin	High	High	Middle	25 to 150
Imipramine	Middle	Middle	High	25 to 150
Tricyclic Secondary Amines				
Desipramine	None	Low	Low	25 to 150
Protriptyline	None	Middle	Low	5 to 30
Nortriptyline	Low	Middle	Low	10 to 35
Tricyclic Dibenzoxazepine				
Amoxapine	Middle	Middle	Low	25 to 150
Tetracyclic				
Maprotiline	Middle	Middle	Low	25 to 150
Other				
Trazodone	Middle	Very Low	Low	50 to 200
Nomifensine	Low	Low	Low	

Source: Ouslander JG, Small GW: Management of depression in the elderly patient with physical illness. *Geriatr Med Today* (Oct) 1984; 3(10):94.

3 weeks to respond to an antidepressant agent. The course of treatment may extend from 6 months to 1 year or longer.

Agitated depressed elders not responsive to the tricyclic class of antidepressants may benefit from a monoamine oxidase inhibitor (MAOI), such as Parnate or Nardil. Tyramine must be eliminated from the diet, and sympathomimetic medications must be discontinued to prevent hypertensive crisis associated with these drugs. For clinical trials of MAOI, lithium, or other psychotropic medications that are particularly challenging to administer and regulate in the elderly, the authors recommend obtaining geropsychiatric consultation.

Electroconvulsant Therapy

The 2- to 3-week lag time between onset of antidepressant drug therapy and symptom relief is a significant liability for severely depressed elders whose health is in danger. When suicide attempt or starvation is a real threat, or when antidepressants are ineffective or contraindicated, electroconvulsive therapy (ECT) should be considered. The main criteria for selecting ECT as the treatment of choice are the severity of depression and the necessity for immediate results (Zung, 1980).

Because of advances in the use of muscle relaxants and anesthesia, ECT is rapidly effective and safe with judicious screening. The unilateral method has been shown to decrease the confusion and recent memory loss associated with this intervention. Essentially, ECT may serve as a lifesaving measure in the elderly, and is especially effective in the relief of delusional depression. Ignorance and negative emotions associated with early, less sophisticated use of ECT should not enter into decisions regarding the appropriateness of this intervention.

CASE STUDY

Nursing Interventions

The nurse met with Mr. R twice a week. Initially she worked toward developing trust and establishing a therapeutic alliance to enable him to work through the grief process eventually and develop more effective coping patterns. She also scheduled meetings with the staff at the facility, which included Mr. R's primary nurse, the dietitian, the social worker, and the activity specialist, so that the interventions developed could be consistently applied and reinforced.

Based on Mr. R's strengths and the assessment outcome, Mr. R was invited to join an assertiveness class. Applying behavioral principles, the nursing home staff consistently identified, praised, and reinforced positive changes in his behavior, assertive interactions, and expression of feelings.

The nurse also worked individually with Mr. R on cognitive restructuring in an effort to reduce his guilt and to encourage expression of feelings by using a "feelings list." This approach eventually helped Mr. R to recognize his own grieving behavior. He was invited, and initially refused, to join a "griever's group" at the nursing home. Despite his reluctance to join the group, nursing staff continued to support Mr. R in the grieving process (see Chapter 43, Dysfunctional Grieving) and to listen to his concerns actively and empathetically.

OUTCOMES

The following short-term and long-term goals can be assessed to evaluate success of the nursing interventions.

Short-Term Goals

1. Patient will begin expressing feelings by identifying one feeling from his feeling list daily.
2. Patient will reduce pacing and combative behavior.
3. Patient will engage in one daily group activity of choice.
4. Patient will express feelings in one-to-one interactions daily with primary care nurses.
5. Patient will accurately appraise coping behaviors.
6. Patient will become more assertive by practicing one assertive interaction every day.
7. Patient will assist in all self-care activities daily (ie, shave self, dress self).
8. Patient will interact with peers informally in activity room.
9. Patient will identify and appraise past adaptive coping mechanisms.

Long-Term Goals

1. Patient will resume former sleep pattern (patient will sleep past 5:00 A.M.).
2. Patient will visit wife, read to her, assist in her care once a week to daily.
3. Patient will attend and participate in "griever's group" weekly meeting.
4. Patient will be prepared for wife's inevitable death by talking about it and expressing feelings.

SUMMARY

The diagnosis Reactive Depression is multifaceted and characterized by a varied constellation of behavior, feelings, and signs. Rarely does depression exist as an isolated clinical entity among the elderly. Rather, biochemical, social, physical, psychologic, and environmental factors present in a complex interplay that makes diagnosis difficult and easy to miss. To aid in this task a series of assessment tools and tips were presented.

The nurse in long-term care settings has a broad armamentarium of interventions to employ. Cognitive and behavioral strategies are particularly effective with depressed elderly. Group and milieu approaches can be very effective in preventing and alleviating depression. The nurse must also be knowledgeable of somatic treatments (eg, medications and ECT), which are often employed as adjunctive treatments with the elderly.

References

American Psychiatric Association: *Diagnostic and Statistical Manual of Mental Disorders*. Washington, DC, 1980.

American Psychiatric Association: *Diagnostic and Statistical Manual of Mental Disorders*, 3d ed. (Revised). Washington, DC, 1987.

Beck AT: *Depression, Clinical, Experimental and Theoretical Aspects*. Harper and Row, 1967.

Brink TL et al: Screening tests for geriatric depression. *Clin Gerontol* 1982; 10:37.

Burnside IM: *Psychosocial Nursing Care of the Aged*, 2d ed. McGraw-Hill, 1980.

Burnside IM: *Working with the Elderly: Group Process and Techniques*. Jones and Bartlett, 1984.

Carroll-Johnson R (editor): *Classification of Nursing Diagnoses: Proceedings of the Eighth Conference*. Lippincott, 1989.

Chaisson GM et al: Treating depressed elderly. *J Psychosoc Nurs* 1984; 22 (5):25–30.

Chaisson-Stewart GM: An integrated theory of depression. In: *Depression in the Elderly: An Interdisciplinary Approach*. Chaisson-Stewart GM (editor). Wiley, 1985.

Durrell L: *Justine*. Dutton, 1957.

Eliot TS: Gerontion. In: T.S. Eliot: *The Complete Poems and Plays 1909 to 1950*. Harcourt Brace, 1971.

Erikson EH: *Childhood and Society*. Norton, 1950.

Freeman N, Bucci W, Elkawitz E: Depression in a family practice elderly population. *J Am Geriatr Soc* 1982; 30(6):372–377.

Freud S: *On psychotherapy* (1904). In: *Collected Papers*, Vol 1. Hogarth Press, 1950.

Gordon M: *Manual of Nursing Diagnosis*. McGraw-Hill, 1982; 166.

Gunderson JG, Will OA, Mosher LR: *Principles and Practice of Milieu Therapy*. Aronson, 1983.

Hill D: Depression: Disease, reaction, or posture? *Am J Psychiatry* 1968; 125:445–457.

Honigfeld G, Gillis RD, Klett CJ: NOSIE-30: A treatment-sensitive ward behavior scale. *Psycholog Rep* 1966; 21:65.

Kendel RE: The classification of depressive illnesses. *Maudsley Monograph* 1968; 18 OUP.

Kneisl CR, Wilson HS: *Handbook of Psychosocial Nursing Care*. Addison-Wesley, 1984.

Kraeplin E: *Manic-Depressive Insanity and Paranoia*. Barclay M, (editor). Livingstone, 1921.

Lazarus LW, Davis JM, Dysken MW: Geriatric depression: A guide to successful therapy. *Geriatrics* 1985; 40(6):43–53.

Lewis AJ: Melancholia: A clinical survey of depressive states. *J Mental Sci* 1934; 80:277–378.

Mapother E: Opening paper of discussion on manicdepressive psychosis. *British Med J* 1926; 2:872–876.

Meyer A: A discussion on the classification of the melancholies. *J Nervous Mental Dis* 1905; 32:114.

Muslin HL: Psychoanalysis in the elderly: A self-psychological approach. Chapter 4 in: *Psychotherapy with the Elderly*. Lazarus LW (editor). Monograph Series of the American Psychiatric Press, 1984.

Rush AJ, Beck AT: Cognitive therapy of depression and suicide. *Am J Psychother* (Apr) 1978; 32(2):201–219.

Seligman M: *Helplessness*. Freeman, 1975.

Selye H: *The Stress of Life*, 2d ed. McGraw-Hill, 1978.

Shader RI, Harmatz JS, Salzman CA: A new scale for clinical assessment in geriatric populations: Sandoz Clinical Assessment-Geriatric (SCAG). *J Am Geriatr Soc* 1974; 22:107.

Stotsky BA: Psychiatric disorders common to psychiatric and nonpsychiatric patients in nursing homes. *J Am Geriatr Soc* 1967; 15(7):664–673.

Thompson LW, Gallagher D: Psychotherapy for late-life depression. *Generations* (Spring) 1986; 38–41.

Whanger AD, Lewis P: Survey of institutionalized elderly. In: *Multidimensional Functional Assessment: The OARS Methodology*. Pfeiffer E (editor). Duke University, 1975.

Williams H: *I'm so lonesome I could cry* (Song). In: *The Best of Hank Williams*. Chappell Music Co., 1982.

Yalom ID: *The Theory and Practice of Group Psychotherapy*. Basic Books, 1975.

Yost EB, Corbishley MA: Group therapy. Chapter 11 in: *Depression in the Elderly—An Interdisciplinary Approach*. Chaisson-Stewart GM (editor). Wiley, 1985.

Zung WWK: Affective disorders. In: *Handbook of Geriatric Psychiatry*. Busse EW, Blazer DG (editors). Van Nos Reinhold, 1980.

36

Body Image Disturbance

Orpha J. Glick, PhD, RN
Linda Eastman, MA, RN

Body image is a multidimensional construct that reflects a composite of an individual's total body experience over time. It represents the cognitive and affective integration of sensory, intrapersonal, and interpersonal information one receives from or about the body. Nurses (Bille, 1977; Fawcett and Frye, 1980; Mabry, 1979; Liviskie, 1973; Wilson, 1981), as well as nuerologists, psychiatrists, and psychologists (Gorman, 1969; Henker, 1979; Lipowski, 1977), have hypothesized that body image is a critical factor in health and illness.

A disturbance in body image is a disruption in the way individuals perceive or experience their bodies. Gordon (1987;184) defines the concept of Body Image Disturbance as "negative feelings or perceptions about characteristics, functions or limits of the body or body parts." This disturbance represents a discrepancy between the individual's perception and reality.

The focus of this chapter is the nursing diagnosis and management of Body Image Disturbance in elderly clients who have or are at risk for developing impairments or alterations in perception or conception of their bodies. The conceptual structure for the discussion of body image is grounded in the complex interplay of neurobiologic and psychosocial phenomena of body experience. The concept of body image is examined as a foundation for understanding the clinical manifestations and etiologies of Body Image Disturbance as well as to establish the relevance of the diagnosis for elderly populations.

BODY IMAGE: A DEVELOPMENTAL PROCESS

Body image as an entity of human experience is difficult to describe because it is a theoretical abstraction of an individual's sensory-perceptual, cognitive, affective, and social experiences with the body. When viewed as a developmental process, body image is fluid and dynamic and changes throughout the lifespan. Some of these changes are very profound and occur rapidly, whereas others evolve more slowly. For example, during childhood and adolescence, there are rapid changes in physical and mental growth as the central nervous system matures and the individual develops physically, emotionally, and socially. As the individual ages, body changes are more subtle and occur gradually through daily life experiences such as body movement, hunger (or satiation), positive (or negative) interpersonal interactions, and intrapersonal reflection. The impact of any of these experiences on the development of body image may or may not be a part of conscious awareness.

Most definitions of body image presented in the literature incorporate perceptual, cognitive, and affective (feelings, attitudes) dimensions. Gorman (1969;17), however, differentiates "precept" (perception) of body from "concept" (conception) of body. He notes, for example, that "body image is the conception of the body rather than a perception." This suggests that it is more a construction of the mind than a sensory image with spatial characteristics that is developed by the visual apparatus.

Shontz (1975) believes that individuals experience their bodies at different levels of perception. He describes four integrated yet distinguishable levels: (a) body schema; (b) body self (boundary); (c) body fantasy; and (d) body concept. Note that these levels are hierarchical in that they become more abstract as they move farther from sensory experience. Further, each level of body experience incorporates phenomena from previous levels. The four levels are described here to provide a conceptual structure for studying and comprehending the complex nature of body image phenomena.

Body Schema

The most fundamental type of body experience is body schema. According to Shontz (1975), body schema has a neurobiologic basis and is "preprogrammed" in the infant's nervous system. It is further developed through physical maturation and processing information received during motor activity and learning (Gorman, 1969; Shontz, 1975).

Body schema incorporates sensory-perceptual information about body structures and functions. It provides the psychobiologic foundation for the development of certain basic psychomotor skills. For example, body schema integrates the wide range of postures for physical activity that are mediated by proprioception. Recall that proprioceptive feedback enables individuals to locate body parts in space and makes it possible for them to assume postures and to sequence movements required for motor function. Body schema also includes a topographic representation of the body. Topographic body schema operates to locate stimuli on or from the surface of the body. This safety mechanism warns the individual about potential injury as well as confirms the body boundary. Although body schemata influence awareness, they usually are not the focus of an individual's awareness. Shontz (1975;64) compares the role of body schema in awareness as the role of "ground" in the view of perception held by Gestalt psychology. He notes that "a body schema is the ground against which stimulation to the body is perceived as the figure."

The significance of body schema in human function was established in the early 1900s by neurologists who observed severe distortions in body perception in patients with brain damage. Gorman (1969) credited Henry Head, a neurologist, with developing the idea of body schema from extensive study of kinesthetic perception and the role of body posture and movement in the evaluation of body schema. The observation that the distortion was most common when the brain lesions occurred in the parietal lobe led to the assumption that brain localization for body image functions was the parietal lobe, particularly the posterior zone of the nondominant hemisphere (Fisher and Cleveland, 1968; Shontz, 1969). This notion is consistent with the knowledge that somatic sensory information is received and processed by regions of the parietal lobe and that it is integrated with sensory and motor signals from other cortical and subcortical brain regions and memory (past experience) in the association cortex (Barr and Kiernan, 1983).

Body Self

The second level of body experience is "self." This level reflects the individual's experiences and perception with the body boundary and the differentiation between the "self" and the "nonself" (Shontz, 1975). Body boundaries are usually described in terms of strength or definiteness in contrast to weakness or indefiniteness (Vinck and Pierloot, 1977). Fisher and Cleveland (1968) are credited with some of the most extensive work on the relationship among body boundary perception and somatic function, psychic function, and personality characteristics. These investigators used projective methods (Rorschach Ink Blot Test) to develop measures of high barrier (strong) versus high penetration (weak) body boundary perceptions. According to Vinck and Pierloot (1977), individuals with definite, clearly articulated body boundaries (high barrier scores) have a "clearer awareness" of body surface and demonstrate more intense reactions to injury of boundary regions (eg, skin or muscle) and less reaction to injury or dysfunction in internal regions of the body. Conversely, persons with less definite, weak body boundary perceptions (higher penetration scores) are more sensitive to internal body regions (eg, cardiac, gastrointestinal) and tend to react more intensely to injury or dysfunction in the internal regions.

The perception of body boundary also influences the definition and use of personal space. This extends the perception of the body boundary beyond the body itself. For example, the differentiation of self from the nonself serves as a reference for perceiving spatial direction such as in front of, behind, and above, as well as distance from the body (Shontz, 1975). These perceptions determine how one relates to other objects in space as well as to individuals in social interaction. Moreover, Gorman (1969) maintains that not only does body image extend beyond the body boundary (when defined as external surface) to external space and protheses, it also extends to tools or vehicles that are intimately associated with the body (eg, leg brace, cane, or wheelchair). This extension of body boundary may also involve body fantasy, a phenomenon discussed in the next section.

In addition to the biologic and psychologic significance of body boundary, the differentiated self involves the social dimension of body image. Schilder, a psychiatrist whose work focused on the influence of visual sensation on the development of body image, is viewed as the first person to address the role of social sanctions and responses in the development of body image (cited in Gorman, 1969). The impact of social responses on individuals' attitudes and beliefs about the appearance and function of their bodies is well known. Murray (1972;617) notes that "we become to a large extent what other people tell us we are." The differentiated self, therefore, is accompanied by self-evaluations and judgments (eg, good vs. bad) depending on the individual's perception of others' reactions. These self-evaluations may or may not be accurate representations of reality.

Although individuals often are not consciously aware of the profound emotional and social significance of body boundary perception, it has been shown that accurate perception and self-differentiation contributes to one's sense of body integrity and safety as well as to selfhood. As previously noted, perceptions of body boundaries can be assessed by projective techniques such as the Rorschach Ink Blot Test. The Draw-a-Person test has also been used and will be described in a later section of the chapter.

Body Fantasy

The fantasy level, the third level of body experience, contains the symbolic content of one's body experience. Fantasies may encompass idealized body appearance or function. For example, elderly individuals with or without compromised health may fantasize their bodies as youthful and healthy. Mabry (1979) postulated that the elderly often perceive their bodies as younger. A body fantasy may also incorporate certain characteristics of an animal that is greatly admired (eg, strength and agility of a lion).

The stimuli for fantasy perceptions can originate from internal responses or from external input from social sources. Shontz (1975) believes that this dimension of body experience embodies the emotional and psychologic content of body image and most likely results from social sanctions throughout life. The fantasy level of body image can also be measured by projective techniques such as the Rorschach and Draw-a-Person tests. Because body fantasy is subjective and represents a more abstract level of body experience, results of projective tests may simultaneously have multiple meanings and be very difficult to interpret (Shontz, 1975).

Body Concept

Body concept, the fourth and most abstract level of body experience, incorporates one's knowledge about body structure and function that is accumulated through learning and life experiences. Although this dimension may be related to health and health practices, it is not essential to the function of body schemata (Shontz, 1975). This level of body experience is frequently used by health professionals to increase clients' comprehension and knowledge of their body functions and the way in which these functions may be altered by pathology and treatment. Hypothesized outcomes of educating individuals about their bodies are increased compliance and self-care, as well as disease prevention and health protection. However, the extent to which knowledge of one's anatomy and physiology actually influences behavior in health or illness has not been consistently documented in the health education literature.

Summary

The preceding description represents body image as a dynamic developmental process that fluctuates and involves the integration of basic levels of sensory experiences and perception (schema, body boundary) and cognitive levels of imagination, information processing and knowledge (fantasy, concept). This results in a unified "gestalt" in the individual's conception of body appearance, structure, and function and the use of the body as an instrument for physical and psychosocial action. Although individuals may have a high level of knowledge about their bodies, it is clear that many of the body experiences described usually are not a part of awareness until body appearance or function is disturbed by developmental changes or by illness, injury, or disability.

The complexity of body image phenomena is further compounded by the interface of the concept with three closely related psychosocial constructs: self-esteem, personal identity, and role performance. *Self-esteem* is the personal judgment of value or worth that individuals have about their body, person, intellect, or performance. Self-esteem is expressed in the attitudes that individuals have toward themselves (Coopersmith, 1967). The significance of self-esteem in human function in health and illness throughout life is well documented. *Personal identity* is defined as the individual's composite view of his or her own physical, intellectual, and emotional attributes, as well as achievements and aspirations. Personal identity is closely related to social *role performance* (Murray, 1972). Conversely, the roles one assumes become a part of personal identity. For example, the role of grandparent incorporates certain personal and social characteristics and expectations. An individual's perception of self-worth and identification with "grandparenting" is intricately related to success and satisfaction in performing that role. Similarly, the perception of adequacy in body function is also linked to the performance of the role.

The constructs of body image, self-esteem, personal identity, and role performance just described and their interrelationships are illustrated as overlapping circles by the North American Nursing Diagnosis Association (NANDA). The size of each component varies with the importance placed on it by an individual at a given time (Kim and Moritz, 1982;308). During the Fourth National Conference (1980), the concepts self-esteem, personal identity, and role performance, previously labeled as individual diagnoses, were added to body image as dimensions of self-concept. The nursing diagnosis label became "Self-Concept, Disturbance in: Body Image, Self-Esteem, Role Performance, Personal Identity" (Kim and Moritz, 1982;391). However, after the Eighth Conference, NANDA again labeled each of these dimensions as separate diagnoses, for example, Body Image Disturbance (NANDA Newsletter, Summer, 1988).

DISTURBANCES IN BODY IMAGE

A disturbance in body image is an impairment in the way an individual perceives or conceives of his or her body. The disturbances may be related to a disorder that affects any level of body experience. It also may or may not carry negative judgments and attitudes toward the body or body function. Historically, the concept of disturbances in body image is not new. Philosophers have reflected on the mind–body connection for centuries. Further, physicians, nurses, family members, and some clients noted changes in body perception that had no apparent basis in reality. Yet, these changes were real in the perceptions of the clients. A frequent example of this is the client who experiences a stroke and requests that "the person" be removed from the client's bed when, in reality, the "other person" is the affected half of the client's own body. This phenomenon represents a disorder of body schema as well as of body self (boundary). Studies have shown that lack of sensation in a body part, as well as perceptual changes due to visual disturbance or loss of position sense, has an effect on one's body image (Shontz, 1969).

Nurses have written about the importance of body image and disturbance of body image in health promotion and in care during illness. One of the earliest studies of body image disturbance was reported by Rubin (1967), who studied body image as a factor in maternal role taking. More recently, the nursing diagnosis Altered Body Image was included in the list of diagnoses generated at the First National Conference on Classification of Nursing Diagnosis in 1973. Since then, the wording of the diagnosis has been changed to Body Image Disturbance (Carroll-Johnson, 1989). According to Metzger and Hil-

tunen (1987) Body Image Disturbance is among the 10 most frequently reported diagnoses.

Prevalence

Although it is commonly believed that elderly individuals are at high risk for disturbances in body image, there is little research that documents the prevalence of these disturbances in the elderly. Moreover, there is little systematic exploration of their responses to alterations in body image. Janelli (1986), for example, reports that only six studies were found that included older adults in the sample. She also noted that the most frequently used instrument was human figure drawings and that many of the studies compared college and grade school children with psychiatric patients and institutionalized older adults. Janelli (1986;8) concluded that "overall, the studies indicated there are differences in body image perception among older adults and young persons as indicated in human figure drawings." The cause of these differences, however, is not clear. Janelli (1986) suggested that more research is needed to determine the effects of variables such as age, health status, and personality on older adults' perceptions of their bodies.

Hoffman (1983) examined perception of body image in the elderly and the effect of stress-related life events on their responses. Contrary to common belief, the subjects in her study (age 65 to 83) demonstrated moderately high (positive) body image scores. When the subjects were divided into two groups (stressed versus nonstressed), there were group differences, with "stressed" subjects being five times more likely to score low on the questionnaire than "nonstressed" subjects. The term *stressed* was operationalized as persons who had experienced severe illness, surgery, or widowhood within the last 5 years. Hoffman (1983) concluded that stress negatively affects body image in that stressed individuals think less positively about their body structure and function. These results, however, are difficult to interpret because sample size and the content of the questionnaire were not included in the report. Issues of validity and reliability also were not addressed.

Norris (1978) suggests it is possible that threats to body image integrity induced by "normal" aging are attenuated by an individual's inner psychologic and intellectual resources. This notion is supported by several researchers who found that age per se is not a risk factor for the development of body image disturbances (Bille, 1977; Hoffman, 1983; Lakin, 1960; Plutchik et al, 1971).

ETIOLOGIES/RELATED FACTORS

Disturbance of body image in the elderly can be caused by a wide range of organic and functional pathology.

As previously noted, for example, organic brain lesions such as hemispheric cerebrovascular accident (CVA) can generate alterations in body schema, particularly when the lesion occurs in the parietal lobe. These disturbances are manifested by inattention to the affected side (unilateral neglect) as well as to the environment (Mesulam, 1985). Body image may also be altered by the presence of pain. For example, an elderly person who has painful joints caused by arthritis may perceive the joint as being huge and overpowering other body parts or functions. Although the individual may be cognitively aware that other people do not perceive the joint in the same way, the presence of pain focuses the joint(s) as the center of his or her world. Moreover, individuals who are experiencing discomfort often feel, behave, or appear differently than their usual pattern (Driscoll, 1985).

Psychopathology may also be a source of body image disturbance. For example, individuals with schizophrenia have described feelings of changed body size or shape, that they have lost a portion of their body or that their body is "permeated" with poison. Depression, on the other hand, may be characterized by expressions of body "deterioration" and "disintegration" (Fisher and Cleveland, 1968).

Disturbance in body image may be caused by inadequate knowledge or inaccurate perceptions about capacity for function. For example, elderly clients may perceive themselves as weak or helpless when actually they are not. Conversely, they may perceive themselves as stronger and more vigorous than they actually are and may overextend themselves physically or socially. The inaccuracy of perception may result from cultural factors such as the current emphasis on being young and slender, or on psychologic factors such as illusions and delusions associated with illness and toxicity of medications. Physical factors such as the loss of a body function or part, or prolonged dependency on a machine (eg, dialysis) may also result in inaccurate perceptions. When physical changes occur suddenly as in traumatic injury, CVA, or surgical excision, time is required to reintegrate sensory experiences as well as the psychosocial impact of change.

Some authors believe that lifesaving technologic advances have allowed more body image problems to surface than previously encountered (Henker, 1979). Similarly, advances in health care have made it possible for the population to age in the absence of epidemics and infections that raised mortality rates for their parents. Increased longevity and changes in lifestyle patterns have increased the incidence and prevalence of the chronic or degenerative diseases associated with age. This, in turn, reduces functional capacity at a time in history when society has turned to a production economy. This means that those who do not produce are devalued. Although elderly persons are becoming more valued as a result of growing social awareness, the American ideal of the independent individual functioning on his or her own

remains (Stanwyck, 1983). This affects the elderly in a fundamental way, since interpersonal feedback is one of the factors involved in the formation and maintenance of one's body image. If the feedback given the elderly is negative and society continues to place greater value on youth and beauty than on the wisdom acquired over a lifetime of experience, it is logical to predict increased risk for negative self-perceptions and attitudes regarding their capacity to function.

In addition to negative societal responses and increased susceptibility to chronic disease, the elderly experience many losses (Murray, 1972; Stanwyck, 1983). These include loss of occupation, role function(s), support systems, and personal items (eg, home, household items, automobile). Retirement brings about a loss of work role as well as social roles and expectations associated with occupational identity and success. In addition to social roles, occupation is integrated into an individual's body image. For example, farmers are often viewed as strong, vigorous, and independent. Murray (1972;621) states that "one's very essence may be felt to be a farmer, miner, musician or nurse." Consequently, retirement or injury requiring the cessation or alteration in work role may pose a threat to body image.

Actual loss or diminution of physical and mental function(s) may also threaten body image wholeness for the elderly. These losses may be induced by normal aging or by illness. Norris (1978) notes that the body "communicates aging." When an individual perceives an aspect of his or her body as inferior, the inferiority is often generalized to the total concept of self (Fisher and Cleveland, 1968). Norris (1978) believes that feelings and perceptions about one's self or body image may define and limit the capacity for function. This suggests that if the elderly are assisted in developing a body image that is consistent with reality and maintaining a body appearance that is consistent with the internalized concept of the body, immobilizing impairments in body image may be reduced or prevented.

In addition to changes in physical appearance of the body, loss of physical or mental functions frequently alters one's ability to control body functions. Developing control of body parts (eg, hands, legs) and functions (eg, dressing, grooming, locomotion) is accomplished through movement and exploration throughout early development. Once the neurobiologic, affective, and cognitive capacity for control is achieved, however, it becomes integrated into one's body image and identity. Only when one is threatened with a potential or actual loss of control of function does it enter conscious awareness and engender a profound effect on body image. Rubin (1968;22) states "To lose or be threatened with the loss of a complex coordinated and controlled functional activity which has been achieved and integrated into the personal system is to lose or be threatened with the loss of self." When this occurs, the mobilization of coping resources is compounded by feelings of inadequacy, shame, and grief. Consequently, efforts to realign body image depend on successful resolution of these and other affective responses.

Another major loss experienced by elderly adults is the loss of their informal support system(s) (Murray, 1972). Informal support systems for the elderly include spouses, children or other family members, neighbors, and friends or peers (Stoller and Earl, 1983). In a sample of 753 noninstitutionalized elderly adults, Stoller and Earl found that a spouse provided the major support for elderly married individuals who were physically impaired. On the other hand, unmarried individuals with few family members relied more heavily on their friends for assistance and support.

The impact on individuals of losing part or all of their support system is less clear than that associated with illness and disability. However, one might hypothesize an indirect effect based on the belief that stress levels increase one's susceptibility to disease and illness and that social support is a resource for stress management. Thomas et al (1985) maintain that social support is becoming accepted as an important determinant of health status in the elderly. They found, for example, that healthy older adults in their sample (N = 256) who had "good" social support systems tended to show lower serum cholesterol and uric acid levels and higher indices of immune function. These findings were independent of age, body mass, tobacco use, alcohol intake, and degree of perceived psychologic distress. These findings suggest that a support system not only ameliorates existing dysfunction from disturbances in body image related to chronic illness or disability but may also serve to decrease the risk of illness and concomitant disturbances in body experiences.

In summary, societal values as well as individual responses to changes in body appearance, structure, and function or control of function in aging and chronic illness or disability may contribute to the incidence of body image disturbances in the elderly. The extent to which these changes cause body image disturbance(s) depends on the rate of onset, severity, visibility, and meaning of the change to the individual (Driscoll, 1985; Lubkin, 1986; Shontz, 1975). Although the amount of research is limited, it is possible that elderly adults, whether or not they reside in their own homes, are at risk for disturbances in body image, which may influence their self-concept and their ability to function in an optimum way.

The etiologies (related factors) of body image disturbances accepted and listed by NANDA are (1) biophysical; (2) cognitive/perceptual; (3) psychosocial; and (4) cultural or spiritual (Carroll-Johnson, 1989;549). Note that these are broad categories of related factors that do not elaborate specific conditions in which disturbance in body image may occur. Although not exhaustive, an expanded list of pathologic, treatment, and psychosocial conditions that affect the elderly and that may alter body image is presented in Table 36.1. The items in this list were

Table 36.1

Pathophysiologic and Psychopathologic Conditions and Therapeutic Measures That May Potentiate Body Image Disturbance

Surgical Excision/Alteration of Body Parts
   Enterostomy
   Mastectomy
   Hysterectomy
   Cardiovascular surgery
   Radical neck surgery
   Laryngectomy
Surgical or Traumatic Amputation
Burn Injury
Facial Trauma
Eating Disorders
   Anorexia nervosa
   Bulimia
Obesity
Musculoskeletal Alteration
   Arthritis
Alteration in Integument
   Psoriasis
   Scars secondary to trauma/surgery
Brain Lesions
   Cerebrovascular accidents
   Dementia
   Parkinson's disease
Affective Disorders
   Depression
   Schizophrenia
Disfiguring Endocrine Disorder
   Acromegaly
   Cushing's syndrome
Chemical Substance Abuse
Diagnostic Procedures
Loss or Diminution of Function
   Impotence
   Movement/Control
   Sensory/perception
   Memory
Treatment Modalities
   High technology (eg, defibrillator implants, joint prostheses, dialysis)
   Chemotherapy
Pain
Psychosocial Changes/Losses
   Voluntary or forced changes in work or social roles
   Significant other support
   Divorce
   Personal possessions (home, household items, finances)
   Translocation/Relocation
Societal Responses to Aging (Ageism)
   Negative interpersonal feedback
   Emphasis on productivity
Knowledge Deficit(s) (personal, caregiver, or societal)

generated from the literature. Although not all clients in these circumstances may experience disturbances in body image, all of them should be assessed to rule out a 0diagnosis of actual or potential Body Image Disturbance.

DEFINING CHARACTERISTICS

The range in manifestations of body image disturbance varies widely and is consistent with the levels of body experience and the wide range of etiologies. Table 36.2 lists the defining characteristics identified and accepted by NANDA (Carroll-Johnson, 1989;549). Note

Table 36.2

Defining Characteristics of Body Image Disturbance as Accepted by NANDA (Carroll-Johnson 1989;549)

Either the following A or B must be present to justify the diagnosis of Body Image Disturbance:
A. Verbal response to actual or perceived change in structure and/or function
B. Nonverbal response to actual or perceived change in structure and/or function
The following clinical manifestations may be used to validate the presence of A or B:

Objective

Missing body part
Actual change in structure or function
Not looking at body part
Not touching body part
Hiding or overexposing body part (intentional or unintentional)
Trauma to nonfunctioning part
Change in social involvement
Change in ability to estimate spatial relationship of body to environment

Subjective

Verbalization of change in lifestyle
Fear of rejection or of reaction by others
Focus on past strength, function, or appearance
Negative feelings about body and feelings of helplessness, hopelessness, or powerlessness
Preoccupation with change or loss
Emphasis on remaining strengths, heightened achievement
Extension of body boundary to incorporate environmental objects
Personalization of part or loss by name
Depersonalization of part or loss by impersonal pronouns
Refusal to verify actual change

that the defining characteristics encompass sensory-perceptual, attitudinal, and emotional responses that may be present.

In addition to listing relevant behavioral manifestations, the NANDA work specifies that in order to justify making the diagnosis Body Image Disturbance, the client must present with a verbal or nonverbal response to actual or perceived changes in structure or function (Carroll-Johnson, 1989;549). These are referred to as "critical" defining characteristics.

Although the NANDA list of defining characteristics is consistent with descriptions of responses associated with disturbances in body image reported in the literature, systematic validation has only begun. Metzger and Hiltunen (1987) conducted a retrospective nurse identification study to examine the content validity of the 10 most frequently reported nursing diagnoses. Fehring's (1986) model for obtaining content validity estimates was used. Five "critical" and 12 "supporting" cues (defining characteristics) were identified for the diagnosis Body Image Disturbance. Critical cues included those items (from the NANDA list) with a validity ratio of .75 or higher, whereas supporting cues were defined as items with ratios between .50 and .75. Items with ratios less than .50 were not included in the report. The critical and supporting cues identified in the study are listed in Table 36.3.

The findings of this study are congruent with the NANDA position that verbal or nonverbal responses to actual or perceived change in structure and/or function are critical defining characteristics that need to be present to make the diagnosis Body Image Disturbance. However, as shown, validity ratios of .75 and above were also obtained for the items "negative feelings about body," "verbalization of: fear of rejection or of reaction by others," and "preoccupation with change or loss." This suggests that there may be additional critical defining characteristics that should be considered requisite for making the diagnosis. Metzger and Hiltunen (1987) suggest that research using large randomly selected national samples be conducted to seek confirmation of the findings. In addition, prospective clinical studies with randomized samples of clients are needed to document the presence of these and presently unknown defining characteristics and etiologies. For example, Driscoll (1985) notes that refusing to wear a prosthesis or use an assistive device may indicate a disturbance in body image. Clinical validation of body image disturbances in elderly clients is critical, since there is little systematic study of body image experiences in this segment of the population.

ASSESSMENT

The assessment of clients for evidence of disturbance in body image includes data collection and analysis

Table 36.3

Critical and Supporting Defining Characteristics of Body Image Disturbance Identified on the Metzger-Hiltunen Study* Ranked by Content Validity Ratio

Critical

Verbal response to actual or perceived change in structure and/or function
Negative feelings about body
Verbalization of fear of rejection or of reaction by others
Preoccupation with change or loss
Nonverbal response to actual or perceived change in structure and/or function

Supporting

Not touching body part
Not looking at body part
Actual change in structure and/or function
Feelings of helplessness, hopelessness, or powerlessness
Verbalization of refusal to verify actual change
Hiding or overexposing body part
Verbalization of focus on past strength, function, or appearance
Change in social involvement
Missing body part
Verbalization of change in lifestyle
Depersonalization of part or loss by impersonal pronouns
Change in ability to estimate spatial relationship of body to environment

*Source: Metzger KL, Hiltunen EF: Pages 148–150 in: *Classification of Nursing Diagnoses: Proceedings of the Seventh Conference.* McLane A (editor). Mosby, 1987.

for the presence of behavior patterns that may indicate actual or potential body image disturbance.

Data Collection

Clinical Interview and Observations Assessment of body image perception and attitudes includes the collection of subjective and objective data. *Subjective data* include clients' verbal statements about their body structure or function as well as their attitudes toward their bodies. For example, statements such as "It feels like my body is separated from me" reflect a distortion in body perception, and labels for body function or appearance such as "dirty," "fat," or "small" may reflect negative feelings about the body. Subjective data are obtained during history-taking interviews or during subsequent interactions with the client. Carpenito (1987;517) suggests several open-ended questions for assessing the various aspects of body image. For example, individuals' attitudes toward their bodies can be assessed by asking "How do you feel about your body?" Perception of body image can be determined by asking "How would you describe your

body?" and "How has getting older made you feel about your body?" Other questions that can be used to assess body image are "Before you were sick (came to the nursing home, and so on) how did you feel about people who were sick (in a nursing home, and so on)?" "How do you feel about not being able to move as well?" (or some other limitation) "What do you think caused your illness? Do you think your family understands what is happening to you?" and "What kind of help is available to you?"

Objective data are composed of the caregiver's observations of behavior, such as the refusal to touch or look at a body part, refusal to discuss or use prosthetic devices, and failure to participate in self-care. Objective data may be obtained during verbal interactions as well as during other care activities with the client.

In addition to interviewing and clinical observation, there are a number of tools that can be used to obtain more formal measurements of body image. Several of these tools can be applied to clinical assessment, whereas others may be more useful when conducting research. A summary of the characteristics of each instrument follows.

Body-Cathexis Scale The Body-Cathexis Scale, developed by Secord and Jourard (1953), is a five-point Likert scale that measures body-cathexis. *Body-cathexis* is defined as the "degree of feeling of satisfaction or dissatisfaction with the various parts or processes of the body" (Secord and Jourard, 1953;343). Individuals are asked to rate their feelings toward 46 body parts (eg, hair, lips, nose, fingers, wrists, legs) and functions (eg, appetite, breathing, elimination, sexual activity). In addition, characteristics such as height, body build, profile, and gender are included. A score of five signifies a strongly positive attitude toward a body part or function, whereas a score of one indicates a strongly negative attitude, and a score of three reflects a neutral attitude. Overall scores that are high indicate a more positive body attitude or image than lower scores.

Although the Body-Cathexis Scale frequently is used in body image research, the validity of the instrument continues to be an issue. Several researchers reasoned that because body image cannot be precisely defined, one cannot know whether the instrument is measuring what it is supposed to measure. However, concurrent validity has been found with other measures of body image such as the Draw-a-Person test and perception of body space (Fawcett and Frye, 1980).

Draw-a-Person Test One of the most widely used body image assessment tools is human figure drawings. Schilder (cited in Gorman, 1969) has been credited with the development of the technique. Several approaches to figure drawing tasks have been used. First, clients have been asked to draw a picture of themselves on a blank piece of paper or within a line frame. This is sometimes referred to as the "self-portrait" and has been used to assess perception of body schema (Bach et al, 1971), perception of body boundary (Fawcett, 1978), and body concept (Silberfarb et al, 1978). In other instances, subjects have been asked to draw a person (Lakin, 1960) or, more specifically, to draw a "figure of a nude male and a nude female" (Plutchik et al, 1978).

In using the Draw-a-Person test, the assumption is made that what a person draws actually represents an image of the person who produced it. This assumption has been challenged by several researchers. In reviewing a series of studies using figure drawing, Fisher and Cleveland (1968) concluded that there has been little success in differentiating characteristics of the drawings that are linked with body image from those that reflect skill in drawing or the testing method (ie, the kind of instructions given to the client or subject). Gorman (1969) notes that in contrast to the criticism of several researchers, clinicians believe that human figure drawings are valuable for diagnosing certain psychologic phenomena. For example, several characteristics of figure drawings suggest disorders of the central nervous system: (1) sketchy, broken, scribbled lines; (2) distortions of "true" anatomic pattern, including loss of symmetry; and (3) the "footing" of the figure appears tentative and insecure. Gorman (1969) maintains that when used with other types of assessment such as interviews, physical and laboratory examination, and medical history, human figure drawings can add useful information about body image, particularly in estimating outlines of the body concept.

The interpretation of figure drawings as a measure of body image disturbances is also compounded by sensory-perceptual disorders such as hemianopsia or some other perceptual-motor dysfunction. Plutchik et al (1978;68) also noted that drawings of normal elderly may be easily confused with those of psychiatric patients regardless of the age of the patient. These investigators compared figure drawings of four groups of subjects: (1) normal adults; (2) adult psychiatric inpatients; (3) senior citizens; and (4) elderly psychiatric patients. They found that there were few differences among normal elderly (senior citizens) and hospitalized elderly psychiatric patients. The drawings of normal elderly and young adult psychiatric patients also showed similar characteristics. These investigators suggested that "norms based upon figure drawings of children or adults may not apply to the elderly and that, therefore, figure drawings may be a less useful diagnostic tool for elderly than they are for children or adults." Although figure drawings may reflect actual perceptions of body image, it would be difficult to determine whether or not the etiology of the disturbance was related to body schema or a higher level of body experience, such as body boundary and personal space.

Baird Body Image Assessment Tool   The Baird Body Image Assessment Tool (BBIAT) is an 11-item Likert scale (1 = strongly disagree, 5 = strongly agree) that is designed to be used at the bedside. Seven of the 11 items are questions that are directed to the client; for example, "Do you perceive yourself differently as a result of this surgical procedure or illness?" The remaining four items are observations regarding the presence of "prominent body feature(s)," "evidence or complaint of pain," "major change in affect," and "equipment present" (Baird, 1985;50). The items for the tool were developed from the literature and the investigator's experience. Ten patients immobilized with orthopedic problems were used for preliminary testing. Although this is a short tool and may be more useful in clinical practice than other measures of body image, further testing and refinement are required to establish the validity and reliability of the measure.

Tennessee Self-Concept Scale   The Tennessee Self-Concept Scale (TSCS) was developed in 1965 by Fitts and has been used extensively to study self-concept. The TSCS consists of 100 self-descriptive statements. Self-perceptions are ranked on a five-point scale, with one indicating an item is completely false as a descriptor and five indicating an item is completely true as a descriptor of self. The items represent three subsets of self-concept: (1) identity, which represents what the individual is; (2) self-satisfaction, which reflects how a person feels about himself or herself; and (3) behavior, which is what an individual does or how she or he acts. Individuals who score high tend to see themselves as valuable people, whereas those with low scores tend to see themselves as less than desirable (Fitts, 1965).

The TSCS is divided into five scales: (1) physical self; (2) moral-ethical self; (3) personal self; (4) family self; and (5) social self. The *physical self* measures the perception that one has of one's body, its function and appearance, and state of health and sexuality. The *moral-ethical self* deals with the moral, ethical, and religious aspects of the self. The *personal self* describes perceptions regarding individuals' personal adequacy, self-respect and self-confidence apart from their body and social relationships. The *family self* describes how individuals see their relationships and role within their group of family and close friends and their sense of adequacy as a member of that group. The *social self* deals with one's sense of worth in relation to other people in general (Fitts, 1965).

Although the TSCS was developed to study self-concept, it has been used to target body image phenomena in a group of people who had rheumatoid arthritis. Eastman (1983) found that the only scale on which the sample consistently scored lower than the norm was on the physical self scale. The mean of her sample fell at the fourth percentile. In addition, results of the physical self scale and scores on the Body-Cathexis Scale were highly correlated in this sample.

Data Analysis

In addition to data collection, assessment incorporates the processes of data analysis and clinical judgment

(Gordon, 1987). Data are analyzed to identify "clusters" or patterns of behavior that support or rule out the diagnosis Body Image Disturbance. The analysis also incorporates judgments about possible etiologies, since nursing interventions should focus on cause(s) of the disturbance (if known) as well as on the body image disturbance itself. Further, identifying and discriminating related or coexisting nursing diagnoses is critical because decisions about nursing interventions are contingent on an accurate diagnosis. Differential diagnosis for body image phenomena is made more difficult by the fusion of the psychosocial processes with other self-concept constructs such as personal identity, role performance and self-esteem. Similarly, affective disorders such as depression may present with negative attributions to body structure or function.

The following case study is presented to illustrate the task of identifying diagnoses that may coexist with body image disturbance. Also note that diagnoses may have multiple etiologies.

CASE STUDY

Body Image Disturbance

Mrs. V is a 72-year-old woman who has cared for her home and husband with the quiet precision she demonstrated for 50 years. She was hurrying in her home when she suddenly tripped, fell, and broke her hip. She was taken to a nearby hospital where her hip was pinned. Her postoperative course progressed well until the third day when she developed a deep vein thrombosis. The thrombosis eventually resulted in a below-the-knee (BK) amputation of the right leg. In a few weeks, Mrs. V went from complete independence to dependence by the loss of her lower extremity.

Mrs. V was transferred to a nursing home where she rarely spoke, made no attempt to learn to use the walker, and refused to go to the dining room to eat or participate in activities. Her husband usually joined her for the noon and evening meal, and she ate well at those meals and chatted with him in her room. She refused to participate in her personal care, including the care of her long hair, which she had worn in a bun for 58 years. Her hair was cut short by the staff to facilitate care. She had no personal items from her home in her room. When staff approached Mrs. V about her apathy and dependency, she responded by saying, "I'm no good without my leg."

A nursing student who asked to care for Mrs. V noted the lack of personal items in Mrs. V's possession, both toiletries and clothing. Mr. V said that his wife did not want to use cosmetics anymore since her surgery, so he took them home. He attributed the lack of personal clothing to weight loss. He explained that Mrs. V had once been a large woman, weighing around 170 lb. Now because she wouldn't eat unless he was there, she weighed closer to

130 lb and "nothing fits her." He also shared with the student the pride Mrs. V had in her long hair and the lovely combs with which she held it in place.

With the help of Mr. V, several new dresses in Mrs. V's favorite color were obtained, and the cosmetics were returned to the nursing home. At the same time, the student began working on modifying the image Mrs. V had developed since her amputation and its concomitant losses. Their daily interactions focused on her feelings about the losses she had experienced, including the loss of her leg. They also discussed ways to view and strengthen the dimensions of her body structure and function that weren't changed by the illness and surgery as well as options for a prosthesis and ambulatory aids. In addition, the student assisted Mrs. V with passive and active knee and hip exercises to maintain joint mobility. In addition to purchasing new clothes, Mr. V brought pictures to hang on the walls of her room and provided new jewelled barrettes to replace the combs in her hair. In the course of several weeks, Mrs. V began to participate in her care, combing her hair, applying makeup, and choosing the clothing she preferred to wear that day. She began to ask for a mirror to check her appearance before she left the room. She still preferred to eat in her own room with her husband, but no longer protested going to the dining room for activities.

Observations (defining characteristics) from the data include:

Refusal to participate in self-care
Refusal to leave her room
Discontinued use of cosmetics and personal clothing
Signs of grief, anger, despair
Preoccupation with disability
Refusal to use walker
Verbalized feelings of worthlessness
Exaggeration of dependence
Change in social activity patterns

TENTATIVE NURSING DIAGNOSES

The tentative nursing diagnoses for Mrs. V include:

1. Body Image Disturbance related to BK amputation
2. Depression related to (a) decreased mobility, (b) disturbance in body image
3. Ineffective Coping related to depression and sensory perceptual alteration
4. Altered Nutrition, Less Than Body Requirements related to ineffective coping or depression
5. Potential Dysfunctional Grieving related to depression

NURSING INTERVENTIONS

Recovery from a body image disturbance requires a reintegration of feelings and body experiences to develop a revised image consistent with reality. Reintegration is a process of recognition, acceptance, and resolution (Carpenito, 1987;520). This implies that an individual must first recognize that a change in body structure, function, or perception has taken place, and these changes must be internalized to resolve the conflict successfully. Liviskie (1973) states that the "old" body image must be discarded and that new perceptions and abilities must be acquired and incorporated.

Although there is agreement that body image disturbances and the attendant emotional responses may impede recovery from the illness or injury and its treatment, nursing research investigating specific interventions to facilitate reintegration of body image is very limited. Consequently, there are few tested guidelines for intervention. The majority of body image literature addressing measures to promote reintegration are based on clinical anecdotes and case studies. These interventions have generally been grounded in the reasoning used to explain the development of body image (ie, touch, vision, and kinesthesia). Others address the need for the client to resolve affective responses to conflicts arising from discrepancies experienced between the internalized model of the body form and the adjustment necessitated by changes in the body or one's control of the body. Four interventions that have been examined clinically or in formal research are described in the sections that follow.

Psychotherapy

One intervention that has been employed in the treatment of body image disturbance is psychotherapy. Henker (1979) maintains that any experience with the body that is not consistent with the individual's internalized image of its form or function evokes a body image disturbance and that this in turn generates anxiety. He presents several guidelines for assisting clients with body image disturbances.

First, Henker (1979) cautions the caregiver that clinical manifestations of body image disturbance may be obscure and may be expressed as anxiety, depression, guilt, fear of rejection, projection, and other emotional responses evoked by a major loss. This means that effective intervention is contingent on an accurate diagnosis. Second, Henker describes three phases of therapy: (1) preparation; (2) encounter; and (3) follow-up. *Preparation* for alterations in body structure or function is a prophylactic measure designed to desensitize individuals to the shock that frequently accompanies sudden change. Although explanation of diagnostic as well as therapeutic measures is a common nursing action, systematic sensory preparation for these experiences as a nursing intervention is a more recent approach and one that has been developed and tested by Johnson (1972).

The *encounter* phase of therapy described by Henker (1979) is a process of facilitating the client's passage through stages of grief and resolution. The process is grounded in crisis theory and includes assisting the person to comprehend and understand the circumstances of the alteration in body image and to explore what she or he is feeling. Addressing the feeling state of the client lowers tension, so that the cognitive elements of information processing can be engaged. Exploring coping strategies and resources is another focus of the encounter phase that assists the client to identify and mobilize adaptive responses. Finally, the client is guided to reenter his or her social system. Henker (1979) believes that clients should be guided to resocialize as early as feasible in their course of recovery, since a pattern of prolonged social isolation is difficult to break.

Long-term *follow-up*, the third phase of treatment for body image disturbance, includes the assessment of physical and psychosocial function. Follow-up should also include provision for reinforcement of acceptance and integration of prostheses or compensatory or alternate ways of performing daily functions. Evidence of regression or lack of progress should be addressed and may require therapy to clarify unresolved emotional conflicts. Wilson (1981) notes that a satisfactory physical outcome is not an indication that the client has resolved emotional conflicts about his or her body. Although working through a period of grief is generally accepted as taking up to a year, some individuals have shown that mourning persists 20 to 30 years after the change in body structure and function (Wilson, 1981).

Sensory Feedback

The significance of sensory experience in the reintegration of body image has been clearly illustrated in a case study reported by Liviskie (1973), who describes this process in a 3-year-old boy during an 11-week hospitalization for a burn injury. A burn injury of the skin directly involves body boundary, not only because the skin surface is disrupted, but also because there is visible loss of fluid from the surface (blood and serum) and pain in those areas. During the course of medical treatment (including whirlpool baths, dressing changes, and, eventually, skin grafts), the child first used vision, then tactile sensation, and finally movement in the process of defining body boundary after a period of refusing to look at or touch his body.

The extent to which the experience of a child can be generalized to older adults who experience similar insults to their bodies has not been investigated. Yet, clinical observation of elderly patients who have experienced the creation of a stoma following rectal surgery suggests that visual and tactile stimulation (ie, looking at and touching the stoma and abdomen) is an essential component of incorporating the new (artificial) opening on the abdominal wall into the body image (McDowell, 1983; Wilson, 1981).

Exercise and Movement Therapy

The role of exercise and movement therapy in maintaining function and well-being of the elderly has been demonstrated (Bassett et al, 1982; Bortz, 1980; Fuller, 1982; Goldberg and Fitzpatrick, 1980). Fuller (1982;82) concluded that the "functional losses attributed to aging alone may, in reality, represent the combined effect of true aging changes, unrecognized incipient disease processes and an increasingly sedentary life style." Bortz (1980), in a review of literature on exercise in the elderly, also speaks to relationships between use of the body and the vitality of body functions.

Although no research was found that tested exercise and movement as interventions for body image disturbance in the elderly, several researchers investigated the effects of exercise on physical as well as psychologic function. It is suggested that if body function is maintained or improved, the risk of body image disturbance and ensuing crippling affective responses could be minimized. Fuller (1982) notes that although exercise doesn't "erase wrinkles," it can improve physical appearance by maintaining muscle tone and decreasing body fat.

Goldberg and Fitzpatrick (1980) used morale and self-esteem as outcome measures for testing the effect of 12 movement therapy sessions (two times per week for 6 weeks) on 30 nursing home residents age 65 and above. Movement therapy was defined as the use of "body motion and language in a dynamic process to meet therapeutic goals" (Goldberg and Fitzpatrick, 1980;342). Morale was measured by the Philadelphia Geriatric Center Morale Scale, a 17-item questionnaire that is divided into high-morale and low-morale responses. Low scores indicate high morale. Self-esteem was assessed with Rosenberg's Self-Esteem Scale, which measures attitudes toward self on a favorable to unfavorable scale. Subjects were randomly assigned to an experimental or control group and tested before and after the exercise program. Although the results showed a trend, there were no statistically significant group differences in self-esteem scores. The experimental group, however, showed "significant improvement" in total morale and in attitude toward their own aging when compared to the control group. Goldberg and Fitzpatrick (1980:344) suggested that "one's attitude toward the life process may be dramatically improved through skilled nursing interventions." Further, they note that these changes occurred even though the subjects' age and disability were advanced, and they recommend movement therapy as a practical nursing intervention to implement.

Bassett et al (1982) studied the effects of a structured exercise program on joint flexibility, quadriceps strength, and balance in 74 elderly subjects aged 62 to 88. Seventeen female volunteer subjects and one male volunteer subject living in a federally subsidized high-rise apartment participated in a 10-week progressive exercise program. The exercises were performed to music three times a week for 30 minutes. Participants exercised with a partner or held a wooden dowel in their hands. These investigators found that shoulder-hip-knee flexibility (measured with a gonimeter) improved significantly on posttest, with shoulder flexibility increasing by 10.5 degrees, hip flexibility by 7.0 degrees, and knee flexibility by 2.4 degrees. Quadriceps strength and balance did not improve. The subjects were retested 12 weeks after the structured exercise program as a control. All three flexibility measurements decreased without the exercise program. However, none returned to preexercise levels, and the only statistically significant decline was a 5-degree loss in shoulder flexibility.

In addition to objective indicators of increased flexibility, subjects reported that they felt better and could get around more easily. The recreation center nurse also reported "improved mental health."

Although sample size in the studies cited above is small, the studies are well designed and represent a beginning in documenting the feasibility and efficacy of specific nursing interventions to enhance the function of elderly adults. Further, improved function can bring about positive change in the way they perceive and feel about themselves. The specific effect of movement or exercise therapy on body image, however, remains an open question.

Patient Education

It has been suggested that knowledge about body structure and function (body concept), as well as attitudes toward one's body and self (cathexis) is basic to self-care practices. Patient education has been viewed as one method of informing individuals about their bodies and health care needs. Although there is widespread use of patient education as a nursing intervention, only two studies were found that explored relationships between patient education and body image phenomena.

Mabry (1979) studied the effects of planned instruction on body image and the use of ambulatory aids by elderly adults living independently. Seventy volunteer subjects age 60 and over who had no known pathology that would preclude their assuming responsibility for their own personal health were randomly assigned to a treatment (n = 24), control (n = 24), or second (placebo) control (n = 22) group. Body image was measured with the Body-Cathexis Scale developed by Secord and Jourard. A structured interview was used to identify the need for and verbal acceptance (or rejection) of ambulatory aids. The planned instruction was composed of a 20- to 30-minute health information class about the correct use of ambulatory aids. Teaching methods included demonstration, lecture-discussion, and modeling. Content of the instruction included body changes accompanying aging, the effect of body changes on locomotion, and the value of supportive devices (canes and walkers) on safety in movement. Results of the study showed that subjects' attitudes toward their body improved (as measured by the Body-Cathexis Scale) in the treatment and control groups, with no gain in the placebo group. There was, however, no significant difference in acceptance of ambulatory aids as indicated by responses to the interview questions. These findings suggest that learning about their body improved the subjects' attitudes toward their body but did not facilitate resolution of emotional responses to the use of ambulatory aids. It is also likely that the emotional impact of requiring the use of assistive devices such as a cane or walker is very profound, and thus requires interventions that go beyond giving information.

Bille (1977) also used the Body-Cathexis Scale to investigate the relationship between body image and learning self-care and subsequent compliance with treatment protocols for myocardial infarction (MI). He reasoned that one way of reducing anxiety generated by an illness such as MI is to learn about the disease or illness. He noted, however, that clients frequently experience a time lag in revising their body image and that failure to internalize body injury (eg, damaged heart) into the body image may impede the learning process. Subjects for the study included 24 male patients age 32 to 75 who were admitted to the hospital with a clinical diagnosis of acute or probable MI. Compliance was measured one month after discharge by a telephone interview. First, patients were asked for their perception of the self-care information given by physicians in eight areas of content (medications, diet, physical activity, stressful situations, work, weight loss, smoking, and use of alcohol). Second, they were asked to estimate the extent to which they followed the advice given in each area during the month following hospitalization. The third part of the interview addressed what areas of difficulty were encountered in following the advice given. No attempt was made to validate patients' perceptions with physicians' perceptions of the instruction. Compliance score ranges based on the interview responses were reported as percentages of the 32 items. Thus, scores could range from 0% to 100% compliance. In addition to compliance scores, a knowledge test composed of 40 items (multiple-choice, true-false, and completion) testing knowledge of the self-care information given for the eight areas was administered.

Results of the study showed no significant correlation between body image as measured by the Body-Cathexis Scale and knowledge scores. Further, there were no significant relationships between amount of learning and ratio of reported compliance. There was, however, a significant correlation between body image scores and compliance. That is, patients who reported a more positive body image also reported higher compliance with posthospitalization prescriptions. Bille (1977) suggested that these patients may place a higher value on caring for their bodies, whereas those who feel more negative may place less value. When body image scores and compliance ratio were analyzed by age, there was no significant relationship between age and satisfaction with body parts and functions (body-cathexis). Similarly, there was no relationship between age and knowledge. On the other hand, age did have a positive effect on compliance behavior. It is not known whether this is a function of value or of more time to carry out the prescribed self-care.

Summary

The nursing interventions just discussed are directed toward biologic, emotional, cognitive, and social dimensions of disturbed body image in elderly clients. Psychotherapy or interpersonal communication addresses emotional responses and perceptual inaccuracies or distortions that may occur with actual or perceived changes in body structure or function. Movement therapy and physical exercise assist in developing muscle strength, joint flexibility, motor control, and endurance required to use the body effectively for independent function in everyday living. When physical exercise is conducted in a group, it offers social stimulation and emotional support. Movement and exercise also provide sensory input and reinforce sensorimotor feedback systems. Finally, client education is used to provide and clarify information about body changes and functions as well as ways the body, even though modified, can be used for self-care and daily activity.

CASE STUDY

Nursing Interventions

The specific nursing interventions for Mrs. V that were illustrated in the case study include:

1. Consulting with the family regarding Mrs. V's past patterns of grooming and dress
2. Engaging Mr. V's assistance in obtaining and encouraging the use of personal items (eg, clothing, makeup, pictures)
3. Engaging in therapeutic (1:1) interpersonal interaction with a focus on clarifying and shaping a realistic image of body form and capacity for function
4. Esthetically enhancing and personalizing the present living environment to increase sensory experience and to reestablish Mrs. V's personal identity
5. Encouraging physical exercise to retain joint mobility and proprioceptive stimulation

It should be noted that the interventions for body image disturbance discussed in this section are not viewed as being comprehensive. Rather, they represent examples of interventions that could be used and tested with elderly clients who have body image disturbances. Shontz (1974) suggests that treatment decisions for body image disturbances should be based on the causes or sources of the disturbance, the level of body image experience that is affected, and the personal or social functions that are altered. He states, "There is no apriori reason to assume that basic sensorimotor capacities need to be enhanced or that intensive psychotherapy is needed; each patient must be understood and treated as an individual" (Shontz, 1974; 469).

OUTCOMES

The paucity of research in the diagnosis and treatment of body image disturbances in the elderly also limits what can be projected as outcomes for the nursing interventions described. In keeping with theoretical as well as clinical notions about body image disturbance, the following broad goals or outcomes are offered:

1. Resolution of the emotional impact of body image changes. Although emotions such as fear and anger may be viewed as "normal" responses to the threat of or actual change in body image, there is agreement that intense, persistent emotional states such as depression impede the cognitive processing that is required for accurate and realistic perceptions of the body or for the body's capacity to function. Stanwyck (1983;12), however, maintains that affective states are "relatively transitory and always open to modification."

2. Reconstruction or realignment of body image consistent with the changes in form and/or function. Reconstruction of body image is accomplished through sensorimotor as well as cognitive and social processes. This is consistent with the interplay between biologic and psychosocial processes that occur in normal development and maintenance of body image.

3. Maintenance or achievement of body control in performing personal and social role functions. The significance of body control in facilitating independent function and self-care is self-evident. It is particularly relevant when autonomy in function is or will be compromised by chronic illness and disability. Lubkin (1986;178) states that "when clients can understand, determine, and participate in self-care, they gain a sense of control over chronic illness and resultant bodily changes."

Individual success in attaining these goals (ie, successful reintegration of body image) depends on the etiology of the body image disturbance and, more important, on the value the individual places on the body part or function

that is altered (Henker, 1979). Lubkin (1986) also suggests that the visibility of the change may affect the outcome.

In addition to characteristics of the body image insult, the client's coping resources will affect the outcomes of intervention. Resources such as a supportive spouse or other significant person(s) may be a key factor in success or failure in the coping process (Wilson, 1981). Variables such as past experience and personality characteristics such as flexibility also can facilitate recovery. For example, in discussing stress responses in elderly clients with changes in body image, Motta (1981;21) states that persons who have lived into old age "have probably been successful in developing strategies to deal with anxiety" and thus have established coping patterns. This is not to say that body image disturbances in the elderly are less profound. Rather, it is possible that longevity is related to the use of successful adaptation to life changes. Finally, it should be noted that in addition to the physical assistance given by professional health caregivers, their unbiased sensitivity to the aged client's body image experiences is a coping resource that contributes to the development of positive feelings, attitudes, and perceptions about his or her body (Esberger, 1978).

SUMMARY

Body image phenomena are of concern to nurses because they have been identified as having a major (although frequently unconscious) impact on health and illness behavior. Yet, there is little concrete knowledge about the nature of body image experiences, particularly in the elderly. The abstract and multidimensional characteristics as well as the psychologic fusion of body experiences with other dimensions of an individual's self-concept render it very difficult to isolate, define, and test clinically. Differential diagnosis is also compounded by obscure clinical manifestations as well as by potential or actual coexisting nursing diagnoses that may be manifested by similar defining characteristics. In Mrs. V's case, for example, coexisting diagnoses may be Reactive Depression, Ineffective Individual Coping, Self-Esteem Disturbance, or Sensory/Perceptual Alterations.

Clearly, the knowledge and clinical expertise required to diagnose and treat body image disturbances in the elderly is more complex and comprehensive than can be illustrated in a simplified case study. In addition to theoretical and clinical knowledge of body image phenomena, knowledge about aging is required to appreciate and become sensitive to the diversity in experiences and needs of elderly individuals. Although there is limited research documenting the nature of body image experiences in the elderly, there is some evidence that aging per se does not induce body image disturbances (Bille, 1977; Lipowski, 1977; Plutchik et al, 1978). What is suggested, however, is that elderly clients who are at risk for or present with disturbances in body image related to pathologic or social events are individuals who, at the same time, may be coping with body and social changes that occur with "normal aging" (Driscoll, 1985; Lubkin, 1986; McDowell, 1983). These changes are often experienced as losses and may compound the responses to and treatment of loss of body image integrity (Lubkin, 1986). Consequently, consideration needs to be given to the function and process of grieving as well as to spontaneous recovery (reintegration) from disturbances in body image. It should also be emphasized that disturbances in body image may range from transient short-term alterations to very profound and chronic changes in perception. Similarly, pathologic and social conditions that cause or contribute to body image disturbance may occur gradually or be very sudden. Wilson (1981;38), for example, noted that 30% of patients with rectal cancer are admitted to hospitals as emergencies. When this occurs, the individual must cope with the emotional impact as well as with the reality of a stoma while in a "crisis situation." This means that nursing diagnosis and treatment of body image disturbance(s) must consider the context of the disturbance as well as the biopsychosocial composition of body image phenomena.

References

Bach P, Tracy HW, Huston J: The use of self-portrait method in evaluation of hemiplegia. *Southern Med J* 1971; 64:1475–1484.

Baird S: Development of a nursing assessment tool to diagnose altered body image in immobilized patients. *Orthop Nurs* 1985; 4:47–54.

Barr ML, Kiernan JA: *The Human Nervous System: An Anatomical Viewpoint*, 4th ed. Harper and Row, 1983.

Bassett C, McClamrock E, Schmelzerm O: A 10-week exercise program for senior citizens. *Geriatr Nurs* 1982; 3:103–105.

Bille DA: The role of body image in patient compliance and education. *Heart Lung* 1977; 6:143–148.

Bortz WM: Effect of exercise on aging—effect of aging on exercise. *J Am Geriatr Soc* 1980; 28:49–51.

Carpenito LJ: Self-concept, disturbance. In: *Nursing Diagnosis: Application to Clinical Practice*, 2d ed. Lippincott, 1987.

Carroll-Johnson R (editor): *Classification of Nursing Diagnoses: Proceedings of the Eighth Conference*. Lippincott, 1989.

Coopersmith S: *The Antecedents of Self-Esteem*. Freeman, 1967.

Driscoll P: Change in body image. Pages 283–293 in: *Rheumatology Nursing: A Problem Oriented Approach*. Pigg J, Driscoll PW, Caniff R (editors). Wiley, 1985.

Eastman L: *Self-Concept, Body Image and the Performance of Activities of Daily Living in Individuals with Rheumatoid Arthritis*. (Master's thesis.) University of Iowa, 1983.

Esberger K: Body image. *J Gerontol Nurs* 1978; 4:35–38.

Fawcett J: Body image and the pregnant couple. *Am J Maternal Child Nurs* 1978; 3:227–233.

Fawcett J, Frye S: An exploratory study of body image dimensionality. *Nurs Res* 1980; 29:324–327.

Fehring R: Validating diagnostic labels: Standardized methodology. Pages 183–190 in: *Classification of Nursing Diagnosis: Proceedings of the Sixth Conference*. Hurley ME (editor). Mosby, 1986.

Fisher S, Cleveland SE: *Body Image and Personality*, 2d ed. Dover, 1968.

Fitts WH: *Tennessee Self-Concept Scale: Manual and Test Booklet*. Nashville: Department of Mental Health, Counselor Recordings and Tests, 1965.

Fuller E: Exercise: Getting the elderly going. *Patient Care* 1982; 16:67–110.

Goldberg WG, Fitzpatrick JJ: Movement therapy with the aged. *Nurs Res* 1980; 29:339–345.

Gordon M: *Nursing Diagnosis: Process and Application*, 2d ed. McGraw-Hill, 1987.

Gorman W: *Body Image and Image of the Brain*. Green, 1969.

Henker F: Body-image conflict following trauma and surgery. *Psychosomatics* 1979; 20:812–820.

Hoffman R: Manifestations of body-image changes in the elderly due to stress and a model for nursing treatment. *New Mexico Nurse* 1983; 28:4–8.

Janelli LM: Body image in older adults: A review of the literature. *Rehabil Nurs* 1986; 11:6–8.

Johnson J: Effects of structuring patients' expectations on their reactions to threatening events. *Nurs Res* 1972; 21:499–503.

Kim MJ, Moritz DA (editors): *Classification of Nursing Diagnoses: Proceedings of the Third and Fourth National Conferences*. Mosby, 1982.

Lakin M: Formal characteristics of human figure drawings by institutionalized and noninstitutionalized aged. *J Gerontol* 1960; 15:76–78.

Lipowski ZJ: The importance of body experience for psychiatry. *Comp Psychiatry* 1977; 18:473–479.

Liviskie S: Definition of boundaries after burn injury. *Maternal-Child Nurs J* 1973; 2:101–109.

Lubkin I: Body image. Pages 167–179 in: *Chronic Illness: Impact and Intervention*. Jones and Bartlett, 1986.

Mabry ER: Effects of planned instruction on body image and the use of ambulatory aids by well-elderly clients. *University Microfilm International*, 1979.

McDowell D: The special needs of the older colostomy patient. *J Gerontol Nurs* 1983; 9:294–296.

Mesulam MM: Attention, confusional states and neglect. In: *Principles of Behavioral Neurology*. Mesulam MM (editor). Davis, 1985.

Metzger KL, Hiltunen EF: Diagnostic content validation of ten frequently reported nursing diagnoses. Pages 144–153 in: *Classification of Nursing Diagnoses: Proceedings of the Seventh Conference*. McLane A (editor). Mosby, 1987.

Motta G: Stress and the elderly: Coping with a change in body image. *J Enterstomal Ther* 1981; 8:21–22.

Murray R: Body image development in adulthood. *Nurs Clin North Am* 1972; 7:617–629.

Norris C: Body image: Its relevance to professional nursing. Pagers 5–36 in: *Behavioral Concepts and Nursing Intervention*, 2d ed. Carlson C, Blackwell B (editors). Lippincott, 1978.

North American Nursing Diagnosis Association (NANDA): *Nursing Diagnosis Newsletter* (Summer) 1988; 15 (1).

Plutchik R, Weiner MB, Conte H: Studies of body image, I. Body worries and discomfort. *J Gerontol* 1971; 26:344–380.

Plutchik R et al: Studies of body image, IV. Figure drawing in normal and abnormal geriatric and nongeriatric groups. *J Gerontol* 1978; 33:68–75.

Rubin R: Attainment of the maternal role. *Nurs Res* 1967; 16:237–245.

Rubin R: Body image and self-esteem. *Nurs Outlook* 1968; 16:20–23.

Secord P, Jourard S: The appraisal of body-cathexis: Body cathexis and the self. *J Consult Psychol* 1953; 17:343–347.

Shontz FC: *Perceptual and Cognitive Aspects of Body Experience.* Academic Press, 1969.

Shontz FC: Body image and its disorders. *Internat J Psychiatry Med* 1974; 5:461–472.

Shontz FC: *Psychological Aspects of Physical Illness and Disability.* MacMillan, 1975.

Silberfarb PM et al: Effects of intestinal bypass surgery on body concept. *J Consult Clin Psychol* 1978; 46:1415–1418.

Stanwyck DJ: Self-esteem through the lifespan. *Fam Community Health* 1983; 11–27.

Stoller E, Earl L: Help with activities of daily life: Sources of support for the noninstitutionalized elderly. *Gerontologist* 1983; 23(1):64–70.

Thomas P, Goodwin H, Goodwin J: Effect of social support on stress-related changes in cholesterol level, uric acid level and immune function in an elderly sample. *Am J Psychiatry* 1985; 142(6):735–737.

Vinck J, Pierloot R: Body image boundary definiteness and psychopathology. *Acta Psychiatrica Belgica* 1977; 77:348–359.

Wilson D: Changing the body's image. *Nurs Mirror* 1981; 152:38–40.

37

Powerlessness

KAREN O'HEATH, MA, RN

POWERLESSNESS CAN HAVE DELETERIOUS EFFECTS ON an elderly individual's physical and emotional states. Although the effects of powerlessness can be seen in all patient populations, the problem of powerlessness is more severe in the elderly, who may have fewer power sources to use. Miller (1983) also identified powerlessness as a precipitant of death. The diagnosis of Powerlessness is dependent on nursing to implement interventions to alleviate it.

Miller (1983;38) defined the concept of powerlessness as "the perception of the individual that one's own actions will not significantly affect an outcome." Powerlessness is a potential problem when one or more of the power resources of physical strength, psychologic stamina, self-concept, energy, knowledge, motivation, and belief system are compromised.

Carpenito (1983;332) viewed powerlessness related to hospitalization as "the state in which an individual perceives a lack of personal control over certain events or situations." She further identified three categories of etiologic and contributing factors for the concept of powerlessness: (1) pathophysiologic, which includes any disease process; (2) situational, which includes a lack of knowledge, personal characteristics that highly value control, and hospital or institutional limitations; and (3) maturational processes along the life span. The North American Nursing Diagnosis Association (NANDA), at the Eighth Conference, defined Powerlessness as the "perception that one's own actions will not significantly affect an outcome; perceived lack of control over a current situation of immediate happening" (Carroll-Johnson, 1989;552).

SIGNIFICANCE FOR THE ELDERLY

The hospitalized or institutionalized elderly person is dependent on the health care system, and this may increase the problem of powerlessness. Powerlessness is also apt to be more problematic for elderly persons because of functional losses and chronic illnesses that often accompany aging.

Control and the Elderly

Langer and Rodin (1976) studied the effects of enhanced personal responsibility and choice on alertness, activity participation, and overall sense of well-being on 91 ambulatory nursing home residents. Subjects in the group that were assigned responsibility were significantly more alert, happy, active, and generally improved as determined by nurses' blind ratings.

Fuller (1978) conducted a study to determine predictors of self-reported morale and found that those residents who perceived greater choice and who spent more time in social interactions reported higher levels of morale. Fuller emphasized that opportunity to make choices is predictive of well-being.

In other studies of locus of control and the elderly, internal locus of control correlated with a positive self-concept (Reid et al, 1977), and external locus of control correlated with depression (Hanes and Wild, 1977). Ziegler and Reid (1979) demonstrated that desired control was significantly negatively correlated with depression and positively correlated with health, knowledge of services, and use of services for 88 elderly community residents. A second sample of 77 elderly men in a chronic care hospital unit demonstrated that desired control was significantly and positively correlated with life satisfaction, tranquility, self-concept, and subject senescence.

To better understand the nursing diagnosis Powerlessness and the consequences for elderly persons, theory and research regarding power, powerlessness, and related concepts are briefly presented prior to a discussion of conceptual development and research on the nursing diagnosis Powerlessness.

POWER

When social psychologists looked to behavior within institutions as the basis for conceptualizing power theory, the connotation of force or coercion began to disappear from the term *power* (Jacobson, 1972). Tawney (1931;23), for example, defined power as "the capacity of an individual, or group of individuals, to modify the conduct of other individuals or groups in the manner in which he desires." Russell (1938) proposed three processes through which one might influence another, two of which did not incorporate the idea of physical force: power by direct physical power, power by rewards and punishments, and power by influence of opinion. Barnard (1938) described power within organizations and made the original distinction between power of position and authority of leadership.

Lewin (1938;383) defined the concept of power as the "psychological force ... a tendency to change some property of the life space." Lewin delineated three types of psychologic force: (1) one's own—the impetus that has its base in one's own needs or anxieties; (2) induced—the motivation originating in the will of another person; and (3) impersonal—environmental influence. Essentially, Lewin proposed that to know the amount of power one person has over another, one must know how much power, or "psychological force," one can exert in relation to the amount of resistance one can expect from the other person.

Experimenters and theorists were also interested in how possession of particular resources affected the operation of power. Dahl (1957;203) wrote that an individual's power is based on "all of the resources—opportunities, acts, objectives, etc.—that one can exploit in order to affect the behavior of another."

Of growing interest to researchers in the 1960s was the long-standing problem of power within organizational structure. McGregor (1960) discussed the assumptions on which power attempts are made, pointing out that there is often a difference between the assumptions about human behavior that guide managerial policies and the findings of social sciences regarding actual human attitudes and behaviors. Thus, the assumptions that people hold about how they can best influence the behavior of others are often erroneous and ineffective.

This brief overview of power demonstrates a lack of consensus of what power is, and, more important, it points out the multiple aspects of power. The nursing diagnosis Powerlessness is discussed as an individual trait or characteristic within individuals, especially the elderly, the ill, and those who are institutionalized.

POWERLESSNESS

Most authors discuss the concept of powerlessness in the context of the absence of power, feelings of powerlessness, or methods of gaining or achieving power, presumably necessary because of a state of powerlessness (Dobb, 1983; Lips, 1981; May, 1972; McClelland, 1975; Winter, 1973).

May (1972;21) noted that feelings of powerlessness occur when "we cannot influence many people; [we feel] that we count for very little; [we feel] that the values to which our parents devoted their lives to are to us insubstantial and worthless; we feel ourselves ... not worth much to ourselves." May discussed the retributions of powerlessness on human beings and society, contending that the state of powerlessness, which leads to apathy and aggression, is the source of violence.

May's (1972) unique perspective of powerlessness and its relation to and potential consequences for society are based primarily on anecdotal accounts. These accounts are primarily of psychotic and neurotic individuals, suggesting that powerlessness is an antecedent or consequence of these disorders.

Seeman (1959) noted that the term *alienation* had been used in a variety of ways in the literature. He then presented research definitions for five basic variants of alienation: (1) powerlessness; (2) meaninglessness; (3) normlessness; (4) value isolation; and (5) self-estrangement.

Seeman (1959;785) defined *powerlessness* as "the expectancy or probability held by the individual that his own behavior cannot determine the outcomes or reinforcements he seeks."

Powerlessness, Social Learning Theory, and Locus of Control

The behavioral significance of powerlessness has been established primarily with respect to social learning. The link between powerlessness, as defined by Seeman (1959), and social learning was built on one of the constructs of Rotter's (1954) social learning theory. This theory contains four basic variables: (1) the potential for behavior to occur; (2) the expectance that behavior will lead to a given reinforcement in a given situation; (3) the value placed on the reinforcement; and (4) the psychologic situation in which the sequence of behavior reinforcement occurs. Expectancy is seen to vary as a function of whether individuals believe future reinforcements are determined by their own actions or by forces that are external to them such as chance, luck, or fate (Rotter et al, 1962).

When the event is interpreted as outside the self, the individual holds a belief in *external control*. If it is believed that the event is contingent on the person's own behavior or relatively permanent characteristics, this is a belief in *internal control* (Rotter, 1966).

It is further hypothesized in social learning theory that when an organism perceives two situations as similar, the experiences for a particular kind of reinforcement will generalize from one situation to another. This does not mean that the expectancies will be the same in the two situations, but changes in the expectancies in one situation will have some small effect in changing expectancies in the other (Rotter, 1954).

The conceptual link between powerlessness and learning thus becomes apparent. Powerlessness, as defined by Seeman (1959), is a perceived lack of personal or internal control of events or in certain situations. Powerlessness can also be equated with perceived external control of events in the learning variable expectancy. Operating as this learning variable, locus of control could be expected to influence learning, either in the sense of acquisition of knowledge or in the sense of developing effective, goal-directed behavior (Johnson, 1967).

There have been a number of studies demonstrating differences in behavior as a function of internal–external locus of control. In one series of investigations, acquisition and extinction of expectancies were shown to vary depending on whether the individual perceives task performance as determined by skill as opposed to chance, luck, or fate (James and Rotter, 1958; Phares, 1957, 1962; Rotter et al, 1961). Concurrent with studies that manipulated skill and chance in a situational context was the development of a scale to measure individual differences in generalized expectancy regarding the nature of causal relationships between behavior and the occurrence of reinforcement (Rotter, 1966). In general, individuals scoring on the internal end of the scale have been shown to differ from those at the external end in the number of shifts in expectancy (Battle and Rotter, 1963); risk taking (Liverant and Scodel, 1960); attempts to control the environment (Gore and Rotter, 1963); degree of conformity (Crowne and Liverant, 1963); preference for skill and chance reinforcements (Rotter and Mulry, 1965); and resistance to subtle influence (Ryckman et al, 1972). In addition, internally controlled people have been shown to be more effective than externally controlled people at seeking and using information relevant to personal decisions (Seeman, 1963; Seeman and Evans, 1962).

These results do not, of course, prove that a sense of internal control causes certain behaviors. The cause–effect relationship could also work in the other direction; for example, effective information-seeking behaviors could lead to an increased belief in internal control.

Health and Locus of Control

Rotter (1975) recognized the need for situation-specific measures relating to a variety of situations when the aim is the prediction of behavior in specific situations. Dabbs and Kirscht (1971) attempted to relate items measuring expectancy of control of health to individuals' tendency to take precautions against influenza, but found, contrary to theoretical predictions, that internally controlled individuals (according to their expectancy measure) took fewer influenza shots than externally controlled individuals. However, the subjects' motivation to exert control over health was measured, and it was found that highly motivated subjects were more likely to take precautions against influenza than less motivated subjects. According to Rotter's (1966) social learning theory, locus of control is an expectancy, as opposed to a motivational construct, and should therefore only be measured by expectancy items. Consequently, information-seeking behavior may be a function of the value an individual attaches to a healthy life, such as the belief that seeking preventive health care information will help maintain health.

Although elderly persons were not the subjects, a study of college students found that seeking information about little-known health-related conditions is a joint function of expectancy. That is, individuals with internal health-related locus of control placed a relatively high value on health (Wallston et al, 1976a). In a second study by Wallston et al (1976b), the health locus control scale (HLC) was developed to measure expectancies regarding locus of control of health-related behaviors. Two experiments demonstrated discriminant validity of the HLC in contrast to Rotter's internal–external locus of control scale. In the first study, HLC internals who valued health highly sought more information than other subjects. In a second study, subjects in weight reduction programs that were consistent with their locus of control as assessed by the HLC were more satisfied with the specific program than other subjects in the program.

These two studies acknowledged the HLC's attempt to operationalize health-related locus of control. The HLC is a generalized measure of expectancy as opposed to beliefs about specific behaviors that could be adapted and tested for use with the elderly.

Johnson (1967) introduced the concept of powerlessness to nursing, noting that perhaps the concept may assist in the understanding of patient behavior. Johnson used Seeman's (1959) definition of powerlessness and identified an association between powerlessness and Rotter's (1954) social learning theory. Johnson (1967;39) contended that for the patients "who do not always behave as expected," the concept of powerlessness offered an additional alternative to be considered in the search for an explanation of behavior.

ETIOLOGIES/RELATED FACTORS AND DEFINING CHARACTERISTICS

NANDA identified the following as etiologies of Powerlessness: health care environment; interpersonal interaction; illness-related regimen; and lifestyle of helplessness (Carroll-Johnson 1989). Defining characteristics of Powerlessness were also identified by NANDA, and are classified as "severe," "moderate," and "low." These characteristics are similar to Miller's (1983) and are primarily operational in nature.

Johnson (1967) noted the need to identify the concept of powerlessness as operative in considering it a determinant of behavior. She identified several problems inherent in this situation. A problem in the assessment area, according to Johnson, is that there is no norm beyond which one can say with certainty that powerlessness is a significant factor in a patient situation. Johnson suggested that norms for powerlessness in the form of probability values could be established.

Johnson (1967) also questioned features of hospitalization that could contribute to a sense of powerlessness. Johnson noted, however, that realistically, health and recovery in many respects cannot be controlled by the individual; the notions of fate and chance are strongly embedded in health care. It is conceivable that individuals who have a high personal control of events may have a high sense of powerlessness in matters of health and illness.

Johnson (1967) asserted that the concept of powerlessness may be used in planning nursing interventions. Knowledge and recognition of the presence of powerlessness could also serve in establishing priorities for the care of patients.

Some of the etiologies of powerlessness that Johnson identified, such as internal locus of control and the institutional and health care environment, are still relevant 20 years after the introduction of the concept of powerlessness into nursing and patient care.

Kritek (1981) used her personal experience as a patient in identifying components of patient power and powerlessness. She kept a diary of her hospitalization for a cholecystectomy and retrospectively analyzed the notes. The theoretical framework employed for this analysis was that of French and Raven (1959), as their definition of power and the power bases they identified were used to guide the analysis of data. Perhaps the biggest limitation was the lack of definition of powerlessness, despite the use of the term. It is inferred that the concept of powerlessness meant a lack of power or bases of power, such as knowledge and information.

Several patient control issues emerged from the data. Subjective experiences of patient powerlessness involved the health care system's control of time, environmental stimuli, information provision, and alteration of the patient's self-concept and role definition. Kritek (1981) suggested that patient power and powerlessness could be studied in relation to other variables as identified in the study. These variables included the amount of nurse-patient contacts, the level of patient sensory deprivation, patients' recovery rate, patients' perceptions of role changes, length of hospitalization, and the nature of patients' illnesses. Thus, the hospital environment, provision of information, and patient control issues emerged from this study as potential etiologies of patient powerlessness or the inability to influence situations regarding care.

Zerwekh (1983) explored some processes that occur with hospitalization that deny power, alternative models for health and nursing, and empowering strategies for the powerless patient. Although powerlessness is not clearly defined, the concept of powerlessness is inferred as the result of denial of power and thus a lack of control. Zerwekh stated that within health care systems, the sources of denial of power for patients are contemporary models of health and illness, institutional and professional caregiving, the sick role, and the helping roles, all of which legitimize and require the assumption of patient powerlessness. Thus, it is the physicians, nurses, and other caregivers who maintain power and control over the elderly person in the health care system.

Institutional and professional caregiving (eg, hospitals, physician offices, and skilled nursing facilities) commonly expect the patient to fit into the existing system, in which caregivers have the power and authority. This system includes predetermined routines standardized according to disease labels; provides little privacy; relies on technology and pharmacology; and demands patient compliance to professional expertise. The sick role assumes exemption from usual role responsibilities. Patients are given no responsibility for healing their condition; their only responsibility is to find competent medical attention and to cooperate (Zerwekh, 1983). "Refusal to play the sick role is essentially a refusal to define oneself in need of help. Learning the sick role requires in essence the relinquishment of rights and duties of normal adult responsibilities and control and entails a desocialization process" (Wu, 1973;168).

Roberts (1976) discussed causes of powerlessness in critical care units of hospitals. According to Roberts, there are two potential causes of powerlessness: loss of control and lack of knowledge.

Loss of control encompasses three categories, which consist of the contributing factors within the physical, psychosocial, and environmental beings of the individual. A fourth category synthesizes what occurs within the physical, psychologic, and environmental categories and signifies how the patient behaviorally manifests loss of control or power. This category contains the patients' mechanisms for coping with powerlessness.

Physiologic loss of control begins when the patient develops an illness and the symptoms of the illness, over which the patient has no power. This usually brings the patient to the hospital. This loss of power over the body is an initial powerlessness episode, and the physical illness may control the patient's consciousness and render the patient powerless to do or think anything else. It is the powerlessness over the body that brings the patient into the health care system, where events may further render the patient psychologically and environmentally powerless (Roberts, 1976).

Psychologic loss of control begins with the admittance procedure of the health care setting. In addition, the loss of control in decision-making matters and of the treatment received is another source of psychologic powerlessness (Roberts, 1976).

Lack of knowledge can also create feelings of alienation and powerlessness. The patient is kept powerless as long as knowledge or information regarding the patient, the illness, and the environment is not provided. Roberts (1976) contended that if the patient does not understand what is occurring, denial may occur. Provision of appropriate information at the appropriate time can result in the reestablishment of the patient's intellectual power.

Miller (1983, 1984) identified defining characteristics of powerlessness. These were determined by 27 graduate students enrolled in a clinical course on chronic illness who made the diagnosis of Powerlessness on 81 chronically ill patients in their caseloads. The signs and symptoms obtained were clustered into 17 broad categories and were then determined to be characteristically "severe,"

"moderate," or "low." When "severe" characteristics were identified it was concluded that the nursing diagnosis was appropriate. The signs and symptoms categorized as "moderate" or "low" are important cues, but Miller felt they could not lead to making the diagnosis of Powerlessness conclusively. Finally, Miller (1983;51) contended:

If powerlessness is not contained, a cycle of lowered self-esteem and depression occurs, followed by hopelessness. The patient is immobilized in terms of solving problems, setting goals, and taking action. If this state is permitted to continue, isolation and death may ensue.

Carpenito (1983) identified two defining characteristics of powerlessness: (1) expressed dissatisfaction over inability to control the situation, and (2) refusal or reluctance to participate in decision making. Associated defining characteristics include apathy, aggression, violent behaviors, anxiety, uneasiness, resignation, acting-out behaviors, and depression. It must be noted, however, that these characteristics are not mutually exclusive for the diagnosis of Powerlessness and could be indicative of many nursing diagnoses.

Patients may have one of two reactions to loss of control. First, the patient may feel guilty over the loss of control. As patients become intolerant of powerlessness, they may exhibit temporary behavior responses. Patients can express themselves in a variety of ways such as anger, hostility, withdrawal, or depression. Thus, patients may not be able to recognize that people in the environment are concerned with their well-being and the restoration of power.

Zerwekh (1983) suggested several symptoms or defining characteristics related to powerlessness. Body language may include shifting eyes, crossed legs and arms, or restless movements. There may be minimal verbalization, or the individual may be demanding or complaining. Swings between retreat and antagonism or passive-aggressive behavior may also be manifestations of perceived powerlessness. However, these may also be manifestations of anxiety or alterations in thought processes. Zerwekh (1983) maintained that those most vulnerable to powerlessness are those whose developmental and situational experiences have led to low self-esteem.

A synthesis of the etiologies and defining characteristics of the nursing diagnosis of Powerlessness identified in the literature is presented in Table 37.1 along with those listed by NANDA (Carroll-Johnson, 1989). It is important to note that these have not been validated, and many could also be indicative of other nursing diagnoses (eg, Noncompliance, Anxiety, Knowledge Deficit).

Differential diagnoses with Powerlessness is not possible because of its lack of refinement/development as a nursing diagnosis. Therefore, several nursing diagnoses are compatible with the diagnosis of Powerlessness (eg, Impaired Mobility, Activity Intolerance, Social Isolation).

Table 37.1

Etiologies/Related Factors and Defining Characteristics Compared With Those Listed by NANDA

NANDA (CARROLL-JOHNSON, 1989)	O'HEATH
Etiologies/Related Factors	***Etiologies/Related Factors***
Health care environment	Health care environment
Interpersonal interaction	Previous experiences
Illness-related regimen	Established health values
Lifestyle of helplessness	Maturational/developmental processes
	Internal control belief
	Perceived or actual loss of control or influence over situation, self, environment, or outcomes
	Lack of knowledge
	Perceived or actual lack of provision of information
Defining Characteristics	***Defining Characteristics***
Severe	Lack of information-seeking behaviors
Verbal expression of no control or influence over situations or outcomes or self-care	Refusal or reluctance to participate in decision-making process
Depression over physical deterioration that occurs despite compliance with regimens	Verbalization of loss of control or influence over situation, self, environment, or outcomes
Apathy	Behavioral responses:
	anger hostility
	apathy resignation
	aggression violent behaviors
	anxiety withdrawal
	depression
Moderate	
Nonparticipation in care or decision making when opportunities are provided	
Behaviors	
Expression of dissatisfaction and frustration over inability to perform previous tasks or activities	
Lack of monitoring progress	
Expression of doubt regarding role performance	
Reluctance to express true feelings	
Fearing alienation from caregivers	
Passivity	
Inability to seek information regarding care	
Dependence on others that may result in irritability, resentment, anger, and guilt	
Lack of defense of self-care practices when challenged	
Low	
Expression of uncertainty about fluctuating energy levels, passivity	

In addition, these diagnoses and their etiologies may be contributing factors to powerlessness, or conversely, powerlessness may be contributing to one of these diagnoses. It must be noted, however, that with any nursing diagnosis made, powerlessness may be present, as the individual may feel a loss of control because of physical and psychologic limitations experienced as a result of illness and being in a health care setting.

ASSESSMENT

According to Carpenito (1983), expressed feelings of powerlessness must be validated by the nurse. Carpenito divides assessment criteria for powerlessness into two areas: subjective data and objective data. The subjective data elicited by the nurse include the patient's decision-making patterns, individual and role responsibilities, and perceptions of control. The data are obtained by asking both closed questions and open-ended questions. The objective data that are to be collected include participation in grooming and hygiene care, information-seeking behaviors, and responses to limits on decision-making and self-control behaviors. This guide is helpful in determining a patient's level of control and decision making and the subsequent effects on the patient if these are lost or given up. However, Carpenito's guide does not indicate those responses or behaviors or their combination that would be indicative of the presence of powerlessness. This limitation in part relates to the fact that the nursing diagnosis of Powerlessness is in the beginning stages of development.

Through clinical study and literature review, Miller and Oertel (1983) developed a behavioral assessment tool that is an observational guide to diagnosing Powerlessness. The tool was developed through field work with the elderly. However, Miller and Oertel feel it is applicable for adults of all ages. The guide contains four categories of assessment data: verbal response; emotional response; participation in activities of daily living; and involvement in learning about care responsibilities.

Potential or actual powerlessness can be determined by scoring 3 or more on a particular item. "Specific nursing interventions to alleviate Powerlessness are needed for a cumulative score of 57 or more" (minimum score is 19; maximum score is 72) (Miller and Oertel, 1983;128). In addition, Miller and Oertel suggested that assessment of changes and losses experienced by the patient is also necessary in making a diagnosis of potential Powerlessness.

Both of these assessment guides are useful in data gathering to determine if powerlessness, or the potential for powerlessness, is present for an individual patient. These guides incorporate both verbalizations of feelings and emotions and behaviors demonstrated by the patient, which are important criteria or cues for the nurse to identify in diagnosing Powerlessness.

CASE STUDY

Powerlessness

Marie is a 73-year-old woman who has been living in a nursing home for the past 6 months. She stated on admission to the nursing home that it was not her choice to live there, but rather the choice of her children, who felt their mother's needs could be better met there. Marie has had arthritis for the past 15 years, and recently, its deteriorating effects have left Marie unable to care for herself. Her children stated they could not take care of her in their own homes and thus decided a nursing home would be the best option for all involved.

On admission to the nursing home, Marie was oriented to her new surroundings. Marie seemed somewhat withdrawn, yet several staff felt this might be Marie's normal personality. However, the primary nurse who would be responsible for Marie's care felt that Marie's withdrawn behavior might be a reaction to Marie losing her home and her level of functioning. While the nurse assisted Marie with unpacking her belongings, Marie made several statements about feeling "helpless" because of her physical condition, her inability to take care of herself, and her lack of input about living in a nursing home. She made comments about nursing homes such as "They are like military camps. No one lets you do anything in one of these places."

Later that day, the nurse assessed and interpreted the statements made by Marie and diagnosed Powerlessness, related to loss of home and perceived and actual loss of control over self, situation, and environment. This diagnosis was evidenced by verbalization of feeling helpless and of having lack of input, withdrawn behavior, and negative comments about lifestyle in a nursing home.

NURSING INTERVENTIONS

If indeed one could carefully assess that powerlessness is operative in a given situation, the question that remains is, "What can be done?" Johnson (1967) argued that because generalized expectancy low personal control is thought to be a permanent personality trait, a high degree of powerlessness may not be rapidly reduced. However, Johnson also pointed out that adult personalities do change and that this could assist in the formulating and testing of modes of interventions that could contribute to change. Furthermore, Johnson contended that people do differ in their degree of powerlessness and this could direct the possibilities for primary and secondary prevention.

Powerlessness can be minimized or even prevented in many situations. Nursing strategies to assist in minimizing powerlessness for the elderly include recognizing the patient's right and need to be included in decision-making processes regarding the health care received, encouraging the patient to participate in the care received, encouraging expression of feelings by the patient, and remembering that hospitalization is usually perceived by most individuals as involving some loss of control. In general, nursing strategies are aimed at preventing loss of involvement and providing adequate information so that the elderly patient can make informed decisions regarding the care received (Carpenito, 1983; Miller, 1983; Miller and Oertel, 1983).

Strategies aimed at preventing powerlessness in elderly patients include involving patients in planning their own care, referring decisions to them to enhance their self-esteem, supplying them with cognitive control through helping them anticipate events and outcomes, and giving them time to adjust to changes (Miller and Oertel, 1983).

Zerwekh (1983) asserted that participation of nurses as partners and catalysts for client health will assist to empower the "powerless patient." Enabling occurs with the application of six strategies: (1) power through attention: the nurse as active listener; (2) power through identity: the nurse fosters insight; (3) power through knowledge: the nurse as teacher; (4) power through active choice: the nurse as advocate; (5) power through sustained network support: the nurse as facilitator; and (6) power through imagination: the nurse as visionary. From these strategies, etiologies of lack of knowledge, lack of opportunity to make decisions, and lack of information can be identified. In addition, nursing interventions can be inferred from the strategies.

In order to assist with the restoration of power, the nurse must provide reassurance concerning how the psychologic systems are regaining control and reaching stability. The nurse must also encourage patients to express feelings, to participate in care, and to make choices and decisions regarding their environment, times of treatment, and the like (Roberts, 1976).

These strategies are aimed primarily at assisting patients to take control of those aspects of care that should have been theirs to begin with, that is, to reinforce to patients that they are the decision makers regarding all aspects of their care, from scheduling of care to treatment choices. It is important that patients be assisted in identifying those factors that they can control. In addition, it is imperative that the elderly patient be given the necessary knowledge to make appropriate decisions regarding care. Further, and perhaps more important, nurses should actively advocate for the elderly client within the system and work to change the system so that the client is not socialized out of the decision-making role.

Advocacy

The strategies or interventions described previously appear to be consistent with the broader intervention of advocacy. To demonstrate this, a brief literature review of advocacy is presented.

An examination of nursing definitions of patient advocacy reveals a wide range of views, from the very simple to the very complex. The major themes that emerge from these definitions include humanism, information giving, human rights, interpersonal relationships, support, and self-determination (Castledine, 1981; Curtin, 1979; Donahue, 1978, 1985; Gadow, 1979, 1980; Kohnke, 1980; Kosik, 1972; Nowakowski, 1977; Thollaug, 1980).

The concept of patient advocacy has received widespread endorsement in the nursing literature. Some authors support the role of the advocate as essential to humanistic care (Christy, 1973; Donahue, 1978, 1985; Kohnke, 1980; Kosik, 1972). Other authors support the justification of the nurse's advocacy role and feel it is implicit in the definition of nursing practice (Anderson, 1977; Fay, 1978; Storch, 1978). Several nurses have proposed specific models in which nurses would assume the role of the patient advocate (Curtin, 1979; Gadow, 1980; Kohnke, 1980). Common to these models is the nurse facilitating the patient's decision-making process by providing information. The information-providing process is what varies with each particular model.

Gadow (1980;84) proposed existential advocacy, which is "based upon the principle that freedom of self determination is the most fundamental and valuable human right." There are five conceptual themes that underlie Gadow's model: self-determination; the patient–nurse relationship; the nurse's values; the patient's values; and individuality. In addition, relevant information is vital to Gadow's model; specifically, the information that is provided is based on how much information the patient feels is needed to make a decision. The nurse as advocate then enables and assists in the patient's self-determined decision-making process.

A third model has been developed by Curtin (1979), who proposed that the nurse advocate is the philosophical foundation and the ideal of nursing. Curtin's model, entitled human advocacy, "is based upon our common humanity, our common needs, and our common rights" (Curtin, 1979;3). Provision of information is crucial to this model. However, Curtin emphasized that how and when patients receive the information, as well as their readiness and ability to assimilate the information, are as significant as what they are told.

In addition to these models, Wilberding (1984) conducted an investigation of 15 nurses' concepts of patient advocacy and how these are used in practice. The behaviors of patient advocacy fell into the two traditional nursing categories of assessment and intervention. Assessment seeks to identify specific problems in the patient's experience that indicate a need for advocacy. Criteria of need for advocacy were found to be a feeling of inferiority, knowledge deficit, lack of understanding, lack of familiarity, fear, nonrecognition of patients' rights, inadequate care, unnecessary treatments, and anger. The nurse advocate assesses the patient by communicating with the patient and observing the patient's behavior.

CASE STUDY

Nursing Interventions

The nurse began immediately to implement the intervention of advocacy by identifying, with Marie, the aspects of life that Marie could still control. These included the environment and Marie's functioning to some extent. The nurse pointed out to Marie that as a patient she, not the staff, decided her daily activity, her meals, the way her room would be set up, and the time that physical therapy would arrive daily. This strategy helped Marie to identify the power she still retained over aspects of her life. In addition, it served as a preventive strategy so that feelings of powerlessness would not be increased, especially over the first week that Marie lived in the nursing home.

The nurse also encouraged Marie to keep up with the exercises prescribed by physical therapy and talked with Marie about the progress she was making in relation to her range of motion and her functioning on a daily basis. In addition, the nurse identified several activities Marie could become involved with at the nursing home.

By the end of the second week, Marie made very positive comments about herself, her physical abilities, and the nursing home. She also stated that she has always been used to making her own decisions and was glad to see that the nursing home did not take that away from her. Marie's physical functioning increased over the next 6 months, and she stated that she had never felt better about herself than she did at that time. Marie also stated that she was lucky to have so many friends at the nursing home, something she missed all those years living alone at home.

Specific desired outcomes of the intervention advocacy that address the etiologies of powerlessness and alter the defining characteristics were defined by the nurse and discussed with Marie. These included:

Outcome	Time Frame
Increased range of joint motion and physical function	End of 2 months
More positive verbalizations about abilities, living environment, and self	End of 1 month
Increased social and recreational activities	End of 3 months
Participation in decisions about own care and living	End of 2 months

Other Interventions Associated With Powerlessness

The intervention of presence may also be appropriate for the diagnosis of Powerlessness. Gardner (1985;321) operationally defined *presence* as follows: "Presence is indicated in the cognitive domain by verbal communication of empathy or understanding of the patient's experience; . . . in the affective domain by a generation of positive regard, trust, and genuineness, which is evidenced by interpersonal rapport; and . . . in the physical domain by being physically available as a helper." The desired patient outcomes identified for the use of presence include comfort, encouragement, motivation, support, and sustained assistance. Presence may be essential to the nurse–patient relationship, and the use of it as an intervention

for powerlessness may assist patients in regaining a sense of control while ill or institutionalized.

Values clarification as an intervention for powerlessness may also be appropriate. The awareness of one's own values and the prioritizing of values are important in decision making. Because patients may be faced with important decisions about their health and health care, and because the need for decision making may contribute to feelings of powerlessness, the nurse may need to intervene to assist the patient with clarification of values. Wilberding (1985) suggested that patients who might benefit from values clarification should be "assessed in terms of the antecedent conditions and behaviors of decision making before the nurse initiates Values Clarification." In addition, the patient's permission to participate should also be sought. Wilberding suggested the clarifying response and the value sheet as two possible techniques when intervening with values clarification.

Bulechek and McCloskey (1985;406) indexed diagnoses and interventions from the contributing authors of their book. The interventions listed for powerlessness include cognitive reappraisal, crisis intervention, culture brokerage, discharge planning, patient advocacy, preparatory sensory information, relaxation training, support groups, and truth telling. As Bulechek and McCloskey point out, these interventions do not constitute a prescription, but rather are suggested by the authors. In addition, "It is apparent that to choose an intervention, the nurse must know more about the cause (etiology)."

SUMMARY

The elderly are at high risk for powerlessness, as multiple losses may be encountered with the aging process. These losses include loss of previous roles, family, health, and functioning. The manifestations of these losses can be seen in the physical, psychologic, and social realms of a person's being. The added stressors of illness and institutionalization only compound feelings of powerlessness within the elderly population.

Perhaps the most startling aspect of powerlessness is that in many cases it can be prevented or minimized by appropriate diagnosis, treatment, and evaluation by the professional nurse. Patients have the need and the right to make decisions that affect every aspect of their lives. Nursing strategies can be employed to decrease patients' sense of loss of control within the environment. Furthermore, patients should be encouraged and allowed to make decisions regarding their health and the health care received. In order to do this, health care professionals must give patients the necessary information to make these decisions. Allowing patients as much control over their environment as possible and allowing them to make decisions that affect their lives diminishes feelings of powerlessness. This constitutes a humanistic approach to nursing care.

The concept of powerlessness is only in the beginning stages of development in relation to etiologies and defining characteristics, as little research has been done in this area. The diagnosis of Powerlessness needs to be further researched in order to document its presence, etiologies, and defining characteristics. Research must focus on the unique components of powerlessness, as many of its characteristics are similar to other diagnoses. Further development of validated assessment tools will also aid in the differential diagnosis of Powerlessness.

The interventions identified that seem appropriate for the diagnosis of Powerlessness also need to be further tested. The interventions of patient advocacy and presence are still being more precisely defined, and the processes to implement them are still quite conceptual in nature. In addition, outcomes of specific interventions need to be defined and measured, and their effectiveness needs to be evaluated.

References

Anderson N: The nurse as a lover of humanity. *Imprint* 1977; 24(4):36–37, 55–57.

Barnard CI: *The Functions of the Executive.* Harvard University Press, 1938.

Battle ES, Rotter JB: Children's feelings of personal control as related to social class and ethnic group. *J Personality* 1963; 31: 482–490.

Bulechek GM, McCloskey JC: Future directions. Pages 401–408 in: *Interventions: Treatments for Nursing Diagnoses.* Bulechek GM, McCloskey JC (editors). Saunders, 1985.

Carpenito LJ: *Nursing Diagnosis: Application to Clinical Practice.* Lippincott, 1983.

Carroll-Johnson R (editor): *Classification of Nursing Diagnoses: Proceedings of the Eighth Conference.* Lippincott, 1989.

Castledine G: The patient's advocate. *Nurs Mirror* (Apr 30) 1981; 14.

Christy TE: New privileges . . . new challenges . . . new responsibilities. *Nurs '73* 1973; 3(11):8–11.

Crowne DP, Liverant S: Conformity under varying conditions of personal commitment. *J Abnormal Soc Psychol* 1963; 66:547–555.

Curtin LL: The nurse as advocate: A philosophical foundation for nursing. *ANS* 1979; 1(3):1–10.

Dabbs JM, Kirscht JP: "Internal control" and the taking of influenza shots. *Psycholog Rep* 1971; 28:959–962.

Dahl RA: The concept of power. *Behav Sci* 1957; 2:201–218.

Dobb LW: *Personality, Power, and Authority: A View from the Behavioral Sciences.* Greenwood Press, 1983.

Donahue MP: The nurse: A patient advocate? *Nurs Forum* 1978; 17(2):143–151.

Donahue MP: Advocacy. Pages 338–351 in: *Nursing Interven-*

tions: Treatments for Nursing Diagnoses. Bulechek GM, McCloskey JC (editors). Saunders, 1985.

Fay P: In support of patient advocacy as a nursing role. *Nurs Outlook* 1978; 26:252–253.

French JRP, Raven B: The bases of social power. Pages 150–157 in: *Studies in Social Power.* D Cartwright (editor). University of Michigan, Institute for Social Research, 1959.

Fuller S: Inhibiting helplessness in the elderly. *J Gerontol Nurs* 1978; 4:18–23.

Gadow S: Advocacy nursing and new meanings of aging. *Nurs Clin North Am* 1979; 14(1):81–91.

Gadow S: Existential advocacy: Philosophical foundation of nursing. Pages 79–101 in: *Nursing: Image and Ideals.* Spricker SF, Gadow S (editors). Springer, 1980.

Gardner DL: Presence. Pages 316–324 in: *Nursing Interventions: Treatments for Nursing Diagnoses.* Bulechek GM, McCloskey JC (editors). Saunders, 1985.

Gore PM, Rotter JB: A personality correlate of social action. *J Personality* 1963; 31(1):58–64.

Hanes C, Wild B: Locus of control and depression among noninstitutionalized elderly persons. *Psychol Rep* 1977; 41: 581–585.

Jacobson WD: *Power and Interpersonal Relations.* Wadsworth, 1972.

James WH, Rotter JB: Partial and 100 per cent reinforcement under chance and skill conditions. *J Experiment Psychol* 1958; 55: 397–403.

Johnson DE: Powerlessness: A significant determinant of patient behavior? *J Nurs Educ* 1967; 6(2):39–44.

Kohnke MF: The nurse as advocate. *Am J Nurs* 1980; 80(11): 2038–2040.

Kosik SH: The nursing profession as health care advocates. *Maine Nurse* 1972; 3(4):12–17.

Kritek PB: Patient power and powerlessness. *Supervisor Nurse* 1981; 12(6):26–34.

Langer E, Rodin J: The effects of choice and enhanced personal responsibility for the aged: A field experiment in an institutionalized setting. *J Personality Soc Psychol* 1976; 34:191–203.

Lewin K: *The Conceptual Representation and the Measurement of Psychological Forces.* Duke University Press, 1938.

Lips HM: *Women, Men, and the Psychology of Power.* Prentice-Hall, 1981.

Liverant S, Scodel A: Internal and external control as determinants of discussion of decision making under conditions of risk. *Psychol Reproduction* 1960; 7:56–67.

May R: *Power and Innocence.* Norton, 1972.

McClelland DC: *Power: The Inner Experience.* Irvington, 1975.

McGregor DM: *The Human Side of Enterprise.* McGraw-Hill, 1960.

Miller JF: Concept development of powerlessness: A nursing diagnosis. Pages 37–57 in: *Coping with Chronic Illness: Overcoming Powerlessness.* Miller JF (editor). Davis, 1983.

Miller JF: Development and validation of a diagnostic label: Powerlessness. Pages 116–127 in: *Classification of Nursing Diag-*

noses: Proceedings of the Fifth National Conference. Kim MJ, McFarland GK, McLane AM (editors). Mosby, 1984.

Miller JF, Oertel CB: Powerlessness in the elderly: Preventing hopelessness. Pages 110-131 in: *Coping with Chronic Illness: Overcoming Powerlessness.* JF Miller (editor). Davis, 1983.

Nowakowski L: A new look at client advocacy. Pages 227-238 in: *Distributive Nursing Practice: A Systems Approach to Community Health.* Hall JE, Wearcer BR (editors). Lippincott, 1977.

Phares EJ: Expectancy changes in skill and chance situations. *J Abnormal Soc Psychol* 1957; 54:339-342.

Phares EJ: Perceptual threshold decrements as a function of skill and chance expectancies. *J Psychol* 1962; 53:399-417.

Reid D, Haas G, Hawkings D: Locus of desired control and positive self-concept of the elderly. *J Gerontol* 1977; 32:441-448.

The Republic. Translated by F.M. Cornforp. Oxford University Press, 1941.

Roberts SL: *Behavioral Concepts and the Critically Ill Patient.* Prentice-Hall, 1976.

Rotter JB: *Social Learning and Clinical Psychology.* Prentice-Hall, 1954.

Rotter JB: Generalized expectancies for internal versus external control of reinforcements. *Psycholog Monographs* 1966; 80:1-8.

Rotter JB: Some problems and misconceptions related to the construct of internal versus external control of reinforcement. *J Consult Clin Psychol* 1975; 43:56-63.

Rotter JB, Liverant S, Crowne DP: The growth and extinction of expectancies in chance controlled and skilled tasks. *J Psychol* 1961; 52:161-177.

Rotter JB, Mulry RC: Internal versus external control of reinforcement and decision time. *J Personality Soc Psychol* 1965; 2:598-604.

Rotter JB, Seeman M, Liverant S: Internal versus external control of reinforcements: A major variable in behavior theory. Pages 473-516 in: *Decisions, Values, and Groups II.* Washburne NF (editor). Pergamon Press, 1962.

Russell B: *Power.* Allen and Unwyn, 1938.

Ryckman RM, Rodda WC, Sherman MF: Locus of control and expertise relevance as determinants of change opinion about student activism. *J Soc Psychol* 1972; 88:107-114.

Seeman M: The meaning of alienation. *Am Sociolog Rev* 1959; 24:783-791.

Seeman M: Alienation and social learning in a reformatory. *Am J Sociol* 1963; 69:270-284.

Seeman M, Evans JW: Alienation and learning in a hospital setting. *Am Sociolog Rev* 1962; 27:772-783.

Storch JL: Nurse as consumer advocate. *AARN Newsletter* 1978; 34(1):12-15.

Tawney RH: *Equality.* Harcourt Brace Jovanovich, 1931.

Thollaug SC: The nurse as patient advocate. *Imprint* 1980; 27(5): 37, 58.

Wallston KA, Maides S, Wallston BS: Health related information seeking as a function of health related locus of control and health values. *J Res Personality* 1976a; 10:215-222.

Wallston BS et al: Development and validation of the health locus of control (HLC) scale. *J Consult Clin Psychol* 1976b; 44(4): 580-585.

Wilberding JZ: *Patient Advocacy as a Role for Staff Nurses: A Descriptive Study.* (Unpublished thesis.) The University of Iowa, Iowa City, IA, 1984.

Wilberding JZ: Values clarification. Pages 173-184 in: *Nursing Interventions: Treatments for Nursing Diagnoses.* Bulechek GM, McCloskey JC (editors). Saunders, 1985.

Winter DG: *The Power Motive.* Free Press, 1973.

Wu R: *Behavior and Illness.* Prentice-Hall, 1973.

Zeigler M, Reid D: Correlates of locus of desired control in two samples of elderly persons: Community residences and hospitalized patients. *J Consult Clin Psychol* 1979; 47:977-981.

Zerwekh J: Empowering the no longer patient. *Washington State J Nurs* (Summer/Autumn) 1983; 12-17.

38

Fear

DIANE CESARONE, MS, RN

THE INITIAL IDENTIFICATION OF FEAR AS A NURSING diagnosis occurred at the First National Conference on Classification of Nursing Diagnoses in 1973. Eight subcategories were also generated. Four of the subcategories represented what was called "functional fear," and four reflected "nonfunctional fear." Each of the four functional and nonfunctional fear subcategories was also qualified by degree, as mild, moderate, severe, or panic. This diagnostic formulation of fear persisted for 7 years.

At the 1982 Fifth National Conference on Nursing Diagnoses, Fear and Anxiety were separated into two distinct categories. Yocom (1984) emphasized that both Fear and Anxiety are separate nursing diagnoses, and further, are not symptoms of other diagnoses. The discussions of the Fifth National Conference also resulted in suggestions that there may be cultural differences related to fear and that fear must be distinguished from phobia. The work of Taylor-Loughran et al (1989) is an effort to differentiate these diagnoses using actual clinical data collected from patients in a tertiary care setting.

FEAR AND ANXIETY

It is necessary to distinguish between fear and anxiety in a discussion on nursing diagnosis. Jones and Jakob (1981) summarized the understandings of fear and anxiety represented in the literature into three major clusters. First, fear and anxiety are used as synonymous, interchangeable concepts. Second, fear and anxiety are distinctly different experiences. Lastly, fear and anxiety become ambiguous in the psychiatric diagnosis of anxiety neurosis, described as a fearful response to a discernible object.

Danesh (1977) described fear and anxiety as similar but different experiences. Yocom (1984) reviewed the literature defining fear and anxiety. Her report supported the notion of fear as a quick and often short-lived response to a specific, identifiable danger.

The common distinction made between fear and anxiety in both nursing and nonnursing literature is the ability to identify the etiologic agent of the fearful response and the inability to specify the cause of anxiety (Barry, 1984; Danesh, 1977; Jones and Jakob, 1981; White and Watt, 1973; Wilson and Kneisl, 1983; Yocom, 1984).

FEAR AND PHOBIA

Just as fear must be distinguished from anxiety, it also must be differentiated from phobia. True phobias are recognized as psychopathologic conditions. The *Diagnostic and Statistical Manual of Mental Disorders* (DSM III) (American Psychiatric Association, 1987;243) described the cardinal feature of simple phobic disorders as "persistent fear of a circumscribed stimulus (object or situation) other than fear of having a panic attack (as in Panic Disorder) or of humiliation or embarrassment in certain social situations (as in Social Phobia)." The phobic individual realizes the fearful response is disproportionately unreasonable in relation to the actual dangerousness of the threat. White and Watt (1973) asserted that a phobia is an irrational dread. This is in direct contrast to the normal fear response, the degree of which is consistent with the actual threat.

THEORETICAL DEFINITIONS OF FEAR: PROBLEM

The problem-etiology-signs/symptoms (P-E-S) system is used as a framework for a more specific discussion of fear as a nursing problem when providing care to the dependent elderly.

The accurate identification of the nursing problem is directly based on an understanding of the meaning of the specific nursing diagnosis. Various theoretical definitions of fear will be reviewed to facilitate a clear, consistent interpretation of the diagnostic concept. Three significant similarities may be noted among the reviewed descriptions of fear (Barry, 1984; Wilson and Kneisl, 1983; Yocom, 1984; White and Watt, 1973). First, fear is a response or reaction. Second, the stimulus for the fearful response is identifiable. Third, an actual and real threat or danger can be identified.

The description of fear presented by Jones and Jakob (1981;23) detailed the threat more clearly. According to them, fear is a "response of focused apprehension toward the presence of a recognized, usually external threat or danger to one's limb, autonomy, self image, or community with others." Krech et al (1974;271) identified fear as primary emotion. They stated that "the key factor for the onset of fear seems to be a lack of power or capability to handle a threatening situation. . . . Fear is induced by . . . feelings of powerlessness in the grip of overwhelming forces." These definitions suggest a focus for nursing assessment and exploration of etiologies in determining a diagnosis of fear.

Kim and Moritz (1982;290) presented the currently accepted nursing definition. "Fear is a feeling of dread related to an identifiable source which the person validates." Gordon (1982) agreed, but specified that the source of fear is perceived as a threat or danger to the self.

ETIOLOGIES/RELATED FACTORS

The origins of fear are potentially limitless. However, a review of the literature on fears of the elderly reveals a small body of information. Although not necessarily different from the fears of other people, the sources of fear in the elderly can be loosely clustered into five major categories. These possible etiologies of fear are presented in Table 38.1 and compared with the related factors proposed by the North American Nursing Diagnosis Association (NANDA) (Carroll-Johnson, 1989).

The fears of physical pain and suffering and incapacitating illness have been cited as occurring in the elderly (Copp, 1981; Eyde and Rich, 1983). These are closely related to fears of dependence, loss of control and becoming burdensome on family and loved ones. Psychologic fears of the elderly have been mentioned by a few writers (Brodie, 1978; Carter and Galliano, 1981; Castles and Murray, 1979; Copp, 1981; Eyde and Rich, 1983). Several authors have described a fear of dying or fears related to dying (Castles and Murray, 1979; Nolan, 1984; Spencer and Dorr, 1975; Williams, 1977). However, most often these fears of dying may be identified more realistically as fear of pain and suffering, fear of loneliness, fear of meaninglessness, fear of the unknown, and/or fear of abandonment. Using a medical model orientation, Roth (1978;557) suggested that "the psychopathology of old age appears to center ultimately on the fear of dying." Wass and Myers (1982) asserted that the aged are no more fearful of death than any other group of individuals, and that often the elderly seem to be less fearful of death than younger persons. Brodie (1978;70) stated "Contrary to the findings of other investigators, the 'most feared' items of retirees did not include death, which was noted as one of the 'least feared' items."

Brodie's (1978) research revealed that the elderly experienced fears related to social interaction and/or significant others. Fear of loss through death or injury of a loved one were disclosed, as was fear of speaking before a group. Carter and Galliano (1981) indicated that withdrawal and social isolation are defense mechanisms used by residents of long-term care facilities. These defenses address the social fears of abandonment and attachment.

The fear of crime and victimization among the elderly has been widely documented (Ebersole and Hess, 1985; Jeffords, 1983; Kennedy and Silverman, 1985; Lebowitz, 1975; Norton and Courlander, 1982; Pollack and Patterson, 1980; Sundeen and Mathieu, 1976). These fears have been studied in elderly who reside in the urban communities, and most often have been shown to be related to the community. It also has been shown that fears of crime and victimization can be reduced when proactive steps designed to increase the elderly individual's sense of security are taken. Closely related to the fear of victimization is the fear of transportation. Commuting (by any modality) places the elderly individual at increased risk for physical mishap and injury or crime (Ebersole and Hess, 1985).

Teri and Lewinsohn (1986) suggested that elderly people may experience a fear of change or disruption of

Table 38.1

Related Factors/Etiologies and Defining Characteristics

NANDA (CARROLL-JOHNSON)	CESARONE
Definition: Feeling of dread related to an identifiable source that the person validates	

NANDA (CARROLL-JOHNSON)

Definition: Feeling of dread related to an identifiable source that the person validates

CESARONE

Possible Etiologies/Sources of Fear in the Elderly

Fears related to the physical body:
   Fear of disease or illness; of pain; of prolonged suffering

Fears related to the psyche:
   Fear of abandonment; of attachment; of "becoming a burden"; of dependence; of failure to adapt; of incompetence; of loss; of "loss of control"; of mental illness

Fears related to dying:
   Fear of death; of loneliness; of meaninglessness; of punishment

Fear related to social interaction and significant others:
   Fear of illness or injury to loved ones; of death of a loved one; of speaking before a group

Other (miscellaneous) fears:
   Fear of change; of crime and victimization; of financial insecurity; of medical/psychiatric diagnostic tests; of transportation; of touch

Defining Characteristic

Ability to identify object of fear (NANDA) (Carroll-Johnson, 1989)*

Common Signs and Symptoms

Subjective Experiences
   Affective/cognitive responses
   Apprehension
   Decreased self-assurance
   Dread
   Expectation of danger to self
   Fright
   Impulsiveness
   Inability to concentrate
   Intense focus on the threat
   Nervousness
   Panic
   Tension
   Terror
Physical sensations
   Palpitations
   Sinking feeling in the pit of the stomach
   Tightness in the throat

Physiologic Responses (Indicate activation of the sympathetic nervous system)
Decreased gastrointestinal activity
Diaphoresis
Dry mouth
Increased blood pressure
Increased heart rate
Increased muscle tension
Increased respirations
Pupil dilation
Superficial vasoconstriction
Urinary frequency

Table 38.1

Related Factors/Etiologies and Defining Characteristics (*Continued*)

NANDA (CARROLL-JOHNSON)	CESARONE
	Behavioral Manifestations
	Avoidance or attack behavior
	Disorganization of speech
	Hand tremors
	Impairment of performance
	Increased alertness
	Increased quantity of verbalizations
	Increased questioning/information seeking
	Increased rate of verbalization
	Motor incoordination
	Narrowed or fixed focus of attention
	Physical flight
	Possible immobilization
	Restlessness
	Voice tremors/pitch changes

*To date, NANDA has developed a definition and one defining characteristic for the nursing diagnosis Fear, but no related factors have been identified (Carroll-Johnson, 1989).

regular routines. Fear of diagnostic tests, especially mental status exams, was also cited. This fear perhaps may be labeled more accurately as a fear of being unhealthy or mentally incompetent or being sent to a nursing home. Copp (1981) suggested that financial fears may be a serious concern for the elderly. Ebersole and Hess (1985) suggested that the institutionalized elderly may be fearful of invasive touching by nurses and other caregivers.

Clearly, it is possible for an elderly individual to be frightened of almost any object or experience that potentially poses a threat. In order to identify the existence of fear, the nurse must know the signs and symptoms that represent it.

DEFINING CHARACTERISTICS

Graham and Conley (1971) stated that both anxiety and fear are accompanied by similar physiologic changes and present in nearly identical ways in a given individual. Wilson and Kneisl (1983;350) indicated that the "experience of fear is inferred from three kinds of data." These data include (1) reports of subjective experiences; (2) physiologic responses representing the activation of the sympathetic nervous system; and (3) observable behavioral manifestations. Gordon (1982) provided a list of defining characteristics for fear. Included in Table 38.1 are the most common assessable signs and symptoms of fear and the NANDA (Carroll-Johnson, 1989) defining characteristic.

The application of Fear as a nursing diagnostic concept that may be used purposefully in clinical nursing practice requires a clear understanding of the problem

(what fear is), an awareness of the signs and symptoms that may indicate the affective occurrence of fear, and the ability to determine the likely etiology or source of the fear. The process of applying the nursing diagnosis formulation requires a multileveled assessment. The nurse must inquire about the elderly client's subjective experiences and must also observe the physiologic behavioral manifestations of the affective state. The assessment must seek to identify the source of the fear. Evaluation of the elderly individual's current life experiences is necessary to hypothesize a fear etiology, since there are no critical signs and symptoms that are universally related to a specific fear-provoking stimulus. Assessment of fear may be successfully accomplished by direct observation and questioning, by indirect measurement of changing physiologic states, or through the use of formal assessment tools.

ASSESSMENT

No formalized nursing assessment tools for the measurement of fear exist at this time. Even in the behavioral science literature, it is not possible to identify a current measure commonly used for fear assessment. Nowhere was there found a fear assessment tool that had real practical clinical relevance for a population of elderly individuals, as most research has used young adult samples. The following review discusses measures of fear that nurses might find useful for the assessment of fear of elderly persons and that should be considered for clinical testing with an elderly population.

Geer (1965) developed the Fear Survey Schedule II, which was patterned after the fear assessment tool developed by Akutagawa (1956). Although Geer (1965;45) reported adequate reliability and validity for the instrument, he acknowledged that his scale was designed primarily for use as a research tool.

Wolpe and Lange (1964) described the Fear Survey Schedule III, which they designed for clinical applications. It is a 72-item measure that the authors suggest is useful in the provision of behavior therapy. They do not indicate how useful it might be in assessing developmentally related fears.

Skidmore (1976) attempted to differentiate "normal" fears from phobic fears. He reported significantly different results on his fear assessment tool between psychiatric and nonpsychiatric samples. Unfortunately, although the author provided a general description of the fear questionnaire, the measure itself and the age range of subjects was not published.

Spiegler and Liebert (1970) presented the only report of assessment of fear in a sample that included senior citizens (age 60 to 85). These researchers used the Fear Survey Schedule III, which assesses primarily unrealistic fears, and a 67-item Supplementary Fear Questionnaire, which they developed. Their results indicated that older men reported themselves to be more fearful than younger adult men and than women of their own age.

Eyde and Rich (1983) described an Affect Abilities Checklist, which is an indirect measure used to assess the ability of the older adult to understand fear as an emotion and to be able to identify various indicators of fear in others, as well as in self.

Although a few fear assessment tools are available, they have little, if any, real application for an institutionalized elderly population. The best approach is multimodal, done by caregivers using direct questions as well as observations of behavioral, physiologic and affective responses.

CASE STUDY

Fear Experienced by an Institutionalized Elder

Mr. and Mrs. R have been married for 56 years. Mr. R is 78 years old and Mrs. R is 74 years old. Two months ago, Mrs. R developed incapacitating physical problems that resulted in her being admitted to a local nursing home. Mr. R tried to visit her regularly, but because he refused to use public transportation, he had to rely on his son to take him to visit his wife. Just recently his son made a job change requiring him to move to another part of the country. Because he would no longer be available to assist his elderly father, the son had Mr. R admitted to the same nursing home in which Mrs. R resides.

Though usually pleasant, Mr. R has seemed upset and angry since coming to live at the long-term care facility. He continuously expresses worry about his wife's condition and once confided in a nurse his own concern about becoming physically or mentally disabled. His son has not contacted him since Mr. R was admitted, and whenever asked about his son Mr. R replies, "Him? Oh, he's the one who forgot about me." A niece calls him frequently and has come to visit, but Mr. R says, "She's a nice girl, very respectful, but I don't want to count on her too much. You know, you just can't tell when she'll lose interest in an old man." Although Mr. R appears to be adjusting to life in the facility, he complained to a coresident, "It's so different living here than at home. I don't think I'll ever get used to it here. And living here costs so much. I never planned for things to happen like this. How do you keep paying?"

Though Mr. R is physically stable, alert, and oriented, and is nearly totally independent in all activities of daily living, he appears nervous and tense and has spells of heart palpitations and urinary frequency that the physician has said have no physiologic cause. The nurse has assessed Mr. R as having several fears of various etiologies. Table 38.2 shows the nursing care plan that was developed for him.

CASE STUDY

Fear Experienced by an Independently Living Elder

Mrs. J is 68 years of age and has been widowed for 5 years. Although Mrs. J has no children, several other widows about her age, including her sister-in-law, live in the same inner-city apartment dwelling and keep an eye on one another. During the past year, however, two widows have died and the apartment dwelling has fallen into the hands of a landlord who is letting the building get very rundown (eg, broken windows and mice). The death of her friends and husband and the decline of her home are daily reminders of her own imminent death, the powerlessness she feels to do anything about the apartment house, and the greater loneliness she can anticipate as more and more losses occur for her.

Mrs. J has had diabetes and hypertension for 10 years, sees a nurse practitioner in an outpatient clinic in a large health care facility regularly, and has been able to control both chronic diseases successfully with diet and medication. In addition to compliance with diet and medication regimens, Mrs. J has always been active and continues to try to walk regularly. A large number of plants in her apartment to tend and lunch daily with at least one of the widows in her social group keep Mrs. J active mentally. Lately, however, Mrs. J's walking has been greatly curtailed, as have her visits to the nurse practitioner, because she and her friends feel unsafe in the neighborhood.

Table 38.2

Care Plan for Mr. R

NURSING DIAGNOSIS, ETIOLOGY, SIGNS AND SYMPTOMS	GOALS:EXPECTED OUTCOMES	INTERVENTIONS
Fear of Mrs. R's death related to her deteriorating physical condition • increased focus on her condition and bodily state • frequent questioning and discussion of her health status, with *all* caregivers • hand tremors, stuttering, and very rapid speech when discussing his wife	Mr. R will express his feelings about his wife's deteriorating condition He will evidence increasing awareness of the ultimate outcome of her illness	Encourage the ventilation of feelings to provide emotional release Facilitate Mr. R's realistic awareness of his wife's impending death by responding to questions as clearly as possible Be truthful about the prognosis for Mrs. R but don't push for acceptance of her death. Allow Mr. R to "pace himself"
Fear of illness and suffering related to his own advancing age and observation of his wife's sickness • intense focus on bodily sensations as indicators of illness • increased questioning of the meaning of different bodily sensations • expressions of apprehension about his "failing health" • verbalizations indicating decreasing self-assurance and self-competence related to taking care of himself	Mr. R will voice his concerns about his own health He will continue to maintain a health-promoting lifestyle He will verbalize less fearfulness about his health	Allow Mr. R to ventilate his fears of deteriorating health Provide validation of his feelings, but reality test with him. Advise him that his current health status is very good; remind him he has no degenerative conditions Encourage him to continue to take good care of himself
Fear of abandonment related to institutionalization and lack of contact from son • complaints of heart palpitations and tightness of throat when talking about his son • facial flushing, rapid speech, and tremors when talking about his son	Mr. R will express his feelings Mr. R will discuss a plan of action that allows him some control and reduces his feelings of being powerless and victimized	Encourage the expression of feelings Assist Mr. R to identify ways of dealing with this issue. Suggest alternatives, if necessary: • Mr. R can call his son • Mr. R can write his son • Mr. R can have social service contact his son
Fear of attachment to niece related to history of perceived abandonment by son • avoidance behavior when niece calls or visits	Mr. R will visit with his niece and will speak with her on the phone	Reality test with Mr. R: Remind him that his niece is freely and willingly coming to see him, that she *wants* to see him Encourage him to visit with her and to express his fears of getting close and then being abandoned by her Continue to provide emotional support
Fear of change related to totally new living arrangements and lifestyle • attention focused on how different his life is at the long-term care facility • difficulty concentrating on current situation; focused on past	Mr. R will become familiar with his new environment and express feelings of increasing satisfaction and control Amount of comparison between present and past living arrangements will begin to decrease	Allow Mr. R to express his feelings Engage him in the long-term care facility's orientation for new residents Consult with Activity Therapy, who may assist him to continue with some of his former interests Encourage the development of new friendships at the facility Suggest that Mr. R make his room more homelike with pictures, etc Encourage him to identify some positive things about his new home and living arrangements

(Continues)

Table 38.2

Care Plan for Mr. R (*Continued*)

NURSING DIAGNOSIS, ETIOLOGY, SIGNS AND SYMPTOMS	GOALS:EXPECTED OUTCOMES	INTERVENTIONS
Fear of financial insecurity related to the unplanned for costs of nursing home living for Mr. R and his wife • frequent focus of discussions with coresidents on money • many questions about the cost of care, supplies, etc • increasing agitation with accompanying increase in vital signs (BP, P, R) when discussing money	Mr. R will discuss his financial concerns with the Social Services Department He will develop a plan for financial maintenance with which he can be satisfied His focus on money will become less frequent	Be empathic to Mr. R's concerns Contact the Social Services Department; ask them to discuss with Mr. R his financial situation and assist him to develop a realistic financial plan
Fear of loss of autonomy/control • expressed worry about wife • expression that son has forgotten him • somatic symptoms	Mr. R will make all decisions about his own care, activities, and financial matters	Nurse should advocate for Mr. R and support him to make decisions about his care and finances

A Social Security check of just less than $300 limits the number of activities that can be sought outside of the apartment house. The fact that her friends and her past are in the neighborhood she has always lived in and loved makes moving, or "flight" from the identifiable source of her fear, an option she does not wish to consider. Meanwhile, Mrs. J attempts to maintain the way of life she has adapted to in the last 10 years despite the feelings of dread, apprehension, and decreased self-assurance she experiences in her apartment and in her "old" neighborhood.

NURSING INTERVENTIONS

Whether intervening with the elderly in institutions or with the elderly living independently at home, "effective care of the fearful client involves identification of the type of etiological factors" (Jones and Jakob, 1981;27). Two broad goals of nursing interventions for fearful individuals are (1) reduce or extinguish the source of fear, and (2) increase coping abilities. The immediate intervention should focus on reducing the affective response, the fear, unless fear is an appropriate response to a threatening stimulus. Additional nursing interventions should promote insight and the development of new styles of problem resolution. The elderly individual's repertoire of coping skills should be increased.

Several intervention strategies for the nursing problem of fear in the elderly have been suggested. Interventions must be based on a comprehensive, individual assessment that includes an evaluation of the elderly individual's usual coping mechanisms. Shipley (1977;86), using principles of classical conditioning, asserted that regardless of the etiology of the fear it "can be reduced or extinguished through repeated or extended exposure to the eliciting conditional stimulus in the absence of any painful event." This individual learns new or different responses (other than fear). Jones and Jakob (1981) also recommended the use of stimulus exposure to reduce fear, citing the preoperative preparation of surgical patients as an example of a nursing application of this principle.

Burke (1982) suggested the value of learning theory as a nursing intervention strategy. She emphasized that by pairing exposure to the fear stimulus with pleasant outcomes the fear can be extinguished. This method is similar to that described by Shipley (1977), but carries it one step further by providing a positive experience in relation to the original fear-provoking stimulus.

General educational interventions that realistically address the fearful response and encourage other reality-based responses may result in an increased sense of personal control and options in the elderly individual. This would culminate logically in a reduction of fear.

Wilson and Kneisl (1983) listed several coping strategies for stress reduction. Some are pertinent as intervention techniques for fear reduction as well. Reliance on self-discipline, personal bravery, or stoicism may make the fearful response manageable by increasing the individual's sense of personal control and capability. Avoidance of or withdrawal from the fear-triggering stimulus also may prove an effective way of dealing with fear in which the etiology is well known and fairly concrete. Likewise, removal of the source of fear, if possible, is an effective intervention approach. Finally, "talking therapy," including clarification and ventilation of feelings, and identification of alternative responses can result in increased insight and new coping styles, simultaneously reducing fearful responses.

OUTCOMES

Whatever intervention strategy may be used, the expected outcomes, or nursing goals, are essentially the same. At least four primary goals can be enumerated. First, fear will be decreased or totally extinguished, and the source of fear will be eliminated, if possible. Second, the elderly individual will develop new coping mechanisms. Third, an increased sense of competency and personal control will emerge. Fourth, new insights and awarenesses will occur. The culmination of the intervention process occurs with evaluation, for it is at this time that the effectiveness of the nursing care is determined. If a formalized assessment tool, such as the Fear Survey Schedule III or some other measure, was used, the assessment can be repeated following the nursing interventions. It would be expected that less fear would be demonstrated on this posttest. Evaluation also includes an assessment for the remission of the subjective and objective indicators of fear. The nurse should look for all the original signs and symptoms that led to the nursing diagnosis of Fear. If the interventions were successful, a reduction in the quantity and quality of these indicators of fear should be found. Finally, a determination of the degree of accomplishment of goals must be made. Successful intervention would evidence itself in accomplishment of goals.

SUMMARY

Fear is an accepted nursing diagnosis. Although there is little documentation about its clinical presentation or measurement in the nursing literature, it is a client problem that every gerontologic nurse will confront. The elderly in the community and in institutions are susceptible to many fears of varying etiologies. The nurse who provides care to older adults must be conscious of fear as a potential nursing diagnosis for clients, must be aware of the definition and defining characteristics of fear, must be familiar with its common etiologies, and must be able to assess its clinical occurrence and intervene effectively. Fear is a very real problem and often is an appropriate nursing diagnosis for the dependent elderly.

References

Akutagawa D: A study in construct validity of the psychoanalytic concept of latent anxiety and test of a projection distance hypothesis. (Unpublished doctoral dissertation.) University of Pittsburgh, 1956.

American Psychiatric Association: *Diagnostic and Statistical Manual of Mental Disorders*: DSM III, 3d ed. (Revised.) Washington, DC: American Psychiatric Association, 1987.

Barry PD: *Psychosocial Nursing: Assessment and Intervention*. Lippincott, 1984.

Brodie JN: Social behavior of the elderly: Effects of fearfulness and perceived locus of control. *Issues Ment Health Nurs* 1978; 1: 64–75.

Burke SO: A developmental perspective on the nursing diagnosis of fear and anxiety. *Nurs Papers* 1982; 14:59–64.

Carroll-Johnson R (editor): *Classification of Nursing Diagnoses: Proceedings of the Eighth Conference*. Lippincott, 1989.

Carter C, Galliano D: Fear and loss of attachments: A major dynamic in the social isolation of the institutionalized elderly. *J Gerontol Nurs* 1981; 7:342–349.

Castles MR, Murray RB: *Dying in an Institution: Nurse/Patient Perspectives*. Appleton-Century-Crofts, 1979.

Copp LA (editor): *Care of the Aging*. Churchill-Livingstone, 1981.

Danesh HB: Anger and fear. *Am J Psychiatry* 1977; 134: 1109–1112.

Ebersole P, Hess P: *Toward Healthy Aging: Human Needs and Nursing Response*. Mosby, 1985.

Eyde DR, Rich JA: *Psychological Distress in Aging*. Aspen, 1983.

Geer JH: The development of a scale to measure fear. *Behav Res Ther* 1965; 3:45–53.

Gordon M: *Manual of Nursing Diagnosis*. McGraw-Hill, 1982.

Graham LE, Conley EM: Evaluation of anxiety and fear in adult surgical patients. *Nurs Res* 1971; 20:113–122.

Jeffords CR: The situational relationship between age and the fear of crime. *Internat J Aging Human Devel* 1983; 17:103–111.

Jones P, Jakob DF: Nursing diagnosis: Differentiating fear and anxiety. *Nurs Papers* 1981; 13(4):20–29.

Kennedy LW, Silverman RA: Significant others and fear of crime among the elderly. *Internat J Aging Human Devel* 1985; 20:241–256.

Kim MJ, McFarland GK, McLane AM: *Pocket Guide to Nursing Diagnoses*, 2d ed. Mosby, 1987.

Kim MJ, Moritz DA (editors): *Classification of Nursing Diagnoses: Proceedings of the Third and Fourth National Conferences*. McGraw-Hill, 1982.

Krech D, Crutchfield RS, Livson N: *Elements of Psychology*. Knopf, 1974.

Lebowitz BD: Age and fearfulness: Personal and situational factors. *J Gerontol* 1975; 30:696–700.

McLane A (editor): *Classification of Nursing Diagnoses: Proceedings of the Seventh Conference*. Mosby, 1987.

Nolan TF: Thanatological counseling of adults and their families. Pages 365–375 in: *The American Handbook of Psychiatric Nursing*. Lego S (editor). Lippincott, 1984.

Norton L, Courlander M: Fear of crime among the elderly: The role of crime prevention programs. *Gerontologist* 1982; 22: 388–393.

Pollack LM, Patterson AH: Territoriality and fear of crime in elderly and nonelderly homeowners. *J Soc Psychol* 1980; 111: 119–129.

Roth N: Fear of death in the aging. *Am J Psychother* 1978; 32: 552–560.

Shipley RH: Applying learning theory to nursing practice. *Nurs Forum* 1977; 16:83–94.

Skidmore D: Measuring fear. *Nurs Mirror* 1976; 143:68–69.

Spencer MG, Dorr CJ: *Understanding Aging: A Multidisciplinary Approach.* Appleton-Century-Crofts, 1975.

Spiegler MD, Liebert RM: Some correlates of self-reported fear. *Psycholog Rep* 1970; 26:691–695.

Sundeen RA, Mathieu JT: The fear of crime and its consequences among elderly in three urban communities. *Gerontologist* 1976; 16:211–219.

Taylor-Loughran AE et al: Defining characteristics of the nursing diagnoses Fear and Anxiety: A validation study. *Applied Nurs Res* 1989; 2(4):178–186.

Teri L, Lewinsohn PM: *Geropsychological Assessment and Treatment.* Springer, 1986.

Wass H, Myers JE: Psychosocial aspects of death among the elderly: A review of the literature. *Personnel Guidance J* 1982; 61:131–137.

White RW, Watt NF: *The Abnormal Personality.* Ronald Press, 1973.

Williams JC: Allaying common fears. Pages 27–32 in: *Dealing with Death and Dying: Nursing Skillbook.* Chaney PS (editor). Intermed Communications, 1977.

Wilson HS, Kneisl CR: *Psychiatric Nursing.* Addison-Wesley, 1983.

Wolpe J, Lange PJ: A fear survey schedule for use in behaviour therapy. *Behav Res Ther* 1964; 2:27–30.

Yocom C: The differentiation of fear and anxiety. Pages 352–355 in: *Classification of Nursing Diagnoses: Proceedings of the Fifth National Conference.* Kim MJ, McFarland GK, McLane A (editors). Mosby, 1984.

39

Anxiety

CONNIE HIGGINS VOGEL, PhD, MA, RN

ANXIETY IS PREVALENT IN ALL AGE GROUPS AND IN A variety of situations. Some authors suggest that anxiety is an ontologic characteristic of life (May, 1982), whereas others identify anxiety as a diagnosable and treatable disorder (Runck, 1984). As a treatable disorder, anxiety is frequently confused with depression (Ayd, 1984) and often accompanies physical disease. As an existential feeling state, it is the topic for discussion by a wide variety of poets and philosophers with a focus on the awareness that one's existence is threatened (May, 1982). None of these ideas are incorrect or even in conflict with each other. For the elderly, in particular, all of these perspectives can be at least partially true and need to be recognized in any meaningful discussion of anxiety among the elderly.

Signs of anxiety are more prevalent among elderly persons than in other age groups and are often expressed through somatic and cognitive symptoms (Conlin and Fennell, 1985). Sallis and Lichstein (1982) report that chronic anxiety is found in 10% of the elderly and that 20% take prescribed anti-anxiety drugs. The elderly are seen as being at risk for depression and anxiety because of disease states, living situations, and beliefs about locus of control (Conlin and Fennell, 1985). Other factors to be considered in a discussion of anxiety among any age group are state and trait anxiety, death anxiety, and differentiation between anxiety and fear (see Chapter 38 on Fear for a discussion of anxiety versus fear).

STATE AND TRAIT ANXIETY

There is often confusion between anxiety as an emotional state and habitual anxiousness or a tendency toward being anxious. State anxiety is characterized by feelings of apprehension and tension and by increased autonomic nervous system activity such as increased heart rate. State anxiety is situational or transient in nature. Trait anxiety is a more firmly entrenched personality characteristic that becomes pronounced when the self-concept of the person is threatened and is often expressed as a particular behavioral pattern (Gomez et al, 1984). Both state anxiety and trait anxiety may be found in the elderly client. Trait anxiety is most often a long-standing character trait, whereas state anxiety may occur in response to environmental or personal stress.

Several tools are available for measurement of state and trait anxiety. The Speilberger State–Trait Anxiety Scale is currently in wide circulation. Although a well-established tool for psychologic assessment, this test is problematic for use with older individuals. In many older individuals as well as others, test anxiety may affect results. This tool also requires specialized training for administration and interpretation, thus limiting its usefulness in nursing assessment (Spielberger, 1975).

Death Anxiety

Although the findings are mixed on the pervasiveness of death anxiety among the elderly, many authors suggest that death anxiety among the elderly is related to the degree the elderly feel their lives are meaningful (de Beauvoir, 1972). Factors to be considered in assessing death anxiety are health, social support, and place of residence. A study by Mullins and Lopez (1982) found that older nursing home residents had higher death anxiety than younger individuals. They also reported that those with poorer functional health, fewer social supports, and longer periods as nursing home residents experienced more anxiety about death. However, Mullins and Lopez (1982) concluded that the elderly, whether institutionalized or not, should be considered a heterogeneous group when examining death anxiety. Death anxiety is present in all individuals as the existential threat to self, but among the elderly, a variety of factors, such as poor health and loss of financial and family supports, may significantly raise the level of conscious death anxiety.

Fear and Anxiety

May (1982) identifies anxiety as characterized by feelings of powerlessness and helplessness that may overcome coping skills and paralyze the individual. He clarifies the difference between fear and anxiety by specifying fear as objective; a specific person or thing is perceived as a threat. Anxiety is a subjective, objectless experience where no specific person or object is perceived as threatening (see Chapter 38 on Fear for further discussion of anxiety versus fear). The intensity and duration of the reaction to anxiety is determined both by the amount of threat perceived and by the duration (Yocom, 1984).

Nursing has had some difficulty deciding the place of Anxiety as a nursing diagnosis, but Jones and Jakob (1984) argue quite persuasively for the addition of Anxiety as a separate diagnosis based on the differentiation of anxiety and fear. Their proposed definition of anxiety is as follows:

> *A vague, uneasy sense of worry and nervousness, anguish or marked ambivalence. The client appears not to have yet expressed the underlying feelings involved, such as fear, grief, conflict, insecurity. . . . Contributing factors may be impaired communication, knowledge deficit, separation from significant other especially a caretaker, ineffective coping, interpersonal transmission, as well as underlying grief, conflict or insecurity (Jones and Jakob, 1984;289).*

ASSESSMENT

Our knowledge of the impact of anxiety on the aged is limited, and caution should be taken in generalizing their responses to anxiety. It is possible that older persons may manifest anxiety in ways that are quite different from the ways manifested by the young. Eisdorfer and colleagues (1981) recommend consideration of three areas in anxiety assessment: (1) overt behavior as reflected in avoidance and inability to make decisions; (2) subjective reports of anxiety; and (3) physiologic manifestations of a state of anxiety, such as increased heart rate, perspiration, and tension. These same three areas are also stressed by Runck (1984), who points out that these responses are only loosely linked and that an intervention may alleviate one area of anxiety while the others are left unchanged. Other authors (Turnbull and Turnbull, 1985) agree that anxiety disturbances may present either as the subjective experiences of worry and nervousness or as somatic symptoms.

In the elderly, a careful assessment process is crucial because of the difficulty of separating subjective complaints of anxiety from depression. It is also often difficult to separate somatic complaints related to anxiety from physical complaints. This is particularly true in the elderly client, who may have numerous preexisting physical problems.

Prompt recognition and intervention in anxiety disorders in the elderly helps to avoid what is sometimes described as the "vicious cycle of anxiety, depression, physical illnesses and other stresses" (Verwoerdt, 1981). Another important aspect of the vicious cycle is the feelings of helplessness that develop in the elderly client, family, and caretaker as anxiety exacerbates physical problems, psychosocial difficulties, and problems in interpersonal relationships (Vogel, 1982).

Two instruments developed by Zung (1971) meet the criteria of being easily administered and interpreted. The Anxiety States Inventory is a 20-item scale covering both affective and somatic complaints. The estimated length of time needed to administer this scale in an interview format is 10 minutes. The Self-Rating Anxiety Scale (SAS) is based on the same 20 items and can be answered by elderly clients responding to how each item on the scale has applied to them in the past week (Zung, 1971).

ANXIETY IN THE ELDERLY

A basic understanding of the dynamics of anxiety is helpful in assessment and in development of a plan to break the cycle. Situations that are not stress producing in other individuals may be stressful for the elderly because of their different perspective and reduced confidence in their abilities to manage particular events. A certain amount of energy is required to cope with anxiety-producing situations, which may further compromise the elderly. The need for increased energy to deal with more frequently occurring anxieties may coincide with decreasing mental and physical energies as a function of the aging process.

All individuals develop unique coping strategies for managing anxiety in the environment (Vogel, 1982). Some of these strategies may be maladaptive but may have worked because of the support of other individuals. A classic example is the older woman who succeeded in getting indulgences from her husband by shedding a few tears. Now, following the death of her spouse, she must deal with her daughters who are less tolerant of "Mama's hysterics." Other coping strategies that may have been effective and healthy for the individual throughout his or her lifetime are no longer feasible because of age-related changes.

ETIOLOGIES/RELATED FACTORS

The etiologies and defining characteristics of anxiety assist in appropriate goal setting and intervention for the elderly client. For the purpose of considering anxiety in the context of the elderly client, it is recommended that the source of anxiety be identified as the etiology. Based on the definition of anxiety presented earlier (Jones and Jakob, 1982) and the discussion of sources of anxiety that follows, the etiologies listed in Table 39.1 are suggested as most applicable to the elderly. Table 39.1 compares etiologies based on the previous discussion with those etiologies recommended by the North American Nursing Diagnosis Association (NANDA) (Carroll-Johnson, 1989).

DEFINING CHARACTERISTICS

Defining characteristics must also be specified to clarify the existence of a nursing diagnosis of Anxiety. The focus of defining characteristics of anxiety in the elderly client should be on the areas identified by Eisdorfer et al (1981). Defining characteristics using this format are contrasted with those suggested by NANDA in Table 39.2.

It is apparent in examining this suggested list of defining criteria that a combination of factors is necessary to substantiate a nursing diagnosis of Anxiety for the elderly client. It is also clear that care must be taken in the assessment process to avoid misdiagnosis and to determine adequately the role of particular defining characteristics in the overall picture. This may be particularly true in the case of physical symptoms of anxiety, such as increased heart rate, that may exacerbate an already preexisting condition. For the elderly client who does not have a preexisting condition, the symptom may be the first sign of an organic problem. Physical assessment skills are crucial in determining the presence of the defining characteristics of a nursing diagnosis of Anxiety in the elderly client, and top priority should be given to a thorough examination of the source of all physical complaints. Physical characteristics, however, cannot be considered alone and must be assessed in combination with subjective symptoms.

Subjective symptoms in any population are difficult to specify, and in the elderly, attention should be given to any significant change in behavior. Such changes should prompt the nurse to consider the possibility of a diagnosis of Anxiety. The case of Mrs. N (see the case study) is an example of the behavioral change being a clue to the problems of anxiety that were developing, with the first clue being that a normally active and alert woman showed

Table 39.1

Related Factors/Etiologies of Anxiety

VOGEL	NANDA ETIOLOGIES (CARROLL-JOHNSON, 1989)
Loss of objects	Unconscious conflict about essential values and goals of life
Loss of external supplies	
Loss of support systems	Threat to self-concept
	Threat of death
	Threat to or change in health status
Loss of sensory function	Threat to or change in environment
Loss of social control	Threat to or change in role functioning
	Threat to or change in interaction patterns
Fear of losses due to the aging process; maladaptive coping strategies	Situational and maturational crises
	Interpersonal transmission and contagion
Declining mental and/or physical abilities; cognitive impairment	Unmet needs

Table 39.2

Defining Characteristics of Anxiety

VOGEL	NANDA CHARACTERISTICS (CARROLL-JOHNSON, 1989)
Pacing	*Subjective*
Hand wringing	Increased tension
Tics or tremors	Apprehension
Repetitive actions, such as twisting or rubbing	Increased helplessness
Elevated blood pressure	Uncertainty
Elevated pulse rate	Fearful
Muscle tension	Scared
Headache	Feelings of inadequacy
Sleeplessness	Shakiness
Facial flushing	Fear of unspecific consequence
	Regretful
Subjective statements such as, "I feel nervous"	Overexcited
Aggressiveness	Rattled
Disturbing dreams	Distressed
Crying	Jittery
Avoidance of decision-making situations and inability to make decisions	*Objective*
Memory impairment	*Sympathetic stimulation—cardiovascular excitation, superficial vasoconstriction, pupil dilation
Inability to focus on content	Restlessness
Obsession with physical complaints	Insomnia
	Glancing about
	Poor eye contact
	Trembling; hand tremors
	Extraneous movements—foot shuffling; hand, arm movements
	Expressed concern regarding changes in life events
	Worried
	Anxious
	Facial tension
	Voice quivering
	Focus on self
	Increased wariness
	Increased perspiration

*Critical defining characteristic.

little response to the offer to buy her home. This was followed by a cessation of usual activities and avoidance of interactions outside her home. Although these changes alone are not enough to indicate a nursing diagnosis of Anxiety, they are sufficient to alert the examiner to the emergence of a problem. Table 39.3 illustrates the process used to arrive at a nursing diagnosis of Anxiety for the elderly client, differentiated from depression, fear, and physical problems.

Framework for Identifying Types of Anxiety

Anxiety as a nursing diagnosis among the elderly requires that efforts be focused toward identifying the

most likely point for intervention. The potential for serious, long-term harm to the elderly client is too great to ignore the value of early and meaningful identification of the source of the anxiety. An effective classification system by Verwoerdt (1981) denotes anxiety in the elderly according to source. The use of this format for identifying types of the nursing diagnosis Anxiety can provide clear implications for nursing interventions.

Depletion Anxiety Depletion anxiety relates to loss of objects and/or external supplies in the environment. Depletion anxiety may be related to grief over the loss of a spouse and/or family members, but may also be seen in any actual or threatened environmental change (Verwoerdt, 1981). Environmental changes may, in addition to

Table 39.3

Differential Diagnosis

SIGNS AND SYMPTOMS	DIAGNOSES RULED OUT	DATA NEEDED
Headache, facial flushing, pacing, hand wringing	Preexisting physical problems	Pulse rate
Obsession with physical complaints, sleeplessness, and disturbing dreams	Depression	Mental status
Verbal complaints of nervousness and muscle tension		
Verbal complaints of dread or apprehension	Fear	Client's awareness and identification of specific source of feelings

increasing anxiety, precipitate or increase depression in the elderly. Increased anxiety may occur from unfamiliarity and variance in favorite rituals resulting from changes in structure (Vogel, 1982). The effect of depletion anxiety is to increase the workload on the body of the elderly person. Among those elderly with impaired physical functioning, there is potential for worsening of problems because of the expenditure of energy associated with increased stress.

CASE STUDY

Depletion Anxiety

Mrs. N was a 78-year-old woman who continued to live alone in her two-bedroom home in the same neighborhood where she had lived with her husband for 40 years. Mr. N died 10 years ago, and Mrs. N's married children, who no longer lived in the community, spoke with pride of their mother's independence and involvement in church and senior citizen activities. The city, determined to build a new recreation facility in the block where Mrs. N lived, offered to purchase her home for a good price. Her children were pleased because they felt this would give their mother an opportunity to live in an apartment, which would be easier to care for. Mrs. N showed little reaction to the offer, although she stopped going to church and was rarely seen outside. Finally, when she did not answer her phone, her children came to see her. They found her unkempt and visibly agitated. They took her to a physician, who found that her pulse and blood pressure were alarmingly elevated. The doctor recognized her anxiety and prescribed an anti-anxiety agent, warning the relatives that this was a temporary measure and that more long-lasting solutions for their mother's anxiety would have to be found.

Helplessness/Powerlessness Anxiety may also be associated with helplessness or powerlessness due to loss of control (Verwoerdt, 1981). Declining physical abilities and loss of sensory functioning may be a major source of anxiety associated with helplessness. In some cases, it is not the actual helplessness that produces anxiety, but a distinct fear of helplessness and powerlessness that occurs with the aging process. Elderly persons often are anxious about actual or potential inabilities to take care of themselves and their affairs, which also makes them less influential over matters that are likely to affect the quality of their lives (see Chapter 37 on Powerlessness).

The loss of physical control is often accompanied by a loss of social kinds of control: Families often make decisions without consulting the older person, or someone else may control finances and property. Older individuals realize they are dependent on others for many of the things that they were very much in charge of a few years earlier. The elderly may feel ashamed of this increased dependency, which affects their self-image. Further, as the image of self as a worthwhile person decreases, feelings of depression may increase. The elderly may also feel shame about declining faculties that are part of the aging process. To those of us in the helping professions, this shame may seem unnecessary, but it must be remembered that older persons may have a different cultural orientation to needing help from others than persons from a generation that accepts "needing a little help from our friends" as a usual part of life (Vogel, 1982).

CASE STUDY

Helplessness-Associated Anxiety

Mrs. W was a capable 72-year-old woman who had experienced no major problems in her declining years until she underwent cataract surgery. Initially, she appeared to be making an excellent recovery, and after spending the first 2 weeks postsurgery at her daughter's home, she returned to her own home some 150 miles away. Late the following week, her daughter called and was surprised to hear her mother's tearful responses. Mrs. W's daughter drove to her mother's home and found her mother's sight was again deteriorating. She was tearful and pacing and repeatedly stated she was going blind. Her anxiety increased until the next day when her daughter took her to visit the eye surgeon. The problem was found and corrected. As Mrs. W's vision returned, so did her usual calm, rational approach to life. Her anxiety was associated with the loss of control and helplessness she experienced when her sight again became impaired.

Chronic Neurotic Anxiety   Chronic neurotic anxiety in the elderly is a manifestation of a basic personality pattern established in young adult years that continues throughout the life span. With aging, the psychodynamics become less important, but the patterns of behavior they have produced are now long standing. The elderly client with chronic neurotic anxiety experiences tension, stress, and often depression without insight into its source (Verwoerdt, 1981). With this type of anxiety, symptoms usually predominate and are often complicated by organic changes and other chronic illnesses that occur as part of the aging process. Persistent physical complaints must be evaluated to determine the need for treatment. Beyond that, a matter-of-fact approach is usually most helpful, by not giving undue attention to the complaints.

The population that experiences chronic neurotic anxiety has failed early in life to develop adequate mechanisms for dealing with everyday stress and anxiety in their lives. It is not uncommon for these individuals to rely heavily on projection as a mental mechanism to explain their unhappiness (eg, spouses' negative characteristics are blamed). In some cases, they may be chronically angry individuals who present particular problems for health care providers. A variety of interventions may be helpful in reducing anxiety by providing purpose and structure in the individual's daily routine. Attempts at education and therapy should be made in an effort to assist elderly individuals in learning strategies for managing stress and anxiety that will contribute to their comfort. It is wise, however, when developing a plan of care, to recognize that therapeutic progress may be limited because of long-standing patterns of behavior and lack of insight.

CASE STUDY

Chronic Neurotic Anxiety

Mr. L is a 70-year-old man brought to live in a residential care facility after the death of his wife. While talking with the staff, his two daughters remarked that, "Mama could manage him, but he does have a temper and is kind of set in his ways." They indicated he often became frustrated and angry in stressful situations. When Mr. L was assigned a room and shown around the facility, he voiced a

number of physical complaints. He seemed complacent, but by the next morning he was loudly complaining about his room. He paced rapidly in the halls with little concern for more fragile residents and became verbally abusive when asked not to do this. He seemed never to be pleased with anything, and when his primary nurse tried to speak with him he again became verbally abusive. His examination indicated no evidence of organic impairment, and staff are beginning to feel frustrated at the lack of success in helping him adjust to the facility.

Psychotic Anxiety   Another group of elderly who often receive little attention are those individuals with psychiatric problems or mental impairment. They constitute a substantial number of nursing home residents, and many, because of deinstitutionalization, may be found living alone in apartments or boarding houses. These individuals have been diagnosed as mentally ill at a young age and, for most, symptoms will have diminished and become less florid over time (Ciompi, 1980). Motor activity associated with psychosis is often reduced, helping the client to manage better in a variety of settings. Another group of individuals who experience mental problems suffer from organic impairment, such as dementia. In the organically impaired group, like those with a functional psychosis, paranoia, restlessness, and agitation may be predominant symptoms.

Anxiety associated with psychosis and mental impairment must be carefully assessed. A useful tool for evaluating mental status in the older person is the FROMAJE. This approach is built around the acronym FROMAJE: F = function, R = reason, O = orientation, M = memory, A = arithmetic, J = judgment, and E = emotional state. This evaluation tool is accurate and rapidly administered by health professionals in the geriatric setting (Libow, 1981). Early recognition of changes in symptoms associated with anxiety may permit alleviation of the problems without increases in medication or movement to a more restrictive environment. In many instances, reduction of stimuli will decrease anxiety that occurs when elderly individuals, because of their impairment, are unable to process all incoming stimuli and react with increased psychotic symptomatology. This problem may be overlooked if anxiety is not seen as the basic difficulty and the assumption is made that an exacerbation of psychosis or mental deterioration is occurring.

CASE STUDY

Psychotic Anxiety

Tom is a 67-year-old man diagnosed with chronic undifferentiated schizophrenia for 42 years. Tom has had multiple hospitalizations, but for the past 6 years has lived in a residential care facility. He has been maintained well on 40 mg of Stelazine per day. Staff are aware that an increase in his medicine produces unpleasant side effects for Tom. Recently, Tom has verbally expressed more feelings of paranoia and is delusional regarding his financial situation. He also is pacing more and picks at his clothes. Staff are aware that the arrival at the home of four wheelchair residents has resulted in less time being spent with Tom as efforts are made to help the new residents adjust. Before considering a medication increase, the staff decide to consider anxiety associated with changes in the environmental setting as the source of the psychotic behavior. Interventions to increase structure and supportiveness in the environment for Tom are successful, and he soon returns to his usual level of functioning.

OUTCOMES

Table 39.4 provides a summary for identification and management of anxiety based on the framework proposed by Verwoerdt (1981). Anxiety as a nursing diagnosis applicable to the elderly needs some refinement to be most useful in goal setting and the development of interventions.

NURSING INTERVENTIONS

The last years of an individual's life have the potential for being as rich and fulfilling as earlier phases.

Table 39.4

Clinical Management of Anxiety

ETIOLOGIES	ASSESSMENT	INTERVENTIONS
Depletion	Self-Rating Anxiety Scale (SAS) or Anxiety Status Inventory	Assess need for support in areas of concern. Use formal sources of support, eg, homemaker services, legal aid, life-line, etc. Encourage informal networking through church and neighborhood systems. Strengthen family support systems through supportive psychotherapy. Use self-help groups, eg, widows' groups, postsurgery groups.
Helplessness	Self-Rating Anxiety Scale (SAS) or Anxiety Status Inventory	Assess need for psychotherapy to enhance adaptation to aging process. Determine environmental changes needed to enhance level of functioning. Encourage regular routines and schedules to increase feelings of control. Assess and obtain treatment as indicated for physical problems. Encourage mobilization and diversions consistent with remaining potential. Encourage relatives and caretakers to anticipate needs, thus reducing frustration and shame. Use social supports and networking as indicated.
Chronic neurotic anxiety	Anxiety Status Inventory	Assess client interest, past as well as present. Determine the client's attention span and physical abilities in relation to environmental setting. Note a preferred time of day, considering nursing schedules, as well as client alertness. Include the client in planning for short-term goals. Review care plan with the client on a monthly basis. Make a list of possible activities, both inside and outside the institution. Aim for activities that do not require problems or deadlines.
Psychotic anxiety	FROMAJE for assessment of mental status	Assess to determine role of anxiety in increased symptoms. Reduce stimuli in the environment. Increase structured activities to release energy. Limit setting to prevent acting-out behavior. Encourage supportive relationships to increase feelings of security.

One aspect of encouraging meaningful old age is to help the older client deal effectively with anxieties that may be unique to the aging process, as well as those that are associated with problems that developed earlier in life. Many of the interventions in the area of anxiety may be considered preventive health care, particularly for those elderly clients who may experience mild chronic illnesses that can be seriously exacerbated with the addition of anxiety. Other goals of intervention aimed at prevention and treatment of anxiety are to reduce dependency and promote self-care in the management of physical, environmental, and psychosocial problems.

Because 94% of the elderly are living outside of institutions, but the remaining 6% who are institutionalized constitute such a major burden for care, it is necessary to focus discussion of interventions for the nursing diagnosis of Anxiety on both populations of elderly clients. The first area of discussion presents interventions aimed at community-dwelling elderly, and the second area focuses on the institutionalized elderly.

Interventions for Community-Based Elderly

Interventions useful in the nursing diagnosis of Anxiety for the elderly client in the community need to be broad based and able to provide input at several points where symptomatology may appear. Because of the often subjective nature of anxiety, it is difficult to define appropriate interventions quantitatively. However, networking, one broad-spectrum intervention used in the reduction of anxiety among the community elderly, has been well researched and shows a strong theoretical base (Dowd, 1975), as well as some empirical evidence of success (Biegel, 1985; Chenitz, 1984; Guttman, 1985).

Networking Social support systems help the elderly person maintain independence and meet needs in times of crisis. These networks may be either formal or informal; the source of the aid is not as important as the effect such aid has on reducing anxiety in the elderly client. The use of networking is particularly useful in depletion of anxiety related to helplessness (see Table 39.4).

Theoretical Base for Networking Dowd (1975, 1980) uses social exchange theory to explain the decreased involvement that sometimes accompanies old age. According to social exchange theory, all social interaction is considered an exchange of rewarding behaviors between two actors, with each individual aiming to maximize rewards and minimize costs. For a relationship to remain mutually satisfying, the value of resources possessed by each actor must be relatively equal. Social exchange theory views the dependence of those with few resources on those with more resources as the source of social power

advantage or disadvantage. Dowd (1975, 1980) believes that social exchange theory is also applicable to the analysis of relationships between members of different age groups. The resources maintained by the elderly in modern society are usually both diminished and of less value than those maintained by younger groups (eg, the elderly's income is reduced). With the onset of retirement, the bargaining position of the older person quickly declines. Other changes, such as widowhood, may also lead to a loss of resources and status.

Being the dependent actor in the exchange situation is uncomfortable and is a clear example of depletion anxiety. The response of the older actor, left with few options in the exchange relationship, is usually to decrease involvement in the relationship. An important factor in the exchange relationship is the presence of reciprocity or balance of resources (Lee, 1985). Actors need to feel that in accepting resources from others they are able to reciprocate; an inability to do so will produce more anxiety. This probably accounts for the reluctance on the part of many elderly to take advantage of formal support groups. If care is not given to considering how the older person can reciprocate or in identifying supports in which this process is already established, the expected solution may only serve to increase already existing anxiety. There are not any clear strategies for resolution, but consideration needs to be given to the issue of reciprocity as part of the planning process to make full use of the potential for support present in informal networks.

Social Support Network Formal networks for social support exist in every community and are easily identified. In many instances such systems provide needed services, and if funding is available to pay for the service, this may be sufficient to meet needs and give the older person the assistance required to deal with anxiety-producing situations. Examples of formal support systems include Meals on Wheels, Lifeline, congregate meals, homemaker and home health aide services, and a wide variety of services designed to cover many contingencies.

There are times, however, when funding is not available or the service provided by the formal system is not comprehensive enough. In these situations, informal networks may be the best source of assistance to the elderly client in the community. It has been well established that families are not alienated from older persons (Shanas, 1979) and that many elderly do receive extensive informal help from their families. However, it is also true that immediate family members frequently live long distances from the older person and most are employed outside the home, thus making them unavailable at various times to the elder.

Neighboring Neighboring and friendships as an intervention to relieve anxiety among the elderly have many advantages. Neighbors and friends may provide an effective support system by promoting socialization, helping the elder to conduct tasks of daily living, and assisting in times of need (Peters and Kaiser, 1985). A large majority of older people continue to live in the same community and maintain ties with friends and neighbors well into later life (Babchek, 1978). The number and kinds of friends reported by older people may vary depending on the size and type of community, but many elderly report stable, long-term relationships often in their immediate residential environment. The type of support obtained from friends and neighbors may vary, but most older people report that friends assist with some chores, provide emergency care, serve as confidants, and act as a security measure. The issue of security is often an area of great concern to older individuals living alone. Daily visits, phone calls, and general alertness to changes in the neighborhood may be very effective in reducing anxiety associated with the elder's living situation and reinforces already existing coping skills.

Another factor to consider in the use of friends and neighbors as a support in reducing anxiety is the area of reciprocity, discussed earlier. The advantage of a support system that has been in place for a long time is that the exchanges have often been reciprocal in the past, and a tradition of helping has been developed that is acceptable to both parties. Power and dependency have not become issues in the relationship, and an imbalance may be tolerated because of the history of the relationship and the intent of the assistance being provided.

CASE STUDY

Nursing Interventions, Mrs. N

Mrs. N responded to the anti-anxiety medications that had been prescribed. Her children were well aware, however, that this was only a temporary response and that they needed a clearer picture of the problem. Unsure of the solution, they asked their family doctor for suggestions. He responded by referring Mrs. N and her family to the local mental health center, where they were seen by a clinical nurse specialist, Miss J. After interviewing Mrs. N it was apparent to Miss J that Mrs. N felt powerless with regard to the sale of her home, and although it would be advantageous financially, it was an emotional disaster to Mrs. N. Several family sessions were held, and Mrs. N was able to tell her children how much her home meant to her in the neighborhood where she had lived for 40 years. She also clearly identified the support that her church, friends, and neighbors were to her. Miss J recognized the value of the social network for Mrs. N as a coping device. She encouraged Mrs. N to consider using the resources that were available for her in the community setting.

While the family was still pondering the best living arrangements for Mrs. N, she arrived at a solution. Mrs. K was also losing her home to the city project, and over coffee in the morning, the two women arrived at the solution of purchasing a small home in the neighborhood together. Their children were at first skeptical, but the social and psychologic support provided for both women by the relationship outweighed their concerns, and the arrangements were made. Mrs. N's ability to find her own solution through the use of the networking prescribed by Miss J increased her feelings of competency. Her symptoms of anxiety, as well as the need for medications, receded.

Interventions for the Institutionalized Elderly

The institutionalized elderly may present with a variety of problems, not the least of which may be anxiety complicated by feelings of helplessness, hopelessness, and dependency. As noted earlier, a careful assessment is needed before any interventions are considered (see Table 39.4). The problem of anxiety among the institutionalized aged is multifaceted, and interventions need to be broad based and capable of dealing with several aspects of the problem.

Theoretical Base Interventions intended to reduce anxiety in the institutionalized client are derived from some basic premises. These premises must encompass (1) the need for autonomy; (2) the need for dignity and respect; (3) the need for identity and individuality; and (4) the need to belong (Kayser-Jones, 1984). Jourard (1958) defined *autonomy* as the ability to make one's own decisions and follow one's own will, not that of others. For most individuals, autonomy is highly valued and closely guarded, but it is sometimes lost in the aging process because of changes in roles, sensory and cognitive changes, and physical impairments. The fact of being a patient is in direct contrast to the desire to maintain independence, and this is particularly true of the chronically sick role (Burnside, 1980). Despite losses and illness, most individuals strive to remain autonomous within their limitations, and institutional settings can encourage this.

To be treated with dignity and respect is necessary to maintain self-esteem. Elderly persons have suffered losses that may have lowered feelings of self-esteem; thus it is particularly important that respect is communicated. Infantilization and dehumanization must be consistently avoided to prevent an increase in dependency and the sick-role image (Kayser-Jones, 1984). One aspect of psychologic health is a sense of personal identity and belief in personal worth (Jourard, 1958). It is more difficult to maintain a strong sense of personal identity in institutional settings because the nature of the institution tends to require conformity (everyone must be treated the same), which contributes to the loss of personal identity. Nursing staff can facilitate an environment that contributes to an atmosphere of autonomy and feelings of personal worth and identity. Wilson and Kneisl (1983) discuss the therapeutic use of empathy as a key to interaction with the institutionalized person and emphasize the impact of viewing the situation from the elderly person's perspective. The nurse who uses empathy effectively is more apt to adjust institution routines, policies, and procedures to accommodate the values of the elder and to maximize the control the elder has over decisions of living.

Nursing Interventions Anxiety among the institutionalized elderly is a complex diagnosis and as such requires a broad-based response. Interventions aimed at manipulating the environment to provide a supportive atmosphere that reduces loss of control experienced by the individual will in turn reduce the anxiety associated with helplessness, chronic neurotic anxiety, and anxiety experienced by the psychotic individual (see Table 39.4). Burnside (1980) emphasizes that planning care and shaping the patient's environment in the institution is an important function of the nurse, and each individual's abilities and needs must be considered in this process.

The client should be helped to recognize and adjust to an appropriate level of functioning. Self-care should be encouraged whenever possible. The client should be allowed to make decisions about care and participate in the development of care plans. Vogel (1982) identifies a number of interventions that may be combined to establish feelings of security and comfort. She suggests measures to reduce dependency and protect the dignity of the individual, such as three-dimensional pictures and signs on bathroom doors to accommodate the failing eyesight of the elderly client.

Elderly clients should be reminded of remaining assets. Mobilization and diversion that are consistent with remaining potential are to be encouraged. The goal must seem worth the effort. Getting out of bed may not in itself be worth the effort, but going outside on a pleasant fall day may be. Nurses are encouraged to talk to the client about areas of interest. Some elderly individuals will have previous interests and areas of expertise that can be used to motivate the elder to participate in specific activities.

Another aspect of this approach is to improve the self-esteem and personal identity of the elderly client through the use of life histories (Butler, 1963). Elderly clients meet in a group led by nursing staff, and the natural tendency of the aged to reminisce is used to help individuals recall the positive aspects of life. In doing so, individuals can understand and evaluate parts of their earlier life, putting this in perspective as part of the total picture. This group approach also adds the benefit of increased socialization.

Physical symptoms such as restlessness are often signs of anxiety in the elderly client, and these may in part be alleviated by an increase in activity, clear expectations for behavior, and a structured environment. Group activities, such as discussion groups or groups that center on exercises involving tactile stimulation, may be effective in reducing anxiety by focusing and diverting attention (Schwab et al, 1984).

CASE STUDY

Nursing Interventions, Mr. L

Mr. L continues to pace the halls rapidly and poses a threat to more fragile residents. He appears to have a short attention span and little evidence of willingness to discuss his concerns. Mrs. Y, his primary nurse, reviews the history provided by the family and his present behavior and determines that Mr. L is experiencing a high degree of chronic, neurotic anxiety exacerbated by his new situation. She develops a care plan focused on manipulating the environment to help Mr. L understand the expectations for his behavior and to provide security through a structured environment. Mrs. Y meets briefly with Mr. L each morning and provides him with an index card with his schedule for the day. This schedule includes a walk outside the institution each morning, participation in a group activity involving tactile stimulation, and an exercise group. Mr. L was also given a choice regarding his diet, and his input was solicited regarding food likes and dislikes. At times when he appeared especially agitated, he was encouraged to go to his room where he could lie down and listen to the country western music he enjoyed. Mr. L did not become a model client, but his verbal abusiveness did decrease, as did the rapid pacing that posed a threat to the more fragile residents. Eventually he was able to go for walks without supervision, and this became an effective means of managing much of his anxiety.

SUMMARY

Anxiety as a nursing diagnosis in the elderly is a complex condition that requires careful assessment with a focus on sources of anxiety. The framework outlined by Verwoerdt (1981) is very helpful in recognizing depletion anxiety, anxiety associated with helplessness, chronic neurotic anxiety, and the anxiety that accompanies psychosis. A clear identification of the etiology of anxiety allows for appropriate goal setting, intervention, and evaluation by the nurse. Defining characteristics that determine the nursing diagnosis of Anxiety in the elderly client should recognize the areas of assessment identified by Eisdorfer et al (1981).

Nursing interventions indicated for the diagnosis of Anxiety in the elderly client need to be broad based and multifaceted to deal effectively with the many aspects of the diagnosis. Because of the subjective nature of anxiety, it is difficult to quantitatively define appropriate interventions, and it is clear that substantial research is needed in this area.

Interventions were identified for both the community-based elderly and the institutionalized elderly. The theoretical basis for the intervention of networking suggested for the community-based elderly was social exchange theory. The institutionalized elderly also need a broad-based approach to interventions that will reduce feelings of hopelessness and dependency that complicate the nursing diagnosis of Anxiety in this population. Interventions that are suggested support autonomy and personal identity.

References

Ayd F: Is it anxiety or depression? *Southern Med J* 1984; 77: 1269–1271.

Babchek N: Aging and primary relations. *Internat J Aging Human Devel* 1978; 9:137–151.

Biegel DE: Application of network theory and research in the field of aging. In: *Social Support Network and the Care of the Elderly*. Sauer WJ, Coward RT (editors). Springer, 1985.

Burnside IM: *Psychosocial Nursing Care of the Aged*. McGraw-Hill, 1980.

Butler R: Life review therapy. *J Gerontol* 1963; 18:46–52.

Carroll-Johnson R (editor): *Classification of Nursing Diagnoses: Proceedings of the Eighth Conference*. Lippincott, 1989.

Chenitz CW: Elders and their family. In: *Mental Health and the Elderly*. Hall BA (editor). Grune and Stratton, 1984.

Ciompi L: Catamnestic long-term study on the course of life and aging schizophrenics. *Schizophrenia Bulletin* 1980; 6:606–616.

Conlin MM, Fennell EB: Anxiety, depression and health locus of control orientation in an outpatient elderly population. *J Florida Med Assoc* 1985; 72:281–288.

de Beauvoir S: *The Coming of Age*. Putnam, 1972.

Dowd JJ: Aging as exchange: A preface to theory. *J Gerontol* 1975; 30:584–594.

Dowd JJ: Exchange rates and older people. *J Gerontol* 1980; 35: 596–602.

Eisdorfer C, Cohen K, Kechieck W: Depression and anxiety in the cognitively impaired aged. In: *Anxiety: New Research and Changing Concepts*. Klein DF, Rabkin J (editors). Raven Press, 1981.

Gomez E, Gomez GE, Otto DA: Anxiety as a human emotion: Some basic conceptual models. *Nurs Forum* 1984; 21:38–42.

Guttman D: Social networks of ethnic minorities. In: *Social Support Network and the Care of the Elderly*. Sauer WJ, Coward RT (editors). Springer, 1985.

Jones PE, Jakob DF: Anxiety revisited—from a practice perspective. In: *Classification of Nursing Diagnosis: Proceedings of the Fifth National Conference*. Kim MJ, McFarland GK, McLane AM (editors). Mosby, 1984.

Jourard SM: *Personal Adjustment: An Approach Through the Study of Healthy Personality*. Macmillan, 1958.

Kayser-Jones JS: Psychosocial care for nursing home residents. In: *Mental Health and the Elderly*. Hall BA (editor). Grune and Stratton, 1984.

Lee GR: Theoretical perspectives on social networks. In: *Social Support Networks and the Care of the Elderly*. Sauer WJ, Coward RT (editors). Springer, 1985.

Libow LS: A rapidly administered, easily remembered mental status evaluation: FROMAJE. In: *The Core of Geriatric Medicine*. Libow LS, Sherman FT (editors). Mosby, 1981.

May R: Anxiety and values. In: *Stress and Anxiety*, Vol 8. Spielberger CD, Sarason IG, Milgram NA (editors). Hemisphere, 1982.

Mullins LC, Lopez MA: Death anxiety among nursing home residents: A comparison of the young-old and the old-old. *Death Educ* 1982; 6:75–86.

Peters GR, Kaiser MA: The role of friends and neighbors in providing social support. In: *Social Support Networks and the Care of the Elderly*. Sauer WJ, Coward RT (editors). Springer, 1985.

Runck C: State of art conference reviews new developments in characterizing and treating anxiety. *Hosp Community Psychiatry* 1984; 35:9–11.

Sallis JE, Lichstein KL: Analysis and management of geriatric anxiety. *Internat J Aging Human Devel* 1982; 15:197–211.

Schwab M, Rader J, Doan J: Relieving the anxiety and fear in dementia. *J Gerontol Nurs* 1984; 11:8–15.

Shanas E: The family as a social support system in old age. *Gerontologist* 1979; 19:169–174.

Spielberger CD: Stress and anxiety. In: *Stress and Anxiety*. Garason IG, Spielberger CD (editors). Hemisphere, 1975.

Turnbull JM, Turnbull SK: Management of specific anxiety disorders in the elderly. *Geriatrics* 1985; 40:75–82.

Verwoerdt A: *Clinical Geropsychiatry*. Van Nos Reinhold, 1981.

Vogel CH: Anxiety and depression among the elderly. *J Gerontol Nurs* 1982; 8:213–216.

Wilson HS, Kneisl CR: *Psychiatric Nursing*. Addison-Wesley, 1983.

Yocom CJ: The differentiation of fear and anxiety. In: *Classification of Nursing Diagnosis: Proceedings of the Fifth National Conference*. Kim MJ, McFarland GK, McLane AM (editors). Mosby, 1984.

Zung WK: A rating instrument for anxiety disorders. *Psychosomatics* 1971; 12:371–379.

40

Self-Esteem Disturbance

ANN L. WHALL, PhD, RN, FAAN

CARLA J. PARENT, MSN, RN

SELF-ESTEEM IS PRESENT TO SOME DEGREE IN EVERYONE. As the *sine qua non* of mental health, low levels of self-esteem accompany mental illness, whereas high levels accompany mental health. Perhaps more than any other concept, self-esteem relates to what it means to be a member of a group or to one's self-evaluation in reference to others. Nurses, therefore, must understand self-esteem in order to facilitate both mental and physical health.

LITERATURE REVIEW

Self-esteem is seen as a positive regard for oneself, as a universal need of every human being, and as a key component in restoring and maintaining mental and physical health (Meisenhelder, 1985). Self-esteem is defined as an individual's self-evaluation that expresses an attitude of approval or disapproval and indicates the extent to which the individual believes himself or herself to be capable, significant, successful, and worthy (Coopersmith, 1967). Branden (1969) states that self-esteem is hard to isolate and identify. Self-esteem affects thinking processes, desires, values, and goals, and it is the single most significant factor in behavior.

Coopersmith (1967) found that people with high self-esteem are generally happier, more independent, more self-confident, less anxious, and more effective in meeting environmental demands than those with low self-esteem. Persons with low self-esteem are likely to be alienated and to feel incapable of controlling their lives (Robinson and Shaver, 1972). Low self-esteem may make a person prone to illness; high self-esteem might contribute to the prevention of illness; and restoration of self-esteem could cure illness. Under certain conditions, self-esteem would be preferred by a deprived person over other aspects of life satisfaction (Goldberg and Fitzpatrick, 1980).

As important as the concept of self-esteem is in the restoration and maintenance of mental and physical health, self-esteem is remarkably neglected in nursing literature and is easily overlooked in clinical practice (Meisenhelder, 1985).

Haber et al (1978) define self-esteem in psychoanalytic terms: Low self-esteem is an outcome of a poorly developed ego that has been additionally traumatized by a failure or loss. Very low self-esteem is equivalent to feeling worthless.

Wilson and Kneisl (1979) view self-esteem from the wellness viewpoint, stating that understanding one's unique personality can contribute heavily to self-esteem. Emotionally healthy people like and accept themselves and are more aware of their feelings and conflicts.

Drawing on the perspective biopsychosocial aspects of sexuality, Hogan (1980) defines self-esteem as the kind of pictures that individuals have of themselves. Self-esteem is based largely on the nature of experiences, both positive and negative, that children have with their bodies and their world. Self-esteem is affected by sociocultural factors such as culture, functional ability, and gender. Murray and Huelskoetter (1983) discuss the gender issue, stating that because women experience more role stress than men, women may experience more self-esteem problems than men. As women age, however, they experience more of a sense of self-satisfaction with life than do men.

Andrews and Roy (1986) state that inherent in the self-concept is the concept of self-esteem. This is the individual's perception of worth. One's level of self-esteem is reflected in behaviors regarding the self. Baker (1985) noted that having a positive self-concept is the key to successful interpersonal relations.

Taft (1985) also defines self-esteem in relation to self-concept. Taft postulates that self-esteem forms the basic foundation for psychosocial health as well as the quality of life. Taft views self-concept as being divided, at least theoretically, into five areas: physical, intellectual, moral-ethical, social, and emotional. When self-concept in any of these areas is devalued by others, self-esteem falters. The aging process often affects the areas related to self-concept, precipitating a sense of lowered self-esteem in the older adult. Institutionalization can adversely affect all of the areas noted by Taft.

SIGNIFICANCE FOR THE ELDERLY

The number of aged individuals, especially the institutionalized aged, has been increasing over the last two decades, and gerontologic research has provided an abundance of information about their characteristics and needs. Many studies describe the psychosocial characteristics of this population as including inactivity, impaired level of overall adjustment, depressive mood tone, low morale, and low self-esteem (Goldberg and Fitzpatrick, 1980).

It has been reported that self-esteem declines with increasing age (Kuhlen, 1960). Rynerson (1972) reviewed the literature regarding self-esteem in the aged. In discussing Maslow, Rynerson stated that inherent in the concept of self-esteem are feelings of adequacy, achievement, mastery, and competence. In discussing Harry Stack Sullivan, Rynerson stated that the development of self-esteem is enhanced through positive interactions with significant others. Sullivan noted the tendency for western culture to worship youth, which leads to the inherent devaluation of the aged. The lack of energy or resiliency perceived in the elderly was viewed as a threat to their self-competence. Some older adults view themselves as useless and experience loss of self-esteem and feelings of

inferiority because they feel that they cannot change or control their life situation (Human, 1973). Conversely, self-defined usefulness, unconfined life space, and positive interactions with others were all associated with positive self-esteem (Rynerson, 1972). It has been suggested that self-esteem is developed and maintained through the successful process of personal interaction and negotiation with the environment.

Age-related events and stresses in late life may alter the older adult's self-esteem, and depending on how successful the older person is in negotiations with the environment, self-esteem may decrease (George and Bearon, 1980). Taft (1985) identified aging experiences that may be related to low self-esteem in the elderly: losses in the areas of health and independence; loss of work and social roles; and loss of support systems. Antecedents of self-esteem, according to Taft, are self-perceptions largely related to efficacy.

A limited number of gerontologic research studies have investigated the relationship between aging and self-esteem. Goldberg and Fitzpatrick (1980) examined the effects of activity on morale and self-esteem in a population of institutionalized aged persons. They concluded that self-esteem may be a more situationally reactive phenomenon than a direct result of aging. Parent and Whall (1984) conducted a research study investigating the relationship between physical activity, depression, and self-esteem in the older adult. The conclusions were similar to those of Goldberg and Fitzpatrick (1980), supporting the contention that self-esteem does not necessarily decline with increasing age. In addition, the findings supported a strong correlation between self-esteem and depression.

Self-esteem and depression are theoretically inversely correlated, and research findings have supported this relationship. When discussing the concept of self-esteem in the elderly, it is important to consider depression and its impact on the older population. Feelings of depression are expressed as sadness, disappointment, and frustration (Jacobson, 1980) and have been demonstrated to be highest in the 65 and older age group (Blazer, 1980; Harris, 1979; Human, 1973), with the suicide rate highest in white men over age 60 (Butler and Lewis, 1982).

Hunter et al (1982) studied the characteristics of elderly persons with high and low self-esteem. Their findings concluded that the elderly with either high self-esteem or low self-esteem did not differ with regard to age. The elderly group with the lowest self-esteem, however, had significantly higher levels of depression, anxiety, and external locus of control.

CRITICAL ATTRIBUTES OF SELF-ESTEEM

Using the concept analysis method of Walker and Avant (1988), the following attributes of self-esteem were extracted from the literature: universal need; self evaluation; and a belief in self-capability. In general, high self-esteem results in feelings of worthiness and a capable self-picture based on life experiences. Low self-esteem is related to a number of losses that have been associated with aging and tend to be situationally dependent in this population. Self-capability, adequacy, competency, interaction with others, and gender can affect self-esteem in the elderly.

GENERAL DEFINITIONS AND CHARACTERISTICS OF SELF-ESTEEM

Self-esteem is defined in several ways:
Universal need
Result of self-evaluation
Result of evaluation by others
A self-picture based on life experiences
Physical, social, moral-ethical, and emotional
  components

The North American Nursing Diagnosis Association (NANDA) has developed a nursing diagnosis of Self-Esteem Disturbance (Carroll-Johnson, 1989). Table 40.1 contrasts the differences and similarities between the

NANDA diagnosis and the diagnosis Self-Esteem Disturbance: Low Self-Esteem developed by Whall and Parent.

When comparing the two approaches, it is apparent that there are many similarities. The contribution of the Whall and Parent approach is that it is more global and comprehensive in attempting to assess the various factors that affect self-esteem in the older adult. Assessment of Self-Esteem Disturbance in the older adult can be difficult because of the multiplicity of factors confronting this population. The following model cases contain all of the attributes of the concept.

CASE STUDY

High Self-Esteem

Mary and John have been married for 55 years, are ages 80 and 71 years, respectively, and are both in good health. They decided that they needed to make their own decisions and to plan for the future. Realizing that they both might need assistance to conduct their lives, they decided to enter a senior citizens residence with a step-up-care alternative. Once in the home, they introduced themselves to others and continued the various activities in which they were interested. "After all," Mary said, "we've been socially active and well accepted by people all our lives."

Table 40.1

Definitions, Related Factors and Defining Characteristics of Self-Esteem

	SELF-ESTEEM DISTURBANCE: LOW SELF-ESTEEM	SELF-ESTEEM DISTURBANCE
	Whall & Parent	NANDA *(Carroll-Johnson, 1989)*
Definition	Negative self-picture based on life experiences having physical, social, moral-ethical, and emotional components; universal need	Negative self evaluation/feelings about self or self-capabilities, which may be directly or indirectly expressed
Related Factors	Disbelief in self-capability and self-adequacy; depression; recent loss	To be determined
Defining Characteristics	Negative view of self	Self negating verbalization; expressions of shame/guilt; evaluates self as unable to deal with events; rationalizes away/rejects positive feedback and exaggerates negative feedback about self; hesitant to try new things/situations; denial of problems obvious to others; projection of blame/ responsibility to others; rationalizing personal failures; hypersensitive to slight or criticism; grandiosity
	Lack of interest in activities; Lack of motivation	
	Neglect of personal appearance	
	Poor eye contact	
	Feelings of sadness and depression	
	Decrease in socialization	
	Feelings of worthlessness	

CASE STUDY

Low Self-Esteem

June had been married for 55 years and is now age 81. Her husband died a year ago, and since then, she has been physically ill and depressed. June's daughters decided she must enter a senior citizen's residence with step-up-care alternatives. June felt that her rights were being taken away from her and that she must indeed be a helpless old lady. Once in the home, she avoided others, feeling that no one would want to associate with her because she was a failure. She cried almost constantly.

In a sense, the model case for high self-esteem is the contrary case for low self-esteem and vice versa. This concept analysis was presented as one way of clarifying self-esteem so that it might be approached in terms of the nursing diagnosis Self-Esteem Disturbance.

TOTAL INSTITUTIONS AND SELF-ESTEEM

In seminal efforts, Becker (1963), Goffman (1961), and Gough (1948) discussed the effects of total institutions on persons. Although their efforts focused on pointing out that symptoms of mental illness may be attributable to the "asylum" itself, their discussion may be used to view the total institutions of homes for the aged.

Goffman (1961) defined a *total institution* as one in which all the needs of the individual are satisfied within that institution. Examples of these needs include meals, living arrangements, health care, and other physical needs as well as social, religious, and work opportunities. In essence, prisons, hospitals, and nursing homes are total institutions. Another aspect of total institutions is that the residence must be relatively permanent with little change occurring for long periods of time.

Researchers have pointed out that the institution's existence depends on keeping large numbers of clients within its walls and that rehabilitation and/or discharge of large numbers of people would be counterproductive to the existence of the institution. In a study of the effects on patients in the asylum, Goffman (1961) identified that one had to become "maladjusted" in terms of outside standards if one was to "adjust" to life in the institution. Persons in asylums thus learned to speak when spoken to, to give the "correct" responses rather than what they felt, and to not express personal demands and needs, thereby placing stress on the system and identifying themselves as "different." Only by "playing by the rules" were they able to survive.

A related notion was that the career of the mental patient (Dimond and Jones, 1983) had a life separate from the patient; that is, no matter how logical the responses of such persons were, all responses were interpreted as the ramblings of a mad person. Once labeled, the mental patient's career was launched, almost separate from the person's characteristics. Moreover, the label took preeminence over reality.

The relevance to nursing homes, senior citizen residences, and other older adult care facilities may not be readily apparent. Some of the commonalities are that nursing homes and the like have not been viewed as places one leaves. The emphasis in the past has not been on maximizing function and returning the elderly person to home or to a less total institution. Rather the emphasis often has been on infantilizing and disenfranchising the patients. Infantile behavior, however, is counterproductive to life on the outside of the institution.

The career of the nursing home resident also appears to be somewhat separate from the person. For example, "ready for a nursing home" has often been equated with senility, and once labeled as such, the patient often has little opportunity to change that stereotype.

High self-esteem or the continued belief in self-adequacy and capability is counterproductive to life in many nursing homes. Rather, not speaking out and conforming are valued. Feelings of worthiness may become shattered as people are infantilized by such phrases as "my baby" or "be a good girl." For the elderly, adjustment to the total institution is related to loss of one's rights, initiatives, feelings, wishes, and desires. In these situations, the patient is "adjusted" when many of the features of low self-esteem are manifested. Thus, total institutions may be counterproductive to high levels of self-esteem, even if the institutional objectives and philosophy indicate otherwise. It is hoped that total institutions that serve the elderly will develop systems in which high levels of self-esteem will be fostered along with the needed care.

THE NURSING DIAGNOSIS: SELF-ESTEEM DISTURBANCE

Gordon (1982) identified the "self-perception–self-concept" pattern as one of the 11 functional health patterns found within the nursing diagnosis system. She further lists the diagnosis of Self-Esteem Disturbance as an accepted diagnosis with the self-concept pattern. The nursing history provides a description of a client's functional health pattern. In terms of the self-perception–self-concept pattern, Gordon (1982;331) stated that one might ask:

How would you describe yourself? Do you feel
    good about yourself most of the time?
Are changes in your body or the things you can do
    a problem for you?

Are there changes in the way you feel about your body or yourself related to recent events?

Do things frequently annoy you, make you fearful, anxious, or depressed? If so, what helps?

ETIOLOGIES/RELATED FACTORS AND DEFINING CHARACTERISTICS

The etiology of Self-Esteem Disturbance may or may not be recognized by the elderly client; that is, sometimes persons do not know why they feel unworthy. The etiology of a condition, however, can be identified in terms of probable cause and probable related causes by the nurse. The defining characteristics are in essence the critical attributes of low self-esteem (see Table 40.1), and a majority of these must be present for the diagnosis to be made. A majority rather than all must be present because everyone does not express disturbances in self-esteem in the same way.

ASSESSMENT

The assessment of Self-Esteem Disturbance draws on these critical attributes:

High self-esteem	Belief in self-capability and self
	Adequacy
	Happiness
	Feelings of worthiness
	Positive self-concept
Low self-esteem	Low morale in terms of ability
	Depression
	Low self-esteem related to losses and to specific situations

To assess these attributes, the nurse could ask:

How does the elderly client view his/her ability to care for or maintain his/her personal needs?

Are there changes or losses that have become problematic for the client?

Does the elderly client believe that he/she has the capacity and capability to make adaptations and adjustments in his/her life to deal better with the loss or change? What things annoy the client or make the client fearful and/or anxious?

These questions, in addition to others, would help explicate the "disturbance in self-esteem" related to the critical attributes of self-esteem.

The assessment of Self-Esteem Disturbance is based on the integration of the nursing diagnosis approach and a nursing mode. For the purpose of this chapter, Roy's adaptation model (1976) will be the nursing theory used.

Roy's adaptation model (1976) views humans as biopsychosocial beings. The person is in constant interaction with a changing environment, confronting physical, social, and psychologic changes. Roy's model offers nursing a framework on which to base the assessment of older adults' capabilities and abilities to adapt to the numerous changes that confront them. Roy (1976) postulates that a person learns or acquires mechanisms that are used to cope with impinging environmental changes. Responding positively to these changes requires adaptation and brings about health. Illness or maladaptation occurs when the person is unable to respond positively to the stimuli.

The stimuli are of three levels:

Focal stimuli—degree of change or stimulus most immediately confronting the person and the one to which the older adult must make an adaptive response. This is the cause of the behavior. An example of a focal stimulus may be an environmental change such as a move to less independent living. It may also include a change in a relationship, such as the loss of a friend through death or relocation. Focal stimuli can have a profound impact on the critical attributes of self-esteem.

Contextual stimuli—all other stimuli present that contribute to the behavior caused by the focal stimuli. Contextual stimuli can be either external or internal, such as developmental age or stresses of illness.

Residual stimuli—factors that may be affecting behavior, but those effects are not validated. Residual stimuli may include beliefs, attitudes, experiences, or traits and cannot be validated by the older adult.

Roy's adaptation model discusses the assessment of the stimuli and the notion that the nurse must also assess the four adaptive modes: self concept, role function, physiologic changes, and interdependence changes. The integration of the nursing diagnosis approach and Roy's adaptation model includes assessing the critical attributes of self-esteem and the older adults' adaptive capabilities. The data obtained from the assessment help the nurse determine the most effective way to change the course of events toward the desired client adaptation. The nurse's mode of intervention is to increase, decrease, or maintain stimulation.

ASSESSMENT TOOLS

The Rosenberg Self-Esteem Scale has been used in several studies to measure self-esteem level. It is unidimensional in nature, designed to measure attitudes toward the self along a favorable-to-unfavorable dimension. Rosenberg defined *self-esteem* as self-acceptance or a basic feeling of self-worth (cited in George and Bearon, 1980). The Self-Esteem Scale consists of 10 items of the Likert type, allowing one of four responses: strongly agree, agree, disagree, and strongly disagree. Integral values are assigned to each scale point, and the total score is obtained by simple summation. The Self-Esteem Scale has been administered to large and diverse samples of all ages. Atchly and Cottrell, Kaplan and Pokory, and Ward (cited in George and Bearon, 1980) have conducted studies using the Self-Esteem Scale with older adults. The scale addresses the critical attributes of self-esteem; a disturbance in maturity would result in a low self-esteem score.

Other types of tests may also be used to assess for the nursing diagnosis Self-Esteem Disturbance. In convergent validity efforts, Rosenberg (cited in George and Bearon, 1980) and Parent and Whall (1984) have suggested the use of the Beck Depression Inventory (BDI), which was developed for the purpose of assessing symptoms of depression. Research findings have supported the inverse relationship between self-esteem and depression in older adults: Therefore, it seems feasible that one could assess depression as an indirect way to assess self-esteem. It is generally best, however, to assess a concept using an instrument developed to measure that specific concept.

There is one caution to the use of any standardized instrument to reach a nursing diagnosis of Self-Esteem Disturbance. A nursing assessment includes the exercise of clinical judgment and the drawing of inferences based on an entire body of knowledge. Therefore, although the instruments may be of value and assistance in the nursing diagnosis of Self-Esteem Disturbance, a more complete assessment is needed.

In summary, the assessment steps are:

1. Interview the older adult using the questions postulated by Gordon (1982) and other appropriate questions to address each of the critical attributes of low and high self-esteem. From these, the focal, contextual and residual stimuli are identified.
2. Use the Rosenberg Self-Esteem Scale or Beck Depression Inventory to confirm the assessment.
3. Assess Roy's (1976) four adaptive modes to identify any related, unidentified disturbances.
4. State the nursing diagnosis in terms of a disturbance in the critical attributes most affected.
5. Validate the diagnosis with the elderly client.

CASE STUDY

Self-Esteem Disturbance

Daisy, age 84, has been admitted to an intermediate care nursing home. Her husband, Peter, who is 90 years old, has congestive heart failure and is no longer able to care for Daisy at home. Their home is an upper flat in a large industrial city in the Midwest. Daisy and Peter are of German extraction and had lived on a farm until 30 years ago. Daisy has been diagnosed as having arteriosclerotic changes in the extremities and can no longer walk, even with assistance. A big woman, 200 lb and 5'10", her care had become increasingly difficult for Peter and a bachelor grandson, Jim, age 30 years, who lives with Daisy and Peter. The two men are managing well now and visit Daisy at least every other day. Their home is located within 4 miles of the nursing home, and Jim works rotating shifts and drives himself and his grandfather to the nursing home in his off hours. Although Daisy's arteriosclerotic changes have caused some degree of multi-infarct dementia, she is still oriented to place and person, and she generally knows the month and the season.

The nursing staff identified several problems in caring for Daisy: She has begun to cry intermittently and is not eating because she says she's "no longer worth anything." Sensing a disturbance in self-esteem and feelings of depression, the clinical nurse specialist in geriatrics began an assessment.

The nurse asked the following questions to assess the attributes of self-esteem. These questions assisted the nurse in identifying the stimuli (related factors) that the interventions will address.

How would you describe yourself? Do you feel good about your abilities, or do you feel saddened or depressed? If so, about what? Are there losses you are concerned about?

Are changes in your capabilities, the things you cannot do, a problem for you?

How do you feel about the changes related to your body and moving into this residence?

What things annoy or bother you or make you feel fearful, anxious, or depressed?

Daisy identified that because she could not walk, she missed getting around outdoors. The loss she was most concerned about was the possibility that she would be confined to her bed. The changes in her body, other than her loss of walking, were not a concern to her, since Daisy had expected these changes with age. The move to the nursing home was a direct result, she believed, of her not being able to walk. Because self-esteem disturbance was evident, but the extent was uncertain, the BDI was administered. Daisy was not suicidal, but was moderately depressed.

Next, the three stimuli were identified. The focal stimulus—the stimulus most immediately confronting the person and the one to which the older adult must make an adaptive response—was the inability to be mobile and more independent. The contextual stimuli—those stimuli that contribute to the behavior caused by the focal stimuli—were identified as feelings of depression, hopelessness, worthlessness, and guilt. The residual stimuli, including beliefs, attitudes, experiences, or traits that cannot be validated, were identified as Daisy's fears that this was the end of her life and that she was worthless.

Roy's (1976) four adaptive modes (self-concept, physiologic integrity, role function, and interdependence) were also assessed to further determine Self-Esteem Disturbance. Physiologically it was uncertain if Daisy could be rehabilitated to walk again, even with a walker. If this was not possible, it was thought that a wheelchair would increase mobility and a greater sense of independence. In assessing interdependence, this adaptive mode was affected in that Daisy no longer felt independent and capable. Daisy also viewed her role function as being greatly compromised in that she was no longer involved in the managing of her home and in the day-to-day care of her husband. In reality, Daisy felt that she no longer had a role or function in life.

Based on the data obtained in the assessment, the nursing diagnosis was stated as follows: Low self-esteem related to loss of the capability to walk (focal stimuli). Daisy validated that not being able to walk was the most upsetting factor immediately present in her life.

NURSING INTERVENTIONS

The interventions described in this chapter are based on Roy's (1976) adaptive model. The interventions involve both the adaptation level of the older adult in the four modes and the stimuli. In order to promote adaptation, other stimuli may also need to be managed. According to Andrews and Roy (1986), management of stimuli involves altering, increasing, decreasing, removing, or maintaining the stimuli. The nursing intervention involves selection of which stimuli to change (ie, focal or contextual) and the approach with the highest probability of bringing about adaptation. Whenever possible, the focal stimulus is the focus of the nursing intervention, but when this is not possible, contextual stimuli must be managed in order to broaden the possible adaptation level. The steps in the nursing intervention, therefore, must serve to increase, decrease, or maintain the stimuli.

The goal of nursing intervention for Self-Esteem Disturbance is to help the client see the focal stimuli as having a positive valuing influence, rather than as being another negative devaluing experience (Roy, 1976). Therapeutic communication is one intervention that may be helpful. The nurse helps the older adult to change his or her view of life. The older adult may need to understand what feelings of sadness, loss, anger, unhappiness, joy, and happiness feel like. The elderly need to understand what these feelings mean personally, from what situations these feelings are derived, and how to express these feelings. Through therapeutic communication, the nurse can help older adults understand what maturational/situational crisis they may be experiencing, what is expected of them, and what they expect of themselves. Older adults need to

understand, define, accept, and try out control of the environment that they identify as comfortable (Driever, 1976). The older adult's self-definition needs to be satisfying and to include a view of self as competent with opportunities to achieve feedback to continue that view. With this kind of positive picture of self, the older adult will be able to change self-views yet still maintain self-esteem and adapt through self-concept (Driever, 1976).

The outcomes of an intervention for Self-Esteem Disturbance would facilitate adaptation of the critical attributes affected. There will be times that all of the critical attributes of self-esteem are the focal stimuli rather than one or two of the attributes having preeminence. When this occurs the nurse would select the attributes that are believed to be maximally affecting adaptation. In reassessing the effectiveness of the intervention, all the critical attributes of self-esteem and perhaps the assessment tools mentioned might be used with the older adult to validate the clinical outcomes.

CASE STUDY

Nursing Interventions

The intervention for Daisy focused on the focal stimuli. The clinical nurse specialist arranged for Daisy to be evaluated by physical therapy to assess her functional potential. It was found that Daisy's muscles had the capability to be strengthened via exercise and that presently she could stand. Walking, however, would require a walker and intensive therapy. Daisy was placed on a reduction diet to facilitate increased mobility and to decrease risk factors. Physical therapy was done on a daily basis.

Other interventions were implemented that dealt with the contextual and residual stimuli. The household residence structure was explored with Peter and Jim to determine if Daisy would be able to use a walker. The nurse discussed with Daisy the meaning of "lack of mobility," and some of the losses Daisy was experiencing were explored. Daisy began to feel that she was worthwhile because someone spent time exploring alternatives and including her in the treatment plan. She followed the reduction diet because she understood that this would help in increasing her mobility potential and was not a punitive measure. Although Daisy needed frequent explanations and encouragement, she did participate in the physical therapy plan and experienced a greater sense of control and self-esteem.

OUTCOMES

Although the outcomes of the physical therapy after 3 months were still in doubt, Daisy could stand and was able to use a walker to transfer from the bed to the chair. This progress had a direct impact on Daisy's self-esteem. The questions that had initially been asked of Daisy were again used to assess Daisy's current level of self-esteem. This assessment noted that Daisy was beginning to exhibit some of the critical attributes of high self-esteem; that is, she felt more worthy and had a positive view of her progress. She continued to have some disbelief in her ability to follow through on the rehabilitation program, but was able to be convinced that progress was both possible and evident. Reassessment with the BDI demonstrated only a mild level of depression at this time. The focal stimuli had thus been modified and the adaptation level increased so that the focal stimuli were within the adaptive range.

This case study is an example of how Roy's adaptation model can be integrated with nursing diagnosis to assess and implement nursing interventions dealing with Self-Esteem Disturbances in the older adult.

SUMMARY

The nursing diagnosis Self-Esteem Disturbance is particularly significant for the dependent elderly and is often associated with depression, anxiety, and other age-related stressors. Because of the multiplicity of factors that may be associated, assessment can be difficult. The Rosenberg Self-Esteem Scale and Beck's Depression Inventory are examples of tools that nurses can use to develop a definitive diagnosis. Nursing interventions are aimed at enhancing the elder's self-adequacy for desired adaptation. The desired outcome is for the elderly person to view focal stimuli (stressors) as positive rather than negative valuing experiences. Nurses are often in a strategic position to intervene with dependent elderly who suffer from Self-Esteem Disturbance.

References

Andrews H, Roy C: *Essentials of the Roy Adaptation Model.* Appleton-Century-Crofts, 1986.

Baker NJ: Reminiscing in group therapy for self-worth. *J Gerontol Nurs* (July) 1985; 11(7):21–24.

Becker H: *Outsiders.* Free Press, 1963.

Blazer D: The diagnosis of depression in the elderly. *J Am Geriatr Soc* 1980; 28:52–58.

Branden N: *The Psychology of Self-Esteem.* Nash, 1969.

Butler R, Lewis M: *Aging and Mental Health,* 3d ed. Mosby, 1982.

Carroll-Johnson R (editor): *Classification of Nursing Diagnoses: Proceedings of the Eighth Conference.* Lippincott, 1989.

Coopersmith S: *The Antecedents of Self-Esteem.* Freeman, 1967.

Dimond M, Jones SL: *Chronic Illness Across the Life Span.* Appleton-Century-Crofts, 1983.

Driever M: Development of self-concept. Pages 180–191 in: *Introduction to Nursing: An Adaptation Model.* Roy C (editor). Prentice-Hall, 1976.

George L, Bearon L: *Quality of Life in Older Persons: Meaning and Measurement.* Human Sciences Press, 1980.

Goffman E: *Asylums.* Doubleday-Anchor, 1961.

Goldberg W, Fitzpatrick J: Movement therapy with the aged. *Nurs Res* 1980; 29:339–346.

Gordon M: *Nursing Diagnosis: Process and Application.* McGraw-Hill, 1982.

Gough H: A sociological theory of psychopathy. *Am J Soc* 1948; 53:359–366.

Haber J et al: *Comprehensive Psychiatric Nursing.* McGraw-Hill, 1978.

Harris C: *Fact Book on Aging: A Profile of America's Older Population.* National Council on Aging, 1979.

Hogan R: *Human Sexuality: A Nursing Perspective.* Appleton-Century-Crofts, 1980.

Human M: The aged psychiatric patient. In: *Psychosocial Nursing Care of the Aged.* Burnside I (editor). McGraw-Hill, 1973.

Hunter KI, Linn MW, Harris R: Characteristics of high and low self-esteem in the elderly. *Internat J Aging Human Devel* 1982; 14:117–126.

Jacobson S: Melancholy in the 20th century: Causes and preventions. *J Psychiatric Nurs Mental Health Services* 1980; 11–21.

Kuhlen R: Aging and life adjustment. In: *Handbook of Aging and the Individual.* Birren JE (editor). University of Chicago Press, 1960.

Meisenhelder JB: Self-esteem: A closer look at clinical interventions. *Internat J Nurs Students* 1985; 22:127–135.

Murray RB, Heulskoetter MMW: *Psychiatric Mental Health Nursing: Giving Emotional Care.* Prentice-Hall, 1983.

Parent C, Whall A: Are physical activity, self-esteem, and depression related? *J Gerontol Nurs* 1984; 10:8–11.

Robinson J, Shaver P: *Measures of Social Psychological Attitudes.* Ann Arbor, Survey Research Center, 1972.

Roy C: *Introduction to Nursing: An Adaptation Model.* Prentice-Hall, 1976.

Rynerson BC: Need for self-esteem in the aged. *J Psychiatric Nurs Mental Health Services* 1972; 10:22–26.

Taft L: Self-esteem in later life: A nursing perspective. *ANS* 1985; 8:77–84.

Walker L, Avant K: *Strategies for Theory Construction in Nursing,* 2d ed. Appleton and Lange, 1988.

Wilson H, Kneisl C: *Psychiatric Nursing.* Addison-Wesley, 1979.

VIII

Role–Relationship Pattern

KATHLEEN BUCKWALTER, PhD, RN, FAAN
MERIDEAN MAAS, PhD, RN, FAAN

Overview

ELDERLY INDIVIDUALS WHO ARE MOVED FROM one location to another may experience stress and have difficulty adapting to the new environment. In Chapter 42, Translocation Syndrome, Remer, Buckwalter, and Maas explore the significance of the diagnosis for nursing practice and for the well-being of institutionalized elderly. The authors review the extensive research documenting the effects of translocation on the elderly and assessing the intervention preparation for relocation. Finally, the authors develop discharge planning as the major nursing intervention for management of Translocation Syndrome among the institutionalized elderly.

In Chapter 43, Whiting and Buckwalter offer a conceptualization of Dysfunctional Grieving that takes issue with the traditional view. The concept is reframed from the point of view of the elderly person who is experiencing grief. The authors argue that a dysfunctional, problem-oriented perspective promotes labeling on the part of caregivers, tends to negate the highly individualized nature of the grief experience, and discourages the use of nursing interventions that provide support and facilitate coping throughout the normal process of grieving. Nursing assessment is described in depth. The

nursing intervention ENUF (empathy, nonjudgment, unconditional positive regard, feeling focus) is recommended as an approach to assist the grieving individual.

In Chapter 44 on Social Isolation, Elsen and Blegen define the diagnosis as a state of being, an actual or perceived separation of the elderly individual from others in terms of interaction, communication, and social and emotional involvement. This definition differs from that currently accepted by the North American Nursing Diagnosis Association (NANDA), which focuses more on the perceptual experience of the individual. Elsen and Blegen report that social isolation is a pressing psychosocial dilemma associated with aging, and they identify many adverse circumstances associated with the diagnosis. A social skills training program and its components are described as one effective intervention that provides an opportunity for elderly persons to improve their social skills and decrease anxiety in social situations. The nurse's role in such a program, including instruction, modeling, feedback, and organizational aspects, is detailed.

The elderly experience a high incidence of cerebral vascular accidents, which may result in impaired verbal communication. Impaired verbal communication often disrupts role behaviors and relationships for the elderly. In Chapter 45, Cusack develops the primary diagnoses of Impaired Verbal Communication: Aphasia and Impaired Verbal Communication: Dysarthria. Three types of aphasia are discussed: expressive, receptive, and global. More specific nursing diagnoses are proposed for each type of aphasia; for example, the diagnoses for expressive aphasia are Impaired Oral Communication and Impaired Written Communication. The important role of the nurse in providing the appropriate environment for language retraining and for reinforcement and assistance with prescribed speech therapy is emphasized.

In Chapter 46, Altered Family Processes: Caring for the Dependent Elderly Family Member, Dixon examines the role of nursing diagnosis and intervention within the context of family and institutionalization of family members. Family structure and process, role relationships, and relationships among family and nurse caregivers are discussed within the frameworks of systems and family theories. Validated family assessment tools are offered for use by nurse case managers. The author uses a case study to illustrate assessment and diagnosis; three subdiagnoses of Altered Family Processes are explicated and interventions for each are described.

In Chapter 47, Potential for Violence: Self-Directed or Directed at Others, Munns and Nolan deal with the phenomenon of violent behavior that is a common concern for health professionals who work with the institutionalized elderly. Using biologic, psychologic, and social framework theories of violence and aggression, the authors focus on etiologic factors that are specific for the elderly who have Potential for Violence including sensory-perceptual alterations, depression, and inability to control behavior. Selection of the most appropriate nursing intervention for a specific etiology is discussed within the framework of eight concepts.

In Chapter 48 on Altered Role Performance: Potential Loss of Right of Self-Determination, Weiler discusses the right of elderly persons to make personal health care decisions. This diagnosis is particularly important because changes in physical and/or mental capacity can subject the elderly to imbalanced power relationships with loss of autonomy when they enter the health care delivery system. Advanced directives, such as the living will and durable power of attorney, are discussed along with the need for nurses to understand the wishes and preferences of elderly persons.

41

Normal Changes With Aging

Donna Bunten, MA, RN
Mary A. Hardy, PhD, RN, C

Definition:

The role-relationship pattern describes the pattern of role engagements and relationships.

The role-relationship pattern describes an individual's perception of his or her major roles and associated responsibilities in his or her current life situation, including whether interactions with others are satisfying. Interaction requires the elderly to have the ability to communicate and to have available opportunities for socialization. Role losses, changes, and threats of loss and change present major challenges for the aging adult.

From a sociologic perspective, three qualitatively different types of loss are associated with normal aging (Bengtson, 1973). First, highly valued social roles such as employee, spouse, or active parent are lost, along with the repertoire of expected behaviors attached to the role. Associated with role loss, then, is the second type of loss—the loss of norms or rules that guide us in acting out each social role. Elderly retirees or widows/widowers have only a vague idea of what is expected of them and how they should identify themselves. The third type of loss is that of reference groups. Reference groups may be work groups, professional groups, religious groups, social groups, or friends. Each of these associations gives people information about the appropriateness of their behavior and reinforces their identity and self-esteem. The elderly feel the impact of changes in all three of these social dimensions.

It is helpful to understand another aspect of the social significance of role loss. Most role changes in early life are voluntary assumptions of increased responsibility. Those changes in roles that occur in later life are often involuntary and involve a loss of responsibility and status. In American society, the importance of roles comes from the prestige, status, wealth, and influence associated with respective roles. The usual positions or roles of the older person are not in themselves viewed as important (Biddle and Thomas, 1966). People do not get wealthy, revered, or influential simply by growing old. As a matter of fact, being defined as old may decrease the value of roles or cause removal from some positions. Many of today's elderly are victims of mandatory retirement policies. They may find themselves without the functional role that contributed to a positive sense of self, justified their social future, and made them feel acceptable to others.

The number and variety of social networks and interactions are reduced for the elderly. As a consequence, a number of elders live very isolated lives (Rathbone-McCuan and Hashami, 1982). According to a 1981 Louis Harris poll (National Council on Aging, 1981), isolation and loneliness are serious problems for about 13% of persons 65 years of age and older. It should be noted that the aged may contribute to their own loneliness by conveying that "I like to be on my own" or "I don't want to be a burden to my children." These expressions of self-determination and independence, predominant among American values, may hinder social integration.

Friendships are subject to erosion over a lifetime as deaths, moving, and retirements occur. The loss of just one long-term friend can be particularly devastating to the older person. Singer (1981) points out that friendship networks help the elderly to maintain autonomy and self-worth and give them an opportunity to gain new roles among peers. Friendships may also fill a void created by the loss of a spouse or other valuable confidant. Unfortunately, many elderly lack income, education, and good health, the resources often required in substituting roles and expanding friendships (Morgan, 1988).

The family is the primary institution in the elderly person's informal social network, particularly for those who have become less active in other institutions. The family has been and continues to be the predominant force in the care of the elderly (Sauer and Coward, 1985). Four of five elderly persons have children. Of these, 18% live in the same household with a child, and another 55% live within 30 minutes of a child. Family members who live in the same community are reported to have daily to weekly contacts, and those separated by long distances have frequent contacts by letter or phone (American Association of Retired Persons/Administration on Aging, 1986; Cunningham and Brookbank, 1988). Siblings and other relatives often play a critical role in the life of the elderly, especially if they have never married or have children (Shaunas et al, 1968).

The loss of physical, mental, social, and/or economic resources may change the position of elderly persons in their social world. The loss of productive roles, of significant others, of self-esteem, and perhaps even of home and possessions puts older persons at risk for anxiety and fear associated with a world that is unfamiliar to them. The provision of opportunities to take advantage of an environment that offers new roles and clearly defined responsibilities will assist the older person to maintain health and a sense of well-being.

References

American Association of Retired Persons and Administration on Aging, Department of Health and Human Services: *A Profile of Older Americans–1986.* American Association of Retired Persons Publication No. PF 3049(1086)–D996, 1986.

Bengtson VL: *The Social Psychology of Aging.* Bobbs-Merrill, 1973.

Biddle BJ, Thomas EJ: *Role Theory: Concepts and Research.* Wiley, 1966.

Cunningham WR, Brookbank JW: *Gerontology: The Psychology, Biology, and Sociology of Aging.* Harper and Row, 1988.

Morgan DL: Age differences in social network participation. *J Gerontol* 1988; 43:5129–5137.

National Council on Aging: *Aging in the 80s: America in Transition.* A survey conducted for the National Council on Aging by L. Harris and Associates. Washington, DC, 1981.

Rathbone-McCuan E, Hashami J: *Isolated Elders: Health and Social Interventions.* Aspen, 1982.

Sauer WJ, Coward RT: *Social Support Networks and the Care of the Elderly.* Springer, 1985.

Shaunas E et al: *Older People in Three Industrial Societies.* Alherton, 1968.

Singer E: Reference groups and social evaluations. In: *Social Psychology: Sociological Perspectives.* Rosenberg M, Turner R (editors). Basic Books, 1981.

42

Translocation Syndrome

Deanne Remer, MA, RN, ARNP
Kathleen C. Buckwalter,
PhD, RN, FAAN
Meridean Maas, PhD, RN, FAAN

The negative impact of moving older people from one living situation to another is called relocation effect, transplantation shock, or translocation syndrome. According to Borup and Gallego (1981), there are four types of environmental change or translocation. They are residential (moving from one residence to another); interinstitutional (transferring from one institution to another); intrainstitutional (moving from one room or unit to another within an institution); and residential/institutional (transferring from a residence to an institution or the reverse). All types of translocation affect the elderly, although the latter three changes are more common among dependent elderly.

DEFINITIONS OF TRANSLOCATION

Translocation is defined as the change in environment that takes place when an individual moves from one location to another. It is a complex sequence of experiences and events that begins with situational changes that precipitate a decision to move, the impact of relocation, and the settling-in process and ends with months of adjustment that follow a move. Translocation Syndrome is manifested by impaired physical health, personal disturbances, and disruption of established behavior patterns and social relationships. Translocation Syndrome has not been accepted for clinical testing by the North American Nursing Diagnosis Association (NANDA) (Carroll-Johnson, 1989). Gordon's (1987;246) definition of Translocation Syndrome as "physiological and psychosocial disturbances due to transfer from one unit of health-care setting to another or from one living situation to another" is similar to but less specific than the definition set forth in this chapter.

Over 200 articles on the effects of translocation have been published, although most of the research in this area was conducted in the 1960s and 1970s. Early in the 1960s, a stream of research began that documented many of the negative effects of translocation. For many elderly, translocation was identified as a stressful life transition for which there was no alternative. The period of preparation, the move itself, and the settling in afterward were all perceived as times of stress (Rosow, 1974). Research subsequent to these early studies was expanded to identify people who were most vulnerable to the translocation effect.

Because of the increasing number of elderly persons, their propensity for illness, and the nature of the health care system, translocation of the elderly from one physical location to another for care has become frequent and will likely become even more frequent in the future (Lentz and Paul, 1971; Paul, 1969). According to Pollack (1976), older people (age 65 or older) have about a one in six chance of being hospitalized during each year. For those under age 65, the chance is one in ten. Older people over age 65 are also three times more apt to have more than one hospitalization in a year than persons under age 65. Once in the hospital, older people stay about four days longer than younger patients (11.7 days versus 7.6 days).

The elderly are thus characterized by high admission and discharge rates, and their tendency toward prolonged hospital stays is shown by the high bed occupancies for this age group. In addition, high-risk elderly patients account for many of the most difficult discharges from the hospital. Patients who are very old or who have had a protracted stay in the hospital are likely to have multiple physical, mental, and social disabilities.

PSYCHOLOGIC ADAPTATION AND COPING

Elderly persons who are relocated most often are forced to do so by circumstances beyond their control. Whatever the reason for the translocation, the elderly person is faced with an event that will likely induce stress and prompt some type of adaptive behavior (Lieberman and Tobin, 1983).

Translocation is a particularly significant and stressful life change for elderly persons who lack the coping mechanisms necessary for a favorable outcome. The stress surrounding translocation arises not only from the impact of the move itself, but also because of the time needed for preparation preceding the move and the period of adjustment that follows. This major life stress requires psychologic adaptation by the elderly person through cognitive appraisal, emotional states, and psychologic coping mechanisms or strategies.

This view of translocation stress, which requires an even greater adaptive ability to meet the new demands of translocation, is especially relevant to elderly persons, whose weakened biologic and psychologic capacity places them at high risk. Unfortunately, elderly individuals often experience these special demands for adaptation at a time when their adaptive capacities are diminishing.

The Effects of Translocation

Translocation implies a crisis for the elderly person. According to Holmes and Rahe (1967), a life crisis is defined in terms of the degree of stress a person experiences as a result of either a sudden onset of events

or the culmination of a gradually developing series of events that produce intense and traumatic changes in the life and experience of the individual.

It has been argued that the elderly may be more susceptible to stress because they undergo many negative life events and experience many losses during a period of concurrent physical decline. According to Sarason and Spielberger (1979), the translocation experience of the elderly often represents a convergence of both slowly accumulating and suddenly traumatic events that can and do produce intense stress for the older person. In the process of aging, basic faculties and functions such as sensory acuity and motor skills often diminish and, as a result, problems relating to the management of one's environment increase.

In addition to the loss of physical functioning, older people suffer other emotionally disturbing losses, such as the death of a spouse, the death of peers, the loss of a job through retirement, and the subsequent loss of income and mental stimulation. It is often the confluence of several or all of these factors that precipitates another crisis—that of changing environment, or translocation. This move from one environment to another is stressful for most elderly people.

For many in this particularly vulnerable group, translocation may manifest itself in undesirable physical, emotional, and social consequences. A number of researchers have reported that extensive environmental change can lead to behavioral, psychologic, and physical deterioration in elderly people (Aldrich and Mendkoff, 1963; Bourestom and Tars, 1974; Kasteler et al, 1968; Killian, 1970; Markus et al, 1972; Miller and Lieberman, 1965; Pablo, 1977).

Mortality

Research has documented many of the negative effects of translocation on the elderly, such as increased mortality and morbidity, increased depression, and decreased activity levels and life satisfaction (Aldrich and Mendkoff, 1963; Bourestom and Tars, 1974; Killian, 1970; Lieberman, 1961; Pino et al, 1978).

In a study of the effects of moving older people to institutional environments, Lieberman (1961) found that negative effects occurred because institutional environments differed radically from previous lifestyles and because the older person's capacity to adapt was overloaded. He found that 24.7% of elderly persons who entered an institution died within the first year as opposed to only 10.5% of elderly persons on a waiting list.

Blenker (1967) reviewed many studies that report an excessive mortality rate among those relocated to nursing homes, as well as excessive mortality for patients transferred between geriatric facilities. There is growing evidence that placement or any abrupt transplantation of elderly people from a familiar surrounding to nursing homes or similar institutions is hazardous and may indeed be a prelude to death (Aldrich and Mendkoff, 1963; Blenker, 1967; Bourestom and Tars, 1974; Jasnau, 1967; Killian, 1970; Pino et al, 1978; Tobin and Lieberman, 1976). However, several studies also have found no increase in mortality among institutionalized elderly (Borup et al, 1979; Miller and Lieberman, 1965; Novick, 1967; Zweig and Csank, 1975). Of the geriatric studies using a control group design, two found increases in mortality (Bourestom and Tars, 1974; Killian, 1970), and one found no significant changes in mortality (Borup et al, 1979). Although the relationship between translocation and mortality is not completely understood, the majority of studies report increased mortality rates following translocation.

SIGNIFICANCE FOR NURSING

Nurses are often involved prior to, during, and following the transfer of elderly persons from one environment to another. Findings reported in the literature strongly suggest that translocation is less stressful and subsequent life satisfaction is greater when translocation takes place gradually, when the degree of change in physical and psychosocial environment is not marked, and when the relocated older person is at the center of the decision making (Borup and Gallego, 1981). It is important for nurses who work with the elderly in institutions and in the community to be aware of translocation stress and be prepared to develop the environmental and procedural changes necessary to help minimize its harmful effects. Once sensitized to the psychologic and physical impact of translocation, nurses can strive for ways to minimize the inherent risks. Nurses who have a basic understanding about the effect of the environment on an individual's mental and physical well-being have much to contribute toward alleviating the patient's translocation stress.

By planning for continuity of care and preparing the patient through discharge preparation, the nurse can often decrease the impact of change and thus minimize the trauma and anxiety generated by translocation.

ETIOLOGIES AND RELATED RISK FACTORS

Many factors increase the probability that an older person will experience at least one type of translocation during his or her lifetime. The most common reasons are financial problems, declining health, urban renewal, and industrial expansion. Changes in the long-term care system and the classification of skilled and intermediate care facilities may also require the elderly to undergo relocation. In addition, the patient's health may improve, thus requiring a less intense level of care, or conversely, a setback in the patient's condition may require more extensive care, making translocation necessary. Furthermore, many elderly persons are destined to experience translocation trauma because professionals often fail to intervene to mitigate the undesirable effects of relocation.

Lazarus (1966) has hypothesized that environmental change is perceived as more stressful and has more drastic consequences for people with few available resources and supports (eg, intelligence, education, finances, relatives, friends) and poorly differentiated or maladaptive coping mechanisms. From this perspective, one might expect more severe reactions to the stress of translocation among the elderly. Variables that are correlated with the probability of being relocated in later life include situational factors, age, physical health, mental health, sex, and income. Identifying etiologic risk factors helps to understand the circumstances under which translocation occurs, why it is stressful, and why elderly individuals often react with decreased life satisfaction to this event (see Table 42.1).

Situational Factors

Situational factors are strongly related to translocation adjustment and have adverse effects on the physical and psychologic well-being of the elderly if the translocation (1) increases the distance to friends and relatives as well as services and facilities; (2) interferes with leisure and social activities; and (3) represents a deterioration in quality of valued attributes (eg, independence, privacy, safety, security, convenience, and familiarity).

Age

The elderly seem to be particularly vulnerable to the adverse effects of translocation. Neugarten (1968) has noted that with increased age there is less energy available for maintaining former levels of involvement with the outside world. In addition, the elderly tend to have less desire to move, less flexibility, and less opportunity for establishing new relationships in a new environment (Goldscheider, 1966).

Physical Health

Several translocation studies of institutionalized populations have looked at the effects of the residents' initial physical health and subsequent adjustment. There is some evidence that among elderly residents, translocation has the worst impact on those who are already in the

Table 42.1

Related Factors/Etiologies and Defining Characteristics of Translocation Syndrome

GORDON (1987)	REMER, BUCKWALTER, MAAS
	Related Factors/Etiologies/Risk Factors
	Transfer from one living or health care environment to another
	Old age
	Poor physical health
	Low levels of socioeconomic resources
	Mental illness
	Confusion
	Social isolation
Defining Characteristics	*Defining Characteristics*
Anxiety, apprehension, vigilance or withdrawal, passivity, change in eating or sleeping habits	Change in living arrangements (residence)
Verbalizations indicating lack of trust in care providers	Pessimism re health
Verbalizations of insecurity in new living situation	Decreased levels of social activity/withdrawal
Presence of dependency	Increased confusion
Change in living situation requiring establishment of new relationships with people and environment	Memory deficits
	Bizarre behavior
	Decreased general activity
	Decreased life satisfaction
	Hyperirritability
	Sleep disturbances
	Disturbed IPRs
	Emotional insulation/detachment
	Decreased trust, insecurity
	Increased stress and anxiety
	Decreased health status
	Increased dependency
	Increased alienation/aggression

poorest physical health (Goldfarb et al, 1972; Heller, 1982; Killian, 1970). Brand and Smith (1974) found that in the community, life satisfaction of elderly persons in poor health was lower among those relocated than those not relocated.

Mental Illness

Because mentally ill people generally have poor coping mechanisms, one might expect them to react adversely to environmental change. Personality factors related to poor coping ability include severe mental or social impairments and organic brain syndrome and depression. Several studies have found that mortality was higher for relocated nursing home residents who were psychotic prior to the move than for nonpsychotic residents (Aldrich and Mendkoff, 1963; Kral et al, 1968). People predisposed to depression or neurosis tend to have more severe reactions to translocation. For depressed and neurotic individuals, translocation may be perceived as more threatening and may overwhelm their adaptive capacities (Heller, 1982).

Sex

Findings of differential impact of translocation by sex are equivocal. Among the elderly, some studies found that women were more negatively affected than men (Brand and Smith, 1974; Bourestom and Tars, 1974), whereas others found that men were more negatively affected (Kral et al, 1968).

Income

Poorly educated and low-income people not only tend to be victims of involuntary translocation, but also are more vulnerable to the adverse effects of translocation (Gurman, 1963). Persons of low socioeconomic status are more likely to be forced from their homes by hunger, eviction, and social unrest.

Kasl (1972;381) summarized research findings that characterize the elderly who are particularly vulnerable to the stress of translocation. These characteristics include being "older, and in poor health; living alone and having few contacts with friends and kin; in poor financial circumstances and of lower social class; having lived in an old neighborhood a long time; of low morale and life satisfaction, reacting to the move with depression, giving up, and hopelessness–helplessness."

DEFINING CHARACTERISTICS

Physical Health

Research findings suggest that institutional translocation either from the community to an institution or from one institution to another is typically accompanied by some deterioration in physical health. Tobin and Lieberman (1976) found that the health of individuals remained stable immediately after they entered a nursing home (during the first 2 months) but deteriorated after 1 year. Studies that examine the effects of translocation from one institution to another report subsequent declines in health including increases in restriction of activity, hospitalization, and health failure (Bourestom and Tars, 1974; Kral et al, 1968; Miller and Lieberman, 1965; Pino et al, 1978).

Kral et al (1968) studied stress reactions following translocation by assessing physiologic functioning as indicated in plasma levels of cortisol. Results showed that (1) men have a significant increase in plasma levels of cortisol (PC) from about 1 week before translocation to about 1 or 2 weeks after; (2) men who had organic brain signs had a larger increase in PC levels; (3) significantly more elderly men than women had died 6 months after translocation; and (4) at the end of 23 months, the death rate for patients with organic signs was higher than for the normal patients. Thus, the stress reaction, as reflected by changes in PC levels, appears to have prognostic value for subsequent morbidity and mortality.

Behavior

The most common signs and symptoms of reported stress reactions to translocation have been emotional, behavioral, and mental health changes. In institutional facilities for geriatric patients, posttranslocation effects have included pessimism with regard to health outlook, decreased levels of social activity (Bourestom and Tars, 1974), and increases in confusion, memory deficits, and bizarre behavior (Miller and Lieberman, 1965). Two studies of involuntary translocation from home suggest that relocated individuals experience a decrease in general activity and life satisfaction (Brand and Smith, 1974; Kasteler et al, 1968). Coleman (1973) identified that translocation stress may be manifested in such behaviors as hyperirritability, sleep disturbances, disturbed interper-

sonal relationships, and ego defense-oriented reactions including emotional insulation and detachment.

According to Bourestom and Tars (1974), relocated patients demonstrate increased pessimism regarding the state of their health, withdraw from activities in which they had formerly engaged, exhibit lower levels of behavior, and are somewhat less inclined to perceive interest or trust on the part of those with whom they come into contact. Other negative effects of translocation include physical changes from decreased activity; stress and anxiety manifestations; decreased health states and health failure; and psychologic behavioral changes including mistrust, insecurity, dependency, withdrawal, and alienation or aggression.

A study by Miller and Lieberman (1965) found that elderly persons who had a negative evaluation of their past life and saw the future in bleak terms demonstrated significantly more negative changes after translocation. According to Pablo (1977), excessively high death rates (during the first 3 months following translocation), decreased activity levels, low morale and life satisfaction, and depression have been attributed to translocation.

With respect to the impact of institutional translocation on self-control, self-esteem, and identity, Gordon and Vinaacke (1973) asked nursing home residents to rate themselves. In all three areas, respondents consistently rated themselves more positively in the past, prior to institutionalization, than during their present institutional state. Leibowitz (1974) found that residents who had no part in making the decisions associated with translocation felt powerless, insignificant, and manipulated.

Borup et al (1979) reported a number of behaviors that result from interinstitutional translocation. Regarding perceived health status, patients demonstrated hypochondria, unwarranted anxiety concerning their health, and behaviors such as violence to self, others, and/or property and forceful aggression with an intent to dominate or control others. The social/psychologic behaviors included alienation or a feeling of being separated and/or isolated from one's social environment. Anxiety was also experienced as an emotional stress, and patients demonstrated this by becoming angry, easily upset, and irritable.

As noted in Table 42.1, there are many similarities between the signs and symptoms reported in the literature and those set forth as defining characteristics by Gordon (1987). It is helpful to consider both categories of criteria when identifying a high-risk patient for relocation preparation or discharge planning (American Hospital Association, 1983;25).

ASSESSMENT

A number of behaviors result from the negative and stressful impact of translocation, including physical changes of decreased health status, health failure, and mortality. Psychologic behavioral changes include mistrust, insecurity, dependency, withdrawal, decreased activity, and alienation or aggression, as well as stress and anxiety manifestations. Nurses should be aware of these serious consequences of relocation. A thorough assessment incorporating the signs and symptoms provides the basis for diagnosis and intervention with potential to prevent adverse sequelae.

There are currently no standardized comprehensive geriatric assessment tools available to use in determining potential for translocation trauma. Remer (1986) developed a predischarge structured interview guide to use with geriatric psychiatric patients at a VA medical center that could be adapted for other geriatric populations. Remer's interview addressed the personal and clinical characteristics of the subjects. The personal characteristics included the age, sex, marital status, educational level, income, religion, and race of the individual patients. The clinical characteristics of the patients included the psychiatric diagnosis, significant others, number of previous psychiatric hospitalizations, length of time since previous hospital discharge, and length of time in present location. Some measure of mental status may also be relevant to determining the efficacy of treatment.

Remer (1986) also used two other standardized assessment tools in her research on the effects of discharge planning on the relocation of geriatric psychiatric patients: (1) The Geriatric Scale of Recent Life Events and (2) The Life Satisfaction Index.

The Geriatric Scale of Recent Life Events

This instrument, developed by Kiyak and Kahana (1975), is a list of life events relevant to the elderly population. The scale estimates the level of stress experienced by the elderly individual. Stress intensity is based on a "life change index," which assumes that the amount of stress a person experiences is related to the number of life change units within a particular period of time.

The Geriatric Scale of Recent Life Events consists of 56 items, 36 of which were taken from the original Social Readjustment Rating Scale developed by Holmes and Rahe (1967). The remaining 20 life change items were obtained from 284 elderly residents in an open-ended questionnaire (Kiyak and Kahana, 1975). These 20 stress-related items were noted to be particularly relevant for an aged sample.

In a personal communication with Dr. Kiyak, the Geriatric Scale of Recent Life Events was identified as a meaningful strategy for assessing life events in the elderly that takes into account age-specific experiences and characteristics. However, the instrument is not perfect because some of the items are not relevant to the relocation of the

dependent elderly. For example, going to jail, menopause, and employment-related items were not identified by the subjects undergoing relocation, whereas change in residence, physical changes, and health-related items were frequently identified factors in the relocation process. A more specific and sensitive instrument with fewer items to measure the impact of relocation on the stress of elderly persons is needed. Such an instrument would more accurately identify pre- and postchanges as a result of this traumatic life experience.

The Life Satisfaction Index (LSI)

This research instrument, developed by Neugarten et al (1961), has been documented extensively in research with elderly populations (Bloom, 1975). Questions on the Life Satisfaction Index center around stresses experienced and perceived by the subject, coping action and emotional patterns, demographic data, and various correlates of adjustment.

Form A (LSI-A) contains 20 statements in which the subject may respond with an agreement, uncertain, or disagreement response to each statement about the respondent's perception of his or her well-being.

Form B (LSI-B) consists of 12 items with two or three response categories for each item. Neugarten et al (1961) define life satisfaction as having five components: zest (versus apathy), resolution and fortitude, congruence between desired and achieved goals, positive self-concept, and mood tone. Thus, a person who is at the positive end of the continuum (1) takes pleasure from the activity that constitutes everyday life; (2) regards his or her life as meaningful; (3) feels that he or she has succeeded in achieving his or her major goals; (4) holds a positive image of self; and (5) maintains happy and optimistic attitudes and moods. This instrument is useful for identifying the elderly person's abilities and characteristics that are likely to be used to cope successfully with translocation or that are more apt to be risk factors for the onset of Translocation Syndrome.

CASE STUDY

Translocation Syndrome

Martha is a 74-year-old widow, hospitalized for gallbladder surgery. Following a successful operation and a 4-day hospital stay, the utilization review committee informed Martha that she had exceeded Diagnostic Related Groups (DRG) guidelines and must be discharged quickly. Martha confided in her nurse that she had no one to care for her after discharge and that she receives only limited Social Security benefits. Martha's medical history consists of high blood pressure and diabetes, which has resulted in a significant loss of vision.

The medical unit's social worker was contacted regarding Martha's case. In this medical facility, the procedure for discharge consisted of calling a list of nursing homes to find an available bed. A frantic and chaotic process ensued to find a suitable facility for Martha. On discharge from the hospital, Martha had not participated in the translocation process, had received little preparation, and had no choice in the placement decision.

Martha was admitted to the Valley View Rest Home following discharge from the medical center. The rest home was located several hundred miles from her only family—a niece and a nephew. The first few days following admission, Martha quietly withdrew to her room and refused to participate in scheduled activities or socialize with other residents.

On day five, Martha reported to the nurse that she felt the other residents were watching her and making "derogatory remarks" because they don't like her. She said that they have, on occasion, followed her on walks. She reported that a man enters her room at night and accuses her of "horrible things." Martha's mistrust of the residents and staff continued. She refused to eat the food, which she said was "poison." She maintained a vigilant state at night and threatened other residents to stay away from her.

The nursing home's consulting physician was notified because of Martha's weight loss, her diabetes test results, and her refusal to take prescribed medications. The staff believed that Martha had "given up on life." The gerontologic nurse specialist conducted an assessment and concluded that Martha was experiencing translocation stress, based on identification of the following behavioral manifestations: (1) withdrawn behavior; (2) decreased participation in social activities; (3) mistrust; (4) disturbed interpersonal relationships; (5) decreased health status; (6) change in eating and sleeping habits.

A number of etiologic factors were also identified that resulted in the development of translocation trauma for Martha: (1) situational factors such as distance from friends and relatives; (2) age; and (3) compromised physical health status postoperatively. Because of the recency of Martha's precipitous move to Valley View, the nurse reasoned that the behaviors exhibited by Martha were indicative of Translocation Syndrome rather than some other nursing diagnosis such as fear, anxiety, reactive depression, activity intolerance, drug toxicity, or fluid volume deficit.

NURSING INTERVENTIONS

Preparation for Relocation

There is some evidence that the stressful effects of translocation can be modified by the degree and perhaps the type of preparation provided prior to the translocation

(Langer and Rodin, 1976; Lieberman et al, 1971; Pastalan, 1976). Pretranslocation preparation as a factor in posttranslocation adjustment has been investigated principally in situations involving involuntary moves from institution to institution.

Studies of programs in which preparation procedures were designed and implemented have shown less negative effects. In general, these studies suggest that the new environment is less threatening and the morbidity outcomes for the relocated patients are less negative when premove special preparation is provided (Bourestom and Tars, 1974; Jasnau, 1967; Novick, 1967; Zweig and Csank, 1975).

Some researchers (Lawton and Yaffe, 1970; Miller and Lieberman, 1965) have shown that negative effects are not exhibited when the elderly are prepared for the move through individual and group counseling, orientation to the new facility (eg, premove visits), participation in the decision-making and planning process, opportunities for choice, continuity of staff, and family and social support.

According to Pino et al (1978), successful adjustment to a new institution appears to be affected by (1) preparation for the move; (2) the patient's attitude toward the move; and (3) the individual's level of mental and physical functioning prior to the move. Such preparation decreases mortality rates (Jasnau, 1967; Pastalan, 1976; Zweig and Csank, 1975), decreases health deterioration, and increases levels of life satisfaction (Pino et al, 1978). A study by Pastalan (1976) suggests that individual preparation is more effective than group preparation, and the effectiveness of translocation-preparation programs depends, in part, on the personal characteristics of the individuals who are relocated.

There is also some evidence that translocation adjustment depends on the degree to which the elderly are "psychologically prepared" for the change. Several institutional translocation programs that did not find any adverse transfer effects provided individualized supportive services, preparatory counseling, site visits, and realistic information about the new setting (Bourestom and Tars, 1974; Jasnau, 1967; Novick, 1967; Zweig and Csank, 1975).

In the Novick (1967) study, staff members prepared residents far in advance of the actual translocation by taking them on frequent bus trips to the new site and by constructing a full-size model of the future bedroom and furniture. Lentz and Paul (1971) found that mental patients who received a preparatory program did not show posttranslocation behavioral decrements, whereas other patients did. The use of preparatory programs may serve to increase predictability and anticipatory coping. Schulz and Brenner (1977) reported that the more predictable the new environment, the less negative the effects of translocation.

Remer (1986) investigated the stressful effects of translocation among geriatric psychiatric patients. Her research concluded that translocation is a stressful event for geriatric psychiatric patients regardless of whether they receive discharge preparation or not. However, patients who received the additional discharge preparation experienced less translocation stress and better life satisfaction.

Several studies suggest that a caring, accepting environment is a key factor in the adjustment and well-being of relocated persons. Slover (1972) reported that decline is greater in relocated elderly who have been placed in environments lacking warmth, individuation, and autonomy. Gurel et al (1972) also report that contact between staff and patients is consistently related to patient outcome. Thus, the special attention of staff who promote a caring and warm environment appears to be a crucial variable in the successful translocation of the elderly mentally ill patient.

Nurses can assist in reducing the stress of translocation and facilitating the adjustment of the elderly following translocation. Preparation is needed to reduce the stress of translocation for elderly persons and subsequently improve their life satisfaction. Bourestom and Tars (1974) suggest that preparatory programs should become mandatory policy prior to involuntary translocation of the elderly.

Discharge Planning

Discharge planning ordinarily refers to the preparation and coordination of care when a person is moved from an institution. Discharge planning has greater relevance for the relocated older (over age 65) population in our country than for any other group and is a crucial element in the care of elderly persons with chronic illnesses. Effective planning should coordinate institutional and community-based care so that continuity of treatment is preserved as the patient moves among settings.

Discharge planning should be a coordinated process of activities that involves various members of an interdisciplinary team, the elderly person, and the family. As a nursing intervention, discharge planning ensures that each patient has a plan for continuing care and/or follow-up that facilitates translocation between units within a setting or from one care setting to another.

Bristow et al (1976;4) state the nurse must use a holistic approach to assist the client and family "to regain as normal and productive a role as possible; providing for

efficient, compassionate, and economical methods for the delivery of health services" in the discharge planning process. According to McKeehan (1981), discharge planning is based on the philosophy of patient care that recognizes that each patient has specific needs for continuing care and continuity of treatment (see Figure 42.1). Elderly patients who experience a major change in lifestyle and support systems through translocation have a great need for discharge planning. Thus, the nurse as a discharge planner is instrumental in assisting elderly persons to be relocated with minimal stress.

Nursing's Responsibilities in the Discharge Planning Process

The professional nurse must be sensitized to the potential outcomes and behavioral manifestations of stress and life satisfaction in relocated dependent elderly. Nurses should understand and expect manifestations of stress and characteristic behavioral symptoms of translocation trauma rather than be alarmed by "acting out" behaviors. Knowledge and understanding of elderly persons and the translocation process will result in more realistic planning of interventions for relocation. Although nurses should play an integral role in discharge planning to reduce translocation trauma, there is currently little nursing research on this phenomenon.

Several nursing responsibilities are critical in the discharge planning process:

1. The nurse shares an obligation with other health care team members to provide the highest possible quality of health care to the patient and family. Advocacy is inherent in this responsibility. The nurse should include the elder in planning in order to prevent or resolve possible conflicts when the elderly person's goals differ from those of the health care team.
2. The nurse must be aware of the available resources for care that exist both within the health care facility and in the community. This responsibility requires a thorough understanding of services offered. A continuing care consultant is an especially valuable resource to facilitate discharge planning.
3. If discharge planning is to be successful, the nurse must establish and maintain collegial relationships with members of other health care disciplines, based on mutual recognition of and respect for each group's

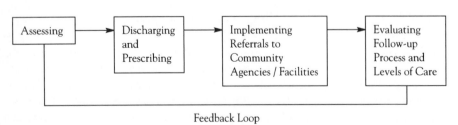

Feedback Loop

Figure 42.1

Discharge planning implementation model. (McKeehan, 1981, p. 12) unique and necessary contribution to the elderly person's well-being. Through cooperative teamwork and open communication the discharge planning process will be facilitated, to the benefit of both the individual and the team.

4. The nurse must develop a clear concept of the roles and responsibilities for discharge planning of the elderly using either functional, team, or primary nursing approaches.

Those elderly persons for whom discharge planning will involve more than routine procedures must be identified. If not correctly carried out, discharge of an elderly individual can result in numerous problems. Early case finding includes identification of high-risk groups based on such variables as diagnosis, age, nutritional status, and combinations of social and economic factors and health status.

Other factors to be considered in developing a post-discharge plan include an assessment of the elderly person's needs for physician services, nursing services, rehabilitation services, clinical laboratory and radiology services, nutritional guidance, social work services, transportation, and financial assistance. Early consultation with the patient's family is also essential.

For each category of need, the assessment must include such specifics as:

Physician Services: Frequency and type (eg, psychiatrist or neurologist) and various sites in which these services can be given (eg, private office, clinic, satellite clinic, hospital, or home)

Nursing Services: Frequency and continuity of availability (eg, regular, part-time, or intermittent); level of needed nursing competence (eg, registered nurse, licensed practical nurse, or aide)

Rehabilitation Services: Specific modalities, frequency, type of equipment used, level of professional supervision required, level of professional skill required, and settings in which the services must be provided

Clinical Laboratory and/or Radiology: Type and frequency of services needed

Nutrition: Type and amount of dietary guidance, supervision, and services (eg, Meals on Wheels) needed; frequency of review or modification; specific guidelines, including food preference; meal plans; short-term and long-term goals; and provisions for follow-up at a nutrition clinic

Social Work Services: Social history, including support system, coping mechanisms, current living situation, counseling needs, and post-hospital plans

Transportation: Frequency, distance, type of conveyance needed, costs, and financial feasibility

Financial Assistance: Availability of third-party coverage and public assistance for needed health care; sources of payment for special needs; family resources; and need for assistance (American Hospital Association, 1973).

By planning for continuity of care between facilities, the nurse can decrease the impact of change and thus minimize the translocation trauma. Based on the elder's condition, any decision for translocation should be made with the elderly person and family in such a way as to provide them with independence and choice.

In addition, nurses should adequately prepare patients for translocation by arranging pretranslocation visits and informing them about various aspects of the new setting that will require personal adjustment. Support systems and counseling should be available to facilitate the process prior to, during, and following relocation as well as during the necessary adjustment period that follows the translocation experience.

Discharge planning also involves the use of a wide variety of community resources to move the elder to the most independent level of living possible within a community. Family should be involved in the discharge planning process, although the degree of involvement may vary with the individual depending on age and mental alertness. Resistance to transfer to a site for care other than home, feelings of rejection if placement at home is not chosen, and fears of new places and personnel are all factors to be assessed carefully. The alternatives to be explored include care at home, day-care centers, foster or boarding home care, and institutional care. Alternatives, as well as a contingency or back-up plan, should be presented to the elderly person and the family.

The discharge plan identifies both short-term and long-term needs and goals and provides for optimum functioning of the patient and family unit. When planning for an alternative to present care, the first consideration is the patient and his or her desires, resources, and capabilities. The second consideration is the family. The family is often not informed about the details of the elderly person's condition nor given ample warning about possible relocation dates and times. Families usually are interested in and have significant influence over the elder's environment, so when the setting requires major modifications, the family should be an integral part of the planning.

Community Resources

Whenever possible, the community resources should be appropriate for the elderly person and his or her family in terms of language and cultural factors, financial ability, age, socialization needs, social and emotional needs and attitudes, medical and nursing needs, and long- and short-term goals. Other important factors in the selection of a community resource are proximity to family and the geographic location with respect to accessibility to needed services, such as home health services or outpatient care.

Referral and Transfer of Information

When the plan for discharge or aftercare requires referral and transfer from one level of care to another, the process must be an organized one with clearly understood procedures. Referrals should be made as early as possible in the planning period. Information about the elderly person's medical condition, care, needs, and social situation should be given to the institution or agency that is being asked to provide care. Whenever possible, arrangements should be made for the elder and the family or other interested persons to see the institution/agency and meet the staff, thus participating actively in the referral process.

Coordination of information from all health care professionals is essential. Information should be clear, concise, and relevant and should include plans for continuing care, as well as diagnostic information, descriptions of treatment procedures and reactions, medication, special care needs, and rehabilitation potential. It should also relate to the elder's and family's present and anticipated level of involvement and expectations.

Follow-Up

Whether elderly persons are transferred to other institutions, relocated within institutions, discharged to outpatient or private physician care, or referred to health and social agencies for continuing services, the degree of responsibility of the nurse for continuity of care can range from follow-up letters to conferences with the interdisciplinary care team where the person is relocated. Completion of the discharge plan may not coincide with the elderly person's discharge. Therefore, follow-up on the care plan to ascertain whether the person has made a satisfactory adjustment and is receiving necessary services should be done.

OUTCOMES

Evaluation of relocation preparation and discharge planning is based on the assessment of beneficial outcomes. According to Bristow and Stickney (1976), beneficial outcomes provide the elderly person with the ability to regain maximum potential for high-level wellness with the least amount of discomfort and emotional stress.

The beneficial outcomes of a coordinated relocation preparation or discharge planning program are threefold: (1) cost containment; (2) improved continuity of care; and (3) minimization or alleviation of negative behaviors associated with translocation trauma.

Because the purpose of nursing intervention is to assist the elderly individual to return to as normal and productive a role as possible, the primary beneficiary of preparation and planning is the elderly person. What the elder and the family learn as they become involved in the relocation process should be lasting. For some persons, the necessary services will enable them to regain, maintain, and even increase their level of functioning.

Another positive outcome is a more efficient patient transfer. The entire procedure can be shortened and made less traumatic. Emphasis is on person-to-person interaction. By planning for continuity of care between settings the nurse, by preparing the patient, can decrease the impact of change and thus minimize the trauma and anxiety often generated by movement from one care setting to another. Ultimately, the nurse must use patient behavioral outcomes to evaluate the effectiveness of relocation preparation and discharge planning. Increased life satisfaction and decreased relocation stress should be observed if the nursing intervention has been successful. More specifically, the nurse should expect the signs and symptoms of Translocation Syndrome, listed in Table 42.1, to be minimized or alleviated unless the behaviors indicate another diagnosis.

CASE STUDY

Nursing Interventions

Referring again to our case example to illustrate the intervention of discharge planning, the nurse at Valley View Rest Home, after consulting with Martha, called Martha's niece and nephew and notified them that Martha was experiencing difficulty adjusting to her new environment after discharge from the hospital. Martha's family members were eager to help in the situation and expressed interest in having Martha relocated nearer to them and her old home. An appointment was scheduled, and the niece and nephew came to Valley View to meet with Martha and the nurse. At that time, Martha was encouraged to participate in the planning process, and her desire to move to a congregate housing site in her former community was a major consideration in development of the discharge plan. The nurse agreed that Martha's health status required some degree of sheltered environment but that nursing home placement was not needed. Martha had often visited friends at the local elderly housing project and was familiar with the setting. Further, the housing site was convenient to the work location of her nephew, who agreed to stop by daily on the way home from work.

The nurse at Valley View called the Council on Aging in Martha's old home town and got her on the elderly housing project waiting list. She also provided Martha's niece and nephew with a list of services she felt Martha would need in order to live independently, including Visiting Nursing Association, Meals-on-Wheels, chore services and a homemaker/home health aide two times per week. The niece and nephew agreed to contact these service providers so that essential services would be in place immediately following Martha's move. Finally, they made arrangements to pick up Martha the following weekend for a premove visit to her proposed housing site.

Three weeks later an opening occurred at the congregate housing site, and Martha's niece and nephew arrived at Valley View to transport her to her new apartment. During this interim period, Martha's paranoid and anxious behaviors diminished dramatically. She began eating again and expressed eagerness to prepare her own meals once again. Her sleep patterns improved somewhat, but she still had problems sleeping in the nursing home. She also expressed some concern that sleep difficulty would continue to bother her in her new apartment because "it just wasn't the same" as her old house.

One month following discharge, the nurse at Valley View called Martha in her new apartment to determine how she was doing postmove. Martha reported she was adjusting well and had begun attending church, visited frequently with friends and family, and was looking forward to planting geraniums in her flower box next spring.

SUMMARY

This chapter reviewed the prevalence and significance of the nursing diagnosis Translocation Syndrome for the elderly. The diagnosis was discussed as a disruptive, stressful, and potentially debilitating event in an older person's life. The period of preparation, the move itself, and the settling in afterward are all times of stress. High-risk factors that contribute to Translocation Syndrome in the elderly population were identified. Relocation preparation and discharge planning were described in detail as the major interventions the nurse should employ to reduce relocation stress. Follow-up evaluation of the interventions was also detailed, including the outcomes that should accrue if interventions are successful.

Findings in the literature reported that proper planning and preparation are helpful in reducing translocation stress and facilitating adjustment of the elderly. Translocation is less stressful when it takes place gradually, when the degree of change in physical and psychosocial environment is not marked, and when the older person is at the center of the decision-making process. There is evidence that preparation for translocation through real-istic information and counseling can help offset some of the stress associated with institutional moves.

The failure to meet the needs of dependent elderly persons adequately is well documented, and the need for discharge preparation is obvious. Ultimately, the quality of care that the elderly receive on relocation becomes the responsibility of the nurse. Thus, the nurse's role in discharge or relocation preparation must be especially effective to ensure acceptable health outcomes.

The concept, process, and implications of relocation preparation and discharge planning were discussed. The nurse's role in achieving continuity of care and specific outcomes for elderly patients involves both independent and collaborative functions with the health care team. As a member of a professional discipline, the nurse diagnoses and treats distinct nursing problems and refers those that are unresolved at discharge or relocation for continued intervention. Because of nursing's holistic focus and continuous presence with the elderly person, nurses are in an ideal position to facilitate the coordination and communication of discharge planning within the health care team. Nursing's specific responsibilities for intervention can be implemented within the framework of the American Nurses' Association *Standards and Scope of Gerontological Nursing Practice* (1987), which reflects the problem-solving steps of the nursing process.

Providing the elderly and their families with the opportunity to be involved in the decision-making process and giving them a sense of control over decisions are major factors to consider in the discharge preparation of the geriatric patient. The purpose of discharge preparation is to assist the elder to return to as normal and productive a role as possible. What the elder learns as she or he becomes involved in the discharge preparation and translocation should be lasting.

References

Aldrich CL, Mendkoff E: Relocation of the aged and disabled: A mortality study. *J Am Geriatr Soc* 1963; 11:185-194.

American Hospital Association: *Statement on a Patient's Bill of Rights.* The Association, 1973.

American Hospital Association: *Introduction to Discharge Planning for Hospitals.* The Association, 1983.

American Nurses' Association: *Standards and Scope of Gerontological Nursing Practice.* ANA Publications, 1987.

Blenker M: Environmental change and the aging individual. *Gerontologist* 1967; 7:101-105.

Bloom M: Evaluation instruments: Tests and measurements in long-term care. In: *Long-Term Care.* Sherwood S (editor). Spectrum, 1975.

Borup JH, Gallego DT: Mortality as affected by interinstitutional relocation: Update and assessment. *Gerontologist* 1981; 21:8-16.

Borup JH, Gallego DT, Hefferman PG: Relocation and its effect on mortality. *Gerontologist* 1979; 19:135–140.

Bourestom, N, Tars S: Alteration in life patterns following nursing home relocation. *Gerontologist* 1974; 14:506–510.

Brand F, Smith R: Life adjustment and relocation of the elderly. *J Gerontol* 1974; 29:336–340.

Bristow O, Stickney C, Thompson S: *Discharge Planning for Continuity of Care.* Publication No. 21-1604. National League for Nursing, 1976.

Carroll-Johnson R (editor): *Classification of Nursing Diagnoses: Proceedings of the Eighth Conference.* Lippincott, 1989.

Coleman LC: Life stress and maladaptive behavior. *Am J Occup Ther* 1973; 27:169–180.

Goldfarb AI, Shahinian SP, Burr HI: Death rate of relocated residents. In: *Research Planning and Action for the Elderly.* Kent DP, Kastenbaum R, Sherwood S (editors). Behavioral Publications, 1972.

Goldscheider C: Differential residential mobility of the older population. *J Gerontol* 1966; 21:103–108.

Gordon D, Vinaake W: Post-hospital discharge, patient care, utilization of services and facilities. *Inquiry* 1973; 10:41–48.

Gordon M: *Manual of Nursing Diagnosis.* McGraw-Hill, 1987.

Gurel L, Linn M, Linn B: Physical and mental impairment of function evaluation of the aged: The PAMIE scale. *J Gerontol* 1972; 27:83–90.

Gurman R: Population mobility in the American middle class. In: *The Urban Condition.* Duhl LJ (editor). Basic Books, 1963.

Heller T: The effects of involuntary residential relocation: A review. *Am J Community Psychol* 1982; 10:321–337.

Holmes TH, Rahe RH: The social readjustment rating scale. *J Psychosomat Res* 1967; 11:213–218.

Jasnau KR: Individualized versus mass transfer of nonpsychiatric geriatric patients from mental hospitals to nursing homes, with specific reference to death rate. *J Am Geriatr Soc* 1967; 15:280–284.

Kasl SV: Physical and mental health effects of involuntary relocation and institutionalization of the elderly—a review. *Am J Public Health* 1972; 62:377–383.

Kasteler J, Gray R, Carruth M: Involuntary relocation of the elderly. *Gerontologist* 1968; 8:276–279.

Killian E: Effects of geriatric transfers in mortality rates. *Social Work* 1970; 15:19–26.

Kiyak AH, Kahana E: *A Methodological Inquiry into the Schedule of Recent Life Events.* Paper presented at the American Psychological Association, New York, 1975.

Kral VA, Grad B, Berenson J: Stress reactions resulting from relocation of an aged population. *Canad Psychiatrist* 1968; 13:201–209.

Langer E, Rodin J: The effects of choice and enhanced personal responsibility for the aged: A field experiment in an institutionalized setting. *J Personality Soc Psychol* 1976; 34:191–198.

Lawton MP, Yaffe S: Mortality, morbidity, and voluntary change of residence by older people. *J Am Geriatr Soc* 1970; 18:823–831.

Lazarus RS: *Psychological Stress and Coping Process.* McGraw-Hill, 1966.

Leibowitz B: Impact of intra-institutional relocation. *Gerontologist* 1974; 14:293–306.

Lentz RJ, Paul GL: "Routine" vs. "therapeutic" transfer of chronic mental patients. *Arch Gen Psychiatry* 1971; 25:187–191.

Lieberman M: Relationship of mortality rates to entrance to a home for the aged. *Geriatrics* 1961; 16:515–519.

Lieberman M, Tobin S: *The Experience of Old Age: Stress, Coping and Survival.* Basic Books, 1983.

Lieberman M, Tobin S, Stover D: *The Effects of Relocation on Long-Term Geriatric Patients.* Final Report Project No. 17-1328. University of Chicago, Illinois Department of Health and Committee on Human Development, 1971.

Markus E, Blenker M, Bloom M: Some factors and their association with post-relocation mortality among institutionalized aged persons. *J Gerontol* 1972; 27:276–283.

McKeehan KM (editor): *Continuing Care: A Multidisciplinary Approach to Discharge Planning.* Mosby, 1981.

Miller D, Lieberman M: The relationship of affect state and adaptive capacity to reactions to stress. *J Gerontol* 1965; 20:492–497.

Neugarten BL: *Middle Age and Aging: A Reader in Social Psychology.* University of Chicago Press, 1968.

Neugarten BL, Havighurst R, Tobin S: The measurement of life satisfaction. *J Gerontol* 1961; 16:134–143.

Novick LJ: Easing the stress of moving day. *Hospitals* 1967; 41:6–10.

Pablo R: Intra-institutional relocation: Its impact on long-term care patients. *Gerontologist* 1977; 17:426–435.

Pastalan L: Report on Pennsylvania nursing home relocation program. Interim research findings. Institute of Gerontology, University of Michigan, 1976.

Paul GL: Chronic mental patient: Current status-future directions. *Psycholog Bull* 1969; 71:81–94.

Pino CJ, Rosica LM, Carter TJ: The differential effects of relocation on nursing home patients. *Gerontologist* 1978; 18:167–172.

Pollack M: Perception of self in institutionalized aged subjects. *J Gerontol* 1976; 17:405–411.

Remer DM: *The Effects of Discharge Preparation on the Relocation of Geriatric Psychiatric Patients.* (Thesis.) The University of Iowa, Iowa City, Iowa, 1986.

Rosow I: *Socialization to Old Age.* University of California Press, 1974.

Sarason IG, Speilberger CD: *Stress and Anxiety,* Vol 6. Hemisphere Publishing, 1979.

Schulz R, Brenner G: Relocation of the aged: A review and theoretical analysis. *J Gerontol* 1977; 32:323–333.

Slover D: *Relocation for Therapeutic Purposes of Aged Mental Hospital Patients.* Paper presented at the meeting of the Gerontological Society, San Juan, Puerto Rico, 1972.

Tobin SS, Lieberman MA: Life satisfaction and social interaction in the aging. *J Gerontol* 1976; 13:344–347.

Zweig J, Csank J: Effects of relocation on chronically ill geriatric patients of a medical unit: Mortality rates. *J Am Geriatr Soc* 1975; 23:132–136.

43

Dysfunctional Grieving

GWEN WHITING, MS, RN
KATHLEEN C. BUCKWALTER,
PhD, RN, FAAN

GRIEF, ALTHOUGH A UNIVERSAL PHENOMENON, HAS been conceptualized in many different ways (Bowlby, 1961; Engel, 1960a; Freud, 1973; Lindemann, 1974; Parkes, 1972) and rarely has been studied systematically. We know little about the time course associated with grief; about the importance, frequency, or manifestations of unresolved grief; or about the morbidity and mortality associated with bereavement (Zisook et al, 1982). Nor do we understand well the natural history of grief in older adults (Dimond, 1981).

Gerontologic nurses and others who work with older adults must understand the process of grieving in order to provide effective support and promote adjustment to loss. Appropriate nursing intervention and guidance during the grieving process is important to prevent grief-related psychiatric disorders, medical illnesses, and social incapacitation (Parkes, 1965; Zisook et al, 1982).

DEFINING GRIEF

Medical and psychiatric models most often have viewed grief as a continuum, with "normal grief" at one end and "pathologic grief reactions" (eg, neurotic and psychosomatic symptoms) at the other end (Volkan, 1970). However, even "normal" grief has been considered an illness because it is a discrete syndrome with predictable symptomatology (Engel, 1960b).

Four related nursing diagnoses were set forth in 1973: arrested grieving; arrested grieving, potential; delayed onset of grieving; and delayed onset of grieving, potential (Kim and Moritz, 1982). In 1980, these diagnoses became synthesized under the diagnostic label "Grieving, Dysfunctional" within the role-relationship pattern (Kim and Moritz, 1982;389).

Gordon (1982) used the term *dysfunctional* to describe any experience that inhibits persons from "going on with their life." McFarland and Wasli (1986;77) defined dysfunctional grieving as being "stuck in one phase of grieving, demonstrating excessive emotional reactions or excessive length of time in a phase." Failure to attain acceptance and successful adaptation; engagement in prolonged, excessive denial; and the development of mental illness, especially depression, were viewed as possible outcomes. Other terms have been used to refer to this same "dysfunctional" element in the grieving process: complicated, unresolved, morbid, neurotic, pathologic, abnormal, deviant, chronic, delayed, exaggerated, atypical, and distorted. The North American Nursing Diagnosis Association (NANDA) has not defined Dysfunctional Grieving. However, Kim et al (1987;22) offer the following definition: "a state in which actual or perceived object loss exists. Objects include people, possessions, a job, status, home, ideals, parts and process of the body, etc." Defining characteristics outlined by NANDA are shown in Table 43.1.

Related factors (etiologies) have been identified by NANDA as actual or perceived object loss, thwarted grieving response to a loss, absence of anticipatory grieving, chronic fatal illness, lack of resolution of previous grieving response, loss of significant others, loss of psychosocial well-being, and loss of personal possessions (Carroll-Johnson; 1989;553–554). Dysfunctional Grieving may be difficult to differentiate from the diagnoses Reactive Depression and Spiritual Distress. To compare the defining characteristics of these diagnoses, see Table 54.3 in Chapter 54 on Spiritual Distress.

The "dysfunctional" approach to grieving considers inappropriate depression, anger, fear, guilt, anxiety, and denial that extend beyond some arbitrarily proscribed time period or level of intensity. Those elderly who do not conform to a "stereotyped set of psychological and physiological reactions in which the three stages of shock, despair, and recovery can be delineated" (Dimond, 1981;462) are often labeled "dysfunctional grievers." Nursing interventions that flow from this dysfunctional framework are often ineffective because they devalue the core level feelings of the older adult.

Compelling research evidence suggests that the grieving process is highly individualized—*not* stereotyped—and

Table 43.1

Grieving, Dysfunctional

NANDA (CARROLL-JOHNSON, 1989)	WHITING/BUCKWALTER
Definition (Kim et al, 1987)*	
A state in which actual or perceived object loss exists (eg, people, possessions, job, status, home, parts and process of body, etc)	Grieving is a normal, functional process that is part of living and is uniquely defined by the person experiencing the loss
Related Factors/Etiologies	
Actual or perceived object loss	Losses/changes inherent in growing older and from chronic illness/disability
Thwarted grieving response to loss	
Absence of anticipatory grieving	Feel/think/act paradigm out of synch
Chronic fatal illness	Inability to fulfill dreams, illusions, fantasies, and projections into the future
Lack of resolution of previous grieving response	
Loss of significant others	
Loss of physiopsychosocial well-being	
Loss of personal possessions	
Defining Characteristics	
Verbal expression of distress at loss	Redefinition, reevaluation, and reattachment in the context of loss
Denial of loss	
Expression of unresolved issues	Depression
Anger	Anger
Sadness	Fear
Crying	Guilt
Difficulty in expressing loss	Anxiety
Alteration in	Denial
Eating habits	Reassessment of attitudes and values
Sleep patterns	Struggle with social, emotional and philosophical structures
Dream patterns	
Activity level	
Libido	
Idealization of lost object	
Reliving of past experiences	
Interference with life functioning	
Developmental regression	
Labile effect	
Alteration in concentration and/or of task	

*NANDA (Carroll-Johnson, 1989) has no definition.

is affected by a variety of social and situational factors, sex roles, and cultural values and practices (Clayton et al, 1971; Faschingbauer, 1981; Glick et al, 1974; Lowenthal and Haven, 1968; Maddison, 1968; Rees and Lufkins, 1967; Vachon, 1976). Systematic assessment efforts confirm a "wide constellation of behaviors, feelings, and symptoms attendant upon bereavement" (Zisook et al, 1982;1591).

This chapter also takes issue with the dysfunctional view of grieving and reframes the concept from the vantage point of the elderly bereaved person. From our perspective, grieving—even prolonged grieving—is part of the process of living, not an impediment to life, as claimed by Gordon. We reject the traditional labels "inappropriate," "negative," and/or "dysfunctional" used to describe the depression, anger, fear, guilt, anxiety, and denial experienced as elderly persons struggle to redefine, reevaluate, and reattach (cope) in the context of their loss.

A physiologic analogy may clarify our approach to this diagnosis. A rise in an elderly person's white blood count (WBC) in response to an infectious process is viewed as part of the body's normal defense mechanisms, not as dysfunctional. If supported by appropriate medical and nursing interventions, the infection resolves and the WBC count lowers.

Despite the commonly accepted nursing diagnostic label Dysfunctional Grieving, we believe that grieving also is a *functional* process. Although grieving can be superimposed on premorbid psychiatric/psychologic problems requiring treatment, most elderly persons experience grieving as a normal, though individually defined, process.

CONCEPTUAL FRAMEWORK FOR GRIEVING

Most studies of grief and bereavement have been based on crisis theory. Unfortunately, this theory is "too narrow in scope and implication" (Dimond, 1981;465) to conceptualize adequately the multidimensional experience of grief among the elderly. Crisis theory implies resolution of a grief reaction in a very short period of time, whereas empirical evidence suggests that grieving requires both time and resources (Dimond, 1981).

Understanding the nursing diagnosis Dysfunctional Grieving can be facilitated with a three-part "feel/think-believe/act" paradigm of change and growth (see Figure 43.1). According to this paradigm, successful change is accomplished when feeling, thinking, and acting are balanced and congruent (Kearney, 1986; Moses, 1985a). However, when persons think without feeling or act without thinking, they may have difficulty coping with changes or losses. This incongruity may lead to the nursing diagnosis of Dysfunctional Grieving. All changes precipitate a grieving process. The changes inherent in

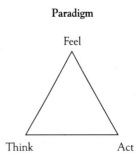

Paradigm

Figure 43.1

Feel/think–believe/act paradigm. (Source: Ken Moses, 1987, Used with permission)

growing older, especially in the presence of chronic illness or disability, have an impact on the dreams, hopes, illusions, and fantasies of aging persons.

THE PROCESS OF GRIEVING

As individuals move through life, they generate many important dreams (Moses, 1985b), including dreams about their later years. Yearnings for completion, peace and contentment, fulfilled responsibilities, financial and material comfort and security, time to be with a partner, and enjoyment of children and grandchildren are only a few of the many intense dreams and fantasies attached to this latter period of life. At the core of these dreams are intense feelings emanating from the elderly individual's unique perception and experience of self and the world.

When core level dreams are threatened, a grieving process begins (Moses, 1983). Death of a spouse, for example, destroys the surviving partner's dreams that depend on the spouse's presence. Degenerative or debilitating illnesses that affect an individual's ability to function physically and/or mentally, affect both the impaired individual and family members. The loss of core level dreams is often so personal that nurses and other health care professionals may not be aware of what is happening. Even the affected elderly individual is frequently confused by the grieving process and the feelings generated.

Through grieving, an individual separates from a significant lost dream, illusion, fantasy, or projection into the future. The individual struggles with social, emotional, and philosophical structures and reevaluates core level attitudes and values in a dynamic "character building" fashion (Moses, 1977). The process supports personal growth and enables the individual to create new, more attainable dreams, even in the face of lost ones.

Grief-related feeling states, including denial, anxiety, guilt, depression, anger, and fear, are often devalued and denigrated, both by the elderly bereaved and by health care professionals. However, feeling level experiences are necessary for successful readjustment in the face of change. In addition, feeling level interactions with a significant other are necessary for the successful evolution of the grieving process (Moses, 1977). In other words, we can't and don't grieve in isolation.

The feeling states of denial, anger, anxiety, depression, guilt, and fear occur in no specific order, and one is not a prerequisite for another. Indeed, the states can be felt simultaneously (Moses, 1981). Grieving is spontaneous, unlearned, and life long (Moses, 1977, 1981). The feelings that result appear to be intrinsic and cross-cultural, and are experienced even in animals (Lewis and Rosenblum, 1974).

Through relationships with caring, supportive, valuing "helpers," elderly individuals can successfully separate from their old dreams and begin to generate new, more attainable dreams. Specific approaches for the nurse to use are presented later in this chapter in the "Interventions" section.

ASSESSMENT

Tools

A psychiatrically based assessment tool, the Inventory of Grief, was initially developed (Faschingbauer et al, 1977) as a 14-item self-report scale with two distinct factors: "present feelings" and "past behavior and feelings immediately following the object loss." The instrument was expanded to 58 items in an effort to measure frequency and time course of grief-related behaviors and feelings (Zisook et al, 1982).

Research using the expanded tool demonstrated that grief did not end at any circumscribed time interval, although most "symptoms" peaked between 1 and 2 years after loss of a loved one. Many behaviors and symptoms appeared to persist indefinitely, and certain preoccupations and painful memories continued to affect bereaved respondents strongly after 10 years.

Zisook and DeVaul (1983) extracted three items from the expanded inventory to create the Unresolved Grief Index. Nine items on the Zung Depression Scale were significantly correlated with items on the Unresolved Grief Index, suggesting a stable (over time) relationship between depression and unresolved grief. However, this research was carried out with middle-aged rather than elderly respondents.

Nursing Assessment

McFarland and Wasli (1986;79) have outlined a 10-point nursing assessment for dysfunctional grieving:

1. Are defining characteristics of dysfunctional grieving present?
2. What is the nature of the loss? When did it occur?
3. How did the patient perceive the loss? Special meaning/value? Significance of loss in relation to patient's perceived and real abilities to meet his or her own needs?
4. What stage of grieving and behavioral manifestations does patient currently present?
5. What is patient's behavior between actual occurrence of loss and present?
6. How has patient coped with loss in the past? What strengths were demonstrated in coping with loss?
7. Is patient at high risk for dysfunctional grieving? Examples of such patients are those with:
   a. Poor relationship with person prior to death
   b. Social isolation of poor social network
   c. History of multiple past losses and use of maladaptive coping strategies.
   d. Presentation of a brave, stoic front
8. What is the nature of the social network present?
9. What is the degree of depression? Are there suicidal tendencies?
10. What are significant others' reactions to patient's response to loss?

Carpenito (1982) set forth five associated defining characteristics of grief: denial, guilt, anger, crying, and sorrow. These signs and symptoms are closely related to those proposed in the conceptual framework of this chapter: denial, anxiety, guilt, depression, anger, and fear.

Denial

Denial is a normal, natural, and necessary part of healthy grieving. Denial keeps elderly persons from having to deal with the feelings associated with the loss experience, and thus from being overwhelmed by the experience.

Four levels of denial might be experienced by elderly individuals encountering loss situations. The individual can deny (1) the existence of the loss or change; (2) the extent and permanence of the loss; (3) the impact of the loss; or (4) the feelings associated with the loss (Moses, 1977, 1981, 1983).

Each level of denial serves the same purpose for the grieving individual. The impact on the nurse, however, can be quite different in each case. Elderly individuals who deny a diagnosis (loss) appear to reject what the health professional has to offer. Health professionals may feel insecure or defensive about the diagnosis or angry that their expertise is being devalued and rejected. The elderly individual often engages in "doctor shopping," looking for an acceptable diagnosis and rejecting those with catastrophic implications.

Denying the permanence of a loss or denying the diagnosis can create confusion among family, friends, and professionals. These older individuals often become vulnerable to "quackery" as they search for and involve themselves in unusual and unorthodox treatments (Moses, 1983).

Elderly individuals who deny the impact of a change may present themselves as having all the necessary resources, knowledge, and attitudes to deal with the loss with no outward manifestation or acknowledgment of stress. Many health professionals encourage this behavior in an effort to minimize the difficulty of implementing necessary treatments.

Elderly individuals who deny feelings acknowledge that a difficult, permanent change has occurred, but claim that "it doesn't matter; it just doesn't upset me," or "I don't know what you're all so upset about." Yet severance of the feeling component doesn't work. The feel/think/act process, whereby "You feel—you think about it—you act on it," offers continuity and congruence to human interactions. Individuals who "jumble" the order (ie, think without feeling, act without thinking, and so on) become incongruent and have trouble coping with whatever change or loss has occurred. Accordingly, elderly individuals who deny their feelings will not experience congruence or successful coping.

Unfortunately, elderly persons at any level of denial will not perceive the need to alter their current attitudes, behaviors, values, or feelings regarding the loss or diagnosis (Moses, 1983). Yet, viewing denial as an impediment to early and effective intervention and treatment devalues the older individual's felt experience and the alliance between the individuals experiencing the loss or change.

Denial provides time to build both internal strength and external supports that facilitate successful coping. Internal strengths include those ego mechanisms that lie dormant in all individuals until they are tested. External supports include friends and family that can be relied on to accept us in our pain. Professionals and the information they provide are important external supports for the elderly. An enormous amount of energy is necessary to accomplish the building of internal and external supports. Older individuals who experience a dramatic loss and the concomitant denial may appear defensive and agitated or rigid and affectless (Moses, 1983, 1985b).

Nurses who attempt to "break through" the denial and convince the denying elderly persons of the fact, permanence, and impact of their loss or to persuade them to follow through on all recommendations will often be frustrated and disappointed. Moreover, forcing an older individual to experience the full force of a loss without internal and external supports in place may result in emotional collapse (Moses, 1983). A more efficient and purposeful approach may be to offer suggestions, recommendations, and information while supporting the legitimacy of the older person's denial. Validating the older

individual's value, even when he or she cannot cope with catastrophic loss, is even more important.

Anxiety

Older individuals who encounter loss and change in long-term care settings may exhibit generalized anxiety. Anxiety develops in response to an imbalance in the individual's thoughts/beliefs, feelings, and actions. Regaining and maintaining balance in the face of the loss or change requires many personal and internal adjustments (Moses, 1983, 1985b), a vast change in knowledge, attitudes, beliefs, and behaviors. This requires enormous energy and skill. Anxiety both mobilizes these energies and focuses them on the important task of reestablishing the balance of thoughts/beliefs, feelings, and actions (Moses, 1983). And yet, sometimes anxiety can be so great that it immobilizes the individual (see Chapter 39, Anxiety).

Attitudes of nurses, family, and friends can strongly affect the pressure that the older individual experiences in the context of the loss. The most important function nurses and other interested helpers can serve is to legitimize anxious feelings. Asking the anxious elder to "calm down" is both futile and counterproductive. Anxiety will continue, even if chemically or psychologically "masked," until it serves its productive purpose. Moreover, anxiety facilitates the restructuring of attitudes necessary to regain balance in the context of loss. The injunction to "calm down" devalues the elderly person's internal experience and the tremendous coping task he or she faces.

CASE STUDY

Denial and Anxiety

Mrs. F, age 66, was suddenly and unexpectedly widowed 6 months ago. She seemed to handle the death of her husband well, living alone in the family home, working part-time, and caring for herself. However, her daughter reportedly noticed piles of unpaid bills for the mortgage and insurance and Social Security forms that had not been filled out. When asked about the papers, Mrs. F would look "blank," then respond, "Oh, they'll be taken care of. Everything will be fine." When pressed further, Mrs. F would grow nervous and change the subject or walk out of the room.

Mrs. F's daughter brought her to a geriatric assessment clinic to talk with a geropsychiatric nurse about her behavior. The nurse spoke briefly with the daughter, who informed her that Mr. F had always handled the couple's finances. Mrs. F used her own paycheck only for "extras." Otherwise, Mr. F took care of everything.

A brief history from Mrs. F concerning her husband's death follows:

NURSE: Mrs. F, tell me a little about why you're here and how you think I can help.

MRS. F: Well (laughs), I really don't know. My daughter thought I needed to come, but she's such a worry wart sometimes. I really don't need to be here at all. (denial of fact and impact)

NURSE: What do you think your daughter is concerned about?

MRS. F: Well, I'm not really sure. She says she's worried about my financial security. I'm *sure* she's just being silly. I've never worried about finances before and everything's been fine.

Guilt, Depression, Anger, and Fear

Existential issues such as adequacy, potency, value, fairness, risk, responsibility, morals, order, causality, and evaluation must be restructured and redefined as part of the task of attaching meaning to life in the face of loss. The feeling states of guilt, depression, anger, and fear assist elderly persons in the task of existential restructuring. These four feeling states are inextricably interwoven, but for purposes of discussion will be treated as distinct elements. Each feeling state corresponds to a major core level element that affects the meaning of life in the following areas: commitment, competence, justice, and love (attachment) (Moses, 1981).

Guilt Guilt is the most difficult and disconcerting of all the grief states. Guilt may be experienced in one of three ways. Older individuals may believe that they caused their own loss experience through poor health habits, smoking, alcohol or drug abuse, contraction of an avoidable disease, or other occurrences that they felt were within their control. This is the most logical manifestation of guilt and therefore is the easiest to accept. Guilt may also be demonstrated in a belief that the loss is fair or just punishment for wrongdoing in the past, even in the absence of any direct connections. This type of guilt has a less logical basis and is easier to counter. Finally, guilt may be evidenced in the philosophical stance that "good things happen to good people; bad things happen to bad people." Thus, the grieving individual is guilty simply because the loss occurred (Moses, 1981).

Guilt is a painful and debilitating feeling state and thus is difficult for both elderly persons and health professionals to view as an acceptable and growth-facilitating experience. Yet, guilt allows grieving individuals to reevaluate their central life commitment—their beliefs about how they affect the world, the validity of their morals, and the usefulness of their ethical structures (Moses, 1983).

How and why one defines certain elements as either their fault or an occurrence of fate is a personal, internal struggle. The goal of this struggle is to develop a functional system that allows the older adult to deal effectively with the vicissitudes of life. A healthy stance avoids both the absurdity of assuming full responsibility for all life events and the equally absurd position of disclaiming responsibility for anything (Moses, 1981, 1983).

The best response to an older individual experiencing guilt as part of the grieving process is to listen sensitively and accept the legitimacy of the guilt feelings. Through empathic listening by a significant other, the grieving individual answers questions regarding causality and impact on the world. Acceptance of the guilt experience of the grieving person as a normal, necessary, and facilitative element of grief provides the basis of a constructive relationship with the older individual. In contrast, viewing guilt as pathologic impedes the helping relationship. Guilt outlives its usefulness only after it facilitates existential restructuring.

Depression Everyone has a need to be competent. Yet definitions of competency change as individuals grow older. Depression helps older individuals confront their definition of competence both within their current life experience and in the context of loss and change affecting that life experience. Three specific facets of competence need to be reworked in the face of loss and change: potency, capability, and criteria for evaluation (Moses, 1981, 1983). Aging persons, particularly those in long-term care settings, may judge themselves as weak (impotent), useless (incapable), and worthless (valueless) because they have no influence or impact in important areas of life.

Although Western culture generally views depression as pathologic, this feeling state can be a normal, necessary, and healthy part of the grieving process. Expressing feelings of "anger turned inward," a sense of impotence and valuelessness, enables the elderly to let go of old definitions of competence and see themselves as competent, adequate, potent, and valuable once again (Moses, 1983). Significant others or health professionals who support, accept, and encourage expression of feelings can help older individuals identify competency issues and establish new evaluative criteria.

Statements that reflect this facilitative attitude can be as simple as "Tell me more about your feelings." "It sounds like you feel helpless/hopeless. Do you, and if so, why?" or "It sounds as if being confined has turned your whole world upside down. Can you tell me how things have changed for you since the doctor told you about this diagnosis?" "Cheering up" or denying the older person the right to their depressed feelings devalues the importance of that individual's struggle to reevaluate essential and core level issues and reinforces the notion that they are indeed inadequate. (For more information on depression see Chapter 35.)

CASE STUDY

Guilt and Depression

Mrs. L, age 73, had been widowed for 10 years. She had one married daughter living in another state and a 40-year-old mentally retarded daughter living with her. Mrs. L initially called her local community mental health center (CMHC) asking for some medication to help her sleep and for assistance with her retarded daughter's "difficult" behavior. Early sessions with both mother and daughter were for evaluation purposes. The daughter was referred for evaluation of her medication and current medical needs and assigned a nurse therapist to assist her with her feeling level issues regarding (1) her retardation; (2) having only her elderly mother as her companion; and (3) the unresolved loss of her father. Because Mrs. L complained of persistent insomnia and anorexia and had lost 15 pounds over the past 2 months, the therapist also evaluated the need for Mrs. L to have assistance in dealing with her own issues regarding her husband, her daughter, and her own anticipated death. Mrs. L had a great deal of difficulty accepting help initially. She tearfully explained that she wanted the nurse-therapist to come, but kept saying, "We should be talking about my daughter, not me. I'll be okay if I just get some sleep and start eating."

Anger Within our culture, strong feelings and expressions of anger are considered immature and inappropriate in the context of "responsible behavior." We work hard to expunge angry expression in all age groups, even in children. At the same time, we have an internalized sense of justice and injustice (Moses, 1977, 1981, 1983). If we treat others fairly, we expect them to reciprocate in kind. Unplanned-for chronic illness or disability violates this sense of justice and fairness in older persons who have worked, saved, and planned for retirement or travel.

Expressions of anger generated by this experience of unfairness are often projected on persons the elderly perceive as the cause of their loss or change. Their "targets" for anger can include physicians, family members, nurses, and others who seem to be the source and/or reminder of the loss and the injustice of shattered dreams. Ironically, the very people on whom the anger is displaced often are most needed by the older person suffering from loss or change. In some cases, older persons may direct their anger at science, God, or life in general. This displacement keeps older persons from confronting their internal values, beliefs, and attitudes regarding fairness and justice and from restructuring core level issues to generate a more reality-based internal sense of fairness (Moses, 1983).

It is crucial that older individuals express the anger they feel in the face of the loss or change. Nurses can assist the elderly in this process by accepting and relating to their anger. Unfortunately, anger often is directed toward the nurse, threatening the nurse's sense of adequacy and value. However, nurses must encourage the elderly person's expression of feelings in order to facilitate the healing interaction and promote the grieving process.

Older individuals who can express their feelings of anger verbally are unlikely to act them out. "Acting out" usually occurs when persons are frustrated in their efforts to express their anger (Moses, 1983). Nurses should understand the underlying dynamics of anger, examine their own motives carefully, and accept the older person's expressions of anger as a preventive measure against the potentially more destructive form of "acting out."

Fear Institutionalized elderly individuals often experience loss of control of their environment, their bodily functions, the expression of their individuality, and the autonomy and intimacy of their relationships with others. They may become painfully aware of their vulnerability, perhaps for the first time, and certainly in a new and unacceptable way. They also may question the wisdom of trying to reattach and reconnect themselves to the world, only to be hurt again (Moses, 1983).

Fear confronts issues of abandonment, vulnerability, and risk in the face of change and loss. New attitudes, beliefs, and definitions concerning the individual's ability to reattach must be formed, knowing the risk inherent in building a new dream (Moses, 1977, 1981, 1983). Our society, through social and political devaluing and abandonment, has fostered an even greater sense of vulnerability among the elderly. In addition, the changes and losses experienced by the elderly further put them in touch with their mortality, sometimes precipitously and often painfully.

Helping older persons face their fears enables them to struggle with reattachment, even in the midst of vulnerability and risk.

CASE STUDY

Anger and Fear

Mr. S, age 70, was released from the hospital following recovery from a myocardial infarction (MI). The extent of the damage was relatively minor, and his physicians gave him permission and encouragement to engage in light activity, especially walking. Prior to his infarction, Mr. S was an active, involved business man. He ran a large corporation, was on the boards of several other large companies, played golf, swam, and traveled a great deal with his wife. His heart attack occurred on the golf course. After his return home, however, Mr. S remained virtually housebound, refusing even to walk around his home. Every time his wife encouraged him or reminded him that the doctor said he should walk he would become angry and say "What does he know" or "I will when I'm ready. Now leave me alone." Then she'd tell him he shouldn't feel angry because the doctors were just doing their job.

The doctor made a referral to a gerontologic nurse practitioner to monitor Mr. S's blood pressure and, more important, to try to assist Mrs. S in dealing with diet and exercise issues. The nurse spent initial sessions listening to Mr. S angrily talk about doctors and "those hospital people" who tell him what to do and "run his life." He snapped at his wife several times when she tried to explain why the doctors were telling him to exercise.

NURSING INTERVENTIONS

ENUF

All interventions with the grieving process are based on the belief that people are best helped by creating an environment in which they can better experience and help themselves. The environment must reflect very specific attitudes toward and values for the older adult, succinctly captured in the acronym ENUF (Moses, 1983).

Empathy is the sharing of an accurate perception of another's experience.

Nonjudgment is an attitude of acceptance, free of evaluation, regardless of content shared.

Unconditional positive regard is a philosophy about the nature of human beings that affirms the value of all people, as they are, simply because they exist.

Feeling focus is the act of emphasizing feelings instead of content in interactions of an emotional nature.

Empathy In everyday interactions, we listen to the feelings, thoughts, issues, and/or concerns of the other person, sift them through our own internal experience of the moment, and share back our feelings, thoughts, issues, and/or concerns. There is relatively equal sharing by both individuals engaged in the interaction. Perceived similarity in feelings results in a mutual sense of support and sympathy.

Very often, however, we approach an interaction struggling with more intense feelings. When we receive a sympathetic response we often come away feeling let down, misunderstood, or even devalued. The core level feeling experience is so intense and unique that the person needs to focus her experience, share it, and know that the experience was understood and valued solely for itself—not because it compared favorably with another's experi-

ence. Sympathetic responses cut off this kind of focused interaction and "muddy the waters" by bringing in the other person's issues and feelings.

Intense feelings are better met through "empathic" responses. Empathy is the sharing of an accurate perception of another's experience—feeding back to the elderly person what was heard, both verbally and nonverbally, and asking whether it was heard accurately. Keeping the focus on the elderly individual allows the intensity of the individual's feelings to be truly experienced and communicated. Focusing back on the elderly person communicates a valuing of his or her felt experience without words. Verifying the accuracy of the perception enhances understanding and allows the elder to continue sharing feelings at this level of intensity. Finally, struggling to achieve accuracy reinforces the intrinsic value of the elderly individual's experience and supports a feeling of trust in the nurse's willingness to listen (Moses, 1981, 1983, 1985a).

Empathy requires nurses to monitor and keep separate their own feelings. Responses such as "I know just how you feel" are devaluing and discounting. The art of empathy is hearing and learning to understand the other's despair, hatred, guilt, fear, or anxiety without "taking it on" yourself or inserting your own experience.

Nonjudgment From birth to death human beings are consistently and constantly judged. Indeed, because of the pervasive experience of being judged, most, if not all, of us become expert at judging others. It is, therefore, difficult and almost paradoxical to be nonjudgmental when hearing the painful core level feelings of others. In addition, being judged makes it hard to expose our own feelings to another's judgment. The immediate reaction to the pain of being "unacceptable" is to pull the feelings back inside until it is "safe" to express them again without fear of rejection.

Nurses must be willing to acknowledge and separate their own feelings, thoughts, and beliefs in order to communicate a value-free attitude of acceptance, regardless of the content shared (Moses, 1983). For example, a nonjudgmental response to "I hate God! The God I believe in never would be this cruel," might be difficult for a strongly religious nurse. A truly nonjudgmental response might be, "If you believe God has caused this to happen, or that He should have kept it from happening, I can understand why you might be feeling so much anger. Tell me more about these feelings and ideas."

The response "You shouldn't blame God" might be perceived as nonacceptance of the elderly person's feelings and devaluation of his pain and struggle. Nurses should not agree or disagree with the content expressed, but rather should accept the elderly person without qualification. The elder, feeling accepted, will be able to continue struggling with incongruent feelings, thoughts, beliefs, and/or actions during bereavement (Moses, 1983).

Unconditional Positive Regard The philosophy of unconditional positive regard, set forth by Carl Rogers (1965), affirms the value of all people, simply because they exist. In other words, "You are valuable just because you are you" (Moses, 1983).

Unconditional positive regard should be communicated throughout interactions in which elderly persons share intense and painful feelings. Unconditional positive regard requires no conditions or criteria to be met or fulfilled by the elder other than humanness. The nurse is not saying "I approve of you as long as you think, feel, believe, or express yourself in ways that I can understand and condone." Rather, the nurse is saying, "Help me understand your feelings, thoughts, beliefs, and actions because they are valuable parts of your humanness." This attitude supports growth by valuing the elderly individual's unique experience.

Feeling Focus In interactions of an emotional nature, there is little purpose in focusing first on the content of the interaction. Unfortunately, because feelings are often painful and undervalued, the elderly disguise them in all types of content-oriented exchanges. Nurses may miss the emotion if only the words are heard. For this reason, intuition is a valuable part of every interaction. What is "felt" while listening to the content? Anxiety? Frustration? Sadness? Consistently sharing back perceived feelings with the elderly person facilitates identification of the felt experience and its meaning within the context of the interaction. Focusing statements emphasize the feeling picked up by the nurse through the content, tone of voice, body language, and facial expressions observed during the interaction. One such response might be, "How does it feel to deal with all these changes you have just described to me?"

Every response to content communications values the content, but more important, the response attempts to assist elderly persons to relate on a feeling level. Elderly are most likely to get "stuck" at an emotional level and be unable to find ways to cope with loss or change (Moses, 1983). Once the elderly allow themselves to struggle emotionally with, redefine, reevaluate, and create new ways of perceiving the issues attached to their feelings, they will be able to cope better with the loss.

As listeners, we might ask ourselves how we are going to get the information we need to help the older person deal with his or her grieving. In particular, we need to know what is getting in the way of this person dealing with his or her grieving. Only the elderly person can answer this question. Feeling level experiences usually take priority over the content-oriented "facts" of the situation and need to be dealt with first. Recognizing the need to revert to a focus on feelings assists the elderly person to cope better at a cognitive and/or functional level.

CASE STUDY

Nursing Interventions (ENUF): Denial and Anxiety, Mrs. F

NURSE: So you've never had to worry before about finances, and it doesn't seem necessary now to start? You believe your daughter is overreacting?

MRS. F: Yes. She makes me so nervous when she keeps talking about it.

NURSE: If *you believe* there is nothing to worry about and talking about it makes you nervous, I can understand why you'd want her to stop talking about the finances. [Empathic and nonjudgmental response]

MRS. F: You do? (Pauses) I don't think my daughter understands. She's always pushing me about these bills. (Starts to cry) I just *hate* it all. I don't *want* to think about it—I *never* had to before. (Crying, but voice sounds angry) [Denial of impact on life—breaking into feelings re impact]

NURSE: You're crying but your voice sounds angry. Do you feel angry when you feel your daughter is pushing you? [Empathy—checking for accuracy]

MRS. F: I guess I do, but I don't know why. She's a good daughter.

NURSE: You just said "I don't *want* to think about it—I never had to before." Tell me about that.

MRS. F: Well, I didn't, I just let my husband. (Looks up, then down, and becomes more agitated) Oh, I wish she'd *stop*. If she just wouldn't push me (angry voice).

NURSE: It feels like your daughter is pushing you, and it makes you feel angry with her?

MRS. F: Yes, I do get angry with her but . . . I guess it isn't her fault.

NURSE: What isn't her fault?

MRS. F: (Long pause) (whispers) That my husband died and I don't know what to do about paying bills. (Starts crying) Nurse moves in to hold Mrs. F's hand and then Mrs. F while she cries.

DISCUSSION

Initially, Mrs. F was in denial concerning the *fact* of a problem with her finances. To acknowledge that there was a problem with her finances, Mrs. F had to acknowledge the painful impact of her husband's death that resulted in the need for change. Her daughter's insistence created the anxiety necessary to begin to deal with the feeling. However, Mrs. F felt no understanding or acceptance from her daughter concerning her pain about changing. When the nurse gently and empathically acknowledged this pain without insisting that she change, Mrs. F felt supported and valued enough to begin to acknowledge the feelings: first anger at the unfairness, then an overwhelming sense of depression concerning her inadequacy to deal with the impact. Empathic support and acceptance allowed Mrs. F to struggle with the issues of fairness and adequacy. She moved quickly into expressing her anger and depression and worked with the nurse, then her daughter, to find alternatives for dealing with her financial situation.

CASE STUDY

Nursing Interventions (ENUF): Guilt and Depression, Mrs. L

NURSE: Mrs. L, you keep saying we should be talking about your daughter. Can you tell me why that seems so important?

MRS. L: Well, she needs help, and it's my job to take care of her, so we should be talking about her.

NURSE: So, you feel responsible for her and her well-being, and talking about other things during our time doesn't feel comfortable for you? [Empathy—checking for accuracy]

MRS. L: Well, I *am* responsible for her. There's no one else. I suppose I should have done something a long time ago. Do you think I was wrong to keep her with me? I probably should have put her somewhere but I couldn't, and then her father took all my time (he was ill a long time before his death). I probably neglected her, and she—you know—regressed or something. . . . (tearful at times) [Daughter graduated from high school but was never placed in any other day programs after high school and remained isolated with mother because few services were available]

NURSE: If I'm hearing you accurately, you have a lot of concerns about the way you've dealt with your daughter over the last 10 to 20 years, lots of questions about the rightness or wrongness of your decisions. Is that correct?

MRS. L: I always worry now about whether I did okay. I feel so bad sometimes. (Cries) What if I made the wrong decisions, and now she has to suffer?

NURSE: (Moving closer and touching Mrs. L's arm while she's crying; sits quietly as she cries) Tell me about your sadness. [Focus on feelings—acknowledges and values them]

MRS. L: I feel like I've done all the wrong things, and if I have—well, what kind of a mother am I? That makes me sad.

NURSE: It sounds like you are questioning your adequacy as a mother.

MRS. L: Yes, I guess I am.

NURSE: What does it mean to you if you made mistakes?

MRS. L: If they were mistakes that she has to suffer for now—well, how can I live with that? Worse, how can I leave her? (Cries some more) It's my fault if her life is awful, and now I can't do anything about it!

NURSE: You're worried that she'll suffer for mistakes you made and you won't be able to help her?

MRS. L: Yes.

NURSE: It looks like those thoughts and ideas are very painful for you. How long have you been this concerned about your decisions concerning your daughter?

MRS. L: I guess I thought the decisions were okay at the time. It felt like I didn't have very many choices, but in the last few years I've been wondering. . . .

NURSE: Any idea what started you wondering?

MRS. L: Oh, talking to other people and trying to plan when I'm gone. (Pause) People just seemed to act like I should have done something sooner.

NURSE: So you started wondering about your decisions when other people seemed to question your choices?

MRS. L: Yes.

NURSE: Were you feeling judged?

MRS. L: Yes—and no one knows how hard it was to make those decisions. But maybe they're right.

NURSE: And if they're "right" does that make it hard to feel like you were a "good enough" mother?

MRS. L: Yes and that was all I had—being her mother. What if I did a terrible job?

NURSE: Being a good mother was the job that gave you a sense of value and worth? And now you're wondering if you still are that valuable person?

MRS. L: Oh yes—if I didn't do it right, how can I look at my life and feel okay about it?

NURSE: If you believe that being a "good and valuable mother" means not making mistakes, I can understand why you feel so sad and depressed when you think about mistakes you may have made. (Pause) Maybe we can look together at the definition you have for being a good enough mother and where it came from to help you deal with this issue.

DISCUSSION

Mrs. L was struggling with feelings of guilt and depression in an attempt to deal with the issues of significance, adequacy and value as a mother and as a human being. Her role as a wife and mother were her major sources of a sense of significance and meaning (hence guilt) and value and adequacy (hence depression). In the face of her own impending death, she was reviewing these issues and struggling with doubts about her significance and adequacy (value). The nurse's responses allowed Mrs. L to examine the definitions and criteria she was using and reevaluate the usefulness of those definitions. If the nurse's reply to Mrs. L had been "Don't feel guilty," the reevaluation process would not have been facilitated.

CASE STUDY

Nursing Interventions (ENUF): Anger and Fear, Mr. S

NURSE: Mr. S, it sounds like you feel you don't have control over your own life anymore. Is that how you feel? [Empathy—checking for accuracy]

MR. S: Well, they'd like to think that they can tell me how to run my life, but I'll be damned if I'll let them.

NURSE: How do you feel when you think about not having control of your own life? [Beginning to *focus on feeling*]

MR. S: Now that's a stupid question. I feel angry, that's how I feel. But it doesn't do any good. They just keep doing it, telling me what to do. It isn't the way I'm used to things being, I can tell you that! [Anger, assisting with issue of unfairness]

NURSE: I can understand if you believe you don't have control of your own life that you might feel angry. It does sound like feeling out of control is not a common experience for you. You're used to being in charge a lot in your business. Is that right? [Expressing attitude of acceptance and valuing even in face of devaluing messages sent to nurse by Mr. S]

MR. S: You're darn right! (Pauses—anger diffused a little)

NURSE: Were there any times in your work life when you felt this kind of anger or "out of control" feeling? [Exploring feelings]

MR. S: (Thoughtfully) Well, sure, I guess when someone messed up a big deal and I was afraid of losing a client or a lot of money. Yeah, I guess the anger felt like I feel now.

NURSE: What would you do in the work situation to deal with your out of control feeling?

MR. S: Well (laughs), I guess I would yell a lot at first at the people who I thought had messed up.

NURSE: What were you most angry about then?

MR. S: (Thoughtfully) I guess at first I was mad because my plan was messed up and it was unfair, but maybe . . . maybe I was scared too. You can lose a lot of money in the deals I'm used to putting together. I never really thought about it. [Fear—dealing with issue of vulnerability]

NURSE: So maybe some of the anger was covering up the scared feeling? It wasn't okay to let anyone know about the scared feelings? [Focusing on feelings]

MR. S: (Laughs again) Oh, yeah, you never let the other guy know you're scared in business deals.

NURSE: Could your anger now have anything to do with being scared? What might you be scared of now?

MR. S: Well, you know that doctor can't give me any guarantees that I won't have another one of these "MIs" even if I do everything I'm supposed to. It feels like a real chancy thing. If I start doing things like exercising, I'm taking quite a chance on having another heart attack.

NURSE: So, it feels like you don't want to take any risks without those guarantees? [Checking for accuracy]

MR. S: Yeah.

NURSE: What do you think would help you decide to take those risks? What helped you in the work situation?

MR. S: (Thoughtfully) Well, I guess I decided what I wanted to achieve was worth the risk and there were some things I *could* do to minimize some of the risks.

NURSE: It sounds like when you decide that going on with your life and enjoying some of your former pleasures are worth the risk, you'll go ahead and do that. Are there any questions I can help you get answered that might help you minimize that sense of risk?

DISCUSSION

Mr. S's struggle was expressed in the feeling states of anger and fear. His anger was necessary to struggle with his sense of unfairness at the events and their impact on his life, and it also masked the more "unacceptable" feeling of fear. The fear, once acknowledged and valued, decreased the need for the anger and allowed Mr. S to use the fear to deal with his sense of vulnerability. By focusing on the fear and anger, the nurse helped Mr. S to identify the issues to which the feelings were attached and to generate ideas and thoughts about how to deal with the situation.

OUTCOMES

Outcomes traditionally associated with resolution of the diagnosis Dysfunctional Grieving have been elaborated by McFarland and Wasli (1986;82). The individual:

1. Engages in normal grief work, that is, works through the phases of normal grieving (eg, denial, anger, bargaining, realization of loss, and acceptance and reintegration)
2. Demonstrates reasonable amount of time in phases of grieving
3. Demonstrates nonexcessive and nonprolonged emotional reactions
4. Restructures and reorders life constructively

However, as shown in Figure 43.2, the grieving process may include movement through the feeling (grieving) states of denial, anxiety, fear, guilt, depression, and anger discussed earlier in this chapter. Using a nursing intervention based on the principles of ENUF, the elderly person is assisted to cope with change and loss.

Coping

Coping is the behavioral (or functional) enactment of attitudinal and philosophic changes that grow out of the grieving process. Although grieving is a prerequisite of coping, both are evident shortly after the onset of a loss. Four issues of coping, not evidenced in any particular order, have been postulated by Wright (1960) and Moses (1983, 1985).

Contain the Impact of the Loss Core level loss affects an older person's whole life. The impact of the loss is generalized, creating the feeling that "everything" is

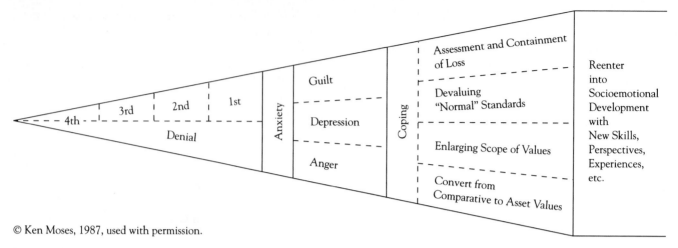

© Ken Moses, 1987, used with permission.

Figure 43.2

An approach to understanding grievous loss.

lost, ruined, or meaningless. Coping with loss requires a careful and accurate assessment of what is actually affected (lost), what is salvageable, and what aspects of life have been unscathed by the loss. Such a sorting process occurs through containing the impact of the loss.

For example, when Mrs. A, a 65-year-old woman, lost her husband, she initially felt that her life was over. "He *was* my life," "I don't have any reason to live without him," "I lived my life for him" were typical statements of her sense of the enormity of her loss. With help to experience and struggle with her feelings she began to see other aspects of her life that remained unchanged (eg, "I'm still a grandmother and a good one," "My friends appreciate and value me," "I can still do a lot of the things I enjoy like playing bridge and going to the symphony with friends." Mrs. A was able to contain the loss to the specific dreams attached to her husband and identify other dreams attached to other aspects of life and to other individuals. In addition, she learned to acknowledge that she had value beyond her abilities as a wife.

Devalue "Normal" Standards Society treats loss as a low-incidence occurrence that only affects certain people. It is not considered "normal" to come from a divorced family, lose your parents, have an impaired child, be wheelchair bound, struggle with a manic-depressive disorder, or suffer with a terminal illness. Indeed, feelings of inferiority on the part of the grieving elder inhibit social integration. Coping requires rejection of "normal" standards that devalue bereaved or afflicted people.

For example, Mr. Y was wheelchair bound and consistently refused invitations to friends' homes or to social events. He saw himself as an "embarrassment," as "a burden," and as "abnormal" because of his wheelchair. These notions were supported at times by nonaccepting and devaluing behaviors of others. Further, the lack of wheelchair-accessible buildings reinforced Mr. Y's feelings

of inferiority. Mr. Y exhibited coping when he devalued the normal standards of society and saw himself as worthy. He insisted that the symphony organization make their building accessible to him, and he had friends assume the responsibility of making their homes accessible to him. He accepted responsibility for letting his needs be known and worked with other responsible individuals to meet those needs.

Enlarge Scope of Values As people grow and develop, they ironically often become more narrow with regard to the values that they hold. When a substantive loss fundamentally shakes their value system, it can enlarge their scope of values and can facilitate their coping.

For example, Mr. P retired from his executive position because of a chronic illness. He had judged his worth on the basis of his career. Defining his value in terms of his job impeded Mr. P's ability to cope. When he enlarged his sense of values to include organizing church fund-raising campaigns and consulting to nonprofit organizations, Mr. P was able to see himself once again as valuable and potent in the world. If he had not enlarged his scope of values, he would have continued to view himself as "washed up" and "over the hill."

Shift From Comparative to Asset Values People appear to be more concerned about how they stand in relation to others than about what assets they are acquiring or accomplishing. This stance becomes intolerable when a loss precludes comparative success. As long as elderly individuals see themselves as valuable only when they "measure up" to others, losses become devastating. Elders who concentrate on their own abilities, accomplishments, knowledge, and experiences can more quickly and easily make use of these assets to assist themselves in creating new dreams.

Therefore, coping with loss includes shifting from comparative to asset values. For example, Miss T was a new resident of a retirement home. She did not know anyone well and, having never been married, did not have children or grandchildren to discuss. She did not play bridge and hated bingo. Miss T felt left out and as though she had nothing of value to share in comparison to those around her. With help from the nurse, she began to recognize her long-term accomplishments as a music and English literature teacher (50 years) and started interacting with others by sharing these experiences. She helped organize a discussion group on current books and began to read books onto tapes for others who were unable to read. She also read to and played music for her fellow residents in special programs and talent shows. Miss T created her "niche" by recognizing her wealth of unique and individual experiences, rather than by trying to measure up to others.

As shown on the right-hand side of Figure 43.2, elderly persons who have successfully coped with loss and change will be able to reenter the world and undertake the developmental tasks of older age with new skills, perspectives, insights, and attitudes. The "hallmark of the resolution of grief is the ability of the bereaved to recognize that they have grieved and can now return to work, re-experience pleasure, and respond to the companionship of love of others" (Zisook et al, 1985;497).

SUMMARY

This chapter has analyzed the grieving process from the perspective that grieving is a *functional*, rather than a dysfunctional, process. Through the feeling states of depression, guilt, anger, fear, and denial, the elderly individual separates from a lost dream. Nurses should support, rather than block, these feelings. Using the principles of ENUF—empathy, nonjudgment, unconditional positive regard, and feeling focus—nurses can assist bereaved elderly to cope better with losses or changes in their lives and environment. Successful movement through the grieving process is accomplished when the older person has achieved a sense of personal growth and can develop new and attainable dreams.

References

Bowlby J: Processes of mourning. *Internat J Psychoanalysis* 1961; 42: 317–340.

Carpenito LJ: *Handbook of Nursing Diagnosis*. Lippincott, 1982.

Carroll-Johnson R (editor): *Classification of Nursing Diagnoses: Proceedings of the Eighth Conference*. Lippincott, 1989.

Clayton P, Halikas J, Maurice W: The bereavement of the widowed. *Dis Nerv System* 1971; 32:597–604.

Dimond M: Bereavement and the elderly: A critical review with implications for nursing practice and research. *J Adv Nurs* 1981; 6:461–470.

Engel GL: Is grief a disease, a challenge? *Psychosomat Med* 1960a; 22:326–327.

Engel GL: Is grief a disease? *Psychosomat Med* 1960b; 23:18–22.

Faschingbauer T: *Texas Revised Inventory of Grief*. Honeycomb Publishing, 1981.

Faschingbauer TR, DeVaul RA, Zisook S: Development of the Texas Inventory of Grief. *Am J Psychiatry* 1977; 134:696–698.

Freud S: Mourning and melancholia. In: *Complete Psychological Works* (1917), Standard ed., Vol 14. Hogarth Press, 1973.

Glick I, Weiss RS, Parkes CM: *The First Year of Bereavement*. Wiley, 1974.

Gordon M: *Nursing Diagnosis: Process and Application*. McGraw-Hill, 1982.

Kearney R: *Intervention Therapy*. Manuscript submitted for publication, 1986.

Kim MJ, McFarland GK, McLane AM: *Pocket Guide to Nursing Diagnoses*. Mosley, 1987.

Kim MJ, Moritz DA (editors): *Classification of Nursing Diagnoses: Proceedings of the Third and Fourth National Conferences*. McGraw-Hill, 1982.

Lewis M, Rosenblum LA: *The Effect of the Infant on Its Caregiver*. Wiley, 1974.

Lindemann E: Symptomatology and management of acute grief. *Am J Psychiatry* 1974; 101:141–148.

Lowenthal M, Haven C: Interaction and adaptation as a critical variable. *Am Sociolog Rev* 1968; 33:20–30.

Maddison DC, Viola A: The health of widows in the year following bereavement. *J Psychosomat Res* 1968; 12:297–306.

McFarland G, Wasli E: *Nursing Diagnosis and Process in Psychiatric Mental Health Nursing*. Lippincott, 1986.

Moses KL: Effects of developmental disability on parenting the handicapped child. In: *Patterns of Emotional Growth in the Developmentally Disabled Child*. Reiff ML (editor). The Julia S. Molloy Education Center, 1977.

Moses KL: The impact of initial diagnosis: Mobilizing family resources. Pages 11–41 in: *Parent-Professional Partnerships*. Mulick JA, Pueschel SM (editors). Academic Guild Publishers, 1983.

Moses KL: Infant deafness and parental grief: Psychosocial early intervention. Pages 86–102 in: *Education of the Hearing Impaired Child*. Powell F et al (editors). College Hill Press, 1985a.

Moses KL: Dynamic intervention with families. Pages 82–98 in: *Hearing-Impaired Children and Youth with Developmental Disabilities*. Cherow E, Matkin N, Trybus R (editors). Gallaudet College Press, 1985b.

Moses KL, Van Heck-Wulatin M: The socio-emotional impact of infant deafness: A counselling model. Pages 243–278 in: *Early Management of Hearing Loss*. Mencher G, Gerber S (editors). Grune and Stratton, 1981.

Parkes CM: Bereavement and mental illness: A clinical study of the grief of bereaved patients. *British J Med Psychol* 1965; 38: 1–15.

Parkes CM: *Studies of Grief in Adult Life.* International Universities Press, 1972.

Rees W, Lufkins SG: Mortality of bereavement. *British Med J* 1967; 4:13–16.

Rogers C: *Client Centered Therapy.* Houghton Mifflin, 1965.

Vachon M: Grief and bereavement following the death of a spouse. *Canad Psychiatric Assoc J* 1976; 21:35–44.

Volkan V: Typical findings in pathological grief. *Psychiatric Q* 1970; 44:231–250.

Wright B: *Physical Disability: A Psychological Approach.* Harper and Row, 1960.

Zisook S, DeVaul RA: Grief, unresolved grief and depression. *Psychosomatics* 1983; 24:247–271.

Zisook S, DeVaul RA, Click MA: Measuring symptoms of grief and bereavement. *Am J Psychiatry* 1982; 139:1590–1593.

Zisook S, Shuchter S, Schuckit M: Factors in the persistence of unresolved grief among psychiatric outpatients. *Psychosomatics* 1985; 26:497–503.

44

Social Isolation

JAN ELSEN, BSN, RN
MARY BLEGEN, PhD, RN

SOCIAL ISOLATION IS DEFINED HERE AS AN ACTUAL OR perceived separation of an individual from others in terms of interaction, communication, and social and emotional involvement (Silverstone and Miller, 1980). This separation can occur for one or more of five general reasons: lack of a shared language, loss of social roles and relationships, anxiety about or deficiency in social skills, decline of the person's physical abilities to contact and communicate with others, and decreased desire to communicate (Ernst et al, 1987; Jones, 1980).

This definition of Social Isolation differs from the one accepted by the North American Nursing Diagnosis Association (NANDA). NANDA defines Social Isolation as "aloneness experienced by the individual and perceived as imposed by others and as a negative or threatening state" (Carroll-Johnson, 1989;533) (see Table 44.1). We view Social Isolation as a state of being as opposed to a perceptual experience. In fact, the definition for the diagnosis Impaired Social Interaction is closer to our concept of Social Isolation. That definition is "the state in which an individual participates in an insufficient or excessive quantity or ineffective quality of social exchange" (Carroll-Johnson, 1989;532). Our definition incorporates aspects of both definitions, includes subjective and objective aspects, and names specific factors deficient in the person's life (Table 44.1). In other words, our definition is written at a higher level of abstraction and is more comprehensive. Later in this chapter we deal with specific aspects of Social Isolation in the elderly by focusing on five classes of etiologic factors. Because the etiologic factors can overlap and combine, we prefer not to distinguish various kinds of social isolation but to include them in a more general concept.

SIGNIFICANCE FOR THE ELDERLY

"Social Isolation has been identified as one of the most pressing psychosocial dilemmas of the aging today" (Ravish, 1985;10). Resources valued by this society include knowledge, skills, power, and position, and the elderly may be ignored because they no longer have these in their control. This lack of control is noted in at least two contrasting views of the elderly. Some members of society view the aging person as free to relax and enjoy freedom from worries and responsibilities. Others see the elderly as being slow and worthless, having nothing to contribute to society. In neither of these views is the older person seen as a contributing member of society. However, this chapter is based on the

Table 44.1

Etiologies/Related Factors and Defining Characteristics of Social Isolation

Diagnosis	Social Isolation (Elsen and Blegen)
Definition	An actual or perceived separation of an individual from others in terms of interaction, communication, and social and emotional involvement
Defining Characteristics	Sad, dull affect, uncommunicative, withdrawn, lack of eye contact, avoidance of social gatherings, preoccupation with own thoughts and memories, and few known visitors or supportive significant others. Expressed feelings of aloneness, rejection, insecurity in social situations, and lack of meaningful relationships
Etiologic Factors	Lack of a shared language. Loss of social roles and relationships. Anxiety about or deficiency of social skills. Decline of physical ability to contact and communicate with others. Decreased desire to communicate

IMPAIRED SOCIAL INTERACTION (NANDA) (CARROLL-JOHNSON, 1989)	SOCIAL ISOLATION (NANDA) (CARROLL-JOHNSON, 1989)
The state in which an individual participates in an insufficient or excessive quantity or ineffective quality of social exchange	Aloneness experienced by the individual and perceived as imposed by others and as a negative or threatening state
Verbalized or observed discomfort in social situations; verbalized or observed inability to receive or communicate a satisfying sense of belonging, caring, interest, or shared history; observed use of unsuccessful social interaction behaviors; dysfunctional interaction with peers, family, and/or others	Absence of supportive significant others; sad, dull affect; inappropriate activities for developmental age/stage; uncommunicative, withdrawn, no eye contact; preoccupation with own thoughts; projected hostility; seeking to be alone, evidence of physical/mental handicap or altered state of wellness; expressed feelings of aloneness, rejection, inadequacy, absence of purpose, inability to meet expectations, insecurity
Knowledge/skill deficit about ways to enhance mutuality; communication barriers; self-concept disturbance; absence of available significant others or peers; limited physical mobility; therapeutic isolation; sociocultural dissonance; environmental barriers; altered thought processes	Immature interests and development; alterations in physical appearance or mental status; unacceptable social behavior or values; altered state of wellness; inability to engage in satisfying personal resources; inability to engage in satisfying personal relationships

assumption that the elderly have much to offer—a lifetime of experiences and knowledge. They should be encouraged to remain actively involved in society and to contribute their experience and knowledge.

The prevalence of Social Isolation among the elderly is difficult to determine from the literature because varying terminology has been used to address the issue and because results of the surveys are varied and contradictory. Rutzen (1980) found no evidence of substantially increased Social Isolation with age. He did find that men were more likely to be isolated than women and that Social Isolation was more prominent in people from lower status occupations. Overall, the greatest Social Isolation was found among those who moved frequently, the foreign-born, the poor, men, and blacks (Rutzen, 1980; 84–85). Silverstone and Miller (1980) list four serious problems of the elderly: fear of crime, poor health, inadequate income, and loneliness. Social Isolation was not listed, but each of these four problems can involve Social Isolation. Riley and Foner (1968) found that more

than 50% of men between the ages of 65 and 85 live with a spouse, whereas only 37.4% of women live with a spouse. This suggests that many women living alone may be experiencing Social Isolation. Although the actual prevalence of Social Isolation is not clear from the literature, we conclude, with these authors, that Social Isolation is a problem for the elderly.

Consequences

One of the consequences of Social Isolation in the elderly is the unfilled need for actual physical assistance from others. Other outcomes include loneliness, lack of social support, and deterioration of social abilities as a result of disuse. Nurses deal with all of these consequences when the elderly are institutionalized.

Without frequent meaningful interaction with others, dependent elderly persons may no longer feel that life is worth living. To have adequate self-esteem, contact with the environment is crucial (Ravish, 1985). Without this contact the elderly may stop trying to stay healthy and active and may suspend contact with the world beyond their bed or chair. The nursing care facility may be perceived as a place for them to be kept out of the way while waiting to die, rather than as a place where they can live to their fullest. Health care professionals, at times, emphasize decline or regression of the elderly rather than growth (Ravish, 1985). Nurses are the health professionals most able to stop this process and perhaps reverse it. By providing the opportunity for meaningful interaction and development of social skills, the nurse can have a significant impact on the elderly person's social involvement.

Significance to Nursing

Intervening successfully in areas that are of central importance to the clients served is of great value to the development of the nursing profession. Social Isolation, as defined here, is an area of central importance in the lives of elderly clients and is an area in which nurses can function independently. In addition to carrying out physical care interventions and attempting to meet psychologic and emotional needs of clients, nurses must design interventions to relieve problems in the social life of clients. Interventions, such as the training group described in this chapter, address often forgotten social needs and can increase the provision of holistic care in the truest sense.

ETIOLOGIES/RELATED FACTORS

Social Isolation can be related to or caused by declining physical abilities, loss of social roles and relationships, anxieties about or deficiencies in social skills, lack of a shared language, and decreased desire to communicate. These etiologic factors are not mutually exclusive causes of Social Isolation. For example, people may reject others because of anxiety about their own social skills, or anxiety about social skills may arise from declining physical abilities. For the elderly, declining physical abilities may occur simultaneously with the loss of social roles and relationships due to retirement and death.

Theoretical Framework

To understand Social Isolation in the elderly person it is necessary to explore the concept's opposite—a socializing person or socialization. A socializing elderly person is one who is communicating with others in ways that are meaningful. Because of the lack of research on the

socialization process in the elderly, a theoretical framework that attempts to integrate pertinent material from several sources is offered. Five equally important requirements of socializing are suggested and discussed in the next section: (1) physiologic abilities to contact and communicate with others; (2) other people with whom to interact; (3) knowledge of the usual methods of communication; (4) a system of language understood by all involved; and (5) and the motivation or desire to interact.

The physiologic abilities necessary for socialization include the physical energy and the mobility to contact other people face to face, over the telephone, or by writing. Although face-to-face communication is the ideal, it requires the most mobility for people who live separately. Telephone and written communication are viable methods of socialization that require other kinds of mobility. The inability to move from one place to another, dial the telephone, or write creates barriers that must be overcome to socialize with others. The neuromotor abilities of speech, vision, hearing, or touch are required to communicate once contact is made. Deficiencies in abilities constitute other barriers to socialization, and the probability of their occurrence increases with age.

Deficiencies in vision, hearing, touch, and mobility are common in the elderly. Usually vision changes occur so slowly that adjustments are made without the individual being aware of the changes, but the decreased ability to see others and the environment may decrease socialization. Difficulties in hearing, including having trouble distinguishing a voice from background sounds and having difficulty hearing higher frequencies, can also decrease involvement with others. Diminished sensations of touch may also inhibit social interaction, and chronic illnesses, which affects many elderly, may limit mobility. Declining physical abilities and sensory losses do not preclude socialization in the elderly; however, these changes often make the process of socialization more difficult.

Having other people with whom to interact is another crucial requirement for socialization. People in our society are seldom totally cut off from others, but the number of people with whom an elderly person can meaningfully interact can vary widely. Family and kinship groups provide the basis for most daily contacts, and work and friendship groups are also of primary importance. Other formal and informal groups that can meet this requirement include neighborhood, church, clubs, and business contacts. Elderly people who have lost family members, friends, and neighbors to death or migration and work contacts to retirement are at particular risk for Social Isolation. Older people who reside in care facilities may be cut off from their remaining family and friends. With the loss of these contacts, the socialization opportunities for the elderly decline and the potential for Social Isolation increases. Fortunately, in long-term care facilities the potential for interaction and socialization activities may actually increase. Nurses can make use of this potential for socialization by facilitating group activities and one-to-one interaction among residents and staff.

The third category, knowledge of the usual methods of communication, is more abstract than the other requirements. This type of knowledge is difficult to specify and includes all those social skills that people learn subconsciously as well as those that may be deliberately taught. Verbal and nonverbal factors are involved, as well as the etiquette of communicating with others, and even the personal space norms of a particular group. The social skills we are concerned with are verbal and nonverbal behaviors that initiate and sustain social interaction. These include making eye contact, making a friendly overture or response, seeking out others for the purpose of interaction, voluntarily joining an informal group, talking about one's ideas and experiences, and asking about the ideas and experiences of others. The ease with which the elderly use these social skills may be a determining factor in their level of socialization. The intervention described later in this chapter addresses these social skills.

The fourth requirement, a shared system of language, is equally important. Individuals in our society who have potential problems regarding a shared language include non-English speaking people, the deaf who use sign language, and the blind who use braille. The varying use of a common language also creates problems. This may occur when an elderly person attempts to communicate with someone much younger. The different uses of common words, slang terms, and different vocabularies may hinder communication. Through spoken words and nonverbal symbols, one person offers another a perspective on an object or idea. If communication occurs, the other person comes to share the perspective, the meaning of the situation. Mead called this sharing of meaning through interaction symbolic interaction (cited in Strauss, 1956). From this process of sharing perspectives, the individual is able to view self and others and thereby develop the sense of social group and self in relation to this group. This is socialization; conversely, the lack of sharing is Social Isolation. Nursing staff in care facilities are often considerably younger than the residents and must remember to communicate as much as possible using terms that are meaningful to both the old and the young to facilitate true interaction.

Finally, the desire to socialize provides the individual with the motivation to contact and interact with others. Without this motivation, interaction may not be attempted even when the other four requirements are met. What provides the desire to socialize? It is most likely that the elderly person either values a specific outcome of an interaction (ie, the answer to a question) or values the process of interaction without a specific outcome in mind. The person then attempts to obtain the valued outcome or process by interacting with another; that is, the individual exchanges communication acts for the other's communication. The "social exchange" approach to be-

havior suggests that people exchange communication for valued rewards, and that they attempt to "profit" from the exchanges. Profit in this sense implies only that the value of the outcome, or the interaction, will be greater than the costs of interacting (Homans, 1974). Barriers to socialization, such as physical problems, decreased contact with others, difficulty with communication, and lack of a shared language, increase the efforts required to interact. If the efforts involved in attempting to interact and the costs of the interaction are higher than the expected rewards from the interaction, the profit and therefore motivation will be low. If the elderly person does not value interaction, perhaps because their recent experiences have not included rewarding interaction, then attempts to communicate may not be made even when the costs are low. Elderly persons can become socially isolated when either the value of the interaction is low or the costs are higher than the perceived value.

Although all five requirements are important to the socialization process, this chapter focuses on only two. We assume that there are other people with whom the elderly client can communicate through a shared language and that the person has the physical ability to communicate. Thus, only the relative lack of social skills and decreased motivation to attempt communication will be addressed. These two factors may be interrelated in many cases. The elderly person who lacks motivation to communicate may have decreased skill through lack of use, and those with inadequate skill may have decreased motivation due to the difficulties encountered in attempting to communicate.

DEFINING CHARACTERISTICS

The defining characteristics of Social Isolation in the elderly include sad, dull affect; uncommunicative and withdrawn behavior; lack of eye contact; avoidance of social gatherings; preoccupation with own thoughts and memories; and few visitors or supportive significant others. In addition, the elderly person may experience feelings of aloneness, rejection, insecurity in social situations, and lack of meaningful relationships.

Social Isolation, as a state of being, can be entered as an active process of withdrawal, as a reaction to events in the environment, or as a passive process as events in the elderly's external or internal environment block avenues of social contact. Some of the defining characteristics are signs of these processes; however, other characteristics reflect the impact of the process on the individual. The impact of being socially isolated can result in depression, hopelessness, and physical and psychologic insecurity, as well as the loneliness pin-pointed in the NANDA definition (Carroll-Johnson, 1989). Table 44.1 presents the definitions, defining characteristics, and etiologic factors of our diagnosis of Social Isolation and the NANDA diagnoses of Social Isolation and Impaired Social Interaction.

ASSESSMENT

A good assessment is necessary for adequate planning of goals and interventions. Next, three general suggestions for assessment of social skills and motivation to interact are made, and an assessment tool is described. First, it is important to determine what the interpersonal difficulties of the elderly resident are. To assess this, the nurse needs to observe the elderly person in a social setting. The nurse should avoid unrealistically high standards and observe for difficulties in asking for help, initiating a conversation, or responding to another person.

Second, it is helpful to collect this information in a systematic manner. Self-report questionnaires give some idea of the resident's perceptions of his or her social skills, but the best assessment is often direct behavioral observations of the patient in interpersonal situations. Assessment Guide 44.1 contains a checklist developed by Durham (1983;61) that organizes observations in a systematic and efficient manner.

Third, the assessment should look for all the potential causes of social isolation (see Table 44.1). For example, in addition to lack of social skills and decreased motivation to interact, there may be decreased physical abilities. Difficulty understanding the language or methods of communication and a lack of other persons to interact with may also affect the elderly's level of social interaction.

After the assessment data are collected, treatment goals should be determined for each resident. These goals should encompass desired changes in the person's social behavior to increase socialization. They should also be designed so that they are compatible with other rehabilitation goals.

CASE STUDY

Social Isolation, Mrs. J

Mrs. J is a 59-year-old widow. One month before admission to a hospital, she was diagnosed with stage IV cervical cancer. She also had a left leg thrombosis. An attempt to save the leg with revascularization surgery failed, and it was amputated at mid-thigh. The loss of her leg makes mobilization difficult for Mrs. J.

Mrs. J is 120 miles away from her friends and family. Because of this distance, her boyfriend has come to visit her only once, and she rarely receives phone calls. She has three children, but they have not made contact with her while she has been hospitalized. Mrs. J seldom initiates conversation and usually will respond only when direct questions are asked. Once a day she sits in a chair for half

an hour. The rest of the time she lies in bed with the television and lights off. Her vision and hearing are not impaired. Attempts to get Mrs. J to discuss her feelings have had minimal effect. She did comment that having her leg cut off would be a waste of money as she would have to throw one of her shoes away every time she went to buy a new pair.

Using the social skills checklist it is observed that Mrs. J avoids eye contact, lacks spontaneity of speech, doesn't hold casual conversations, shows no interest in general appearance, keeps all feelings inside, and won't ask for help when needed. After these assessments, we look for the possible cause(s) of her problems: loss of usual social contacts due to a new environment; decreased mobility, as well as grief, fear, poor body image with the loss of her leg, and a diagnosis of cancer; possible lack of social skills (we don't have premorbid data on this factor); and decreased desire to communicate. Approaching Mrs. J to determine what she felt her problems were was unsuccessful.

CASE STUDY

Social Isolation, Mrs. M

Mrs. M, a 78-year-old widow, has lived in the nursing home for 4 years. She has mild chronic obstructive pulmonary disease (COPD) and an old hip fracture. Mrs. M has difficulty walking more than 20 feet with her walker. She spends most of the day in a geriatric chair, alone in her room watching television. She has one daughter who lives in town and visits her once every 2 weeks. Her other daughter lives 400 miles away and visits her once a year.

Her vision is good with glasses, and her hearing is only slightly diminished. She goes to the dining room for her meals and visits a little with her tablemate. Although responsive to questions, Mrs. M seldom makes eye contact and gives only yes or no answers. Mrs. M refuses to participate in group activities. She denies loneliness but appears depressed most of the time.

Mrs. M doesn't have as many problems as Mrs. J, but difficulty with movement, lack of eye contact, social distancing, lack of spontaneity of speech, and inability to hold casual conversation are barriers for her. Possible causes may be loss of usual social contacts, decreased mobility, and decreased desire to interact with others.

Nursing Diagnoses

After all the information has been obtained, nursing diagnoses are made to get a clear picture of each person's problem and what the causal factors are. For example, Mrs. J's nursing diagnoses would be Social Isolation related to decreased desire to communicate, impaired physical mobility and state of wellness, loss of usual social contacts, and possible lack of social skills, as evidenced by sad, dull affect; uncommunicative and withdrawn behavior; lack of eye contact; avoidance of social gatherings; no visitors; and inability to move purposefully because of loss of leg and weakness. Mrs. M's nursing diagnoses would be Social Isolation related to loss of usual social contacts, decreased mobility, decreased desire to communicate, and possible lack of social skills, as evidenced by sad, dull affect; withdrawn behavior; lack of eye contact; avoidance of social gatherings; and few visitors.

From this information, determining specific goals and planning specific interventions can proceed. Specific goals for Mrs. J include expressing ideas and feelings, increasing eye contact, and holding casual conversations with others. Goals for Mrs. M are to increase eye contact, to increase time spent outside of her room, to attend and actively participate in at least one group activity per week, and to increase time spent in conversation with those around her.

NURSING INTERVENTIONS

In designing an intervention that will increase both elderly clients' social skills and their desire to communicate, two things are needed. First, a list of needed social skills must be determined. Second, an understanding of the acquisition of this kind of knowledge provides guidance for the process. Together these describe the intervention proposed here—a social skills training program.

The first component of a social skills training program is the content to be learned. Many articles discuss social skills in broad terms, but few actually define them. Robinson (1988), Gutride et al (1973), and Durham (1983) define social skills to a greater extent. Social skills encompass a wide variety of actions, behaviors, and postures that can vary with different cultures and relationships. According to Robinson (1988;60), social skills are personal characteristics that predispose one to develop a functional social network and include "(1) introducing self to others; (2) making phone calls to initiate social contact; (3) participating in groups; (4) using assertive behavior to meet needs; (5) engaging in self-disclosure; and (6) being responsive."

Body language/appearance, the type and characteristics of speech, and conversation behavior are part of social skills. Having no eye contact with the speaker, laughing or smiling when the speaker is sharing a sad story, being extremely tense, backing away from the speaker, sitting on hands, having both arms and legs crossed tightly, and being extremely close or far away from the speaker are considered inappropriate body language. On the other hand, when the speaker is relating a sad story, appropriate body language includes maintaining a serious facial expression and even shedding a tear, making eye contact, leaning forward slightly, and reaching out to touch the other.

The types and characteristics of speech considered socially proper include using appropriate tone and volume while initiating and responding to conversation, and talking for more than 10 consecutive seconds (Gutride et al, 1973). Making meaningful conversation (ie, talking of more than the weather), being spontaneous, showing interest in the environment and others, being alert, expressing feelings, asking for help when needed, giving and accepting compliments, and cooperating with others are all types of social skills (Durham, 1983). Social skills we wish to promote include increased eye contact, speech appropriate to the situation, nonverbal behavior congruent with the situation, initiation and response to interactions with others, and participation in groups.

The second component of the social skills training program is the process of learning the skills. Bandura's (1977) social learning theory maintains that learning is a process of pairing behaviors with rewards and that rewarded behaviors are repeated. Bandura goes beyond classical conditioning in describing observational learning. Observational learning occurs when a person watches others perform behaviors that are rewarded and then reproduces these behaviors for external or internal reinforcement. The social learning analysis of the modeling phenomenon (Bandura, 1977) proposes that a model's behavior is a source of information for the observer. The observer perceives and then processes the modeled behavior. The information is processed through symbolic and cognitive organization, actual motor reenactment, and pairing of the behavior to a reward. Symbolic repertoires of behavior are built through the observation of others' behavior. The next step is a cognitive one in that the observed information is retained. Finally, the observer enacts learned behaviors that are appropriate for his or her situation.

For the intervention proposed here, the nurse initially serves as the model, and elderly residents are the observers. As the observers enact social behaviors, they become models as well. The elderly members of the social skills group do not simply mimic the nurse's actions; they actively process the information provided and then convert what was learned through observation to action. In general, people don't enact everything they process; they enact only the behaviors that fit and that they expect to be rewarded. Thus, they may change the observed action to one that fits them. The modeled behavior, in the case of social skills training, should be social skills that the elderly can use successfully to communicate with others and be rewarded for using.

To summarize, several things are needed for effective learning of social skills. First, the learner must observe other people (models) using the social skills. Second, these skills should be used in a setting or interaction that is similar to the learner's setting and potential interactions. Third, the learner should observe the role model receiving a positive reward for using the social skill. Fourth, the learner should be able to process the observations and enact them. Lastly, to maximize potential learning, the observer–learner should be rewarded when he or she has enacted the social skill.

In the past, social workers, psychologists, and recreational and occupational therapists have all worked with socialization and social skills training programs on a formal level. Jones (1980;209) feels that social skills training groups are vehicles "for providing practice in social behavior in a relatively realistic, yet non-threatening setting" and that these groups also function to form relationships and social contacts. Nurses should be at the forefront of social skills programs in long-term care facilities. This chapter describes one training program that nurses can use for their elderly institutionalized clients.

The social skills training program provides an opportunity for elderly persons to improve their social skills and decrease their anxiety in social situations through the observation of modeled behavior and feedback of the group leader and group members. The formal part of the program takes place in a group of 5 to 10 people discussing topics of interest. According to Bandura's (1977) theory, through observation of the social behavior of others in the group and through actual discussion of actions and feelings appropriate for certain situations, the person internalizes new behaviors. The informal part of the program occurs when the new behaviors are acted out and approval or disapproval is given by others (ie, staff or fellow residents). Instruction and modeling are necessary for behavioral change; practice and positive feedback are necessary for lasting change.

Organizing the Group

The nurse needs to ask four basic questions before a socialization group is established. First, what is the philosophy of rehabilitation in the elderly person's living area and in the institution as a whole? High morale among staff, good communication, and clear treatment goals make it easier to establish a socialization group. If these elements are lacking, the training group could still be formed; however, interventions that increase morale and communication and that establish clearer goals may also be necessary.

The second question pertains to how the living unit is organized. Social skills training requires the ward staff to keep actively involved with patients in order to reinforce and maintain the social skills learning from group sessions. Activities to meet staff needs should include emotional support, involvement with decision making, clear responsibilities, and clear communication between staff members so that staff morale and a therapeutic atmosphere can be maintained.

Third the nurse should determine whether recreational and social opportunities are available on the unit. Some elderly persons may be able to function at a higher level

than observed if there are social opportunities available to them. Other elderly residents may have difficulty in even simple social activities. Having social activities on the ward gives the nurse a chance to assess how well each resident is getting along and what interventions are needed, as well as providing residents with the opportunity to practice the social skills they have learned. If there is a lack of social activities, this should be corrected before starting the social skills training group.

Finally, what is the staffing situation for the unit? Because nursing works on a rotating shift system, at least three nurses will be needed as group leaders so that continuity can be maintained and mutual support can be given. The nurses also need to be permanent staff members so that consistent therapeutic interactions can take place while in and out of the formal group situation. If the care facility does not have RN coverage on every shift, LPNs can be trained in therapeutic interactions.

Once these questions have been answered, group participants can be selected. The nurse, who sees the elderly residents day after day and interacts with them the most, is in the best position to make this selection. The 5 to 10 persons selected for the group should have some conversational skills and be motivated to attend without excessive prompting. They clearly should have interpersonal difficulties but also should have some social awareness.

In general, two meetings per week for 3 to 4 months are recommended. Although a duration of 45 minutes is approximately the right length, the meeting time could be extended or shortened as needed. When deciding how often the group should meet, three things should be considered. First, it is difficult to maintain continuity if the group meets less than once a week. Second, although meeting twice a week is desirable, the meeting should occur regularly. If meetings occur irregularly, then once a week would be better. Third, the number of staff willing to lead the group needs to be taken into consideration. The group should run for about 3 or 4 months and then have a month or two off. This prevents burnout of the group leaders and loss of interest among group members.

A conversational theme or topic helps to stimulate group discussion. Consideration of current events or seasonal activities are timely topics, or common problems of the group may be discussed. Setting up an agenda one month ahead may be helpful for group leaders, as they would not feel pressured for a topic the day of the group. Other possible topics include growing older, how to get involved, handling losses, meeting new people, striking up a conversation, and reminiscences.

Implementation

Before the social skills group session starts, the leaders must choose the discussion topics, review what happened during the last session, and review the specific goals for each patient. This in turn may lead to some ideas for directing the group.

At the beginning of each session, the leaders should introduce themselves and have each of the members introduce himself or herself. Having the members shake hands with the persons next to them increases interaction. Following the introductions, a review of the last session and homework assignments could be done. If the group members have something specific to discuss, this could be done next; if not, bring up the topic for discussion. Throughout the session, the most important tasks of the leader are to model social skills and to encourage the group to talk about and practice good social skills.

Each group session should concentrate on a particular social skill and a specific discussion topic in which to use the skill (eg, using direct eye contact while discussing the problems one has with growing older or initiating conversations while discussing meeting new people). Other possible combinations of social skills and discussion topics might be responding to interactions and opinions about television shows and participating in larger groups combined with playing games. Many different combinations are possible. The important point is to present and practice a social skill in a way that is enjoyable and meaningful to the elderly participants.

To close the session, the leader should summarize the key points of the discussion. The leader could also shake hands with or even hug each of the members, thanking them for coming and for something they contributed during the group meeting (eg, "Thank you Mrs. M for sharing your fears on . . ."). The group should be told when the next group meeting will be held and encouraged to attend. After the session, the nurse leaders should discuss how the group meeting went and offer constructive feedback. This is a good time for mutual support, especially if it was a difficult group meeting.

Group leaders should also consider several other factors. Leaders should maintain a minimal level of self-participation in the group by devising ways of encouraging the participation of all group members. This can be accomplished by structuring the exercises, such as asking specific questions or giving specific tasks to be completed. Leaders should create an atmosphere that is warm and supportive but balanced with task orientation. Reinforcing learning attempts, even if unsuccessful; focusing on the assets as much as the deficits; using humor; and having a style of interaction that is nondefensive, positive, and open to feelings and concerns create a caring, positive atmosphere. Leaders should establish expectations that positive changes will occur. This can be accomplished by setting realistic goals and rewarding behavior that is a step toward these goals. Leaders should practice what they teach. For example, when encouraging eye contact with others the leader should model the behavior by making

eye contact with group members. This modeling should take place both in group meetings and on the unit.

The learning of social skills should not terminate at the end of each session but should be integrated with the daily interactions between staff and patient. To promote this informal learning, the entire staff should know which of the elderly persons are involved in the group and should be taught the process of modeling and rewarding the desired social skills. In fact, the key to ensuring treatment gains is through positive social interaction among all team members and residents.

Based on their assessment data, Mrs. M and Mrs. J would both be candidates to attend a social skills training group. Group discussions on losses, body image, decreased mobility, how to hold a conversation, and sharing feelings and ideas are some of the topics that would benefit them. Starting with less stressful topics would give them a chance to relate experiences that are less threatening than their current problems. After the group members feel more at ease with each other, the topics can be directed toward more stressful topics.

CASE STUDY

Nursing Interventions

Mrs. J and Mrs. M were two of seven people in a social skills training group. At the first meeting, held around a circular table, everyone introduced themselves. Mrs. J and Mrs. M were given the tasks of serving coffee and cookies to the rest of the group members. Discussion centered on favorite cookies and drinks, with each member sharing a specific memory associated with their favorite cookie. At the end of the meeting a game was played to see if each member's favorite cookie could be named. For homework, each member was asked to approach two other people before the next meeting to find out what cookies they like best.

The socialization group met twice a week. Members took turns serving the refreshments. At the beginning of each meeting homework assignments were discussed. Each meeting included a light subject, such as each member's favorite type of music at a party, and a social skill, such as what topics are discussed at parties. At the end of 3 months the group members held a party for the rest of the residents.

Both Mrs. M and Mrs. J attended the socialization groups during the 3-month period. Mrs. M reluctantly attended meetings at first but near the end was arriving an hour early. She began attending other activities and held conversations with her tablemates at mealtimes. Her daughter, who lived in town, noticed a dramatic difference in her mother over the 3-month period. Before the social skills training, Mrs. M had little to say during her daughter's visits, but by the end of this time, she held lively conversations and asked her daughter to help her bake cookies at her home.

Mrs. J also showed improvement in her social skills, though not as marked as Mrs. M's improvement. Mrs. J became interested in what she wore, especially on meeting days. She also started communicating more with the staff, though mostly on the pretense of carrying out homework assignments. At group meetings, Mrs. J seemed to enjoy serving refreshments. Initially she quietly passed around the refreshments, but by the end, she made sure everyone received seconds and increased her eye contact with other people.

OUTCOMES

The basis for evaluation of the effectiveness of the group should be the achievement of individual treatment goals. This is done by reassessment to see if any improvements were made. If no improvements are made in a reasonable time period, adjustments may be needed in the interventions or goals.

Evaluation of the elderly resident's social skills needs to extend to interactions with staff and other residents outside of the group meetings. Ongoing social activities once again provide the opportunity for practice of social skills and for evaluation of the elderly resident program.

Evaluation of the socialization group as a whole should be done at the end of each 3- to 4-month period by both staff and participants and yearly to assess the costs and benefits of the program. Evaluation at these intervals allows the program to be improved on an ongoing basis.

SUMMARY

Social Isolation is recognized as an important concept for nursing, but has not been fully developed as a nursing diagnosis. A·revised definition is offered in this chapter and compared to two concepts, Social Isolation and Impaired Social Interaction, the diagnoses accepted by NANDA (Carroll-Johnson, 1989). Many etiologic factors can be involved when social isolation develops. These factors must be identified and used to determine the appropriate nursing goals and interventions. The concept of Social Isolation, as developed in this chapter, is accompanied by a list of five etiologic factors. This revision

may be helpful in the process of further developing the concept of Social Isolation and applying it to assist the elderly.

The theoretical framework for Social Isolation used in this chapter emerged from the concept of socialization. Factors that are needed for socialization include the physical ability to contact and communicate, other people to interact with, social skills, a shared language, and motivation or desire to interact. The elderly are at a greater risk for Social Isolation because of deficiencies in vision, hearing, touch, and mobility that may occur as one ages. Elderly people are also more likely to experience Social Isolation because of loss of friends and family to death, retirement, or migration. Relocation to a care facility, for example, can disrupt elderly persons' ties with their remaining social contacts. Declining desire to socialize and a decrease in social skills may also occur.

A social skills training group intervention using Bandura's theory of social learning as a guide was described. The purposes of the training group are to improve social skills, to decrease anxiety in social situations, and to increase the motivation to interact. The social skills training group is designed especially for institutionalized elderly persons. In the training group 5 to 10 elderly residents discuss topics of interest with the group leader, who models appropriate social skills. The session also includes time for practicing the skill. Recreational or occupational therapy, social clubs, and even physical therapy may also be used to intervene in social isolation caused by other factors.

Group training in social skills represents a positive step toward holistic nursing. By incorporating socialization goals in care plans, nursing can include this important area in the care of elderly people. Nursing can also carry out what was taught in the group to the whole unit, reinforcing and modeling the social skills of the particular socialization group as well as letting the rest of the residents benefit from it.

Socialization and social skills programs have been in existence for more than two decades. These programs have been most often used for nonpatients in such areas as assertiveness training, communication, and sexuality. Nursing has a pivotal role in the socialization and social skills training groups for the elderly. Nurses can also benefit professionally from developing the program, since it requires expanding knowledge and leadership skills through leading the group, giving support and guidance, and being a model for other nurses. Most important, however, are the social health improvements made available to the elderly people participating in the socialization groups.

ASSESSMENT GUIDE 44.1

Social Skill Checklist

Please assess the following aspects of the resident's social behavior in terms of the categories below:

1. serious difficulty in this area, disturbing to others;
2. general difficulty in this area, interferes with social interaction;
3. difficulty in some situations or with some people;
4. generally appropriate, does not interfere with social interaction;
5. very appropriate, definite asset.
N.O. not observed.

Your assessment should be based on observations of the resident's behavior in a number of different settings over a period of 2 weeks. Remember to add comments as necessary and to summarize the information at the end.

Nonverbal behavior	*Category*	*Comments*

1. Facial expression
2. Eye contact
3. Body posture
4. Body movements
5. Social distance
6. Tone of voice
7. Loudness of speech
8. Speed of speech
9. Spontaneity of speech
10. Hesitations in speech
11. General appearance
12. Holding casual conversations
13. Showing interest in what other people say
14. Expressing feelings appropriately
15. Disagreeing with people without getting upset
16. Keeping symptoms from being intrusive
17. Asking for help when needed
18. Accepting compliments
19. Cooperating with others
20. Responding to criticism
21. Other problems (please specify)

Please also comment on the following:

22. Social supports in the community
23. Friendships in the hospital
24. Degree of social anxiety
25. Response to organized social activities
26. Interest in social activities

Summarize key areas in need of some intervention:

References

Bandura A: *Social Learning Theory.* Prentice-Hall, 1977.

Carroll-Johnson R (editor): *Classification of Nursing Diagnoses: Proceedings of the Eighth Conference.* Lippincott, 1989.

Durham R: Long-stay psychiatric patients in hospital. In: *Development in Social Skills Training.* Spence S, Shepherd G (editors). Academic Press, 1983.

Ernst P et al: Isolation and the symptoms of chronic brain syndrome. *Gerontologist* 1987; 18:468–473.

Gutride M, Goldstein A, Hunter G: The use of modeling and role playing to increase social interaction among asocial psychiatric patients. *J Consult Clin Psychol* 1973; 40:408–415.

Homans G: *Social Behavior, Its Elementary Forms,* rev. ed. Harcourt Brace Jovanovich, 1974.

Jones B: Social isolation: How can we help? *Nurs Times* 1980; 76: 208–209.

Ravish T: Prevent social isolation before it starts. *J Gerontol Nurs* 1985; 11:10–13.

Riley M, Foner A: *Aging and Society: An Inventory of Research Findings,* Vol 1. Russell Sage Foundation, 1968.

Robinson K: A social skills training program for adult caregivers. *ANS* 1988; 10:59–72.

Rutzen S: The social distribution of primary social isolation among the aged: A subcultural approach. *Internat J Aging Hum Dev* 1980; 11:77–87.

Silverstone B, Miller S: Isolation in the aged: Individual dynamics, community and family involvement. *J Geriatr Psychiatry* 1980; 13:27–47.

Strauss A: *George Herbert Mead on Social Psychology.* Chicago Press, 1956.

45

Impaired Verbal Communication

DONELLE CUSACK, MS, RN

THE USE OF VERBAL LANGUAGE TO COMMUNICATE meanings is a characteristic that distinguishes humans. An individual who loses the ability to use verbal language is isolated and unable to send and/or receive messages to let others know of personal discomforts, opinions, or preferences. Unable to formulate and/or interpret verbal messages, the victim naturally experiences great anxiety, embarrassment, and frustration and becomes agitated. If physical strength permits, the person may become aggressive to the point of violence (Cusack, 1984). As feelings of helplessness and hopelessness mount, depression usually sets in (Heilman, 1980). Most sad, the individual is deprived of the means of sharing deepest feelings of endearment with loved ones. For elderly persons, the loss of ability to communicate verbally is especially problematic and often compounds other losses of cognitive and functional abilities that accompany aging.

In many cases the individual can no longer contribute to the family's financial or functional support or participate fully in family decisions. Rather, the person with impaired verbal communication often becomes dependent on other members of the family, which markedly changes family roles and relationships. These circumstances are likely to result in institutionalization of elderly victims because of the higher incidences of loss of family and other social support, loss of self-care abilities, and loss of economic independence.

DEFINITION OF IMPAIRED VERBAL COMMUNICATION

Communication

In order to judge an elderly patient's verbal communication pattern as "normal" or "impaired," nurses must have an understanding of the process of communication. Generally, it involves seven components : (1) a sender; (2) an encoding action; (3) a message; (4) a channel (medium); (5) a decoding action; (6) a receiver; and (7) feedback (Samovar and Rintye, 1979).

The code is the embodiment of language—the system of symbols by which messages are transmitted. Language is usually transferred in two expressive codes (speech and script) and is interpreted in two receptive modes (listening and reading). In verbal communication, words are the code symbols by which the language is communicated. The names and corresponding meanings of the symbols are stored in the dominant cerebral hemisphere of the brain. Words are produced by speech (forcing exhaled air through the vocal cords), by script (imprinting on paper), or by body signing/language. The message thus encoded is ultimately decoded by listening or reading.

Obviously, the two communicators (sender and receiver) must have a mutual understanding of the meanings of the code symbols. Concordant information must be established for both the sender and the receiver to attain confirmation and gratification (McFarland and Naschinski, 1985).

Impaired Verbal Communication: Aphasia

The diagnosis Impaired Verbal Communication was accepted in 1982 by the North American Nursing Diagnosis Association (NANDA) and is used on current lists of accepted nursing diagnoses. Although it may require further specificity in the future, it is a useful diagnosis, especially when paired with specific etiologies. Table 45.1 illustrates the current NANDA definition, related factors/ etiologies, and nursing diagnosis of Impaired Verbal Communication (Carroll-Johnson, 1989) compared with related factors and defining characteristics from other sources discussed in this chapter.

Any inability to send or receive the message through word symbols results in impaired verbal communication. The loss of the use of language due to disruption in the neurocirculation of the dominant cerebral hemisphere of the brain is a serious handicap. This disturbance in the conduction of messages through the neural pathways interferes with analysis and synthesis of verbal codification—recognition, retrieval, and reconstruction of words (Cermak et al, 1984). Difficulty in processing and/or using language symbols has, for the past century, commonly been called *dysphasia* or *aphasia*. Those terms have come to be used more or less interchangeably, although there is a basic etymologic distinction according to the prefixes: The literal translation of *dysphasia* means "difficulty in utterance and/or comprehension," whereas *aphasia* is "the total absence of the ability to articulate ideas verbally." However, *aphasia* commonly is used to indicate either partial or complete loss of language ability. Therefore, the term *aphasia* will be used with both meanings in this chapter.

Table 45.1

Definition, Related Factors, and Defining Characteristics of Impaired Verbal Communication

---

Definition: A state in which an individual experiences a decreased or absent ability to use or understand language in human interaction

NANDA (CARROLL-JOHNSON, 1989)	OTHER SOURCES DISCUSSED IN THIS CHAPTER
Related Factors/Etiologies	*Related Factors/Etiologies**
Decrease in circulation to the brain	Vascular
Physical barrier, brain tumor, tracheostomy, intubation	Hemorrhage
Anatomic deficit, cleft palate	Embolism
Psychologic barriers, psychosis, lack of stimuli	Thrombosis
Cultural difference	Spasmodic occlusion
Development or age-related	Neoplasmic
	Traumatic
	Infectious
	Dementias
Defining Characteristics	*Defining Characteristics*†
‡Speaks or verbalizes with difficulty	Decreased meaningful use of verbal language
‡Unable to speak dominant language	Decreased comprehension of verbal messages
‡Does not or cannot speak	Decreased auditory and/or visual perception
Stuttering; slurring	Inappropriate outbursts of automatic phrases
Inappropriate verbalization	Emotional lability (sudden weeping or laughing)
Dyspnea	Depression
Disorientation	
Difficulty expressing thought verbally	
Difficulty forming words or sentences	

---

*Darley, 1975.
†Campbell, 1978; Carpenito, 1983; Gordon, 1982.
‡Critical defining characteristic.

The five general causes of aphasia due to neural disruption in the brain are listed in Table 45.1 along with common defining characteristics. Dementia is a common cause among elderly persons (see Chapter 29 on Altered Thought Processes). The particular symptomatology depends on the site of the brain involved and on the size of the area. The neuroanatomic location of the brain damage, not the causative agent, is the key to the aphasic symptomatology. Totally different pathologic states can and do produce identical aphasic syndromes (Benson, 1979).

SIGNIFICANCE FOR THE ELDERLY

The brain has been likened to a computer (Burck et al, 1983; Maranto, 1984). The total number of nerve cells has been estimated at 14×10^9. It has been estimated that only 10% of the brain is used, even by academicians.

Any disturbance, obstruction, or destruction of the cortical neural structure is devastating. Spontaneous hemorrhage, infarction, or occlusion are among the leading challenges to geriatricians today.

Ironically, stroke, with its resulting impairments of aphasia and dysarthria, strikes persons in their later years when they have the greatest need for effective communication to adapt and cope with environmental, physiologic, psychologic, and sociocultural conditions (Hagen and Horning, 1984; Shadden and Raiford, 1984). Voices also tend to weaken as individuals age because of reduced strength and increased fatigability in the muscles of the chest and throat (Wilder, 1984).

Of the stroke survivors, 80% have residual neurologic impairment but are not totally disabled (Steinberg, 1986). Those persons may be able to benefit from nursing rehabilitative interventions.

Trauma is another leading cause of neurologic disability. Remarkably similar symptoms result from destruction of neural tissue in victims of both traumatic accidents and cerebrovascular accidents. Advances in modern health care sciences have resulted in declining mortality rates. This means that more persons are surviving, but most of them are burdened with severe residual communication deficits. Modern surgery is able to perform remarkable physical repair, but many survivors are subjected to a long life of communication impairment.

In cases of injury to neural tissues, the activity of the adjacent as well as the immediate areas of the brain are disrupted. Tissue surrounding the disturbed site is subject to involvement because of loss of circulation and oxygenation when blood vessels are interrupted.

Edema is a common cause of interference with the usual neural connections. An excessive accumulation of fluid in the intracellular tissue spaces results from increased permeability of the capillaries due to anoxia, trauma, tumors, and so on (Matthews and Glaser, 1979).

The growth of neoplastic tumors in the brain is extremely serious. They are space displacing and exert pressure on all tissue within the cranium, influencing function of all brain cells, even cells not a part of the tumor per se.

The fourth common causative classification of neural disruption is infections. Irreversible residual damage often results from the invasion and multiplication of microorganisms that produce intracellular injury (Benson, 1979; Matthews and Glaser, 1979).

HISTORY OF IMPAIRED VERBAL COMMUNICATION

Since the beginning of recorded time, interest has been expressed in the tragic phenomenon of loss of language. The cause was attributed variously to demons, disfavor of the gods, disorders of the tongue, and so on. Greek philosophers attempted to balance the humors in an effort to relieve the obvious distress (Critchley, 1970; LaPointe, 1984).

Johann Wolfgang von Goethe, German poet, dramatist, novelist, lawyer, and philosopher, is remembered for his masterpiece "Faust" (Critchley, 1970). But, his description of motor aphasia in "Wilhelm Meisters Lehrjahre" bears an infinitely more urgent message of the need for therapeutic care of the victim of apoplexy (an archaic term for cerebrovascular accident).

Dr. Arthur L. Benton, eminent professor of neurology and psychology at The University of Iowa, conducted scholarly surveys of the literature from the earliest medical writings (Hippocratic Corpus, 400 B.C.) to modern times (cited in Benton and Joynt, 1960). He found that our present knowledge of aphasic disorders is the product of an evolution that spans millennia. Most of the writings before the 19th century are of a descriptive nature. Several physicians of the Renaissance era recorded particularly vivid, though brief, detailed observations.

Johann Augustin Philipp Gesner (1739–1801), a prolific medical writer, presented a conceptualization of anatomic and physiologic correlates of what he termed "speech amnesia" or "forgetting of speech." He was the first to publicize the rupture between abstract thought and linguistic symbols.

Until rather recently, the brain has not been readily observable. Only after brutal trauma (as in war) were significant numbers of living brains available for direct examination. Dr. Pierre Paul Broca, a French anatomist and surgeon during the Franco-Prussian war, brought order and scientific observation to the study of the brain (Geschwind, 1970). Later, during World War I, another army surgeon, this time in England, made fortuitous use of the tragic devastation. Dr. Henry Head studied a number of healthy, intelligent, brain-injured young men manifesting a diversity of disorders of speech (Head, 1926).

Because of the large numbers of brain-injured, speech-disabled servicemen during World War II and the social obligation to rehabilitate them, there was renewed interest in aphasia, as it had come to be called by that time. A Russian surgeon–neurologist seized the opportunity of war to observe the ravages of brain damage in an effort to solve the enigma of brain functions. As a result, Alexander Romanovitch Luria emerged as a preeminent figure in international aphasiology (Luria, 1977).

Post-World War II, Dr. Harold Goodglass led a multidisciplinary study at Boston University to develop an assessment of neuropathologic functioning of aphasic persons in order to achieve a psycholinguistic analysis of each individual's aphasic language. The Boston Diagnostic Aphasia Examination has proved to be an accurate, comprehensive instrument for speech/language diagnoses (Goodglass and Kaplan, 1983) (see the section on Assessment for further discussion of this tool).

Greater visualization of interior areas of the human body is now possible because of exciting advances in technology. Computerized tomography (CT) (Matthews and Glaser, 1979), positron emission tomography (PET), magnetic resonance imaging (MRI), evoked response (ER), blood flow studies, quantitative autoradiography, magnetoencephalography (MEG), and so on are expensive but effective developments that enable investigators to establish increasing knowledge of cytoarchitecture, interrelationships, and neurotransmitters.

Localization of central nervous system functions was originally confirmed primarily by means of electrical stimulation mapping studies, as first conducted by Penfield and Roberts (1959) during craniotomies on conscious patients under local anesthesia.

Cerebral localization was fiercely contested by eminent authorities for over a century. Opponents of the localization theory held that mental capability (evidenced by language facility) was the product of total brain activity. In 1861, Dr. Broca observed concomitant speech impairment and right hemiplegia in cases in which postmortem examination revealed neural damage in the left frontal lobe.

Further support of localization in the left cerebral hemisphere was presented in 1874 when Dr. Carl Wernicke published his classic text *The Symptom Complex of Aphasia: A Psychological Study on an Anatomical Basis.* He differentiated the aphasias of the left temporal lobe ("Wernicke's aphasia") and the aphasias of the left frontal lobe ("Broca's aphasia") (cited in Springer, 1981). Prestigious investigators over the years presented evidence on both sides of the controversy.

Semmes (1968) published indirect evidence that sensory and motor functions are focally organized into discrete, relatively nonoverlapping zones in the left or

dominant hemisphere, but are diffusely organized in the right hemisphere (Borod and Goodglass, 1980; Semmes, 1968). However, one would expect the reverse to be true of about 40% of those persons who are left-handed (7% of total population) who have a dominant right hemisphere, or approximately 3% of the total population (Brain, 1961).

TYPES OF APHASIA

The impairment of verbal communication is manifested in the following commonly used classifications of aphasia, each of which will be discussed in detail:

Expressive Aphasia
    Impaired oral communication
        Broca's aphasia
        Wernicke's aphasia
        Transcortical motor aphasia
    Impaired written communication (agraphia)
Receptive Aphasia
    Impaired auditory perception
        Pure word deafness
        Semantic aphasia
    Impaired visual perception
    Impaired comprehension
Global Aphasia

Expressive Aphasia

Impaired Oral Communication Halting, labored, telegraphic oral use of verbal language results from involvement of the posterior–inferior area of the frontal lobe of the left hemisphere, anterior to the Sylvian fissure. This has come to be called "Broca's aphasia" after the French doctor who first circumscribed this area (Geschwind, 1970) (see Figure 45.1). Although the speech is nonfluent, the person's comprehension is impaired and the ability to hear and read with understanding is retained. The difficulty is in the motor activity of producing language verbally. Impulses in this area of the brain activate vocalization—the coordination of the lips, tongue, and throat muscles. If the impulses are not transmitted to the adjacent moror cortex, the appropriate muscles are not activated (Bloom et al, 1985). This results in knowing what one wants to say but not being able to say the words fluently.

A completely different decrease in oral use of verbal language (decrease in content) results from involvement of the posterior–superior temporal lobe of the left hemisphere, posterior and inferior to the Sylvian fissure. This has come to be called "Wernicke's aphasia," since it was first described in 1874 by Dr. Carl Wernicke (cited in Geschwind, 1970). This speech is fluent (Boller, 1981) and circuitous, but the intended precise words are not readily retrievable. The sentences may contain nonsense and nonexistent words that render the conversation meaningless (Buckingham and Kertesz, 1976). Rhythm, intonation, and grammatical forms may be perfect, but comprehension and the ability to read and write are impaired. This person does not understand much of what is being said, nor what should be said. The elderly individual does not understand what is received, nor can the individual monitor what he or she is saying.

Because the sites of pathology of both Broca's aphasia and Wernicke's aphasia are located on opposite sides of the Sylvian fissure of the dominant hemisphere, they are known as the "perisylvian aphasic syndromes."

There are a number of other aphasic syndromes in which repetition of spoken language remains normal. The sites of pathology of these aphasias are located outside the perisylvian region in the vascular border zone between the middle, anterior, and posterior cerebral arteries. They have been called "transcortical motor aphasia" (TCM) for over 100 years. The term *transcortical* is archaic, but in this case it is universally recognized and accepted (Benson, 1979). The spontaneous speech of TCM is nonfluent, highly simplified, and produced with considerable effort. Most patients with TCM attempt to facilitate their speech production with gross motor assistance such as hand waving, walking, and so on. There is a tendency toward stumbling, perseverative, stuttering, spontaneous output. The ability to repeat words and phrases is remarkable in TCM. Series speech is performed surprisingly well once the series (chronologic numbers, days of the week, months, prayers, poems, nursery rhymes, and so on) is initiated. Comprehension of spoken language and written material is usually very good, but most patients with TCM have difficulty reading aloud.

Impaired Written Communication The loss or impairment of the ability to produce written language due to brain damage is called *agraphia*. It always accompanies oral aphasia in some degree. Writing difficulties fall roughly into four groups:

1. The quality of handwriting (calligraphy)
2. Visual spacial attributes
3. Spelling (orthography)
4. Appropriate choice of words. Written output in Broca's aphasia is very sparse, whereas the messages written in Wernicke's aphasia may be wordy, empty paragraphs.

Because language disruption characteristically occurs in conjunction with hemiparesis of the dominant side, some distortion in formulation of handwriting may be erroneously attributed to the awkwardness of learning to use the nondominant hand. However, persons forced to use a nonfavored hand in cases of injury rapidly develop a facility seldom achieved in aphasic agraphia.

Occasionally, a patient may retain the ability to legibly perform an automatic, highly overlearned bit of writing such as a signature. Accurate assessment of writing ability should include progressively more difficult testing, such as dictation of a sentence including some numbers, the copying of a short paragraph (with assessment of comprehension of it), and, if the patient successfully accomplishes these, an original brief narrative report.

Receptive Aphasia

Impaired Auditory Perception Sounds are received in the primary auditory cortex (verified by audiometric testing), but the messages are not transmitted through the Wernicke's area for understanding as language. It is not the hearing mechanism that is impaired; rather, it is the internal translating abilities of the brain that impair reception as well as expression of language.

"Pure word deafness" is a syndrome in which understanding of written language is normal, but there is severe disability in understanding spoken language due to disruption in the Wernicke's area (posterior temporal area of the dominant hemisphere).

Semantic aphasia is the term applied to the condition in which patients receive auditory signals well, as evidenced in the ability to repeat language spoken to them, but are unable to extract meaning from the words. The area involved is outside the perisylvian area in the parietal-temporal border zone.

"Broca's aphasia" is the classic condition in which there is understanding of single words but not of extended sentence-length material. Pathology is in the traditional Broca's area (posterior–inferior area of the frontal lobe of the left hemisphere, anterior to the Sylvian fissure).

Impaired Visual Perception Sight of written words is received in the primary visual cortex but not transmitted as language through the Wernicke's area.

Global Aphasia

A profound diminution of all functions of communication (both expressive and receptive) has come to be called *global aphasia*. It is marked by extreme reduction of verbal output, anomia (loss of the power of naming objects or ideas) and comprehension deficits. It is frequent consequence of a massive lesion in the left hemisphere or in softening in the entire territory of the Sylvian artery (DeRenzi, 1980). Some globally aphasic persons produce only one recurring consonant vowel (CV) syllable. Fortunately, prosody is usually preserved—different shades of meaning are conveyed by variations in pitch, rhythm, and emphasis (Poeck et al, 1984).

Dysarthria

In addition to aphasia, verbal communication may be impaired mechanically by disturbance in the articulation and phonation of language. *Dysarthria* is an impairment of motor control of the speech musculature due to neurologic dysfunction. "Internal speech" (the language of thought) is unaffected. It does not cause a disturbance in ideation. There is comprehension of spoken and written language. Intelligence is unimpaired. Only the neuromuscular mechanics of the coordination of movements of respiratory, laryngeal, pharyngeal, lingual, and labial muscles are involved. (Many of the same muscles are also used in swallowing, so swallowing is usually impaired as well.)

Dysarthria is often associated with right-sided paralysis. Spastic hemiplegia is most frequent, in which cases the speech is characterized by slow rate, imprecise articulation, effortful phonation, and harsh, low-pitched tonality. In flaccid hemiplegia, the dysarthria is usually breathy with audible (stridorous) inspiration. The hypernasal quality and distinctive pronunciation of dysarthric speech cannot be imitated by a normal speaker. The most common causative condition seems to be cerebrovascular accident (CVA), especially embolization of the subcortical tissue below the Broca's area. It can be visualized by CAT scan. Dysarthric speech is also heard in cases of poliomyelitis, tumor, and Parkinson's disease.

ASSESSMENT

The bedside assessment for impaired verbal communication must be as physiologically and psychologically systematic and comprehensive as possible in order to establish a data base on which all further activities will be built (Benson, 1979; Cusack, 1986; Hausman et al, 1985; Sahs, 1974). A referral to the speech pathologist/therapist is recommended for further and more definitive assessment.

The nurse's initial approach to the patient must be reassuring and nonthreatening. Because of the patient's inability to provide verbal information, it may be necessary for the nurse to rely on family members for the health history and other perinent data. Take care not to talk about patients as though they are an inanimate object, a child, or deceased, but rather include them in the conversation, directing questions to them and allowing adequate time for their replies.

Comprehension

Understanding can be assessed first by conversation. Response to simple, straightforward commands is a standard start, such as: "Please open your mouth," or "Close your eyes," or "Let me see your hand." Ask the patient to point to familiar objects—the window, television set, and so on. *Apraxia* (inability to carry out purposeful movements that can be accomplished automatically) may impede the patient's motor response to commands. Therefore, yes/no questions may be the most accurate method of checking comprehension. The questions must be straightforward and simple, containing only common words. Try asking: "Is your name (the nurse then says the person's name)?" Later, recheck the answer by repeating the questions with an inappropriate name. Often this delights the patient and leads him or her to say the correct word (Agranowitz and McKeown, 1966).

If the patient is unable to verbalize "yes" or "no" intelligibly, the nurse should establish some other sign, such as closing the eyes for "no." If possible, be assured of the patient's premorbid ability to speak, read, and write English.

If the patient answers "yes" to everything (often erroneously), the possibility should be considered that this may be an effort to please the questioner (Agranowitz and McKeown, 1966).

Comprehension is seldom completely present or completely absent. Where there is aphasia, there is usually a certain degree of deficit, although most aphasics are able to understand at least some conversation. Comprehension may seem to be heightened at some times more than others; for example, fatigue has a depressing effect.

Fluency/Nonfluency

The presence or absence of the quality of smooth, easy flow of conversation is significant in assessment of the type and severity of aphasia. This distinction can be immediately determined by the following criteria.

Rate of Speech   Normally, Americans speak at 100 to 150 words per minute. In Broca's aphasia, the output is usually less than 50 words per minute and often less than 10. In Wernicke's aphasia, the rate may be more than 200 words each minute.

Phrase Length   In Broca's aphasia, answers may be as short as a single word, whereas in Wernicke's aphasia, the circumlocution may be an endless maze of empty five-word phrases, with short infrequent pauses for futile anomic word searches.

Prosody   Broca's aphasia is characterized by awkward, nonmelodic dysrhythmia, whereas Wernicke's aphasia has a melody of speech.

Effort   For the patient suffering Broca's aphasia, speaking is an obvious struggle with facial grimacing, tense body posturing, labored deep breathing, groping gestures of the nondominant hand, and, most important, urgent eye contact. Typically, the patient with Wernicke's aphasia speaks effortlessly, unaware of the meaningless sentences.

Information   The few words transmitted in Broca's aphasia will be nouns and action verbs with few adjectives, adverbs, or conjunctions. Conversely, the Wernicke's aphasia sentences will be a proliferation of meaningless phrases and nonsense words (neologisms).

Repetition   The ability to repeat, exactly, the words presented by the examiner is significantly abnormal in both Broca's aphasia and Wernicke's aphasia. Testing should begin with simple monosyllabic words, advancing to complex sentences. The remarkable ability of patients suffering transcortical motor aphasia to exhibit superior repetitive spoken language enables the examiner to make the differential diagnosis from Broca's aphasia.

Word Finding   Inability to call forth well-known nouns (anomia) is a universal deficit in aphasia. It can be tested by requesting the patient to name visually presented objects, pictures, geometric shapes, and so on; to name objects from verbal descriptions of their function; and to name objects in a given category (animals, fruits, and so on). In each case, the examiner should supply the words immediately after testing to eliminate further frustration.

Definitive aphasia testing can be conducted by the speech/language pathologist in order to diagnose the presence and type of aphasia syndrome, to measure performance levels (initial and through changes over time), and to assess assets and liabilities in all language areas as a guide to therapy. The Boston Diagnostic Aphasia Examination is a comprehensive battery of tests formulated in 1972 by Harold Goodglass, PhD with the collaboration of Edith Kaplan, PhD (Goodglass and Kaplan, 1983).

CASE STUDY

Impaired Verbal Communication

Mr. O was born April 1, 1919, the youngest of four children of a harnessmaker. He enjoyed a happy, normal childhood; graduated from high school; and for the next 40 years was an industrious head of household.

In May 1978 he suffered a cerebrovascular accident. The medical diagnosis at that time read "Right hemiplegia with aphasia secondary to CVA." On the speech/language Boston Diagnostic Aphasia Examination z-score rating (a 6-point scale from 0 [most severe] to 5 [mild], Mr. O's profile was plotted at "minus .5—problems across all language modalities" (Goodglass and Kaplan, 1983).

Mr. O is presently a resident in a nursing home. He requires assistance for all aspects of activities of daily living. The staff are attentive to his needs and attempt to engage him in conversation, but his few verbal expressions are essentially unintelligible. When asked a question offering him an opportunity to express a choice of "yes" or "no," he appears to have a preference (by emotive facial animation), but the response is usually an unrecognizable grunt. He is heavily medicated for hypertension (both diastolic and systolic readings are customarily above normal limits).

Mr. O had received speech/language therapy for 5 years. However, the phonetic exercises conducted three times per week in the clinic had not been fruitful. When it became apparent that his language abilities had not improved, his name was removed from the roster of active speech therapy candidates. He continued to be tested annually.

The following assessment data were noted:

68-year-old man whose central nervous system had heretofore enjoyed normal perception, communication, rhythmicity, learning ability, self-concept, and health

Neurocirculatory disruption of dominant left cerebral hemisphere of brain due to cerebrovascular accident

Requires assistance with all activities of daily living

Inability to answer "yes" or "no" to questions appropriately

Verbal expressions unintelligible

Loss of acuity, right visual fields

Responds with facial animation to verbal cues

Appears frustrated/agitated when attempts to communicate

NURSING DIAGNOSES

Impaired Verbal Communication related to left CVA, evidenced by loss of language/speech skills: articulation, word finding, fluency, serial speech, auditory comprehension.

Sensory Perceptual Deficit related to left CVA, evidenced by right homonymous hemianopsia.

NURSING INTERVENTIONS

Process of Speech Recovery

There are many explanations of the mechanisms of the recovery process. Miller (1984) classifies them into three major groups: (1) artifact theories, (2) anatomical reorganization, and (3) functional adaptation.

Artifact Theories   Secondary deficits of a temporary nature are among the physiologic changes following any brain insult. Edema is a prime example. Extracellular fluid increases the tissue volume, causing deficits immediately after the cerebrovascular event. However, the excess fluid eventually withdraws, bringing about an improvement in the patient's condition.

A different example is *diaschisis*, a form of shock, originally explained by von Manakow in German publications in 1914 (Feeney and Baron, 1986; Finger, 1978). The Russian explanation of amorphous inhibition of brain activity, possibly due to reduction of acetylcholine at the synapse, is a similar theory (Luria, 1977).

In all examples in the artifact group, whatever is recovered was never really lost.

Anatomic Reorganization   Recovery from brain damage can occur by means of other sections of the brain taking over for the damaged area. This often occurs spontaneously in young children as a result of endogenous development of alternative growth patterns.

Exercises to stimulate more development can be conducted by means of a tachistoscope, a machine by which a three-dimensional image can be briefly (about one-tenth of a second) flashed on a screen to only one precise visual field. The subject is directed to look continuously at a small black dot in the center of the screen. To stimulate more development of verbal functions in the right hemisphere, the image is flashed to the left of the dot. The subject does not have time to move the eyes away from the dot; only the one hemisphere views the image (Bloom et al, 1985).

Functional Adaptation   By application of speech/language methodologies, the patient can be assisted to reattain function. Relearning has been achieved through psychologic practices such as tactile and proprioceptive feedback.

Measurable improvement in speech/language skills can be achieved through consistent exercise. Essential components are precise diagnosis of the speech/language deficits; establishment of an individualized therapy program of effective exercise; and continuous implementation of the activities prescribed by the speech/language pathologist as discussed in the research example presented later. Cooperation of those persons in direct attendance (nursing personnel and family members) is vital (David et al, 1979; Wertz et al, 1986). Patients can be enabled to meet their personal needs, and even the most severely handicapped can progress. For some, the achievement of being able to express a clear, deliberate "yes" or "no" liberates them from a lonely life devoid of choices.

Speech Therapy Enhancement Program (STEP)

One quasi-experimental study tested nursing interventions designed to remediate communication deficits in elderly institutionalized patients with a diagnosis of aphasia, dysarthria, or both (Buckwalter, 1986). Phase I of the study tested the effectiveness of an individualized speech/language therapy program (STEP) devised by speech therapists and implemented by nursing staff on a daily basis in a therapeutic care environment (TCE) (discussed later). Phase II included family involvement by providing memorable pictures/photographs accompanied by in-person or taped (audio and video) reminiscences and also incorporated evaluation of the treatment by family members.

Study results suggested that the STEP intervention significantly improved communication ability on targeted speech tasks but had minimal influence on standardized measures of global speech ability. In addition to speech, subjects also improved on goals related to socialization and positive interpersonal behaviors. Subjects were most satisfied with the segment Systematic Attention, which entailed a staff member simply talking (not speech therapy) to the patient for brief (10 minutes) periods twice a day. This finding coincided with findings on affective and behavioral improvements. Family members involved in the STEP Phase II study were significantly more satisfied with all aspects of care, which generalized to their reported desire to become more involved in the patient's care in the institutional setting as well as after discharge.

Therapeutic Care Environment (TCE)

The nurse's first responsibility in the care of the patient suffering Impaired Verbal Communication is to create a "therapeutic environment." Insofar as possible, the atmosphere must be controlled to be consistently comfortable. All supportive conditions and influences must be mobilized to exert a positive effect. Nursing staff and family members who are understanding can do much to console and strengthen patients and enable them to reach their optimum level of improvement. The surroundings must be safe, clean, pleasant, and well-ventilated at the proper temperature. Sufficient, unobtrusive, nonglaring lighting must be provided. No disturbing, distracting sounds should be allowed. A quiet, relaxed atmosphere puts patients at ease and facilitates their advancement.

All conversation regarding patients that is conducted within their range of hearing should be expressed directly to them. Care must be taken not to talk about them as though they were an inanimate object or child. They should be addressed on an adult level both in vocabulary and in subject interests.

It is imperative that the speaker position himself or herself within clear view of the patient before initiating a conversation. The rate of speaking should be slow and even, with distinct natural enunciation. The choice of words should be from familiar, commonly used vocabulary. Key words can be emphasized and reinforced by gestures and pantomine movements. The speaker's voice should not be loud unless the patient has a hearing impairment.

Emotional and controversial subjects should be avoided as well as abstract concepts. Only one clear idea should be presented at a time. In giving directions, involve only one movement, motion, or activity. Construct questions to allow "yes" or "no" answers.

Patients must never be hurried in expressing their thoughts. Time should be allowed for them to scan their store of memories, plan their reply, and find the precise words of choice ("response latency") (Portnoy, 1984). Acceptance is encouraging. Accept every effort. Try to decode all the messages that are sent. Convey the realization that the patient's frustration is understood even if his or her speech is not. Say: "I know this is difficult for you, but we'll all get used to it" (Darley, 1975). Overlook all mistakes, profanity, jargon, outbursts of weeping, and inappropriate words.

Persons suffering nonfluent (Broca's) aphasia retain comprehension and, therefore, sink into a justifiable depression when contemplating their plight ("catastrophic reaction"). Persons suffering fluent (Wernicke's) aphasia often seem unaware of their disabilities.

Good humor smooths most tense situations. If aphasic patients can recognize their own errors, they are sometimes amused (Agranowitz and McKeown, 1966). Laugh *with* them, but beware of the appearance of laughing *at* them. Loving laughter is a form of communication.

Use tact and avoid tasteless, thoughtless remarks. It is better to refer to the patient's affected side as his "weaker" side, rather than as his "bad" side.

Help the patient to avoid fatigue. Short, frequent, meaningful conversations are the most productive. Shield the patient from long tiring visits, especially in large groups of persons competing for attention and conversation.

Once the therapeutic care environment is established, multidisciplinary rehabilitation can be conducted. Nursing will be able to give continuity and meaningful practice to the individualized exercises prescribed by the speech/language pathologist.

Language Rehabilitation

Wepman (1953), a psychologist who devised one of the early and most enduring tests for evaluating and understanding aphasics, has also developed a conceptual model for processes involved in recovery from aphasia. Three concepts—stimulation, facilitation, and motivation—form the constructs that are inextricably interrelated in the recovery process. *Stimulation* is the outside persuasion that is conducted externally to heighten the patient's efforts. *Facilitation* assists, enables, and creates the proper stage. *Motivation* is the goal-directed behavior of patients based on their background, interests, capabilities, drives, and so on.

The nurse and the family members who spend the most time with the patient (Cusack, 1984) and on whom the patient depends are in the best position to combine these three constructs. Their innate interest enables them to provide the courage and support the aphasic individual needs. It is hoped that nurses and family members will avoid overprotection, which would invalidate and infantilize the patient, and that they will enable the victims to work their way through feelings of futility and worthlessness to regain as much autonomy as possible.

Because professional speech/language sessions are usually scheduled for only a few hours a week, arrangements should be made for the nursing staff and family to provide continuation of the prescribed activities in all interactions with the patient. The speech/language pathologist who tests the patient and establishes the speech diagnosis should educate the nursing staff and family in administration of the repetitive exercises and should regularly monitor their progress. In this way, the influence of the speech/language therapy can continue uninterruptedly on a round-the-clock daily basis (Cusack, 1984).

Recent studies indicate that improvement in communication results from the support and encouragement provided in a one-to-one therapeutic relationship, rather than from any specific skills relating to speech therapy (David et al, 1979; Lincoln et al, 1984; Shewan and Kertesz, 1984). In the event that the services of a speech/language pathologist are not available, the nurse can structure therapeutic communication according to the characteristics of the therapeutic care environment described earlier.

One of the most effective means of encouraging a reluctant speaker is to set the stage for reminiscence. Providing photographs, audiocassettes, and, most important, in-person visits of family and friends enables the re-creation of memorable events of earlier years (Buckwalter, 1983). The recall of intense experiences arouses strong needs to express appropriate comments. In many elderly patients, long-term memories are usually more accesible than recent memories. Reflections of the "good old days" may bring a sense of well-being in the realization of a accomplishments during those active days. Recounting experiences to receptive listeners enhances the patient's feelings of self-worth. Staff appreciation and admiration result in multiple benefits to the patient. Spontaneous social conversation based on meaningful memories is an infinitely more effective exercise than hours of monotonous drills.

Musical Speech Interventions

Appreciation and production of musical experience involves a variety of brain functions. Untrained melody recognition and enjoyment probably takes place in the right temporal lobe. Training—analysis of pitch, rhythm, tempo—for most persons takes place in the left temporal lobe (Kirshner, 1986).

Music with a cheerful, strong rhythm creates a positive atmosphere that raises spirits, blots out distracting noise, gives ordered regularity, and uses anatomic reorganization to call forth language in the right hemisphere. Aphasic patients can often recall and sing the words of old familiar songs completely. They may easily sing the familiar kindergarten song "Good Morning to You," whereas they are unable to say "Good morning" (Agranowitz and McKeown, 1966). Luria has written of intrasystemic reorganization—transferring control either downward or upward within the system. Melodic intonation therapy (MIT) has been extremely successful in aphasic populations (Johns, 1978). Starting with unison singing, using strong rhythm and intonation patterns, patients progress through a repetition of phrases in normal intonation to production of sentences in response to questions.

General Considerations

Supportive care of the person suffering from Impaired Verbal Communication must be individualized. No two cases are identical, although some may appear to be superficially similar. Patients' personalities will differ according to their experiential and educational background, intellectual potential, and so on. However, one commonality experienced by all individuals with impaired verbal communication is frustration.

The impaired person should be enabled to develop alternative means of expression, such as paper and pencil notes (if writing skills are intact). Self-cueing exercises can assist a determinedly self-reliant person. Category names help enlarge the number of retrievable, often-used words. Gestures should be encouraged. However, there is often a limitation in gesturing ability, which corresponds to the limitations in expressive language (Glosser et al, 1986).

Some persons with Impaired Verbal Communication become adept at "Amerind"—American Indian sign language. Gestures represent objects, actions, direction, and descriptions. Amerind was adapted by speech therapists to enable people suffering severe oral–verbal apraxis to express their thoughts more freely. Some patients have developed spontaneous word production synchronously with the use of these signs. Another of the most exciting possibilities for transfer of information is the computer. Computer programs can be specifically planned for use by the cognizant verbally impaired (Fisher, 1986).

CASE STUDY

Nursing Interventions

Staff nurses, concerned by Mr. O's frustration, devised simple games in an effort to relieve his anxiety and to help him develop speech skills. They took every

opportunity while administering his regular nursing care to establish a therapeutic care environment by (Cusack, 1984):

1. Positioning themselves within his limited view
2. Establishing eye-to-eye contact
3. Conversing with Mr. O on an adult level on topics of interest to him
4. Conversing with Mr. O at a relaxed, slow rate, allowing him plenty of time to repond
5. Enunciating clearly and naturally
6. Using common concrete words in simple sentences (no abstract thoughts)
7. Employing gestures to support messages
8. Encouraging Mr. O to gesture with his left arm and hand
9. Discussing pleasant, positive topics (no controversy or emotionalism)
10. Keeping the volume of their voices at a normal level

OUTCOMES

All patients suffering from Impaired Verbal Communication give evidence of increased emotional tension resulting from inability to express thoughts verbally. Therefore, the first priority in the elderly person's care must be to relieve her anxiety and frustration, both immediately and as a long-term goal. Concomittantly, the perception and production of language must be fostered.

Therefore, the outcome criteria for the elderly suffering from Impaired Verbal Communication are focused on three areas: (1) decreased frustration; (2) increased understanding; and (3) increased speech or compensatory ability to communicate needs and feelings.

Complete restitution, especially in older persons, is seldom possible. Amelioration of the devastation is a more attainable goal (Sarno et al, 1970). The patient will experience satisfaction in the realization of being assisted, accepted, understood, and respected by the nurse and others (Wilder, 1984).

CASE STUDY

Outcomes

Within a week following initiation of the nursing interventions, Mr. O exhibited signs of relaxation: His diastolic and systolic blood pressure readings were routinely at least 15 points lower. His countenance changed from a habitual brow-furrowed frown to a smile, and he often chuckled during conversation. Mr. O became able to articulate a consistently appropriate, recognizable "Yes!" His family was delighted in his obvious increase in contentment.

SUMMARY

The development of Impaired Verbal Communication (aphasia) disturbs a person's personality and ability to interact socially. Loss of the use of language can be occasioned by vascular, neoplasmic, traumatic, and infectious causes. The most common etiologies are cerebrovascular accidents ("stroke") and traumatic accidents. The specific symptomatology depends on the site of the brain involved and on the size of the area. Throughout the history of mankind, there has been fascination with this phenomenon, but only in recent years has technology provided the means to confirm the physiologic basis of the problem visually.

Although complete remediation of the handicap is seldom possible, the frustration can be lessened by enabling increased communication skills of both expression and understanding. Consistent exercise, based on precise diagnosis of the deficit and conducted by those persons in constant attendance (nursing personnel and family), enhances verbal facility.

References

Agranowitz AL, Mckeown MR: *Aphasia Handbook* (2nd printing). Thomas, 1966.

Benson DF: *Aphasia, Alexia and Agraphia.* Churchill Livingstone, 1979.

Benton AL, Joynt RJ: Early description of aphasia. *Arch Neurol* (Aug) 1960; 3:205–221.

Bloom FE, Lazerson A, Hofstader L: *Brain, Mind and Behaviour.* Freeman, 1985.

Boller F: Strokes and behavior: Disorders of higher cortical functions following cerebral disease (disorders of language and related functions). *Current Concepts of Cerebral Vascular Disease: Official Journal American Heart Association* 1981; 16:1–4.

Borod JC, Goodglass H: Hemispheric specialization and development. Chapter 7 in: *Language and Communication in the Elderly.* Obler LK, Albert ML (editors). Lexington Books, DC Heath, 1980.

Brain WR: *Speech Disorders: Aphasia, Apraxia and Agnosia.* Butterworth, 1961.

Buckingham HW Jr, Kertesz A: Neologistic jargon aphasia. In: *Neurolinguistics.* Hoops R, Lebrun Y (editors). Swets and Zeitlinger, 1976.

Buckwalter KC: Remediation of communication deficits in elderly post-CVA patients. (Abstract.) Robert Wood Johnson Foundation, 1983.

Buckwalter KC: Annual progress report Year 2 to: Robert Wood Johnson Foundation for grant #9062. *Increasing Communication Ability in Stroke Patients,* 1986.

Burck B, Gillman D, Ose P: Brain research for educators. *J Contin Educ Nurs* 1983; 15(6):195–204.

Campbell C (editor): *Nursing Diagnosis and Intervention in Nursing Practice.* Wiley, 1978.

Carpenito LJ: *Nursing Diagnosis: Application to Clinical Practice.* Lippincott, 1983.

Carroll-Johnson R (editor): *Classification of Nursing Diagnoses: Proceedings of the Eighth Conference.* Lippincott, 1989.

Cermak LS, Stiassny D, Uhly B: Reconstructive retrieval deficits in Broca's aphasia. *Brain and Language* 1984; 21:95–104.

Critchley MD: *Aphasiology and Other Aspects of Language.* Edward Arnold LTD, 1970.

Cusack D: Increasing communication ability in stroke patients. *Staff Education Model.* The University of Iowa, 1984.

Cusack D: *Neurological Assessment Module of Physical Assessment Series.* Veterans Administration Medical Center, 1986.

Darley FL: Treatment of acquired aphasia. Pages 111–145 in: *Advances in Neurology,* Vol 7. Freidlander WJ (editor). Raven Press, 1975.

David RM, Enderpy P, Bainton D: Progress report on an evaluation of speech therapy for aphasia. *British J Disorders Communication* 1979; 14(2):85–88.

DeRenzi E: Aphasia in the elderly. Pages 198–204 in: *The Aging Brain.* Barbagallo-Sagiorgia G, Exton-Smith AN (editors). Plenum, 1980.

Feeney DM, Baron JC: Diaschisis. *Stroke* (Sept-Oct) 1986; 17: 817–830.

Fingers (editor): *Recovery from Brain Damage.* Plenum, 1978.

Geschwind N: The organization of language and the brain. *Science* 1970; 170:940–944.

Goodglass H, Kaplan E: *The Assessment of Aphasia and Related Disorders,* 2nd ed. Lea and Febiger, 1983.

Gordon M: *Manual of Nursing Diagnosis.* McGraw-Hill, 1982.

Hagen C, Horning KL: Communication disorders. *Generations* (Summer) 1984; 26–29.

Hausman KA, Hartshorn J, Evans JA: *Analyzing Neurological Status.* Resource Applications, 1985.

Head H: *Aphasia and Kindred Disorders of Speech.* Macmillan, 1926.

Heilman KM, Valenstein E: Emotional disorders caused by CNS dysfunction. *Geriatrics* (Jan) 1980; 35:70–86.

Johns DF (editor): *Clinical Management of Neurogenic Communicative Disorders.* Little, Brown, 1978.

Kirshner HS: *Behavioral Neurology.* Churchill Livingstone, 1986.

LaPointe LL: Approaches to aphasia treatment. Volume 42 in: *Advances in Neurology: Progress in Aphasiology.* Rose FC (editor). Raven Press, 1984.

Lincoln NB et al: Effectiveness of speech therapy for aphasic stroke patients. *Lancet* (June 2) 1984; 1197–1200.

Luria AR: Neuropsychological studies in aphasia. In: *Neurolinguistics.* Hoops R, Lebrun Y (editors). Swets and Zeitlinger, 1976.

Maranto G: A mind within the brain. *Discover* (May) 1984: 34–43.

Matthews WB, Glaser GH (editors): *Recent Advances in Clinical Neurology* (No.2). Churchill Livingstone, 1979.

McFarland GK, Naschinski CE: Impaired communication. *Nurs Clin North Am* (Dec) 1985; 20(4):775–785.

Miller E: *Recovery and Management of Neuropsychological Impairments.* Wiley, 1984.

Penfield W, Roberts L: *Speech and Brain Mechanisms.* Princeton University Press, 1959.

Poeck K, DeBleser R, VonKeyserlingk DG: Neurolinguistic status and localization of lesion in aphasic patients with exclusively consonant-vowel recurring utterances. *Brain* 1984; 107: 199–217.

Portnoy EJ: Communication connections and aging. *Geriatr Care* (Oct) 1984; 16(10).

Sahs AL et al: *Essentials of the Neurological Examination.* Smith Kline and French Laboratories, 1974.

Samovar LA, Rintye ED: Group communication: Theory and practice. *Small Group Communication: A Reader,* 3rd ed. Brown, 1979.

Sarno MT, Silverman M, Sands E: Speech therapy and language recovery in severe aphasia. *J Speech Hearing Res* 1970; 13:607–623.

Semmes J: Hemisphere specialization: A possible clue to mechanism. *Neuropsycologia* 1968; 6:11–26.

Shadden BB, Raiford CA: The communication education of older persons: Prior training and utilization of information sources. *Educ Gerontol* 1984; 10(1–2):83–97.

Shewan CM, Kertesz A: Effects of speech and language treatment on recovery from aphasia. *Brain and Language* 1984; 23: 272–299.

Springer SP: *Left Brain, Right Brain.* Springer and Deutsch, 1981.

Steinberg FU: Rehabilitating the older stroke patient: What's possible? *Geriatrics* (Mar) 1986; 41(3):85–91.

Wepman JM: A conceptual model for the processes involved in recovery from aphasia. *J Speech Hearing Disorders* 1953; 18:4–13.

Wertz RT et al: A comparison of clinic, home and deferred language treatment for aphasia (a Veterans Administration cooperative study). *Arch Neurol* (July) 1986; 43:653–658.

Wilder CN: Management of speech and language disorders in the elderly: Some general considerations. In: *Aging and Communication Problems in Management.* Wilder CN, Weistein BE (editors). Haworth Press, 1984.

46

Altered Family Processes: Caring for the Dependent Elderly Family Member

MARGUERITE DIXON, PhD, RN

THE NURSING DIAGNOSIS ALTERED FAMILY PROCESSES means that the normal or usual function of the family is changed. This diagnosis has been accepted for clinical testing by the North American Nursing Diagnosis Association and is defined as "the state in which a family that normally functions effectively experiences a dysfunction" (Carroll-Johnson, 1989; 535).

This chapter examines the roles of nursing diagnosis and intervention within the context of family and dependent elderly family members. Topics include an overview of family systems theory, in particular, family assessment; the nurse and the family of the institutionalized senior member; nursing diagnoses that are more specific forms of Altered Family Processes; and relevant nursing interventions and outcomes for evaluation.

THE PERSPECTIVE OF THE FAMILY AS A SYSTEM

Conceptualization of the family as a unit for study and treatment became popular at the end of World War II because of available funding for and research in schizophrenia. Professional awareness of the family as an interpersonal network in which each member influences, and is influenced by, every other member was established and energized by theorists such as Nathan Ackerman (1958); Virginia Satir (1967); Gregory Bateson, John Weakland, Jay Haley, and Don Jackson (1956); Murray Bowen (1966, 1978); and Salvador Minuchin (1967). Although it is usually discussed and applied to families with children of infant through adolescent years, family theory is germane for older families as well.

Traditionally, a family is viewed as a group of persons united through marriage, birth/blood, or adoption. From a general systems perspective, a family system is a set of intimately related persons. Because the system's components are interdependent, a change or movement in any part of the system affects all other parts (Buckley, 1967; Hazzard, 1971; Miller, 1965; and VonBertalanffy, 1968). The degree and nature of the interdependencies of the family system vary over time (Aldous, 1978). Examples of this include the role reversal experienced by many parents and children in older age because of failing abilities that may occur in old age, or the loss of role of breadwinner because of retirement. The ease with which these changes take place within the family system is determined by the adaptability and flexibility of the system. Conceptualizing the family as a system places emphasis on its wholeness as a unit and also focuses attention on the interconnectedness of family members and their feelings, thoughts, and behaviors, which have reciprocal influence on each other. Any system, including the family system, functions within an identifiable boundary (Buckley, 1967). The extent of the family boundaries are characterized by terms such as *nuclear family, extended family, adopted family* and *marital dyad*.

SIGNIFICANCE FOR THE ELDERLY

Family members assume or are delegated interdependent roles within the family organization. Criteria for assignment of roles may be based on gender, age, current societal role expectations that prescribe certain behaviors and prohibit others, or any combination of these. Cultural mores are also influential. For example, a culture or society that reveres its aged is apt to pamper grandparents and allot them special psychologic and tangible space and little responsibility. In another society the elders—notably older women—may be expected to rear grandchildren, do housework for younger family members, or share other responsibilities. In a culture that regards them as useless, elders may be excluded from family and societal activities. In this situation elders may have to fend for themselves and may be left to die alone.

A range of cultural practices related to the elderly are found in the United States. The status and roles of the aged reflect changing societal values, expectations, and attendant constraints. Constraints are often economic in nature. Social Security, private insurance, and retirement plans assure some income for those who are eligible. When these sources of income are inadequate, the senior adult, who may have enjoyed social and economic independence as a younger person and who may have been relied on even into retirement years by other family members for some measure of economic sustenance, becomes dependent on family or government resources.

Drastic changes in an individual's usual role can be psychologically damaging at any age. The elderly are particularly at risk for role change. Those who live long enough to be considered "old" experience losses, sometimes several major losses within a relatively brief period in almost every aspect of their lives. These losses include *social* (eg, employment, income, death of some family members and friends); *physical* (eg, body changes, acute or worsening chronic illness(es) and/or dysfunction); and *psychologic* (eg, loss of the perception of being personally productive, needed, wanted, valued). As the family's older members become gradually or suddenly incapacitated by physical infirmity or illness or become financially dependent, members of the immediate or extended family network or public or private agencies may need to intervene in a helping way. This period can be one of social and psychologic discomfort and stress for the older person, for the responsible and caring adult children, and for other relatives (Cicirelli, 1981). This can also be a time of reaffirmation of interpersonal bonds as family members support one another. These altered roles can precipitate feelings of meaninglessness and depression or can be an impetus for positive change and redefinition of self. The losses associated with old age can result in positive or negative changes in body image, self-identity, and responses to life events.

Intergenerational Relationship Patterns

Increased longevity of the United States population has altered the structure of families so that multigenerational families are becoming increasingly common. Currently about half of all persons age 65 and older have great-grandchildren and about 10% of the age group have a child who is also 65 or older (National Institute of Aging, 1982). According to the American Association of Retired Persons (AARP) (*A Profile of Older Americans,* 1987), in 1986 about 67% of noninstitutionalized older persons lived in family settings, and about 28% lived alone. With advancing age, particularly for older women, the percentage of persons living in intergenerational households increases (*Aging America,* 1984). The majority of elderly remain in the community in which they lived most of their lives, have strong ties with family, and prefer to live separately from offspring (Eliopoulos, 1987). Relationships between older spouses and siblings tend to become stronger and more stable later in life. Fewer than half of all elderly have no family or live alone.

Elderly living in institutions, primarily nursing homes, compose about 6% of the population (*A Profile of Older Americans,* 1987). When the elderly of minority and some immigrant groups are considered, the statistics are different. For example, a slightly higher proportion (96%) of black elderly live in the community; slightly less, about 3%, live in institutions. Likewise, about 97% of Hispanic elderly live in households in the community, and about 3%, live in nursing homes (*A Portrait of Older Minorities,* 1985). This contrast between the reference population's and minority population's living arrangements may imply sociocultural differences in attitudes about institutionalization versus home care of the elderly. Decisions regarding living arrangements are also influenced by economic resources and the perceived health or physical status of the individual. Apart from the implied cultural belief is the economic constraint. On the whole, black families have less income when compared with the majority population, and because nursing homes cost money, black families choose to maintain their elderly members in households. When members of the household are unable to provide care, or if the physical condition of the aged member makes home care impractical, institutionalization may be favored despite cultural beliefs and customs that oppose this action. The unique situation, policies, beliefs, customs, and goals of each family are intertwined in the decision-making process.

The "Absent" Older Member

Older persons vary in the number of years they can safely live independently. When the individual's ability for total self-care diminishes, family members, friends, or agencies may find it advisable to assist the aged person to make alternative living arrangements. The elderly person may move into someone else's home, share their own home with others, or go to a long-term care facility.

No household is exempt from stresses emanating from external or internal sources. For example, an elder member's progressively deteriorating physical illness or cognitive impairment may strain family financial resources and relationships. Family social, economic, and restorative capabilities are likely to become taxed to the point that the family's equilibrium is severely threatened or damaged. Mitigative influences are the quality of family members' past interpersonal relationships, the role and extent of participation of the elder member in the family structure, the family's beliefs and attitudes about aging and the elderly, economic conditions and resources, and current societal mores (Cox, 1984). When family traditions have favored retaining and nurturing elderly members under any and all circumstances, that family may be expressly resistive to considering institutional care for parent, grandparent, or another aged family member, even when the family has decided that it can no longer provide adequate or appropriate care in the home.

Consider the Granville family. Mrs. Ceola Granville had been widowed about 30 years when, at age 82, previously observed signs of memory disturbance, confusion, and personality disorder became more disabling for her. She lived with her eldest child, an unmarried daughter (a high school principal) in an apartment building owned by three of her five children. Mrs. Granville had been a homemaker into her late 70s. Because Mrs. Granville was alone during the day and required some assistance, her children pooled their monies and hired a housekeeper–companion to be with their mother. This arrangement continued through several years when Mrs. Granville needed more intensive help with bathing, dressing, toileting, feeding, and general safety.

Family members rotated responsibility among themselves to care for her on weekends. Finally, it became necessary to hospitalize Mrs. Granville. She died during the third week of hospitalization.

The Granvilles exemplify those families whose members coalesce to support and care for their elderly. Each adult child was involved in planning, and then facilitating

the plan, for their mother. As her cognitive abilities deteriorated, she was "absent" in the sense that she became very different from the person she had been. Although periods of nonrecognition occurred, she usually recognized one or all of her children.

When persons who have been an integral part of the family group become cognitively impaired or are physically removed from the family, a void is created: They are "missed." Their absence may, in turn, create ambivalent reactions of sadness and mourning, or relief, as if a burden has been removed.

Family Policies and Practices

As noted earlier, during the course of a year, approximately 6% of all elderly persons are in long-term care facilities (*A Profile of Older Americans*, 1987); about one third have been there for less than 1 year, one third for 1 to 3 years, and one third for 3 or more years (National Center for Health Statistics, 1978). Nine percent of all older people will spend time in a nursing home during the course of a year, and 23% to 38% of people age 65 years and more will spend time in a nursing home before death (Health Care Financing Administration, 1981). Brody et al (1978) and others (Health Care Financing Administration, 1981; Tobin and Kulys, 1980) corroborate that most families have a commitment to, and behave responsibly toward, their elderly relatives. Moreover, when the elderly belong to a family, they are less likely to be placed in an institution. When institutionalization appears necessary, placement is often delayed until there is no other reasonable alternative. Families tend to maintain the individual in the home for as long as necessary, based on their psychologic and financial circumstances and reserves. From their study of urban noninstitutionalized elderly and of elderly who made a decision to be institutionalized, Brock and O'Sullivan (1985) suggest that old age and lack of a social support network are major predictors of institutionalization rather than health or other social variables.

ROLE OF THE PROFESSIONAL NURSE

The professional nurse who has educational and clinical preparation in family assessment and intervention in combination with a good foundation in gerontology is equipped to intervene with dysfunctional family processes due to actual or potential institutionalization of an elder member. The nurse can motivate a family to examine its care-providing capacity, to determine intra-family conflict and support pattern(s), to identify current and long-term expectations, and to actuate problem-solving potential and skills. Using written records, observation, and interviews, the nurse assesses family needs and the scope of their problems. As an advocate and helper, the nurse assists the family to apportion its resources, both tangible (eg, financial assets, space/property) and intangible (eg, commitment, interpersonal bonds, emotional energy), to promote self-maintenance and to provide the best possible care for the ailing member.

Typically the family and the nurse are brought together through intermediaries, such as service agency intake workers or linkages within the health systems network, because of a family problem or crisis. In this client–helper situation, learning (or relearning) of social and management skills may occur. If the nurse and family begin as strangers, some time will be needed to build the reciprocal trust that is essential for a working relationship. Doubts and fears about the elder member's physical and/or mental condition and his or her capabilities for managing the situation may pervade the family. Painful interpersonal conflicts within the family system that hinder problem-solving tactics may be uncovered. Psychologic pain and social discomfort is amplified if there are other coincident family problems such as financial, health, or marital problems among the adult children. The nurse processes and integrates all of this information with knowledge of family theory and dynamics. The diagnostic process has begun.

ASSESSMENT

The nurse must obtain and review recorded data and information and observe and interview family members individually and as a group. These measures provide the basis for (1) assessing the family system; (2) circumscribing the presenting problem(s); (3) developing an action plan; and (4) implementing appropriate support and problem-solving strategies to alleviate and/or solve the problem(s). Etiologies and defining characteristics for Altered Family Processes are contained in Table 46.1. Answers to the following questions provide a data base from which the nurse can develop nursing diagnoses and interventions:

Which family member(s) presents the issue(s)/ problem(s)?

Which other members are identified as being clearly involved in the situation; which members are not involved; and what criteria are offered for the designations "involved" and "not involved"?

How do members describe the family in terms of environment, communication and cooperation, intrapersonal relationships, and roles?

What subsystems appear to be operating within the family?

What is the family's income level and sense of its adequacy?

What is its racial, ethnic, and cultural identification and sense of identity and belonging?

What is its religious identification and connection to significant norms, value systems, and practices?

What unique factors (eg, economic, social) appear to be linked to the current situation?

To conduct an effective and accurate assessment the nurse must have knowledge of family theory. Observations of interactions, determination of family boundaries, and adaptability are imperative. The nurse must become familiar with the individual family structure and roles in addition to available economic and psychosocial resources. Through continued interaction with the family, the nurse can determine family values and goals and assess the strengths and weaknesses of the system. A careful history of significant life events such as death of a family member, major health problems, and previous coping strategies can prove invaluable in formulating the family portrait.

ASSESSMENT TOOLS

A number of well-validated family assessment tools are available in the literature. These include (1) Family Adaptability and Cohesion Evaluation Scales (FACES) (Olsen et al, 1978); (2) Family Environmental Scale (Moos et al, 1974); (3) Family APGAR (Smilkstein, 1978); and (4) Family Functioning Index (Pless and Satterwhite, 1973). These instuments cover issues relevant to family dynamics such as boundary maintenance, authority, and dominance, but not necessarily from a holistic nursing perspective. The Family Dynamics Measure (Lasky et al, 1985) has relevance for nursing. Nurse researchers developed this tool to measure family functioning objectively during both health and illness.

NURSING DIAGNOSIS

Nursing diagnoses are the result of systematizing data collection and analyses for informed practice. Shoemaker (1984;94) defines nursing diagnosis as "a clinical judgment about an individual, family, or community which is derived through a deliberate, systematic process of data collection and analysis. It provides the basis for prescriptions for definitive therapy for which the nurse is accountable. It is expressed concisely and it includes the etiology of the condition when known." Table 46.1

Table 46.1

Etiologies/Related Factors and Defining Characteristics of Altered Family Processes

NANDA (CARROLL-JOHNSON, 1989)	DIXON
Definition: The state in which a family that normally functions effectively experiences a dysfunction	The state in which a family that normally functions effectively experiences altered and dysfunctional roles and relationships
Etiologies/Related Factors	
Situation transition and/or crises Development transition and/or crises	Situational transition and crises (eg, financial dependence); sociocultural differences in attitudes, values, goals; lack of social support network; physical and cognitive losses of aging; institutionalization of elderly family member
*Defining Characteristics**	
Family system unable to meet physical needs of its members	Family system unable to meet physical needs of a member
Family system unable to meet emotional needs of its members	Family members unable to relate to each other
Family system unable to meet spiritual needs of its members	Family equilibrium threatened or damaged because of altered family structure, function, roles
Parents do not demonstrate respect for each other's views on childrearing practices	Family has doubts and fears about elder member's physical and/or mental capabilities
Inability to express or accept wide range of feelings	
Inability to express or accept feelings of members	
Family unable to meet security needs of its members	
Inability of family members to relate to each other for mutual growth and maturation	
Family uninvolved in community activities	
Inability to accept or receive help appropriately	
Rigidity in function and roles	
Family does not demonstrate respect for individuality and autonomy of its members	
Family inability to adapt to change or to deal with traumatic experience constructively	
Family fails to accomplish current or past developmental task	
Ineffective family decision-making process	
Failure to send and receive clear messages	
Inappropriate boundary maintenance	
Inappropriate or poorly communicated family rules, rituals, symbols	
Unexamined family myths	
Inappropriate level and direction of energy	

*The first 13 defining characteristics are specifically from Otto H: Criteria for assessing family strengths. *Fam Process* (Sept) 1963; 2:329–338.

compares NANDA's etiologies and defining characteristics for the diagnosis Altered Family Processes with the etiologies and defining characteristics proposed in this chapter.

CASE STUDY

Altered Family Processes

When Mrs. Edith Dodds entered Mayfair Health Center for the Elderly—a long-term nursing care facility—

she was 87 years old and had been widowed for 5 years. Mr. Dodds had died of cancer. Mrs. Dodds's diagnoses were Parkinson's disease, hypertension, and localized neuropathy. She had been in failing health for approximately 7 years but was alert and conversed with relatives and visitors during that time. Occasionally she "saw things . . . mysterious forms" around her bed. During the 2 years prior to admission to Mayfair, she required total care in bathing, dressing, feeding, and toileting, and she was hospitalized twice. Her sons, Leonard, Raynard, James, and Kevin, and one daughter, Lindsay (the youngest of her children), were in their 40s and 50s. The eldest and youngest sons, Leonard and Kevin, resided in the same city as their mother; the other children lived in three other states. When it became obvious that Mrs. Dodds, who had been an industrious, hardworking woman, was physically unable to be alone, her youngest son and his wife, Karen, and their four children who ranged in age from 16 to 21, took Mrs. Dodds into their home. Karen voluntarily resigned from her job to care for Mrs. Dodds and was paid by the family.

By consensus, each of her children was to contribute monthly to assist with payment of Mrs. Dodds's expenses. Two of the five children were irregular contributors: This caused some family discord. It had been agreed among the children that Raynard would collect the monthly assessments (which were based on each child's income in order to make it a fair arrangement), pay his mother's bills, deposit and withdraw from her bank account as necessary, and provide periodic financial reports to his brothers and sister. James verbally agreed to this arrangement but also expressed some anger toward Raynard: He was vague about the source of his anger.

Mrs. Dodds was taken to the Mayfair Health Center when Karen became ill and was no longer able to care for her mother-in-law. Mrs. Dodds resided at the Center for about 4 months before lapsing into a coma. She died 2 days later.

The Dodds family narrative is an example of a situational transition and crises: her supportive (family) network was in place, but a major component in that network, Karen, was suddenly withdrawn. Because Karen's role had been vital to the family plan for maintaining Mrs. Dodds at home, an alternative plan, perceived by the family as undesirable but necessary, was implemented: When Mrs. Dodds's physical needs could no longer be met at home, she was taken to an extended care facility.

The diagnosis Altered Family Processes is applicable to the Dodds family's actual and potential problems related to home care and subsequent institutionalization of the senior, Mrs. Dodds. Three subdiagnoses are identified and discussed: (1) Altered Family Structure and Roles; (2) Altered Family Function; and (3) Altered Human and Economic Resources. Table 46.2 outlines these subdiagnoses, interventions and outcomes.

ALTERED FAMILY STRUCTURE AND ROLES

This subdiagnosis repesents a modification or change that occurs when a family member becomes dependent, is institutionalized, or dies. The structure changes if the member(s) had assigned or assumed roles that were important to the family (eg, breadwinner, cook, family negotiator, scapegoat), roles that likely would be reassigned or some other accomodation made to fill the void. A role that is viewed as less important or dispensable might be banished from the family or, if maintained, its presence might be diminished. The roles of the other family members and their satisfaction or dissatisfaction with them is also included in this diagnosis. The diagnosis becomes more complex when external forces are involved, such as change in employment or a death in the family, which may affect roles, income, and so on. Internal forces such as inability to meet role expectation or inheriting a role that is unwanted are also at issue.

Although Mrs. Dodds had been independent and active, had been a homemaker and good cook, and had been involved in church and community organizations, she had not functioned in these roles for several years prior to her illness. However, she was revered as the family matriarch—a position that could be filled by no other member. In contrast, Karen's roles had a more direct day-to-day effect on the family: She was wife, mother, homemaker, and nurse. When her own responsibilities enlarged, Karen's husband and children expanded their roles by performing more housekeeping tasks. Mrs. Dodds's children modified their lives to permit them to travel frequently to visit Mrs. Dodds. Each person was affected by, and reacted to, changes in family structure and roles.

ALTERED FAMILY FUNCTION

Altered Family Function and the previous diagnosis, Altered Family Structure and Roles, are closely associated. The difference is that function is related to specific responsibilities associated with roles. The function of the family may change with the abilities and adaptability of the family. Willingness to assume a new function is considered, as well as ability to assume the new function. Normal functioning of a family will be more intensively and probably adversely affected by clustering or "pileup" of problems, which involves the occurrence of many stressors simultaneously or nearly simultaneously (Burnside, 1988). Coping ability may be affected by "pileup" so careful and detailed assessment of family life events is imperative. A change in one individual's place or job influences every other person's place or job within the family. Notable is the adjustment that must have been needed when Mrs. Dodds became part of Kevin's and Karen's household. Because Karen no longer worked outside of the home and was home all day, every day, her family may have changed in their expectations of how she would meet their nurturant needs: Indeed, she may have changed how she met those needs. When their mother's physical condition necessitated changes in residence and physical care, they were required to function differently with their mother and with one another: They had to agree on plans for her care and their individual contributions. Whereas before their mother became dependent, they had functioned to maintain only themselves and their own families, their mother was now included in their planning and their budgets. The family function was revised or altered.

ALTERED HUMAN AND ECONOMIC RESOURCES

Losses experienced by the aged include loss of financial resources through loss of employment, a reduced and fixed income, or overwhelming health care costs. Just the routine health care costs for the aged require a substantial financial outlay. These include purchase of dentures, hearing aids, and medication prescribed for multiple chronic conditions. It is unfortunate that these expenses occur at a time when income is lower and fixed. Reforms in Medicare and Medicaid coverage limit the amount paid for by these governmental agencies.

In addition, family members may be faced with financial problems. Children of the young old are frequently finishing raising a family, perhaps with children in college, and children of the frail elderly are faced with the beginnings of their own old age and perhaps the onset of their own health problems and losses associated with aging.

The matriarchal head of the family was "lost" as an active family resource when Mrs. Dodds became an invalid. Karen became the self-selected human resource that was temporarily "lost" to the family system when she became ill. As a result of these losses, Mrs. Dodds's care was transferred from the home to the nursing care center. Economic assets, particularly financial, were not unlimited for individual members. Placing Mrs. Dodds in a long-term care facility caused her children to reassess costs and resources. They had to decide what they were going to do, who was going to do it, and how it would be accomplished. There was change in human and economic resources.

NURSING INTERVENTIONS

From the data, one could conclude that the Dodds family system appears to have few problems (eg, the variable participation of two offspring and one brother's anger of unclear origin), but their circumstances suggest *potential* difficulties. The role of the nurse would be supportive and the nurse's goal would be to intervene to prevent occurrence of major problematic situations. One preventive strategy would be use of anticipatory planning. Although each subdiagnosis has more than one articulated intervention, for purposes of this chapter only one intervention for each diagnosis is highlighted.

Interventions for Altered Family Structure and Roles

Ideally, family issues are addressed by convening all members or as many members as possible. The objective is to assess family dynamics and style and, using the acquired data, to stimulate, teach, and encourage effective interaction among family constituents. Assessment is the precursor of change and provides information that assists the nurse to point the family toward meaningful learning and change. Knowledgeable and responsive family members may use this opportunity to assess family operations. Another purpose for convening families is to energize awareness, sensitivity, and insight toward developing or sustaining behaviors that support effective relationships. For families that function well—the Dodds family is an example—the nurse may serve to enhance their capabilities. A desirable outcome is enrichment of interpersonal relationships. The Dodds family had been engaged in a process to combine and actuate their resources to provide the best care possible for their mother. Their strengths were demonstrated in their ability to "take charge": They met, discussed their predicament, and made workable decisions regarding their mother's care. Face-to-face discussion affords opportunity to verify impressions and to clarify communication immediately. Convening the Dodds family might assist James to express and deal with his anger in a more productive manner.

Interventions for Altered Family Function

The assessment process should provide information about the kind and level of the family's behavior and mode of operation. The experience and interpersonal talents that the nurse brings to the setting should be supportive of a comfortable exchange between people. Each member of the Dodds family, for example, would be encouraged to share her or his perception of the situation and its personal impact. The nurse supports the efforts of individuals and the family unit to cope with a taxing circumstance. He or she assists the members to articulate what has changed and what they want reality to be like; how they have managed other and similar situations; and what has "worked" or not "worked." The nurse serves as a receptive sounding board for the family and is a conduit for expression. In the process, nurses should avoid taking over the family members' lives. Nurses can best assist family members by providing an understanding and supportive climate.

Family therapy may be indicated and is strongly recommended by many authorities. Gerontologic nurses trained in family therapy would be an excellent choice. Some of the complexities in the Dodds family's interactions may be worked out in family therapy. Karen Dodds, who is not a blood relative of the elder Mrs. Dodds, gave up her job in order to care for her mother-in-law. Family therapy could assist in determining how Karen felt about this and her subsequent health problems, allowing her to ventilate her feelings and providing a more constructive context for family interactions.

James may be able to express the source of his anger. Perhaps he was the scapegoat of the family and had feelings of resentment toward his mother. Perhaps he has overwhelming problems of his own. Allowing James the opportunity to vent and explore his feelings would be an effective method of helping him deal with his anger and would also assist the family in observing, understanding, and placing his anger in perspective. Family therapy could facilitate decision making regarding the changed roles of family members.

Interventions for Altered Human and Economic Resources

Mrs. Dodds's children pooled their monies to provide for her. This strategy prevented burdening only one person. Moreover, because it was the family's idea, the strategy had a better chance of success than if it had been suggested by someone external to the family.

If the need exists, the nurse can assist the grown children to explore alternative care arrangements. He or she can provide information about public and private policies related to extended care and funding and make appropriate referrals.

The nurse can assist the family in seeking governmental agencies that provide funding for the aged. Medicare and Medicaid programs are available throughout the country, since they are federal programs. Many communities offer a wealth of services for the aged such as meals, transportation, wellness clinics, vision screening, and respite care at low costs. The nurse can refer the family to the agency social worker for assistance in this area. Table 46.2 presents the diagnoses discussed in this chapter and summarizes nursing interventions and outcomes.

OUTCOMES

Outcomes related to the nursing diagnosis Altered Family Processes can be specified according to subdiagnoses, as illustrated in Table 46.2. For example, when family structure and roles have been altered, the nurse would document degree of role adaptability in maintaining the integrity of the family system. Flexibility and capability for decision making, short- and long-term planning, and implementation of plans should be evaluated. Outcomes

Table 46.2

Expected Outcomes and Nursing Interventions for Altered Family Processes Diagnoses

DIAGNOSES	NURSING INTERVENTIONS	EXPECTED OUTCOMES
Altered family structure and role	Convene the family one or more times; interview family	Demonstrate role adaptability for maintaining family integrity
	Assess family process/dynamics, presenting problem	Demonstrate flexibility and capability for short- and long-term planning and action
	Encourage, support discussion of family and individual views	
	Explore role changes caused by Mrs. D's changed physical condition	
	Develop goal-oriented plans, short- and long-term, alternative plans	Demonstrate effective family decision making
	Encourage communication of unexpressed grief, anger, joy, fear, perceived losses	Demonstrate comfort with own feelings
Altered family functioning	Encourage each person to identify family strengths/weaknesses	Demonstrate awareness of family operations, individual perceptions
	Discuss how family coped prior to Mrs. D's physical change and since	Getting "in touch" with factors that can/cannot be controlled, managed
	Explore perceptions of what has and has not changed since Mrs. D's illness and since her residency in an extended care facility	
Alteration in human and economic resources	Assist family to assess "person" and financial/economic resources; review present and anticipated expenses	Demonstrate anticipatory preparation for contingency events
	Encourage/support problem-solving and self-help tactics; discuss linkages to and procedures for contacting helpers (person, agencies) as needed	Maintenance of present skills
		Knowledge of available services

associated with altered family functioning include family awareness of how it operates as a system as well as recognition of the perceptions of individual family members. Family members should be able to identify factors that affect family functioning and understand which factors can be managed or changed. In a situation in which human and economic resources have been altered, the nurse should evaluate the family's ability to prepare or plan in advance for events such as institutionalization of an older member, as well as their awareness of treatment and service options available to them.

SUMMARY

This chapter analyzed the nursing diagnosis Altered Family Processes related to institutionalization of an elderly family member. The subdiagnoses Altered Family Structure and Roles, Altered Family Function, and Altered Family Human and Economic Resources are explicated from the more general diagnosis, Altered Family Processes. Assessment guidelines are presented and four validated family assessment tools are described. Assessment and diagnosis are illustrated using a case study. An intervention strategy is discussed for each of the specific altered family processes diagnoses. Finally, evaluation of desired outcomes is described for each subdiagnosis.

References

Ackerman N: *Psychodynamics of Family Life.* Basic Books, 1958.

Aging America: Trends and Projection. U.S. Senate Special Committee on Aging and the American Association of Retired Persons, 1984.

Aldous J: *Family Careers.* Wiley, 1978.

Bateson G et al: Toward a theory of schizophrenia. *Behav Sci* 1956; I:251–264.

Bowen M: The use of family therapy in clinical practice. *Comp Psychiatry* 1966; 7:345–374.

Bowen M: *Family Therapy in Clinical Practice.* Jason Aronson, 1978.

Brock AM, O'Sullivan P: A study to determine what variables predict institutionalization of elderly people. *J Adv Nurs* 1985; 10:533–537.

Brody SD, Poulshock SW, Masciocchi CF: The family care units: A major consideration in the long-term support system. *Gerontologist* 1978; 18:556–561.

Buckley W: *Sociology and Modern Systems Theory.* Prentice-Hall, 1967.

Burnside IM: *Nursing and the Aged: A Self-Care Approach,* 3d ed. McGraw-Hill, 1988.

Carroll-Johnson R (editor): *Classification of Nursing Diagnoses: Proceedings of the Eighth Conference.* Lippincott, 1989.

Cicirelli VG: *Helping Elderly Parents: Role of Adult Children.* Auburn House, 1981.

Cox H: Family patterns in later life. Chapter 8 in: *Later Life: The Realities of Aging.* Prentice-Hall, 1984.

Eliopoulos C: *A Guide to the Nursing of the Aging.* Williams and Wilkins, 1987.

Hazzard ME: An overview of systems theory. *Nurs Clin North Am* (Sept) 1971; 7:385–393.

Health Care Financing Administration. *The Medicare and Medicaid Data Book.* U.S. Government Printing Office, 1981.

Lasky P et al: Developing an instrument for the assessment of family dynamics. *West J Nurs Res* 1985; 7(1):40–57.

Miller IG: Living systems: Basic concepts. *Behav Sci* (July) 1965; 10:193–237.

Minuchin S et al: *Families of the Slums: An Exploration of Their Structure and Treatment.* Basic Books, 1967.

Moos R, Insel P, Humphrey B: *Preliminary Manual for Family Environmental Scales.* Consulting Psychologists Press, 1974.

National Center for Health Statistics: *An Overview of Nursing Home Characteristics: Provisional Data from the 1977 Nursing Survey.* Advance Data, No. 35. U.S. Public Health Service, 1978.

National Institute of Aging: *Population Aging.* American Council of Life Insurance and Health Insurance Corporation of America, 1982.

Olsen D, Bell R, Portner J: Faces: Family adaptability and cohesion evaluation scales. Unpublished technical report, Family Social Services, University of Minnesota, 1978.

Otto H: Criteria for assessing family strengths. *Fam Process* (Sept) 1963; 2:329–338.

Pless IB, Satterwhite B: A measure of family functioning and its application. *Soc Sci Med* 1973; 7:613–621.

A Portrait of Older Minorities. American Association of Retired Persons, 1985.

A Profile of Older Americans. American Association of Retired Persons, 1987.

Satir V: *Conjoint Family Therapy.* Science and Behavior Books, 1967.

Shoemaker J: Essential features of nursing diagnosis. Page 94 in: *Classification of Nursing Diagnoses: Proceedings of the Fifth National Conference.* Kim MJ, McFarland GK, McLane AM (editors). Mosby, 1984.

Smilkstein G: The family apgar. *J Fam Pract* 1978; 6:1231–1239.

Tobin SS, Kulys R: The family and services. Pages 370–399 in: *Annual Review of Gerontology and Geriatrics.* Springer, 1980.

VonBertalanffy L: *General Systems Theory.* George Braziller, 1968.

47

Potential for Violence: Self-Directed or Directed at Others

DIANNE MUNNS, MA, RN
LUCYANNE NOLAN, MSN, RN

THE PHENOMENON OF VIOLENT BEHAVIOR IS ENCOUNtered daily by health care professionals in all specialties and with all age groups. Methods to assess, predict, and prevent violence in patient populations require ongoing study. This chapter will explore those aspects of violent behavior that are specifically seen in the elderly and will develop the nursing diagnosis Potential for Violence including interventions relevant to the elderly population. Aggressive and potentially harmful behavior is a continuing cause for concern among those who care for the institutionalized elderly.

PREDICTION OF VIOLENCE

Prediction of violence, which is the basis for formulating the nursing diagnosis Potential for Violence, is contingent on an understanding of the three basic conceptual approaches to aggression: the biologic approach, the psychologic approach, and the sociologic approach.

The biologic theories suggest that aggression comes from innate biologic drives and that all violent behavior stems from these drives, which at one time were necessary for survival (Fields and Sweet, 1975; Lorenz, 1966; Mark and Erwin, 1970; Sadoff, 1978).

Psychologic approaches propose that explanations for violence and aggression lie in the interaction of the individual with the social environment, and locate the source of violence in relationships, learning processes, and self-attitudes. Social framework theories examine social structure or arrangements such as norms, values, organizations, and systems to explain individual violence. The three approaches to violence and aggression are closely intertwined, and aspects of each complement the other. All three functions of an individual are in constant interaction in the production of behavior, and one particular approach may be applicable for one individual at a given time but totally inappropriate for another.

SIGNIFICANCE FOR THE ELDERLY

Potential for Violence is related to underlying psychopathology in elderly patients and can generally be classified as:

1. Impaired judgment and violent behavior as a manifestation of a pathophysiologic dysfunction

2. Violence as a component of psychiatric impairment
3. Violence as a response to sociocultural and environmental factors

Petrie et al (1982), in a study of 222 consecutive admissions to the geriatric service of a state psychiatric hospital, noted a distinct difference in psychopathology between violent patients and aggressive patients. In this study, violence was defined as acts committed or threatened that involved weapons. However, aggression can be described as physical violence without weapons or as verbal threats.

Petrie and his colleagues (1982) found that the medical diagnoses for the violent groups were primarily functional diagnoses of late paraphrenia, schizophrenia, or mania. These patients experienced paranoid delusions, hallucinations, or both and believed that they were in danger of being attacked.

The aggressive groups of patients showed a much greater occurrence of senile dementia. Disorientation was common with this group, especially to place and time, and disorganization and diffuse cognitive decline were evident to such a degree that outbursts were less likely to be dangerous than with the violent group. Within the aggressive groups, patients with mixed or structural organic lesions proved more unpredictable and dangerous than patients with primary degenerative dementia (Petrie et al, 1982;444).

These findings underscore the importance of identifying etiologic/risk factors before establishing the nursing diagnosis Potential for Violence. Although defining characteristics may be the same or similar, determining a specific etiology is important for interventions.

DEFINITION OF POTENTIAL FOR VIOLENCE

Potential for Violence, accepted by the North American Nursing Diagnosis Association (NANDA) in 1980, is one of the few diagnoses with the qualifier "potential," indicating the presence of risk factors (Kim and Moritz, 1982;281). A review of the etiology/risk factors and defining characteristics leads to a definition close to that given for aggressive behavior (see Table 47.1). Carpenito (1983;501) defines Potential for Violence as "a state in which an individual experiences aggressive behavior that is or can be directed either at one's self or others."

ASSESSMENT

In assessing Potential for Violence, the single most valid predictor is a past history of violent and criminal acts (Monahan, 1984). Other areas proposed for evaluation of Potential for Violence include life experiences that have created bitterness and resentment, frequent quarrels with family, associations with significant figures who are themselves violent, and an interest in weapons (Kalogerakis, 1971). There is a positive association between a history of brain dysfunction and violent behavior, and severe headaches and convulsions are frequently found in violent groups (Bachy-Rita, 1971; Climent, 1972). A history of opiate and/or alcohol abuse is cited as a Potential for Violence throughout the literature (Monahan, 1981; Rubin, 1972).

Coping patterns, maturity level, and predisposition to anxiety and anger are cues for potentially violent behavior. Rothenberg (1971) states that violence occurs when anger is unexpressed and threats that caused the anger cannot be removed. "It is a consistent observation that the most truly violent people are those who have difficulty dealing with angry feelings" (Rothenberg, 1971;92).

Behavioral characteristics indicative of increased hostility due to repressed anger are increased irritability; verbal outbursts against others; self-destructive acts; testing-out behavior; and other evidence of an increased anxiety level (Geurguis, 1978; Rothenberg, 1971). Persons who are predisposed to cope with stress in a violent manner will exhibit an acute state of emotional arousal and readily express violent fantasies against others (Monahan, 1981). Nonpurposeful motor activity that indicates a loss of conscious control over motor behavior because of mounting tensions is mentioned as an important physiologic manifestation of potential action (Clunn, 1975).

Environmental factors are also discussed as elements that contribute to violent behavior. Overcrowding in institutional settings, staff attitudes, presence of other violent or potentially violent patients, feelings of boredom, and helplessness are all present in hospitals and long-term care facilities and are identified by Kalogerakis (1971) as indicators for violence.

ETIOLOGIES/RISK FACTORS AND DEFINING CHARACTERISTICS

Munns (1985), in a study on the validation of the defining characteristics, provides literature support and validation for all etiologic/risk factors and defining characteristics as published by NANDA (see Table 47.1).

The following are the most commonly occurring etiologies/risk factors identified as contributing to Potential for Violence in an elderly population and the defining characteristics for each. Table 47.2 contains a detailed summary of these indicators for assessment.

Table 47.1

Potential for Violence: Self-Directed or Directed at Others

NANDA (CARROLL-JOHNSON, 1989)

Risk Factors

Antisocial character
Battered women
Catatonic excitement
Child abuse
Manic excitement
Organic brain syndrome
Panic states
Rage reactions
Suicidal behavior
Temporal lobe epilepsy
Toxic reactions to medication

Defining Characteristics

Body language: clenched fists, facial expressions, rigid posture, tautness indicating intense
    effort to control
Hostile threatening verbalizations; boasting of prior abuse to others
Increased motor activity, pacing, excitement, irritability, agitation
Overt and aggressive acts; goal-directed destruction of objects in environment
Possession of destructive means: gun, knife, or other weapon
Rage
Self-destructive behavior and/or active, aggressive suicidal acts
Substance abuse/withdrawal
Suspicion of others, paranoid ideation, delusions, hallucinations

Other Defining Characteristics

Increasing anxiety levels
Fear of self or others
Inability to verbalize feelings
Repetition of verbalizations: continues complaints, requests, and demands
Anger
Provocative behavior: argumentative, dissatisfied, overreactive, hypersensitive
Vulnerable self-esteem
Depression (specifically active, aggressive, suicidal acts)

Potential for Violence Related to Sensory-Perceptual Alteration Secondary to Acute Dementia-Delirium

In managing elderly, confused, or aggressive patients, a detailed assessment must be performed to determine the etiologies of the aggressiveness. Elderly persons' physiologic and social integrity has a narrow range for adequate function (Morrant, 1983; Wolanin, 1983). Therefore a slight deviation in either functional area may be significant enough to cause a change in mental status.

The nurse, in developing the nursing diagnosis, would observe for posture, facial expression, and affect. Deter-mining additional history of depression, coping patterns, and substance abuse will assist in differentiating the diagnosis.

Elderly persons are more susceptible to the toxic effects of medications as a result of the liver's decreased ability to metabolize drugs and the decrease in binding sites for drugs. Adverse behavioral effects may be precipitated by inappropriate drug use or by interacting medications (Buckelew, 1982; Freedman, 1983).

If the patient is taking an anticholinergic drug and signs of central nervous system toxicity such as confusion, disorientation, restlessness, agitation, visual hallucinations, and memory impairment, especially of recent memory, are observed, anticholinergic toxicity should be suspected (Todd, 1984). All medications must be reviewed for

Table 47.2

Occurrence of Defining Characteristics: Potential for Violence

Defining Characteristics	ETIOLOGIES/RISK FACTORS				
	Delirium	Dementia	Depression Possible	Paranoid Present	Distrust/ Frustration/ Anxiety Possible
Body Language:					
Clenched fists	No	No	/	/	/
Facial expressions	No	No	/	/	/
Rigid posture	No	No	/	/	/
Tautness	No	No	/	/	/
Hostile, threatening verbalization	No	No	Possible	Present	/
Boasting of prior abuse	No	No	/	Present	/
Increased Motor Activity			Possible	Present	/
Pacing	Possible	Possible	/	/	/
Excitement	Present	Possible	/	/	/
Irritability	Possible	Possible	/	/	/
Agitation	Present	Present	/	/	/
Overt and Aggressive Acts					
Goal-directed destruction of objects in environment	No	No	/	/	Possible
Possession of weapon	No	No	Present	Possible	/
Rage	No	No	Possible	Possible	/
Self-destructive behavioral/active, aggressive suicidal acts	No	No	Present	Possible	/
Substance abuse/withdrawal	Possible	Possible	Present	Possible	/
Suspicions of others, paranoid ideations		Possible	Possible	Present	/
Delusions	Present	Present	/	/	No
Hallucinations	Present	Present	/	Possible	No
Increased anxiety levels	Possible	Possible	Present	Possible	Present
Fear of self or others	Present	Possible	Present	Present	Possible
Inability to verbalize feelings	Present	Present	Present	Present	/
Repetition of verbalization	No	No	Possible	Present	/
continued complaints	No	No	/	/	/
requests, demands	No	No	/	/	/
Anger	Present	Possible	Present	Present	Present
Provocative behavior			Possible	Present	Possible
argumentative	Possible	Possible	/	/	/
dissatisfied	Present	Possible	/	/	/
overreactive	Possible	Possible	/	/	/
hypersensitive	Possible	Possible	/	/	/
Vulnerable self-esteem	No	No	Present	Possible	Present
Depression (specifically) active, aggressive suicide acts	Possible	Possible	Present	Possible	Possible

possible toxicity for interaction (Goldenberg and Chiverton, 1984; Todd, 1984).

Potential for Violence Related to Altered Thought Processes Secondary to Organic Brain Syndrome-Dementia

Differentiating between delirium and dementia as etiologies/risk factors requires a detailed assessment of defining characteristics. The demented elderly patient exhibits personality changes, loss of memory, and disturbed affect before any other signs are apparent. Onset is insidious, and the course of the illness is exorably progressive, often over many years. History of substance abuse, previous violence, and long-term disorientation can be present in demented persons, and in general, there is a slower onset of the symptoms described for delirium. The demented individual usually cares little for personal appearance and will appear unkempt. The individual is also unaware of forgetfulness, and entire events are permanently forgotten (Freedman, 1983). Although delirious persons may manifest many of the same symptoms as demented individuals, a delirium is an acute and reversible confusional state, with rapid onset, frequently related to adverse medication responses or acute infectious processes in the elderly. An acute confusional state (delirium) may be superimposed on a chronic confusional state (dementia), especially during an illness or surgical experience. The defining characteristics (such as boasting of prior abuse, or continued complaints, requests, and demands), that are more frequent in the potentially violent younger individual are usually absent in the demented or delirious elderly patient.

Set Test The Set Test (Goldenberg and Chiverton, 1984) is an easily administered quantitative verbal strategy method used with the elderly to screen for mental status changes. It neither replaces a full mental status exam nor pinpoints lesions in the brain. Results can be used to prevent overuse of medications such as psychotropic drugs, failure to control for environmental factors and safety measures, premature closure of diagnosis, prolonging hospitalization, and an attitude of complacency on the part of the staff (ie, confusion is "normal" with the elderly). The Set Test cannot be used with patients who are aphasic or unable to follow simple directions. To conduct the Set Test the patient is asked to name as many items as possible in each of four sets: animals, cities, colors, and fruits. One point is scored for each correct item. The maximum score in each category is 10; the maximum total score is 40. The test is conducted in a relaxed atmosphere, and the time limit is determined by the clinical judgement of the nurse based on the state of the patient. A score of less than 15 on the Set Test correlates with other validated diagnostic measures for dementia. A score of 15 to 24 indicates possible dementia, and a score greater than 24 indicates no dementia. Persons with depression score higher on this test than do individuals with dementia, and it can therefore be administered by nurses to help determine a differential diagnosis.

Violence in the demented individual results from impaired judgment and is accompanied by confusion and loss of emotional control. The aggressive act is usually sudden and impulsive and occurs if the patient is frustrated or confused. Unfamiliarity with surroundings, new routines, and new people can precipitate an incident. Night is usually the time of maximal confusion, giving rise to the term *sundown syndrome* (see Chapter 27). In a state of confusion, the patient wanders through halls attempting to orient himself or herself. The patient may rummage in others' belongings, precipitating a violent incident with other patients, some of whom may also be confused (Petrie, 1984).

Again, differentiation of etiologies/risk factors based on presence or absence of defining characteristics is illustrated in Table 47.2.

Potential for Violence Related to Depression

Depression is the most common psychiatric illness in the elderly, as well as in the general population. Anxiety and anger are always linked to hurt, and depressed patients may display violent behavior toward self or others. Recognizing depression in the elderly is sometimes difficult, as it may present as vague problems like lethargy, anorexia, or insomnia. Any change in usual behavior in an elderly person should always be taken as a serious possibility of depression (Morrant, 1983).

Gage (1973) describes a process that differentiates depression in the aged person from normal mourning. This process includes love-object loss, withdrawal of libido, cathexis of own ego, identification of ego to the lost object, feelings of sadness that result in a decrease in interest in the outside world, decreased capacity to love, and a decrease in activity. Gage also identifies a decrease in self-esteem, a verbalization of self-reproach, and a need for punishment. Punishment of self can terminate in suicide, and violent behavior toward others is often part of the suicidal phenomenon.

To assess violence potential in a depressed elderly individual, the nurse must have a knowledge of the elder's previous coping mechanisms and of how the elder has responded in the past to frustrations and stressors. If the elder has had some recent series of frustrations and if he or she is confused or showing signs of impaired judgment, potential for violence is more likely.

Unlike the demented person, a depressed elderly individual may possess a weapon. Other cues that may be present include signs of anxiety such as rigid posture, hypersensitivity, dissatisfaction, and hostile sarcastic verbalizations. Vulnerable self-esteem and signs of depression such as active aggressive suicidal acts warn of the potential for further violence.

Potential for Violence Related to Altered Thought Processes Secondary to Paranoid Ideations

In the study by Petrie et al (1982) of geriatric admissions to a state psychiatric hospital, the diagnosis of late paraphrenia or late onset schizophrenia was significantly associated with the violent groups.

Another group that surfaces frequently in studies of violence in psychiatric settings are the schizophrenic patients who have been ill for many years. Both of these groups present predominantly paranoid ideations, that are not accompanied by confusion or disorientation (Petrie, 1984;113).

In the late onset groups, a delusional state arises in a clear consciousness, and hallucinations and ideas of reference may also be present. Patients in this group usually are strongly committed to their delusions and will act on them. All paranoid individuals will exhibit some of the other classic defining characteristics of Potential for Violence before a violent episode. Body language, including rigid posture, angry facial expressions, and clenched fists, is often an early indication of impending aggression. Hostile verbalizations, repetition of complaints, demands, pacing, agitation, and rage should all be viewed as indicative of impending violence. Past behavior should always be a major consideration in establishing a diagnosis with this group.

The nursing diagnosis of Potential for Violence related to altered thought processes secondary to paranoid ideations is based on the defining characteristics that are consistent with those listed in Table 47.2.

Potential for Violence Related to Inability to Control Behavior Secondary to Distress/Frustration/Anxiety

Distress, frustrations, and anxiety are very real and common conditions in the elderly. Losses related to aging can be catastrophic to the person experiencing them. Having to depend on others for such intimate functions as toileting, or having to cope with wheelchairs, catheters, and protheses, produces a degree of anger and anxiety in most persons. If the individual has coped with anger through aggressive behavior as a young person, that pattern will continue with aging. Blurring of the senses and slowing of thought processes can further contribute to the inability to cope with a situation and potentiate the possibility of violent behavior.

Defining characteristics for this diagnosis may be limited to hostile gestures toward others, hostile affect, or simple lashing out during frustrating situations. An astute diagnostician will recognize the situation that produces this phenomenon. Is too much being expected of the elderly patient? Is he or she being patronized or pushed by staff or family? Is this a person who normally mistrusts everyone anyway? Has he or she experienced a recent, disturbing change in lifestyle? Is the attitude of the staff toward this individual one of dislike or mistrust? Consideration of these and similar questions can alert the nurse to a potentially violent individual before injury or harm is done.

ASSESSMENT TOOLS

Reliable and valid assessment instruments have not as yet been researched. A number of questions must be answered before a valid tool can be produced. Which defining characteristics always occur with which etiologies? How often must a defining characteristic occur before a violent act in order to be classified as a valid cue?

How many defining characteristics must be present for the nursing diagnosis Potential for Violence to be made? These points will be clarified as the diagnostic entities are further developed and defined.

Table 47.2 contains a differentiation between etiologic/risk factors through clustering of defining characteristics. The characteristics indicated usually occur with the etiologic/risk factor, but no individual characteristic is known to occur 100% of the time.

NURSING INTERVENTIONS

When evaluating Potential for Violence, the nurse must assess for signs, symptoms, and risk factors predictive of potential for suicide, self-directed violence, and aggression and violence toward others or the environment. When the diagnosis Potential for Violence has been established, an assessment for Disturbance in Self-Concept is recommended. Although no correlational studies have been published, clinical practice suggests that negative responses to one or more of the four aspects of self-concept as described by Kelly (1985) will also be present.

Interventions for this diagnostic category can be proactive and/or reactive. Because one goal of nursing intervention is to prevent complications (ie, aggression or violence toward self, others, or the environment), emphasis is placed on proactive interventions. The word *potential* implies that violence is not occurring and may be preventable. The purpose of comprehensive training for the prevention and management of aggressive and violent behavior in the institutionalized elderly is to increase the effectiveness of nurses working with this patient population (Blake and Taylor, 1977; Turner, 1984).

In situations of inevitable or spontaneous physical acting out, there are physical techniques appropriate for controlling and moving a patient who is destructive to self, others, or the environment. These techniques should be employed only as a last resort when proactive interventions have been ineffective. Physical interventions and mechanical restraining should be used as a therapeutic modality and not as a punishment. Verbal interventions should continue during the physical intervention to provide reassurance and security. Nurses must use good clinical judgment and the minimal amount of physical action necessary to achieve control. Whenever physical intervention is used there is always the potential for injury of the persons involved in the restraining process.

Concepts Underlying Choice of Intervention

An understanding of the following eight concepts will enable the nurse to assess the Potential for Violence and plan appropriate interventions: types of aggressive and violent behavior; components of a therapeutic institution; cycle of aggression; anger continuum; locus of control; proxemics: space and territory; communication model; and guidelines for dealing with an angry person. Any number of proactive interventions can be effectively employed.

Types of Aggressive Behavior   Aggressive and violent behavior is motivated by a desire to punish or to protect, either of which may be expressed directly or indirectly. Although maladaptive behavioral responses may be identical regardless of the motivation, interventions vary based on the intent. It is essential for the nurse to assess accurately the intent of the maladaptive response prior to prescribing interventions. An appropriate intervention for one type of aggression may negatively escalate another type (Blake and Taylor, 1977; Lippincott, 1982;923).

Components of a Therapeutic Institution   The patient, the staff, and the environment all interact to determine the level of aggressiveness. After analyzing the factors influencing each component of the institution and the additive effect of their interaction, the nurse will be better able to plan interventions to decrease or eliminate some or all of the identified stressors (Blake and Taylor, 1977; Buckelew, 1982; Freedman, 1983; Goldenberg and Chiverton, 1984; Palmore, 1980).

The following case study illustrates the use of the interventions exercise, environmental structuring, and reminiscence.

CASE STUDY

Potential for Violence, G.R.

G.R., an 82-year-old man, 6'2'' tall, was transferred from a community nursing home to a long-term care facility for management of combative behavior. According to the nursing transfer summary, G.R. attacked peers and staff for "no apparent reason." An assessment of role relationships revealed that G.R. had been incarcerated for a period of 5 years after an armed robbery conviction. He was observed on several occasions threatening an unsuspecting, weak, and nonassertive debilitated patient. G.R. moved quickly across the dayroom, pounding one clenched fist on the palm of the other hand, with an angry hostile expression on his face. As he neared the unsuspecting victim he drew back his arm and fist as if he were going to strike him. The nurse made direct eye contact and in an authoritative tone said "Stop!" Fortunately this intervention was effective. When confronted with the behavior G.R. said that the intended victim reminded him of somebody who had wronged him

in prison and he wanted him out of there, but he did not want to go back to jail for assaulting another person. G.R. said that if he didn't have to be with this person all of the time he thought he could control his aggressive urges. The diagnosis Potential for Violence related to altered thought processes secondary to paranoid ideation was made. Mr. G.R.'s behavior was goal directed and indicated nursing interventions that involved G.R. in more off-ward activities that were as physically demanding as he could tolerate. When on the unit G.R. and the other man were placed in different areas for eating, socializing, and sleeping. Reminiscence therapy on an individual basis was another effective intervention for this person, as he could talk about his earlier life with the primary therapist.

Cycle of Aggression   An act of aggression or violence is usually preceded by a predictable sequence of events. A stressor or a series of stressors is followed by a negative subjective response/feeling, then by behavioral responses that escalate to anger if the stressor(s) continues to increase in duration, intensity, or number (Brigman et al, 1983; Freedman, 1983; Goldenberg and Chiverton, 1984; Ochitill and Krieger, 1982; Rada et al, 1985; Todd, 1984).

Anger Continuum   Most aggressive or violent persons have demonstrated a series of observable negative behaviors that have escalated over a period of time. Human beings develop habitual behavioral response patterns. The nurse must document the behavioral responses with appropriate interventions and a complete diagnostic statement on the nursing care plan (eg, Potential for Violence toward others related to inability to control behavior; signs and symptoms: argumentative with peers and staff, volume of voice increasing, tone becomes demanding, hyperverbal, and pacing) (Burnside, 1980; Turner, 1984).

The following case study illustrates several of the concepts underlying choice of the intervention environmental structuring and timing.

CASE STUDY

Potential for Violence, F.C.

F.C., an 87-year-old man, was identified as a combative patient by the nursing staff. The nurses reported that this patient would strike peers and staff "without warning and without apparent provocation." Assessment included a detailed description of events preceding the assaultive incidents. It was determined that all of the assaultive acts occurred on returning to the unit from the dining room. Further, the combativeness was evident only after nursing staff had attempted to feed F.C. his meal or to usher him out of the dining room. The social history revealed that F.C. came from a home where all meals were prepared and served in an elegant fashion by a live-in chef. He dined in a leisurely fashion at each meal. Mr. F.C.'s habitual behavioral response pattern—that is, becoming combative on return from the dining room—indicated that breaking the cycle of aggression or anger continuum through environmental structuring was the intervention appropriate for the diagnosis of Potential for Violence related to inability to control behavior, secondary to distress or frustration. Acting on this information the nursing staff implemented environmental structuring and timing by taking F.C. to the dining room first, assigning him an individual table where peers could not disturb him by snatching food from his tray, and allowing him to eat at his leisure. With these interventions the combative behavior disappeared.

Locus of Control   When the elderly act in a physically aggressive manner, the nurse must use external controls to ensure safety. While physical or mechanical restraints, seclusion, and medications are being used, the nurse must continue to use verbal interventions to provide reassurance and to assist the patient to regain internal control and channel aggressive feelings adaptively.

Proxemics   The boundaries of personal space and physical territory are distinct throughout the life span (Hall, 1966). Personal space and distance are distinguished by the senses and may change as one ages because of the changes in the acuity of the senses and the narrowing of physical territorial boundaries (Blazer and Siegler, 1984; Esberger, 1982). There is a marked difference between the physical territory of a home or an apartment and the personal area assigned to the elderly in an institution. Nursing procedures and institutional activities invade these zones. The nurse must develop a sensitivity to and respect for space and territory to maximize the efficiency and effectiveness of nursing procedures and proactive nursing interventions (Burnside, 1980; Hein, 1980).

Communication Model   Frequently the elderly have neither a voice in decisions affecting them nor control over the multiple physiologic and psychosocial losses experienced with advancing age. They may demonstrate hostile and aggressive behavior in response to feelings of powerlessness, separation, loneliness, confusion, and helplessness. In order to respond and intervene appropriately, the nurse must actively listen to be able to restate the content/intent of the verbalization and accurately identify the feeling state. The guidelines for interacting with an angry person as presented in Veterans Administration medical centers (VAMC) throughout the country are listed in Table 47.3.

Active Listening   Treating a patient with the diagnosis Potential for Violence effectively depends on the nurses' knowledge base and active listening ability to recognize, interpret, and respond accurately to cues that indicate a change in behavior in either a positive direction or a negative direction. Helms (1985) described active listening as both an assessment technique and an intervention technique. Although active listening per se is not research based, there is support in the literature for positive outcomes resulting from listening as an assessment strategy and as an intervention.

Active listening includes skill in interpreting the patient's verbal, paraverbal, and nonverbal behavior and in responding effectively (Helms, 1985). Skills used in active listening, interview, observation, and inspection are identified as methods of data collection used for the initial, interim, and update nursing assessments. According to Warden (1984), the nursing history contributes 80% of the data used in the nursing assessment. Inspection, a specific method of observation, can yield 90% of all the information of a physical examination (King, 1984). In addition, Birdwhistle (1979) estimated that only 35% of the meaning of social interchange is conveyed verbally. Nonverbal messages are generally clear and truthful, conveying feelings and emotions more accurately than words. The significance of active listening and observing in conducting a nursing assessment is clearly established.

An interview is a goal-directed communication between the patient and the nurse; that is, either the patient or the nurse has a specific purpose in mind. The goals of communication are (1) to gain information; (2) to give information; and (3) to motivate. When intervening with a patient with the diagnosis Potential for Violence, the goal of nursing intervention is to motivate the patient to move in a positive direction.

Active listening and responding should be continous to evaluate Potential for Violence accurately and to evaluate the effectiveness of the verbal intervention or the nonphysical management. In the prevention and management of aggressive behavior, the nurse has to listen actively to restate the content and identify feelings expressed by the angry patient.

Most complaints about medical care concern a lack of individual attention and personal interest. In an address to a group of physicians, a defense lawyer urged them to "talk to your patients!" Most charges of malpractice are based on a lack of communication and not on substandard care. Gazda et al (1982) assert that effective communication is a dynamic means of preventing misunderstanding and aggression, making human relations training proactive and preventive rather than reactive and remedial.

The following case study illustrates the use of communication and active listening.

Table 47.3

Guidelines for Interacting with an Angry Person

1. Intervene as soon as you think or feel something is wrong.
2. Listen actively to the content person is saying and feeling.
3. Listen nonjudgmentally to the person.
4. Do not make negative consequences for feeling angry.
5. Do not take anger personally and become defensive.
6. Do not ignore an individual's anger to calm yourself down.
7. Enlist the individual's help in selecting appropriate channels to direct the anger.
8. Sometimes it is best to insist that an angry person regain control before discussing the issue.
9. Do not make promises you cannot keep.
10. Do not corner physically or psychologically; avoid verbal and physical power struggles, Win-Lose, Right-Wrong situations.
11. Level with the person without leveling him or her.
12. Timing.
13. Focus on what the individual can do (positive) rather than what they cannot do (negative).
14. Reinforce attempts and successes at self-control.
15. Be descriptive rather than evaluative.
16. Be specific rather than general.
17. Discuss only one behavior at a time.
18. Avoid using *always* and *never*.
19. Use a positive tone of voice rather than a demanding or cajoling one.
20. Set limits on actions not on feelings.
21. Actions speak louder than words: Aggression (on the part of the staff) begets aggression.
22. The stressed person's ability to reason abstractly disintegrates and response is to isolated stimuli rather than to the context of the situation.
23. Assaultive individuals are looking for controls and reassurances that they will receive help and will not have to do anything that they will be ashamed of or embarrassed about later.
24. Document objective facts regarding frequency, context and behavior of incident.

Source: Prevention and Management of Aggressive Behavior Training Manual, VAMC Augusta, Georgia, 1983.

CASE STUDY

Potential for Violence, Mr. R.M.

Mr. R.M., age 72, was becoming an increasing management problem on a busy medical-surgical unit. He had been admitted with acute chronic obstructive pulmonary disease (COPD)/pneumonia. As his respiratory condition seemed to improve, his acceptance of treatment and care seemed to deteriorate. He had been involved in four aggressive incidents in 3 days. He attempted to punch a lab technician when she tried to draw blood from him and had difficulty inserting the needle. The next day he reached up and shoved a nurse when she opened the curtain around his bed in the four-bed ward. That same afternoon, he threatened to strike a nurse's aide who was looking through his bedside stand for his bath basin.

Mr. R.M. went to the dayroom for a cigarette several times a day, although his physician and the nursing staff told him he should not be smoking. On his last trip to the dayroom, he struck another patient who was sitting in his favorite chair.

Mr. R.M.'s primary nurse tracked all the incidents and spoke to Mrs. R.M. about her husband's history of coping with anger and frustration. Based on his behavior and a history of anger in response to feelings of powerlessness and helplessness, the nursing diagnosis Potential for Violence related to depression and secondary to frustration and anxiety was made. The nursing staff was instructed to be very aware of Mr. R.M.'s surroundings, to ask permission and explain before beginning procedures or treatments, and to give Mr. R.M. choices regarding his care. A more respectful approach to his regimen was implemented along with instructions on controlled breathing and other stress management techniques. No other aggressive incidents occurred during Mr. R.M.'s hospitalization, and he was discharged smiling, with a stable respiratory picture.

SUMMARY

Most incidents of aggressive and violent behavior are predictable and therefore preventable. Some incidents such as those resulting from closed head trauma, Alzheimer's disease, or substance-induced delirium are unpredictable and necessitate the staff being prepared to respond at all times (Ochitill and Krieger, 1982; Turner, 1984). With comprehensive education and training planned to address the special management problems of the aggressive elderly, proactive interventions can be emphasized, keeping the focus on the potential rather than on the maladaptive aggressive or violent responses.

References

Bachy-Rita G: Episodic dyscontrol: A study of 130 violent patients. *Am J Psychiatry* 1971; 127:1473–1478.

Birdwhistle RL: *Kinesics and Context: Essays on Body Motion Communication*. University of Pennsylvania Press, 1979.

Blake K, Taylor C: *The Prevention and Management of Aggressive Behavior*. South Carolina Department of Mental Health, 1977.

Blazer D, Siegler I: *A Family Approach to Health Care of the Elderly*. Addison-Wesley, 1984.

Brigman C, Dickey C, Zeeger L: Agitated aggressive patient. *Am J Nurs* (Oct) 1983; 1409–1412.

Buckelew B: Health care professionals vs. the elderly. *J. Gerontol Nurs* (Oct) 1982; 560–564.

Burnside I: *Psychosocial Nursing Care of the Aged*. McGraw-Hill, 1980.

Carpenito L: *Nursing Diagnosis: Application to Clinical Practice*. Lippincott, 1983.

Carroll-Johnson R (editor): *Classifications of Nursing Diagnoses: Proceedings of the Eighth Conference*. Lippincott, 1989.

Climent C; Historical data in the evaluation of violent subjects. *Arch Gen Psychiatry* 1972; 27:621–625.

Clunn P: Nurses' Assessment of a Person's Potential for Violence. (Doctoral dissertation, Teachers College, Columbia University, 1975.) Dissertation Abstracts International 27, B 2770B (University Microfilm No. 71-27, 7000).

Esberger KR: Stalking a claim. *Geriatr Nurs* (July/Aug) 1982; 246–247.

Fields W, Sweet W: *Neural Bases of Violence and Aggression*. Warren H. Green, 1975.

Freedman ML: Organic brain syndromes in the elderly. *Postgrad Med* 1983; 74:165–176.

Gage F: Depression in the aged. Pages 44–51 in: *Psychosocial Nursing Care of the Aged*. Burnside I (editor). McGraw-Hill, 1973.

Gazda GM, Childers WC, Walter RP: *Interpersonal Communication : A Handbook for Health Professionals*. Aspen, 1982.

Geurguis E: Management of disturbed patients. An alternative to the use of mechanical restraints. *J Clin Psychiatry* 1978; 39: 295–299.

Goldenberg B, Chiverton P: Assessing behavior: The nurse's mental status exam. *Geriatr Nurs* (Mar/Apr) 1984; 94–98.

Hall ET: *The Hidden Dimension*. Doubleday, 1966.

Hays A: The Set Test to screen for mental status quickly. *Geriatr Nurs* (Mar/Apr) 1984; 96–97.

Hein EC: Sociocultural influences. Chapter 12 in: *Communication in Nursing Practice*, 2d ed. Little, Brown, 1980.

Helms J: *Active Listening in Nursing Interventions: Treatment for Nursing Diagnoses*. Saunders, 1985.

Kalogerakis M: The assaultive psychiatric patient. *Psychiatric Q* 1971; 45:372–381.

Kelly MA: *Nursing Diagnosis Source Book*. Appleton-Century-Crofts, 1985.

Kim MJ, Moritz D: *Classification of Nursing Diagnosis*. McGraw-Hill, 1982.

King RC: Refining your assessment techniques. *RN* (Feb) 1984; 46:43.

Lippincott Manual of Nursing Practice. Lippincott, 1982.

Lorenz K: *On Aggression*. Harcourt Brace Jovanovich, 1966.

Mark V, Ervin F: *Violence and the Brain*. Harper and Row, 1970.

Monahan J: *Predicting Violent Behavior*. Sage, 1981.

Morrant JC, Ablog J: The angry elderly patient. *Postgrad Med* 1983; 74:93–102.

Munns D: A validation of the defining characteristics of the nursing diagnosis "Potential for Violence." *Nurs Clin North Am* 1985; 29:711–721.

Ochitill N, Krieger M: Violent behavior among hospitalized medical and surgical patients. *South Med J* 1982; 75:151–155.

Palmore E: The facts on aging quiz: A review of findings. *Gerontologist* 1980; 20:669–672.

Petrie W: Violence: The geriatric patient. Pages 110–111 in: *Violence in the Medical Care Setting*. Turner J (editor). Aspen, 1984.

Petrie WM, Lawson EC, Hollender MH: Violence in geriatric patients. *J Am Med Assoc* 1982; 248(4):443–444.

Rada J, Doan J, Schwab S: How to decrease wandering: A form of agenda behavior. *Geriatr Nurs* (July/Aug) 1985; 196–199.

Rothenberg A: On anger. *Am J Psychiatry* 1971; 128:86–92.

Rubin B: Prediction of dangerousness in mentally ill criminals. *Arch Gen Psychiatry* 1972; 27:397–407.

Sadoff R: *Violence and Responsibility: The Individual, the Family and Society*. S.P. Medical and Scientific Books, 1978.

Todd B: Central anticholinergic syndrome. *Geriatr Nurs* (Mar/Apr) 1984; 117–119.

Turner JT: *Violence in the Medical Care Setting*. Aspen, 1984.

Veterans Administration Medical Center, Augusta GA: *Prevention and Management of Aggressive Behavior Training Manual*, 1983.

Warden LS: The nursing history. In: *Nursing Assessment: A Multidimensional Approach*. Ballack J (editor). Wadsworth, 1984.

Wolanin M: Scope of the problem (confusion) and its identity. *Geriatr Nurs* (July/Aug) 1983; 227–230.

48

Altered Role Performance: Potential Loss of Right of Self-Determination

KAY WEILER, MA, JD, RN

THE NURSING DIAGNOSIS ALTERED ROLE PERFOR-mance: Potential Loss of Right of Self-Determination focuses on the factors that may affect an elderly person's ability to exert self-determination in health care treatment decisions. These include the elderly person's physical and/or mental capacity; the presence or absence of an advance directive for health care; and a health care provider's respect for the elderly person's right of self-determination. Nursing interventions may be implemented if an elderly person's right of self-determination in health care treatment decisions is threatened.

The right of a competent older American to accept or to reject medical care is based on the common law right to self-determination and the constitutional right to privacy.[1]

No right is held more sacred, or is more carefully guarded, by the common law, than the right of every individual to the possession and control of his own person, free from all restraint or interference of others, unless by clear and unquestionable authority of law.[2]

The origin of this right has been described as: "Every human being of adult years and sound mind has a right to determine what shall be done with his own body."[3] Simply stated, it is the right of the person "to be let alone."[4]

The right of an elderly person to make health care decisions is protected by the constitutional right to privacy. This right has been found within the penumbra or zone of rights in the ninth[5] and fourteenth amendments.[6] Although the constitution does not explicitly state the right to privacy, the Supreme Court has determined that this right is implied in the intent and wording of the constitution.[7] This right recognizes the individual's interest in preserving "the inviolability of his person."[8] The New Jersey Supreme Court has found that the constitutional right to privacy is "broad enough to encompass a patient's decision to decline medical treatment under certain circumstances"[9] even if that personal decision would foreseeably result in death.

Although the common law right to self-determination and the constitutional right to privacy have been established, these rights are not absolute.[10] These personal rights are balanced against societal interests in (1) preservation of human life; (2) prevention of suicide; (3) protection of the interests of innocent third parties; and (4) preservation of the integrity of the medical profession.[11]

The first societal interest is in the preservation of life, and it is generally considered the most significant of the four state interests. It expresses the societal belief in the sanctity of all human life. It is predicated on the belief that the existence of all human life should be protected.[12] However, this abstract interest has often yielded to the personal interest that the individual has in directing his or her own life.[13]

Prevention of suicide, the second societal interest, is an important consideration when attempting to determine whether the elderly individual who is refusing medical care wants to exert the right to self-determination or wants to implement self-destruction.[14] The critical differences between the refusal of health care and suicide are (1) in refusing treatment the person does not wish to die; and (2) even if death is desired, the cause of death is natural and is not from self-inflicted injuries.[15]

The third societal interest is the need to protect innocent third parties. This interest has been recognized when the needs and interests of dependent children are balanced against an adult's right to self-determination in a health care decision.[16]

This interest has also been considered when a patient with a communicable disease has made a health care decision that was considered a harmful risk to the community.[17] The protection of innocent third parties is an important societal interest; however, it has not generally been a relevant factor in the consideration of health care decisions made by or for the elderly.

The fourth societal interest, preservation of the integrity of the medical profession, has been a significant issue when patients have asserted their right to self-determination in a direction contrary to the physician's or health care provider's professional judgment.[18] Questions regarding this issue have arisen from patients who have sought to compel health care providers and institutions to take specific health care treatment measures. Concerns have also arisen from health care institutions who have sought to clarify their position, specifically when there has been a question about the capacity of the individual to forego treatment.[19]

This interest has been countered with two responses: (1) "(m)edical ethics do not require medical intervention in disease at all costs,"[20] and (2) the right to make an individual health care decision is only valid when there is a right to refuse health care treatment.[21] This final issue, the refusal of available health care, has raised difficult and complex ethical and legal questions.

The balancing that occurs in each specific case will vary with the facts of the case. The analyses, deliberations, and considerations that have been employed in the reported cases may help to resolve present and future controversies prior to a judicial determination.

SIGNIFICANCE FOR THE ELDERLY

The elderly are often subjected to sociocultural impediments in performing their usual roles because of the loss of work roles and income, loss of monetary assets, and loss of social and family relationships.

A change in physical and/or mental capacity can subject the elderly to imbalanced power relationships with loss of autonomy when they enter the health care delivery system. The Retirement Research Foundation's Personal Autonomy in Long-Term Care Initiative program found that although there seems to be general agreement that institutionalized elderly are entitled to maximum self-determination and dignity, caretakers often tend to make a variety of decisions for them, resulting in erosion of the elder's usual role performance and autonomy.[22] Nursing, medical, and other "helping" interventions for the frail or physically and/or mentally incapacitated elderly are often judged by the goals, values, and motivations of the helper rather than by the preferences of the elderly patient.

Multiple factors affect the health care system and make health care decisions difficult and complex for all members of our society. No one person or profession has all of the answers.[23] Therefore, all professions—nurses, physicians, social workers, attorneys, and judges—must work together to ensure that the elderly individual's rights to privacy and self-determination within the health care decision-making process are preserved.

Nurses in the emergency room, acute care treatment centers, senior citizens centers, nursing homes, and hospices interact with the elderly in situations in which they must make health care decisions. Potential areas of concern for nurses are the adult's legal rights in accepting or refusing health care interventions; the means available to the elderly to effectuate their health care decisions; the specific rights of the dependent elderly; and the special vulnerability of the elderly.

CURRENT STATUS OF THE DIAGNOSIS

Altered role performance is defined as "disruption in the way one perceives one's role performance."[24] The North American Nursing Diagnosis Association (NANDA) has not described related factors/etiologies for this diagnosis. However, Table 48.1 compares NANDA's defining characteristics and related factors of Altered Role Performance with the defining characteristics and related factors of Altered Role Performance: Potential Loss of Right of Self-Determination presented in this chapter.

CASE STUDY

Lane vs. Candura[25]

This case concerns a 77-year-old widow, Mrs. Rosaria Candura, of Arlington, who is presently a patient at the

Table 48.1

Comparison of NANDA Etiologies/Related Factors and Defining Characteristics for Altered Role Performance With Those Proposed by Weiler for Altered Role Performance: Potential Loss of Right of Self-Determination

NANDA (CARROLL-JOHNSON, 1989)	WEILER
Definition	*Definition*
Disruption in the way one perceives one's role performance	Potential loss of an individual's right to make personal health care treatment decisions.
Related Factors/Etiologies	*Related Factors/Etiologies*
To be developed	Change in physical and/or mental capacity Institutionalization Lack of advance directive
Defining Characteristics	*Defining Characteristics*
Change in self-perception of role Denial of role Change in others' perception of role Conflict in roles Change in physical capacity to resume role Lack of knowledge of role Change in usual patterns or responsibility	Negative attitude/knowledge of caregivers re right of self-determination Change in others' perception of role Change in usual patterns of responsibility Lack of knowledge re right of self-determination Lack of advocates, social support Lack of social contacts/interactions Incongruence of patient/client's stated/documented wishes re treatment prescribed/provided by health professionals/caregivers Family members/caregivers uncertainty re client's competence Loss of autonomy/decision-making authority

Symmes Hospital in Arlington suffering from gangrene in the right foot and lower leg. . . . Her daughter . . . filed a petition in Probate Court for Middlesex County seeking appointment of herself as temporary guardian with authority to consent to the operation on behalf of her mother. An order and a judgment were entered in the probate court to that effect, from which the guardian ad litem appointed to represent Mrs. Candura has appealed. . . .

The principal question arising on the record before us, therefore, is whether Mrs. Candura has the legally requisite competence of mind and will to make the choice for herself. (The trial court) decision does not include a clear-cut finding that Mrs. Candura lacks that requisite legal competence. . . .

We hold that Mrs. Candura has the right under the law to refuse to submit either to medical treatment or to a surgical operation, that on the evidence and findings in this case the decision is one that she may determine for herself, and that therefore her leg may not be amputated unless she consents to that course of action.

DISCUSSION

Mrs. Candura was a 77-year-old widow who had a history of an infected toe on the right foot in 1974, which

had became gangrenous and was amputated. Mrs. Candura reinjured her right foot in 1977, gangrene resulted, and a portion of the right foot was amputated. In 1978, after a difficult recovery, Mrs. Candura injured the right leg again, and the surgical decision was to amputate the remainder of the right foot. Mrs. Candura originally consented to and then refused the surgery.

Formally stated, the nursing diagnosis is Altered Role Performance: Potential Loss of Right of Self-Determination related to change in physical capacity, evidenced by daughter's uncertainty regarding mother's competence and change in patterns of responsibility.

The trial court found that Mrs. Candura was disappointed in the failure of the earlier operations to arrest the gangrene. The court determined that she did not believe that the operation would cure her and that she did not want to live as an invalid in a nursing home. Furthermore, the court stated that she did not fear death but welcomed it. She was described as stubborn, somewhat irascible, hostile to certain doctors, and occasionally combative in response to questions. Her conception of time was distorted; however, overall she demonstrated a high degree of awareness and acuity in response to the question of her possible surgery. She was clear in her decision to refuse the surgery even though it could lead to her death.

Each adult is presumed competent to make personal health care decisions unless evidence demonstrates that the person is incompetent. The burden is not on the patient to establish competence but on the petitioners to establish incompetence. The court in Mrs. Candura's case decided that there was not sufficient evidence to defeat the presumption of competence. The choice of refusing the surgery may have been medically irrational; however, that did not justify a conclusion of incompetence.

Mrs. Candura suffered a change in her physical capacity, refused surgery, and contradicted her daughter's wishes for her to have surgery. Therefore, her daughter questioned Mrs. Candura's decision-making ability and petitioned the court for the right to make personal care decisions for her mother. Mrs. Candura demonstrated the ability to appreciate the nature and consequences of her act and, therefore, she retained the right of self-determination and the freedom of individual choice.

Cases such as this one have arisen when an elderly person suffers from such extreme physical disability that following his or her directives would result in death. However, failure to follow the expressed wishes would eviscerate the elderly person's right to self-determination.

ALTERED ROLE PERFORMANCE: POTENTIAL LOSS OF RIGHT OF SELF-DETERMINATION WITH ADVANCE ORAL AND WRITTEN DIRECTIVES

Advance Directives

Individuals who anticipate the need for future health care decisions may communicate their treatment preferences through a variety of means. Verbal comments, a living will, and a durable power of attorney have been recognized as valid advance directives for future health care treatment decisions.

Oral Directives

One method of communication of treatment preferences is the use of oral statements made by the elderly person in relation to potential health care problems and possible treatment decisions. Verbal comments indicating a thoughtful and consistent approach have been recognized by the courts as valid indicators of the person's preferred approach to potential treatment alternatives.[26] However, the limitations of verbal comments are apparent, as illustrated in the following case study.

CASE STUDY

Brophy vs. New England Sinai Hospital, Inc.[27]

Paul E. Brophy, Sr. (Brophy) was afflicted on March 22, 1983, by the rupture of an aneurysm located at the apex of the basilar artery. Prior to that time, Brophy had been a healthy, robust man, who had been employed by the town of Easton as a fireman and emergency medical technician. He enjoyed deer hunting, fishing, gardening, and performing household chores. At about midnight on March 22, 1983, he complained to his wife, Patricia, of a severe, "splitting" headache. He became unconscious. His wife called the Easton fire department, and Brophy was transported to Goddard Hospital. An angiogram . . . revealed the eneurysm. Surgery . . . was not successful. He has never regained consciousness. Brophy is now in a condition described as a "persistent vegetative state." He is unable to chew or swallow, and is maintained by an artificial device . . . known as a gastrostomy tube (G-tube) through which he receives nutrition and hydration. . . .

Brophy is not terminally ill nor in danger of imminent death from any underlying physical illness. It is true, however, that his life expectancy has been shortened by his physical affliction. . . .

(The question was) . . . whether the substituted judgment of a person in a persistent vegetative state that the artificial maintenance of his nutrition and hydration be discontinued shall be honored. . . .

The judge found on the basis of ample evidence, which no one disputes, that Brophy's judgment would be to decline the provision of food and water and to terminate his life. In reaching that conclusion, the judge considered various factors . . . (1) Brophy's expressed preferences; (2) his religious convictions and their relation to refusal of treatment; (3) the impact on his family; (4) the probability of adverse side effects; and (5) the prognosis, both with and without treatment. . . .

(The question that remained) was whether the Commonwealth's interests require that his judgment be overridden. . . .

(W)e conclude that the State's interest in the preservation of life does not overcome Brophy's right to discontinue treatment. Nor do we consider his death to be against the State's interest in the prevention of suicide . . . (and) so long as we decline to force the hospital to participate in removing or clamping Brophy's G-tube, there is no violation of the integrity of the medical profession. . . .

(The hospital was ordered) to assist the guardian in transferring the ward to a suitable facility, or to his home, where his wishes may be effectuated.

DISCUSSION

Mrs. Patricia Brophy, Brophy's wife and guardian, had asked the physicians and the hospital to discontinue the gastrostomy tube feedings that were used for the maintenance of nutrition and hydration. His guardian based this request on her substituted judgment of what Mr. Brophy's decision would have been in this situation.

Mr. Brophy's nursing diagnosis is Altered Role Performance: Potential Loss of Right of Self-Determination related to change in physical and mental capacity, evidenced by incongruence of patient's stated preferences for health care treatment and the prescribed treatment.

The principle of substituted judgment in a health care decision for an incompetent person was introduced in *Superintendent of Belchertown vs. Saikewicz.*[28] It is a subjective test "to determine with as much accuracy as possible the wants and needs of the individual involved."[29] It is not based on what a reasonable person would choose in similar circumstances; it is a test based on what the patient would have chosen if he had been competent to make the decision.[30]

In the Brophy case, Mr. Brophy had been a competent communicative individual prior to his ruptured aneurysm. He had discussed his thoughts and preferences related to possible health care treatment decisions; however, he had not expressed his thoughts in a written form. His wife, serving as his court-appointed guardian, asked the court to respect and honor his decision even though it was not in a written form.

Based on the substituted judgment test, the court granted his guardian the authority to discontinue the artificial tube feedings. The court did not require the hospital to assist in the treatment decision; however, the court did require the hospital to assist Mrs. Brophy in transferring Mr. Brophy so that the treatment decision could be carried out.

The change in Brophy's physical and mental capacity, his wife's attempts to have his verbal directions followed, and the hospital's refusal to honor his verbal directive all demonstrate factors that may affect an individual's ability to assert the right to self-determination. The Brophy decision identifies that verbal comments can form the basis for a substituted judgment. However, numerous problems arise in applying the principle of substituted judgment: (1) the determination of what the patient would have chosen is difficult and time consuming; (2) the nature, content, and depth of previous comments must be examined to make current health care treatment decisions; (3) the current circumstances must be analyzed to determine if they are comparable to situations that the patient anticipated; and finally (4) court approval must be sought in order to carry out the substituted judgment. These potentially serious problems demonstrate the advantages of more formal treatment directives.

Written Advance Directives

Two forms of formal written advance directives have recently become important in health care decision-making situations: the living will and the durable power of attorney. Both provide future guidelines in the event that the elderly person is incapable of participating in the decision-making process.

CASE STUDY

Bartling vs. Superior Court[31]

Mr. Bartling was 70 years old and suffered from emphysema, chronic respiratory failure, arteriosclerosis, an abdominal aneurysm . . . and a malignant tumor of the lung. Mr. Bartling also had a history of . . . "chronic acute anxiety/depression" and alcoholism. . . .

(Mr. Bartling) was placed on a ventilator. . . . (He) remained on the ventilator until the time of his death, and efforts to "wean" him from the machine were unsuccessful. . . .

A living will, signed by Mr. Bartling with an "X" and properly witnessed . . . stated in part: "If at such time the situation should arise in which there is no reasonable expectation of my recovery from extreme physical or mental disability, I direct that I be allowed to die and not be kept alive by medications, artificial means or heroic measures."

A "Durable Power of Attorney for Health Care," executed by Mr. Bartling . . . stated in part: "I do not wish to continue to live under these conditions. It is therefore my intent to refuse to continue on ventilator support and thereby to permit the natural process of dying to occur—peacefully, privately and with dignity." . . .

The trial court . . . findings, includ(ed): (1) Mr. Bartling's illnesses were serious but not terminal; . . . (2) although Mr. Bartling was attached to a respirator to facilitate breathing, he was not in a vegetative state and was not comatose; and (3) Mr. Bartling was competent in the legal sense. . . .

There is no question in our minds that Mr. Bartling was, as the trial court determined, competent in the legal sense to decide whether he wanted to have the ventilator disconnected. . . .

Having resolved the threshold issue of whether or not Mr. Bartling was legally competent, we turn to the major issue in this case: whether the right of Mr. Bartling, as a competent adult, to refuse unwanted medical treatment is outweighed by the various state and personal interests. . . .

In California, "a person of adult years and in sound mind has the right, in the exercise of control over his own body, to determine whether or not to submit to lawful medical treatment."

DISCUSSION

Mr. William Bartling was a 70-year-old man with an extensive medical history who was admitted to a private religious hospital for treatment of his depression. On admission, a routine chest x-ray identified the presence of a lung tumor. The tumor was examined by a needle biopsy, which resulted in a collapsed lung. The lung did not reinflate; therefore, a tracheostomy tube was placed, and respiratory support with a ventilator was provided. Mr. Bartling's physicians identified that he was seriously ill; however, he was not terminally ill, and death was not imminent.

There was no disagreement between Mr. Bartling, his wife, the physician, the hospital, or the court that Mr. Bartling was competent to make his health care decisions. Mr. Bartling wanted to live, but he preferred death to his life with a ventilator. In the event that Mr. Bartling became incompetent to make health care treatment decisions, he executed a written living will that stated his desire to cease his daily struggle with life. He also made and signed a durable power of attorney naming his wife as the attorney-in-fact.

Mr. Bartling tried to detach the ventilator from the tracheostomy tube himself. He was subsequently restrained with soft restraints so that he could not accidentally or intentionally disconnect the ventilator.

The hospital sought an injunction to prevent Mr. Bartling or his representative from disconnecting the ventilator. The hospital argued that as a religious hospital it could not ethically participate in this patient's suicide. The hospital also expressed concern about potential civil and criminal liability if they disconnected the respirator.

The nursing diagnosis for Mr. Bartling is Altered Role Performance: Potential Loss of Right of Self-Determination, evidenced by change in physical condition, by lack of caregiver's knowledge regarding his right of self-determination, by change in caregiver's perceptions of his role, and by incongruence between Mr. Bartling's documented wishes and prescribed treatment.

The question before the court was whether a competent adult's right to refuse unwanted medical treatment is outweighed by the various state interests. The court decided that an adult has the right to determine whether or not to accept medical treatment. The **Bartling** decision is viewed as extending the right to self-determination to situations in which there is a serious illness that is not a terminal illness.

The relevant factors in evaluating Mr. Bartling's right of self-determination included Mr. Bartling's change in physical capacity; his questionable change in mental capacity; the hospital's refusal to follow his verbal or written directives; and the hospital's application for a court injunction. All of these were important in evaluating Mr. Bartling's potentially altered role performance and his right of self-determination.

Mr. Bartling verbally expressed his present decision regarding his health care treatment and provided two written advance directives that were to be followed in the event that he was no longer able to communicate those wishes personally. He did not rely on the ability of another person to make his decision. In this situation, he did not become mentally incapacitated, and there was no need to refer to the living will or the durable power of attorney for directions. However, these written directives had been communicated to his guardian, the physicians, the hospital, and the court. They served as verification of his verbal statements regarding his health care treatment decision.

Living Will A living will serves as an advance directive for a health care treatment decision. Forty states and the District of Columbia have enacted living will legislation.[32] This legislation authorizes an adult to control decisions regarding the administration of life-sustaining treatment.[33] The individual leaves directions to be followed in the event that he or she is in a terminal condition and unable to participate in medical treatment decisions.

Living will legislation is limited to situations in which **life-sustaining measures** are being considered for an adult who (1) has an incurable or irreversible condition; (2) is unable to participate in the treatment decisions; and (3) is likely to die soon.[34] It does not apply to life-sustaining measures for (1) minors, (2) adults who have not written a living will, or (3) treatment decisions made by a proxy decision maker.[35] The specific characteristics of these variables will differ in each state jurisdiction.

The living will declaration becomes effective when (1) the declaration has been communicated to the attending physician; (2) the declaring adult is determined by the attending physician to be in a terminal condition; and (3) the declaring adult is incapable of making a health care treatment decision.[36] The living will may be revoked at any time by the declarant, and the revocation is effective when the attending physician is notified of the revocation.[37]

Living will legislation is particularly appropriate in view of the multiple health care needs and concerns of the elderly. It is one form of future directive.[38] It does not rely on another person to form the substituted judgment of that decision. It depends on health care personnel, especially physicians and nurses, to carry out the decision.[39]

One final concern in applying a living will is whether court approval is necessary before withdrawal of life support systems. The Florida Supreme Court was presented with the following questions:

> In the case of a comatose and terminally ill individual who has executed a so-called "living" or "mercy" will, is it necessary that a court appointed guardian of his person obtain the approval of a court of competent jurisdiction

before terminating extraordinary life support systems in order for consenting family members, the attending physicians, and the hospital and its administrators to be relieved of civil and criminal liability?[40]

The Florida Supreme Court determined that a prior court approval to terminate care was not required. The court reviewed the rights that a competent adult would have to refuse treatment and recognized that "there must be a means by which this right may be exercised on their behalf, otherwise it will be lost."[41] Even though Florida had not enacted living will legislation, the living will that had been executed was viewed as persuasive evidence of the incompetent person's intention and was given great weight by the person who substituted his or her judgment on behalf of the incompetent patient.

Durable Power of Attorney for Health Care The traditional power of attorney is a private agreement between parties that authorizes one person (the agent) to act in the place of or on behalf of another person (the principal).[42] The traditional power of attorney explicitly becomes ineffective if the principal becomes mentally incapacitated.[43] This specific characteristic of the traditional power of attorney rendered this relationship inappropriate for health care decisions. The situation of diminished or lack of capacity is precisely when an agent for decision making is needed. Therefore, some states have enacted legislation that provides for the creation of a relationship that remains in effect even if the principal becomes mentally incapacitated and unable to make decisions. This "durable" power of attorney is especially important in health care decisions related to the elderly.

The characteristics of a durable power of attorney are (1) the principal must be mentally competent at the time that the relationship is created; (2) it is a private written agreement between two persons in a principal–agent relationship; and (3) the document creating the relationship must contain words showing that the principal intended that the authority conferred would be exercisable even if the principal became incapacitated or disabled.[44] Words that may be used to indicate the durability of this document include "This power of attorney shall not be affected by subsequent disability or incapacity of the principal."[45]

The Uniform Durable Power of Attorney Act provides that the principal–agent relationship may be in either of two forms.[46] In the first form, the relationship is created on execution of the document and continues in effect if the principal becomes incapacitated.[47] The second form of the relationship is a springing durable power of attorney. The springing power becomes effective only if and when the principal becomes incapacitated.[48] This type of relationship allows the principal to identify and stipulate the conditions that activate the agent's power.

ALTERED ROLE PERFORMANCE: POTENTIAL LOSS OF RIGHT OF SELF-DETERMINATION WITH NO ADVANCE DIRECTIVES

The most difficult health care decisions arise in situations in which the individual who is in need of health care treatment is unable to participate in the decision-making process and has not clearly indicated his or her preferences in health care treatment decisions.[49] Therefore, when the time for a decision comes, questions arise regarding who should make the decision for the patient; what information should be considered in making the decision; and what standard should be used in determining the balance between (1) the patient's needs; (2) the benefits of the treatment; and (3) the costs (physical, emotional, and financial) of the treatment.

CASE STUDY

Matter of Conroy[50]

In 1979 Claire Conroy, who was suffering from an organic brain syndrome that manifested itself in her exhibiting periods of confusion, was adjudicated an incompetent and plaintiff, her nephew, was appointed her guardian. . . .

Ms. Conroy was no longer ambulatory and was confined to bed, unable to move from a semi-fetal position. She suffered from arteriosclerotic heart disease, hypertension, and diabetes mellitus; her left leg was gangrenous to her knee; she had several necrotic decubitus ulcers (bed sores) on her left foot, leg and hip; an eye problem required irrigation; she had a urinary catheter in place and could not control her bowels; she could not speak; and her ability to swallow was very limited. On the other hand, she interacted with her environment in some limited ways: she could move her head, neck, hands, and arms to a minor extent; she was able to scratch herself, and had pulled at her bandages, tube, and catheter; she moaned occasionally when moved, when fed through the tube, or when her bandages were changed; her eyes sometimes followed individuals in the room; her facial expressions were different when she was awake from when she was asleep; and she smiled on occasion when her hair was combed, or when she received a comforting rub. . . .

This case requires us to determine the circumstances under which life-sustaining treatment may be withheld or withdrawn from an elderly nursing home resident who is suffering from serious and permanent mental and physical impairment, who will probably die within approximately one year even with the treatment, and who, though formerly competent, is now incompetent to make decisions about her life-sustaining treatment and is unlikely to regain such competence. Subsumed within this question are two corollary issues: what substantive guidelines are appropriate for making these treatment decisions for incompetent patients, and what procedures should be followed in making them. . . .

This starting point in analyzing whether life-sustaining treatment may be withheld or withdrawn from an incompetent patient is to determine what rights a competent patient has to accept or reject medical care. It is therefore necessary at the onset of this discussion to identify the nature and extent of a patient's rights that are implicated by such decisions. . . .

The right of a person to control his (or her) own body is a basic societal concept, long recognized in common law. . . . The right to make certain decisions concerning one's body is also protected by the federal constitutional right of privacy. . . .

In light of these rights and concerns, we hold that life-sustaining treatment may be withheld or withdrawn from an incompetent patient when it is clear that the particular patient would have refused the treatment under the circumstances involved.

DISCUSSION

Miss Conroy was an 84-year-old woman who, because of her many physical problems, was confined to her nursing home bed. She had an extensive medical history. She had a very limited ability to respond to her environment, and a limited life expectancy; however, she was not brain dead, comatose, or in a chronic vegetative state. She had one living relative, her nephew. She had never married nor had children; her siblings were deceased; and she had no close friends. The question was whether her nephew, as her guardian, had the authority to withhold nasogastric feedings from her.

The changes in Miss Conroy's physical and mental capacity, her lack of advance directive, her institutionalization, and her lack of advocates and social support may have led her nurses to the identification of the diagnosis Altered Role Performance: Potential Loss of Right of Self-Determination.

The court identified several factors that distinguished Miss Conroy's situation from the well-known Quinlan case.[51] Miss Quinlan was a 19-year-old comatose woman, seemingly dependent on a respirator, in an acute care hospital. Her family, physicians, and the hospital prognosis committee were in agreement that the respirator should be discontinued. In contrast, Miss Conroy was 84 years old and was not comatose, but had serious mental and physical impairments. Miss Conroy did not have an extensive family unit to identify and protect her interests or desires. Miss Conroy was in a nursing home in which there was no team of physicians or a hospital ethics committee to review the decision to withhold or withdraw life-sustaining treatment.

The court in **Conroy** particularly noted that nursing home patients have special needs for health care, and their right to make health care treatment decisions must be protected. Miss Conroy continued to receive the nasogastric feedings but died during the court proceeding. Despite her death, the court decided that the issue was not moot and proposed resolutions for future situations.

In resolving the central question, the court identified two corollary issues: (1) What guidelines are appropriate for making treatment decisions for incompetent patients? and (2) What procedures should be followed in making decisions? The court stated that the guidelines for making the treatment decisions were (1) the established rights of competent and incompetent adults to refuse health care treatment, and (2) a balancing of the patient's right to self-determination with the interests of society.

The court decided that an adult, regardless of competency, has the right to accept or refuse medical care. Therefore, Miss Conroy had the right to refuse the nasogastric tube feedings. The court balanced her right of refusal against the four societal interests discussed previously: (1) preservation of life; (2) prevention of suicide; (3) protection of innocent third parties; and (4) protection of medical profession. The court concluded that none of these societal interests outweighed Miss Conroy's interest in refusing the treatment.

Determining that Miss Conroy had the right to refuse the medical treatment did not, however, provide a procedure for the resolution of whether a specific incompetent individual would choose to accept or refuse a proposed health care intervention. The court developed three tests and identified that the level of guidance available from the individual determined which test would be used. The three tests were the subjective test, the limited-objective test, and the pure-objective test.

The subjective test asks What would this particular patient have done if he had been able to choose for himself? As noted in **Brophy,** if the incompetent patient, during competency, has clearly indicated a refusal of similar interventions under similar circumstances, the substituted decision for the person may be to withhold or withdraw the treatment from the patient. The substitute decision maker is required to synthesize all of the relevant information in an attempt to determine and effectuate the patient's right to self-determination.

The subjective test cannot be applied if the incompetent patient has left only limited information or no information regarding preferences or directions for future administration of health care. In that case the substituted decision maker must use a test that would meet the best interests of the individual. The court did not want to "foreclose the possibility of humane actions, which may involve termination of life-sustaining treatment"[52] for persons who had not indicated prior choices. Therefore, the court identified two tests based on the **parens patriae** power of the state. This **parens patriae** power is derived from societal interest in protecting those who cannot or will not protect themselves.[53]

The limited objective test requires some trustworthy evidence that the patient would have refused the treatment. This evidence may include comments or reactions by the patient to other individuals and their medical conditions.

This evidence would provide some indication of the individual's preferences in the treatment decision. The substituted decision maker's choice to accept or reject treatment is determined by considering that the patient:

will continue to suffer throughout the expected duration of his life, unavoidable pain, and that the net burdens of his prolonged life . . . markedly outweigh any physical pleasure, emotional enjoyment, or intellectual satisfaction that the patient may still be able to derive from life.[54]

The pure-objective test is to be applied if there is no evidence that the patient would have declined the treatment. Under this test, the life-saving treatment could be withheld if "the net burden of the patient's life with the treatment should clearly and markedly outweigh the benefits that the patient derives from life."[55] Thus, the life-sustaining treatment would be withheld if the patient would suffer recurring, unavoidable, and severe pain and if the effect of the treatment would be to extend life in an inhumane fashion. If the patient had expressed a wish to be kept alive regardless of his or her physical status, the life-sustaining treatment would be implemented and would not be withdrawn.

The court's rationale for the three tests was that Miss Conroy, as an elderly nursing home patient, had needs that differed from patients in acute care settings. Miss Conroy had suffered significant changes in physical and mental capacity: she had not indicated advance oral or written directives; her nephew had petitioned the court for removal of the nasogastric tube feedings; and she had limited access to an institutional review of that treatment decision.

NURSING INTERVENTIONS AND OUTCOMES

The problems presented in Miss Conroy's situation are not unique. Many elderly Americans must make serious and often life-sustaining health care treatment decisions with minimal family or social support while suffering from disabling physical impairments. It is vital that nurses understand the wishes and preferences of elderly patients. As a primary caregiver, the nurse is often in a unique position to communicate with the patient both verbally and nonverbally. Nurses are especially well qualified to identify and document the stated wishes or reactions of the patient to health care problems and interventions. Nurses are also qualified to identify and

document changes in the patient's physiologic or psychosocial responses to the health care process.

Nurses are possibly the "last friend" of the elderly client.[56] This bond may serve to comfort or support the patient at a time of stress or crisis. Nurses are more visible at the bedside and may have intimate and influential contact with the client at the critically important decision-making moment.[57] Thus, nurses must recognize the right of an elderly person to self-determination and facilitate an exploration of advance directives for health care treatment decisions.

SUMMARY

Many questions may arise when the patient must make health care treatment decisions. These questions are:

1. Is the patient able to make health care treatment decisions?
2. If not, has the patient made prior written or oral statements regarding potential health care treatment decisions?
3. If there are no directives to indicate the patient's wishes, then how are those health care treatment decisions to be made?

Nurses are in a unique position to identify and document information to resolve these questions. This chapter discusses the role of the nurse in assisting the dependent elderly to exercise the right of self-determination. Nurses must understand the right of privacy, the use of advance directives, and the role of substitute decision makers.

Endnotes

1 Matter of Conroy, 98 N.J. 321, 486 A.2d 1209 (1985).
2 Matter of Conroy, 98 N.J. 321, 346 486 A.2d 1209, 1221 (1985). *Citing* Union Pacific Railroad Co. v Botsford, 141 U.S. 250, 251, 11 S.Ct. 1000, 1001, 35 L.Ed. 734, 737 (1891).
3 Schloendorff v. Society of New York Hospital, 211 N.Y. 125, 129-130, 105 N.E. 92, 93 (1914).
4 TM Cooley, A Treatise On The Law Of Torts (National Textbook Series) 29 (1930).
5 Griswold v Connecticut, 381 U.S. 479, 85 S.Ct. 1678, 14 L.Ed.2d 510 (1965).
6 Roe v Wade, 410 U.S. 113, 93 S.Ct. 705, 35 L.E.2d 147 (1973).
7 Griswold v Connecticut, 381 U.S. 479, 85 S.Ct. 1678, 14 L.Ed.2d 510 (1965).
8 Superintendent of Belchertown v Saikewicz, 370 N.E.2d 417, 424 (Mass. 1977) *quoting* Pratt v Davis 118 Ill.App. 161, 166 (1905), aff'd 224 Ill. 300, 79 N.E.562 (1906).
9 Matter of Quinlan, 70 N.J. 10, 40, 355 A.2d 647, 663 (1976).

10 Brophy v New England Sinai Hosp., Inc., 398 Mass 417, 497 N.E.2d 626 (Mass. 1986).

11 Id.

12 Matter of Conroy, 98 N.J. 321, 486 A.2d 1209 (1985); President's Commission for the Study of Ethical Problems in Medicine and Biomedical and Behavioral Reseach, Deciding to Forego Life-Sustaining Treatment [hereinafter President's Commission] 32 (1983); Matter of Spring, 380 Mass 629, 405 N.E.2d 115 (1980); Superintendent of Belchertown v Saikewicz 370 N.E.2d 417 (Mass. 1977).

13 Somers, *In re Conroy: Self Determination: Extending the Right to Die*, 2 Journal of Contemporary Health Law and Policy 351, 361 (1986).

14 Matter of Conroy, 98 N.J. 321, 351, 486 A.2d 1209, 1224 (1985).

15 Superintendent of Belchertown v Saikewicz, 370 N.E.2d 417 (Mass. 1977); Matter of Quinlan, 70 N.J. 10, 355 A.2d 647 (1976); President's Commission, supra note 12 at 38 (1983).

16 Matter of Conroy, 98 N.J. 321, 353, 486 A.2d 1209, 1225 (1985); Application of President and Directors of Georgetown College, Inc. 331 F.2d 1000, 1008 (D.C.Cir), *cert. denied*, 377 U.S. 978, 83 S.Ct. 1883, 12 L.Ed.2d 746 (1964).

17 Jacobson v Massachusetts, 197 U.S. 11, 25 S.Ct. 358, 49 L.Ed. 643 (1905).

18 President's Commission, supra note 12 at 40 (1983).

19 Id.

20 Matter of Conroy, 98 N.J. 321, 352, 486 A.2d 1209, 1224 (1985).

21 Id at 352–353, 1225.

22 Hoffland, *Autonomy in long term care: Background issues and a programmic response. Gerontologist* (June) 1988; 28 (supplementary issue): 3.

23 Matter of Conroy, 98 N.J. 321, 344, 486 A2d 1209, 1220 (1985).

24 Carroll-Johnson R (editor): *Classification of Nursing Diagnoses: Proceedings of the Eighth Conference.* Lippincott 533 (1989).

25 Lane v Candura, 6 Mass. App. 377, 376 N.E.2d 1232 (1978).

26 In re Storar, 52 N.Y.2d 363, 420 N.E.2d 64 (1981).

27 Brophy v New England Sinai Hospital, Inc., 398 Mass 417, 497 N.E.2d 626 (1986).

28 Superintendent of Belchertown v Saikewicz, 370 N.E.2d 417 (Mass. 1977).

29 Id at 430.

30 Id.

31 Bartling v Superior Court, 163 Cal. App. 3d 186, 209 Cal, Rptr. 220 (1984).

32 Society for the Right to Die, Newsletter, Spring 1989.

33 Uniform Rights of the Terminally Ill Act (U.L.A.).

34 Id at prefatory note.

35 Id.

36 Id at § 3.

37 Id at § 4.

38 Id at prefatory note.

39 Cohn, *The Living Will from the Nurse's Perspective.* 11 Law, Medicine & Health Care 121 (1983).

40 John F. Kennedy Memorial Hosp. v Bludworth, 452 So.2d 921, 922 (Fla. 1984).

41 Id at 926.

42 Restatement, Second, Agency § 1.

43 Id at § 133.

44 Uniform Durable Power of Attorney Act (U.L.A.) § 1 and comments.

45 Id at § 1.

46 Id.

47 Id.

48 Id.

49 Marzan, the *"Uniform Rights of the Terminally Ill Act"*: A *Critical Analysis* 1 Issues in Law and Medicine 441 (1986).

50 Matter of Conroy, 98 N.J. 321, 486 A.2d 1209 (1985).

51 Matter of Quinlan, 70 N.J. 10, 355 A.2d 647 (1976).

52 Matter of Conroy, 98 N.J. 321, 364, 486 A.2d 1209, 1231 (1985).

53 Kapp M.: *Preventing Malpractice in Long-Term Care: Strategies for Risk Management* 114 (1987).

54 Matter of Conroy, 98 N.J. 321, 365, 486 A.2d 1209, 1232 (1985).

55 Id.

56 Grant and Forsythe, *The Plight of the Last Friend: Legal Issues for Physicians and Nurses in Providing Nutrition and Hydration* 2 Issues in Law and Medicine 277, 1987.

57 Kapp M, Bigot A:*Geriatrics and the Law*, 1985.

IX

Sexuality–Reproductive Pattern

KATHLEEN BUCKWALTER, PhD, RN, FAAN
MERIDEAN MAAS, PhD, RN, FAAN

Overview

IN CHAPTER 50, KERFOOT, BUCKWALTER, AND Maas analyze the often ignored diagnosis of Sexual Dysfunction in the institutionalized elderly. From the perspective that dysfunction can be determined only by the individual, the authors examine the psychologic, physiologic, and cultural roots of this diagnosis. They thoroughly explain normal changes in sexual responsiveness associated with aging, emphasizing that these changes do not necessarily denote dysfunction. Myths and misinformation surrounding the topic of sexuality and older adults are debunked, and several interventions to facilitate healthy sexual expression in the elderly are set forth. These include sexual counseling; sex education for the elderly, their partners, family members, and staff; and environmental restructuring.

49

Normal Changes With Aging

DONNA BUNTEN, MA, RN
MARY A. HARDY, PhD, RN, C

Definition:

The sexuality-reproductive pattern describes clients' satisfaction and dissatisfaction with sexuality pattern; it also describes reproductive patterns.

THE ELDERLY ARE DEALT A GREAT INJUSTICE BY A society that believes that sex is not desired, necessary, or possible in advanced age. It is not "normal" or "nice" for older persons to be interested in sex or having intercourse (Lobsenz, 1981). In a time when more tolerant attitudes toward sexual self-determination are becoming prevalent, the elderly are perceived differently. We are all familiar with the "dirty old man" and the more recent "dirty old woman" jokes and other disparaging stories about geriatric lovemaking. Yet, young people do not have a monopoly on sexuality. Societal attitudes may cause the elderly to shut off sexual feelings out of shame and embarrassment about having them or because they fear the ridicule or censure of younger persons.

Four major studies of human sexual behavior (Kinsey et al, 1948, 1953; Masters and Johnson, 1966; Pfeiffer et al, 1968) demonstrated that a majority of men and women in later years want and are able to have a satisfying sexual life. The studies also indicated that those persons who were most sexually active during their youth and middle years are more likely to retain their sexual interest and vigor longer into old age. Masters and Johnson (1966, 1982) clinically tested older persons regarding their sexual responses to get a detailed picture of the aging body's physiologic reactions. They found that aging does slow down a man's capacity for erection and climax and a woman's capacity to achieve orgasm, but none of these responses are ended by the aging process. Moreover, it was discovered that these changes may increase an older person's pleasure in sexual activity.

Assuming that older people are in reasonably good health, the main factors responsible for any loss of sexual responsiveness are primarily social or psychologic. Byers (1983) identified six categories of barriers to sexuality: (1) monotony of a repetitious sexual relationship; (2) mental or physical fatigue; (3) overindulgence in food or drink; (4) preoccupation with career or economic pursuits; (5) physical or mental infirmities of either partner; and (6) anxiety about performance related to any of the above. Biologic changes do occur in both the female and male reproductive systems with advancing age, but none of the changes should negate the possibility of the elderly achieving a satisfying sexual life if they have the desire and a partner.

Many of the physical changes in the reproductive system of older women are related to a decrease in the output of female sex hormones after menopause. A reduction in circulating estrogen levels causes less acidic vaginal secretions and a thinning of the vaginal walls. Lubrication of the vagina may be reduced during sexual excitement because there are fewer and less effective Batholin glands. The vagina itself is shorter and the lumen is smaller because of reduced elasticity of the structural walls. As muscle tone diminishes generally in the aging body, reduced estrogen contributes to atrophy in the breasts, vulva, and clitoris. Other changes that are apparent in the external genitalia include less pubic hair, less subcutaneous fat, and flattened labial folds. None of these changes should preclude sexual gratification if the elderly woman is at ease with her sexuality.

Changes that occur in men as they age include reduced testoterone, prostatic hypertrophy, and sclerosing of penile arteries and veins. Although more time is required to achieve a full erection, there is no evidence that a normally healthy man loses his ability to achieve and maintain erection during coitus solely as a result of aging. On orgasm, the older man ejaculates a smaller amount of seminal fluid with less forcefulness. Forty-eight percent of sperm-producing tubules in men between 80 and 90 years of age produce potent spermotozoa (Rockstein and Sussman, 1979). The time it takes for a man to have another erection and climax after ejaculation increases with age. As is the case with many other physiologic changes that are seen with aging, most causes of sexual dysfunction in the male are due to iatrogenic factors like drugs and surgery (Burnside, 1988).

Demographics and cultural standards combine to affect the ability of some subgroups of the elderly to express and fulfill sexual needs. Older women are especially at risk. U.S. Department of Census data show that half of all older women in 1985 were widows and that there were over five times as many widows as widowers (American Association of Retired Persons/Administration on Aging, 1986). In terms of sheer availability of partners, older men have a far better statistical opportunity for sexual expression. It is also important to consider that elderly cohorts have grown up in an era when men took the sexual initiative, when nonmarital sex was more available to men, and when "illicit" sex was a transgression that was not as serious for a man as for a woman. Cultural patterns of youth tend to follow a person into advanced years.

Institutionalized elderly are at high risk of finding themselves in an environment that is not conducive to sexual expression. Institutional rules, governmental regulations, and staff attitudes combine to limit opportunities for fulfillment of the need for intimacy and other desires. These factors are critical when one considers that 35% or

more of older adults are estimated to be at a risk of being institutionalized at some time (Liang and Tu, 1986). Sexuality must not be entirely equated with coitus. The more basic need for intimacy (physically maintained through touching, stroking, patting, hugging, and emotionally maintained by sharing joy, sorrow, affection, ideas, and values) is lifelong (Abbink, 1983). Health care providers must understand and respect the elderly's need for intimacy and provide opportunities for the fulfillment of this aspect of sexuality (Allen, 1987; Travis, 1988).

References

Abbink C: Adult development and the impact of disruption. In: *Medical Surgical Nursing.* Lewis S, Collier I (editors). McGraw-Hill, 1983.

Allen ME: *Holistic Nursing Practice.* Aspen, 1987.

American Association of Retired Persons and Administration on Aging, Department of Health and Human Services: *A Profile of Older Americans—1986.* American Association of Retired Persons Publication No. PF 3049(1086)-D996, 1986.

Burnside IM: Intimacy and sexuality. *Nursing and the Aged,* 3d ed. McGraw-Hill, 1988.

Byers JP: Sexuality and the elderly. *Geriatr Nurs* 1983; 4: 293-297.

Kinsey AC et al: *Sexual Behavior in the Human Male.* Saunders, 1948.

Kinsey AC et al: *Sexual Behavior in the Human Female.* Saunders, 1953.

Liang J, Tu E: Estimating lifetime risk of nursing home residency—a further note. *Gerontologist* 1986; 26:560-563.

Lobsenz NM: Sex and the senior citizen. In: *Aging in America: Readings in Social Gerontology.* Kart CS, Manard BM (editors). Alfred, 1981.

Masters W, Johnson V: *Human Sexual Response.* Little, Brown, 1966.

Masters W, Johnson V: Sex and the aging process. *Med Aspects Human Sexuality* 1982; 16(6):40-57.

Pfeiffer E, Verwoerdt A, Wang HS: Sexual behavior in aged men and women. *Arch Gen Psychiatry* 1968; 19:753-758.

Rockstein M, Sussman M: The reproduction system. In: *Biology of Aging.* Rockstein M, Sussman M (editors). Wadsworth, 1979.

Travis SS: Older adults' sexuality and remarriage. *J Gerontol Nurs* 1987; 13(6):9-14.

50

Sexual Dysfunction in the Elderly

Karlene M. Kerfoot, PhD, RN

Kathleen C. Buckwalter, PhD, RN, FAAN

Meridean Maas, PhD, RN, FAAN

FOR US

Sex after sixty a delightful pleasure,
To be sipped, enjoyed and savored at leisure.
No tearing away at undershorts, zippers,
No frantic fumbling of hooks and grippers.
Time to explore those still unknown—
Each and every erogenous zone.
No fretful, teething baby's cry
To interrupt a lover's sigh.
Just the warmth of each other's embrace,
Fingers tracing a familiar face.
No more worry about periods due,
We've indulged before, but forever it's new.
And when we total up the accounts,
It's quality, not quantity, that counts.

(Friedlander in Hays, AM,
Journal of Geriatric Psychiatry 1984; 17:161–165

OUR SOCIETY FOSTERS THE COMMON STEREOTYPE that sexuality ends as aging progresses (Walz and Blum, 1987). Many young people mistakenly assume that their elders are not sexually active, and some have difficulty imagining that their parents or other respected older adults actually make love. Puritanical approaches to senior citizens, dormant Oedipal fears, and incest taboos associated with sexual expression in our parents and grandparents may inhibit acceptance of sexuality in the aging population (Falk and Falk, 1980).

Love and sex between people of disparate ages are often not accepted. Relationships between older women and younger men are judged particularly harshly. Family members may wrongfully assume that financial exploitation is involved or neurotic needs are the motivation for these relationships. However, May–December relationships can flourish quite successfully.

Our Social Security and retirement systems, by levying financial penalties, encourage older adults to cohabit rather than marry. Widows in particular face loss of pensions and other benefits if they remarry. Children occasionally have difficulty accepting their parent's choice of lifestyle, making the older cohabiting couple uncomfortable and inducing tremendous guilt.

Attitudes toward sexuality can hamper health care outcomes (Walz and Blum, 1987). Health practitioners frequently have difficulty addressing the sexual needs of the older person. The older patient, in turn, often has difficulty discussing sexuality and can easily repress sexual feelings or feel shame and embarrassment about having these feelings (Woods, 1979). Many older people believe that sexual exertion is dangerous to their health. They may also fear the ridicule and censure of younger people if they display interest in sexuality.

Individuals in retirement communities and nursing homes are usually faced with prescriptive regulations about sexual expression (Walz and Blum, 1987). If health professionals and administrators felt more comfortable about the elderly's sexuality, then more privacy for petting, uninterrupted time for masturbation, and the support of warm, affectionate relationships between people in nursing homes could be provided.

SIGNIFICANCE FOR THE ELDERLY

Classic studies by Kinsey (1948, 1953) and Masters and Johnson (1966, 1970, 1981) showed that older people in good health were physiologically able to maintain satisfying sexual relationships. The most important determinant of satisfying sexual activity in older adulthood was an active sexual lifestyle in the younger years.

Older people have the freedom to explore a wider emotional range of sexuality unencumbered by considerations of birth control and the drive for purely physical pleasure. Sexual activity can be an opportunity to experience communication at its intimate best, a transformation of sexuality and communication into a higher state of awareness. Sexual intimacy can include touching, holding, caressing, massaging, and sexual teasing. Orgasm may or may not be part of this communication (Comfort, 1976).

William Masters and Virginia Johnson first documented the physiology of the sexual response cycle in older people. Their most important finding was that sexual responsiveness was physiologically possible throughout the older years. According to Masters and Johnson (1966), reaction time to sexual stimuli slowed as men aged. Men who had responded to physical caressing with an erection within 30 seconds when younger could require 3 minutes or longer for a similar response to appear as they aged. However, erections could be sustained for longer periods of time. Preejaculate fluid diminished and eventually disappeared, and the ejaculate contained less seminal fluid and semen. Orgasm often was shorter in duration, and the feeling of ejaculatory urgency diminished. Older males experienced more rapid loss of erection after orgasm and were unable to sustain a second erection as readily. The time between orgasms lengthened to several days, and ejaculation was not achieved with each session of intercourse. However, an ejaculate was likely to occur within three intercourse experiences. Older males also were subject to fatigue as an inhibitor of sexual responsiveness.

Masters and Johnson (1966) also found that with the onset of menopause, women experienced some changes due to alterations in hormone levels. Response time became slower, vaginal lubrication took longer, and the vagina became smaller and less elastic and expanded more slowly to accommodate the penis. The walls of the vagina became thin and smooth, and the external genitalia became soft and less structured. Older women complained of pain with intercourse because their abdominal organs were not cushioned by thick vaginal walls. Although clitoral size and the number of contractions at orgasm reduced, older women were able to become orgasmic and were more satisfied because of their male partner's ability to sustain erection for longer periods of time. Some older women reported uterine spasm that appeared as pain in the lower abdomen and radiated down the legs. Irritability and pain in the bladder and urethra and an urgency to urinate immediately after intercourse also occurred.

For women with severe physiologic changes, steroid replacement may increase vaginal thickness and lubrication and decrease uterine spasms. Lubrication of the vagina to replace the normal lubrication is indicated (Walz and Blum, 1987). Different positions of intercourse and alternate sexual techniques can solve most related problems.

SEXUAL DYSFUNCTION IN THE ELDERLY

At the Seventh Conference, the North American Nursing Diagnosis Association (NANDA) proposed that the nursing diagnosis Sexual Dysfunction be defined as "the state in which an individual experiences a change in sexual function that is viewed as unsatisfying, unrewarding or inadequate" (McLane, 1987;493).

The key to understanding this diagnosis is to consider the perspective of the older person. People who have never been comfortable with sex, who were not sexually active in their younger years, and who express no desire for a sexual relationship might regard themselves as perfectly normal. In contrast, older persons who are sexually active might be considered dysfunctional by their peers because they do not support the concept of diminishing or absent sexuality. Therefore, it behooves the nurse to consider the older person's definition of healthy sexuality before evaluating degree of health or dysfunction (Eliopoulos, 1979).

ETIOLOGIES/RELATED FACTORS

Sexual Dysfunction in the elderly can be associated with multiple etiologies, including psychologic, sociologic, and institutional changes. Table 50.1 contrasts the factors related to Sexual Dysfunction suggested by NANDA (Carroll-Johnson, 1989) with those set forth in this chapter.

Sexual Dysfunction can have both physiologic and psychologic origins. A physiologic slowing down of sexual response time is normal in the aged. An acceptance of

Table 50.1

Etiologies/Related Factors of Sexual Dysfunction in the Elderly

NANDA (CARROLL-JOHNSON, 1989)	KERFOOT
Related Factors	*Etiologies*
Biopsychosocial alteration of sexuality	Institutionalization
Ineffectual or absent role models	Sensory-perceptual
Physical abuse	Decreased mobility
Psychosocial abuse, eg, harmful relationships	Decreased self-care ability
Vulnerability	Social isolation
Misinformation or lack of knowledge	Grieving/loss of partner
Values conflict	Disturbance in self-concept
Lack of privacy	Illness/drugs
Lack of significant other	
Altered body structure or function:	
pregnancy, recent childbirth, drugs, surgery, anomalies,	
disease process, trauma, radiation	
Misinformation or lack of knowledge	

slower response time can enable older couples to express sexuality in a variety of ways. Without this acceptance couples may react with panic, become emotionally distraught, and be unable to perform.

Sexual function is also clearly related to cultural and personal expectations. Psychologic Sexual Dysfunction induced by peer pressure, assignment of stigma, and lack of support in this culture for sexual activities among the aged can create physiologic changes as well.

Sexual Dysfunction Related to Institutionalization

Many hospitals, residential homes for older people, and nursing homes do not support and foster healthy sexual expression in the elderly. Institutional staff frequently believe the elderly are asexual and reflect this belief in their environments (Walz and Blum, 1987; Wasow and Loeb, 1979).

Rarely do institutions provide privacy for older persons to touch and hold one another, to participate in masturbation, or to explore any other means to gain intimacy, relatedness, and a sense of self-esteem. Access to partners for intimate and emotional sexual contact also can be lost with institutionalization, resulting in sexual dysfunction and depression.

Sexual expression encompasses touching, holding, cuddling, the intimacy of personal relationship, and the relaxation that comes from a companion's massage, as well as intercourse. Institutions and the staff who work in them need to support these activities so that residents can find more fulfillment in their later years.

Sexual Dysfunction Related to Sensory-Perceptual Deficits

Loss of sensory-perceptual clues to the environment progresses with age, blunting perception of sexual cues. As hearing decreases, the ability to assimilate romantic innuendos decreases. Stronger and more frequent touch is often necessary to arouse the same amount of stimulation as in younger years. The overpowering sexual impact of another person lessens, and the lack of stimulation can cause sexual dysfunction.

Sexual Dysfunction Related to a Decrease in Physical Mobility and Self-Care Deficit

Many medical and psychologic conditions can result in permanent handicapping. When physical mobility is limited by assistive devices or frailty, both self-care ability and self-esteem can diminish. Accepting and loving one's body in spite of the alterations that handicapping conditions can bring is critical to sexual health in the later years (Verkuyl, 1975).

Sexual Dysfunction Related to Social Isolation

The lack of available partners and negative proscriptions regarding sexuality often lead to social isolation and consequent sexual disturbance. This is somewhat of a gender-specific issue in that men have access to younger partners more readily than do older women. The high percentage of widows among the elderly means a decreased number of partners for older women. Further, older women are not valued as sexual partners by younger men to the extent that older men are valued by younger women. Many older people, especially women, long for touch, intimacy, caressing, and holding, and they feel unfulfilled without intimacy. This isolation may worsen with advancing decades.

Sexual Dysfunction Due to Grieving or Loss of Partner

Loss of a partner also can produce Sexual Dysfunction problems. During the grief process, interest in sexual activity may decline secondary to reactive depression. When sexual activity is initially resumed, lack of practice and fear of failure and the appearance of anxiety can interfere with sexual functioning. The guilt experienced with renewed sexual activity can also inhibit strong sexual feelings and responses. With continued engagement in sexual activity, however, satisfactory responsiveness returns (Masters and Johnson, 1981).

Sexual Dysfunction Due to a Disturbance in Self-Concept

Elderly persons must reconcile their self-image with age-related bodily changes. Perceptions of changes in sexual organs and responses to those changes can be either positive or negative. For some people physiologic changes greatly interfere with their perception of themselves as sexual persons. Sexual Dysfunction therefore can result from decreased self-concept and body image changes. Chapter 36 on Body Image Disturbance and Chapter 40 on Self-Esteem Disturbance expand on these problems for the elderly.

Sexual Dysfunction Related to Illness or Drugs

Many illnesses directly affect older persons' ability to engage in sexual activity. Chronic conditions such as arthritis, hypertension, and cardiac problems may require changes in the technique of sexual expression. In addition, many medications taken by the elderly affect sexual ability (Kaplan, 1974). Yet, with appropriate assessment, rehabilitation, and counseling, sexual activity can continue in spite of health-related problems.

ASSESSMENT

Specific techniques and principles for history taking in sexuality can be used with elderly clients (Hogan, 1980). The nurse must obtain information about sexual beliefs and practices and about psychologic, physiologic, sociologic, environmental, and medical treatment factors that will influence sexuality. Once the nurse has obtained this information, a determination of the presence of Sexual Dysfunction can be made (Wilson, 1975).

The ability to conduct a sexual interview with an older person is a skill that can be learned. Interviewers must be aware of their own feelings about sexuality in the aged and not project their personal attitudes and beliefs onto others. Nurses must display willingness to discuss sexuality and an acceptance of the older person's sexual lifestyle. It also is important for the nurse conducting an assessment to communicate in words the older person is most comfortable using. For example an older person might prefer the term *sleeping together* to *intercourse*.

The nurse must be knowledgeable about ways that illness and drugs affect sexuality in order to assess elderly persons effectively. Many clients expect that health professionals will ask questions about sexuality and are surprised when they do not. However, the following techniques are suggested by Green (1975) to assist in discussion of sexuality with elderly people:

1. When the interview is initiated, the nurse should tell the elderly person that sexuality is an important part of life and that illness, medications, and stress often alter sexual functioning.
2. Tell the elder that questions about sexuality will be asked and that the nurse will answer any questions about sexuality.
3. Using prefaces to questions that let the elder know that many elderly persons experience what is being discussed.
4. Begin with least sensitive topics and proceed to more sensitive ones.
5. Summarize the interview to reinforce the elder's learning and leave ample time for questions.

The nurse must be sensitive to the elder's feelings in deciding what questions should be asked and how probing the questions should be. A belief that sexuality is a normal, everyday part of life; knowledge and practice with interviewing; and knowledge of how illness and treatments can affect sexual function are essential for the nurse to be able to assess and intervene for the problem of Sexual Dysfunction in the elderly.

Walz and Blum (1987) have suggested that persons working with the elderly can increase their understanding of sexuality in this population through a personal knowledge assessment tool they developed, the Adult Sexuality Knowledge and Attitude Test (ASKAT) (Walz and Blum, 1986).

The defining characteristics of Sexual Dysfunction in the elderly are listed in Table 50.2 and contrasted with those cited by NANDA (Carroll-Johnson, 1989).

CASE STUDY

Sexual Dysfunction

Mr. Ames was admitted to the hospital at the age of 78 for a heart attack. His 72-year-old wife stayed with him throughout his hospitalization. After 1 week, he was discharged and recovered well from his illness.

Mr. and Mrs. Ames had enjoyed an active sexual lifestyle, including nightly backrubs and massages before retiring, caressing and holding each other, and verbally expressing sexual innuendos. Intercourse had continued into their older years, although orgasm was not experienced on every occasion. Mrs. Ames perceived herself as someone who enjoyed sex and needed the closeness of a physical relationship.

Mrs. Ames believed that her interest in sexuality had placed strain on Mr. Ames, precipitating the heart attack. She was unable to discuss her thoughts with anyone during his hospitalization and assumed that sexual activity could never again be a part of their lives. She became fearful of future heart attacks and ceased any activities that she thought might put stress on her husband's heart. As Mr. Ames recuperated, he sought out the close touching and massage activities he had enjoyed before. Mrs. Ames would neither participate nor verbalize her fears. Mr. Ames interpreted her behavior as lack of interest in him, and his self-esteem diminished.

NURSING INTERVENTIONS

Sexocentrism is the belief that one way to express sexuality is best and that individuals who deviate from that standard are not sexually healthy. Sexocentrism has led health professionals to make themselves the "ethical gurus" of our society (Szasz, 1974). Yet the definition of sexuality is culturally and personally specific. Professionals should concentrate on the health aspects of sexuality and let specialists in ethics and religion recommend societal norms. Avoiding judgment and working within the individual's personal choices and preferences are prerequisite to intervening in the area of sexuality. The interventions most appropriate for nurses to use are sexual counseling, sex education, and environmental structuring.

Sexual Counseling

Sexual counseling is a broad approach that includes assessment, active listening, encouragement of effective coping mechanisms and use of humor, reinforcement of healthy sexual practices, and identification of medications and health deviations that may affect sexuality and body image. A critical aspect of assessment is to determine the older person's attitudes and willingness to discuss sexual beliefs, values, and behaviors. This nursing intervention is distinguished from sexual therapy techniques such as systematic desensitization that require expertise with specific sexual disorders. Nurses should assess sexual functioning and counsel regarding feelings, behaviors, and myths (Kaplan, 1974), and refer elderly clients who require more specialized treatment to a sexual therapist (Kerfoot and Buckwalter, 1985).

Sexual counseling should first focus on encouraging persons to disclose their beliefs and feelings of guilt. The nurse can clear up beliefs that are myths and provide encouraging support. However, premature reassurance should be avoided. It is not helpful to interrupt or terminate the disclosure of guilt feelings by reassuring elderly clients that they have done nothing wrong. Persons with dysfunctional guilt should be encouraged to consider referral for psychotherapy or for counseling by a member of the clergy.

Table 50.2

Defining Characteristics of Sexual Dysfunction in the Elderly

NANDA (CARROLL-JOHNSON, 1989)	KERFOOT
Verbalization of problem	Verbalization of problem
Alteration in achieving perceived sex role	Actual or perceived inability to perform
Actual or perceived limitation imposed by disease and/or therapy	Lack of access to sexual partner
Conflicts involving values	Actual or perceived limitation imposed by disease and/or therapy
Alterations in achieving sexual satisfaction	Recent loss of spouse or sexual partner
Inability to achieve desired satisfaction	Verbalization of "myths" or misinformation about sexual activity by elderly
Seeking of confirmation of desirability	
Alteration in relationship with significant other	
Change of interest in self and others	

For a more detailed discussion of the nursing intervention sexual counseling, including specific counseling techniques, the reader is referred to Kerfoot and Buckwalter's chapter on sexual counseling in Bulechek and McCloskey's (1985) book *Nursing Interventions: Treatments for Nursing Diagnoses.*

Sexual Education

Nurses also need to provide information that will prevent future sexual problems for the elderly. Information to dispel commonly shared myths can prevent or correct misunderstandings about healthy sexual behavior. Older people need to know that sexual drive can remain into the seventies and beyond. They should be aware that sexuality is healthy and normal, something to be enjoyed. Specific techniques such as alternate positions can be taught to senior citizens to enhance their enjoyment of sexuality.

Older people need access to information about how to cope with illness and medication-related problems in order to preserve and enhance their sexual lifestyle. Some persons might decide to quit taking medications that interfere with sexual performance. The nurse needs to be alert to this possibility when treatment regimens appear to be failing. If an accurate assessment is done and side effects that interfere with sexual activity are discovered, the nurse should confer with the physician to seek another equally beneficial medication or arrange for an alternative administration schedule.

Education of the spouse or sexual partner is also important. Both the sexually impaired person and the partner need to be informed about options such as caressing, massaging, and masturbation, so that they can enjoy mutually agreeable alternatives. Sexual partners can have varying perceptions of the appropriateness of sexual activities. Their divergent belief systems must be negotiated so that they can engage in a mutually agreeable set of activities. Intensive educational work is often indicated for children, grandchildren, or other relatives who attempt to dictate forms of sexual expression to their elderly kin (Guarino and Knowlton, 1980).

Environmental Structuring

The environment can play a critical role in the inducement or prohibition of sexual expression, especially in long-term care institutions. Lack of privacy and negative staff attitudes inhibit satisfying sexual expression. The nurse is in a critical position to structure the environment appropriately for each elderly person (Griggs, 1978; Kas, 1978).

Group living does not encourage sexual expression and enjoyment. Staff need to arrange and assure privacy for elderly couples as well as for individuals who prefer to express their sexuality alone. The provision of sexual aids such as vibrators should also be considered.

Walz and Blum (1987) recommended areas with softer lighting, quiet spaces, and artwork depicting older persons enjoying intimacy. They also suggested candlelight meals with adult decorations, and perhaps even a cocktail hour to put elders in a more romantic mood (Walz and Blum, 1987:86).

CASE STUDY

Nursing Interventions

A nurse provided sexual counseling and sexual education to both partners in the case study situation. During a routine checkup visit, the nurse asked the Ames if they had questions about sexuality and the effect of the heart attack. Mr. Ames answered, "I'm all washed up. The heart attack did me in." The nurse pursued this theme and included Mrs. Ames in the conversation. Mr. Ames elaborated that people now treated him as an invalid and commented "Even my wife thinks I'm an old has-been." The nurse responded, "After a bout of illness many people believe that they cannot continue with the activities they were involved in prior to hospitalization. They are fearful to resume exercise, hobbies that gave them pleasure, sexual activities, and other interests. Have you had fears and questions about any of these areas?" Mrs. Ames began to cry and talked about fearing another heart attack. The nurse had given the couple an opportunity to discuss a serious matter for them. The nurse then discussed alternate positions and activities and assured them that sexual activities would not stress the heart further if proper precautions were respected. On subsequent visits, the Ames reported they had resumed their sexual activities without problems.

OUTCOMES

Outcomes must be negotiated with clients and measured in terms of client desires and lifestyle. Outcomes can take the form of maintaining the current level of health and sexual activity, restoring the client to a former state of functioning, or helping the client cope with deficits that cannot be prevented or ameliorated.

Evaluation of outcomes is a mutual process between the nurse and the client, with the client's viewpoint serving as the basis for evaluation. Failure to establish mutually agreed on outcomes and an evaluation procedure results in loss of progress and a sense of disillusionment.

SUMMARY

Aging can be a time of great growth and creativity or a time of hopelessness and depression. Intimacy and relatedness are important and essential aspects of all persons' lives. Nurses have the opportunity to help older people experience healthy sexual function, vigor, and fullness. As nurses work with community-dwelling persons and their families, and as they structure environments and cultures in nursing homes, they can help preserve the older person's self-esteem and access to sexuality. Addressing the sexual needs of older persons is an integral component of comprehensive nursing care.

References

Bulechek G, McCloskey J (editors). *Nursing Interventions: Treatments for Nursing Diagnoses*. Saunders, 1985.

Carroll-Johnson R (editor): *Nursing Diagnoses: Proceedings of the Eighth Conference*. Lippincott, 1989.

Comfort A: *A Good Age*. Crown, 1976; 195–197.

Eliopoulos CK: *Gerontological Nursing*. Harper and Row, 1979; 322–326.

Falk G, Falk UA: Sexuality and the aged. *Nurs Outlook* (Jan) 1980; 28:51–55.

Green R: *Human Sexuality: A Health Practitioner's Text*. Williams and Wilkins, 1975.

Griggs W: Staying well while growing old: Sex and the elderly. *Am J Nurs* (Aug) 1978; 1353–1354.

Guarino, SC, Knowlton CN: Planning and implementing a group health program on sexuality for the elderly. *J Gerontol Nurs* 1980; 6(10):600–603.

Hogan RM: *Human Sexuality: A Nursing Prospective*. Appleton-Century-Crofts, 1980; 403.

Kaplan HS: *The New Sex Therapy: Active Treatment of Sexual Dysfunction*. Brunner/Mazel, 1974.

Kas MJ: Sexual expression of the elderly in nursing homes. *Gerontologist* (Aug) 1978; 18:372–378.

Kerfoot K, Buckwalter KC: Sexual counseling. In: *Nursing Interventions: Treatments for Nursing Diagnoses*. Bulechek G, McCloskey J (editors). Saunders, 1985.

Kim M, McFarland T, McLane A: *Pocket Guide to Nursing Diagnoses*, 2d ed. Mosby, 1987.

Kinsey AC: *Sexual Behavior in the Human Male*. Saunders, 1948.

Kinsey AC: *Sexual Behavior in the Human Female*. Saunders, 1953.

Masters WH, Johnson VE: *Human Sexual Response*. Little, Brown, 1966.

Masters WH, Johnson VE: *Human Sexual Inadequacy*. Little, Brown, 1970.

Masters WH, Johnson VE: Sex and the aging process. *J Am Geriatr Soc* (Sept) 1981; 29(9):385–390.

McLane A (editor): *Nursing Diagnosis: Proceedings of the Seventh Conference*. Mosby, 1987.

Szasz T: *The Myth of Mental Illness*. Harper and Row, 1974.

Verkuyl A: Some neuromotor syndromes and their sexual consequences. Pages 173–179 in: *Human Sexuality: A Health Practitioner's Text*. Money J, Musaph H (editors). Williams and Wilkins, 1975.

Walz T, Blum N: *Adult Sexuality: Knowledge and Attitude Test*. University of Iowa, 1986.

Walz T, Blum N: *Sexual Health in Later Life*. Heath, 1987.

Wasow M, Loeb MB: Sexuality in nursing homes. *J Am Geriatr Soc* (Feb) 1979; 27:73–79.

Wilson RR: *Introduction to Sexual Counseling*. Carolina Populations Center, 1975.

Woods N: Sexuality in aging. Pages 151, 156–159 in: *Current Practice in Gerontological Nursing*. Reinhardt AM, Quinn MD (editors). Mosby, 1979.

X

Coping–Stress Tolerance Pattern

KATHLEEN BUCKWALTER, PhD, RN, FAAN
MERIDEAN MAAS, PhD, RN, FAAN

Overview

OLD AGE, ALONG WITH OTHER STAGES OF LIFE, involves adaptation to many changes. For the elderly, successful coping with losses of functional abilities can often avoid further losses such as forced removal from one's own home. In Chapter 52, Wilberding critically examines the nursing diagnosis Ineffective Individual Coping in terms of the validity of defining characterisics, suggesting that the diagnosis needs further development and clinical validation for maximum usefulness. Wilberding provides additional indicators and a conceptual basis for the diagnosis from a review of literature. He suggests that many coping behaviors may appear to be ineffective for certain persons when they are in fact effective for others. Cognitive reappraisal is discussed as an intervention to improve coping and offers outcomes that take the subjective nature of coping into account for evaluating the efficacy of nursing approaches.

51

Normal Changes With Aging

DONNA BUNTEN, MA, RN
MARY A. HARDY, PhD, RN, C

Definition:

The coping-stress pattern describes the general coping pattern and effectiveness of the pattern in terms of stress tolerance.

LOSSES OF FAMILY, FRIENDS, INCOME, AND SELF-WORTH that are common to aging can become overwhelming when they happen so close in time that coping mechanisms have not been internalized or when accompanied by declining cognitive status and health, diminishing support systems (Russell, 1986), and fading sensory perceptions (Nesbitt, 1988). Holmes and Rahe (1967) reported susceptibility to physical and mental health diseases as a result of being faced with these life stresses. Finally, the ever-increasing proximity to death that accompanies aging is a threat.

Views regarding the coping abilities and mechanisms of the elderly vary considerably. Jarvik and Russell (1979) suggested that neither fight nor flight are appropriate to the stresses of aging, and that aside from the fact that these responses are not usually available, the most likely response for the elderly is to "freeze." This view is contrasted with the assertion by Eisdorfer and Wilkie (1977) that studies of stress consistently suggest that relatively healthy aged individuals can and do successfully cope with the most stressful situations that occur in life. Although some may experience low morale and depression following a major life change, most eventually find a solution to problems.

Labouvis-Vief et al (1987) found that the ability to cope with stress was a function of developmental maturity rather than stressful situations or chronologic age. Dohrenwend and Shrout (1985) reported that a related variable, individual personality disposition, was one important component of life stress. These views are important in the treatment of stress in the elderly because coping with stress is viewed as a lifelong process one learns in order to adjust his or her needs to the demands of the environment. Thus, stress in and of itself should not be taken as detrimental to well-being. When an individual, by virtue of early developmental processes and other life experiences, is able to cope with the demands of life events, especially life changes (including daily hassles), stress may well be associated with growth. In fact, the experience of successfully coping with stress may be a precondition to the development of a mature personality and, hence, good mental health.

Older persons, like younger persons, have differing capacities for coping with life stresses and for coming to terms with their changing life situations. Given a supportive environment, older persons, like younger ones, will choose combinations of activities that offer the most ego involvement and that are most consonant with their self-concepts. As Havighurst (1968;67) states:

From a social psychological perspective aging is better viewed, not as a process of engagement or disengagement, but as a process of adaptation in which personality is the key element. The aging individual not only plays an active role in adapting to biological and social changes that occur with the passage of time, but in creating patterns of life that will give him the greatest ego involvement and life satisfaction.

References

Dohrenwend BP, Shrout PE: "Hassles" in the conceptualization and measurement of life stress variables. *Am Psychologist* 1985; 40:780–785.

Eisdorfer C, Wilkie F: Stress, disease, aging and behavior. In: *Handbook of the Psychology of Aging.* Birren JE, Schaie KW (editors). Van Nos Reinhold, 1977.

Havighurst RJ: A social-psychological perspective on aging. *Gerontologist* 1968; 8:67.

Holmes TH, Rahe RH: The social readjustment rating scale. *J Psychosomat Res* 1967; 11:213–218.

Jarvik LF, Russell D: Anxiety, aging, and the third emergency reaction. *J Gerontol* 1979; 34:197–201.

Labouvis-Vief G, Hakin-Larson J, Hobart C: Age, ego level, and the life-span development of coping and defense processes. *Psychology Aging* 1987; 2:286–293.

Nesbitt B: Nursing diagnosis in aggregated changes. *J Gerontol Nurs* 1988; 14(7):7–12.

Russell DW: *Stress, Social Support, and Physical and Mental Health Among the Elderly: A Longitudinal Causal Model.* Paper presented at the annual meeting of the Gerontological Society of America, Chicago, IL, 1986.

52

Ineffective Individual Coping

JAMES Z. WILBERDING, MA, RN

EACH STAGE OF LIFE PRESENTS CHANGES AND CHALlenges to which people must adapt. Old age is no exception. Elderly persons often face diminishing sensory capacities as well as changes in physical strength and agility. In a culture that values youth and physical strength as highly as ours does, normal changes of aging can be stressful. Additional adjustments to losses that often accompany aging can also be stressful (eg, moving out of one's home, facing institutionalization, and accepting care from younger people). *Coping* is a common term for successful adaptation to difficult or stressful conditions or events. In this chapter the nursing diagnosis Ineffective Individual Coping, as defined by the North American Nursing Diagnosis Association (NANDA), is examined, especially as it relates to the institutionalized elderly (Carroll-Johnson, 1989). The concept of coping is explored as a foundation for a discussion of the diagnosis and an appropriate intervention.

STRESS, ADAPTATION, AND COPING

Coping is directed toward adaptation in the face of a stressful problem. The terms *adaptation* and *stress* are often found together in the same context, which suggests that they are both related to the struggle for survival (Lazarus, 1966). Of stress, Lazarus (1966;27) wrote: "It seems wise to use 'stress' as a generic term for the whole area of problems that includes the stimuli producing stress reactions, the reactions themselves, and the various intervening processes." He further pointed out that stress may be sociologic, psychologic, or physiologic.

Selye (1956), an endocrinologist, approached stress from a biologic perspective and linked it with adaptation. Once stress has become operative in the biologic realm, the organism responds with adaptation. Stress causes the adaptation (Selye, 1956). Selye described two types of adaptation syndrome: the local adaptation syndrome (LAS) and the general adaptation syndrome (GAS). The LAS is a response to stress in a specific organ or tissue such as the inflammation of an eye caused by a toxic substance. The GAS consists of an alarm reaction, a stage of resistance, and finally a stage of exhaustion. LAS and GAS are interdependent, therefore activation of the LAS in a number of parts of the body can induce the GAS to function. Thus adaptation is carried out locally as long as the organism's requirements are met, but when the requirements involve a larger segment of body organs, the general adaptation syndrome is activated. Biologic adaptation, then, is characterized by both local and general syndromes of adaptation to stress or nonspecific changes in the biologic system (Selye, 1956;64).

The experience of stress has also been examined from a psychologic perspective. Janis (1958) described three phases of psychologic stress:

1. The *threat* phase, during which persons perceive signs of oncoming danger and/or receive communications of warning that are likely to arouse anticipatory fear

2. The *danger impact* phase, during which persons perceive that physical danger is actually at hand and realize that their chances of escaping intact depend partly on the protective actions executed by the self or by other people who are in a position to help them

3. The *postimpact victimization* phase, during which persons perceive the losses they have sustained and, at the same time, undergo some severe deprivations that continue for a varying length of time after the acute danger has subsided

Lazarus (1966;29) described psychologic stress as being indicated by "four main classes of reaction: reports of disturbed affects, motor-behavioral reactions, changes in the adequacy of cognitive functioning, and physiological changes, both biochemical and autonomic." Lazarus, like Janis, saw threat as intrinsic to psychologic stress. Threat involves appraisal or judgment, "is anticipatory or future-oriented, and . . . is brought about by cognitive processes involving perception, learning, memory, judgment, and thought" (Lazarus, 1966;30).

White (1974) gave emphasis to threat and looked at adaptation as a broad response to life conditions, delineating three variables of adaptation. The first is an appropriate amount of information necessary for action, with neither underload nor overload being desirable. Second, there should be physical and affective internal organization of the individual. Third, autonomy or freedom of action is important.

Whereas White (1974) outlined coping, mastery, and defense as strategies of adaptation, Lazarus (1966) focused primarily on coping as the mechanism of adaptation. As noted earlier, Lazarus emphasized the cognitive process of appraisal of a situation to determine the existence of threat. With regard to coping, Lazarus (1966;155) used the term *secondary appraisal*, which is "the cognitive process which determines the form of coping." He postulated a reappraisal process in which one's original perception of the situation is altered (Lazarus et al, 1974). Thus, appraisal determines whether adaptation is necessary (ie, whether threat exists), and secondary appraisal determines what type of adaptation (ie, coping strategy) would be effective. Reappraisal may eventually change one's original feeling of threat.

ADAPTATION TO SOCIAL STRESS

With regard to social stress, Levine and Scotch (1970;13) identified the following sources of stress: "the family, the work setting, social class position, and degree of urbanization." Outcomes in response to stress are physical, psychologic, and social in nature. Factors that Hinkle (1974) found to be related to health status were changes in activities, habits, ingestants, exposure to disease-causing agents, or physical characteristics of the environment.

In summary, stress or threat is present in the biologic, psychologic, and sociologic spheres of life. Adaptation is a response to these stressors or threats, and coping is one form of adaptation.

COPING

Coping is the behavior that people adopt when confronted with problems that place a greater than usual burden on their adaptive capabilities (Lazarus, 1966; Weisman, 1979; White, 1974). Opinions differ concerning whether coping includes the defense mechanisms such as denial, projection, or repression. Lipowski (1970) focuses on coping with illness and differentiates coping style from coping strategy. He includes defense mechanisms under the heading of coping style.

> *Coping style* refers to an individual's enduring disposition to deal with challenges and stresses with a specific constellation of techniques. This aspect includes both the tendency to the predominant use of certain defense mechanisms as well as manifestations of the individual's cognitive and perceptual styles (Lipowski, 1970;93).

Coping style is further differentiated as cognitive and behavioral coping styles. The cognitive styles consist of minimization of consequences through ignoring, denial, rationalization, and vigilant focusing. The behavioral coping styles consist of tackling, capitulating, and avoiding (Lipowski, 1970).

Lazarus et al (1974;250–251) defined coping as problem-solving efforts made by individuals when the demands they face are highly relevant to their welfare and when these demands tax adaptive resources. He believes there are two modes of expression of coping: "those that fundamentally entail direct action on the self or the environment, and those that function primarily through intra-psychic processes" (Lazarus et al, 1974;261). Several coping strategies fall within these modes. For example, an elderly person with diminishing vision may have the walls of her home painted a color that greatly contrasts with that of the floors to minimize confusion that could cause a fall. This would be acting on the environment. An elderly man may blame relatives for unintelligible mumbling in the face of audiometric tests indicating hearing loss. This coping strategy involves the intrapsychic processes of denial and projection.

Weisman (1979) differs with Lipowski in his attitude toward defense mechanisms. He writes: "A prerequisite for coping is to have a recognized problem which needs to be dealt with. In contrast, most people when they are being defensive do not realize what they are fending off " (Weisman, 1979;41). The distinction, then, between coping and use of defense mechanisms would depend on the user's recognition and acknowledgement of a problem, which seems to imply a value judgment on the use of defense mechanisms. This may also imply that if coping abilities become exhausted one falls back on defensive behaviors. Although such distinctions and implications are of theoretical interest, they may be of limited value clinically. If one believes that "coping may be defined as what one does about a problem in order to bring about relief, reward, quiescence, and equilibrium" (Weisman, 1979;27), then denial in some situations would seem to provide relief. As a matter of fact, Moos and Tsu (1977) list denial as one of seven coping skills used with physical illness.

Whether one separates defense mechanisms from coping mechanisms is often a moot point in clinical work with the elderly, who are faced with numerous losses and the changes of aging that place new demands on them. Nurses must be primarily concerned that the elderly client copes effectively.

ETIOLOGIES/RELATED FACTORS

Definitions

The Fourth National Conference on the Classification of Nursing Diagnosis defined four diagnoses related to coping: Coping, Ineffective Individual; Coping, Ineffective Family: Compromised; Coping, Ineffective Family: Disabling; and Coping, Family: Potential for Growth (Hurley, 1986). This discussion focuses on Ineffective Individual Coping, keeping in mind that most elderly people are part of some sort of kinship system that functions as a family. In practice it may be difficult to sort out Ineffective Individual Coping from the ineffective functioning of a family system. (See Chapter 46 on Altered Family Processes.)

The purpose of coping is adaptation and effective functioning in a threatening situation. In a discussion of ineffective coping, the first question that should be posed is, What indicates that coping is ineffective? Weisman (1979) has written that there are three essential facets of coping. First, there is a recognized problem from which one seeks relief, respite, and resolution. Second, what one does or does not do about that problem constitutes how one copes. Third, there is an outcome; however, there are no permanent guarantees about the long-term effectiveness of the coping strategy (Weisman, 1979;27).

The literature mentions very little, if anything, about determining the effectiveness of coping. Perhaps the unwritten assumption is that one casts about for a coping strategy until one finds something that eases the existential discomfort of the threat. This leads to the question, Is the effectiveness of a person's coping judged subjectively by that person, or can an objective assessment of its effectiveness be carried out by another person?

The North American Nursing Diagnosis Association (NANDA) has provided an answer to some of these questions in the definition, etiologies, and defining characteristics proposed for Ineffective Individual Coping. NANDA defines this diagnosis as "impairment of adaptive behaviors and problem-solving abilities of a person in meeting life's demands and roles" (Carroll-Johnson, 1989;538). This definition seems to place the problem in the coping behaviors, apparently reasoning that if the coping behavior is impaired, the result will be less-than-satisfactory adaptation. The NANDA etiologies are listed in Table 52.1 and compared with those of McFarland and Wasli. McFarland and Wasli (1987;158) provide a definition of Ineffective Individual Coping that is more in keeping with the theoretical bases of stress and adaptation; that is, "The patient is unable to formulate a useful appraisal of the stress, does not have an adequate response repertoire, and does not deploy his coping resources." They also delineate many more (eight versus three) etiologies for this nursing diagnosis, as listed in Table 52.1.

DEFINING CHARACTERISTICS

Verbalization of inability to cope or inability to ask for help and inability to problem solve are considered critical defining characteristics of this diagnosis (McLane, 1987). However, there may be circumstances in which withdrawal from a situation in which one could not problem solve would be effective coping. For example, a 72-year-old woman living in a home that is in need of multiple repairs may say, "I just don't know what to do about all of these things that need fixing." She may give up, sell the house, and make arrangements to live with one of her children, finding this solution satisfactory. She could not solve the problem, but by withdrawing, she solved it indirectly. Indeed, such withdrawal leads some elderly people to choose institutionalization. The point of this discussion is not to belittle nor vitiate this nursing diagnosis but rather to point out that it is not inherently valid or comprehensive in its present form. In fact, the diagnosis depends greatly on subjective value judgments.

Table 52.1

Ineffective Individual Coping

CARROLL-JOHNSON (1989)

Etiologies/Related Factors

Situational crises
Maturational crises
Personal vulnerability

Defining Characteristics

Verbalization of inability to cope or inability to ask for help
Inability to meet role expectations
Inability to meet basic needs
Inability to problem solve
Alteration in societal participation
Destructive behavior toward self or others
Inappropriate use of defense mechanisms
Change in usual communication patterns
Verbal manipulation
High illness rate
High rate of accidents

McFARLAND AND WASLI (1987)

Etiologies/Related Factors

Crisis, situational or maturational
Poor self-concept
Nervous system impairment (ie, sensory, perceptual, cognitive)
Severe pain
Conflict
Lack of social support system
Continued stress over period of time
Memory loss or memories of past stressful experiences, particularly negative ones

Defining Characteristics

Verbalization of inability to cope or inability to ask for help
Inaccurate cognitive appraisal
   Inability to recognize source of threat
   Inability to redefine or interpret threat correctly
   Inability to find meaning for the event
   Inability to identify the skills, knowledge, and abilities self has to cope with the threat
   Inability to formulate goals or outcomes
   Inability to make valid appraisal of the threat in context
Inadequate response repertoire
   Difficulty in expressing feelings, especially anger, fear, and guilt
   Use of behaviors destructive to self or others, such as suicide attempts, aggressive acts toward others, and use of alcohol and illicit drugs
   Inability to seek out or learn new skills and knowledge needed to resolve stress
   Inability to deal with tangible consequences of stress
   Increasing emotional responsiveness or lack of objective responsiveness
   Defensive avoidance of dealing with threatening situations
   Lack of assertive behaviors
   Impaired communication skills
   Lack of palliative skills
Inappropriate deployment of coping resources
   Inability to develop alternative goals, plans, actions, and rewards
   Lack of ability to transfer knowledge and/or skills to actual problem resolutions
   Relinquishment of hope and spiritual values
   Social withdrawal
   Difficulty in using problem-solving or decision-making skills
   Concerns and/or fears about initiating action
   Lack of an appropriate coping response because there is not a cognitive cue to act
   Lack of supportive social network
   Overuse of certain defense mechanisms, such as denial, projection, distortion, hypochondriasis, fantasy, intellectualization, repression, dissociation, and reaction formation
   Use of inappropriate behaviors, such as acting out, passive aggressiveness, and dependency
Inability to recover from stress episode
   Overdependence on significant others or professional help or institutions
   Nonproductive lifestyle
   Nonperformance of activities of daily living
   Lack of functioning in usual social roles
   Inertia or apathy
   Hypervigilance

Nevertheless, the etiologies and defining characteristics in Table 52.1 are what we currently have to work with.

One validation study of this diagnostic category has been published (Vincent, 1985). Ninety-four percent of the respondents (psychiatric clinical specialists) identified anxiety as "nearly always to frequently present" in people who are coping ineffectively, and 84% reported life stress in clients with ineffective coping. In response to an open-ended question, the clinical specialists identified depression and inability to sleep or eat properly as defining characteristics. Vincent (1985;637) concluded that "rather than eliminating any currently accepted behaviors from the category, the list can be expanded" to include anxiety, reported life stress, depression, and inability to sleep or eat properly. This presents an interesting situation in that she has included a psychiatric diagnosis, depression, as a defining characteristic of a nursing diagnosis (see Chapter 35). It may seem redundant to list impaired eating and sleeping as defining characteristics of the nursing diagnosis since they are symptoms of depression anyway. However, it is possible to have impaired eating and sleeping without depression, so they are not necessarily redundant. This discussion points out some of the difficulties involved in sorting out the phenomena distinctive to nursing. (Depressive behaviors such as anorexia and insomnia are also subjective and objective behavioral data that can indicate other nursing diagnostic phenomena.)

ASSESSMENT

Validation of the defining characteristics of the diagnosis Ineffective Individual Coping is important if clinicians are to assess elderly clients accurately. Wegmann (1984) briefly describes 10 different instruments purported to measure various aspects of coping. The research tools she describes are directed at determining what coping styles a subject uses rather than the effectiveness or ineffectiveness of coping. In this same vein Miller et al (1982) studied the reliability and validity of a semantic differential tool designed to measure the attitudes of cardiac patients toward their prescribed medical regimen. Because attitudes affect compliance, they suggest that the tool could be used with myocardial infarction (MI) patients to assist them to gain insight into their motivations and values regarding health behavior, and to assist in compliance. One of the subscales of the tool measures stress response, and coping is regarded as a stress response. Thus, this tool may contribute to the search for a clinical assessment tool.

Bedsworth and Molen (1982) used a four-question, open-ended interview in a qualitative study of psychologic stress in spouses of patients with myocardial infarction. The interview was clearly designed to elicit information about how the spouses coped. Again, however, the effectiveness of coping responses was not addressed.

Moving from the arena of research to clinical practice, Johnson-Saylor et al (1982) described a self-administered assessment form for determining patients' health status and coping responses that the authors used in their primary care practice. Although they expressed positive feelings about using the tool, they offered no empirical evidence of its validity or reliability. Thus, the value of the tool is uncertain.

Jalowiec et al (1984;157) constructed a 40-item coping scale "to provide a means of examining the coping methods used by hypertensive and emergency room patients." The authors reported satisfactory levels of reliability, content, and construct validity, while acknowledging the need for further testing. They stated that "unique educational opportunities exist when patients can be informed of the practical significance of inappropriate coping and its subsequent impact on health" (Jalowiec et al, 1984;160–161). The question must be asked, What is inappropriate coping? Jalowiec and colleagues do not make this concept clear. Their tool would be useful in assisting clients to identify what they are doing to cope, but the appropriateness or effectiveness of their behavior depends ultimately on the outcome, and the Jalowiec scale does not measure that aspect.

King (1985) addressed the outcomes of coping behavior. She studied 50 patients undergoing coronary artery bypass grafting to explore the coping strategies they used and their effectiveness. King found that the subjects' views of the effectiveness of strategies changed over time.

Vincent (1985) believes that a tool for assessing coping may be developed in the future. Ideally, such a tool would be brief enough to fit into a general nursing assessment. Numerous tools exist, but they may be directed at answering research questions rather than solving clinical problems (Bedsworth and Molen, 1982; Wegmann, 1984). Nevertheless the open-ended approach of Bedsworth and Molen (1982) could be advantageous in the richness and depth of information it elicits. It would be helpful, however, to have a clear measure of effectiveness, such as provided by King's (1985) instrument. There is no reason why clinicians could not combine these qualitative and quantitative approaches. Indeed, given the complexity of coping, such an approach should be encouraged. It is doubtful that assessment of the effectiveness or ineffectiveness of an individual's coping activity will ever be simple. The defining characteristics (see Table 52.1) should be kept in mind by the clinician, but determining their presence or absence must be the result of a process that is as objective as possible. It is also essential to consider the client's cultural and value orientation in making this type of assessment. McFarland and Wasli (1987) recommended that the nursing assessment identify the nature of the stress and how the patient interprets the stress, assess the patient's coping responses, and note their evaluation of the situation. Effective coping will be determined by the client's subjective evaluation, the accuracy of the client's appraisal of threatening stimuli, and the client's use of constructive behaviors and resources to deal with stress or threats. For example, the social withdrawal of an elderly person living alone in a dangerous neighborhood may be coping effectively by accurately noting the dangers of social interaction in the neighborhood. Another example of what might ordinarily be considered maladaptive behavior is decrease in sexual activities (libido) reported by many elderly widows. In these circumstances, without an available partner, diminished sexual interest may be considered an effective coping strategy.

Coping in the Elderly

It is reasonable to question whether coping changes with aging. At this time there has not been any published study of the nursing diagnosis of Ineffective Coping in the elderly. There have been other related studies, however.

McCrae (1982) reports two different studies that look for possible changes in coping that occur with age. Coping actions that decreased with age were self-blame, withdrawal, assessing blame, hostile reaction, positive thinking, humor, escapist fantasy, sedation, and self-adaptation. Use of faith increased. Defense mechanisms such as altruism, suppression, anticipation, and sublimation did not increase with age. Withdrawal in some circumstances may be indicative of the ineffective coping defining characteristic alteration in societal participation, and self-blame and hostile reaction are part of destructive behavior toward self and others (see Table 52.1).

McCrae (1982) suggests that in light of these results, stress associated with aging changes (ie, the challenges diminish and threat and loss increase). This may account for the changes in coping observed in the elderly. To investigate this, he examined the previously mentioned age effects using statistical controls for type of stress. The result was that the decreases previously found in self-blame and withdrawal were no longer significant. Thus, the greater use of these mechanisms by younger persons may be due to a disproportionate number of challenges in earlier periods of life (McCrae, 1982).

In a second study, McCrae (1982) assessed coping methods used with one event in each of three categories: coping with harm or loss; coping with threat; and coping with challenge. Six significant effects were found. As age increased, the use of hostile reaction, positive thinking, escapist fantasy, restraint, self-adaptation, and humor decreased. These results supported those of the first study.

There is evidence that depression may affect coping in the elderly. Foster and Gallagher (1986) found that although depressed elderly persons do not differ significantly from the nondepressed in terms of coping strategies used, they do use emotional discharge significantly more. Depressed elderly also found all coping strategies to be significantly less helpful than their nondepressed counterparts.

The elderly do not appear to be greatly different from other age groups with respect to coping methods. It is reasonable to question whether cognitive, sensory, and physical changes associated with aging have an impact on choice of coping method.

The nursing diagnosis Ineffective Individual Coping is a difficult diagnosis to make because it relies on rather subjective value judgments. Whether the defining characteristics of the diagnosis as set forth by NANDA can be objectively measured is open to question. Nevertheless, Vincent's (1985) research indicates that the clinical experience of a sizable sample of psychiatric clinical specialists points to the existence of a phenomenon called Ineffective Individual Coping. The following case study illustrates how this nursing diagnosis may manifest itself in an elderly client.

CASE STUDY

Ineffective Individual Coping

Mrs. G was a 65-year-old retired school teacher who was hospitalized for invasive adenocarcinoma of the colon, which filled her pelvis and had been judged inoperable. A colostomy had been created and radiation treatments initiated to shrink the tumor. Mrs. G's postoperative course was medically unremarkable except for a brief period of sepsis and a problem with anemia. The rectal pain she had experienced diminished as the radiation shrank the tumor. Mrs. G's husband and family visited often. They tried to be cheerful and nonchalant.

Mrs. G's colostomy was to be permanent. No one in the family ever mentioned it, nor did she speak of it to them. When nursing staff gave her skin care and changed the collection bag, Mrs. G closed her eyes. A nursing student caring for Mrs. G frequently provided broad openings for her to express her feelings about her situation, but she had little to say. When asked directly about how she felt about the colostomy, Mrs. G stated, "It's just something I have to have. I have to live with it."

Eventually Mrs. G and her family had to think about discharge planning. They unanimously decided that she would move to a nursing home because her colostomy care could not be managed at home. This decision was made in spite of the fact that her husband was healthy and cognitively intact and Mrs. G was ambulatory and without cognitive impairment.

Mrs. G was coping ineffectively with her situation. Her colostomy was so repugnant to her that she could not look at it, nor would she even attempt to learn to care for it. Her family mirrored her response, so placement in a nursing home was proposed. Thus Mrs. G was unable to meet her basic need for colostomy care. Her only way to solve this problem was to elect institutionalization, which would radically alter her pattern of social interaction and family life. In this case, three of the NANDA defining characteristics of Ineffective Individual Coping were present: inability to meet basic needs; inability to problem solve; and a potential alteration in societal participation.

Mrs. G eventually returned home. The administrator of the nursing home would not accept her application and wisely referred her to a home health agency that provided supportive counseling in addition to the necessary colostomy care.

NURSING INTERVENTIONS

The goals of nursing intervention for clients experiencing Ineffective Individual Coping include (1) assisting them to perceive themselves as able to cope with stress; (2) developing an objective appraisal of the situation; (3) developing an awareness of their emotional reaction to the situation; (4) developing coping responses to the objective features of the situation; (5) developing plans and actions in response to the situation; (6) developing coping responses to the emotional reactions of the situation; and (7) evaluating the impact of the coping response (McFarland and Wasli, 1987).

Scandrett (1985) recommends cognitive reappraisal as one intervention for Ineffective Individual Coping. Cognitive reappraisal is a process whereby patients are assisted to examine their beliefs and perceptions carefully in order to alter their response to life events. The premise for this is the belief that affective and/or psychophysiologic reactions to our experiences are strongly influenced by our beliefs, perceptions, and expectations. Scandrett (1985) lists five basic assumptions that, according to Childress and Burns (1981), underlie cognitive theory:

1. Adaptive and maladaptive behavior and affective patterns are developed through cognitive thoughts.
2. Moods and feelings are influenced by current patterns.
3. Cognitions include inner dialogue, perceptions, and fantasies, which represent meanings the client attaches to experiences.
4. Pessimistic thoughts that cause anxiety are frequently unrealistic, illogical, and distorted.
5. Many clients have underlying assumptions or cognitive schemes that predispose them to anxiety or depression.

These assumptions echo those of Lazarus (1966) discussed earlier—that cognitive appraisal is necessary both to determine that a condition of threat exists and to choose a form of coping. Indeed, this intervention is targeted at the phase of reappraisal that Lazarus proposed as a part of coping.

Cognitive reappraisal is a five-step program. Step 1 is stress identification. The "stresses, fears, hurts, and problems of the client" are identified (Scandrett, 1985;52). Step 2 is stress evaluation. The nurse and client explore "incidence of stressors, frequency of occurrence, meaning of the stressor to the client, pervasiveness of threat or amount of actual risk to client's well-being, and the placement of stimuli in relation to other things in life" (Scandrett, 1985;52). Step 3 is the development of a stress hierarchy. The client organizes stressors along a continuum from most upsetting to least upsetting. Assessment of coping is Step 4. Here clients explore the ways in which they manage stressors. They may be helped by the nurse to learn new coping responses. The client also is helped to sort out what aspects of the stressor are amenable to change and which are not. Step 5 is the acquisition of behavior management techniques such as extinction procedures, persuasion, vicarious experiences, imagery, and problem solving. Cognitive reappraisal can help elderly clients to view their experiences more realistically and then respond with more appropriate and effective coping behaviors.

CASE STUDY

Nursing Interventions

In the case of Mrs. G, the intervention of cognitive reappraisal was helpful. Her colostomy was so threatening to her that she could neither look at it nor speak of it comfortably. She thought of it as dirty and was disgusted by it. The colostomy was also a constant reminder of her cancer. This type of reaction to loss of normal body function and disfigurement is not unusual given our cultural devotion to cleanliness and body image. Mrs. G was helped to identify what it was about the colostomy that was stressful. This required some mild confrontation of her nonverbal behavior (ie, not looking at the colostomy). She was then guided through an examination of how truly threatening the colostomy was and assisted to prioritize the stressors. The nurse then assisted Mrs. G to look at her reaction to the colostomy to see whether it was in proportion to the severity of the stress. Finally, Mrs. G benefited from a desensitization program to reduce the feeling of threat. This program involved several components. As Mrs. G became more accepting of the thought of the colostomy, the nurse introduced her to other ostomates who were coping well. She then set some goals with Mrs. G that involved progressively greater contact with the colostomy: for example, looking at the colostomy with the bag attached, looking at it without the bag, touching the bag, touching the skin adjacent to the ostomy, and finally touching the ostomy itself. Each of these steps was accompanied by assisting her to relax, discussing her feelings about the ostomy, encouraging her to see the colostomy as something that assists her to maintain a body function, and offering support and encouragement as she practiced the behaviors.

Such a program of cognitive reappraisal relies heavily on the nurse's interpersonal skills, since it is conducted primarily via verbal and nonverbal communication. The development of a strong trusting relationship between nurse and client is a necessary prelude to the intervention, since it requires the patient to take actions that are likely perceived as risks.

OUTCOMES

McFarland and Wasli (1987) delineate four major outcome criteria, indicating that the elderly client can (1) accurately appraise stress; (2) demonstrate adequate emotional and cognitive responses; (3) use adequate coping resources; and (4) resolve stress-producing episodes.

A positive outcome with cognitive reappraisal, for example, would be a reduction in stress as clients meet the challenges presented to them. More specifically, desired outcomes would be reversal or elimination of the defining characteristics of ineffective coping. Clients might be able to seek help, meet role expectations, meet basic needs, problem solve, participate in usual social interactions, exhibit nondestructive behavior toward self and others, and use appropriate defense mechanisms when confronted with stressors.

SUMMARY

The nursing diagnosis Ineffective Individual Coping is as yet poorly defined; the defining characteristics are rather vague and somewhat difficult to measure. The whole notion of judging particular coping behaviors as ineffective needs to be examined. Clearly any behavior that is directly self-destructive may be considered ineffective, but other behaviors are less easily judged. Even in the case reviewed earlier in this paper, it is arguable that Mrs. G had a right not to look at her colostomy and to deny its existence completely. After all, it's her body and her life.

In time, Ineffective Individual Coping will become a more useful and usable nursing diagnosis. As it is currently developed, the diagnosis is useful to assist the nurse to identify behaviors that the elderly use when confronted by stressors that may not allow them to maximize personal autonomy and control over their lives.

References

Bedsworth JA, Molen MT: Psychological stress in spouses of patients with myocardial infarction. *Heart Lung* 1982; 11:450–456.

Carroll-Johnson, R (editor). *Classification of Nursing Diagnoses: Proceedings of the Eighth Conference.* Lippincott, 1989.

Childress AR, Burns DD: The basics of cognitive therapy. *Psychosomatics* 1981; 22:1017–1020, 1023–1024, 1027.

Foster JM, Gallagher D: An explanatory study comparing depressed and non-depressed elders' coping strategies. *J Gerontol* 1986; 41:91–93.

Hinkle LE: The effect of exposure to culture change, social change, and changes in interpersonal relationships on health. In: Dohrenwend BS, Dohrenwend BP (editors). *Stressful Life Events: Their Nature and Effects.* Wiley, 1974;9–44.

Hurley ME (editor): *Classification of Nursing Diagnoses.* Mosby, 1986.

Jalowiec A, Murphy SP, Powers MJ: Psychometric assessment of the Jalowiec coping scale. *Nurs Res* 1984; 33:157–161.

Janis IL: *Psychological Stress.* Academic Press, 1958.

Johnson-Saylor MT, Pohl J, Lowe-Wickson B: An assessment form for determining patients' health status and coping responses. *Top Clin Nurs* 1982; 4:20–33.

King KB: Measurement of coping strategies, concerns, and emotional response in patients undergoing coronary artery bypass grafting. *Heart Lung* 1985; 14:579–586.

Lazarus RS: *Psychological Stress and the Coping Process.* McGraw-Hill, 1966.

Lazarus RS, Averill JR, Opton EM: The psychology of coping: Issues of research and assessment. In: *Coping and Adaptation.* Coelho GV, Hamburg DA, Adams JE (editors). Basic Books, 1974;249–315.

Levine S, Scotch N: *Social Stress.* Aldine, 1970.

Lipowski ZJ: Physical illness, the individual and the coping processes. *Psychiatry Med* 1970; 1:91–102.

McCrae RR: Age differences in the use of coping mechanisms. *J Gerontol* 1982; 37:454–460.

McFarland G, Wasli E: *Nursing Diagnoses and Process in Psychiatric Mental Health Nursing.* Lippincott, 1987.

Miller P et al: Development of a health attitude scale. *Nurs Res* 1982; 31:132–136.

Moos RH, Tsu VD: *The Crisis of Physical Illness: An Overview in Coping With Physical Illness.* Moos RH (editor). Plenum, 1977; 3–21.

Scandrett S: Cognitive reappraisal. In: *Nursing Interventions.* Bulechek G, McClosekey J (editor). Saunders, 1985; 49–57.

Selye H: *The Stress of Life.* McGraw-Hill, 1956.

Vincent KG: The validation of a nursing diagnosis. *Nurs Clin North Am* 1985; 20:631–640.

Wegmann J: Instruments that measure coping. *Oncol Nurs Forum* 1984; 11(14):119–120.

Weisman AD: *Coping with Cancer.* McGraw-Hill, 1979.

White RW: Strategies of adaptation: An attempt at systematic description. In: *Coping and Adaptation.* Coelho GV, Hamburg DA, Adams GE (editors). Basic Books, 1974; 47–68.

XI

Value–Belief Pattern

KATHLEEN BUCKWALTER, PhD, RN, FAAN

MERIDEAN MAAS, PhD, RN, FAAN

Overview

BECAUSE OF LOSS OF CONTROL, THE RELATIVE imminence of death, and loss of traditional support systems, the institutionalized elderly are particularly susceptible to Spiritual Distress. In Chapter 54, Fehring and Rantz argue that later life does not have to involve a loss of hope, peace, and meaning of life, but can be a time of spiritual fulfillment and well-being. Emphasizing the highly individual nature of spirituality, the authors explore the concept as a major way of coping with the stresses that often accompany institutionalization. The research base for the diagnosis Spiritual Distress, quantified tools for assessment, and differential diagnosis from depression and grieving are discussed. The nurse's role in implementing and evaluating the intervention healing of memories is described.

53

Normal Changes With Aging

Donna Bunten, MA, RN
Mary A. Hardy, PhD, RN, C

Definition:

The value–belief pattern describes patterns of values, beliefs (including spiritual), or goals that guide choices or decisions.

Values and beliefs guide the choices we make throughout our life span whether we are consciously aware of it or not. Our perception of whether events are stressful is affected by our beliefs and values. This holds true and may become even more important as the elderly address developmental tasks associated with later adulthood. The neo-Freudian work of Erik Erikson (1963) is a benchmark in describing the challenges of old age. Erikson believed that in the last stage of life, before satisfaction can be experienced, an individual must put his or her life into perspective, accept the good and bad about life, and find that life had meaning and usefulness. If this task, called "ego integrity," cannot be successfully accomplished, the aging person will experience despair. Eliopoulos (1987) also points out that acceptance of choices and "life as lived" is the key to inner peace. The elderly need to seek satisfaction not only from the life they have lived but from other tasks that need to be accomplished during aging, including learning to live with infirmities and preparing for death (Butler and Lewis, 1982). Realization of the short time left to work through unresolved feelings can be emotionally crippling. Recognition and validation by others of accomplishments will benefit the older person's self-esteem and help him or her face the task of dealing with other unfinished issues.

Religion provides many people with a baseline and framework from which to establish values and beliefs. Elderly persons who have not been religious in earlier life are not likely to become religious in late life, but those who are religious seem to have a greater sense of meaning or purpose in late life (Forbis, 1988). Although Spiritual Distress is rarely diagnosed and reported in institutionalized settings, the potential for this diagnosis is great among elderly residents. Separation from traditional religious and cultural support systems, lack of purpose and meaning at the latter stage of life, lack of forgiveness from friends and family, anger over past life hurts, and the prospect of imminent death can contribute to an elderly resident's distress of the spirit.

References

Butler RN, Lewis MI: *Aging and Mental Health: Positive Psychosocial and Biomedical Approaches*, 3d ed. Mosby, 1982.

Eliopoulos C: *Gerontological Nursing*, 2d ed. Lippincott, 1987.

Erikson E: *Childhood and Society*, 2d ed. Horton, 1963.

Forbis PA: Meeting patients' spiritual needs. *Geriatr Nurs* 1988; 9:158–159.

54

Spiritual Distress

RICHARD J. FEHRING, PhD, RN
MARILYN RANTZ, MA, RN

ELDERLY PERSONS ARE AT RISK FOR SPIRITUAL DISTRESS because of the loss of independence, the inevitability of death, the loss of traditional support systems, and the possibility of institutionalization.

Spiritual Distress, however, does not have to be an inevitable course for the elderly person. Later life can be a time of peace, hope, meaning and even a time of accepting death as part of living life to the full (Bianchi, 1985; Hulme, 1986). This chapter will address the concepts of Spiritual Distress and spiritual well-being (SWB) and illustrate some of the interventions that nurses caring for dependent elderly in the home and institutional settings can use to prevent and treat Spiritual Distress.

Spirituality can be devoid of a religious context and simply be an "affirmation of life"—life lived fully. Spirituality is also a belief in something beyond the physical nature, a sense of a force beyond oneself, a life-giving and integrating force. Egan (1984) described the striving to be in union with this force as a mystery.

Banks (1980) conducted a survey among 76 health education professionals to determine the meaning of spirituality. She discovered four major themes that were common to the understanding of spirituality. Spirituality (1) is a unifying force; (2) provides meaning in life; (3) is a common bond between individuals; and (4) is based on individual perceptions, values, and faith.

If spirituality is a life force, an affirmation of life, what is Spiritual Distress? It can be a sense of not having purpose and meaning, not having harmony with a life force, and/or not being bonded with other individuals. It can include experiencing a moral crisis and questioning a belief in a deity, self, and others. Spiritual Distress, however, does not necessarily mean that a person has given up on life or despairs about life. It can mean that the individual is struggling with the meaning and mystery of life. This struggle can be a positive experience if it brings a person to a deeper understanding of life and a deeper sense of peace, meaning, and purpose. However, when the struggle or distress leads one to feel abandoned, isolated, or without hope, then it can be a negative experience.

SIGNIFICANCE FOR THE ELDERLY

Spirituality is an important dimension of well-being for the elderly. As an elderly person's physical and mental capacities decline, spirituality can grow and develop (Dunn, 1977; Hunglemann, 1985; Ruffing-Rahal, 1984). For the elderly person, spirituality can bring relief from anxiety and can provide a sense of purpose, meaning, and integration. It can be a source of personal self-esteem and can help the elderly individual prepare for death (Hulme, 1986; Moberg, 1980). A number of studies have consistently detected the importance of spirituality for people who are coping with chronic health problems (Baldree et al, 1982; Miller, 1983; O'Brien, 1982a).

A number of studies have used a tool developed by Paloutzian and Ellison (1982) to measure spiritual well-being. Kohlbry (1985) recently discovered an inverse relationship between SWB and hopelessness in people with chronic illness. The SWB index also has been applied to elderly populations. Leasor (1983) found that there was a negative relationship between SWB and negative mood states in elderly patients coping with chronic obstructive pulmonary disorder (COPD). Miller (1985) found that an elderly population of patients coping with arthritis had higher levels of SWB and less loneliness than a younger population of healthy college faculty.

Spirituality may also be a key to effective management of stress. Selye (1979) has said that the best way to manage stress is to develop a belief system. He suggested a belief system that values charity and selflessness and lessens the value of competing for the top spot at all costs. Likewise, Hulme (1986) concludes that as one gets older in wisdom of the spirit, material goods, workaholism, and unhealthy competition are no longer valued or are valued less. A nonmaterial and less competitive belief system helps an older person to keep life in perspective and to manage stress. According to Tubesing (1980) the source of stress is the lack of a spiritual outlook on life.

Recent writers in the fields of psychology and coping are rediscovering that the spiritual dimension is necessary for holistic healing. May (1982) has stated that psychology can go only so far in helping people with the stress of life; then the spiritual dimension must take over. Carl Jung, the Swiss psychologist, has been frequently quoted as saying that he never found an elderly individual "whose problem in the last resort was not that of finding a religious outlook on life . . . and none of them really has been healed who did not regain his religious outlook" (cited in Tubesing, 1982; 94). Jung also believed that religion often provided a complete holistic system of mental health and healing. Kelsey (1986) has used the basis of Jungian principles to place modern psychologic, cognitive, and behavioral therapies in a religious framework.

The use of the spiritual dimension as a major way of coping with stress has relevance to the elderly and especially to institutionalized elderly. Elderly individuals who have developed spirituality throughout their lives will be able to cope better with the changes that aging entails and to the stress of living in a long-term care facility (Hulme, 1986; O'Driscoll, 1985). It will help elderly persons to cope with their many losses and changes, to interpret life experiences meaningfully, and to prepare for death.

PREDISPOSITION OF ELDERLY TO SPIRITUAL DISTRESS

For some elderly, affirmation of life in the face of change and loss, the thought of death, and the experience of living in a nursing home will be difficult. For others, Spiritual Distress will be a result of not having or of losing a sense of purpose and meaning in life. Spiritual Distress might also be a result of a challenged belief system or the loss of or removal from past religious and cultural support systems. For the elderly person who relied on the spiritual dimension to manage stress throughout life, this will be a time of struggle, but it will also be a time of spiritual growth. At times of crisis or stress persons with a well-developed spiritual system will continue to need spiritual support to help them grow from the experience and to achieve higher levels of well-being.

For others the experience of change and loss and the use of the spiritual dimension will be new. The elderly person who does not have an established spiritual dimension might develop this affirmation of life though the stimulus of aging and the struggle of life in the nursing home. This will more likely happen if the nursing home has a support system of pastoral care and a nursing staff that is attuned to the phenomenon of Spiritual Distress and the assessment factors and interventions appropriate for this diagnosis. Emphasis on the spiritual dimension of nursing has been stimulated by the focus provided by the nursing diagnosis movement, as well as by the rising interest in humanistic values, holistic health care, and total "wellness."

ETIOLOGIES/RELATED FACTORS AND DEFINING CHARACTERISTICS

In 1973, at the First National Classification Conference, four spiritually oriented nursing diagnoses were presented and included in the original nursing diagnoses classification system.

At the Fourth National Classification Conference in 1980 the only spiritual diagnosis to remain on the official list was Spiritual Distress or Distress of the Human Spirit (Kim and Moritz, 1982). Eight of the etiologies for Spiritual Distress were also dropped at this time. The definition, the etiologies/related factors, and the defining characteristics of Spiritual Distress that were refined and developed at the Fourth National Classification Conference are the ones in current use (Carroll-Johnson, 1989). They can be found in Table 54.1.

Although there have been no changes in the diagnosis of Spiritual Distress since the Fourth National Classification Conference in 1980, participants at the Fifth National

Table 54.1

Definitions, Etiologies/Related Factors and Defining Characteristics of Spiritual Distress

DEFINITIONS

A disruption of the life principle that pervades a person's entire being and that integrates and transcends one's biologic and psychosocial nature (Kim et al, 1984a)

The state in which the individual experiences or is at risk of experiencing a disturbance in his/her belief or value system that is his/her source of strength and hope (Carpenito, 1985)

A feeling of despair or alienation related to religious, moral, or other beliefs/values (Kelly, 1985)

ETIOLOGIES/RELATED FACTORS
(CARROLL-JOHNSON 1989)

Separation from religious and cultural ties
Challenged belief and value system

ETIOLOGIES/RELATED FACTORS (CARPENITO, 1985)

Loss of body part or function
Terminal disease
Debilitating disease
Death or illness of significant other
Embarrassment at practicing spiritual rituals
Hospital barriers to practicing spiritual rituals
Conflicts to belief system
Beliefs opposed by family, peers, health care providers

RISK FACTORS (KELLY, 1985)

Disruption in usual religious activity
Personal and family disasters
Loss of significant others
Behaviors contrary to society/cultural norms

DEFINING CHARACTERISTICS (CARROLL-JOHNSON, 1989)

Expresses concern with meaning of life and death and/or belief system
Anger toward God (as defined by the person)
Questions meaning of suffering
Verbalizes inner conflict about beliefs
Verbalizes concern about relationship with deity
Questions meaning for own existence
Unable to choose or chooses not to participate in usual religious practices
Seeks spiritual assistance
Questions moral and ethical implications of therapeutic regimen
Displacement of anger toward religious representatives
Description of nightmares or sleep disturbances
Alteration in behavior or mood evidenced by anger, crying, withdrawal, preoccupation, anxiety, hostility, apathy, etc

DEFINING CHARACTERISTICS (CARPENITO, 1985*)

Experiences a disturbance in belief system
  Questions credibility of belief system
  Is discouraged
  Is unable to practice usual religious rituals
Expresses concern (anger, resentment, fear) about meaning of life, suffering, and death
Requests spiritual assistance for a disturbance in belief system

DEFINING CHARACTERISTICS (KELLY, 1985*)

Feeling separated or alienated from deity
Dissatisfaction with personal past/present
Depression
Crying
Self-destructive behavior/threats
Fear
Feelings of abandonment
Feelings of hopelessness

---

*Not included in Fehring and Rantz validation study (Fehring and Rantz, 1987)

Conference suggested that the labels of Spiritual Distress related to forgiveness, love, hope, trust, and meaning and purpose be considered as separate diagnostic labels. These new labels were suggested based on the work of Flesner (1981), whose research entailed the development of a tool to measure Spiritual Distress. Her tool was based on the five categories of basic spiritual needs: love, hope, forgiveness, meaning and purpose, and trust.

Other nursing authors have suggested different labels, definitions, etiologies/related factors, and defining characteristics for Spiritual Distress. O'Brien (1982b) presented seven nursing diagnoses related to spiritual integrity for consideration: spiritual pain, spiritual alienation, spiritual anxiety, spiritual guilt, spiritual anger, spiritual loss, and

spiritual despair. O'Brien developed these spiritual nursing diagnoses from data she gathered for developing a spiritual assessment guide.

Kelly (1985) and Carpenito (1985) have developed their own definitions, etiologies/related factors, and defining characteristics of Spiritual Distress (Table 54.1). Kelly included risk factors and differential diagnoses for Spiritual Distress, and Carpenito summarized contributing factors.

There have been several chapters about spirituality or Spiritual Distress in medical-surgical textbooks. Stallwood (1975) developed a model of spirituality with the spirit as the core or center of a person. The intellect and the physical being emanate from that core. This model has been used as the conceptual framework for two masters theses (Kohlbry, 1985; Leasor, 1983). Stallwood's (1975) chapter also provides the nurse with information on the use of prayer and scripture as nursing interventions.

An important book on spirituality and the nurse's role in spiritual care has been written by Fish and Shelly (1978). Although the book does not directly address the diagnosis of Spiritual Distress, it does include a chapter on three key spiritual needs: the need for meaning and purpose, the need for love and relatedness, and the need for forgiveness. These needs, if not met, could lead to Spiritual Distress in patients. These three spiritual needs are also similar to the defining characteristics of Spiritual Distress. Fish and Shelly (1978) discuss how the nurse can be a channel in helping patients to meet spiritual needs, and they give many case examples.

RESEARCH BASE FOR THE DIAGNOSIS

Several studies have been done to measure or validate Spiritual Distress (Flesner, 1981; Weatherall and Creason, 1986). The authors of this chapter used Fehring's (1986) diagnostic content validity (DCV) model for validating defining characteristics of the nursing diagnosis Spiritual Distress. According to Fehring's (1986) model, the defining characteristics are more valid as they approach a value of 1.0. Defining characteristics with a value of 0.75 or greater can be considered critical indicators of that diagnosis.

The NANDA indicators of Spiritual Distress (Table 54.1) yield a high average DCV score (0.767), providing evidence from a retrospective clinical analysis that this is a valid diagnosis.

ASSESSMENT

A number of approaches and tools have been developed to assess or measure the diagnosis Spiritual Distress. Assessment of spirituality by a nurse can be controversial. Some nurses, patients, and members of other professions (particularly the clergy) might question the appropriateness of nurses attempting to assess spiritual matters (DeYoung, 1984). Another more basic controversy is whether the spiritual dimension can be assessed and measured (Fehring and McLane, 1986; Moberg, 1984). Some people believe if you can measure it, it is not spiritual. However, this objection could be used for many of the "soft," abstract phenomena that nurses and therapists consider part of their domain, such as depression, powerlessness, and hopelessness. Essentially what a nurse or other professional does when assessing or

measuring a phenomenon is to identify indicators (defining characteristics) of that phenomenon. Similarly, when assessing any spiritual phenomenon, indicators of that phenomenon are being identified (Moberg, 1984). The difficult part is establishing evidence that the indicators truly reflect the phenomenon that is being measured. It is imperative to develop measurement tools and diagnostic characteristics that are valid and reliable.

Tools to Assess Spirituality

A number of methods of assessing a person's spirituality or spiritual needs have been reported in the literature. These methods are not specific for the nursing diagnosis Spiritual Distress, but they give some indications of spiritual problems that might reflect or precipitate Spiritual Distress. (See Table 54.2 for a summary of these assessment tools.) Stoll (1979) postulated four basic areas that could guide the nurse in doing a spiritual assessment: (1) concept of God or deity; (2) sources of strength and hope; (3) religious practices; and (4) relationship between spiritual beliefs and health. Using these as a guide, the assessment would include identifying the patient's (1) concept of a transcendent being or life force; (2) persons and practices that provide strength and hope; (3) important religious practices and symbols; (4) uses of prayer or meditation; and (5) alteration of religious practices by illness. The process of the assessment should be open ended and nonthreatening, allowing patients time to express themselves and at the same time allowing the nurse to be aware of sensitive areas of discussion.

O'Brien (1982b) developed a spiritual assessment guide based on empirical data gathered from chronically ill hemodialysis clients. The tool has questions that cover six areas of spirituality: (1) general spiritual beliefs; (2) personal spiritual beliefs; (3) identification with institutionalized religion; (4) spiritual/religious support systems; (5) spiritual/religious rituals; and (6) spiritual deficit/distress. The area of Spiritual Distress in the assessment guide includes questions to assess spiritual pain, alienation, anxiety, guilt, anger, loss, and despair. She advised that a spiritual assessment be undertaken by a nurse only when a need or concern has been "clearly articulated by the client himself" (O'Brien, 1982b;100).

Although O'Brien's spiritual assessment guide is longer than Stoll's and includes many more questions, it would be appropriate to gather the information the tool provides over a period of time for residents in a long-term care setting. If a nurse is to give holistic nursing care, and if the spiritual dimension is important to that care, then it is imperative that spiritual information be obtained. O'Brien's assessment guide appears to be an empirically grounded tool that can provide important information about a resident's spiritual health.

Table 54.2

Tools for Spiritual Distress

ASSESSMENT TOOLS	COMPONENTS
(Indicators of spiritual problems that might reflect or precipitate Spiritual Distress)	
Stoll (1979): Guidelines for spiritual assessment	Concept of God or deity Sources of strength and hope Religious practices Relationship between spiritual beliefs and health
O'Brien (1982b): Spiritual assessment guide	General spiritual beliefs Personal spiritual beliefs Identification with institutionalized religion Spiritual/religious support system Spiritual/religious rituals Spiritual deficit/distress
Tubesing and Tubesing (1983) : "Spiritual pilgrimage"	Raising consciousness about spiritual health and affirming life experiences that have shaped spiritual development
Personal reflection guide	Values, beliefs, commitments Central spiritual truths and beliefs Aspects of the spirit that are missing What (if any) religious rituals are meaningful How these rituals can increase a healing effect Advice to give a younger person on developing a richer spiritual life

QUANTIFYING TOOLS	COMPONENTS

Paloutzian and Ellison (1982): Spiritual Well-Being (SWB) Index	Dimensions of spirituality
	   Religious: based on a person's relationship with God or a supreme being
	   Existential: based on a person's satisfaction, meaning, and purpose in life

Flesner (1981): Spiritual Distress Index	Forgiveness, love, hope, trust, meaning/purpose

Tubesing (1980, 1982) and Tubesing and Tubesing (1982, 1983) have developed several tools and questions to assess spiritual outlook. These could be used to determine whether a person is in Spiritual Distress or not. One of the assessment processes is called a "spiritual pilgrimage" (Tubesing and Tubesing, 1983). The purpose of the pilgrimage is to raise consciousness about a person's spiritual health and to affirm life experiences that have shaped a person's spiritual development. The process can be used either with individuals or with groups. The spiritual pilgrimage entails drawing a timeline (or graph) of one's spiritual pilgrimage from birth to the present and then extending the timeline into the future according to how a person sees his or her spiritual growth. The timeline includes the highs and lows of spiritual health that are stimulated by significant life events, such as, "times of clear (or clouded) purpose, value conflicts, awe inspiring experiences, shifts in religious beliefs or practices, major commitments, significant rituals/celebrations, dry spells, difficult choices, moments of doubt" (Tubesing and Tubesing, 1983;95). The final

step of the spiritual pilgrimage is to ask participants to give themselves an overall grade for their spiritual health based on the ups and downs of their timeline. The spiritual pilgrimage could be an excellent, nonthreatening process for individuals or groups of elderly people to raise their consciousness about spiritual health. The process would also allow the nurse to enter into a dialogue with the individual or group about past spiritual hurts and about how the nurse could aid further spiritual growth.

Tubesing and Tubesing (1983) also have formulated a personal reflection guide on spiritual health and spiritual outlook. The personal reflections focus on (1) values, beliefs, commitments; (2) central spiritual truths and beliefs; (3) aspects of the spirit that are missing; (4) what (if any) religious rituals are meaningful; (5) how these rituals could increase a healing effect; and (6) advice to give a younger person about how to develop a richer spiritual life. A nurse could use this personal reflection guide with an elderly person to stimulate spiritual dialogue and to get a sense of the person's spiritual health.

Tools to Quantify Spiritual Distress

Several measurement tools have been developed that nurses can use to quantify levels of Spiritual Distress (see Table 54.2). Before using these tools, the nurse should have knowledge of tests and measurement, be sensitive in the administration of the tools, and be knowledgeable about the limitations of paper and pencil measurement tools. If used correctly they can be a valuable source of information.

Paloutzian and Ellison (1982) have developed a 20-item Likert-scaled tool to measure spiritual well-being (SWB). The Spiritual Well-Being Index was designed to reflect two dimensions of spirituality: (1) a religious dimension based on a person's relationship with God or a supreme being and (2) an existential dimension based on a person's satisfaction and meaning and purpose in life. The tool has been shown to be reliable (Ellison, 1982) and valid (Fehring and Frenn, 1986, 1987). Although SWB is not the same as Spiritual Distress, low scores on the SWB Index may indicate that the person's low SWB is a result of Spiritual Distress. The source of Spiritual Distress (eg, a poor relationship with a supreme being or God or an unclear purpose and meaning in life) may also be determined.

The SWB tool developed by Paloutzian and Ellison (1983) was stimulated by Moberg's call for development of a measure of SWB and by his theoretical dimensions (religious and existential) of SWB. Through factor analysis of survey research data Moberg (1980, 1984) developed seven indices of SWB: Christian faith, self-satisfaction, personal piety, subjective spiritual well-being, optimism, religious cynicism, and elitism. He also constructed three indices of personal volunteer activity: political, charitable, and religious involvement. In subsequent research he found that these indices correlate highly with Paloutzian and Ellison's SWB Index among subjects from diverse, but mostly elderly, populations. Before and after measures might give a nurse, chaplain, pastor, pastoral team, or other caregivers some indication of the effectiveness of various religious services and practices, spiritual disciplines, or pastoral and nursing care for residents' SWB. These tools also could be helpful to clinical psychologists and others in the helping professions.

Flesner (1981) developed a quantifiable measure of Spiritual Distress. The Spiritual Distress Index is a 22-item Likert-type scale based on five areas in which a person can experience Spiritual Distress: (1) forgiveness; (2) love; (3) hope; (4) trust; and (5) meaning and purpose. The five areas were extrapolated from the nursing literature. The tool has high test–retest reliability coefficients and consistently shows high positive correlations with Paloutzian and Ellison's SWB Index.

The authors of this chapter administered Paloutzian and Ellison's SWB Index and Flesner's Spiritual Distress Index to 28 nonconfused residents in a nondenominational county-run nursing home. The residents' mean age was 83 years; four of the subjects were men, and all reported some type of Christian religion. The residents' Spiritual Distress scores on the Flesner tool showed a high significant negative correlation with the SWB scores (r = – 0.85, p – 0.001). These tools need further testing with non-Christian populations.

Differential Diagnosis

In assessing the elderly, the nurse should keep in mind that other diagnoses are closely related to Spiritual Distress, especially Depression and Dysfunctional Grieving. Although closely related, they are not the same. In order to differentiate Spiritual Distress from Depression and Dysfunctional Grieving, a nurse should be aware of the differences in defining characteristics and etiologies/related factors (Table 54.3). Although both Depression and Dysfunctional Grieving have a spiritual dimension if viewed from a holistic perspective, and although many of the defining characteristics are the same (such as crying, sadness, and anger), there are some differences. The defining characteristics of Spiritual Distress focus more on anger toward a deity, conflicts with values and beliefs, and the meaning of suffering and death. Also, the etiologies of Spiritual Distress are more related to conflicts with religious/cultural beliefs and value conflicts. Depression, on the other hand, is defined by low self-worth and anger toward self and may be caused by a sense of powerlessness.

Grieving is related to a loss or perceived loss and the resultant anger and sadness. Expressions of grief do not necessarily pertain to a conflict with belief systems, values, beliefs about a supreme being, or meaning and purpose in life. However, a person who is grieving may experience Spiritual Distress, and grief may be reinforced by Spiritual Distress. Precipitation of Spiritual Distress by grief is most likely to happen if the grief focuses on anger toward a deity or results in the loss of a sense of meaning and purpose, and if there is inability to derive satisfaction from usual spiritual practices and support systems.

Future validation studies of Spiritual Distress should include measurements and defining characteristics of depression and dysfunctional grieving in order to cross validate and differentiate these diagnoses from Spiritual Distress (see Chapter 35, Reactive Depression and Chapter 43, Dysfunctional Grieving).

CASE STUDY

Spiritual Distress

The following case study of an elderly resident in a nursing home illustrates the diagnosis of Spiritual Distress, some nursing interventions that can be used to treat a

Table 54.3

Differential Diagnosis

ETIOLOGIES/RELATED FACTORS

Spiritual Distress	*Reactive Depression*	*Dysfunctional Grieving*
Separation from religious and cultural ties (Kim et al, 1984; Gordon, 1986)	Perceived powerlessness (Gordon, 1986)	Actual or perceived object loss (Kim et al, 1984)
Challenged belief system (Kim et al, 1984; Gordon, 1986)	Physical: aging, hormonal imbalance, medication reaction, etc. (Gettrust et al, 1985)	Unavailable support system (Gordon, 1986)
	Emotional: environmental changes, developmental crisis, loss of significant other, etc. (Gettrust et al, 1985)	Loss or perceived loss/change (Gordon, 1986)

DEFINING CHARACTERISTICS

Spiritual Distress (Kim et al, 1984; Gordon, 1986)	*Reactive Depression (Gordon, 1986; Gettrust et al, 1985)*	*Dysfunctional Grieving (Kim et al, 1984; Gordon, 1986)*
Expresses concern with meaning of life and death and/or belief system	Expresses hopelessness, despair	Verbal expression of distress of loss
Anger toward God	Inability to concentrate	Denial of loss
Questions meaning of suffering	Change in usual activities	Expression of guilt
Alteration in behavior or mood as evidenced by anger, crying, withdrawal, preoccupation, anxiety, hostility, apathy, etc.	Continual questioning of self-worth, self-esteem	Expression of unresolved conflicts
Displacement of anger toward religious representation	Feeling of failure (real or imagined)	Anger
	Withdrawal from others to avoid possible rejection (real or imagined)	Sadness
	Misdirected anger toward self	Crying
		Difficulty expressing loss
		Interference with life functioning
		Alteration with life functioning
		Alteration in concentration and/or pursuit of tasks

person with Spiritual Distress, and how the interventions for Spiritual Distress can be evaluated.

Millie Brown is an 83-year-old white woman with the medical diagnosis of cancer of the lungs. Her cancer has been treated in the past with chemotherapy and radiation. The doctors have told her that she has a life expectancy of about a year. At present, she is in no pain but needs periodic oxygen and is confined to a wheelchair. Her husband died 12 years ago from heart failure. She has lived in her own home until 2 years ago when she was hospitalized for her cancer and subsequently placed in a nursing home. Millie has two daughters who briefly visit her several times a month.

Since Millie moved into the nursing home, she has been despondent, cries often, and only rarely interacts with the other residents or participates in recreational activities. The nurses who care for her have indicated that she is depressed, complains of having no energy or desire to do anything, and feels lonely. When family or friends visit, however, she interacts very little. She also has expressed that she is afraid of dying and is angry with God. She blames God for all the suffering she is going through and for her meaningless existence over the past 2 years. Even though Millie expresses fear of dying, she often states she just wants to be left alone to die. Her room is usually very dark with the shades drawn.

Nurses and members of the pastoral team who have talked to her have suggested the use of prayer and have encouraged her to attend church services. She says that she is too angry to pray and refuses to go to church services, saying that they are a waste of time. Millie lists her religion as Lutheran. According to her daughters, she was very active in her church but has not gone to church for the past 12 years since her husband died. She says that when her husband was in the hospital the minister in her church never bothered to visit him. She is still angry about that incident. The geriatric clinical specialist of the nursing home administered the Flesner Spiritual Distress Scale and Paloutzian and Ellison's SWB Index. Millie's scores for both scales were in the low 50s, indicating that she had low SWB and was spiritually distressed.

NURSING INTERVENTIONS

Although the use of prayer by elderly people often brings peace, meaning, and purpose to life (Davidson and MacDonald, 1983), the fact that Millie was angry with God, had past life hurts related to formal religion, and could not find any meaning in her suffering, illness, and approaching death prevented her from being able to pray. Her past life hurts were blocking any attempt to try to find relief through either prayer or formal religious beliefs and practices. To help relieve the distress of the human spirit that Millie Brown was experiencing, the nurse would first have to assist with healing past hurts, help to relieve her anger with God, and help her to find some meaning in her illness, suffering, and approaching death.

The primary interventions that will be discussed as appropriate to relieve or treat Spiritual Distress of an elderly person are inner healing through prayer, imagination, and healing of memories. Before beginning a discussion of the use of these nursing interventions, it is necessary to point out that spirituality is not the same as religion and belief in God. For some people spirituality can be dealt with in a purely generic fashion devoid of religious connotations. However, a nurse would be remiss to avoid the religious component of spirituality. This does not mean that nurses should force their beliefs on patients or that patients must have any certain belief or religion. Rather, in order to be most effective in giving holistic care, nurses must take a patient's belief system into account, whatever those beliefs may be.

The nurse who is treating a person with Spiritual Distress will have to choose an intervention that will not offend the patient's belief system. This might seem an impossible task with the great variety of religious and spiritual expressions in the United States. One way of not offending a person's faith system would be to use interventions that are devoid of any religious context. For example, the interventions of prayer and healing of memories could be simply the use of meditation, imagery, and reminiscence. However, Benson (1985) and others (Propst, 1980) have found that cognitive/behavioral interventions are often more effective when they include the individual's faith system. For example, Benson (1985) advocates that instead of using the word *one*, a person could use a word or phrase (eg, *shalom* or *The Lord is my shepherd*) from his or her individual faith system to focus on. The relaxation technique then becomes more meaningful for the person and will more likely be used. Combining the relaxation technique with the individual's belief system is what Benson calls the "faith factor."

Healing of Memories

The use and method of healing of memories has been developed and popularized by two psychotherapists (Linn and Linn, 1978) and a nurse (Schleman et al, 1980). The healing of memories process is based on the use of imagery and the healing power of prayer for persons who are known to pray. Linn and Linn (1978) viewed inner healing of memories as a twofold process: (1) seeking forgiveness for self and (2) forgiving others. This process also entails going through five stages of healing life's hurts that are similar to the five stages of acceptance of dying. As

a person works through the stages of denial, anger, bargaining, depression, and acceptance of life's hurts, the feelings of anxiety, anger, fear, and guilt are relieved. Past life hurts eventually become integrated with the person's present life. If the person is healed totally, the past life hurts will become the person's strengths or "gifts." The healing of past memories and integrating of the past hurts into the present and future is particularly important for elderly persons (Austin, 1986). This integration helps the elderly person find meaning in the past life and a sense of harmony with the past, present, and future.

The healing of memories process, which results in the eventual integration of past experiences, is strikingly similar to reminiscence therapy as promoted by Butler in the 1960s (King, 1982). (See Chapter 25, Diversional Activity Deficit, for further discussion of reminiscence therapy.)

Dobson (1982) viewed inner healing from a theologic perspective as essentially the continuity of the creative powers of God—that is, a daily flow of divine energy that repairs our brokenness, frees our inner selves, and truly heals past hurts. Inner healing is a day-to-day process of growing closer to God. Healing prayer is a means by which God gives one the power to heal specific memories and to grow spiritually.

Linn and Linn (1978) felt that the process of healing life's memories through the five stages of forgiveness was a means of not only spiritual growth but also of emotional and physical healing. They produced a movie, *The Power of Healing Prayer*, that demonstrated a controlled experiment in which 24 patients with medically incurable illness were prayed over by a team of a nurse, a priest, and two other individuals. A physician who examined the patients found significant improvement in 21 of the 24 patients and attributed the improvement to prayer (Dobson, 1982;202).

There are few research studies examining the effects of healing of memories or the inner healing process. Schlientz (1981), a nurse, investigated the use of healing of memories on the emotion of anger. She found that subjects who used a healing of memory process, prayer, and imagination through past common developmental stages had less anger than a control group. Propst (1980) compared the effectiveness of religious and nonreligious imagery on treating mild depression in religious individuals. She found religious imagery to be significantly more effective in decreasing depression than nonreligious imagery. The religiously oriented cognitive therapy might have been more effective because the subjects were older people. With older people the religious dimension is often very strong, so integrating a faith system or religion into therapy may be therapeutic.

A number of books and workbooks describe the process of inner healing, healing of memories, and praying with another for healing (Dobson, 1982; Linn et al, 1983, 1984). Fish and Shelly (1978) provide an excellent in-depth approach to the use of spiritual care through the nursing process that is sensitive to individuals' faith systems. They also provide chapters on the use of prayer and Scripture. Shelly (1978) wrote a workbook on spiritual care that provides nurses with practical exercises. The Linns also have a number of tapes and films that can be rented or purchased; nurses can use them to learn and become comfortable with prayer in the healing process.

Linn et al (1984) also describe how to pray with another for healing. They have chapters on preparation, on follow-up, and on how to manage the blockages to healing prayer. The prayer process that they describe includes group, individual, and home spiritual experiences. The chapters end with suggestions for daily home prayer experiences, daily journal keeping of personal reflections, and Scripture readings. Journal keeping is a form of written prayer in which a person keeps a daily record of insights, prayers, spiritual intuitions, significant events, and other products of the inner self. Dobson (1982;59) defined journal keeping as "a material or physical sign of the movements of our minds and spirit . . . and the result of God's grace in our lives." Simon's (1976) book describes how to keep a personal journal.

Many home experiences, brief Scripture readings, and "contemplation in action" prayers could easily be incorporated into the dependent elderly's care plan. As a Christian example, Linn et al (1983;11) suggested doing a two-step prayerful relaxation visit as follows: "(1) Pray by enjoying the presence of Jesus as you enjoy a close friend. Visit a close friend or recall a previous visit with someone you felt especially close to; and (2) Then ask Jesus to be even closer to you than your friend, and just spend a few minutes relaxing and enjoying Jesus' presence."

Davidson and MacDonald (1983) also have written a book that nurses can use as a guide to praying with an elderly resident. Their book illustrates many simple types of traditional and newer types of prayer forms, including non-Christian yoga, Zen prayer, and transcendental meditation.

Many of the prayer and healing processes described by the Linns centered on a belief in God and trust in Jesus Christ. Although most elderly in the United States believe in God and profess some form of the Judeo-Christian religion, spiritual interventions obviously must be modified for atheists, Buddhists, Jews, Moslems, and other religious beliefs; each individual's belief system must be respected. Elderly clients who do not believe in God can use imagery, relaxation techniques, and cognitive techniques without a religious underpinning to help decrease their distress. Bulechek and McCloskey (1985) also recommend reminiscence therapy and music therapy (see Chapter 25, Diversional Activity Deficit, for further discussion).

Audio tapes are available that might help lift the spirit. Halpern's (1984) antifrenetic music or selective classical music might be uplifting. Tubesing (1982) has an audio tape of "spiritual centering" (a combination of guided relaxation and spiritual imagery) that uses mental imaging and is nonthreatening to an individual's belief system. Geiger (1983) also prepared a tape series of music, guided imagery, and voice based on scriptural passages that have been selected to help people of any faith with various mood states, such as depression, anxiety, and tension.

OUTCOMES

Davidson and MacDonald (1983) mentioned a number of benefits that occur as a result of prayer. These include a cure for worry, a decrease in anger, more energy, greater self-esteem, decreased depression, a better sense of purpose in life, and a sense of peace and joy. They also caution that peace and inner strength do not automatically occur when a person prays. The benefits of prayer often happen only slowly after a period of time. Prayer requires persistence and patience, and it may produce results that do not meet our expectations.

The primary goal for the elderly who believe in God but are spiritually distressed would be to help them find and develop a satisfying relationship with their God and a sense of meaning and purpose in life. Other desirable outcomes are decreased anger; a sense of peace; integration of past life experiences, joys, and hurts with the present; and satisfaction with the future even in the face of death.

One way that a nurse could evaluate whether goals or outcomes were met would be through qualitative observations of the elderly person's behaviors and verbal responses. A patient's verbalizations of having or experiencing satisfaction in prayer and having a deeper relationship with God are some indications of decreased Spiritual Distress. Observations of decreased anger and bitterness and increased socializing with family, friends, or other residents if in an institution would be other indicators. Friends, family, and other residents may not want to be with or visit an elderly resident who is spiritually distressed and bitter about life. However, if the person exhibits a sense of peace, inner joy and satisfaction with life, then other people may want to be with her or him. The nurse could also complete a spiritual timeline (spiritual pilgrimage, see previous discussion of Assessment of Spiritual Distress) with the resident as illustrated by Tubesing and Tubesing (1983). If the timeline increases upward in projections into the future, this is another indication of decreased Spiritual Distress.

Two quantitative measures could be used to indicate whether the elderly person's Spiritual Distress was relieved and if he or she was having a greater sense of purpose in life and a better relationship with God or a supreme being. One measure is Paloutzian and Ellison's (1983) Spiritual Well-Being Index. Total scores of 80 or more on the index would indicate fairly high levels of

SWB and, conversely, lack of Spiritual Distress. The subscores of religious well-being (RWB) and existential well-being (EWB) give the nurse some indication of the elderly's feelings about their relationship with God and their sense of meaning and purpose in life. RWB and EWB scores of 40 and more are indications of a good relationship with a higher being and a good sense of meaning and purpose in life.

The other quantitative measure that a nurse could use to evaluate the outcomes of prayer and healing of memories interventions is Flesner's (1981) Spiritual Distress Index. Although norms for this tool have not been established for elderly residents in long-term care settings, the authors of this chapter have found that the tool correlates highly with the SWB Index and that scores of 90 and above are good indications that the person is not in Spiritual Distress. Individual items of the scale can be observed for levels of distress related to love, trust, meaning and purpose, hope, and faith.

These quantitative indexes, however, need to be used with caution with the elderly. They could be upsetting if administered improperly. Furthermore, the scores are only approximate indications of the elderly person's spiritual state. The scores of the two quantitative tools give the nurse considerable information regarding the state of an elderly person's SWB. This information, along with a prolonged qualitative assessment, provides a thorough means of evaluating the effects of healing prayer or other therapies.

CASE STUDY

Nursing Interventions

Millie Brown, the elderly women with Spiritual Distress described earlier in the case study, slowly decreased her distress over a period of time. The primary nurse responsible for her care first had to gain Millie's trust through her caring presence, empathetic listening, and patience. The nurse discussed some of Millie's past hurts with her and especially her feelings toward religion and God since the death of her husband. The nurse obtained some simple traditional Lutheran prayers and a daily Lutheran meditation prayer booklet in large print from the pastoral minister of the nursing home. Millie refused the prayers until the nurse assured her that it was all right to be angry with God and to express those angry feelings in the form of prayer. The nurse also suggested that each day she would read to Millie one of the prayers from the daily meditation guide and discuss the short story or parable that accompanied it.

Millie began to look forward to these short prayerful encounters with the nurse and at times expressed how comforting they were to her. After a time, the nurse mentioned to Millie that there were some special prayers and meditations that could help her with some of the anger she had from past life events. At first the nurse used Lesson 7 of the prayer guide developed by Linn et al (1983), which includes healing through the five stages of forgiveness. After Millie was comfortable with the format of the prayers for healing, the nurse suggested that other people might participate to help her with the healing process. Eventually the primary nurse, the pastoral minister from the nursing home, other residents from the nursing home, and occasionally family members participated in the prayer and discussion sessions.

As the months progressed, the prayer, discussion, healing, and life review sessions became part of the nursing home's activity. Many residents participated, and many life hurts, fears of death, and angry feelings with God were discovered and healed. Millie looked forward to these prayer and healing sessions, and when she felt she had enough physical energy, she became a prayer leader. Millie shared her past life hurts and testified how, through prayers, sharing, and the caring presence of the nurse, she was able to transcend that anger and distress. After about a year, Millie died from her cancer, but she died peacefully and lived life fully until the end.

SUMMARY

Although Spiritual Distress is rarely diagnosed and reported in institutionalized settings, the potential for having Spiritual Distress is great among elderly persons. Spiritual Distress is rarely diagnosed because many nurses are not attuned or sensitized to the spiritual dimension, do not view the spiritual dimension as part of their domain, are unaware of methods and tools to measure it, or are unfamiliar with interventions for the diagnosis of Spiritual Distress.

Spiritual Distress of elderly individuals is an important human response that professional nurses must be prepared to manage. As a person gets older, the potential for spiritual growth, unlike physical growth, continues. If the elderly person's spiritual self does not continue to grow or is blocked by some past life hurt, then the nurse is often in an ideal position to develop a trusting therapeutic relationship for that elderly person and to aid him or her in healing the past hurt and reaching higher levels of spiritual well-being. The use of prayer, the process of inner healing, the healing of memories, and other interventions have great potential for treating the distress of the human spirit. We hope that this chapter will stimulate nurses to be more sensitive to and aware of Spiritual Distress in elderly persons, to use prayerful therapeutic relationships to heal and be healed, and to call on appropriate professional or volunteer resources to meet spiritual needs that are appropriate to each person under their care.

References

Austin J: Regrets: They can be diminished by reviewing the past. *Milwaukee Sentinel* (July 11) 1986; Part 1:10.

Baldree KS, Murphy SP, Powers MJ: Stress identification and coping patterns in patients on hemodialysis. *Nurs Res* 1982; 31:107–112.

Banks R: Health and the spiritual dimension: Relationships and implications for professional preparation programs. *J School Health* 1980; 50:195–202.

Benson H: *Beyond the Relaxation Response.* Berkeley Books, 1985.

Bianchi EC: Death preparation as life enhancement. Pages 150–178 in: *Affirmative Aging: A Resource for Ministry.* Episcopal Society for Ministry on Aging (editor). Winston Press, 1985.

Bulechek G, McCloskey J: *Nursing Interventions: Treatments for Nursing Diagnoses.* Saunders, 1985.

Carpenito LJ: *Handbook of Nursing Diagnosis.* Lippincott, 1985.

Carroll-Johnson R (editor): *Classification of Nursing Diagnoses: Proceedings of the Eighth Conference.* Lippincott, 1989.

Davidson GJ, MacDonald M: *Anyone Can Pray: A Guide to Methods of Christian Prayer.* Paulist Press, 1983.

DeYoung S: Perceptions of the institutionalized elderly regarding the nurse's role in supporting spiritual well-being. Pages 10-1 to 10-10 in: *Spirituality: A New Perspective on Health.* Fehring RJ, Hunglemann JA, Stollenwerk RA (editors). Marquette University Continuing Education in Nursing, 1984.

Dobson TE: *How to Pray for Spiritual Growth.* Paulist Press, 1982.

Dunn HL: What high-level wellness means. *Health Values: Achieving High-Level Wellness* 1977; 1:9–16.

Egan K: Spirituality: Life to the full. Pages 1-1 to 1-16 in: *Spirituality: A New Perspective on Health.* Fehring RJ, Hunglemann JA, Stollenwerk, RA (editors). Marquette University Continuing Education in Nursing, 1984.

Ellison CW: Spiritual well-being: Conceptualization and measurement. *J Psychol Theol* 1983; 11:330–340.

Fehring RJ: Validating diagnostic labels: Standardized methodology. Pages 183–190 in: *Classification of Nursing Diagnoses.* Hurley ME (editor). Mosby, 1986.

Fehring RJ, Frenn M: Nursing diagnoses in a nurse-managed wellness resource center. Pages 401–407 in: *Classification of Nursing Diagnoses.* Hurley ME (editor). Mosby, 1986.

Fehring RJ, Frenn M: Holistic nursing care: A church and university join forces. *J Christian Nurs* 1987; 4:25–28.

Fehring RJ, McLane AM: Spiritual distress. Pages 1843–1857 in: *Clinical Nursing.* Thompson JM et al (editors). Mosby, 1986.

Fehring RJ, Rantz M: Validation of the diagnosis of spiritual distress. Unpublished study, 1987.

Fish S, Shelly JA: *Spiritual Care: The Nurse's Role.* InterVarsity Press, 1978.

Flesner RS: *Development of a Measure to Assess Spiritual Distress in the Responsive Adult.* (MSN Essay.) Marquette University, College of Nursing, December, 1981.

Geiger LJ: *The Journey Tapes.* Lura Media, 1983.

Gettrust KV, Ryan SC, Engelman DS (editors): *Applied Nursing Diagnosis: Guide for Comprehensive Care Planning.* Wiley, 1985.

Gordon M: *Manual of Nursing Diagnosis.* New York: McGraw-Hill, 1986.

Halpern S: *Halpern Sounds.* Wadsworth, 1984.

Hulme WE: *Vintage Years—Growing Older With Meaning and Hope.* Westminster Press, 1986.

Hunglemann JA et al: Spiritual well-being in older adults: Harmonious interconnectedness. *J Religion Health* 1985; 24:147–153.

Kelly MA: *Nursing Diagnosis Source Book.* Appleton-Century-Crofts, 1985.

Kelsey M: *Christianity As Psychology.* Augsburg Publishing House, 1986.

Kim MJ, McFarland GK, McLane AM: *Pocket Guide to Nursing Diagnoses.* Mosby, 1984.

Kim MJ, Moritz DA (editors): *Classification of Nursing Diagnosis: Proceedings of the Third and Fourth National Conferences.* Mosby, 1982

King K: Reminiscing psychotherapy with aging people. *J Psychosoc Nurs Mental Health Services* (Feb) 1982; 20:21–25.

Kohlbry PW: *The Relationship Between Spiritual Well-Being and Hope/Hopelessness in Chronically Ill Clients.* (MSN Thesis.) Marquette University, College of Nursing, 1985.

Leasor M Sr: *Spiritual Well-Being and Psychological Mood States in Patients With Chronic Obstructive Pulmonary Disease.* (MSN Thesis.) Marquette University, College of Nursing, 1983.

Linn D, Linn M: *Healing Life Hurts: Healing Memories Through Five Stages of Forgiveness.* Paulist Press, 1978.

Linn D, Linn M, Fabricant S: *Prayer Course for Healing Life Hurts.* Paulist Press, 1983.

Linn D, Linn M, Fabricant S: *Praying With Another For Healing.* Paulist Press, 1984.

May GG: *Will and Spirit: A Contemplative Psychology.* Harper and Row, 1982.

Miller JF: *Coping With Chronic Illness: Overcoming Powerlessness.* Davis, 1983.

Miller JF: Loneliness and spiritual well-being. *J Professional Nurs* 1985; 1:45–49.

Moberg DO: Social indicators of spiritual well-being. Pages 20–37 in: *Spiritual Well-Being of the Elderly.* Thorson JA, Cook TC (editors). Charles C. Thomas, 1980.

Moberg DO: Subjective measures of spiritual well-being. *Rev Religious Res* 1984; 25:351–364.

O'Brien ME: Religious faith and adjustment to long-term hemodialysis. *J Religion Health* 1982a; 21:68–80.

O'Brien ME: The need for spiritual integrity. Pages 85–116 in: *Human Needs 2 and the Nursing Process.* Yura H, Walsh MB (editors). Appleton-Century-Crofts, 1982b.

O'Driscoll TH: Aging, a spiritual journey. Pages 1–11 in: *Affirmative Aging.* Episcopal Society for Ministry on Aging (editor). Winston Press, 1985.

Paloutzian R, Ellison C: Loneliness, spiritual well-being and quality of life. Pages 227–237 in: *Loneliness: A Sourcebook of*

Current Theory, Research, and Therapy. Peplau L, Perlmann D (editors). Wiley, 1983.

Propst LR: The comparative efficacy of religious and non-religious imagery for the treatment of mild depression in religious individuals. *Cognitive Ther Res* 1980; 4:167–178.

Ruffing-Rahal MA: The spiritual dimension of well-being: Implications for the elderly. *Home Health Care Nurse* (Apr) 1984; 12–16.

Schleman BL, Linn D, Linn M: *To Heal as Jesus Healed.* Notre Dame, IN: Ave Maria Press, 1978.

Schlientz MA: *A Study of the Decrease of Unresolved Anger Through a Teaching Protocol and Healing Prayer as a Nursing Intervention in Spiritual Care.* (PhD Dissertation.) University of Pittsburgh, 1981.

Selye H: Self-regulation: The response to stress. Pages 59–84 in: *Inner Balance: The Power of Holistic Healing.* Goldwag EM (editor). Prentice-Hall, 1979.

Shelly JA: *Spiritual Care Workbook.* InterVarsity Press, 1978.

Simons G: *Keeping Your Personal Journal.* Paulist Press, 1976.

Stallwood J: Spiritual dimension of nursing practice. Pages 1086–1098 in: *Clinical Nursing.* Beland I, Passos JY (editors). Macmillan, 1975.

Stoll RI: Guidelines for spiritual assessment. *Am J Nurs* 1979; 79:1574–1576.

Tubesing DA: Stress, spiritual outlook and health. *Specialized Pastoral Care J* 1980; 3:17–22.

Tubesing DA: *Spiritual Centering Tape.* Whole Person Press, 1982.

Tubesing DA, Tubesing NL: *The Caring Question.* Augsburg Publishing House, 1983.

Tubesing NL, Tubesing DA: *Structured Exercises in Wellness Promotion.* Whole Person Press, 1982.

Weatherall J, Creason N: Validation of the nursing diagnosis spiritual distress. Abstract presented at the Seventh Conference on Classification of Nursing Diagnosis, St. Louis, 1986.

Future Directions for Research and Practice

KATHLEEN C. BUCKWALTER,
PhD, RN, FAAN
MERIDEAN MAAS, PhD, RN, FAAN
DOLORES ROSE, MA

MUCH WORK REMAINS TO BE DONE IN THE CONCEPtual development and testing of nursing diagnoses and interventions. Some of these issues which arose during this writing include the lack of (1) complete explication and standardization of nomenclatures for both nursing diagnoses and interventions; (2) clinically validated assessment tools for the study of diagnoses; (3) funding and administrative support for clinical research regarding identification, development, and validation of diagnoses, interventions, and patient outcomes; and (4) knowledge regarding the application of nursing diagnoses among nurse administrators, educators, and clinicians in a variety of settings.

The problem of incomplete development and standardization of nomenclatures has been noted by several nurse scholars and clinicians (Aydelotte and Peterson, 1987; Bulechek and McCloskey, 1990; Gordon, 1982; Maas, 1986; Warren, 1985). We regard this as a natural part of taxonomic development in a discipline. Some North American Nursing Diagnosis Association (NANDA) diagnoses (especially those in the psychosocial and health promotion/wellness domains) are less well developed than others and need input from practitioners in these areas as well as more qualitative and quantitative research to develop and validate diagnostic concepts. Many diagnostic and intervention labels are vague, ambiguous, and synonymous, representing various levels of abstraction. However, we encourage nurses to resist the temptation for premature closure and undue criticisms of the issues of emerging nursing diagnosis and interventions taxonomies. This book is intended to be heuristic in that it will help clarify some of the concepts for taxonomy development. It is intended to stimulate clinical researchers to identify, define, and validate additional nursing diagnostic and intervention concepts, as well as to conduct studies that compare diagnoses and interventions across a variety of client populations and settings. Clearly, nursing needs to continue the development and testing of taxonomies, both inductively from practice and deductively from theories, using qualitative and quantitative research strategies.

The rapid development of computerized data bases to support nursing assessment, diagnosis, intervention, and outcome evaluation modeling makes it imperative that standardized nomenclatures be validated and used. Although much in this area remains to be done, the nursing diagnosis movement, led by NANDA, has and will continue to make great strides for the profession. Particularly encouraging are efforts spearheaded (1) by the American Nurses' Association (ANA) and NANDA to test taxonomies for the diagnosis, intervention, and outcome elements of the nursing process (incorporating the NANDA taxonomy for nursing diagnoses); (2) by Sigma Theta Tau to develop an international classification of nursing research; and (3) by Harriet Werley in establishing the Nursing Minimum Data Set (Werley and Lang, 1988; Werley et al, 1986). Use of the Minimum Data Set should improve the documentation and research efforts of nurses in a variety of practice settings and the overall quality of care provided to clients, including the elderly. While these taxonomies are evolving, they may appear to be incompatible. However, the editors anticipate that in time, and with refinement, these various approaches and taxonomies will ultimately coalesce into meaningful and related concepts that validly describe and explain nursing phenomena.

There is a need for the development of a number of resources to support clinical research of nursing diagnoses and interventions. Although much of organized nursing recognizes the need for taxonomies of nursing phenomena (eg, ANA Social Policy Statement, Sigma Theta Tau research taxonomy), funding agencies for the most part have not included this area of research in their initiatives. The National Center for Nursing Research (NCNR) funding of research to classify nursing interventions is one notable exception (McCloskey and Bulechek, 1990). Further, such research is often not viewed as a priority in practice settings, even those affiliated with academic settings. In addition to the opportunity for dissemination of research through NANDA's new journal, *Nursing Diagnosis*, nursing journals, especially research journals, need to expand opportunities for nurses to publish the results of studies that validate nursing diagnoses and the efficacy of interventions for achieving specific patient outcomes.

Many nurses have minimal exposure to nursing diagnosis and research. Thus, there is a need for nurses to gain knowledge and skill with diagnosis and diagnostic concepts and with related research strategies. Educational programming (generic, graduate, and continuing education) is required so that nurses are prepared to use nursing diagnoses in their practice and conduct or participate in research to validate concepts and test the linkages among diagnoses, interventions, and desired outcomes. To this end, nursing textbooks in general and nursing research texts in particular should include more information about nursing diagnoses and a variety of methods for conducting research on these phenomena. For example, most research texts currently used in graduate nursing programs do not emphasize content on how to conduct rigorous qualitative or quantitative validation studies or on the many difficult methodologic dilemmas encountered in doing nursing diagnosis research. Courses and texts on nursing theory development should incorporate nursing diagnoses, intervention, and outcomes in discussions and exercises of concept and theory development.

Nursing diagnosis for the elderly is a particular challenge because of the complex interplay among physical, mental, social, spiritual, and environmental factors in this population. At present, many care settings do not use nursing diagnoses. Yet nursing diagnoses can be the keystone to both the administration of these practice settings and the practice of nursing itself (Maas, 1986). Indeed, nursing diagnoses can provide the language whereby communication is enhanced between nurse practitioners, administrators, and members of other health disciplines regarding the health problems of their clients. Nursing diagnoses also enable nursing administrators to identify more clearly the clinical foci for programming, such as quality assurance and staff education. Recently, nursing diagnoses have shown promise for costing out nursing services in acute care settings (Halloran and Halloran, 1985). This effort needs to be extended to a variety of practice settings, especially long-term care institutions and community settings.

In the final analysis, whatever nursing hopes to accomplish is predicated on its ability to demonstrate and document that nursing provides a valuable and needed service. This will require a greater emphasis on research and the use of data-based findings in clinical practice. We are optimistic that the future will bring a proliferation of research designed to validate diagnostic and intervention concepts and to test the effects of interventions to treat specific diagnoses and achieve specific patient outcomes. This will require that nurses in academia and those practicing in clinical settings become involved. A good first step is to join NANDA. Although this book is not endorsed by NANDA, a NANDA enrollment form is provided (Figure 1). We hope this book will stimulate nurses who work with the elderly to be part of this much needed effort.

At the 1988 NANDA conference, 14 new nursing diagnoses were accepted for clinical testing and added to the taxonomy (Table 1) (Carroll-Johnson, 1989). Particu-

Table 1

Nursing Diagnoses Approved at the 1988 NANDA Conference (NANDA, 1988)

Potential for Aspiration
Colonic Constipation
Perceived Constipation
Health-Seeking Behaviors (Specify)
Chronic Low Self-Esteem
Situational Low Self-Esteem
Defensive Coping
Ineffective Denial
Potential for Dysreflexia
Fatigue
Ineffective Breast Feeding
Parental Role Conflict
Potential for Disuse Syndrome
Decisional Conflict

larly noteworthy are the diagnoses that describe states of wellness and those that further explicate previously approved diagnoses. This illustrates the evolving nature of the taxonomy and the need for further development through research and comparisons with existing diagnoses. Not all of the new diagnoses are relevant to the elderly (eg, Ineffective Breast Feeding). Although it would have been ideal to have included each of the new diagnoses that are relevant for the elderly in this book, the publication deadlines and lack of information regarding the structures of the diagnoses precluded doing so. We encourage the readers to reflect on these new diagnoses while reviewing the content of chapters that discuss closely related diagnoses in the appropriate health patterns.

References

Aydelotte M, Peterson KH: Keynote address: Nursing taxonomies—state of the art. In: *Classification of Nursing Diagnoses: Proceedings of the Seventh Conference.* McLane A (editor). Mosby, 1987.

Bulechek GM, McCloskey JC: Nursing intervention taxonomy development. In: *Current Issues in Nursing.* McCloskey JC, Grace HK (editors). Mosby, 1990.

Carroll-Johnson R (editor): *Classification of Nursing Diagnoses: Proceedings of the Eighth Conference.* Lippincott, 1989.

Gordon M: *Nursing Diagnosis: Process and Application.* McGraw-Hill, 1982.

Halloran EJ, Halloran DC: Exploring the DRG nursing equation. *Am J Nurs* 1985; 85(10):1093–1095.

Maas M: Nursing diagnoses in a professional model of nursing: Keystone for effective nursing administration. *J Nurs Admin* 1986; 16(12):39–42.

McCloskey JC, Bulechek, GM: *Classification of Nursing Interventions.* National Center for Nursing Research (NR02079), 1990.

Warren J: Accountability and nursing diagnosis. *J Nurs Admin* 1985; 13(10):34–37.

Werley HH, Lang NM (editors): Identification of the Nursing Minimum Data Set. New York: Springer, 1988.

Werley HH, Lang NM, Westlake SK: Brief summary of the Nursing Minimum Data Set Conference. *Nurs Management* 1986; 17(7):42.

Werley HH, Lang NM, Westlake SK: The Nursing Minimum Data Set Conference: Executive summary. *J Prof Nurs* 1986;2:117.

MEMBERSHIP APPLICATION

Date: _____ Status: _____ New _____ Renewal To apply for year 19 _____

TYPE: Member (enclose $25.00 U.S. funds)   Associate Member (non-nurse or not licensed $12.50 U.S. funds)

Name: _____

Last   First   Middle Initial

Home Address: _____

Street   City/State   Zip Code

Position/Title: _____ Home Phone: _____ Business Phone: _____

Place of Employment: _____ Business Address: _____

_____

Current license: _____   _____

Number   State/Province

(Check One In Each Category)

Initial Nursing Education	**Highest Degree Held**	**Primary Function**	**Area of Specialization**
01. Diploma _____	01. BSN _____	01. Administrator _____	01. Community Health ____
02. AD _____	02. MS _____	02. Clinician _____	02. Maternal/Newborn ____
03. BSN _____	03. MSN _____	03. Consultant _____	03. Medical/Surgical _____
04. Other _____	04. PhD _____	04. Educator _____	04. Nursing of Children ___
	05. DNSc _____	05. Researcher _____	05. Psych/Mental Health ___
	06. EdD _____	06. Other _____	06. Other _____
	07. Other _____		07. List any Subspecialties: _
			_____

Local NrDx Group *(if applicable):*

_____

_____

PR Code: _____

NANDA Committee Interest *(Please check no more than 3):*

01. Diagnosis Review _____	05. Publications _____
02. Membership _____	06. Public Relations _____
03. Nominations _____	07. Research _____
04. Program _____	08. Taxonomy _____

The membership list with names and addresses is made available to individuals/groups with an interest in nursing diagnosis.

Please complete this application form and return it with payment. Please indicate the method of payment you have chosen. *(Checks should be made payable to NANDA.)*

Check _____ Money Order _____ Charge Card _____

If using credit card, complete:

MasterCard _____ or, VISA _____

Card Number: _____ Exp Date: _____

Authorizing Signature _____

Return to: **NORTH AMERICAN NURSING DIAGNOSIS ASSOCIATION**

St. Louis University School of Nursing

3525 Caroline St.

St. Louis, MO 63104

Upon receipt of this completed application and the appropriate dues, new members will be sent a copy of the association bylaws and a membership certificate.

Membership year: January 1 – December 31. (All members must renew by February 15.)

ACTIVITY AND INTEREST FORM

Identify your general emphasis in nursing diagnosis:

(01) ☐ Critical Care
(02) ☐ Long Term Care
(03) ☐ Mental Health
(04) ☐ Nurse Practitioner
(05) ☐ Agency Implementation/Quality Assurance
(06) ☐ Family Health
(07) ☐ Curriculum/Educational Implementation
(08) ☐ Research
(09) ☐ Computerization
(10) ☐ Wellness
(11) ☐ Taxonomy
(12) ☐ Direct Payment for Nursing Service
(13) ☐ Acute Care
(14) ☐ Ambulatory Services

Frequently the Association has requests for names of individuals who have special clinical or research expertise in certain diagnoses. List (by their code number*) no more than five diagnoses in the category which describes your activity best.)

Clinical Expert _____

Research in Progress _____

Research Completed _____

Publication _____

01 Activity Intolerance
28 Activity Intolerance, Potential
00 Adjustment, Impaired
02 Airway Clearance, Ineffective
29 Anxiety
01 Body Temperature, Potential Alteration in
03 Bowel Elimination, Alteration in: Constipation
30 Bowel Elimination, Alteration in: Diarrhea
04 Bowel Elimination, Alteration in: Incontinence
31 Breathing Pattern, Ineffective
05 Cardiac Output, Alteration in: Decreased
32 Comfort, Alteration in: Pain
02 Comfort, Alteration in: Chronic Pain
06 Communication, Impaired: Verbal
33 Coping, Family: Potential for Growth
07 Coping, Ineffective Family: Compromised
34 Coping, Ineffective Family: Disabling
08 Coping, Ineffective Individual
35 Diversional Activity, Deficit
09 Family Process, Alteration in
36 Fear
10 Fluid Volume Alteration in: Excess
37 Fluid Volume Deficit, Actual
11 Fluid Volume Deficit, Potential
38 Gas Exchange, Impaired

012 Grieving, Anticipatory
039 Grieving, Dysfunctional
103 Growth and Development, Altered
013 Health Maintenance, Alteration in
040 Home Maintenance Management, Impaired
104 Hopelessness
105 Hyperthermia
106 Hypothermia
107 Incontinence, Functional
108 Incontinence, Reflex
109 Incontinence, Stress
110 Incontinence, Total
111 Incontinence, Urge
112 Infection, Potential for
014 Injury, Potential for: (poisoning, potential for; suffocation, potential for; trauma, potential for)
041 Knowledge Deficit (specify)
015 Mobility, Impaired Physical
042 Noncompliance (specify)
016 Nutrition, Alteration in: Less than Body Requirements
043 Nutrition, Alteration in: More than Body Requirements
017 Nutrition, Alteration in: Potential for More than Body Requirements
044 Oral Mucous Membrane, Alteration in
018 Parenting, Alteration in: Actual
045 Parenting, Alteration in: Potential
114 Post Trauma Response
019 Powerlessness
046 Rape Trauma Syndrome
020 Self-Care Deficit; feeding, bathing/hygiene, dressing/grooming, toileting
047 Self-Concept, Disturbance in body image, self-esteem, role performance, personal identity
021 Sensory-Perceptual Alteration: visual, auditory, kinesthetic, gustatory, tactile, olfactory
022 Sexual Dysfunction
115 Sexuality Patterns, Altered
048 Skin Integrity, Impairment of: Actual
023 Skin Integrity, Impairment of: Potential
049 Sleep Pattern Disturbance
116 Social Interaction, Impaired
024 Social Isolation
050 Spiritual Distress (distress of the human spirit)
117 Swallowing, Impaired
118 Thermoregulation, Ineffective
025 Thought Processes, Alteration in
119 Tissue Integrity, Impaired
051 Tissue Perfusion, Alteration in: cerebral, cardiopulmonary, renal, gastrointestinal, peripheral
026 Urinary Elimination, Alteration in Patterns
120 Urinary Retention
052 Violence, Potential for: self-directed or directed at others
027 Other (specify) _____

(*This numerical code is for NANDA's computer purposes, it does not relate to the Taxonomy.)

Epilogue: Implications for Policy, Theory, Research, and Practice

ADA JACOX, PhD, RN, FAAN

THE EVOLUTION OF NURSING DIAGNOSIS HAS CHRONIcled the problems and progress of nursing over the past 40 years, and in particular the past 20. The concept was first mentioned in the literature in 1950 by McManus (cited in Gordon, 1985) and is part of the intellectual and professional heritage of nurses teaching and studying at Teachers College, Columbia University in the post-World War II era. Serious attention to nursing diagnosis, however, was not given until 1973, with the First National Conference on the Classification of Nursing Diagnoses, which brought together a diverse and self-selected array of clinicians, researchers, educators, and theorists. Some of the participants had already studied and written about various aspects of nursing diagnosis, and others were interested in the potential that the idea had for organizing knowledge in a way useful to nurses in their quest for defining a more independent profession.

Those developing nursing diagnoses today and the issues they confront represent a microcosm of contemporary nursing, which is reflected in this book on nursing diagnoses and intervention for the dependent elderly. In describing common clinical problems and interventions, the editors and authors further stake out the domain of nursing practice and take responsibility for clarifying and extending its research base. They have selected a high-risk and basically neglected population for study—the dependent elderly—and developed nursing diagnoses most relevant to that population. Although the editors used Gordon's Functional Health Patterns as an overall organizing framework, they did not adopt any single nursing theory because of their belief that an eclectic theoretical approach will best further the development of nursing diagnoses. They wisely encourage nurses to resist the temptations of premature closure in selecting taxonomies for nursing diagnoses and interventions on the one hand, and of undue criticism of emerging nursing diagnoses and interventions on the other.

Thus, the issues dealt with in the book include those related to:

- *Policy*: For what problems are nurses responsible, and for what problems do they share responsibility with physicians and others?
- *Theory*: What are the important concepts (nursing diagnoses and interventions), and how are they related?
- *Research*: What are the appropriate methods for identifying, describing, and validating the concepts?
- *Clinical practice*: What are the clinical problems characterized as potential and actual threats to health; what assessment tools are clinically

useful; and what are appropriate interventions for nurses to take?

The editors are firmly grounded in gerontologic practice and research and share a vision of a strong and autonomous nursing profession. This book is another sign of a maturing profession in its confident, nondefensive, and straightforward statement of nursing's claim to a particular area of practice.

One of the most refreshing features of this book is its balanced critical stance toward nursing diagnosis and intervention. A number of years ago Madeleine Leininger (1968), writing presumably in response to the intensely negative tone that characterized critiques of research then, produced an excellent discussion of the nature and art of critique. In it, she emphasized that a useful critique not only points out weak aspects of the research, but also acknowledges its strengths and contributes to its further development. It is this balanced and reasoned tone of criticism that the editors and authors bring to their readers. They try to hasten the evolution of nursing diagnoses by relating their work to the work of the North American Nursing Diagnosis Assocation (NANDA), neither embracing NANDA's work as Holy Writ, nor rejecting it because of its inadequacies. Instead, they compare their work with NANDA's, pointing out when it supports NANDA's work and offering explanation for when it differs. They expand on NANDA's accepted list of diagnoses, develop subcategories to make the diagnoses more relevant to the population of institutionalized elderly, add new diagnoses, and offer numerous suggestions for how NANDA's work can be improved. This kind of constructive, rigorous criticism, coupled with experienced professional judgment and the presentation of new research findings, will put the study and use of nursing diagnosis on a solid foundation.

This book makes a major contribution not only to our understanding of nursing problems of the dependent elderly, but to knowledge of the kinds of activities necessary for the sophisticated development of nursing diagnoses. It serves as a useful model for those interested in developing nursing diagnoses and related interventions in other areas of practice. Some of the many issues raised in the book are further explored here.

IMPLICATIONS FOR POLICY

The American Nurses' Association's (1980) Social Policy Statement defines nursing as concerned with the potential and actual responses of people to threats to their health and asserts that nurses diagnose the problems for which they are accountable and carry out interventions intended to resolve the problems. This definition of nursing has been incorporated into nurse practice acts in several states and is widely cited as an acceptable definition of nursing. As the editors of this book point out, nursing must demonstrate and document that it provides a valuable and needed service. A policy statement regarding the domain of the field is a useful and necessary starting point for conceptualizing the field. It requires, however, a considerable amount of research and interpretation to make real the abstract concepts reflected in the social policy statement. Unless there is substance to support the policy statement, in the sense of identifying and studying nursing diagnoses, interventions, and intended patient outcomes, implementing the definition of nursing will in the long run be unsustainable. The desire to have a more autonomous discipline of nursing and to have that acknowledged by public and private policy-making bodies requires clear and persuasive demonstration that nursing has the necessary knowledge to carry out its work.

Another policy area related to how nursing is defined is reflected in the scope of practice described for nursing. Some persons in the nursing diagnosis movement argue that the concepts that nursing defines must be uniquely its own and not overlap with medicine or other disciplines. They eschew a concern with pathology and focus narrowly on those phenomena they determine to belong to nursing. Although it is important to identify those areas for which nurses have primary responsibility, it also is necessary to reflect the reality of nursing practice in the taxonomical schemes that classify its practice. The editors of this book note the NANDA taxonomy's predominantly illness orientation, suggesting that this may be criticized. The editors and authors, most of whom are experienced clinicians, have selected some of the most common problems with which nurses caring for the dependent elderly must deal. Although attention is given to health promotion and to psychosocial and spiritual aspects of health, heavy emphasis also is placed on physiologic and pathologic aspects. This reflects the clinical reality within which these and many other nurses practice, and it is a disservice to practicing nurses not to acknowledge major components of their work as legitimate and in need of a strong research base.

This same point was made by Cathie Guzzetta (1987), an experienced clinician in cardiovascular nursing, who observed that:

> On any given day in critical care, for example, only 10% of our day may include the so-called independent role of the nurse. If most of our day involves interdependent functioning, then it is clear that nursing diagnoses do not capture the essence of critical care practice. The current accepted list of nursing diagnoses poorly describes the scope of responsibilities and the major contribution of the critical care nurse in changing patient outcomes. It does not permit critical care nurses to document their role in preventing the catastrophic complications of injury and disease.

Definitions of nursing that limit practice to independent functions needlessly constrain nurses. Policy statements and taxonomies must be visionary, but they must also acknowledge the reality in which practitioners operate. Additionally, it is important to use language understandable to nurses, physicians, and others, avoiding needlessly esoteric jargon in the interest of clear communication about patients in their care.

Another important policy area addressed in this book is the target population—the dependent elderly—a group at high risk for many of the nursing diagnoses identified thus far. It is a neglected population, many of whom are in nursing homes that resemble warehouses more than humane care facilities. How to provide care to the elderly is an increasing problem for this society and one that is appropriate for nurses to confront. This book describes and explains many of the problems faced by the elderly, including normal aging, the potential for serious injuries and other health problems, role changes, sexual dysfunctioning, and spiritual distress. The comprehensive scope of problems dealt with in the book and the editors' observation that these represent only some of the more common problems faced by the elderly are indication of the enormous amount of effort that must go into developing a better knowledge base for providing care to this group.

Many of the book's contributing authors have an association with the Iowa Veteran's Home, an institution that has a history of 20 years of progress in developing an enlightened and autonomous organizational model for professional practice (Maas and Jacox, 1977; Maas et al, 1975). Nurses working at that facility acknowledged in the late 1960s that if nursing was indeed the major service delivered to the clients, then nurses had an obligation to develop a better knowledge base. A few dozen nurses at this long-term care setting established, among other things, a set of bylaws for the nursing department that specified authority for nursing care, a peer review system, and a committee to do research in gerontologic nursing, at a time when these ideas were just beginning to take root in nursing. Their clearly stated policy was that nursing is the most essential service provided to institutionalized elderly, and they have continued over time to improve that service. The kind of knowledge represented in this book puts substance in a policy statement that names nursing as having primary responsibility for care of the institutionalized elderly.

Finally, there are other public policy implications of nursing diagnosis. One is the choice of measures for determining nurses' workload and reimbursement. As Halloran (1988) and others have argued, case mix as measured by Diagnostic Related Groups (DRGs) does not explain all the variability in the cost of treating hospitalized patients, particularly variability in nursing costs. Halloran (1980) showed that DRGs predicted only 26% of nursing resources used, whereas the number of nursing diagnoses predicted 52%. Halloran (1988), Vice President

for Nursing at Case Western Reserve University Hospital, described use of a nursing diagnosis-based patient classification instrument to measure patients' dependency on nurses for care. Using documentation of nursing diagnoses, he illustrates a method of determining the cost of nursing care based on the number of patient conditions. Having patient classification systems that accurately reflect patients' needs for nursing care is prerequisite to establishing accurate measures of nurse workload and reimbursement policies for nursing services.

IMPLICATIONS FOR THEORY CONSTRUCTION

The theoretical perspective adopted by the editors in organizing this book was Gordon's Functional Health Patterns and the criteria for selection of interventions were based on the work of Bulechek and McCloskey (1985). Although the editors note the desirability of maintaining theoretical eclecticism, their adoption of one organizing conceptual framework (Gordon's) reflects an important issue in the development of nursing diagnoses— the relationship between the development of nursing diagnosis taxonomy and nursing theories. As Gordon (1982) notes, the First National Conference on Nursing Diagnoses was called by Gebbie and Lavin of St. Louis University because of their concern with clinical issues. Their interests were in identifying the nurse's role in an ambulatory care setting and in deciding what clinical problems would be recorded in a computerized record-keeping system. Much of the impetus for the development of nursing diagnoses thus came from clinicians, who took an essentially inductive approach in identifying the nursing problems for which they were accountable. The organizing framework for the first nursing diagnoses developed was the alphabet. At the Third and Fourth National Conference (1978 and 1980), efforts were made to adopt a conceptual framework for nursing diagnoses, which resulted in a "unitary man" framework. One clinician's response (Stafford, 1982) to the unitary man framework expresses the frustration of trying to relate broad theoretical formulations to specific practice.

Philosophically, I reject the framework and clinically (at least at this writing) I find it ineffective, cumbersome, and time-consuming, a futile exercise in words and an exercise lacking in specificity. It does not provide a means of accountability or a method of communication. How can we be held accountable for something which is so nebulous, so ill defined? How can we communicate to others what we ourselves do not understand? Peer review in this framework would have no meaning, as each of us could differ in our perceptions of the appropriate pattern placement. And third party payment, or fee for services, would legitimately raise the question: what services?

There seems to be serious interest on the part of clinicians and theorists to work together to make nursing diagnoses both clinically relevant and theoretically organized. Previous attempts to develop global conceptual frameworks in nursing have been viewed by many clinicians as having little relevance for what they do in their day-to-day practice. This is so because conceptual frameworks, by their nature, are broad and abstract, and until recently there have been few middle-range theories in which the applicability to nursing practice is more readily apparent. A recent analysis of the nursing diagnosis literature reported that of the nurse authors, 57% were academics and 43% were clinicians (Turkoski, 1988). The author, however, noted the lack of evidence of academic and clinical collaboration in the nursing diagnosis literature. A field in which both clinicians and theorists are so active would seemingly constitute natural common ground for collaboration in developing middle-range theories with applicability to clinical practice. It may be that the continuing dialogue between clinicians and theorists promoted by NANDA and other groups concerned with development of nursing diagnoses will enable such eventual collaboration by clinicians and theoreticians.

The problem seems to be to find ways to organize nursing diagnoses that are coherent and relevant to practice without prematurely committing to any particular theory. Organizing nursing diagnoses alphabetically is certainly theoretical but does not provide much of an underlying rationale for the organization. Perhaps the next most neutral way of organizing nursing diagnoses is in the work being done to develop a nursing minimum data set (Werley and Lang, 1988). In this classification scheme, nursing care elements (nursing diagnoses, nursing interventions, patient outcomes, and nurse staffing) are based on the nursing process, which is a broad type of conceptual framework. Werley and Lang (1988;405) define nursing diagnosis as "a clinical judgment made by a nurse about a human response to an actual or potential health problem, the intervention for which nurses are accountable." The nursing diagnoses are those taken from NANDA or other "recognized diagnostic systems" representing an organizing framework limited only by a rather broad definition of nursing. Examples of other ways of organizing nursing diagnoses are represented in Gordon's Functional Health Patterns, used in this book, and the unitary man theory, adopted by NANDA, both of which reflect assumptions about the nature of human beings and nursing that are more specific than the nursing minimum data set.

The controversy regarding selection of organizing frameworks reflects the issues involved in theory construction more generally. This is so because taxonomies are a type of conceptual framework. Kritek (1982) argued that classification of nursing diagnoses reflects theory at the factor-isolating level, and the classification should be completed before higher-level theories are developed. This argument ignores the intertwining of concept and theory development that actually occurs as theories are developed (Suppe and Jacox, 1985). The theory deductively (even when the theory is broad) provides direction for the concepts (nursing diagnoses) to be included and studied, and inductive study of the concepts in turn yields findings that modify the theory.

Therefore, acknowledging the difficulty in arriving at a consensus regarding a framework acceptable to a majority of people working in the nursing diagnosis area, agreement on a broad conceptual organizing framework such as the nursing minimum data set may represent a sufficiently neutral framework within which to organize nursing diagnoses. Those interested in particular areas of practice, such as care of the institutionalized elderly or care of the critically ill, may develop middle-range theories, selecting those concepts most relevant for practice in this population. Such middle-range theories should make explicit the assumptions made as the basis for concept selection. In this book, for example, the selection of nursing diagnoses clearly reflects a holistic approach, with priority given to those commonly experienced diagnoses that in the editors' professional judgment most need to be developed and shared by nurses working with the dependent elderly. The combination of considerable looseness and generality in the overall conceptual framework with specificity of assumptions and concepts for middle-range theories may be the most productive way for work to proceed in the development of taxonomies for nursing diagnoses and interventions.

IMPLICATIONS FOR RESEARCH

In the previous chapter of this book, Buckwalter et al note the need for resources to support clinical research in nursing diagnoses and interventions. They cite the lack of priority given to the study of nursing diagnoses by funding agencies, limited opportunities to publish results of nursing diagnosis validation studies in nursing research journals, and general lack of discussion in graduate nursing research texts regarding methodologic problems in doing research relevant to nursing diagnoses. This lack of support by research institutions was substantiated by Gordon's (1985) review and critique of research on nursing diagnoses between 1950 and 1983. Gordon identified only eight studies of identification and validation of nursing diagnoses, none of which were published in research journals.

That funding agencies, journals, and texts have been slow to incorporate the study of nursing diagnoses into their priorities is not surprising. Kuhn (1960) described the conservatism of the research enterprise in trying to maintain the status quo in what is accepted as legitimate science. Those making decisions regarding expenditure of research funds and dissemination of ideas related to research feel more confident in supporting areas that are already generally accepted. Any new idea, including that of taxonomies for nursing diagnoses and nursing interventions, has considerable difficulty in breaking through the belief systems regarding what makes up legitimate science. It does seem, however, that sufficient study has been done in nursing diagnoses, and that the concept has such meaning for clinicians and clinical practice, that it ought now to be viewed by the research community as a legitimate area of study. There is likely sufficient expertise and interest in those studying nursing diagnoses to justify the establishment of a new research journal dedicated to that area. Such a journal would have on its editoral board and review panel professionals with the wide range of opinion and expertise in nursing diagnoses and research methods necessary to do adequate critiques and research reports.* This would not, of course, preclude publication in other research journals, but may serve to hasten the dissemination of needed knowledge.

Many methodologic issues are involved in the study of nursing diagnoses. Much work related to those issues has been done in other fields and needs to be adapted to the study of nursing diagnoses. To this end, the involvement of researchers with strong preparation in traditional research methods, such as characterizes the editors of this book, will bring much needed methodologic rigor to this area. Additionally, some of the approaches described by Norris (1982) and Walker and Avant (1983) would be useful adjuncts to the study of nursing diagnoses.

IMPLICATIONS FOR PRACTICE

Much of the discussion of implications for policy, theory, and research also is related to clinical practice issues. It was noted that the interest in nursing diagnoses arose from clinicians and that clinicians contribute in a major way to the literature. The chord that nursing diagnosis has struck among clinicians says much regarding its usefulness to them. Nursing diagnosis offers a way for practicing nurses to conceptualize and focus on the clearly nursing components of their practice.

The incorporation of numerous practical assessment tools in this book and the case studies given to illustrate how the nursing diagnoses and interventions can be used should be most helpful to clinicians. Additionally, the authors in the book acknowledge the need for nurses to understand both medical and nursing interventions but emphasize the latter in their chapters. For example, in Chapter 17 of this text, Specht et al say:

For most nurses, prescriptive authority still rests with their medical colleagues. For this reason, the medications used to treat urinary incontinence will be discussed only as they relate to nursing and not medical interventions. Similarly, although nurses will play a part in the accurate diagnosis of clients who require surgical intervention . . . these treatments are essentially medical in nature and will not be discussed in this chapter. . . . However, a number of interventions are available to nurses that do eliminate or control the number of incontinent episodes a client experiences.

The need for nurses to understand related and overlapping aspects of practice as well as understanding nursing practice is an important issue for those dealing with nursing diagnoses. Nursing diagnoses are an essential part of what a nurse needs to know, but as clinicians point out, as presently conceptualized, they do not include all that nurses need to know. The development of nursing diagnoses must acknowledge the clinical reality in which nurses practice. The editors and authors of this book clearly have taken a major step in clarifying that reality and in offering the promise of improved care for the dependent elderly.

References

American Nurses' Association: *Nursing: A Social Policy Statement.* Publication No. NP-63 20M 9/82R, 1980.

Bulecheck G, McCloskey J (editors): *Nursing Interventions: Treatments for Nursing Diagnoses.* Saunders, 1985.

Gordon M: *Nursing Diagnoses: Process and Application.* McGraw-Hill, 1982.

Gordon M: Nursing diagnosis. Pages 127–146 in: *Annual Review of Nursing Research,* Vol III. Werley HH, Fitzpatrick HH (editors). Springer, 1985.

Guzzetta C: Nursing diagnoses in nursing education: Effect on the profession. *Health Lung* 1987; 16(6):634.

Halloran EJ: Analysis of variation in nursing workload by patient medical and nursing condition. *Dissertation Abstracts International,* 41-093. University Microfilms #8106567, 1980.

Halloran EJ: Conceptual considerations, decision criteria, and guidelines for development of the nursing minimum data set from an administrative perspective. Pages 48–66 in: *Identification of the Nursing Minimum Data Set.* Werley HH, Lang NM (editors). Springer, 1988.

Kritek P: The generation and classification of nursing diagnoses: Toward a theory of nursing. Pages 18–29 in: *Classification of Nursing Diagnoses: Proceedings of the Third and Fourth National Conferences.* Kim MJ, Moritz DA (editors). McGraw-Hill, 1982.

Kuhn T: *The Structure of Scientific Revolutions,* 2d ed. Holt, Reinhart, and Winston, 1960.

Leininger M: The research critique: Nature, function and art. Pages 20–32 in: *Communicating Nursing Research,* Vol 1. Batey MV (editor). WICHE, 1968.

---

* Editors note: Subsequent to the writing of this chapter, the journal *Nursing Diagnosis* was published by NANDA in 1990.

Maas M, Jacox A: *Guidelines for Nurse Autonomy/Patient Welfare.* Boston: Appleton-Century-Crofts, 1977.

Maas M, Specht J, Jacox A: Nurse autonomy: Reality not rhetoric. *Am J Nurs* (Dec) 1975; 2201–2208.

Norris CM: *Concept Clarification in Nursing.* Rockville, MD: Aspen, 1982.

Stafford M: Responses of clinical specialists to the unitary man framework. Page 268 in: *Classifications of Nursing Diagnoses: Proceedings of the Third and Fourth National Conferences.* Kim MJ, Moritz DA (editors). McGraw-Hill, 1982.

Suppe F, Jacox AK: Philosophy of science and the development of nursing theory. Page 250 in: *Annual Review of Nursing Research,* Vol III. Werley HH, Fitzpatrick JJ (editors). Springer, 1985.

Turkoski BB: Nursing diagnosis, 1950–1985. *Nurs Outlook* 1988; 36(3):142–144.

Walker L, Avant KO: *Strategies for Theory Construction in Nursing.* Appleton-Century-Crofts, 1983.

Werley HH, Lang NM. *Identification of the Nursing Minimum Data Set.* Springer, 1988.

Index

Table Credits

Tables 2.1, 2.2, 4.1, 5.1, 9.2, 11.1, 12.1, 14.3, 15.2, 16.1, 17.1, 19.1, 21.1, 23.1, 30.1, 32.1, 36.1, 37.1, 40.1, 43.1, 44.1, 45.1, 46.1, 47.1, 50.1, 50.2.   Reproduced by permission from North American Nursing Diagnosis Association. *Classification of Nursing Diagnoses: Proceedings of the Seventh Conference* (McLane, Audrey M, Editor). 1987. St. Louis: The C.V. Mosby Co.

Table 2.2.   Carpenito, LJ *Nursing Diagnosis: Application to Clinical Practice,* 1st ed. 1983, Philadelphia: J.B. Lippincott.

Table 15.1.   Adapted from Krejs, D, Fordtran, J. Diarrhea, *Gastrointestinal Disease: Pathophysiology, Diagnosis Management,* 3e, 1983. Philadelphia: W.B. Saunders.

Table 17.5.   Ouslander, J et al. *Technologies for Managing Urinary Incontinence.* Office of Technology/Health Case Study 33. July 1985. U.S. Government Printing Office.

Table 23.2.   Adapted from Frances K. Milde, Physiological Immobilizations, *Concepts Common to Acute Illness,* Hart, Fehring, Reece (Eds.) 1981. St. Louis: Mosby.

Table 24.3.   From Implementing Nursing Diagnosis Through Integration with Quality Assurance, AE McCourt, *Nursing Clinics of North America 1987.* 22(4): 89-904. Used with permission of A.E. McCourt.

Tables 29.2 and 29.3.   Hall, G & Buckwalter, K. Progressively lowered stress threshold: A conceptual model for care of adults with Alzheimer's Disease. *Archives of Psychiatric Nursing.* December 1987; 1(6):399-406.

Table 33.3.   Reprinted with the permission of the American Association of Diabetes Educators from M McSweeney, Measuring the effect of patient teaching. *The Diabetes Educator* 1981;7(3):9-15.

Tables 35.1 and 42.1.   Reproduced by permission from Gordon, Marjory: *Manual of nursing diagnosis, 1988-1989.* 1989. St. Louis: The C.V. Mosby Co.

Table 35.3.   American Psychiatric Association: *Diagnostic and Statistical Manual of Mental Disorders, Third Edition, Revised.* 1987. Washington, D.C.: American Psychiatric Association.

Table 35.4.   Adapted from Zung, WWK. Affective Disorders, *Handbook of Geriatric Psychiatry,* Busse, EW & Blazer, DG (Eds) p. 357. 1980. Van Nostrand Reinhold. Reprinted by permission of the publisher. All Rights Reserved.

Table 35.5.   Adapted from Yost, EB, Corbishley, MA. *Depression in the Elderly—An Interdisciplinary Approach.* Chassion–Stewart (Eds) 1985. John Wiley & Sons.

Table 35.6.   From J Gunderson, O Will and L Mosher, *Principles and Practice of Milieu Therapy.* Copyright 1983. Jason Aronson Inc. Reprinted with permission of the publisher.

Table 35.7.   Adapted, with permission, from Ouslander JG, Small GW, Management of Depression in the Elderly Patient with Physical Illness. *Geriatric Medicine Today* 1984: 3(10):90.

Figure Credits

Figure 10.2.   Reprinted from *AMERICAN FAMILY PHYSICIAN.* 1980; 17:84-95. Published by the American Academy of Family Physicians.

Figure 14.3.   Reproduced by permission from North American Nursing Diagnosis Association. *Classification of Nursing Diagnoses: Proceedings of the Seventh Conference* (McLane, Audrey M, Editor). 1987. St. Louis: The C.V. Mosby Co.

Figure 29.1.   From Wolanin, M & Phillips, L, Etiologies of Alternation in Thought Processes. *Confusion: Prevention and Care.* 1981. St. Louis: Mosby, p. 5.

Figure 30.1.   Stewart, M.L. Measurement of Clinical Pain. 1977. In Jacox, A. (Ed.) *Pain: A Source Book for Nurses and Other Health Professionals*

Figure 42.1.   McKeehan, KM (Ed.) *Continuing Care: A Multidisciplinary Approach to Discharge Planning.* 1981. St. Louis: C.V. Mosby. p. 12.

Figure 43.2.   Ken Moses, Ph.D., handout for conference in Chicago, IL April 23-24, 1987. Resource Networks, Inc.

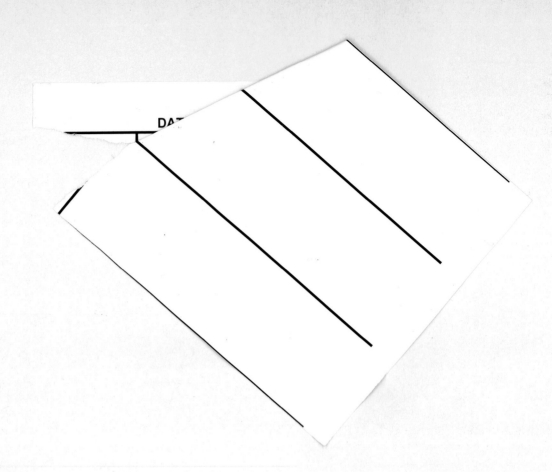